W9-CZK-897

Health Assessment

A NURSING APPROACH

edition 3

Health Assessment

A NURSING APPROACH

▲ **JILL FULLER**, RN, PhD
Vice President
Patient Services
Winona Community Memorial Hospital
Winona, Minnesota

▲ **JENNIFER SCHALLER-AYERS**, RNC, PhD
Assistant Professor
College of Nursing
University of Arkansas for Medical Sciences
Little Rock, Arkansas

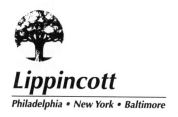

Lippincott

Philadelphia • New York • Baltimore

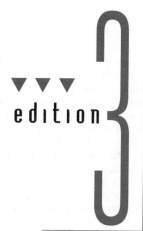

▼▼▼
edition 3

Acquisitions Editor: Ilze Rader
Assistant Editor: Dale Thuesen
Senior Project Editor: Tom Gibbons
Senior Production Manager: Helen Ewan
Production Coordinator: Michael Carcel
Design Coordinator: Carolyn O'Brien
Indexer: Ellen Murray

3rd Edition

Copyright © 2000 by Lippincott Williams & Wilkins
Copyright © 1994, 1990 by J. B. Lippincott Company. All rights reserved. This book is protected by copyright. No part of it may be reproduced, stored in a retrieval system, or transmitted, in any form or by any means—electronic, mechanical, photocopy, recording, or otherwise—without the prior written permission of the publisher, except for brief quotations embodied in critical articles and reviews. Printed in the United States of America. For information write Lippincott Williams & Wilkins 227 East Washington Square, Philadelphia, PA 19106.

Library of Congress Cataloging in Publications Data

Fuller, Jill.
    Health assessment : a nursing approach / Jill Fuller, Jennifer
Schaller-Ayers. — 3rd ed.
        p.   cm.
    Includes bibliographical references and index.
    ISBN 0–7817–1566–0 (cloth : alk. paper)
    1. Nursing assessment.   2. Physical diagnosis.   I. Schaller
-Ayers, Jennifer.   II. Title.
    [DNLM: 1. Nursing Assessment.   WY 100.4 F966h 2000]
RT48.F85   2000
616.07′5—dc21
DNLM/DLC
for Library of Congress   99–31261
                              CIP

Care has been taken to confirm the accuracy of the information presented and to describe generally accepted practices. However, the authors, editors, and publishers are not responsible for errors or omissions or for any consequences from application of the information in this book and make no warranty, express or implied, with respect to the contents of the publication.

The authors, editors and publisher have exerted every effort to ensure that drug selection and dosage set forth in this text are in accordance with current recommendations and practice at the time of publication. However, in view of ongoing research, changes in government regulations, and the constant flow of information relating to drug therapy and drug reactions, the reader is urged to check the package insert for each drug for any change in indications and dosage and for added warnings and precautions. This is particularly important when the recommended agent is new or infrequently employed drug.

Some drugs and medical devices presented in this publication have Food and Drug Administration (FDA) clearance for limited use in restricted research settings. It is the responsibility of the health care provider to ascertain the FDA status of each drug or device planned for use in their clinical practice.

DEDICATION

To Doug, for all his love and support.

And to our precious sons, Max and Jase, for keeping everything

in perspective.

J.F.

For James—the presence of your love and support

is always near and appreciated

Johana—let your dreams and your hopes carry you anywhere

and everywhere

Otto and Geneva—thanks for being there

J.S.A.

Handwritten margin notes:

Dx Concussion

Head-
c/o Hit Ⓡ forehead while Roller blading
Ⓡ forehead discoloration, mod bruising & swelling
a loss of conscience, SI HA.

- Ice on & off 20min x for 24°.
- HOB T
- Return to ED in any changes in mental status, vomiting or T HA;
✓ Cranial Nerve Assessment

Dx - URI

Reop - c/o of cold sxs w/ coughing @ noc.   Afebrile. USS. Sputum clear, Chest x-ray - Neg.
                                             nonproductive cough   Lateral
- T Fld Intake   Ø SOB   "A/P"
- Tylenol Q4° 2 tabs as needed discomfort   ✓ pneumonia.
- Robitussin AC @ noc.
- Rest

Heart - c/o "Burning pressure of the chest"   Assess CUS
   Dx - GERD   Chemistry
      Sent home on Mylanta.   EKg
                                               CXR
   D/c Home Zantac 150mg PO BID   CPK/tropi
                                               6 I Cocktail

EARS -

C/o - ⊕ ear pain for 2 days. Afebile.
    Relieved with Tylenol 2 tabs every 4 hours 650mg's

    Whispered Voice

Eyes

S - "I got poked in the eye. It feels like my eye is scratched."
    Ø fever VSS.

    Tx - Send them home on erithromycin for 10 days.
         WARM Compresss as needed for comfort.

ABD -

C/o - "I ate chicken @ a seafood restaurant 3 days ago. C/o n/v for 24°.

BS normal , Ø constipation

- 1 dose of compazine suppository

 - Sips of water if tolerated

 - START Brat diet - bananas, rice, applesauce & toast.

Musc   ASS mSS

Hit ⓡ shoulder on the ~~fire~~.   X-ray ordered - Results Neg.
Ice on & off @ 70 min for 24 hrs. Tylenol for discomfort. Q 4hr 2 tabs 650mg's.

PREFACE

Abd

> B*ut if you cannot get the habit of observation one way or another, you had better give up the being a nurse, for it is not your calling, however kind and anxious you may be.*
>
> **Florence Nightingale**

Health Assessment: A Nursing Approach is a modern-day textbook designed to teach the nurse the "habit of observation," the skills of inquiry and investigation, and the aptitudes required for clinical judgment. It provides a strong foundation for assessment and diagnosis, integrating the nursing process, interviewing techniques, health history taking, diagnostic study interpretation, physical examination skills, environmental evaluation, and growth and development concepts. But this text is more than a book of assessment skills and techniques. It is a foundation for clinical practice that illustrates the scope and responsibility of today's professional nurse with emphasis on nursing's distinctive domain in health care.

CONCEPTUAL FRAMEWORK

Health Assessment: A Nursing Approach is a unique text that provides a nursing model for health assessment. This text will clarify the relationship of assessment to nursing diagnosis and nursing process to medical treatment. It uses the frameworks of *functional health* and *nursing diagnoses* while incorporating traditional physical examination techniques and clinical problem identification. The intent is to prepare a practitioner who can effectively evaluate persons in a variety of practice settings. The health assessment process is presented in a way that is congruent with the nursing goals of gathering and analyzing data about a person's state of *wellness, functional ability, physical status, strengths,* and *responses to actual or potential health problems.*

The conceptual framework of functional health and nursing diagnoses is appropriate regardless of the nurse's philosophy or practice setting because it represents a way of organizing the nursing data base, regardless of the theoretical model used for practice. This conceptual frame-

work also ensures a *holistic* approach to assessment with consideration of all aspects of human function. This text provides the traditional emphasis on assessing *physical health status* as well as other dimensions of health, including *health perception and health management, sleep and rest, self-concept, roles and relationships, sexuality, stress and stress responses,* and *values and beliefs.*

As nursing evolves as a discipline with a unique body of knowledge, nurses are increasingly questioning traditional assessment methods based primarily on a medical model and the relevance of such methods for nursing. *Health Assessment: A Nursing Approach* is committed to refining and evolving a distinctive nursing approach to health assessment.

ORGANIZATION

The text is organized in three main sections: Unit I, *Overview of Health Assessment and Clinical Competencies;* Unit II, *Health Assessment of Human Function;* and Unit III, *Health Assessment Across the Life Span.*

Introduction to Health Assessment

Unit I presents a foundation of professional and clinical concepts required for health assessment, including a discussion of the nature and scope of a nursing health assessment; the principles of interviewing and history taking; basic physical examination techniques and instrumentation; the sequence and documentation of a comprehensive physical examination; diagnostic reasoning and documentation guidelines; and vital sign assessment techniques.

Chapter 1, "Introduction to Health Assessment," emphasizes *critical thinking* as the basis for health assessment. Diagnostic reasoning is presented as an intellectual process for formulating judgments about health status based on assessment data. Subsequent chapters apply the critical thinking concepts presented in Chapter 1 through discussions of nursing diagnosis and clinical problem identification as well as through discussion questions in the critical thinking exercises at the end of each chapter.

The Physical Examination

Chapter 3, "The Physical Examination," presents an overview of a complete physical examination, including a *full-color photo presentation of a head-to-toe physical examination.* This sets the stage for subsequent chapters in which procedural aspects of the physical examination are discussed in detail. The student is shown the "big picture" and how the various elements of the physical examination fit together before learning detailed examination procedures and the relationship of the data to clinical diagnosis. Chapter 3 also illustrates how functional health as an assessment data collection framework can be easily and comfortably interchanged with traditional methods of body systems and head-to-toe examination sequences.

Functional Health Patterns

Unit II presents guidelines for assessing functional abilities and physiologic status. The chapters are organized according to 11 functional health areas rather than by body systems or as a sequential head-to-toe method of physical examination. This approach was chosen because nurses today collect assessment data to focus on nursing diagnoses, level of wellness, personal strengths, and physiologic alterations as manifestations of the patterns of human function. Guidelines are presented for evaluating human function using interview data, nursing observations, results of diagnostic studies, and physical examination data.

The organization of all Unit II chapters is similar. Each chapter begins with an **introductory overview** that describes the **assessment focus** for the functional area being discussed and lists the **nursing diagnoses** that might be identified after thorough evaluation of that particular function. The assessment focus describes what the nurse assesses to evaluate a particular functional area thoroughly. If all of the areas presented in the chapter are assessed, the nurse has screened for the signs and symptoms associated with the nursing diagnoses listed in the chapter.

The next section of each chapter is called the **knowledge base for assessment.** This section provides the theoretical basis for assessing a particular functional pattern. The knowledge base section presents definitions of terms and concepts and reviews pertinent physiologic processes or theoretical underpinnings. For example, in Chapter 11 "Assessing Self-Concept," this discussion highlights the definition of self-concept proposed by nursing and other disciplines. In addition, variables that may affect the development of self-concept are identified. The knowledge base in Chapter 6, "Assessing Nutrition and Metabolism," focuses primarily on reviewing the physiologic processes involved in nutrition and metabolism. In all chapters, knowledge base concepts lend greater significance to the assessment data obtained through the methods highlighted in each chapter.

Assessment methodology in each Unit II chapter begins with a discussion of the **health history** that is required to gain a thorough understanding of the functional health area being discussed. Interview guidelines are provided in each chapter to assist the nurse in obtaining data corresponding to indicators for each nursing diagnosis listed at the beginning of the chapter. Situations in which it would be appropriate to use screening questions in place of a comprehensive interview are identified. The significance of the types of data obtained by interviewing is discussed in detail in the text.

A discussion of the **diagnostic studies** that may contribute to an overall understanding of a particular functional area follows the health history discussion. Pertinent diagnostic studies may focus on the significance of laboratory values, special imaging, or psychometric measurement. For example, in Chapter 6 the laboratory studies used to make judgments about nitrogen balance, an indicator of protein metabolism, are discussed. In Chapter 10, "Assessing Sleep and Rest," particulars of a sleep laboratory evaluation are highlighted. In Chapter 14, "Assessing Stress and Coping," the diagnostic study section focuses on surveys or questionnaires the nurse might use to evaluate stressors and the stress response.

Each chapter then discusses the pertinence of observational or physical examination data to the functional area. This section is indicated by the headings **physical examination techniques** in Chapter 6 through 9 and 13, and **nursing observations** in Chapters 5, 10 through 12, 14, and 15. In addition to the types of general appearance observations that are helpful in determining a person's level of functioning in a particular area, detailed **assessment guidelines** are presented for this section of Unit II. The examination guidelines may focus on physical examination techniques or specific types of observations that are informative for a particular functional area.

Following each examination guideline is a discussion that focuses on **documenting examination findings.** Examples are provided to assist the nurse with the documentation of both normal and abnormal findings. Finally, the **nursing diagnoses** and **clinical problems** associated with data that may be obtained from each examination process are discussed. This section focuses on how data are used to identify and support a particular clinical diagnosis.

Each chapter concludes with a **case study** and a **critical thinking exercise.** The clinically oriented case study presents a situation related to the functional area examined in the chapter. A brief clinical scenario introduces a person with functional alterations. The critical thinking required to arrive at conclusions about the person's profile is then discussed. This serves to illustrate concepts presented in Chapter 1, "Introduction to Health Assessment." The critical thinking exercise provides additional material related to the chapter content and uses discussion questions to further stimulate higher-level cognitive processes relevant to assessment.

Special Situations in Health Assessment

Unit III presents specialized aspects of health assessment, including approaches that should be used for different age groups—infants, children, adolescents, and the elderly—and those that apply to different practice settings and contexts. Chapter 16, "Assessing Infants, Children, and Adolescents," and Chapter 17, "Health Assessment of Elderly Persons," focus on normal age-related physical findings, examination skill modifications for different age groups, and growth and development concepts in relation to functional areas. Chapter 18, "Assessing in Special Situations," provides specific guidelines for assessment in the acute care setting, trauma assessment, assessment in the chemical dependency treatment setting, and assessment in bladder retraining programs. The intent is to illustrate the types of modifications and special skills that might be required in a variety of different practice settings. For example, in the acute care setting, nurses conduct bedside head-to-toe examinations to screen for illness complications and to monitor treatment responses. Additionally, the nurse requires special skills for evaluating the technology that is often associated with medical treatment in this setting. Chapter 18 provides practical guidelines for modifying assessment techniques learned in Unit II to fit with the real, and often hectic, world of nursing practice.

KEY FEATURES

Health Assessment: A Nursing Approach presents the essential concepts, processes, and skills that help students build a solid foundation for a nursing-oriented health assessment pertinent to a variety of health care settings. To achieve this goal, the text emphasizes the following key features:

- *A strong nursing process and nursing diagnosis framework.* Assessment is viewed as the initial step in the nursing process that concludes with the diagnosis of a person's health or illness status. The relevance of assessment data to nursing diagnoses is highlighted throughout the text.

- *A holistic and transcultural approach to health assessment across the life cycle.* By using the framework of 11 functional health areas, students learn the focus of a holistic assessment that emphasizes physical status as well as psychosocial and cultural aspects of the person. Developmental concepts are presented to illustrate assessment strategies applicable across the life span.

- *Health and wellness.* A specific chapter emphasizing the assessment of health perception and health management practices helps the student relate health and wellness concepts to assessment. The nature of normal findings is emphasized throughout the text to further illustrate these concepts.

- *Varied data collection methods, including interviewing, diagnostic testing, observation, and physical ex-*

amination. The approach to health assessment advocates the use of multiple and varied data sources and methods. The relevance of diagnostic test findings to the interpretation of health status is added to the traditional armamentarium of interviewing and physical examination.

- *Clinical relevance.* Special assessment methods are provided to guide the nurse in the evaluation of common or special clinical concerns, including edema, wound healing, suicide potential, crisis, pain, physical changes of pregnancy, and equipment functioning.

PEDAGOGIC FEATURES

To reinforce and enhance learning and involve the student in the learning process, numerous pedagogic aids summarize or highlight text information.

- *Interview Guides* for each functional area indicate the types of questions the nurse should ask when eliciting a health history.

- *Anatomy and Physiology Overviews* precede each physical examination section to enhance understanding of physical examination techniques and findings. Assessment Guidelines are arranged in an easy-to-read two-column format: the left column outlines the step-by-step procedure for conducting the examination, and the right column highlights the clinical significance of various aspects of the physical examination, including normal findings and deviations from normal.

- *Displays of Abnormal Findings* expand on the material in the examination guideline section to help the student recognize, sort, and describe abnormal findings. An extensive collection of original art illustrates these displays.

- *Documentation Samples* of normal and abnormal findings illustrate the language that may be used to ensure complete yet brief descriptions of findings. A variety of formats are illustrated, including narrative, SOAP, and charting by exception.

- *Nursing Diagnosis and Clinical Problem sections* provide additional discussion of factors to consider when making a diagnosis.

- *Case Studies* present clinical scenarios and take the student through the clinical thinking processes required for formulating accurate and valid nursing diagnoses.

- *Critical Thinking Exercises* provide discussion topics that require the application of higher-level cognitive processes such as application, analysis, synthesis, and evaluation.

- *Abundant illustrations and photographs* clarify the text and enhance understanding.

Jill Fuller, RN, PhD
Jennifer Schaller-Ayers, RN,C, MNSc, PhD

ACKNOWLEDGMENTS

We are grateful to the many people who lent their support, help, and inspiration to this project. We acknowledge the following persons with special appreciation:

The nursing students to whom we have taught health assessment and other clinical courses, and our nursing colleagues in Minot, North Dakota, and the University of Arkansas for Medical Sciences (especially Cheryl Rhoads, Cheryl Schmidt, Richard Smith, Sue Huskey, and Michelle Grey) and the University of Texas at El Paso (especially Patricia Fowler, Sandra Montgomery, and Tanya Probaseo)

Friends in North Dakota (especially Larry and Paula Johnson who provided a quiet retreat for writing at Dougl Bay)

The reviewers of the first edition and second edition manuscript, whose insights helped us to improve our product

Brad Nelson from Medical Illustration at the University of Utah Medical Center, Salt Lake City, for his excellent photography; and Larry Ward for his artistic talent with the line illustrations

Ilze Rader and Dale Thuesen for their editorial support and insights. Their interest, expert guidance, and encouragement were essential for the completion of this project.

The many experts behind the scenes at Lippincott Williams and Wilkins, especially Tom Gibbons and Michael Carcel.

CONTENTS

UNIT ONE

Overview of Health Assessment and Clinical Competencies   1

CHAPTER 1   Introduction to Health Assessment   3

Health Assessment in Nursing Practice   4
Purpose of Health Assessment   10
Health Assessment Processes   10

CHAPTER 2   The Health Assessment Interview and Health History   23

Introductory Overview   24
Knowledge Base for Assessment: Interviewing   25
▼ ASSESSMENT GUIDELINES: The Initial Health Assessment Interview   35
▼ ASSESSMENT GUIDELINES: The Medical History   40
▼ ASSESSMENT GUIDELINES: The Medication and Substance Abuse History   44
Documentation: The Health History   45

CHAPTER 3   The Physical Examination   59

Introductory Overview   60
Knowledge Base for Assessment   61
▼ ASSESSMENT GUIDELINES: The Complete Physical Examination   77
▼ ASSESSMENT GUIDELINES: The General Survey   91
Documentation: The Physical Examination   94

CHAPTER 4   Assessing Vital Signs   99

Introductory Overview   100
Interpretation of Vital Signs   100
Body Temperature   101
▼ ASSESSMENT GUIDELINES: Body Temperature   104
Arterial Pulse   108
▼ ASSESSMENT GUIDELINES: Arterial Pulse   109
Respiratory Rate and Pattern   111

▼ ASSESSMENT GUIDELINES: Respiratory Rate and Pattern   112

Blood Pressure   113

▼ ASSESSMENT GUIDELINES: Blood Pressure Measurement   117

UNIT TWO

Health Assessment of Human Function   121

CHAPTER 5   **Assessing Health Perception and Health Management   123**

Introductory Overview   124

Assessment Focus   125

Knowledge Base for Assessment   126

Health Perception—Health Management Pattern Assessment   131

▼ ASSESSMENT GUIDELINES: Health Perception Interview (Health History)   135

▼ ASSESSMENT GUIDELINES: Health Maintenance—Health Perception:
Physical Assessment   139

CHAPTER 6   **Assessing Nutrition and Metabolism   153**

Part 1 Assessing the Pattern   154

Introductory Overview   154

Assessment Focus   154

Knowledge Base for Assessment   155

▼ ASSESSMENT GUIDELINES: Nutrition Interview (Health History)   165

▼ ASSESSMENT GUIDELINES: Diet Evaluation   169

▼ ASSESSMENT GUIDELINES: Diagnostic Studies of Nutrition Status   172

▼ ASSESSMENT GUIDELINES: Anthropometric Assessment   174

▼ ASSESSMENT GUIDELINES: Interpreting Physical Examination Findings Related
to Nutrition   178

Part 2 Physical Examination Techniques   181

Integumentary System: Skin, Hair, and Nails   181

▼ ASSESSMENT GUIDELINES: Skin   183

▼ ASSESSMENT GUIDELINES: Wound Assessment   191

▼ ASSESSMENT GUIDELINES: Hair   194

▼ ASSESSMENT GUIDELINES: Nails   195

The Jaw and Oral Cavity   200

▼ ASSESSMENT GUIDELINES: Jaw and Oral Cavity   204

The Abdomen   212

▼ ASSESSMENT GUIDELINES: Abdomen   215

▼ ASSESSMENT GUIDELINES: Evaluating Abdominal Fluid   223
The Thyroid Gland   226
▼ ASSESSMENT GUIDELINES: Thyroid Gland   227
The Lymphatic System   229
▼ ASSESSMENT GUIDELINES: Lymphatic System   231

CHAPTER 7   Assessing Elimination   237

Part 1 Assessing the Pattern   238
Assessment Focus   238
Knowledge Base for Assessment   239
▼ ASSESSMENT GUIDELINES: Bowel Elimination Interview (Health History)   243
▼ ASSESSMENT GUIDELINES: Bladder Elimination Interview (Health History)   247
▼ ASSESSMENT GUIDELINES: Diagnostic Studies of Elimination   251
▼ ASSESSMENT GUIDELINES: Stool   254
▼ ASSESSMENT GUIDELINES: Urine   259
▼ ASSESSMENT GUIDELINES: Interpreting Physical Examination Findings Related
   to Elimination   263
Part 2 Physical Examination Techniques   268
Anus and Rectum   268
▼ ASSESSMENT GUIDELINES: Anus and Rectum   271

CHAPTER 8   Assessing Activity and Exercise   281

Part 1 Assessing the Pattern   282
Introductory Overview   282
Assessment Focus   282
Knowledge Base for Assessment   283
▼ ASSESSMENT GUIDELINES: Activity and Exercise Interview (Health History)   289
▼ ASSESSMENT GUIDELINES: Diagnostic Studies for Evaluation of Activity
   and Exercise Functions   291
▼ ASSESSMENT GUIDELINES: Interpreting Physical Examination Findings Related to Activity
   and Exercise   293
Part 2 Physical Examination Techniques   296
Cardiovascular System   296
▼ ASSESSMENT GUIDELINES: Heart and Precordium   304
▼ ASSESSMENT GUIDELINES: Arterial Pulses   312
▼ ASSESSMENT GUIDELINES: Neck Veins   318
Respiratory System   322
▼ ASSESSMENT GUIDELINES: Nose and Sinuses   326
▼ ASSESSMENT GUIDELINES: Lungs and Thorax   329
Musculoskeletal System   338
▼ ASSESSMENT GUIDELINES: Bones, Joints, and Muscles   344

CHAPTER 9   **Assessing Cognition
and Perception   369**

Part 1 Assessing the Pattern   370
Introductory Overview   370
Assessment Focus   370
Knowledge Base for Assessment   371
▼ ASSESSMENT GUIDELINES: Cognition and Perception Interview (Health History)   377
▼ ASSESSMENT GUIDELINES: Mental Status Evaluation   382
▼ ASSESSMENT GUIDELINES: Diagnostic Studies for Evaluation
  of Altered Mental Status   389
▼ ASSESSMENT GUIDELINES: Interpreting Physical Examination Findings Related to Cognition
  and Perception   389
Pain   392
▼ ASSESSMENT GUIDELINES: Pain   398
Part 2 Physical Examination Techniques   401
The Cranial Nerves   401
▼ ASSESSMENT GUIDELINES: Cranial Nerves   403
Motor System and Reflexes   407
▼ ASSESSMENT GUIDELINES: Deep Tendon Reflexes   409
▼ ASSESSMENT GUIDELINES: Superficial Reflexes (Optional)   411
Sensory System and Cerebellar Functions   413
▼ ASSESSMENT GUIDELINES: Sensory System and Cerebellar Functions   418
The Eyes and Vision   422
▼ ASSESSMENT GUIDELINES: Eyes   425
▼ ASSESSMENT GUIDELINES: Testing Visual Acuity   435
The Ears and Hearing   438
▼ ASSESSMENT GUIDELINES: Ears   442
▼ ASSESSMENT GUIDELINES: Hearing   444

CHAPTER 10   **Assessing Sleep and Rest   453**

Introductory Overview   454
Assessment Focus   454
Knowledge Base for Assessment   455
▼ ASSESSMENT GUIDELINES: Sleep and Rest Interview (Health History)   461
▼ ASSESSMENT GUIDELINES: Sleep Laboratory Evaluation   465
▼ ASSESSMENT GUIDELINES: Interpreting Physical Examination Findings Related to Sleep
  and Rest   466
▼ ASSESSMENT GUIDELINES: Sleep Pattern Observation   467

CHAPTER 11   **Assessing Self-Concept   475**

Introductory Overview   476
Assessment Focus   476

Knowledge Base for Assessment   477

▼ ASSESSMENT GUIDELINES: Self-Concept Interview (Health History)   482

▼ ASSESSMENT GUIDELINES: Self-Concept: Physical Assessment   484

CHAPTER 12   **Assessing Roles and Relationships   491**

Introductory Overview   492

Assessment Focus   492

Knowledge Base for Assessment   493

▼ ASSESSMENT GUIDELINES: Roles and Relationships Interview (Health History)   500

▼ ASSESSMENT GUIDELINES: Roles and Relationships: Physical Assessment   503

CHAPTER 13   **Assessing Sexuality and Reproductive Patterns   513**

Introductory Overview   514

Assessment Focus   514

Knowledge Base for Assessment   516

▼ ASSESSMENT GUIDELINES: Sexuality and Reproduction Interview (Health History)   522

▼ ASSESSMENT GUIDELINES: Sexuality and Reproduction: Physical Assessment   531

The Female   532

▼ ASSESSMENT GUIDELINES: Female Genitalia: Physical Assessment   535

Breasts and Axillae   551

▼ ASSESSMENT GUIDELINES: Breasts: Physical Assessment   553

Physical Changes During Pregnancy   560

▼ ASSESSMENT GUIDELINES: Physical Examination of Fundal Height, Fetal Heart, and Fetal Lie   565

The Male   570

▼ ASSESSMENT GUIDELINES: Male Genitalia: Physical Assessment   573

CHAPTER 14   **Assessing Stress and Coping   583**

Introductory Overview   584

Assessment Focus   585

Knowledge Base for Assessment   585

▼ ASSESSMENT GUIDELINES: Stress and Coping Interview (Health History)   594

▼ ASSESSMENT GUIDELINES: Suicide Potential   599

▼ ASSESSMENT GUIDELINES: Interpreting Physical Examination Findings and Stress Responses   600

CHAPTER 15   **Assessing Values and Beliefs   607**

Introductory Overview   608

Assessment Focus   609

Knowledge Base for Assessment   609

▼ ASSESSMENT GUIDELINES: Values and Beliefs Interview (Health History)   618
▼ ASSESSMENT GUIDELINES: Values and Beliefs Pattern   621

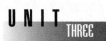

UNIT THREE

Health Assessment Across the Life Span   625

CHAPTER 16   **Assessing Infants, Children, and Adolescents   627**

Introductory Overview   628
Assessment Focus   628
Knowledge Base for Assessment   629
▼ ASSESSMENT GUIDELINES: Pediatric Interview (Health History)   642
▼ ASSESSMENT GUIDELINES: Physical Examination of Newborns   646
▼ ASSESSMENT GUIDELINES: Physical Examination of Infants   663
▼ ASSESSMENT GUIDELINES: Physical Examination of Young Children   670
▼ ASSESSMENT GUIDELINES: Physical Examination of Older Children and Adolescents   675

CHAPTER 17   **Health Assessment of Elderly Persons   685**

Introductory Overview   686
Assessment Focus   686
Knowledge Base for Assessment   687
▼ ASSESSMENT GUIDELINES: Elder Interview (Health History)   689
▼ ASSESSMENT GUIDELINES: Physical Examination   695

CHAPTER 18   **Assessing in Special Situations   703**

Introductory Overview   704
Special Situations and Different Assessment Approaches   704
▼ ASSESSMENT GUIDELINES: Bedside Head-to-Toe Examination   706
▼ ASSESSMENT GUIDELINES: Chest Tubes   709
▼ ASSESSMENT GUIDELINES: Nasogastric Tubes   711
▼ ASSESSMENT GUIDELINES: Enteral Feeding Tubes   713
▼ ASSESSMENT GUIDELINES: Intravascular Pressure Monitoring   714
▼ ASSESSMENT GUIDELINES: Oxygen Therapy   716
▼ ASSESSMENT GUIDELINES: Urinary Catheters and Bladder Irrigation Systems   718
▼ ASSESSMENT GUIDELINES: Intravenous Therapy   719
▼ ASSESSMENT GUIDELINES: Cardiac Monitoring   721
▼ ASSESSMENT GUIDELINES: Pulse Oximetry   722
▼ ASSESSMENT GUIDELINES: Trauma   724

▼ ASSESSMENT GUIDELINES: Substance Abuse   730

▼ ASSESSMENT GUIDELINES: Bladder Retraining   733

Appendices   737

Appendix A   Recommended Daily Calorie Intake for Adults According to Body Weight and Activity Levels as Defined by the World Health Organization   739

Appendix B   Recommended Daily Dietary Allowances (RDAs)   741

Appendix C   Height and Weight Tables for Adults   745

Appendix D   Denver Developmental Screening Test II (DDST2) and Denver Articulation Screening Examination   747

Appendix E   Infant and Child Growth Charts   753

Appendix F   Flowsheet for Documenting Assessment Findings in the Acute Care Setting   763

Appendix G   Trauma Flowsheet   767

Index   771

A color insert, "Ophthalmoscopic and Otoscopic Examination," appears between pages 428 and 429.

UNIT ONE

Overview of Health Assessment and Clinical Competencies

1. Introduction to Health Assessment

2. The Health Assessment Interview and Health History

3. The Physical Examination

4. Assessing Vital Signs

CHAPTER 1

Introduction to Health Assessment

CHAPTER ORGANIZATION

Introductory Overview

**Health Assessment
in Nursing Practice**
- Florence Nightingale
- Expanded Nursing Roles
- The Nursing Process
- Nursing Diagnosis
- Functional Health Patterns

**Purpose of Health
Assessment**

**Health Assessment
Processes**
- Data Collection
- Documentation
- Diagnostic Reasoning
- Classification and Naming
  of Health Status

INTRODUCTORY OVERVIEW

For nurses, *health assessment* can be defined as a process of systematically collecting and analyzing data to make judgments about health and life processes of individuals, families, and communities. The nurse engages in the health assessment process by making accurate and relevant observations, drawing inferences from those observations, and making judgments. These individual elements of the assessment process require skill in the basic techniques of data collection and the critical thinking abilities known as diagnostic reasoning. Knowledge of classification systems for nursing diagnoses and other health problems provides a method for identifying and labeling the nurse's judgment about an individual, family, or community as a response to health and life processes.

The focus of this book is on the health assessment of individuals who receive nursing care, with an emphasis on teaching the skills and techniques of data collection. Additionally, emphasis is placed on the interpretation of clinically significant findings.

Nurses have used the terms *person, client,* or *patient* to refer to individual recipients of nursing care. The assessment of individuals by nurses has traditionally been associated with different modifiers. The terms *patient assessment,* or even *physical assessment,* reflect nursing's alignment with the medical sciences that focus on the collection and analysis of clinical data. *Clinical data* refers to material or facts obtained by direct observation of a person in a patient care setting such as an outpatient facility or a hospital. In these settings, clinical data are collected and analyzed to determine patient care and treatment needs.

But nurses also care for persons in nonclinical settings, including an individual's home and community. The assessment of individuals by nurses in nonclinical settings may still be called *patient assessment,* or other variations may be used, including *client assessment* or *nursing assessment.* In all settings, nurses assess individuals to determine care and treatment needs as well as overall health status, health promoting factors, and health risk factors. We believe the term *health assessment* depicts this broader connotation of assessment as part of the nursing process. But regardless of the semantics associated with the various modifiers for the assessment process performed by nurses, the important thing to understand is that assessment, in any setting, provides the foundation for nursing care.

HEALTH ASSESSMENT IN NURSING PRACTICE

Florence Nightingale

Florence Nightingale (1820–1910), widely regarded as the founder of modern nursing, considered assessment an essential nursing function and referred to this activity as "observation of the sick." She stressed the importance of nursing observation and reporting because the physician was not constantly at the patient's bedside as the nurse was. Nightingale believed nurses needed to develop technical data collection skills such as the ability to measure and record vital signs and observe vital physical functions. She also emphasized the importance of interviewing patients to obtain pertinent information about health and illness. Moreover, she believed in assessing the environment and living conditions of the patient. In her writing, Nightingale stressed that assessment required data collection as well as analysis and interpretation of the data.

Nursing historians state that Florence Nightingale was well ahead of her time, for although her nursing peers had begun to discuss the importance of nurses' observational skills, patient assessment and the analysis of any clinical observations were considered more within the domain of medicine than nursing.

Expanded Nursing Roles

Nursing roles continued to expand in the late 19th century as more hospitals were built in the United States in response to urban and industrial growth. As the need for nurses in hospitals increased, so did the number of nurse training programs. Public health nursing, which developed in the early 1900s, was also experiencing growth as a nursing specialty. Public health nurses practiced independently in homes and in the community to promote health, provide preventative health care, and identify problems requiring nursing intervention. Consequently, they needed additional assessment skills to more effectively screen people for health problems. Postgraduate courses were developed to emphasize health assessment of environments, families, groups, and individuals.

Nursing roles continued to develop in the postwar years of the mid-20th century. Expansion of acute care hospitals after World War II created a greater need for nurses with specialized assessment skills. More than ever before, physicians relied on hospital nurses in constant attendance at the patient's bedside to be responsible for ongoing clinical assessment. In the 1970s, the development of the first intensive care units (ICUs) expanded nursing roles to include even greater surveillance of patients with acute pathologic conditions. Nurses were expected to make on-the-spot clinical judgments about a patient's physiologic statistics.

The advanced practice nurse practitioner role emerged during the same period as a result of two projects initiated in 1967: a nurse-run outpatient clinic at the University of Kansas Medical Center and the first pediatric nurse practitioner graduate education program, established at the University of Colorado. The nurse practitioner role evolved to include providing primary health care to certain underserved groups, especially children and women, rural communities, and elders. In providing primary health care, nurse practitioners began performing comprehensive physical examinations addressing all the major body systems. This type of assessment activity—the comprehensive physical examination of a patient—previously had been considered a medical function. Increasingly, nurses began using the physical examination methods of medicine to collect data pertinent to providing nursing care in many settings.

Whether a nurse should perform a comprehensive physical examination and whether the resulting data contributed to nursing's goals was debated during this time by both nurses and physicians. Many nurses believed the use of the physical examination methods traditionally considered part of the exclusive domain of medicine to collect data was appropriate as long as the nurse's findings from the physical examination were used to make judgments that were pertinent to providing nursing care. Kramer (1971) framed the issue by the following observation published in *Nursing Outlook:*

> The real question is not whether the nurse should check a child's ears with an otoscope (that is, a means), but what is her purpose (her end) in doing so?

In response to expanding nursing roles, nursing education programs in the 1970s began to place a greater emphasis on teaching nurses data collection skills and methods, including those needed to perform a comprehensive physical examination. Influenced by nurse practitioner programs, most undergraduate nursing programs used a medical model to teach patient assessment. This model focused on assessing the status of body systems to evaluate the physiological effects and complications of disease and the effectiveness of disease management. The medical model of assessment was well standardized and included a specific interview format to elicit data (chief complaint, history of the current illness, medical history, family history, review of systems) followed by a physical examination emphasizing body systems. Although the medical assessment model enabled nurses to identify and monitor disease processes, it did not provide a means of systematically assessing a person's need for nursing care. Nevertheless, the medical assessment model dominated nursing education, literature, and clinical practice during the 1970s and into the present.

The Nursing Process

Lydia Hall first conceptualized nursing as a process in the 1950s. Thereafter, many nurse scholars began to describe nursing activities in the context of a nursing process. Yura and Walsh (1967) defined the components of the nursing process as assessment, planning, implementation, and evaluation. Since then, each nursing process component has been extensively discussed and developed in the context of nursing as a unique discipline with its own body of knowledge, and assessment has been reclassified as assessment and diagnosis.

During a 1967 national conference on nursing process, nurses presented papers dealing extensively with the assessment concepts. Black (1967) stated that a nursing assessment was focused on assessing "patient needs." Nursing needed greater guidance, however, if such assessments were to be useful and accurate. Merely saying that patients had physical, psychological, social, and spiritual needs ". . . fails to point to particulars that are specific enough to guide us in a detailed assessment of needs" (Black, 1967, p. 1). Black advocated adopting Maslow's (1968) hierarchy of needs as a framework to guide nursing assessment, and specified assessment parameters for each of Maslow's categories. When assessing physiologic needs, for example, the nurse should collect data about food and fluid intake, oxygenation, rest, physical activity, waste elimination, and sexual satisfaction.

At the same conference, Harpine (1967) emphasized that nursing assessment should actively involve the person being assessed whenever possible. Only after making observations about the person, and then exploring those observations with the person as a means of validating the nurse's perceptions, should the nurse begin to make clinical judgments.

Consequently, certain principles about the assessment of individuals by nurses have been established:

Principles of Assessment of Individuals by Nurses

- Assessment initiates the nursing process.
- Assessment is a systematic, deliberate, and interactive process.
- A health assessment conducted by nurses focuses on specific individual characteristics, especially functional abilities and the ability to perform activities of daily living.
- Data are collected from several sources by various methods.
- The health assessment process includes data collection, clinical judgment, and validation of perceptions.

Nursing Diagnosis

Many conceptual models of nursing emerged in the 1960s and 1970s. These models represented efforts to define the essential substance of nursing as an autonomous professional discipline as well as to direct the restructuring of nursing curricula to support professional education. Although many of these models stimulated progress toward the goal of articulating nursing's unique identity, these so-called "grand theories" of nursing did not significantly shape nursing practice or stimulate significant research programs.

In the early 1970s, nursing began to adopt another approach to defining its essential substance as a discipline. Rather than focus on developing broad theories of nursing, this approach focused on defining and classifying the unique clinical judgments that nurses could independently formulate and manage through nurse-prescribed interventions. In other words, what was that part of nursing that could be independently evaluated and managed by the nurse without the supervision or direction from another group of professionals, such as physicians? The classification of this aspect of nursing practice was undertaken to further define nursing's unique identity and to contribute to the health care of individuals, families, and communities. This was the birth of what will be known in nursing's history as the *"Nursing Diagnosis Movement."* The aim of this movement was to formally classify and label what had been loosely structured in the past and known by a variety of terms such as "patient care needs," "nursing problems," or "patient problems."

Technically, this type of classification work is referred to as taxonomy development. A *taxonomy* is a type of classification system that results in the assignment of descriptive labels to various related entities. A well-developed taxonomy includes a description of the theoretical basis behind the classification system, including the principles, procedures, and rules for how to classify and identify the components within the system. In nursing, this type of taxonomic work resulted in what are today known as nursing diagnoses. *Nursing diagnoses* are labels that represent nursing judgments about individuals, families, and communities (Display 1-1).

In 1973, the *North American Nursing Diagnosis Association (NANDA)* was chartered, initiating the development of a formal nursing diagnosis taxonomy. At the first national NANDA conference, nursing diagnoses were defined as human responses to actual or potential health problems that nurses were qualified to manage independently within the scope of their practice. This definition was incorporated into the definition of nursing included in a seminal publication by the American Nurses Association (ANA) in 1980, called *Nursing: A Social Policy Statement.* In this document, ANA defined *nursing* as ". . . the diagnosis and treatment of human responses to actual or potential health problems" (ANA, 1980). To many, the work of this era meant that nursing had come of age and was clearly able to articulate its unique identity, and describe a nursing approach to health care that was distinctive and separate from medicine.

The development of a taxonomy for nursing diagnosis provided a language for nurses to use in clinical practice to better describe their focus and contributions to patient care. In addition to developing a formal language of nursing diagnosis labels, nursing also focused on determining what criteria must be met for a particular nursing diagnosis label to be used. This stimulated research by nurses to identify and validate criteria that would be used to establish various nursing diagnoses. These criteria are known as the *defining characteristics* for the diagnosis. Defining characteristics are the material or facts on which a final diagnosis is based.

This work is of great significance to nursing. Through the development of a nursing diagnosis taxonomy, including nursing diagnosis labels with their associated defining characteristics, nursing had for the first time in its history, collectively and systematically, determined what data would be relevant to collect in the course of assessing individuals to determine overall health status, and especially, the person's need for nursing care. The nature and content of a clinical database that would logically lead to establishing nursing diagnoses had finally been defined. That database would include indicators and information relevant to the nursing diagnoses included in this new taxonomy.

Functional Health Patterns

The content of a clinical database relevant to nursing should include information about the presence or absence of the indicators suggested by the defining characteristics of nursing diagnoses. A nursing clinical database includes information relevant to confirming or ruling out the indicators of a particular nursing diagnosis. The next challenge for nursing was to determine a standard method for generating this type of clinical database.

As work on nursing diagnosis progressed and nurses started to evaluate the use and application of nursing diagnosis in clinical practice settings, nurses observed difficulty in formulating nursing diagnoses. Some of this difficulty was attributed to using the traditional body systems model of medicine as the format for conducting an assessment and organizing assessment data. Although the body systems format worked well to guide the nurse in the collection of data necessary for the identification of clinical problems or medical diagnoses, it did not help nurses to collect data in a manner that would routinely lead to the identification of nursing diagnoses. Nursing began to look for a process that would generate a clinical database relevant to nursing and lead more directly to nursing diagnoses. Efforts were directed toward developing an assessment framework for nursing analogous to the chief complaint and body systems framework that was so well established for medicine.

Gordon (1987), who participated in much of the early work on nursing diagnosis, proposed a framework for data collection and data base organization with a strong nursing perspective called *Functional Health Patterns (FHPs).* The categorization schema of Functional Health Patterns addresses 11 aspects of human health and life

DISPLAY 1.1

Nursing Diagnoses, North American Nursing Diagnosis Association

BY FUNCTIONAL HEALTH PATTERN CATEGORIES.

Health Perception and Health Management

Aspiration, Risk for
Infection, Risk for
Injury, Risk for
Poisoning, Risk for
Suffocation, Risk for
Trauma, Risk for
Growth and Development, Altered
Growth, Altered, Risk for
Development, Altered, Risk for
Health Maintenance, Altered
Therapeutic Regimen: Individual, Ineffective Management of
Therapeutic Regimen: Family, Ineffective Management of
Therapeutic Regimen: Community, Ineffective Management of
Therapeutic Regimen: Individual, Effective Management of
Protection, Altered
Health-Seeking Behaviors
Noncompliance (Specify)
Latex Allergy Response
Latex Allergy Response, Risk for
Energy Field Disturbance
Failure to Thrive, Adult
Disorganized Infant Behavior, Risk for
Disorganized Infant Behavior
Organized Infant Behavior, Potential for Enhanced

Nutrition and Metabolism

Nutrition, Adequate
Nutrition, Altered: More Than Body Requirements
Nutrition, Altered: Less Than Body Requirements
Nutrition, Altered: Risk for More Than Body Requirements
Infant Feeding Pattern, Ineffective
Swallowing, Impaired
Self-Care Deficit, Feeding
Fluid Volume Excess
Fluid Volume Deficit
Fluid Volume Deficit, Risk for
Skin Integrity, Impaired
Skin Integrity, Risk for Impaired
Tissue Integrity, Impaired
Dentition, Altered
Oral Mucous Membrane, Altered
Body Temperature, Risk for Altered

Hypothermia
Hyperthermia
Thermoregulation, Ineffective

Elimination

Constipation
Constipation, Perceived
Constipation, Risk for
Diarrhea
Incontinence, Bowel
Urinary Elimination, Altered
Incontinence, Stress
Incontinence, Reflex
Incontinence, Urge
Incontinence, Urge, Risk for
Incontinence, Functional
Incontinence, Total
Urinary Retention

Activity and Exercise

Activity Intolerance
Activity Intolerance, Risk for
Diversional Activity Deficit
Home Maintenance Management, Impaired
Physical Mobility, Impaired
Walking, Impaired
Wheelchair Mobility, Impaired
Transfer Ability, Impaired
Bed Mobility, Impaired
Self-Care Deficit, Bathing/Hygiene
Self-Care Deficit, Dressing/Grooming
Self-Care Deficit, Feeding
Self-Care Deficit, Toileting
Fatigue
Tissue Perfusion, Altered (Specify Type) (Renal, Cerebral, Cardiopulmonary, Gastrointestinal, Peripheral)
Fluid Volume Excess
Fluid Volume Imbalance, Risk for
Cardiac Output, Decreased
Gas Exchange, Impaired
Airway Clearance, Ineffective
Breathing Pattern, Ineffective
Spontaneous Ventilation, Inability to Sustain
Ventilatory Weaning Response, Ineffective
Peripheral Neurovascular Dysfunction, Risk for
Perioperative Positioning Injury, Risk for
Surgical Recovery, Delayed

(continued)

DISPLAY 1.1

Nursing Diagnoses, North American Nursing Diagnosis Association (continued)

Cognition and Perception

Knowledge Deficit (Specify)
Thought Process, Altered
Confusion, Acute
Confusion, Chronic
Memory, Impaired
Environmental Interpretation Syndrome, Impaired
Verbal Communication, Impaired
Sensory–Perceptual Alterations (Specify) (Visual, Auditory, Kinesthetic, Gustatory, Tactile, Olfactory)
Unilateral Neglect
Injury, Potential for
Dysreflexia
Autonomic Dysreflexia, Risk for
Pain
Pain, Chronic
Nausea

Sleep and Rest

Fatigue
Sleep Pattern Disturbance
Sleep Deprivation

Self-Perception and Self-Concept

Body Image Disturbance
Personal Identity Disturbance
Self-Esteem Disturbance
    Self-Esteem, Chronic Low
    Self-Esteem, Situational Low
Anxiety
Death Anxiety
Fear
Hopelessness
Powerlessness
Self-Mutilation, Risk for
Violence: Self-Directed, Risk for

Roles and Relationships

Family Processes, Altered
Family Processes: Alcoholism, Altered
Parenting, Altered
Parenting, Risk for Altered
Parent–Infant Attachment, Risk for Altered
Parental Role Conflict
Chronic Sorrow

Grieving, Anticipatory
Grieving, Dysfunctional
Role Performance, Disturbances in
Social Isolation
Relocation Stress Syndrome
Loneliness, Risk for
Caregiver Role Strain
Caregiver Role Strain, Risk for
Social Interaction, Impaired
Verbal Communication, Impaired
Violence: Directed at Others, Risk for

Sexuality and Reproduction

Sexual Dysfunction
Sexuality Patterns, Altered
Breast-Feeding, Effective
Breast-Feeding, Ineffective
Breast-Feeding, Interrupted
Rape-Trauma Syndrome
Rape-Trauma Syndrome:
    Compound Reaction
    Silent Reaction

Coping and Stress Tolerance

Coping: Individual, Ineffective
Adjustment, Impaired
Coping, Defensive
Denial, Ineffective
Coping: Family, Ineffective
    Disabling
    Compromised
Coping: Family, Potential for Growth
Coping: Community, Potential for Enhanced
Coping: Community, Ineffective
Decisional Conflict (Specify)
Grieving, Dysfunctional
Grieving, Anticipatory
Post-trauma syndrome
Post-trauma syndrome, Risk for

Values and Beliefs

Spiritual Distress (Distress of the Human Spirit)
Spiritual Distress, Risk for
Spiritual Well Being, Potential for Enhanced

processes. The 11 functional health patterns include the following:

Functional Health Pattern Categories

- **Health Perception and Health Management:** A person's perceived level of health and well-being and their practices and behaviors related to maintaining health
- **Nutrition and Metabolism:** The pattern of food and fluid consumption relative to metabolic need and nutritional processes
- **Elimination:** Bowel and bladder elimination functions and patterns
- **Activity and Exercise:** A person's abilities to engage in activities of daily living as well as their responses to activities requiring energy, endurance, physical conditioning, and coordination
- **Cognition and Perception:** Patterns of sensory experiences and cognitive functions
- **Sleep and Rest:** Sleep, rest, and relaxation patterns
- **Self-Perception and Self-Concept:** A person's attitudes toward self including identity, body-image, and sense of worth
- **Roles and Relationships:** A person's roles in life and the nature of their relationships with others
- **Sexuality and Reproduction:** Patterns of sexuality and sexual identity, sexual behaviors, and reproductive functions
- **Coping and Stress Tolerance:** A person's perception of stress and their own coping abilities as well as their responses to stress
- **Values and Beliefs:** A person's values, beliefs, and spirituality

These 11 categories make possible a systematic and standardized approach to data collection and analysis with a clear nursing focus. The use of FHPs as an assessment format and content organizer further emphasizes the nursing process and encourages critical thinking and clinical reasoning. Gordon illustrates these principles with her contemporary model of the nursing process (Fig. 1-1).

According to the nursing process model shown in Figure 1-1, assessment begins by deciding what aspects of the person should be the framework for data collection. Gordon (1987) uses functional health patterns as this framework. Gordon defines *pattern* as a sequence of behavior across time. The nurse would proceed by evaluating the function of an individual in relation to each pattern and would make one of the following determinations:

Classification of Patterns

- **Functional:** The individual is at an optimal level of

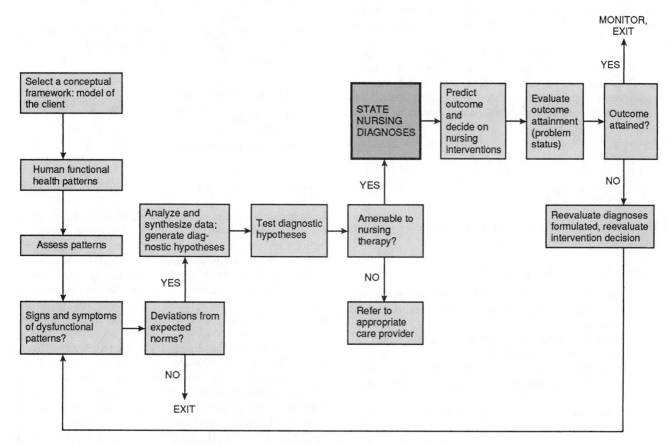

FIGURE 1.1 The nursing process. A nursing process model advocating the use of a nursing conceptual framework (functional health patterns) to direct data collection and assessment (Gordon, M. [1987]. *Nursing diagnosis: Process and application* [2nd ed.]. New York: McGraw-Hill)

functioning. This represents an individual strength or state of health and wellness.

- **Dysfunctional:** The individual is assessed and found to have deficits, health problems, or illness.
- **Potentially dysfunctional:** The individual is vulnerable to developing a dysfunctional state. There is risk for disability and illness.

Whenever a dysfunctional or potentially dysfunctional state is identified, the nurse will need to determine whether the problem can be addressed or treated by the nurse. As a result of this analysis, the nurse will classify the problem in one of the following ways:

Classification of Problems

- **Nursing diagnosis:** The problem *can be independently managed* by the nurse within the scope of nursing practice
- **Clinical problem:** The problem *cannot be independently managed* by the nurse even though the nurse may have a significant role in monitoring the problem or the nurse may participate with other healthcare providers in the management of the problem. Various terminologies may be used to refer to clinical problems that cannot be independently managed by nurses, including *collaborative problem* or *medical diagnosis.*

The use of functional health patterns as a format for the collection of data during the assessment process is not as universally applied by nurses as medicine's chief complaint and body systems format is by physicians conducting the medical assessment process. Even so, the functional health pattern framework is continuing to gain widespread use as a framework for assessing individuals to determine their overall health status and nursing care needs.

PURPOSE OF HEALTH ASSESSMENT

The purpose of health assessment of individuals by nurses includes the following:

Purpose of Health Assessment

- To gain an *understanding* of the person's experience of *health and life processes,* including health, illness, and recovery
- To *identify strengths* that promote health or need to be enhanced for optimal functioning
- To *identify needs, clinical problems, or nursing diagnoses* that form the basis of nursing care and intervention
- To *evaluate* the effects of therapeutic plans and interventions

Nursing is a discipline that focuses on understanding health and life processes of individuals. The work of nursing is to provide care for persons during their experience of life processes associated with health and illness. Because of nursing's history and tradition of alignment with medical science, nursing's approaches to assessment have focused on understanding how people respond physically to illness and health problems. But in relating to the health and illness phenomena of the human experience, nursing must focus, as well, on understanding and evaluating the broader perspectives people have about health and illness, including basic beliefs about health, health promotion, and the meaning of illness; the impact of these human experiences on the sense of self as well as on relationships with others; and the individual's capacity for dealing with stress and adaptation. This broader perspective of health assessment is difficult to encompass using the traditional methods of clinical assessment—brief, focused measurement techniques to determine the clinical status of various body systems at a particular time. Taken by themselves, these traditional methods are limited to defining the physical manifestations of pathologic conditions. Therefore, these methods should be viewed as only one of several approaches that may be used to know the individual in the context of the human health experience.

HEALTH ASSESSMENT PROCESSES

Health assessment processes aimed at the identification of an individual's responses, strengths, problems or needs include the following:

Health Assessment Processes

- Data collection
- Documentation
- Diagnostic reasoning

Data Collection

Data collection refers to the process of obtaining uninterpreted material, facts, or clinical information about an individual such as body temperature, blood pressure, height, weight, medications used, personal habits, heart and lung sounds, or skin color. Until this material is analyzed and interpreted, it is known as *data.* Data collection can be thought of as a health assessment activity of observing or obtaining measurements related to an individual's health status.

Data collection is driven by knowledge of what is being observed or measured. For example, to measure blood pressure, the nurse needs an understanding of the vascular sounds associated with systole and diastole. Data collection also requires skill in the various methods of clinical observation and measurement. Continuing with the example of blood pressure measurement, the datum blood pressure is obtained by applying procedural skills that include the correct application and inflation of the blood pressure cuff.

Data Collection Methods

During the health assessment, the nurse will collect data through interaction with the individual being assessed, their significant others, and other healthcare providers, when appropriate. A variety of methods may be used to collect data during the health assessment process, including the following:

Data Collection Methods

- The assessment interview
- Physical examination
- Review of records

Assessment Interview. The *assessment interview* is a structured, goal-directed conversation between the nurse and an individual for the purpose of yielding information about the person, their health perceptions, functional status, and other factors relevant to health, healing, and illness. The assessment interview is often considered the best source of data about an individual, and the assessment process often starts with an interview. A general approach to the assessment interview is described in Chapter 2. In addition, guidelines for assessing an individual in relation to each FHP are described throughout this book.

Physical Examination. A *physical examination* is the observation of an individual in which the nurse uses the senses of sight, hearing, touch, and smell and the observation techniques of inspection, palpation, percussion, and auscultation. The nurse's perceptions during the physical examination are interpreted in light of the nurse's knowledge of normal and abnormal anatomy and physiology. The nurse's perceptions are also interpreted in the context of functional health patterns, nursing diagnoses, and clinical problems. A general approach to a complete physical examination is described in Chapter 3. Specific and detailed techniques for the examination of various body systems or body areas are introduced throughout this book in relation to FHPs for which physical examination findings are interpreted to make judgments about functional status. For example, the evaluation of the skin is discussed in the context of nutrition and metabolism; and the examination of the eyes and ears are discussed with the assessment of cognition and perception.

Review of Records. The *review of records* most pertinent to health assessment involves a review of the patient's medical record (also known as the *chart, health record,* or *clinical record*). The medical record is an account of the person's health status that is compiled by various healthcare providers, including physicians, nurses, dieticians, physical therapists, social workers, and others. Data included in a medical record include the patient's medical history, descriptions of illness and details of treatments or interventions, findings from physical examinations conducted by various practitioners, reports of diagnostic tests, findings and conclusions from special technical examinations, and medications that have been prescribed. If a medical record is available, nurses and other healthcare providers will often review the record early in the health assessment and data collection process. Throughout this book, the significance of medical record data, especially the reports of diagnostic tests and medications, is discussed in relation to assessing functional status.

Subjective and Objective Data

Data are usually classified as subjective or objective. *Subjective data* are data that are not readily quantified or measured, such as personal opinions, values, or social relationships. In health assessment, subjective data relate to perceptions held by the individual being evaluated and not to the perceptions held by the nurse. For example, descriptions of pain are considered subjective data because pain is described from the perspective of the person experiencing the pain. Other examples of subjective data might include a person's description of symptoms such as nausea or dizziness, or the descriptions of feelings such as fear or anxiety.

Objective data refers to facts that are determined by direct observations such as quantitative measurements (*e.g.,* blood pressure), physical examination (*e.g.,* heart sounds), or sensory observation (*e.g.,* seeing or smelling). Objective data are usually made without personal bias or opinion and can be verified by another observer. Examples of objective data include a grimace during a dressing change, a serum potassium level measurement of 4 mEq/L, crackles heard during lung auscultation, and a decubitus ulcer measuring 4 cm in diameter.

Scope of Data Collection

Depending on the setting for providing nursing care, the individual's needs, or the overall assessment objectives, the scope of data collection activities may vary. The scope of data collection activities can be distinguished on the basis of intensity and complexity and classified in the following manner:

Scope of Data Collection

- Screening
- Comprehensive
- Focused

Screening Assessment. *Screening* involves the collection of very specific data to identify an occurrence or state that requires further evaluation. Screening does not provide sufficient amounts of data to establish a diagnosis. Screening may be performed to determine whether the individual is in need of additional services, evaluation, or testing. For example, patients admitted to hospitals may be screened to determine whether their nutritional status is at risk or impaired. The nurse may collect minimal amounts of data to complete the nutritional screening process. If the screening criteria indicate any abnormalities with nutritional processes, a clinical dietician may be consulted, and a more comprehensive assessment of nutritional status may be initiated. Similarly, the American Cancer Society recommends a number of screening activities to identify persons at risk for cancer. To screen for colorectal cancer, a stool specimen may be collected and the presence of occult blood determined. The presence of occult blood is the screening finding that will initiate a more comprehensive assessment. As another example, blood pressure screening involves the measurement of blood pressure, and, on the basis of the results of this single data collection activity, the practitioner will make referrals for additional evaluation and testing.

Comprehensive Assessment. Comprehensive nursing care requires complete and ongoing collection of data about the individual's health status. A *comprehensive initial health assessment* is usually conducted during the initial encounter between the nurse and the client to identify the person's needs for nursing care. This may be part of the admission process in a hospital or long-term care setting or the focus of the first visit between the nurse and an individual in a home setting. An ongoing assessment process would then continue as long as the nurse continued to provide nursing care. Often, this type of comprehensive initial assessment is a prerequisite to establishing a nursing care plan.

The type of data that should be collected to initiate a comprehensive initial health assessment is often specified by the assessment format that is being used. For example, the use of FHPs as an assessment format directs the nurse to systematically collect data on all 11 FHPs. In addition, the format may specify that certain other data be collected, such as demographic data, including date of birth, residence, and occupation. The particular format used for the initial data collection process may be dictated by professional standards or organizational policy and further indicated by standardized forms that may be used for recording data. The assessment standard for General Professional Nursing Practice developed by the American Nurses Association provides additional direction regarding the initial comprehensive assessment of an individual (Display 1-2).

Focused Assessment. Data collection activities are *focused* when the goal is to identify and evaluate a specific problem, to evaluate a person's response to treatment procedures, or to detect significant changes in status. For example, a focused data collection process may be appropriate during the initial or ongoing evaluation of specific health problems such as pain, urinary incontinence, or impaired skin integrity. The amount of data that might be collected to determine whether a person had a therapeutic response to a pain medication is considerably less than the amount of data collected to determine the person's overall needs for nursing care. Moreover, the results of a focused data collection process are likely to be recorded differently in the medical record than the information developed from a comprehensive initial assessment.

Prioritizing Data Collection Activities

The prioritization of data collection activities should always be determined by the individual's immediate condition or needs. Even though the nurse may want to conduct a comprehensive assessment, the person's immediate needs may be more pressing. If an individual is in pain, in need of sleep or rest, or at immediate risk for adverse physiologic or psychological events, it may be best to postpone a comprehensive health assessment and narrow your data collection efforts based on prioritization of the person's needs. For example, a patient recently admitted to a coronary care unit with a medical diagnosis of acute myocardial infarction may have immediate needs for pain relief, medication administration, and electrocardiographic (ECG) monitoring. Data collection efforts should focus on obtaining the information needed to make judgments about the effectiveness of the medical treatment plan. In this case, the nurse would direct his or her data collection efforts toward vital signs, ECG recordings, and other pertinent diagnostic data. It would be appropriate to postpone a lengthy assessment interview until such time as the patient's condition has stabilized.

Another common example that calls for the practitioner to prioritize his or her data collection efforts occurs during the care of patients presenting to a hospital emergency department with major trauma. Trauma care standards specifically prioritize assessment procedures with guidelines for conducting the primary and secondary survey of the trauma patient. During the primary survey, evaluation is focused on the status of the patient's airway, breathing, circulation, and cervical spine. The primary survey is conducted immediately and is completed within minutes. The secondary survey is conducted next and takes into account the status of the major body systems. The intent is to quickly collect data to determine whether there are life-threatening injuries. In this setting, because of the patient's most immediate needs, the process of collecting data to establish a comprehensive clinical database is postponed.

The nurse also may encounter individuals who have no interest in being interviewed or examined until a more pressing concern is addressed. In this case, you should attempt to determine the person's immediate need before initiating a more extensive data collection process. A simple way to proceed in this type of situation is for the nurse to simply say, "Tell me what's most important for you to talk about now."

Frequency of Data Collection

If an individual is receiving nursing care on an ongoing basis, data should be collected in such a manner to assure that assessment is ongoing and based on up-to-date material and facts. Data collection also should be conducted at appropriate intervals to reasonably detect changes in a person's status that would require changes in the nursing plan of care. This implies a process of ongoing assessment and reassessment of the individual. The frequency of data collection will be determined by a numbers of factors, including the following:

Factors Influencing the Frequency of Data Collection

- The person's *diagnosis*
- The *level of care* that is being provided
- *Responses* to treatments

A Clinical Database

A clinical *database* is an organized collection of data documented in a standardized format. Clinical databases may

DISPLAY 1.2

Assessment Standard for General Professional Nursing Practice

STANDARD I

The collection of data about the health status of the client/patient is systematic and continuous. The data are accessible, communicated, and recorded.

Rationale

Comprehensive care requires complete and ongoing collection of data about the client/patient to determine the nursing care needs of the client/patient. All health status data about the client/patient must be available for all members of the health care team.

Assessment Factors

1. Health status data include
   - Growth and development
   - Biophysical status
   - Emotional status
   - Cultural, religious, socioeconomic background
   - Performance of activities of daily living
   - Patterns of coping
   - Interaction patterns
   - Client's/patient's perception of and satisfaction with his or her health status
   - Client/patient health goals
   - Environment (physical, social, emotional, ecological)
   - Available and accessible human and material resources
2. Data are collected from
   - Client/patient, family, significant others
   - Health care personnel
   - Individuals within the immediate environment and/or the community

3. Data are obtained by
   - Interview
   - Examination
   - Observation
   - Reading records, reports, etc.
4. There is a format for the collection of data that
   - Provides for a systematic collection of data
   - Facilitates the completeness of data collection
5. Continuous collection of data is evident by
   - Frequent updating
   - Recording of changes in health status
6. The data are
   - Accessible on the client/patient records
   - Retrievable from record-keeping systems
   - Confidential when appropriate

(American Nurses Association. [1991] Standards of clinical nursing practice. Washington, D.C.: ANA.)

---

vary in content, type of information contained, and design, depending on the objectives of the practitioners having input to the database. A common denominator of any database that would be useful to nurses should be that it contains content that can logically lead to the formulation of nursing diagnoses. In general, the following type of information would be included:

Components of a Clinical Database

- **Identifying Information:** name
- **Vital Statistics:** birth date, address, significant others, religious background, allergies
- **Relevant Medical History:** illness, operations, injuries, previous hospitalizations
- **Medication and Substance Use History**
- **Functional Health Patterns:** indicators of functional and dysfunctional patterns
- **Physical Examination:** normal and abnormal findings

The database should be organized so that it is accessible, retrievable, and confidential when appropriate.

Documentation

Health assessment data are documented for several reasons. Documentation of data, information, and health assessment conclusions provide the following:

Purpose of Documentation

- A written display of findings and observations used as the basis for clinical judgments and diagnoses
- A method to make data and information accessible to other providers, using the medical record contributing to continuity of care
- A legal record of events and findings
- A record that may be used to justify the provision of services

Documentation Guidelines

In general, health assessment requires documentation of the nurse's findings from the data collection process. This documentation may consist of a series of observations the nurse writes on a standardized form using a fill-in-the-blank format. Or the nurse may record assessment findings in a brief narrative-style progress note. In any case, certain documentation guidelines should be applied to ensure objectivity, accuracy, clarity, and efficiency.

1. Avoid recording inferences and judgments when documenting data.

    An inference is a judgment based on the examiner's observation of the facts. If your intent is to objectively document your findings, then stick to the facts. For example, *do not* write, "Oral examination reveals receding gum lines, food debris, and halitosis, *indicating poor oral hygiene.*"

    Avoid value-laden language or opinionated statements. For example, the following written statement is inappropriate: "Patient requests for pain medications are too frequent."

    Record any inferences or judgments only after the data have been collected and analyzed. Professional judgments may appear in the record as nursing diagnoses, as problem statements, or as assessment notes such as those appearing in SOAP-style progress notes (see following section—"SOAP Documentation Format").

2. Record findings rather than techniques.

    Avoid a detailed discussion of how the data were obtained. For example, *do not* write, "The ear examination was conducted by inserting otoscope speculum after pulling the auricle upward and backward. Once the tympanic membrane was visualized, it was noted to be pearly gray with a light reflex." This entry is time-consuming to write and read and may discourage careful reading of the examiner's findings.

3. Record the individual's perceptions.

    The individual's perceptions are significant because they reveal what the person believes about their health status or experience. The person's responses to any problems or concerns and expectations in relation to health care are also significant.

4. Write concisely and efficiently.

    Avoid redundant statements that are both annoying to read and time-consuming to write. Examples of redundant statements include "Visible by inspection," "Heard on auscultation," and "Bilaterally symmetric." It is also considered redundant to write, "The patient . . ." (or "the client") in the medical record, because the patient is always assumed to be the subject of the record.

    Summarize and condense the individual's statements whenever possible. For example, you do not need to record verbatim a person's 5-minute description of chest pain, but rather, you may write, "Substernal chest pain occurred three times today, with each episode lasting 5 minutes and relieved by sublingual nitroglycerin. Pain pressure-like without radiation. No shortness of breath, nausea, diaphoresis, palpitations, or lightheadedness during pain."

    Finally, avoid superfluous data. For example, *do not* write, "Able to drive car to work. Drives a red convertible."

5. Record the relevant details.

    All relevant data should be recorded, including both positive and negative findings that might either confirm or rule out a diagnosis. For example, you may observe an individual who is short of breath and has some difficulty walking without a walker. You may be considering a diagnosis of self-care deficit. But if your observations are also recorded to indicate that the person can independently carry out all activities of daily living, the diagnosis of a self-care deficit may not be appropriate.

    Also, record normal findings when abnormal findings might be expected. For example, normal heart sounds and the absence of ankle edema in a person with congestive heart failure should be duly noted.

6. Describe normal findings.

    Your observations should be recorded in specific, descriptive terms. Many nurses find it easier to describe and document abnormal findings than normal findings. Using terms such as *normal, within normal limits,* or *negative* are not recommended because they do not describe your observations as much as reflect your judgment. To substantiate your judgments, you should document your observations. Describe normal findings in terms of what you observe and note through inspection, palpation, percussion, and auscultation. Rather than writing "lung sounds normal," you should write "Lungs clear to auscultation and percussion."

    An exception to the practice of thoroughly describing normal findings may be noted with the documentation method known as "charting by exception." (See Chapter 3 for sample documentation.) If you are charting by exception, only abnormal findings are addressed by the examiner in a medical record entry.

7. Organize and format the data in a logical fashion.

    Record the health assessment data in a systematic and logical manner. Generally, the findings from the health assessment interview will be recorded before the physical examination findings. Printed forms provided by the healthcare organization, such as admission forms and flowsheets, may clearly indicate how the data should be organized and recorded. Such forms often include headings to indicate the subject matter to be recorded and provide spaces for recording specific findings. If a printed form is not available, you may create your own headings to promote easy readability and organization.

    Health assessment data may be logically organized in different ways by different healthcare providers. For example, physicians organize assessment data in relation to illness and symptoms (chief complaint, history of the current illness), medical history, and body systems (review of systems). Nurses may organize assessment data according to FHPs so that relevant data are grouped together in a way that facilitates the diagnostic reasoning involved in making a nursing diagnosis.

Finally, health assessment data relating to a person's health status and health history should be organized in some form of chronological order to facilitate easy retrieval and understanding. Record current concerns or problems chronologically, beginning with the time of onset. List past surgeries or hospitalizations in order, from the earliest occurrence to the most recent. For each entry, specify the date, event, and significant consequences.

8. Use appropriate grammar and punctuation.

Complete sentences should have subjects and verbs. Phrases may be used in place of complete sentences if you carefully consider the punctuation. Commas, dashes, periods, and semicolons give specific indications of how words are related to each other. Correct spelling as well as correct use of abbreviations are expected in a professional record.

SOAP Documentation Format

SOAP Progress notes are a method of conceptualizing and recording information in a problem-oriented medical record. A problem-oriented medical record is a type of medical record in which a patient's health history, physical examination findings, laboratory results, and other clinical data are organized according to problems such as "Impaired skin integrity," or "Chest pain," or "Anxiety." SOAP is an acronym for the following categories of information:

S = Subjective Data. In a SOAP note, *subjective data* refers to data obtained from the patient or a representative of the patient. Subjective data indicates the patient's perceptions and may be recorded as a direct quote, such as, "My mouth hurts." Alternatively, the nurse may summarize or paraphrase the patient's perceptions, such as "States he is worried about surviving heart surgery." The latter approach may be used to condense a lengthy discussion about fears related to surgery.

O = Objective Data. This part of the SOAP entry designates objective data obtained by observation, physical examination, and diagnostic studies. Examples include, "Crying after wife's visit," "Ulcerated lesion ½ cm in diameter on mucosa inside left cheek," and "White blood cell count 15,000."

A = Assessment. This part of the SOAP note refers to assessment of the patient's status based on the previously recorded subjective and objective data. This statement may be a brief statement of status but should not be a restatement of the problem being referred to in the SOAP note. The assessment component should represent the examiner's analysis of the clinical findings in relation to the individual's problem. In the assessment component of the SOAP note, documentation also may include reference to causative factors, the clinical course of the problem, pertinent prognostic indicators, and any notable responses to interventions. An assessment statement incorporating these elements might appear as follows: "Altered oral mucosa related to

mechanical trauma from oral suction catheter; no longer requires oral suctioning and can maintain own oral hygiene; no signs of infection such as redness or drainage; should heal spontaneously as long as hydration and nutrition are maintained."

P = Plan. The plan is not "health assessment" documentation per se, but rather a brief statement of the therapeutic plan for the resolution or management of the problem. For example, the following plan was noted in a patient with potential for impaired skin integrity, "Assist with repositioning every 2 hours. Reevaluate effectiveness of turning schedule by inspecting pressure points with each position change. Modify turning frequency if indicated. Instruct regarding (1) the importance of position changes and (2) how to shift weight with the aid of overhead trapeze."

Narrative-Style Documentation

Health assessment information also may be recorded in a narrative style on the medical record. Various logical organizational approaches are acceptable. For example, health assessment data may be recorded in a progress note to reflect the application of the nursing process. In this case, all of the available assessment data would first be recorded in the nursing progress note. Then the nurse would record additional analysis and interpretation of the data, and interventions and the person's response to interventions. This narrative approach is conceptually similar to the SOAP documentation format. Another organizational approach involves arranging facts and findings according to body systems. For example, you may record your observations in relation to each of the major body systems. Examples of these documentation styles are presented on Display 1-3.

Documentation of a Comprehensive Initial Assessment

A comprehensive initial assessment data base may be recorded in either a narrative or "fill-in-the blank" style. The "fill-in-the blank" style has been modified and adapted for clinical practice and FHPs. A number of sample forms can be found in various healthcare organizations and in the nursing literature. Examples of documentation of the initial comprehensive assessment are displayed in Chapters 2 and 3.

Diagnostic Reasoning

The final assessment process that should be considered in addition to data collection and documentation is diagnostic reasoning. *Diagnostic reasoning* involves the ability to think critically about the assessment process and your findings and make appropriate clinical judgments. It involves the ability to make accurate and relevant observations and to draw inferences from those observations. Diagnostic reasoning skills are explicitly required when the person's clinical picture or pattern does not "fit the box." In that type of situation, the nurse truly needs to be a

DISPLAY 1.3

Documentation—Narrative Style

NARRATIVE NURSING PROGRESS NOTE

"States that he was first diagnosed with 'sugar diabetes' at age 15. Has been independently managing diet, medications, and blood sugar monitoring. States he checks blood sugar routinely, twice a day, and more frequently if indicated. States he wants to manage disease optimally so he can 'be a normal kid' at school. Able to verbalize insulin routine, including method of site rotation. Utilizing exchange diet plan. Able to verbalize appropriate modifications he would make at fast food restaurant, friend's home, or camp-out. Motivated, appropriate health management behaviors, and high self-esteem. Will continue to reinforce present management plan and introduce additional educational materials for continuing reinforcement of healthy behaviors."

NARRATIVE DOCUMENTATION OF BODY SYSTEM FINDINGS

Cardiovascular

Denies chest pain or pressure. Heart rhythm regular, no murmurs or extra heart sounds. All peripheral pulses palpable and equal intensity. Skin warm and pink.

Respiratory

Denies dyspnea. No reports of coughing. Breath sounds clear in all lobes and equal bilaterally.

Neurological

Alert and oriented. Speech clear and appropriate. Follows commands; behavior is appropriate to situation. No reports of pain, paresthesia, or numbness.

Integumentary

No current skin problems reported. Skin is warm and dry and without lesions. Well-healed old surgical incision line in right upper quadrant of abdomen from previous gallbladder surgery.

Gastrointestinal

Denies any nausea, heartburn, or problems with eating and disgestion. Active bowel sounds in all abdominal quadrants. Abdomen soft, nondistended, and nontender.

---

problem solver, a diagnostician, and a critical thinker capable of diagnostic reasoning. The components of the diagnostic reasoning process that lead to the formulation of nursing diagnoses and other clinical judgments include the following:

The Diagnostic Reasoning Process

- Collecting relevant data
- Organizing data so it has meaning
- Drawing a conclusion

Collecting Relevant Data

The diagnostic process begins with the nurse collecting data and identifying clinically significant information—that is, information that indicates normal or abnormal conditions or changes in the person's condition or data that informs the nurse of the person's overall health status in relation to functional capacities.

Data are collected during the assessment process, evaluated by the practitioner, and recorded on assessment forms. Assessment forms usually contain prompts or cues that influence the type of data that are collected and the way in which information is analyzed for clinical signifi-

cance. The nurse also may be prompted to collect certain data or make additional observations by the context of the situation, experience, or the input of other practitioners. Any of these factors may influence the nurse to collect more data based on developing perceptions about the person's health status. The development of a relevant and significant database is enhanced by a systematic and thorough data collection process guided by the nurse's clinical knowledge of human responses to health and illness.

1. Begin With an Adequate Database. It is important that the nurse collect enough data to provide an adequate indication of the person's overall health status. The initial admission assessment, conducted when a nurse first meets the individual, initiates the assessment process and the formation of the clinical *database*. A clinical database organized by FHPs should include pertinent information about all 11 functional areas and become the basis for comparison when evaluating any changes in the person's condition. It is important to use a thorough and systematic approach in developing the database, so that important material or facts are not omitted or overlooked. A random approach to data collection is not advised because of the risk of inadvertently omitting important data. Conducting a systematic head-to-toe physical examination that includes vital signs and inquiries regarding all 11 functional areas greatly increases the probability of obtaining sufficient information to identify significant problems as well as healthy behaviors and sources of strength for the individual.

The following scenario describes a situation in which the nurse initially overlooked an important and crucial piece of information relevant to the person's health and well-being. This emphasizes the importance of thorough and systematic data collection process to ensure that all pertinent information is considered.

Nurse: Aside from doing vital signs and asking a few questions from our hospital's admission form, I never really used to do what I would call a thorough nursing assessment. I tended to skip over the psychosocial parts and only listen to the heart and lungs. I was taking care of an elderly lady who had been very intoxicated on admission. She had been admitted with hypothermia after being found lying in a neighbor's yard. I kept coming out of her room saying, "Something's being missed here" or "Something's not right." I told another nurse about it, and she said, "Well, did you ask her if something triggered her drinking?" or "Did she have problems that were difficult to deal with?" I had never routinely assessed how people were coping or what type of problems they were facing outside the hospital. After talking with her, I found out that she had no history of alcohol abuse but that 2 days ago she had been notified that the drunk driver who had killed her husband 5 years ago in a hit-and-run accident had been released from prison. She talked about how difficult this was to deal with and how she was "falling apart." Now rather than saying, "I think something's wrong," I routinely conduct a thorough assessment so I can get a better idea of the patient's condition.

This example illustrates the importance of assessing all 11 functional pattern areas during the health assessment process. In this case, a more thorough assessment of patterns such as coping and stress tolerance probably would have provided the nurse with information about significant stresses in the person's life as well as her reactions to the stresses.

2. Draw on Clinical Knowledge and Experience. The type of data that you collect and begin to recognize as significant will be influenced by your own knowledge base. If you are a novice nurse, you tend to rely on knowledge gained through study and other educational activities more than experience in providing nursing care. Conversely, if you are an experienced clinician, you draw more on what you know firsthand from clinical situations. You may even have developed an intuitive knowledge of clinical situations and how individuals might respond given different circumstances.

Nurses require extensive knowledge about individuals and families and their responses to different health problems or life processes to make sound clinical judgments. For example, a nurse caring for postoperative patients will see what he or she expects to see based on knowledge about postoperative nursing care that is stored in memory. The nurse might recall his or her academic training related to the care of operative patients and their needs for oxygenation, mobility, safety, and pain control. Drawing on this stored knowledge and being able to anticipate the problems most commonly encountered in a particular context enables the nurse to focus on collecting pertinent data and recognizing patterns that either confirm or rule out all the potential problems the nurse is knowledgeable about. Note how the nurse in the following example draws on both academically and clinically acquired knowledge when assessing the patient.

Nurse: I knew that even though this man was only recovering from surgery under a local anesthetic, he was at risk for developing respiratory problems. His chart indicated that he had a long history of chronic obstructive pulmonary disease (COPD), he was elderly, and he had the appearance of someone with long-standing COPD—he had the barrel chest, he was very thin, and he started to get short of breath with only minimal activity and even resorted to pursed-lip breathing. Then his wife told me that he had not taken his theophylline that morning because he was supposed to be NPO for surgery. Knowing what I did about the disease process, I decided I had better do more than just routine postoperative vital signs, so I carefully listened to his lungs and observed his ventilatory effort and skin color. I also assessed him more often than what was considered routine for a surgical outpatient. He had very little air exchange and was working very hard to breathe. I immediately notified the physician. If this man had been assessed "routinely," with no consideration of his underlying disease process, he may not have received the early and aggressive intervention he needed.

Expertise in the diagnostic reasoning process is enhanced as you add to your clinical experience or theoretical base. Analysis of health assessment data requires special knowledge of health and life processes. For example, an analysis of the finding "lung crackles" requires knowledge of normal and abnormal lung sounds as well as clinical problems that might be associated with lung crackles.

If you have not had adequate education or experience and cannot rely on memory to supply the necessary knowledge about a particular type of patient, especially in relation to pertinent physiological, psychological, or developmental factors, you should consult appropriate references or knowledgeable colleagues.

Organizing Data for Meaning

The next step in the diagnostic process involves the ability to organize or cluster data so that patterns begin to emerge. Rarely is a sound diagnosis ever made on the basis of a single, isolated bit of data. Diagnostic conclusions are usually based on interpreting patterns consisting of a cluster of data.

1. Group Together Related Data. As data are assembled, note which elements seem to "fit" together and indicate a particular problem. Data are clustered to suggest certain diagnostic possibilities. For example, you may note that a new mother (a) states that she is disappointed that her newborn baby is a girl, (b) leaves the room as the baby begins to cry, (c) does not make eye contact with the baby when she holds her, and (d) verbalizes feelings of fatigue. Items a, b, and c seem to be related because they are indicators of the mother's relationship with her baby. This cluster of data, considered as a whole, indicates a potential problem more clearly than any single item considered alone. These data serve as a set of indicators that match the defining characteristics associated with the nursing diagnosis "altered parenting."

Grouping the data together helps assure that the "match" was not made just on the basis of one fact or observation that may or may not be sufficient to establish the correct diagnosis.

2. Use an Appropriate Framework for Collecting, Recording, and Organizing Data. Two frameworks that might be used to guide the collection and recording of data have already been mentioned in this chapter—FHPs and Body Systems. The reason to use a particular framework is to help organize information to provide clarity and to achieve a particular outcome. For example, if your goal is to arrive at a medical diagnosis, a physiologic framework, such as body systems, would be a logical choice for directing data collection and documentation because medical diagnoses are based on dysfunctions in body systems. If your goal is to arrive at a nursing diagnosis, however, you should use a different framework, such as FHPs, that groups indicators of related nursing diagnoses. Each of the 11 functional health patterns is associated with a list of primary nursing diagnoses. If a dysfunctional pattern exists, the indicators for the associated diagnoses will usually appear together as you evaluate the data associated with a particular functional area. For example, in the course of evaluating the nutritional–metabolic pattern, you may observe a cluster of indicators of abnormal nutrition and an actual or potential health problem that is on the list of primary nursing diagnoses associated with the nutritional–metabolic pattern. Once a fit can be established between the data cluster and the defining characteristics associated with a particular diagnosis, you are ready to state the diagnosis.

Drawing a Conclusion

Data analysis is the process of interpreting the raw data and drawing a valid conclusion leading to a diagnosis or clinical judgment. Data that have been transformed by analysis and interpretation into a form that may be used to draw conclusions and make decisions are now referred to as information. For example, interpretation of the blood pressure data, 185/102, may lead to the conclusion that the individual is experiencing an abnormal elevation of both the systolic and diastolic blood pressures. The use of the term *abnormal* illustrates interpretation and judgment of the data.

Once data are clustered and interpreted, the conclusion that is drawn should be given a name. That name could represent a need or problem, a medical diagnosis, or a nursing diagnosis. Any of these conclusions should be considered tentative until you are certain that it is the best interpretation of the data. The diagnostic process continues until you are certain that your conclusions are valid. This involves considering all other possibilities and, often, collecting additional data to support your conclusions. Your ability to draw conclusions based on clusters of data will be enhanced by your knowledge of various diagnostic indicators that might be associated with specific clinical problems or diagnoses. Moreover, the accuracy of your conclusions will be enhanced by considering other competing diagnoses before making a definitive diagnosis. Finally, you should validate your final diagnosis by check-

ing the fit between the diagnostic indicators and the actual data one more time.

1. Become Familiar with Diagnostic Indicators. A nursing diagnosis is formulated based on a cluster of data indicating various defining characteristics or criteria for the diagnosis. To arrive at a diagnosis, the nurse must ensure that there is a similarity or match between the clustered data and those known indicators for the diagnosis. The North American Nursing Diagnoses (NANDA) Taxonomy I, Revised, lists all of the official nursing diagnoses with all of the associated defining characteristics or indicators for each diagnosis. Nurses should become familiar with these defining characteristics, which can help them learn to cluster findings appropriately and recognize a match between data cluster and diagnosis. This process of data collection and clustering occurs repeatedly during the diagnostic process. Nurses do need to have knowledge of the signs and symptoms from various disease processes, but certainly for the professional nurse, emphasis should also be on knowing the indicators or defining characteristics for various nursing diagnoses.

An example of how the clustering of data can help lead to the appropriate diagnosis is illustrated using the preceding example of mother/baby interaction and noting the process:

Steps in the Diagnostic Process: Example

- The nurse assesses the functional area—roles and relationships.
- Data are collected and significant findings are grouped.
  - Mother states she is disappointed her newborn baby is a girl.
  - Mother leaves the room as baby begins to cry.
  - Mother does not make eye contact with her baby when holding her.
- The diagnosis is proposed—Altered parenting.
- The defining characteristics are compared with the data cluster for "fit":
  - Verbalization of resentment toward the infant
  - Lack of parental attachment behaviors
  - Inappropriate visual, tactile, and auditory stimulation

The diagnostic process may or may not follow such a logical, sequential process. Some nurses, especially experienced nurses, will quickly form an impression and make a diagnosis without going through the steps listed above. For example, an experienced ICU nurse may quickly make a diagnosis of activity intolerance with very little attention to a formal data collection process. However, in retrospect, it is likely that some or all of the indicators of this diagnosis were observed by the nurse making this diagnosis.

In addition to identifying general defining characteristics for each nursing diagnosis, NANDA is working toward identifying the critical defining characteristics or "critical indicators," which would be those signs and symptoms that *must be present* to formulate a particular nursing diagnosis.

2. Treat Your Conclusion as a Working Hypothesis Until You Have Ruled Out Other Possibilities. Initially, it is best to consider all diagnostic conclusions tentative, like a hypothesis, until you effectively rule out any competing possibilities. Resist the temptation to settle for the first diagnosis that comes to mind. Investigate further to determine whether your hypothesis is valid. You can investigate by collecting additional data related to your initial conclusion. For example, you may use the protocol for symptom analysis described in Chapter 2, or, if you have data indicating altered elimination status, you may do a more exhaustive examination of the person's elimination pattern to better understand the nature of the problem. Consider the meaning of disconfirming data or data that have been uncovered that clearly do not support your hypothesis. Avoid the tendency to ignore disconfirming data just so you can draw a conclusion and bring the process to closure.

3. Evaluate Your Conclusion. Once you have investigated further and concluded that your final diagnosis is valid, consider again the quality of the match between the data and the indicators for the diagnosis. Remember that even your final conclusion is, at best, a conjecture.

Classification and Naming of Health Status

The *classification and naming of the individual's health status* follows the data collection and data analysis processes. The nurse makes a determination of the individual's health status and communicates significant conclusions by naming the conclusion a patient care need, clinical problem, or nursing diagnosis. Factors contributing to a final diagnosis or problem also may be identified and stated as causative factors and included in the diagnostic statement.

A variety of classification and naming systems are used by the various disciplines that provide health care. In general, classification and naming systems are designed to reflect a particular healthcare discipline's unique body of knowledge as well as that discipline's scope of clinical practice.

Classification refers to the systematic arrangement of health status concepts in groups or categories according to established criteria or based on relationships between concepts. The classification system used by physicians is known as medical diagnosis. The specific classification and naming of diseases is addressed by the more detailed nomenclature known as the *International Classification of Diseases, Tenth Revision (ICD-10)*. The ICD-10 is a comprehensive list of diseases and medical treatments with corresponding codes compatible with the World Health Organization's list of disease codes.

Medical diagnoses are labels for specific disease states or pathophysiologic processes. For example, myocardial infarction is a medical diagnosis and denotes cardiac pathology that can be identified on the basis of defined clinical signs and symptoms.

Nurses make use of medical diagnoses when providing patient care. Knowing the medical diagnosis gives the nurse the necessary conceptualization of the patient's risk for physiological complications that are monitored and treated as a part of nursing practice initiating both nurse-prescribed and physician-prescribed interventions. These physiologic complications as well as medical diagnoses that are monitored and evaluated and collaboratively managed by nurses with other providers such as physicians are referred to as clinical problems. Generally, it is outside of the nurse's defined scope of practice to independently diagnose, manage, and treat clinical problems. Instead, the nurse's role in patient care will be collaborative and interdependent with other health professionals.

Other types of clinical judgments that nurses make about individuals, such as judgments about individual responses to health problems and life processes, are more appropriately classified and named to reflect nursing's body of knowledge and scope of practice using the nomenclature of nursing diagnosis. The North American Nursing Diagnosis Association (1996) defines nursing diagnosis as "a clinical judgment about individual, family, or community responses to actual and potential health problems/life processes. Nursing diagnoses provide the basis for selection of nursing interventions to achieve outcomes for which the nurse is accountable." A patient with a myocardial infarction may be evaluated and assessed by the nurse who makes the following clinical judgments about the person's responses that are stated as nursing diagnoses: activity intolerance; decreased cardiac output; and defensive coping. Not only is it within the nurse's defined scope of practice to independently make these clinical judgments, but the nurse also can manage and treat these responses by independently initiating nurse-prescribed interventions.

The specific nomenclature of nursing diagnosis has been developed by NANDA and is known as *NANDA Taxonomy I, Revised*. Eventually, nursing diagnosis nomenclature may be included in a standardized vocabulary being developed by the International Council on Nursing called the *International Classification of Nursing Practice (ICNP)*. In fact, as clinical practice continues to move toward a true interdisciplinary, patient-focused care environment, the standardized vocabularies of all health care–related disciplines may be incorporated into an overall standardized vocabulary. NANDA supports this effort but wants additional development of nursing's standardized diagnosis language to precede inclusion into any type of standardized classification system.

Although the use of nursing diagnosis language has largely replaced the naming of health assessment conclusions in the form of patient needs, the identification of needs still may be an outcome of the health assessment process. There is no standard classification system to name patient needs. Needs are defined as some thing or action that is essential, indispensable, required, or cannot be done or lived without. Examples would include "need for fall precautions" or "need for oxygenation." Nursing is moving away from the practice of naming needs, largely because of the development of a more universal and accurate clinical language embodied in NANDA Taxonomy I.

CHAPTER 1	S U M M A R Y

Health Assessment

Health assessment is a process of systematically collecting and analyzing data to make judgments about health and life processes of individuals, families, and communities.

Health Assessment in Nursing Practice

Health assessment has evolved in nursing practice since Florence Nightingale emphasized the importance of clinical observation by the nurse providing care at the patient's bedside. The following factors have influenced the evolution of health assessment in nursing practice:

- Expansion of nursing roles—public health, acute hospital care and intensive care, advanced nurse practitioner roles
- Theoretical work related to nursing process
- The "Nursing Diagnosis Movement" and development of a nursing diagnosis taxonomy
- The development of nursing frameworks for health assessment including Functional Health Patterns

Purpose of Health Assessment

The purpose of health assessment of individuals by nurses includes the following:

- To gain an *understanding* of the person's experience of *health and life processes* including health, illness, and recovery
- To *identify strengths* that promote health or need to be enhanced for optimal functioning
- To *identify needs, clinical problems, or nursing diagnoses* that form the basis of nursing care and intervention
- To *evaluate* the effects of therapeutic plans and interventions

Health Assessment Processes

The three processes of health assessment include data collection, documentation, and diagnostic reasoning.

Data Collection

Data collection refers to the process of obtaining uninterpreted material, facts, or clinical information about an individual. Data are classified as subjective or objective. The primary methods of data collections in health assessment include the following:

- The assessment interview
- Physical examination
- Review of records

Data collection activities can be prioritized depending on the person's immediate condition or needs. The frequency of data collection activities depends on the person's diagnosis, the level of care that is being provided, and the individual's response to treatments. The scope of data collection varies and can be classified on the basis of intensity and complexity of the situation in the following manner:

- Screening
- Comprehensive
- Focused

A clinical database is an organized collection of data documented in a standardized format. The clinical database includes identifying information about the individual, the relevant medical history, the medication and substance use history, information about functional health patterns, and the results of the physical examination.

Documentation

Documentation of data, information, and health assessment conclusions provides the following:

- A written display of findings and observations used as the basis for clinical judgments and diagnoses
- A method to make data and information accessible to other providers using the medical record, contributing to continuity of care
- A legal record of events and findings
- A record that may be used to justify the provision of services

Documentation should be conducted in a manner that ensures objectivity, accuracy, clarity, and efficiency. Various documentation styles are acceptable, including the use of SOAP progress notes, narrative-style documentation, and "fill-in-the-blank"–style documentation.

Diagnostic Reasoning

Diagnostic reasoning involves the ability to think critically about the assessment process and the findings and make appropriate clinical judgments. The diagnostic reasoning process has the following components:

- Collecting relevant data
- Organizing data so it has meaning
- Drawing a conclusion

Critical Thinking Exercise

Assessment is a key process of professional nursing practice. Nursing, as a discipline, has developed the assessment process to determine people's needs for nursing care, to monitor responses to illness and intervention, and to evaluate overall health and well-being. Data collection, documentation, and diagnostic reasoning skills are important health assessment processes.

1. There are various models for health assessment, including Functional Health Patterns, NANDA's Unitary Human Framework, and the traditional body systems model.

   Defend the use of a conceptual model to guide the health assessment process.

   How important is it to have one model of health assessment to guide nursing practice? How has this issue been addressed in the nursing literature?

   What are the alternatives to adopting one model for health assessment?

   If you had to design an organizing framework to guide nurses in the process of health assessment, describe what it would look like.

2. You have been asked to develop a new documentation system for your facility to use for recording data obtained during the comprehensive initial patient assessment.

   Develop the overall goals that will guide you through this process.

   Develop an outline for any standardized forms that will be included in your system.

   Describe the strengths and weaknesses of your proposed system.

3. Explain how you would guard against drawing premature conclusions about an individual during the health assessment process.

   Describe an example in which you reached a conclusion about another person that was not accurate. What would you have done to prevent this from happening?

   Describe a clinical situation (or work with an example provided by your instructor or colleagues) and provide two or more initial hypotheses that you could explore as you try to establish a diagnosis.

BIBLIOGRAPHY

American Nurses' Association. (1980). *Nursing—A social policy statement*. Washington D.C.: American Nurses' Association.

American Nurses Association. (1991). *Standards of clinical nursing practice*. Washington, D.C.: American Nurses Association.

Benner, P. (1984). *From novice to expert*. Menlo Park, CA: Addison-Wesley.

Black, K.M. (1967), Assessing patients' needs. In H. Yura & M.B. Walsh (Eds.). *The nursing process: Assessing, planning, implementing, evaluating*. Washington, D.C.: The Catholic University of America Press.

Burke, L.J., & Murphy, J. (1995). *Charting by exception applications: Making it work in clinical settings*. Albany, NY: Delmar Publications.

Carnevali, D.L. et al. (1984). *Diagnostic reasoning in nursing*. Philadelphia: J.B. Lippincott.

Carnevali, D.L., & Thomas, M.D. (1993). *Diagnostic reasoning and treatment decision making in nursing*. Philadelphia: J.B. Lippincott.

Chase, S.K. (1997). Charting critical thinking: Nursing judgments and patient outcomes. *Dimensions of Critical Care Nursing, 16*(2), 102–111.

Field, L., & Winslow, E. (1985). Moving to a nursing model. *American Journal of Nursing, 85,* 1100–1101.

Field, P. (1987). The impact of nursing theory on the clinical decision making process. *Journal of Advanced Nursing, 12*(5), 559–562.

Fitzmaurice, J.B. (1987). Nurses' use of cues in the clinical judgment of activity tolerance. In A.M. McLane (Ed.). *Classification of nursing diagnoses: Proceedings of the seventh conference*. St. Louis: C.V. Mosby.

Fitzsimmons, V.M., & Gallagher, L.P. (1978). Physical assessment skills: A historical perspective. *Nursing Forum, 4*(17), 345–355.

Ford, L., & Silver, H. (1967), The expanded role of the nurse in child care. *Nursing Outlook, 15,* 43–45.

Gebbie, K. & Lavin, M.A. (1974). Classifying nursing diagnoses. *American Journal of Nursing,* 250–253.

Gebbie, K. & Lavin, M.A. (Eds.). (1975). *Classification of nursing diagnoses: Proceedings of the first national conference*. St. Louis: C.V. Mosby.

Gordon, M. (1987). *Nursing diagnosis: Process and application* (2nd ed.). New York: McGraw-Hill.

Gruber, M., & Benner, P. (1989). The power of certainty. *American Journal of Nursing, 89*(4), 502–503.

Guzzetta, C.E., Bunton, S.D., Prinkey, L.A., et al. (1989). *Clinical assessment tools for use with nursing diagnoses.* St. Louis: C.V. Mosby.

Guzzetta, C.E., & Kinney, M.R. (1986). Mastering the transition from medical to nursing diagnosis. *Progress in Cardiovascular Nursing, 1,* 41.

Hammond, K.R., Kelly, K.J., Scheider, R.J., & Vancini, M. (1966). Clinical inference in nursing: Analyzing cognitive tasks representative of nursing problems. *Nursing Research, 15,* 134.

Harpine, F.H. (1967). Assessing the needs of the patient. In H. Yura & M.B. Walsh (Eds.). *The nursing process: Assessing, planning, implementing, evaluating.* Washington, D.C: The Catholic University of America Press.

Hartman, D., & Knudson, J. (1991). A nursing data base for initial patient assessment. *Oncology Nursing Forum, 18*(1), 125–130.

Henning, M. (1991) Comparison of nursing diagnostic statements using a functional health pattern and a health history/body systems format. In R.M. Carroll-Johnson (Ed.). *Classification of nursing diagnoses: Proceedings of the ninth conference* (pp. 278–279). Philadelphia: J.B. Lippincott.

Jacoby, M.K., & Adams, D.J. (1981). Teaching assessment of client functioning. *Nursing Outlook, 29*(4), 248–250.

Kim. M.J., McFarland, G.K., & McLane, A.M. (1984). *Classification of nursing diagnoses: Proceedings of the fifth national conference.* St. Louis: C.V. Mosby.

Kramer, M. (1971). Team nursing: A means or an end? *Nursing Outlook, 19*(10), 648–652.

Lewis, C., & Resnik, B. (1967). Nurse clinics and progressive ambulatory patient care. *New England Journal of Medicine, 227,* 1236–1241.

Lunney, M. & Paradiso, C. (1995). Accuracy of interpreting human responses. *Nursing Management, 26*(10), 48h–48k.

Lynaugh, J.E., & Bates, B. (1974). Physical diagnosis: A skill for all nurses? *American Journal of Nursing, 74*(1), 58–59.

Marrellin, T.M. (1996). *Nursing documentation handbook.* St. Louis: C.V. Mosby.

Maslow, A.H. (1968). *Toward a psychology of being* (2nd ed.). New York: Van Nostrand and Reinhold.

Morrissey, R.M. (1988). Documentation: If you haven't written it, you haven't done it. *Nursing Clinics of North America, 23*(2), 363–371.

Murphy, J., & Burke, I.J. (1990). Charting by exception: A more efficient way to document. *Nursing, 20,* 65–68.

Newell, A., & Simon, H. (1972). *Human problem solving.* Englewood Cliffs, NJ: Prentice-Hall.

Nightingale, F. (1992). *Notes on nursing: What it is and what it is not.* Philadelphia: J.B. Lippincott.

North American Nursing Diagnosis Association. (1996). *NANDA nursing diagnoses: Definitions and classification 1997–1998.* Philadelphia: NANDA.

O'Connell, B. (1995) Diagnostic reliability: A study of the process. *Nursing Diagnosis, 6*(3), 99–107.

Padrick, K.P., et al. (1987). Hypothesis evaluation: A component of diagnostic reasoning. In A.M. McLane (Ed.). *Classification of nursing diagnoses: Proceedings of the seventh conference.* St. Louis: C.V. Mosby.

Putzier, D.J., Padrick, K., Westfall, U.E., & Tanner, C.A. (1985). Diagnostic reasoning in critical care nursing. *Heart and Lung, 14*(5), 430–437.

Radwin, L.E. (1995). Knowing the patient: A process model for individualized interventions. *Nursing Research, 44*(6), 364–370.

Rew, L. (1988). Intuition in decision making. *Image: Nursing Scholarship, 20*(3), 150–154.

Rhodes, A.M. (1986). Principle of documentation. *Maternal Child Nursing Journal, 11*(6), 381.

Rossi, L. (1987). Organizing data for nursing diagnosis using functional health patterns. In A.M. McLane (Ed.). *Classification of nursing diagnoses: Proceedings of the seventh conference.* St. Louis: C.V. Mosby.

Rossi, L. (1992). Evaluating the patient with coronary artery disease. *Nursing Clinics of North America, 27*(1), 171–188.

Strader, M., Moore-Greenlaw, R.C., & Decker, P.J. (1994). Nurses and patient assessment. *Journal of Nursing Administration, 24*(12), 17–19, 58.

Tanner, C.A. (1982). Instruction in the diagnostic process: An experimental study. In M.J. Kim, & D. Moritz (Eds.). *Classification of nursing diagnoses: Proceedings of the third and fourth national conferences.* New York: McGraw-Hill.

Tillis, M.S. (1986). What do you say when you can't say normal. *Nursing Success Today, 3*(6), 29–30.

Vincenz, M.C., & Siskind, M.M. (1994). Functional health patterns: A curricular course model for adult acute care. *Nursing Diagnosis, 5*(2), 82–87.

Weed, L.L. (1970). *Medical records, medical evaluation, and patient care.* Chicago: Year Book Medical Publishers.

Westfall, U.F., Tanner, C.A., Putzier, D., & Padrick, K.P. (1986). Activating clinical inferences: A component of diagnostic reasoning in nursing. *Research in Nursing and Health, 9,* 269–277.

Westfall, U.F., Tanner, C.A., Putzier, D., & Padrick, K.P. (1987). Errors committed by nurses and nursing students in the diagnostic reasoning process. In A.M. McLane (Ed.). *Classification of nursing diagnoses: Proceedings of the seventh conference.* St. Louis: C.V. Mosby.

Whiteside, C. (1997). A model for teaching critical thinking in the clinical setting. *Dimensions of Critical Care Nursing, 16*(3), 152–162.

Wurzbach, M.E. (1991). Judgment under conditions of uncertainty. *Nursing Forum, 26*(3), 27–34.

Yura, H., & Walsh, M.B. (Eds.). (1967). *The nursing process: Assessing, planning, implementing, and evaluating.* Washington, D.C.: The Catholic University of America Press.

Yura, H., & Walsh, M.B. (1988). *The nursing process* (5th ed.). Norwalk, CT: Appleton-Lange.

CHAPTER 2

The Health Assessment Interview and Health History

ASSESSMENT GUIDELINES

- The Initial Health Assessment Interview
- The Medical History (Past Health History and Review of Systems)
- The Medication and Substance Use History

CHAPTER ORGANIZATION

Introductory Overview

Knowledge Base for Assessment: Interviewing
- The Purpose of the Health Assessment Interview
- The Interview Process
- Therapeutic Communication
- Interview Challenges

Documentation: The Health History

INTRODUCTORY OVERVIEW

In Chapter 1, the primary data collection methods used by nurses to conduct a health assessment of individuals were identified as the following:

Data Collection Methods for Health Assessment

- Assessment Interview
- Physical Examination
- Review of Records

The data obtained by these methods are organized in a clinical database used by the nurse to evaluate and address nursing care needs. The two main components of a clinical database include the following:

Components of a Clinical Database

- Health history
- Physical examination

The focus of this chapter is to further explore the basic concepts and skills required for the development of an individual's health history. The essential content of the health history and interviewing skills are presented.

The *health history* consists of data and information about health status, present and past, obtained by direct inquiry or review of records. The inquiries about the individual's health status may be conducted in several ways—the person may be interviewed, the person's family or others may be interviewed, a questionnaire may be completed, or other healthcare providers may be consulted. In addition to these types of primary inquiries, information may be obtained from secondary sources such as records of health care, including the chart or medical record.

Before you initiate an interview, you should understand the fundamental concepts of interviewing as a health assessment method. The general principles of the health assessment interview process and effective communication techniques should be considered before you begin to interview a person about specific functional areas such as coping patterns, nutritional practices, or sexuality. In addition, you should be prepared to manage a number of challenging interview situations, including the interview of a person from a different cultural background from your own, as well as the challenges presented by age differences, discussing sensitive topics, and the presence of strong emotions.

The richest source of data for the health history is often from *primary sources,* where data are obtained directly from an individual through the interview. The interview provides an excellent opportunity for building a relationship between the nurse and the individual that encourages disclosure and sharing of information. Interviewing also provides the opportunity to explore topics in greater depth. Of all the techniques for obtaining a health history, interviewing often demands the greatest skill because of the interpersonal interaction and communication expertise required. Interviewing also requires critical thinking skills so that the nurse may thoughtfully explore information provided during the interview process in greater depth to determine the significance of the information.

Primary source information is also obtained when the individual completes a questionnaire designed to elicit data about health status. In some healthcare settings, a person is asked to complete a questionnaire about their health status before being interviewed by a nurse or other provider. Questionnaires provide several advantages. First, the questionnaire is an efficient way to obtain preliminary data, including identifying information about the person, medical history, and lifestyle. In addition, some people may feel more comfortable answering questions of a personal nature (such as questions about drug and alcohol use, bowel habits, or sexually transmitted diseases) by filling out a questionnaire. However, the nurse should review the information recorded on a questionnaire with the individual to provide additional clarification and to discuss significant findings in more detail. Questionnaires need to be written so that the meaning of the questions is clear and medical jargon is avoided.

Health history information also may obtained through *secondary sources,* including other professionals involved in an individual's health care, or from the clinical record. If the individual or their significant others cannot be a primary source of information, the record and accounts of other providers may be the only resources available for establishing a health history. Records can provide some of the same types of information that may be obtained through an interview, such as a general description and chronology of events related to an individual's health status. Records also may identify the professional judgments of others such as clinical problem lists or diagnoses. Clinical records also may contain the results of various diagnostic tests and procedures, such as laboratory tests, radiographs, or surgical procedures. All of these types of information may be incorporated into a comprehensive health history.

Comparison of data obtained from primary and secondary sources should occur whenever possible as a means of validating information. *Validation* refers to establishing the accuracy and truth of information.

KNOWLEDGE BASE FOR ASSESSMENT: INTERVIEWING

Basic knowledge and skills are required to successfully complete the health assessment interview. The nurse's knowledge base should include an understanding of the purpose of the health assessment interview, the phases of the interview process, and therapeutic communication techniques. Knowing how to vary your interview style and communication techniques depending on the person's age, cultural considerations, or cognitive and behavioral factors is also important. Applying this type of knowledge during the interview process will be as important as the specific questions you ask during the interview to actually elicit data.

The Purpose of the Health Assessment Interview

The health assessment interview is a structured, goal-oriented conversation between the nurse and an individual for the purpose of yielding information about the person, their health perceptions, functional status, and other factors relevant to health, healing, and illness. The assessment process usually starts with an interview, and often, an accurate diagnosis may be made solely on the basis of observations you make during the interview, including the overall appearance of the individual and the actual data elicited as responses to your questions.

The assessment interview also provides the opportunity to establish a positive, therapeutic relationship between the nurse and the individual. Rapport, trust, and a feeling of care and concern characterize a therapeutic relationship. This type of relationship is the basis for promoting health and wellness; establishing hope; finding understanding in the experiences of illness, pain, or anxiety; and providing emotional or spiritual support.

Indicators for nursing diagnoses or other clinical problems may be identified through the interview process. The assessment interview provides the opportunity to identify the person's special concerns and perceptions about health, illness, health management practices, and health care. The interview is also a means for obtaining demographic data as well as data pertaining to social background and support systems. The data and information gleaned from the assessment interview provides the foundation for clinical judgment and diagnostic reasoning.

The Interview Process

The assessment interview may be formal and structured to collect a wide range of information, or informal and focused on a specific area of concern. An admission assessment interview is usually formal and structured to establish a comprehensive nursing data base. During an informal interview, you may discuss specific concerns with the person while providing nursing care. Data collection through interviewing and questioning should be a continuous, ongoing process, lasting as long as you and the person interact.

The health care setting may influence the scope of the assessment interview. In well-child clinics, for example, the interview usually focuses on routine health practices, nutrition, and normal growth and development, whereas in the intensive care unit, data collection focuses on physical symptoms and responses to threatening conditions.

Three interrelated phases constitute an effective interview: the introductory phase, the working phase, and the termination phase (Display 2-1).

DISPLAY 2.1

The Interview Process: Clinical Profile

Mrs. Jones, age 26 years, comes to the health clinic as a potential participant in the nurse-operated weight reduction program. Mrs. Jones is worried she will not be accepted for the program because she does not meet weight and height criteria for being overweight. Although she is reluctant to discuss it, Mrs. Jones explains that her weight stays as low as it does because she induces vomiting after eating.

THE INTRODUCTORY PHASE

Nurse: Good afternoon, Mrs. Jones. I'm Mrs. Klein, one of the registered nurses associated with the weight program. (Smiles and extends hand.)

Client: Hello. Please call me by my first name. (Accepts handshake but avoids eye contact.)

Nurse: I'd like to discuss the program you are interested in. Then, I'd like to ask you some general health and nutrition questions so you and I can decide if our program meets your needs. We have about 30 minutes. (States purpose, implies a mutual decision-making process, and states time limitations.)

Client: You probably won't take me into the program.

Nurse: You seem worried about not getting the kind of help you need.

At this point, the nurse focuses on the client's feelings, which should be clarified before questioning and data collection continue.

THE WORKING PHASE

The nurse is concerned with obtaining additional information about the client's nutritional practices and weight perceptions. Asking numerous questions may intimidate the client, especially Mrs. Jones, who is initially reluctant to share information. Note the techniques the nurse uses.

Nurse: So, you are interested in the weight reduction program.

Client: Yeah, I've heard from a couple of friends how successful it is. And the people are caring no matter how much or how little you need to lose.

Nurse: Yes. We try to help people achieve realistic goals and feel good about themselves in the process. To do this, I need to find out a little more about your goals and how you feel about your present weight. These are personal questions, but your answers will help me plan an individualized program.

Client: Well, I guess I only need to lose about 10 to 20 pounds. I'm not sure. My husband is upset with the way I look in a bathing suit—especially compared to his friends' wives or girlfriends.

Nurse: So your husband's reactions are one reason for coming here.

Client: Yeah, but I have been dieting and keeping my weight controlled. I just don't feel very healthy anymore.

Nurse: Most people I talk with use several methods for weight control. Some are successful and others aren't, and as you mention, feeling healthy is an important factor. Tell me more about some of your experiences.

The nurse is gathering data by techniques other than direct questioning. She is also careful to avoid judgmental questions or statements such as, "Why would you want to lose weight?" or "Your husband is wrong." Such statements will probably inhibit honest disclosure.

THE TERMINATION PHASE

The nurse is able to discuss the client's weight perceptions and to obtain data about her eating disorder during the working phase. The client is accepted into the weight reduction program with the understanding that weight maintenance, healthy eating habits, and self-esteem will be emphasized. After 25 minutes, the nurse initiates the termination phase.

Nurse: I see we have only 5 minutes left today. Before we finish, I'd like to review your situation and make plans for you to start the program.

Client: Okay.

Nurse: You are concerned that you weigh too much, although we haven't yet explored why in great detail. You usually watch your diet but sometimes engage in binge-type eating. When you binge, you purge. You see your behavior as unhealthful and desire to change. We discussed the goals of your plan and agreed to discuss how to proceed at the beginning of the program, 1 week from now.

Client: I feel ready to start this program. It's not going to be easy, though.

Nurse: Um-hmm. (Silence.) Let me give you an on-call number. If talking to someone on our staff will help before next week, please call. Or call if you have questions.

The nurse terminates with summary statements, and follow-up plans are made. Finally, the nurse shakes hands with the client and thanks her for her participation.

The Introductory Phase

The introductory phase sets the tone and direction of the interview and establishes a mutual understanding of the purpose of the exchange. The purposes of the introductory phase are as follows:

- To establish rapport
- To ensure a comfortable setting
- To state the purpose of the interview

Establishing Rapport. Rapport between nurse and client is an essential component of the helping relationship. Establishing rapport begins with demonstrating respect for the client as a person with problems, rather than regarding the person as a problem to be solved.

You should demonstrate respect at the beginning of the interview by extending a cordial greeting, addressing the person by name, and then introducing yourself by name and title. You should not address an adult with his or her first name unless invited. Offering to shake hands is one way of demonstrating warmth and acceptance.

Nonverbal behaviors, especially on your part, also may help build rapport. Mutual respect can be expressed best when you and the person face each other and maintain eye contact. If possible, you should avoid standing over the person because this may be intimidating. Of course, such a position may be appropriate if you are informally interviewing the person while providing care. If the interview is conducted at the bedside, you should sit beside the bed with the siderail down, leaning slightly toward the person. Nonverbal behaviors such as expressions of disgust, boredom, or impatience may interfere with establishing rapport or may imply lack of interest.

The interview should be conducted in a manner that implies you have adequate time to spend with the person. For example, do not say to the person, "I have to ask you all these questions before I finish my shift."

Beginning the interview with a brief, casual conversation that focuses on the person may help dispel tension or awkwardness. If your comments are predominantly self-centered, the person may feel neglected or unimportant.

Ensuring Comfort. If possible, you should conduct the interview in a private setting, free from interruptions or distractions. When privacy is difficult to maintain, such as in acute care settings, you can at least close the door or wait until other people have left the room before initiating the interview. Pulling the curtains or moving to the corner of the room also helps to promote a sense of privacy, even though these gestures may not necessarily prevent others from hearing what is said.

You should take every effort to assure the confidentiality of the information provided by the person. This includes limiting discussion of the information to appropriate persons and limiting access to the record.

Stating Purpose. State your purpose at the beginning of the interview. Tell the person you want to discuss his or her health to determine how, as a nurse, you can help. Encourage the person to participate in the interview. The person who answers questions, responds honestly, and shares relevant personal information is most likely to benefit from the health assessment interview.

The Working Phase

During the working phase of the interview, which is the most time-consuming phase, you should collect data that are pertinent to the person's overall health status. Such information will be invaluable in forming an appropriate care plan. Record both verbal responses and nonverbal behavior. The purposes of the working phase are as follows:

- To collect biographic data
- To collect data pertinent to the client's health status
- To identify and respond to the client's needs

The Structured Interview. A structured interview may be used to facilitate data collection during the working phase. Familiarity with the forms before the interview will enable you to concentrate on the person's responses. Formats for structured interviews vary. Traditionally, nurses have followed a medical model in conducting health assessment interviews. However, nursing models are now being used in many settings.

The structured interview usually begins with biographic information, including name, age and birthdate, sex, address, birthplace, marital status, and occupation. Although asking about previously recorded biographic information is unnecessary, you should always record such data because they are relevant to the person's social identity and self-concept.

The next portion of the structured interview concentrates on determining the person's functional status. (Subsequent chapters discuss specific interview guidelines for each functional area.) You can proceed smoothly from one topic to the next by using transitional phrases such as "Now I'd like to discuss how you feel about your sleep habits," or "Now I'd like to ask you some questions about your bowel and bladder functions."

The structured interview should proceed from general to specific. Gather general biographic information and data pertaining to health perceptions before discussing sexuality, personal values, and relationships. You must establish trust and rapport before discussing intimate topics.

If the person is reluctant to discuss specific topics, you should provide an opportunity to talk about what he or she feels is most important. Use broad opening statements such as, "Why don't you begin by telling me what brings you here," or "What's troubling you today?" Once the person has expressed immediate concerns, he or she is more likely to discuss other subjects.

View the structured interview as a guide rather than a rigid series of questions that must be asked in a set order. Excessive questioning may undermine rapport, inhibit responses, and encourage the person to assume a passive role of merely answering questions. Applying principles of therapeutic communication rather than direct questioning may result in a more productive interview, as is discussed in more detail in the next section. Such techniques encourage free expression about the topics raised.

Communication is also enhanced when both you and the client speak the same "language." The terminology used should be simple and appropriate and not based on medical jargon. When necessary, define terms and structure questions to allow time for the person to respond thoughtfully and meaningfully.

Completing the health assessment interview in one session may not always be possible. If the person shows signs of fatigue or a limited attention span, bring the interview to a close. Trying to continue under these circumstances would be nonproductive.

The Termination Phase

The termination phase serves to end the interview. Saying how long the interview will last at the beginning will prevent the person from experiencing a sense of premature closure at the end of the interview.

Presummary, summary, and follow-up techniques may be incorporated into the termination phase. Presummary involves providing cues to indicate that the interview is coming to an end. For example, you could say, "I see that we only have 10 minutes left. Is there anything else you would like to discuss before our time is up?" or "There are three more questions I'd like to ask." Planning additional interview sessions may be necessary if all relevant topics have not been adequately discussed.

Next, a brief summary of the points covered will allow both you and the client a chance to validate perceptions. Specific plans for follow-up or additional interviewing are discussed at this time.

Therapeutic Communication

Therapeutic communication is purposeful, goal-directed, and always focused on the client. Therapeutic communication, which includes both verbal and nonverbal interaction, will result in an open and authentic exchange of information through the development of rapport. If the nurse's goal is assessment, the health assessment interview is conducted using therapeutic communication techniques.

In the spirit of therapeutic communication, the interview should be conducted so that general questions are followed by specific questions, and less intrusive questions precede questions of a more personal nature. Personal questions should be asked only after some rapport and trust is established through the interview process. In general, you should always give the person adequate time to respond to questions, never answer your own questions, and avoid asking loaded or judgmental questions. Adjust the level of vocabulary to match that of the person being interviewed and avoid using healthcare jargon. The individual may be hesitant to tell you he or she does not understand your questions and may even cover up this fact by answering questions incorrectly. Choose your words carefully, and remember that the person may easily misinterpret your comments.

You should be attentive to your general appearance and demeanor as you interview the person. Your appearance should be professional including dress that is appropriate to the clinical setting and appropriate grooming. Hairstyles that are extreme should be avoided, as should excessive jewelry.

Your general demeanor should indicate interest and focus on the person being interviewed. You should always greet the person in a professional manner and avoid talking to others once you have started the interview. Being too formal may give the person the impression that you do not have time or genuine concern. Conversely, an overly casual approach may fail to instill confidence.

Effective Communication Techniques

A number of communication techniques can help you conduct an effective assessment interview. The application of these techniques varies considerably among clinicians. Overuse or forced use of the techniques may actually stifle communication. Practice is the key to using communication techniques naturally and effectively.

Personalize the Interview. As you interview, remember that you are not only eliciting information but also establishing a helping relationship. To do this, you must personalize the interview by conveying sincerity and focus on what the person is saying rather than on a form that needs to be completed. The best approach would be one in which the nurse glances at the questions on the form, establishes eye contact with the person while asking questions, looks at the person while the person is answering, and offers clarification of responses and additional probing when needed (Fig. 2-1). The worst approach would be one in which the nurse does not look at the client but looks down at the form to be filled out and reads the questions verbatim from it, without providing any clarification of answers or without probing for further clarifica-

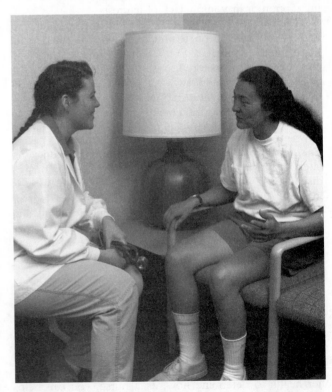

FIGURE 2.1 Establishing eye contact during an interview is an important communication technique.

tion from the client. Note the approaches used in the following examples:

Example 1: Poor Technique

Nurse: Do you have any problems with your usual activities, such as walking, housework, or shopping?
Client: No, not really.
Nurse: Do you have enough energy to do your daily activities?
Client: Yes.
Nurse: Are you independent in all your daily acitivities?
Client: Yes.

Example 2: Good Technique

Nurse: You mentioned before that you were concerned about your recovery from your knee surgery you had 3 months ago. How are things going for you?
Client: I initially seemed to be improving a little each day, but now I think I've reached a plateau.
Nurse: That must be frustrating for you. Tell me what you mean by reaching a plateau.
Client: I seem to have made progress since my surgery, but now I think I'm not making any more improvements, and I have more problems getting around than I did before surgery. It's especially hard to go down stairs and get up from a chair.
Nurse: What happens when you do these things?
Client: I need to use my arms to help me get up from a chair. I have to either pull myself up or push up off the chair with my arms. I go down stairs only one stair at a time and have to walk kind of sideways.
Nurse: That sounds awkward and uncomfortable. What concerns do you have about your safety as you move around?

Clearly, the nurse in example 2 is using better communication techniques to interview the client about activity and exercise patterns. Attempts are made to personalize the interview. The nurse begins by linking the questions to something the client had already talked about. Making these transition statements as you proceed through a lengthy interview helps keep the person focused.

Use Open-Ended Questions. Verbal therapeutic communication techniques are most effective if the questions asked are open-ended rather than closed-ended. Open-ended questions usually prompt full answers and provide more information, whereas closed-ended questions can be answered in one word, either "yes," "no," or "okay." The following are examples of open-ended questions:

"Tell me about your family."
"What are some of your concerns about caring for your new baby?"
"What do you do to stay healthy?"

You can see that these questions could not be answered by a simple "yes" or "no" but require that the person tell the interviewer more specific information. In example 1 (poor technique), you can see that every question was a closed-ended question. Although using closed-ended questions is often necessary, using all closed-ended questions makes the interview very impersonal and gives only a very limited picture of the individual's health. Closed-ended questions do not allow the interviewer and client to develop any personal rapport. In example 2 (good technique) the interviewer asks open-ended questions, which elicit much more helpful specific information and also allow more interaction between the interviewer and the client, which is conducive to more open communication. Open-ended questions that ask "why" should be avoided because the person might feel threatened or intimidated and, thus, give a defensive response. For example, if parents who have brought a young child with an elevated temperature to the emergency department are asked, "Why didn't you bring your child to the hospital sooner?", they might feel that the health care provider is blaming them for the problem or accusing them of not acting in a responsible manner.

In certain circumstances, such as when requesting biographic information such as name, occupation, address, and marital status, closed-ended questions are appropriate. They are also appropriate in emergency situations, when quick responses are required. For example, if a person arrives in the emergency room wheezing and out of breath, you would ask, "Do you have asthma? Are you allergic to anything?" rather than, "Tell me about your shortness of breath."

Make Broad Opening Statements. Broad opening statements may be especially helpful in the earliest stages of the interview, but may be used at any time. This technique allows the client to play an active role in the interview and to establish the priorities for discussion. Examples of this kind of statement are as follows:

"Tell me about your accident."
"What brings you to the clinic today?"
"What would you like to discuss today?"

Use Reflection. Reflection is the technique of repeating or paraphrasing a person's words or questions to promote further explanation and discussion. For example:

Client: My skin is driving me crazy.
Nurse: Driving you crazy?
Client: Yes. For the last week it's been itching and burning.
Nurse: Itching and burning for 1 week?
Client: Well, not constantly. And it seems to itch more than burn. I think it burns only after I've been scratching it.

Verbalize Implied Ideas. This technique involves restating what the client has said and adding some interpretation. As with reflection, the purpose is to encourage further discussion to amplify the problem being explored. This technique also gives the client an opportunity to verify the meaning of what he or she has said. For example:

Client: I don't know what's wrong with me. I used to sleep 6 or 7 hours a night without awakening.

Nurse: You're concerned because you've noticed a change in your sleeping habits?

Client: Yes, I've always been a good sleeper. Now I'm up and down all night.

Nurse: This seems unusual to you?

Client: Yes, even though I don't feel tired or take naps during the day.

Nurse: You're getting enough sleep but you're still bothered by nighttime awakenings?

Client: Yes. The nights are so long—just lying there, awake in bed, when I should be sleeping.

Provide General Leads. Another method for keeping the conversation going in a specific direction is to inject certain leading phrases or responses, such as "Go on," "Um-hmm," "Oh?", "And then what happened?" or "How did you feel about that?"

Seek Clarification. Occasionally, the person being interviewed will make a vague or confusing statement. In such instances, it is important to clarify what has been said before continuing with the interview. A suitable response might be, "I'm not sure I understand what you're trying to say," or "What do you mean by unbearable?"

Use Silence. At times during the interview, the most appropriate response is silence. Silence allows you a moment to organize your thoughts and also indicates that talking is not necessarily a criterion for nurse–client interaction. Some interviewers, however, feel uncomfortable when nothing is being said. Self-confidence is needed to use this technique effectively. Periods of silence offer an opportunity to observe nonverbal cues such as posture, facial expressions, and body movements.

Use Open Body Language. You should also use nonverbal cues as a method of communication. Maintaining eye contact or sitting in a relaxed, nonthreatening posture conveys a sense of interest in what the client is saying. Sit with your arms unfolded and your body slightly relaxed, and lean toward the client. Keep your facial expression interested but neutral, avoiding expressions of disgust, anger, or boredom.

Listen Actively. Listening is a communication skill that enhances assessment because it concentrates attention on what the client is saying and enables you to consider subtle messsages that the client may be conveying. Effective listening involves blocking out environmental distractions as well as your own prejudices. Attentive behavior and occasional verbal responses assure the client that you are listening.

Share Perceptions. It often helps to share your observation with the person to prompt further discussion. Statements such as, "You appear to have some physical discomfort today," or "I notice that you bring up you boyfriend frequently," or "It seems to me that you . . ." may open the conversation to a greater expression of feelings.

Confront Contradictions. When inconsistencies arise between the person's statements and behavior, you should explore the contradiction directly, as, for example, in the following statements: "You tell me that you're not upset about it, but you look like you're about to cry," or "You tell me that you are not tired but it looks like it's becoming more of an effort to keep talking."

Review the Discussion. Therapeutic interactions, especially health assessment interviews, should always close wih some type of summary. The main points should be discussed and reviewed in relation to the goals of the interview. For example, you could briefly review the person's health strengths, perceptions, and any identified health problems.

Communication Patterns to Avoid

Displaying Inappropriate Body Language. You should be sensitive to the amount of eye contact you make during the interview and also remember that different people will be comfortable with different levels of eye contact. In general, continuous eye contact should be avoided, because it may be perceived as too intrusive and intimidating. Make eye contact when the person is answering your questions. You can naturally break eye contact by looking at your notes from time to time. Some people will be most comfortable with little or no direct eye contact. Variations are often best understood by considering cultural norms and behaviors.

Avoid facial expressions of alarm, anxiety, or anger during the interview. The other person, who may feel you are being judgmental or condescending, may negatively perceive displaying such expressions.

Finally, avoid standing over the person as you interview. Standing over the other person portrays inequality and domination.

Proceeding Too Quickly. Avoid rushing the person through a long list of questions. If you proceed too quickly, the person may feel that you do not have a genuine interest in him or her as an individual. This, in itself, may stifle open communication and disclosure about important issues. You also may entirely miss the opportunity to obtain important information if you hurry through the interview. If you are in a hurry, you may not adequately reflect on what the person's responses to your questions are and you may fail to ask appropriate follow-up questions.

Offering Advice. Giving the person advice or voicing opinions is generally not helpful and may discourage decision making. Often when the person asks, "What would you do?", he or she is seeking assurance that you would do the same thing in the same situation. If your advice differs from what the client wants to hear, it may stir feelings of ambivalence. A request for advice can be turned into a therapeutic exchange with a response such as, "What would you like to do?" or "It sounds like you need more information to make this decision. Let's talk about it some more."

Abruptly Changing Subjects. It is generally not a good idea to change subjects too quickly. Doing so can be disconcerting and can disrupt rapport. Pausing frequently during the interview and using transitional phrases when moving from one subject to another provide opportunities to think through responses and reactions.

Acting Defensively. If the person being interviewed lashes out at other members of the staff or even family members or friends, it is best not to defend the people being criticized. To do so would imply judgment and inhibit further expression of feelings.

Minimizing Feelings. Disagreeing with a person's feelings about a situation succeeds only in denying the person the right to his or her own feelings. It is equally nonproductive to insist that there is nothing to worry about when, in fact, the person is expressing concern. Such a response demonstrates a lack of understanding or empathy.

Offering False Assurance. Offering false hope or promising quick solutions to complicated problems is unfair and unrealistic. Saying "Everything will be okay" denies the reality of the situation and frequently forces the person to hide fear and anxiety, which are human responses that require nursing intervention.

Jumping to Conclusions. You should never make an assumption and act on that assumption without first checking out the facts. For example, you should not assume that a person who is overweight wants to lose weight; neither is it wise to assume that a person who has breast cancer will automatically agree to the traditional treatment. Such conclusions represent your personal values and judgments and may serve to antagonize the client.

Interview Challenges
Cultural Considerations

Culture has a profound effect on the way people communicate. Therefore, sensitivity to culture should influence how the interview is conducted. Cultural differences that have the greatest impact on communication are language, verbal communication patterns, and nonverbal communication patterns. Cultural variations that are especially significant when you are evaluating health status include beliefs about health and illness, culturally accepted ways to express pain and emotions, and the manner of decision making about health and health care. People from the same culture will usually recognize and conform to the various forms of both verbal and nonverbal communication that exist in that culture. People from two different cultures, however, may have different "rules" for interaction and therefore may misunderstand or offend each other by their different communication styles. If misunderstanding or other barriers to communication are apparent, you should consult with colleagues who may have a better understanding of the person's cultural norms or language, if applicable.

Communication Guidelines for Cultural Variations

Use Translators. You may need to interview a person who does not speak your language. In that case, you will need to obtain the assistance of a translator. Many hospitals and clinics maintain a roster of translators who can be called on to interpret different languages. Family members or friends also may serve as translators but may not always be objective in what they communicate between the parties. Moreover, the individual being interviewed may be reluctant to translate personal information through a family member—especially if the translator is the person's child, a different gender, or from a different age-group. Furthermore, when family is asked to translate, the individual's right to a private and confidential discussion is compromised.

Avoid Slang Expressions and Jargon. Be careful to avoid the use of slang expressions or healthcare jargon, especially with non-native speakers. A non-native speaker may have an adequate understanding of proper language but be confused by slang expressions. Jargon can be confusing to people who speak the same language but do not belong to a certain group. For example, terms commonly used by healthcare providers, and especially acronyms, are often misunderstood by persons without a healthcare background. The person may feel uncomfortable because they do not understand you but yet be reluctant to admit misunderstanding. This interferes with the establishment of rapport and may prevent you from obtaining important data about health status.

Observe Appropriate Personal Space. How close people stand or sit near one another is determined by the way their culture defines personal space. In many Middle Eastern cultures, people stand close when talking to one another, whereas Anglo-Americans prefer to maintain a greater distance when engaged in conversation. Touch may be perceived differently among different cultural groups. Touching may be an accepted part of everyday interaction in some cultures; others consider touching among casual acquaintances to have a sexual connotation. Even individuals with similar cultural backgrounds may vary considerably in their perceptions and receptivity to touch. It is best to avoid using touch during the initial healthcare interview to maintain your professional demeanor as well as to avoid making the other person uncomfortable or self-conscious.

Use Appropriate Eye Contact. In many Western cultures, direct eye contact may indicate interest and attentiveness. In other cultures, eye contact may be viewed as rude, intrusive, or immodest. In some cultures, eye contact may be acceptable between persons of the same gender, but in others it may be considered disrespectful for a woman to make direct eye contact when speaking to a man.

Interpret Nonverbal Behavior. One way to determine whether the other person is having difficulty understanding you is to watch for verbal and nonverbal cues, such as a frown or a blank stare. In such a case, you may say, "I'm not sure you understand what I mean when I ask you if you have been dieting. Let me explain."

Understand Cultural Variations in the Expression of Emotion and Pain. Cultural variations may influence the person's willingness to openly express their emotions or pain. Similarly, how an individual will verbally respond to the experience of pain may also be culturally determined. For example, many Anglo-Americans and Native Americans are taught not to cry in response to pain because crying is considered to be childish or self-indulgent. Conversely, Latin Americans are permitted by their culture to respond to pain in a physical and vocal manner.

Understand Cultural Variations in Disclosing Personal Information. Although you may believe that you will obtain pertinent information about health status through direct questioning, you should know that some cultures view direct questioning about personal matters by strangers as intrusive, rude, or embarrassing. Rather than respond to your questions, you may observe an overall reluctance to participate in the interview or vague responses to your questions in an attempt to avoid embarrassment or confrontation.

Determine Family Decision-Making Processes. As you interview the individual and their family, you should determine how decisions about health care are made and by whom. If family members are present, note who responds to questions on behalf of the person being interviewed, who asks for more information, and who individuals look at as decisions are made.

Developmental Considerations

The age of the person being interviewed affects the way you should conduct the interview. Special consideration should be given to the conduct of the interview with children and elders.

Communication Guidelines for Children

Identify the Child's Age and Stage of Development. Childhood stages are classified in the following manner:

Premature neonate—born before 40 weeks' gestation
Newborn—birth to 30 days
Infant—1 to 12 months
Toddler—1 to 3 years
Preschooler—3 to 6 years
School age—6 to 12 years
Adolescent—12 to 18 years

The degree to which a child can participate in an interview will depend on the child's age and verbal communication skills and attention span. For a child younger than 6 years of age, it is usually necessary to interview a parent or guardian, although the child's behavior should be observed during the interview for relevant cues to health status. Interviewing a parent or guardian involves employing communication techniques similar to those used when interviewing any adult. Be aware that children as young as 2½ to 3 years of age may be capable of comprehending what is being said in their presence.

In general, toddlers have short attention spans and may not understand how to cooperate with an interview. A child older than 6 years of age can be interviewed directly; play and picture drawing are alternative means to elicit data. Asking the child to draw a picture illustrating his or her experience in the hospital, a picture of a family member, or a self-portrait can serve as a basis for discussion. Adolescents, as they become more independent from parents, may not want their parents to answer health-related questions on their behalf. In fact, adoles-

cents may feel stifled in the presence of a parent during the health assessment interview.

Establish Rapport. Regardless of the child's age, you should always make an effort to address the child directly as well as people accompanying the child during the interview. Through such direct verbal interaction, you can convey interest in the child as well as communicate comfort and safety. When the child is a newborn or infant, you will usually greet and introduce yourself to the parents first. For school-age children and adolescents, who may participate actively in the interview process, you should address the child first.

Introductions should be sufficient to establish your name, title, and role; the child's name and any preferred nicknames; and the identity and relationships of people accompanying the child. If parents are not accompanying the child, it is important to determine the reason.

Both verbal and nonverbal communication influence the establishment of rapport. Take care that verbal and nonverbal behaviors communicate to the child that the surroundings are safe. Many children feel threatened by white uniforms or lab coats, strange equipment, or harsh lighting. As when interviewing adults, you should maintain eye contact and assume a position that does not intimidate the child. Be careful not to "talk down to the child" or treat the older child like a baby or toddler.

A hurried, abrupt, uncaring attitude may be threatening to the child. Praising the child during the health assessment process is one way to make the child feel more comfortable (*e.g.,* "You're helping by holding so still" or "Thank you for telling me that story").

You should make a special effort to establish an atmosphere that is nonjudgmental and noncritical. This effort is especially important when establishing rapport with those accompanying the child. Parents may feel guilty if their child becomes sick or injured and may actually blame themselves for the child's illness. In such instances, you should use nonjudgmental questions to elicit pertinent data. Questions such as "When did you first notice signs of fever?" are much more appropriate than "Why didn't you bring him to the clinic sooner?" If the parents feel guilty or inferior, they are less likely to share their perceptions with you. Providing support and reassurance by empathizing with the parent's concerns (*e.g.,* "You seem very worried") may encourage a more open response and encourage the sharing of additional information.

Observe Family Interactions. Parents or guardians may or may not be present when you interview a child. If a parent is present, you are afforded an opportunity to observe family interactions. If parents or guardians are not accompanying the child, it is important to determine the reason. If the parent is dominating the conversation, or coaching or coercing the child to make certain responses, you should address the child directly with comments such as, "Now I'd like to hear how you feel about the situation."

Communication Guidelines for Elders

Establish Rapport. The older person will probably be more willing to share pertinent information in an atmosphere that encourages trust or mutual respect. Open the interview courteously and give your name, title, and purpose of the interview. Do not assume that the older person will be able to read such information from your nametag. Determine how the person wishes to be addressed—for example, use of first name versus being called Mr. or Mrs. Smith (many elders prefer Mr. or Mrs. Smith but may say "you can call me Dale," knowing that this is the current social custom).

Explain the purpose of eliciting information. Some elders have been conditioned to keep personal matters to themselves and may be hesitant to answer some questions. Ask the person's permission to record interview data and explain the purpose of such records. Some people may be suspicious that written records will be used against them in insurance claims.

Evaluate Hearing Acuity. Not every person becomes hard of hearing with advancing age, but hearing impairment is among the most common reasons for communication problems between nurses and elders. The type of hearing loss most prevalent in elders results in difficulty perceiving high-pitched sounds. Loud voices can be distressing and even offensive. If you detect a hearing loss, speak slowly with a low voice tone. Speaking rapidly tends to run words together, and raising the voice only increases the pitch. Make sure before the interview begins that the person is wearing his or her eyeglasses or hearing aids. Face the person directly and provide adequate lighting for lip-reading. Eliminate any extraneous sounds, such as from telephones, televisions, radios, or background conversations.

Allow Adequate Time. Obtaining a complete health history from an elder can be a challenge, especially if the person has had multiple hospitalizations, illnesses, or is taking many medications. Allow more time when interviewing an older person. More than one interview session may be necessary to collect all of the appropriate data. An elderly person usually has more health and illness information to share than a younger person does. Conversely, elders may tend to underreport or refrain from revealing pertinent symptoms, because they may consider the symptoms to be a part of aging and therefore unimportant.

The older person may require more time to process questions and formulate thoughts and answers. You may be asking the individual for information about events occurring 40 or 50 years ago. Give the person time to answer one question before asking the next question. Otherwise the person may feel rushed, depersonalized, and hesitant to share important information. Allow the person to finish statements, and avoid interrupting. Family members, if present, may tend to respond for the older person. Avoid this situation by interviewing the older person and the family separately.

Allow the Person to Reminisce. The interview process and your questions may stimulate past memories, which can be therapeutic for the elder and instructive for the nurse. For example, the person may discuss methods of handling problems that will give you insight into a partic-ular coping style. You will need to establish a balance between the person's need to reminisce and your need to collect health assessment data in a timely manner.

Show Respect. It is important that you do not use disrespectful communication techniques such as an overuse of medical jargon or modern slang, talking down to the elder, or yelling when you think the person cannot hear you. Physical aging does not mean the person is cognitively impaired or unable to understand you. Establish trust with the elder and keep any information you obtain during the interview private and confidential.

Complicated Interview Considerations

Occasionally, individuals may be "difficult" to interview because of cognitive barriers or because of emotional or behavioral factors, or the subject matter may involve the discussion of a sensitive topic. Not every person you interview you will be willing to participate, and not everyone will understand the relevance of the interview, especially if the person has been subject to several interviews and examinations with physicians, residents, medical students, and others. There may be other reasons an interview does not proceed smoothly. The person may be angry or depressed or simply not feeling well enough to participate. There may be barriers to communicating verbally, or the person may have impaired cognitive abilities.

Cognitive Limitations. If the person is unable to communicate verbally, you should first determine whether alternative methods for communication would work. The inability to speak does not necessarily mean that the person is cognitively impaired; it may be due to other factors such as hearing impairments, speech disorders, or language barriers. You should determine whether alternative methods, such as using a pencil and paper or a sign language interpretor, could facilitate the exchange of information.

The person with true cognitive impairment may be limited in his or her ability to answer questions or otherwise participate in the interview. Cognitive impairment may be secondary to some type of organic brain syndrome, metabolic disorders, drug use, or extreme sleep deprivation. The person may be labeled a "poor historian" in the medical record, and the traditional interview may be impossible to conduct. You will need to obtain information from other sources, including other medical records, family members, and your own observations of the individual. Your observations should include the person's grooming, motor coordination, orientation to time, person, and place, attention span, and level of consciousness.

Anger. A person may express anger in a number of ways, including verbal or physical abuse, being uncooperative with medical procedures or treatments, being overly controlling, or even by becoming overly dependent. People who are ill may feel frustration, a loss of control, and eventually, anger at others, including nurses. If additional stresses are present, such as financial difficulties or family problems, illness and health problems may contribute even more to an angry presentation.

You should avoid reacting to the angry person with your own anger because this usually will make the other person angrier. Approach the person with a calm, in-control demeanor. Allow the person to express their anger in nondestructive ways, including the ventilation of feelings. Do not discount the person's feelings. The interview may proceed more smoothly once feelings are expressed. If the person is out of control, you should avoid arguing or touching them and provide adequate personal space so that the person does not feel threatened. If you have concerns about your safety, you should seek help from others.

Anxiety. The anxious person may be apprehensive, frightened, or feeling uneasy. The person may not even be able to identify the source of their anxiety. An anxious person may speak rapidly or be restless, inattentive, and irritable. Nurses frequently encounter people who may be anxious because of the threats associated with a change in health status. These threats include changes in self-concept, threats of pain or death, changes in roles, and feelings of loss of control because of an inadequate understanding of events or medical procedures.

To effectively interview the anxious person, you should use a simple and organized approach. It is important not to hurry because the anxious person may have a harder time taking in and processing information. There may be a greater need to know why you are asking certain questions, so you should explain your role and purpose as you proceed throughout the interview.

Depression. Depression may be a common response in persons experiencing major changes in their health status, or depression may represent a more established condition. The depressed person will appear withdrawn and listless. In addition, speech may be slow, body movements may lack spontaneity, eye contact may be avoided, and crying may be observed. The depressed person may suffer from sleep disturbances and a lack of appetite. As you interview the depressed person, you may detect themes of hopelessness and helplessness, low self-esteem, and suicide ideation.

Interviewing the depressed person may be emotionally draining for the nurse. The person may not actively participate in offering information about themselves, especially in response to open-ended questions you may ask. As a result, you may feel that you have to drag information from the person. In this case, you should ask more directive questions, such as "Tell me when this happened" versus an open-ended questions such as "Tell me about your illness."

Avoid the tendency to give the person false hope or reassurance. If you say things such as, "Tomorrow will be a better day" or "it can only get better," the person may think you are insincere and do no really understand their feelings. You should use a more neutral and empathetic approach, such as "I understand you are worried about how things will turn out."

Manipulation. Manipulation is a type of coping mechanism people use when they need to feel control over a situation or others and have no other methods for gaining control. Manipulative people may appear overly dramatic or insincere. Manipulation is expressed by lying, by flat-tery, or by playing one staff person against another. For example, the person may tell you that you are the only nurse who knows how to effectively carry out procedures or get things done. Although you may find this type of behavior flattering, it is important to recognize that you are being manipulated. In general, if it feels to you that you are being manipulated, then, most likely, you are. Other ways in which manipulative behavior is expressed is by the person appearing helpless, intimidated, or making threats to harm themselves.

The most effective way to deal with manipulation is to first recognize that it is occurring. Then it becomes important to provide structure and set limits on the person's behavior to control the manipulation. Avoid the tendency to become angry with the manipulator. If you feel you are being manipulated and cannot control the situation, ask for the help of a colleague to restore your perspective.

Seductive Behavior. Seductive behavior may represent a regressive coping mechanism for the person facing physical threat or illness, or it may be a more established personality pattern. In the first case, you may observe more childlike than sexual behaviors, such as idealizing or flattery in an attempt to win you over. In the latter case, you may see behavior that is more flirtatious, sexual innuendoes, or even overt sexual behavior such as fondling or sexual propositions.

You should use a similar approach as you would with the manipulator, First, recognize that the behavior is occurring. Then set clear limits with the person and let him or her know you will not tolerate overt sexual behavior. Less obvious sexual innuendoes should be ignored.

Discussions About Sexuality. Obtaining information about sexual topics is an important component of a comprehensive health history. Many people experiencing chronic illness such as heart disease, hypertension, or diabetes may experience changes in their sexual practices either directly as a result of the illness or because of the effects of medication used in the treatment of their illness. Or the person you interview may have questions about sexual practices, be carrying or at risk for a sexually transmitted disease, or have other issues related to sexuality. In any case, sexuality is an integral consideration in health and illness.

An individual may feel fear, anger, or embarrassment when discussing sexual topics with healthcare providers. You need to ask questions simply and use a straightforward and nonjudgmental approach. Try to help the person understand why your questions are relevant to nursing care. Provide a private environment for the discussion and consider the impact of culture and religious values on your discussion.

If you feel uncomfortable discussing sexual topics with the person, you should make a referral to another qualified provider so that the individual's concerns and questions are addressed. As you increase your own knowledge base about the impact of health and illness on human sexuality, you will find sexual topics easier to discuss.

Discussions About Terminal Illness. Nurses who work in hospitals or nursing homes frequently come in contact with persons who have terminal illnesses. Frequent contact, however, does not always mean that nurses are comfortable in their interactions with dying patients. In fact, nurses may even avoid using the word "death" or "dying." More than likely, this is because of the nurse's own fears or failure to come to terms with feelings about death.

When you are interviewing a person with a terminal illness, it is helpful to know whether the person has been told about their prognosis. Most patients will have had a discussion with another healthcare provider or family members. In some cases, the person may not have been told directly about their illness, but they may accurately sense that their illness is fatal by observing the way people are treating or avoiding them or the person may even have an intuitive sense of the situation.

The person may respond differently at different times during their illness with typical manifestations of grief, including denial, anger, bargaining, and acceptance. At any time, the person may need to ventilate feelings or discuss their situation more fully. Providing the person with emotional support should be a nursing priority.

You will communicate most effectively with the dying person by taking care not to avoid contact and allowing the person to discuss what is important to them without changing the subject or offering false reassurance. It is important that you provide direct and honest information if the person requests it. If you feel uncomfortable talking to the person with a terminal illness, you should make an appropriate referral to another colleague.

▼ ▼ ▼

GUIDELINES

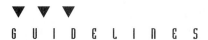

Assessment Guidelines The Initial Health Assessment Interview

General Approach

Understand the Scope of the Initial Health Assessment Interview. The health assessment process usually starts with an interview. To assess an individual's need for nursing care, the initial assessment interview should be comprehensive and include questions that will help identify specific nursing care needs. An interview with questions designed to obtain data pertaining to the 11 Functional Health Patterns provides the appropriate focus for determining nursing areas of concern. In addition, most initial assessment interviews are designed to elicit basic demographic data, the person's reasons for seeking health care, medical history, and current medication use history. The interview presented in this guideline provides a general approach to the content of the questions you should ask during the initial comprehensive interview. The interview guidelines for specific functional health patterns presented in Chapters 5 through 15 present more detailed approaches for evaluating functional health status, including the interpretation of normal and abnormal findings.

Review the Purpose of the Initial Assessment Interview. An initial assessment interview addressing all 11 functional health patterns, reasons for seeking health care, medical history, and medication history helps to elicit basic information about health status and establish the database necessary for initiating nursing diagnosis and care planning.

Coordinate Data Collection. A number of healthcare providers may be interested in interviewing the individual seeking health care. This is especially true in settings in which health care is provided by a multidisciplinary team, such as a hospital. To avoid overwhelming the person and subjecting him or her to repetitive requests for data, you should make every attempt to coordinate the collection of essential data with other providers. For example, a physician may elicit data pertaining to the person's medical history. If these data are available on the medical record, you may choose not to conduct another detailed interview regarding medical history. You should review these data, however, and discuss significant findings as appropriate with the person during your interview to determine nursing care needs. For example, if you note on the medical history that the person has diabetes, you should address how the person manages their overall health, diet, and skin care as well as their understanding of their medications.

Use Therapeutic Communication. Throughout the interview, apply therapeutic communication techniques (see "Knowledge Base for Assessment: Interviewing").

Prepare the Interview Environment. The ideal interview environment is one in which the nurse and the individual face each other in a quiet room without the common interruptions that might be experienced in some healthcare settings, such as noisy or busy nursing stations, intercom systems, ringing call lights or telephones, noisy equipment, or other distractions. In

▼ ▼ ▼

an ideal setting, both the nurse and the client would have unlimited time and few other responsibilities. Unfortunately, the ideal environment is seldom the case in the real world. However, you can strive toward the ideal by doing the following:

- For hospitalized patients, try to schedule the interview for a time when the patient will not be called away for tests or other procedures. Choose a time when you do not expect to be called away suddenly for an emergency or situation with another patient.
- For outpatient surgery patients, try to schedule the interview before the day of surgery. Otherwise, the interview will be conducted the morning of the procedure, which is the least optimum time because the patient and family are usually under stress. Stress may interfere with a person's ability to provide complete and accurate information.
- Do what you can to promote privacy. Close the door or bedside curtain. Consider moving to a private conference room to conduct the interview if the person is mobile and the space is available.
- Eliminate other unnecessary distractions such as televisions or radios playing in the background.
- Get focused. Sit as close to the individual as is comfortable and in a position to make eye contact. Convey a sense of priority and interest toward the individual.

Explain your Purpose and Format. You know that you are going to ask the person questions about general medical history and 11 areas of functional health and that you will be following a logical format of proceeding from one topic to the next and from one functional health pattern to the next. It is important that you explain the overall purpose of the interview and why you need the information to the individual in familiar language. This will help the person accept what might otherwise seem like a lengthy barrage of unrelated questions.

- Develop a concise, opening statement that will not confuse or bore the person. For example, you may open the interview by saying the following: "I would like to ask you some general questions about your health so I can understand better how you and I might approach your health care. I will be asking questions about a number of topics. It should take me about 30 minutes."
- During the interview, use appropriate introduction phrases and transition phrases to help the person understand your logic and sequence. You can start the interview by saying: "First, I would like to ask you for general information. . . ."
- When you change the subject from one topic to another, make appropriate transition statements such as the following:
  - "I'm going to ask you some questions about how you feel about your general health . . ."
  - "Now I'd like to talk about diet and nutrition. . . ."
  - "That completes the questions I have about nutrition. Now I'd like to talk about bowel and bladder functions. . . ."

Make Appropriate Modifications for Elders. When assessing elders, provide a comfortable environment for the health assessment interview. The room should be well lighted, and the room temperature should be adjusted to the person's comfort. Chairs should be easy to get in and out of. Allow sufficient time for the interview, because elders may talk and move at a slower pace than other age-groups. If the person has a hearing impairment, be sure to face the individual and speak in a strong, low-pitched voice because the person may have difficulty hearing high-pitched sounds.

Make Appropriate Modifications for Children. When assessing children and their families, you should determine the following about the parents or guardian: reading level, understanding of the child's health status, and their ability to reinforce health-related education with the child.

In addition to the health status data you would obtain by asking the child or another person questions about the 11 functional health patterns, the following data should be collected and clearly displayed on the database:

- Family status—parent's marital status, custodial parent, guardian, usual caregiver, siblings
- Developmental level—premature neonate, newborn, infant, toddler, preschooler, school age, adolescent
- Response to separation
- Security objects
- Immunization status
- Recent exposure to communicable and infectious diseases
- Childhood diseases
- Previous hospitalizations

Review Identifying Information. Basic demographic or biographical information about the individual may be obtained during the initial health assessment interview. If someone else obtained this information, you do not need to ask for the information a second time, but you should ascertain the accuracy of the information as necessary. You should review this information because it can give important cues about the person's cultural, religious, and social background.

Perform Symptom Analysis. In medicine, a *symptom* is considered an indicator of a physical disorder or disease. For example, a headache is a symptom of many diseases, ranging from migraine to meningitis. As you interview the person, you may be informed of problems or symptoms that the person is experiencing. For example, the person may tell you about pain in a certain area of the body, nausea, dizziness, difficulty swallowing, or shortness of breath.

Symptom analysis is a common technique used by clinicians to further evaluate symptoms in a systematic and standardized manner. The technique of symptom analysis is most applicable to the analysis of physical problems and helps the clinician differentiate one physical problem from another in the course of arriving at a final diagnosis. The process of analyzing information to choose from among several diagnostic possibilities is referred to as *differential diagnosis.*

Symptoms may be analyzed by systematically asking about the following characteristics:

Criteria for the Analysis of a Symptom
- *Onset:* When did you first notice the symptom or problem (time and date)? Was the onset sudden or gradual? Has this symptom (problem) occurred at other times in the past? What circumstances precipitated the symptom onset?
- *Location* (applies to the evaluation of pain): Where did you feel the pain? (Ask the person to point to the exact location.) Does the pain radiate (move away from a central point)?
- *Quality:* Describe the way you feel when you experience this symptom (problem).
- *Quantity:* How intense was the symptom/problem? (Pain can be rated on a scale of 1 to 5). Did the symptom/problem interfere with your usual activities such as talking, walking, or sleeping?
- *Frequency and Duration:* How often do you experience the symptom/problem and how long does it last?
- *Aggravating and Alleviating Factors:* What makes the problem worse or better?
- *Associated Factors:* Have you noticed any other problems in relation to this symptom/problem? (Hint: Ask about factors normally associated with the symptom, such as nausea with chest pain.)
- *Course:* How has the symptom/problem changed or progressed over time?

Interview Content and Questions

The general types of questions you may want to ask about the 11 functional health patterns

▼ ▼ ▼

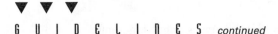

G U I D E L I N E S *continued*   The Initial Health Assessment Interview

during the working phase of the interview are presented in this section. These questions will direct you in the collection of data about the person's overall health status.

To obtain more information, especially about a potentially dysfunctional pattern, the nurse needs to ask additional questions and encourage additional discussion by the individual being interviewed. Refer to the chapters in Unit II for additional interview guidelines specific to a particular functional health pattern.

Identifying Information: Content for the Initial Assessment Interview

- Name
- Religion
- Residence
- Marital status
- Age
- Occupation
- Date of birth
- Health insurance
- Place of birth
- Nationality
- Gender

Additional Identifying Information for Children

- Primary caregiver (parent, guardian, other)
- Parent's marital status
- Custodial parent (if applicable)
- Developmental level

Functional Health Patterns: Sample Interview Questions

Health Perception and Health Management

- How would you describe your present state of health?
- What kinds of things do you do to maintain or improve your health?
- Have you made any changes in your lifestyle to improve your health in the past 2 years?
- What goals do you have for improving your health?
- When was your last visit to a healthcare provider? For what reason?
- Have you had any problems following a healthcare provider's advice?

Additional Questions for Persons Who Are Managing Chronic Diseases

- What do you know about your illness (condition; disease)?
- What kinds of questions do you have about your illness?
- What kind of changes do you think you will have to make because of your illness?
- How have you been able to make the changes in diet, exercise, medication, etc. that you need to make?
- (If applicable) How are you managing with the new equipment/devices you have had to learn to use to take care of yourself?

Additional Questions for Children

- What immunizations has the child had? Is the child up to date now?
- Has the child had recent exposure to communicable and infectious diseases?
- What childhood diseases, such as measles or mumps, has the child had?

Nutrition and Metabolism

- What is your current height?
- What is your current weight?
- Have you experienced any recent weight gain or weight loss? Any recent change in appetite?

▼ ▼ ▼

- Describe a typical day's menu (include content of meals and snacking patterns).
- Are you on a special diet? What is it? How closely do you follow it?
- Are there any foods you avoid? For what reason?
- Do you use any vitamin supplements?
- Do you have any problems with chewing or swallowing; indigestion; sore mouth; dental work? If so, describe.
- Do you have dentures?
- Have you noticed any changes in your hair, nails, skin?

Elimination
- How often do you have a bowel movement?
- Do you have any problems with diarrhea; constipation; loss of control?
- Do you take any medications if these changes occur?
- Have you noticed changes in your bowel movement patterns?
- Describe your usual pattern of urine elimination. How often do you void during the day? At night?
- Do you ever lose urine when you cough, sneeze, or laugh?
- Do you have problems with passing urine when you don't want to?

Activity and Exercise
- Describe the type, frequency, and amount of physical exercise you engage in on a regular basis.
- What are your leisure activities?
- How are you able to do the following: Feeding yourself? Bathing? Dressing and grooming? Toileting? Transferring? Ambulating? Stair climbing? Shopping? Cooking? Home maintenance?

Cognition and Perception
- Do you have any problems with hearing? Vision?
- Do you use a hearing aid? Right, left, or both ears?
- Do you wear glasses? Contact lenses?
- Do you have any problems reading educational materials?
- What is the best way for you to learn new things? Reading? Demonstration? Videos?
- Are you experiencing pain? How is pain controlled?

Sleep and Rest
- Do you feel well rested after sleep?
- Are you experiencing any sleep problems? Difficulty falling asleep? Difficulty staying asleep? Other?
- What helps you sleep well?

Self-Concept
- How do you feel about yourself, in general?
- What do you identify as your strengths and weaknesses?
- What most concerns you about your health/illness/hospitalization?

Roles and Relationships
- Are you employed? Unemployed? Disabled?
- What do you do for a living?
- (if retired) What was your past occupation? How do you feel about being retired?
- What kinds of relationships do you have with your co-workers?
- Do you live alone or with others?
- Whom do you rely on for support?
- What kinds of relationships do you have with spouse or partner, children, or other family members?
- How does your health/illness affect family or significant others?

▼ ▼ ▼

G U I D E L I N E S *continued*   The Initial Health Assessment Interview

---

- Are you a caregiver for anyone else? Spouse, child, parent, other? What happens if you are not available for this person?

Sexuality and Reproduction
- Do you have any concerns regarding your sexual health? (body image? male/female roles?)
- Are there any recent changes in your health that have affected your sexual health/roles?
- Have you had any sexually transmitted diseases? If yes, describe.

Additional Questions for Women
- When was your last menstrual period?
- What was the year of your last menstrual cycle/menopause (if applicable)?
- Do you have any menstrual problems?
- Have you ever been pregnant? Number of pregnancies; number of live births; number of stillbirths; number of abortions/miscarriages?
- Did you have any pregnancy or delivery complications? Describe.

Coping and Stress Tolerance
- How would you rate your current level of stress? High? Average? Low?
- What do you do when you are under stress?
- What major life changes or stresses have you experienced in the last year?
- Have there been any recent losses in your life?

Values and Beliefs
- What is most important in your life?
- Do you have a religious affiliation? Is this important to you?
- Do you have any special requests related to your religion that healthcare providers should know about?
- Do you have values or beliefs that healthcare providers should consider in providing your care?

Concluding the Initial Assessment Interview

Always conclude by asking the person whether there is anything else they would like to discuss or share with you during this initial interview process. Also, ask the person whether they have any questions they would like to ask you.

Summarize what you think are the most significant issues or findings encountered during this initial assessment interview. As appropriate, make plans to address any issues or problems.

▼ ▼ ▼

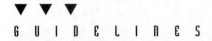

Assessment Guidelines   The Medical History (Past Health History and Review of Systems)

General Approach

The *medical history* or *past health history* includes information about the person's history of illnesses, surgical and other clinical procedures, hospitalizations or other types of health care, and previous accidents or injuries. An inventory of the health status of body systems known as the *review of systems (ROS)* also may be included. A good medical history can almost always provide additional information that will help you better understand a person's overall health status and nursing care needs.

The procedure for obtaining the medical history is presented as a separate guideline to highlight the key elements of a medical history. Often, the medical history is also recorded on the medical record as a separate and readily identifiable section of the database. If a thorough medical history is documented and available elsewhere, it may not be necessary to repeat the process of taking the entire medical history again with the individual. However, you should verify the accuracy of the information contained in the medical history in the course of your ongoing relationship with the individual.

The medical history is often relevant to an individual's functional status. Therefore, in subsequent chapters in Unit II that provide more detailed guidelines for evaluating functional status, frequent references are made to medical history.

As you gain experience with the framework for assessing health status in relation to the eleven functional health patterns, you will begin to integrate an analysis of the medical history with the analysis of a particular functional health pattern.

Obtain a Complete Medical History. Many people may believe that surgery or illness that occurred many years ago is not important and may not mention distant events when giving a medical history. For example, a person who is asked whether they have high blood pressure, heart problems, or diabetes may say no, believing that it is under control and therefore not a problem. Skillful questioning is required to obtain a complete medical history. If the medical history is obtained by asking the person or family to complete a form, the wording must be in terms that are readily understood by the general public.

Ask for Lists. If the person has had numerous surgical or medical procedures and the circumstances allow, ask the person to bring a list of these procedures to the interview. A list may provide more complete recall than asking the person to name procedures at the time of the interview. If you are asking for a list, it should include the name of the procedure, the date it was performed, the reason, the clinician who performed it, and the facility. Alternatively, you can ask for lists of events as you interview the person.

Present Data in Sequence. Use a consistent approach and sequence when you ask for and record information about past procedures. Ask the person to provide information in chronological order. For example, "Tell me about all your hospitalizations, starting with the earliest one and ending with the most recent one."

Review Data Obtained from Questionnaires with the Individual. You should always review data recorded as a response on a questionnaire or standard form with the individual you are assessing or a member of their family to ensure that the information is accurate, thorough, and truly reflects the individual's medical history. Discuss any data that conflict with other information in greater detail. For example, if the person reports taking a medication for high blood pressure but checks "no" to a question inquiring about high blood pressure, discuss this in more detail with the individual.

Make Appropriate Modifications for Elders. Approximately 86% of people older than age 65 years report having one or more chronic diseases, the most common being arthritis, hearing impairment, hypertension, and heart conditions. Obtaining a complete medical history from an elder may be a challenge, and some elders may not consider certain chronic diseases significant. To avoid an incomplete history, you may have to specifically ask about these types of diseases.

Conduct a Review of Systems. The ROS is always included in the history obtained and recorded by clinicians whose primary focus is on the natural history of disease, such as physicians. Nurses may not always choose to conduct an ROS, depending on the overall assessment goals. For example, nurses may have a greater interest in the person's response to a disease process than the disease process itself. Alternatively, the nurse may review systems

▼ ▼ ▼

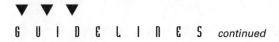

G U I D E L I N E S *continued*   The Medical History (Past Health History
                                                    and Review of Systems)

---

during the course of the physical examination by asking the person questions about each system as the examination is being conducted. The review of systems is conducted to secure additional pertinent details about the health status of each body system.

When documenting an ROS, you should only record the data provided as the individual's responses to your questions during the interview. A common mistake by beginning practitioners is to record findings of the physical examination with the documentation of the review of systems.

An ROS is an interview that is conducted in a roughly head-to-toe sequence. The sample interview questions in the next section illustrate the main topics to review and a typical sequence.

Interview Content and Questions

The general types of questions you would ask to obtain a medical history and ROS are presented in this section.

Medical History: Sample Interview Questions

Allergies
- Do you have any allergies to food, medications, dyes, or other substances?
- If yes, list and describe the type of reaction to each substance listed.
- Have you ever been identified as being sensitive or allergic to latex?

Injuries and Disabilities
- Have you ever been in an accident or injured?
- If yes, describe each incident, starting with the first one.

Chronic Disease Processes/Significant Illnesses/Hospitalizations
- Have you ever been hospitalized?
- If yes, list each hospitalization, starting with the earliest, and identify date, place (facility), reason, and doctor.
- Other than what you already mentioned, have you had any other diseases or illnesses?
- If yes, list and identify any continuing problems or medical treatment.
- What diseases did you have as a child (e.g., measles, mumps, chicken pox)?
- Have you ever been treated for emotional or mental problems?

Surgical Procedures
- Have you ever had surgery?
- If yes, identify date, place, procedure, doctor.

Other Types of Invasive or Diagnostic Procedures
- Have you had any other major types of medical procedures (cancer treatment, heart procedures)?
- When was the last time you had a chest x-ray, electrocardiogram, and laboratory tests?
- What was done and why?

Review of Systems (ROS): Sample Interview Questions

Skin, Hair, Nails
- Have you had any problems with skin (lesions, excessive dryness, rashes, sweating, excessive bruising, eczema, psoriasis, hives)?
- Have you noticed changes in skin color? In the appearance of moles?
- Have you experienced recent hair loss? Changes in hair texture? Dandruff?
- Any changes in the shape, color, or brittleness of the nails?

Head and Neck
- Have you had any problems with severe or frequent headaches, dizziness, or vertigo?

▼ ▼ ▼

The Medical History (Past Health History and Review of Systems)

- Any history of head injury?
- Have you experienced neck pain or stiffness; difficulty swallowing; sore throat; goiter, lumps, or swelling; enlarged or tender nodes?

Eyes
- Have you had any difficulty with your vision (decreased acuity, blurring, blind spots, double vision)?
- Any history of glaucoma or cataracts?
- Do you experience any of the following eye problems: redness, pain, watering, or discharge?

Ears
- Do you have any problems with your hearing (decreased acuity, ringing or buzzing)?
- Do you have problems with earaches, infections, discharge, vertigo (dizziness)?

Mouth, Nose, Throat, and Sinuses
- Do you experience mouth pain, frequent sore throats, dysphagia?
- Any problems with the condition of your teeth or gums? Any bleeding?
- Do you experience frequent or unusually severe colds? Any nasal or sinus discharge? Any sinus pain?
- Any problems with nasal obstructions, nosebleeds, allergies, or hay fever?
- Have you noticed any alterations in taste or smell?

Thorax and Lungs
- Have you had any lung diseases (asthma, emphysema, bronchitis, pneumonia, and tuberculosis)?
- Have you experienced chest pain with breathing? Wheezing? Shortness of breath during routine activity? Cough or sputum production? Coughing up blood?

Breasts and Axilla
- Do you perform monthly self-breast examinations?
- Have you ever noticed lumps or discharge from nipples? Swollen or tender nodes in the axilla?
- Do you have any history of breast disease or breast surgery?

Cardiovascular
- Have you experienced chest pain? Palpitations? Shortness of breath on exertion? Edema?
- Do you have any history of hypertension? Coronary artery disease? Heart attack? Anemia? Heart murmur?

Peripheral Vascular
- Have you experienced swelling of the legs and feet?
- Have you experienced any leg pain, cramping, tingling, numbness? Any sores or lesions on the legs?
- Do you have varicose veins?
- Do you have any history of intermittent claudication? Thrombophlebitis?

Gastrointestinal
- Do you have any problems with indigestion, nausea, abdominal pain, gas, vomiting, vomiting blood?
- Do you have any history of ulcers? Liver or gallbladder problems? Rectal conditions?
- Have you noticed any changes in bowel habits or stool?
- Any problems with constipation? Diarrhea? Rectal bleeding?

Male Genital System
- Do you have any problems with urination?

▼ ▼ ▼

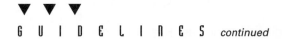

G U I D E L I N E S   *continued*

The Medical History (Past Health History and Review of Systems)

- Have you had any sexual problems? Are you aware of any contact with a partner who has a history of a sexually transmitted disease?
- Have you noticed any penile drainage, pain, hernia, or swelling in the scrotum?

Female Genital System

- Do you have any problems with urination?
- Have you had any sexual problems? Are you aware of any contact with a partner who has a history of a sexually transmitted disease?
- Do you have any problems with menstruation? What was your age of menarche? Age of menopause? Any postmenopausal bleeding?
- Have you been pregnant? Any problems?
- Have you noticed any vaginal itching, drainage, painful intercourse?

Musculoskeletal

- Do you have any problems with mobility? Joint stiffness, swelling, deformity?
- Have you experienced muscle or joint pain?
- Do you have a history of arthritis or gout? Disc disease?

Neurologic

- Have you experienced headaches, seizures, blackouts?
- Have you experienced any weakness, tics or tremors, paralysis, or coordination problems?
- Have you experienced any numbness or tingling?
- Have you experienced any memory problems?
- Have you experienced mood changes? Nervousness? Depression?

▼ ▼ ▼

G U I D E L I N E S

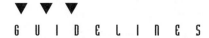 The Medication and Substance Use History

General Approach

The *medication and substance use history* focuses on the various medications and substances the individual is ingesting.

The procedure for obtaining the history of medication and substance use is presented as a separate guideline to highlight the key elements. As is the case with a medical history, the medication history may be recorded on the medical record as a separate and readily identifiable section of the database. If a thorough medication history is documented and available elsewhere, it may not be necessary to repeat the process of taking the entire medication history again with the individual. You do need to evaluate the person's understanding of their medications. You should verify the accuracy of the information contained in the medication history if you are reviewing a history documented by another clinician.

The medication history is often relevant to an individual's functional status. Some medications are taken to improve or maintain function. Other medications may have adverse effects on functional status. As you gain experience with the framework for assessing health status in relation to the 11 functional health patterns, you will begin to integrate an analysis of the medication history with the analysis of a particular functional health pattern.

Make Direct Observations. Ask the person to bring current medications with them to the interview or a list of all medications being used. A person may not always remember all the medications they are taking, their names, or their dosages.

▼ ▼ ▼

Consider Polypharmacy. *Polypharmacy* refers to the practice of prescribing and ingesting more than one type of medication. This practice is especially prevalent in elders. Some studies have been conducted showing that elders ingested an average of eight different types of prescription and over-the-counter medications. The more drugs a person takes, the greater risk of harmful drug interactions and adverse drug effects. When you assess an individual who is taking a number of different substances, you should determine who prescribed each medication and whether the person's primary healthcare provider has knowledge of all substances an individual is taking. If multiple providers have been prescribing for the person, the risks of adverse effects and drug interactions are increased.

Assess for Adverse Drug Reactions. As you obtain a medication history, and throughout the interview process, be alert to any signs and symptoms of adverse drug reactions. An adverse drug reaction is an undesirable response associated with the use of a drug that either compromises the therapeutic effect of the drug, enhances the drug toxicity, or both. Many adverse drug reactions manifest through nonspecific symptoms that may be associated with other conditions such as confusion, dizziness, fatigue, or constipation.

Interview Content and Questions

General Questions to Identify Medications and Other Substances

- What medications are you taking that have been prescribed by your doctor or another healthcare provider?
- Are you taking any medications that you can purchase over-the-counter at a drug or grocery store?
- Why do you take it and how often?
- Does your physician or healthcare provider know about all the drugs that you are taking, including over-the-counter preparations?
- Do you drink beer, wine, or other alcoholic beverages? If so, how much?
- Have you ever used, or do you now use, illicit (illegal) drugs?

For Each Medication Identified, Determine the Following

- Who prescribed it and why?
- When was the prescription last filled?
- What dosing instructions were provided? In particular:
  - How many times a day were you instructed to take the medication?
  - What time of day were you told to take the medication?
  - When do you take the medication in relation to meals?
- Do you follow the dosing instructions provided?
- Do you follow any advised dietary restrictions or modifications related to using this medication?
- Do you feel the drug is helping?
- Have you experienced any adverse effects from this medication?

  Note: You may need to review the common adverse effects listed in the prescribing information to determine whether there are adverse effects.

DOCUMENTATION: THE HEALTH HISTORY

Two basic approaches may be used to document the health history. Regardless of the approach used, the recorded health history should include basic identifying information about the client as well as any relevant demographics such as religious affiliation, marital status, and occupation.

Two Approaches for Documenting the Health History

- Narrative style documentation
- Standardized form completion

Narrative style documentation allows the nurse to summarize the interview findings in a series of narrative paragraphs. Although narrative-style documentation may appear "free-form," you should still present the information in a logical and organized manner so that it is easy to understand, retrieve, and communicate findings to others. Display 2-2 shows a narrative-style documentation of an initial health assessment interview using the functional health pattern framework.

More frequently, in healthcare settings, you are likely to see the health history recorded on a standard form created to include all the necessary information. A number of sample forms may be found in various health care organizations and in the nursing literature. Display 2-3 illustrates a form that may be used to document the health history.

The documentation example presented in Display 2-2 and the form presented on Display 2-3 illustrate that data obtained from interviewing and physical examination are often presented together. Although the discussion in this chapter has focused on the process for developing the health history by interviewing, with minimal reference to the physical examination, it is common to see displays of data obtained from interviewing and physical examination on clinical records.

DISPLAY 2.2

Sample Health Assessment Data Base: Functional Approach

DEMOGRAPHIC DATA

Mr. Arnold K., 956 Cedar Lane, Mann City
46 years old, steel plant worker (welder)

REFERRAL

Required annual physical for work.

CURRENT MEDICATIONS

1. Acetaminophen or aspirin for headaches (occasional use)
2. Dihydroxy aluminum sodium carbonate (Rolaids) tablets for indigestion (2 to 3 times/month)
3. Clonidine hydrochloride (Catapres) prescribed for hypertension; does not know dosage and does not take as prescribed

PAST MEDICAL—SURGICAL HISTORY

1. Hypertension—diagnosed 1 year ago during routine physical; has not had routine blood pressure measurements since.
2. Fractured right wrist in industrial accident, 1984; treated with cast; healed with no residual problems.
3. Hemorrhoidectomy, 1982; recovery uncomplicated; no recurrence of hemorrhoids.

HEALTH PERCEPTION AND HEALTH MANAGEMENT

Views self as healthy. Greatest concern is that present examination may reveal something is wrong with him. Being healthy means "not having to go to the doctor and not having to take any pills." Engages in no scheduled health screening activities except annual physical required by employer. Comprehensive health insurance provided by employer. Clonidine was prescribed 1 year ago for hypertension but he states he only takes it when he feels his BP is high—"when I get headaches." Reasons for not taking Catapres: "I don't like pills"; "I don't think my blood pressure is high"; cost. No regular blood pressure screening.

ILLNESS AND INJURY RISK FACTORS

1. Family health history (see diagram at right).
2. Exposure to health and safety risks: Does not smoke cigarettes, drink alcohol, or use illegal drugs; has been exposed to asbestos through work; no pulmonary function testing to date; result of chest x-ray 1 year ago was normal (verified by record).
3. Safety measures: Wears safety glasses at work and while doing yard work; wears seatbelt on freeways or rural highways but not for city driving. Wears helmet for dirt biking and requires same of children.

OBJECTIVE DATA

BP 144/88 (LA)
BP 140/90 (LA—repeated 10 minutes after first measurement)

NUTRITION AND METABOLISM

Sees self as 20 pounds overweight because of sedentary lifestyle and "love of food." Views weight gain as "part of life" and has no desire to reduce. Good appetite, likes most foods, no food allergies, no special diet, and no problems with eating. Wife does shopping and cooking. Eats out once per week.

SAMPLE DIET

- Breakfast—Black coffee, 2 doughnuts, orange juice
- AM break at work—coffee, sweet roll
- Lunch—Ham and cheese sandwich, soda, potato chips, fruit
- Dinner—Chicken, steak, or hamburger; cooked vegetable; potato with butter and sour cream; cookies or pudding
- Evening snacks—Chips or cookies; milk before retiring

(continued)

Sample Health Assessment Data Base: Functional Approach continued

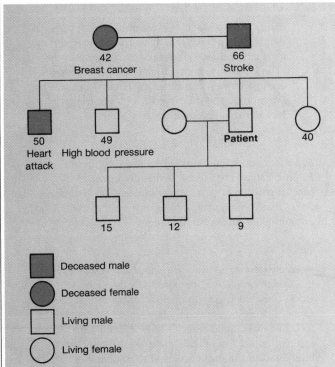

- ■ Deceased male
- ● Deceased female
- □ Living male
- ○ Living female

OBJECTIVE DATA

Height 6'0" Weight: 230 lbs.
Ideal weight (large frame): 168–192 lbs.
Triceps skinfold: 17.5 mm
Skin: Intact; no lesions except for old scars from minor trauma.
Oral cavity: Moist oral mucosa. No lesions.
Cranial nerves IX, X, XII intact.
Abd and Thyroid

ELIMINATION

- Urinary: No problems with voiding. Has never had hesitancy, burning, or urgency.
- Bowel: Usually has daily bowel movement after breakfast.
- Occasional constipation (once per month) when regular schedule is disrupted. Takes magnesium hydroxide (Milk of Magnesia) for constipation—"If I let it go, I think my hemorrhoids would be back." Currently no problems with hemorrhoids. Result of stool test for occult blood was negative 1 year ago; no gross blood noted in stools.

OBJECTIVE DATA

Rectal exam: No masses or tenderness. Prostate without enlargement or nodules, firm. Soft brown stool, negative for occult blood.

ACTIVITY AND EXERCISE

Drives to work. Occasionally heavy lifting but otherwise little exertion required for work activities. Engages in yard work nightly after work (spring and summer) to maintain garden. Other leisure activities—fishing from boat once per week; watching TV; dirt bike riding with family once per week; camping; spectator sports. No regular exercise—views camping, fishing, and biking as exercise.

Self-care: Independent in all ADLs.

Denies any cardiovascular or musculoskeletal symptoms in relation to activity—no chest pain, dyspnea, leg, joint, or back pain.

OBJECTIVE DATA

Musculoskeletal system: Full range of motion; muscle strength 3 on 5-point scale. Steady gait. No observed deficits in general mobility. No joint deformities.

Cardiovascular system: Regular heart rhythm. Pulse 88. Clear S_1 and S_2—no extra heart sounds or murmurs. No dependent edema. PMI 5th ICS at the MCL.

Respiratory system: Equal and full chest expansion. Lungs resonant. Breath sounds clear without adventitious sounds.

COGNITION AND PERCEPTION

Trade school graduate. Learns easily by "seeing something done and then doing it."

Special senses: Wears reading glasses; last eye exam 4 years ago; not sure if he was tested for glaucoma. No problems with hearing or other senses.

Frontal headaches every 2 to 3 months; takes aspirin or acetaminophen (Tylenol) and if unrelieved takes clonidine (Catapres) "since it might be my blood pressure."

OBJECTIVE DATA

Eyes: Vision 20/30 (OD) and 20/40 (OS); reads telephone print with reading glasses. Full peripheral vision by confrontation. PERRLA. Conjunctiva pink and moist; cornea and lens clear. No AV nicking, fundal lesions, or fundal edema.
EARS

SLEEP AND REST

Usually sleeps 6 to 7 hours per night (10:30 PM–5:30 AM); stays up later and sleeps in on weekends. No problems falling asleep or maintaining sleep. Sleeps in king-size

(continued)

Sample Health Assessment Data Base: Functional Approach continued

bed with wife. Presleep activities include watching television news and saying prayers.

SELF-CONCEPT

Views self as needing to be in control of own life and family's emotional and financial security. Wants to be strong and healthy for his family—"I feel like I'd be letting them down if I got sick." States he is a good husband and father, and dependable, skilled worker. Mostly positive about self and life. Describes self as religious.

OBJECTIVE DATA

Relaxed during interview except when questioned about medications and blood pressure. Well-groomed with greasy hands and fingernails from working with engines. Maintains eye contact.

ROLES AND RELATIONSHIPS

Family: Wife and children healthy and family relationships close and happy. Three sons—ages 15, 12, 9. Family goes camping and biking every weekend during summer. Takes sons deer hunting with friends every fall. States sons are "good boys" and active in church and sports. Family discusses social issues and uses religious concepts to guide life. States he would worry more about his sons if they weren't active in church activities. Wife works part time as receptionist.

Social: Socializes with other church members. Family-style get-togethers with friends once every 2 to 3 weeks. All close friends are part of this group. Compatible with coworkers but minimal interaction outside work.

Work: Enjoys work but worries that it is "a young man's job" and he may have trouble with physical demands in a few years. Is being considered for foreman position but not pursuing aggressively—"The job looks like too much trouble—I make enough money to support my family." Belongs to labor union "because it goes with the territory." Not active in union affairs.

SEXUALITY AND REPRODUCTION

Reports no problems with sexual relationship but states BP medication affected his sexual performance. No problems when not taking medication. Three sons. States that commitment, monogamy, and "obeying God" are important for sexual fulfillment.

COPING AND STRESS TOLERANCE

Feels greatest stressor is worrying about work—feels that health or age may unexpectedly threaten ability to work. Concerned about potential loss of income because "I don't have much money stored away even though I make good wages." Work-related pension considered helpful but not adequate to maintain current lifestyle. States he has done little to resolve this problem except "worry about it."

VALUES AND BELIEFS

Family and religion most important to him. Describes self as "born again Christian." Attends church regularly with family except during summer when camping. Family Bible studies conducted weekly. Believes that persons with dissimilar beliefs need to "be saved" but generally avoids people with different beliefs. Describes social and political views as conservative. Believes strongly in afterlife, which gives him a sense of peace and satisfaction.

Documentation Form for the Clinical Database

This is an actual form used by nurses and other health care providers at Presbyterian Medical Center in Philadelphia, PA. Data pertaining to status of Functional Health Patterns are recorded along with a medical history, medication history, diagnostic test results, and physical examination findings. This form also includes space for a screening tool to determine risk for skin integrity impairment. It is common practice for health care organizations to develop forms that are relevant to their patient population, organizational policies and procedures, and patient care philosophy. The interdisciplinary nature of this form supports the team approach to patient care.

NAME	DATE	TIME	AGE

CONTACT PERSON	PHONE #	GUARDIAN

INFORMATION OBTAINED FROM: ☐ PATIENT ☐ OTHER _____ ☐ FAMILY/SIGNIFICANT OTHER PARTICIPATED
RELIABILITY: ☐ GOOD ☐ POOR ☐ NON-COMMUNICATIVE

ADMITTED FROM: ☐ HOME ALONE ☐ HOME WITH RELATIVES ☐ HOME OF ANOTHER ☐ HOMELESS ☐ LONG TERM
CARE FACILITY ☐ BOARDING HOME ☐ ED ☐ HOSPITAL _____ ☐ OTHER _____

CODE STATUS: ☐ ADDRESSED ☐ FULL CODE
☐ NOT ADDRESSED REASON _____

PRIMARY CARE PHYSICIAN _____ **PHONE NO.** _____

CHIEF COMPLAINT (DURATION): _____
_____
_____
_____

HISTORY PRESENT ILLNESS: _____
_____
_____
_____
_____
_____
_____
_____
_____
_____
_____
_____

MEDICATION (ALSO OTC)	DOSAGE	LAST DOSE	PURPOSE	LEARNING NEEDS: Y ☐ N ☐

ALLERGIES (INCLUDE FOOD, DRUG, LATEX & OTHER)	REACTION	LEARNING NEEDS: Y ☐ N ☐

PHYSICIANS MUST COMPLETE SHADED AREAS ADDRESSOGRAPH

UNIVERSITY OF PENNSYLVANIA HEALTH SYSTEM
PRESBYTERIAN MEDICAL CENTER

MULTIDISCIPLINARY ADMISSION ASSESSMENT

722086 (1/97) PAGE 1

NAME: _____ MR# _____

PAST MEDICAL & SURGICAL HISTORY: (REVIEW OF PAST MEDICAL RECORDS IF APPROPRIATE) _____
_____
_____
_____
_____
_____
_____
_____
_____
_____
_____
_____

FAMILY HISTORY: _____
_____
_____
_____
_____
_____
_____

REVIEW OF SYSTEMS:
SKIN: _____
HEENT: _____
ENDOCRINE: _____
CARDIOVASCULAR: _____
RESPIRATORY: _____
GASTROINTESTINAL: _____
LYMPHATIC: _____
NEUROLOGIC: _____
MUSCULOSKELETAL: _____
PERIPHERAL VASCULAR: _____
HEMATOLOGIC: _____
URINARY TRACT: _____
REPRODUCTIVE/SEXUAL:
SEXUAL ACTIVITY: _____ VENEREAL DISEASE: _____

    FEMALE
    IS THERE ANY CHANCE YOU MIGHT BE PREGNANT? _____YES _____NO
    MENSTRUATION HISTORY: FDLMP: _____
    MENARCHE: _____ MENOPAUSE: _____
    PREGNANCIES: _____
    LAST PAP SMEAR: _____ RESULTS: _____
    LAST MAMMOGRAM: _____ RESULTS: _____
    MALE
    LAST PROSTATE EXAM: _____ RESULTS: _____
    PSA TEST: _____ RESULTS: _____
PSYCHIATRIC: _____
_____
_____

HIV RISK FACTORS: _____

SEXUALITY/REPRODUCTIVE PATTERN

	LEARNING NEEDS:
	Y N

MENSTRUAL PROBLEMS ☐ YES ☐ NO SPECIFY: _____   ☐ ☐
_____

BIRTH CONTROL ☐ YES ☐ NO TYPE _____ WOULD YOU LIKE INFORMATION: ☐ YES ☐ NO
MONTHLY SELF-BREAST/TESTICULAR EXAM ☐ YES ☐ NO
INFORMATION GIVEN: _____
SEXUAL CONCERNS RE ILLNESS ☐ YES ☐ NO SPECIFY: _____

PHYSICIANS MUST COMPLETE SHADED AREAS

PAGE 2

NAME: _____ MR # _____

☐ NOT APPLICABLE	☐ BCG _____, 19___	☐ HEPATITIS _____, 19___
☐ INFLUENZA _____, 19___	☐ TUBERCULIN _____, 19___	☐ TETANUS _____, 19___
☐ PNEUMOCOCCAL _____, 19___	☐ – ☐ + _____ MM INDURATION	☐ OTHER _____, 19___

PHYSICAL EXAMINATION

	DESCRIPTION
VITAL SIGNS:	
SKIN:	
HEENT:	
(OPHTH. EXAM):	
NECK: TRACHEA	
CAROTID BRUIT	
VEINS	
NODES	
THYROID	
OTHER	
CHEST:	
HEART: AUSCULTATION	
RHYTHM	
PMI	
ABDOMEN:	
MUSCULOSKELETAL/JOINTS:	
LYMPH NODES:	
NEUROLOGIC:	
MENTAL STATUS	
CRANIAL NERVES	
MOTOR	
SENSORY	
CEREBELLAR (GAIT)	
DTR'S	
OTHER	
EXTREMITIES:	

PERIPHERAL VASCULAR:	L	R	
RADIAL			
BRACHIAL			
FEMORAL			
POPLITEAL			
DORSALIS PEDIS			
POSTERIOR TIBIAL			

BREASTS:	
GENITALIA:	
RECTAL:	
PROSTATE	
HEME:	☐ NEG ☐ POS

NAME: _____ MR # _____

NUTRITIONAL/METABOLIC PATTERN

LEARNING NEEDS:
Y N
☐ ☐

HEIGHT: _____ WEIGHT: _____

MEALS/SNACKS #_____ /DAY SPECIAL DIET/SUPPLEMENT _____

COMPLIANCE ☐ PREVIOUS DIETARY INSTRUCTION _____

PROBLEM OBTAINING/PREPARING FOOD ☐ NO ☐ YES* EXPLAIN: _____

APPETITE: ☐ NORMAL ☐ INCREASED ☐ DECREASED ☐ DECREASED TASTE

☐ NAUSEA ☐ VOMITING > 3 DAYS* ☐ STOMATITIS ☐ MINIMAL PO INTAKE > 5 DAYS*

FLUID INTAKE: (8 OZ. GLASSES/DAY) REQUEST DIETARY TEACHING/VISIT ☐ YES ☐ NO

☐ RESTRICTED ☐ 0-5 GLASSES ☐ 5-10 GLASSES ☐ > 10 GLASSES

WEIGHT FLUCTUATIONS: ☐ NONE ☐ GAIN ☐ LOSS > 10 LBS LAST 3 MONTHS*

SWALLOWING DIFFICULTY: ☐ NONE ☐ SOLIDS* ☐ LIQUIDS* ☐ CHEWING DIFFICULTIES ☐ MEAT ☐ RAW FRUIT & VEGETABLES

DENTURES: ☐ NONE

☐ UPPER ☐ PARTIAL ☐ FULL WITH PATIENT? (Y or N)

☐ LOWER ☐ PARTIAL ☐ FULL WITH PATIENT? (Y or N)

SKIN/HEALING PROBLEMS: ☐ NONE ☐ LESION ☐ ABNORMAL HEALING ☐ RASH

*ITEMS REQUIRE CONSULT WITH NUTRITION SERVICE ☐ BRUISE EASILY ☐ DRYNESS ☐ EXCESSIVE PERSPIRATION ☐ PRURITUS

ELIMINATION PATTERN

LEARNING NEEDS:
Y N
☐ ☐

BLADDER ☐ NORMAL ☐ FREQUENCY ☐ URGENCY ☐ DYSURIA ☐ REQUEST ET VISIT
☐ RETENTION ☐ HEMATURIA ☐ INCONTINENT ☐ NOCTURIA ☐ YES ☐ NO

INCONTINENCE ☐ N/A ☐ TOTAL ☐ DAYTIME ☐ NIGHTTIME ☐ OCCASIONAL
☐ INABILITY TO PERCEIVE BLADDER CUES ☐ DIFFICULTY DELAYING VOIDING

GU ASSISTIVE DEVICES ☐ NONE ☐ INTERMITTENT CATHETERIZATION ☐ OSTOMY: TYPE _____
☐ INDWELLING CATHETER: DATE INSERTED _____ ☐ INCONTINENT BRIEFS ☐ EXTERNAL CATHETER
☐ PENILE IMPLANT: TYPE _____

BOWEL _____ # OF BMs/DAY _____ DATE LAST BM _____ LAXATIVES/ENEMAS?
☐ NORMAL ☐ CONSTIPATION ☐ DIARRHEA > 5 DAYS* ☐ INCONTINENT ☐ PATTERN CHANGE
☐ COLOSTOMY ☐ ILEOSTOMY APPLIANCE _____ SELF-CARE ☐ YES ☐ NO

ACTIVITY/EXERCISE PATTERN

LEARNING NEEDS:
Y N
☐ ☐

SELF-CARE ABILITY:	0	1	2	3	4	5
EATING/DRINKING						
BATHING						
DRESSING/GROOMING						
TOILETING						
BED MOBILITY						
TRANSFERRING						
AMBULATING						
STAIR CLIMBING						
SHOPPING						
COOKING						
HOME MAINTENANCE						

0 = INDEPENDENT
1 = ASSISTIVE DEVICE
2 = ASSISTANCE FROM PERSON
3 = ASSISTANCE FROM PERSON AND EQUIPMENT
4 = DEPENDENT/UNABLE
5 = CHANGE IN LAST WEEK

ASSISTIVE DEVICES ☐ NONE ☐ CANE ☐ WHEELCHAIR ☐ WALKER ☐ CRUTCHES
☐ SPLINT/BRACE ☐ TRAPEZE ☐ BEDSIDE COMMODE ☐ OTHER _____

ACTIVITY TOLERANCE ☐ NORMAL ☐ WEAKNESS ☐ VERTIGO ☐ UNSTEADY GAIT ☐ DYSPNEA ON EXERTION
☐ ANGINA ☐ DYSPNEA AT REST ☐ INTERMITTENT CLAUDICATION
☐ REST PAIN ☐ OXYGEN USE ☐ OTHER _____

SLEEP/REST PATTERN

HABITS ☐ NONE ☐ < 8 HRS/NIGHT ☐ 8 HRS ☐ > 8 HRS ☐ AM NAP ☐ PM NAP
PROBLEMS ☐ UNRESTED AFTER SLEEP ☐ EARLY WAKING ☐ INSOMNIA ☐ NIGHTMARES ☐ ORTHOPNEA

SUBSTANCE USE

TOBACCO: ☐ < PK/DAY ☐ 1-2 PKS/DAY ☐ > 2 PKS/DAY PK/YR HX _____
☐ PIPE ☐ CIGAR ☐ CHEW ☐ QUIT ☐ NONE

ALCOHOL: ☐ < 3 CANS BEER/DAY ☐ 3-6 CANS BEER/DAY ☐ > 6 CANS BEER/DAY ☐ WINE
☐ < 1 PT/DAY ☐ 1-2 PTS/DAY ☐ > 1 QT/DAY ☐ NONE

OTHER DRUGS ☐ YES ☐ NO ☐ WOULD YOU LIKE REHAB INFORMATION? ☐ YES ☐ NO
TYPE/FREQUENCY _____ DATE LAST DRINK/DRUG _____

PHYSICIANS MUST COMPLETE SHADED AREAS

NAME: _____ MR # _____

COGNITIVE/PERCEPTUAL PATTERN

| | | | | LEARNING NEEDS: Y ☐ N ☐ |

MENTAL STATUS
- ☐ ALERT   ☐ UNRESPONSIVE   ☐ RESTLESS   ☐ ORIENTED
- ☐ RECEPTIVE APHASIA   ☐ COMBATIVE   ☐ LETHARGIC   X _____
- ☐ CONFUSED: ☐ INTERMITTENT   ☐ NIGHTTIME   ☐ TOTAL

HEARING
- ☐ NORMAL   ☐ IMPAIRED: ☐ LEFT   ☐ RIGHT   ☐ HEARING AID
- ☐ TINNITUS   ☐ DEAF: ☐ LEFT   ☐ RIGHT

VISION
- ☐ NORMAL   ☐ EYE GLASSES   ☐ CONTACT LENSES   ☐ PROSTHESIS
- ☐ IMPAIRED: ☐ LEFT   ☐ RIGHT   ☐ BLIND: ☐ LEFT   ☐ RIGHT
- ☐ CATARACT: ☐ LEFT   ☐ RIGHT   ☐ GLAUCOMA

SPEECH
- ☐ NORMAL   ☐ SLURRED   ☐ GARBLED   ☐ EXPRESSIVE APHASIA
- ☐ LANGUAGE/BARRIER: ☐ SPOKEN LANGUAGE _____   ☐ INTERPRETER

DISCOMFORT/PAIN   ☐ NONE   ☐ ACUTE   ☐ CHRONIC

DESCRIPTION (USE PAIN SCALE ALSO) _____
_____

PAIN MANAGEMENT _____

COPING/STRESS TOLERANCE

LEARNING NEEDS: Y ☐ N ☐

MAJOR CONCERNS REGARDING HOSPITALIZATION/ILLNESS

SPECIFY: _____

COPING STRATEGIES: ☐ TALKING TO OTHERS   ☐ DRUGS/ALCOHOL/TOBACCO (CIRCLE)   ☐ PHYSICAL ACTIVITY
☐ AVOIDANCE   ☐ OTHER: _____   ☐ BEING ALONE

COPING ABILITIES ARE EFFECTIVE AGAINST CURRENT STRESSORS: ☐ YES   ☐ NO

LIFE CHANGES: ☐ NONE   ☐ CHANGE IN RELATIONSHIP   ☐ CHANGE WITH JOB   ☐ FINANCIAL
☐ DEATH OF PARTNER   ☐ BIRTH OF A CHILD   ☐ MOVE   ☐ O THER: _____

CONSULT: ☐ SOCIAL WORK DATE _____   ☐ PSYCH CNS DATE _____
☐ PASTORAL CARE DATE _____

IF YOU SUSPECT AN INDIVIDUAL MAY HAVE BEEN ABUSED, ASK THE FOLLOWING QUESTIONS: VIOLENCE/ABUSE IS AN INCREASING PROBLEM IN OUR SOCIETY. HAVE YOU EVER BEEN A VICTIM OF VIOLENCE OR ABUSE?   ☐ YES   ☐ NO   IF YES: WOULD YOU LIKE TO HAVE INFORMATION ABOUT AGENCIES OR INDIVIDUALS THAT COULD ASSIST YOU?   ☐ YES   ☐ NO   SOCIAL WORK CONSULTED DATE: _____

VALUE/BELIEF PATTERN

LEARNING NEEDS: Y ☐ N ☐

ARE THERE ANY RELIGIOUS OR CULTURAL PRACTICES THAT MAY BE AFFECTED BY THIS HOSPITALIZATION:
(DIETARY RESTRICTIONS, BLOOD TRANSFUSIONS, ETC.)   ☐ YES   ☐ NO   SPECIFY: _____
_____

REQUEST CHAPLAIN VISIT AT THIS TIME   ☐ YES   ☐ NO
RELIGIOUS AFFILIATION: ☐ NONE ☐ CATHOLIC ☐ JEWISH ☐ PROTESTANT ☐ ISLAMIC ☐ JEHOVAH WITNESS ☐ OTHER
SPECIFY DENOMINATION: _____
ORGAN DONATION INFORMATION: ARE YOU AN ORGAN DONOR: ☐ YES ☐ NO   WOULD YOU LIKE INFORMATION: ☐ YES ☐ NO

ADVANCE DIRECTIVES:
HAVE YOU EVER RECEIVED INFORMATION ABOUT ADVANCE DIRECTIVES: ☐ YES   ☐ NO
IF NO, PEASE PROVIDE INFORMATION.   DATE _____
DO YOU ALREADY HAVE A LIVING WILL/ADVANCE DIRECTIVE AND/OR DURABLE POWER OF ATTORNEY FOR HEALTH CARE? ☐ YES ☐ NO
IF YES, COPY OF PATIENT DOCUMENT ATTACHED TO CHART. ☐ YES ☐ NO
NAME OF PERSON WITH DURABLE POWER OF ATTORNEY: _____
REFERRAL MADE TO REQUESTED PARTY: _____   DATE: _____

ROLE/RELATIONSHIP PATTERN

OCCUPATIONAL HISTORY: _____

EMPLOYMENT STATUS
- ☐ EMPLOYED   ☐ UNEMPLOYED   ☐ SHORT TERM DISABILITY
- ☐ LONG TERM DISABILITY   ☐ RETIRED   ☐ NONE

SUPPORT SYSTEM
- ☐ SPOUSE/SIGNIFICANT OTHER   ☐ NEIGHBORS/FRIENDS   ☐ FAMILY NOT PRESENT
- ☐ FAMILY IN SAME RESIDENCE   ☐ FAMILY IN SEPARATE RESIDENCE
- ☐ NONE   ☐ OTHER _____

UTILIZATION OF COMMUNITY RESOURCES: ☐ HOME CARE/HOSPICE ☐ MEALS ON WHEELS ☐ ADULT DAY CARE ☐ HOMEMAKER AIDE
☐ OTHER _____   ☐ NONE ☐ CHURCH GROUP   ☐ COMMUNITY GROUP
TRANSPORTATION ARRANGEMENTS FOR DISCHARGE:
FAMILY CONCERNS - HOSPITALIZATION ☐ YES ☐ NO SPECIFY: _____
_____
_____

NAME: _____ MR # _____

INTEGUMENTARY ASSESSMENT

☐ INTACT ☐ CONTRACTURES
☐ WOUND CARE CONSULT ≥ STAGE III
☐ NUTRITION CONSULT ≥ STAGE III

INDICATE STAGE & LOCATION OF:

LESIONS, ULCERS, SCARS, RASHES,
INCISIONS ON BODY CHARTS

AMPUTATION(S): _____
LOCATION: _____
_____
_____

WOUND STAGE

STAGE I - REDDENED INTACT SKIN
STAGE II - EPIDERMIS IS REMOVED, BLISTER
STAGE III - SUBCUTANEOUS TISSUE IS VISIBLE
STAGE IV - MUSCLE & BONE ARE VISIBLE

LOCATIONS/STAGE	SIZE (cm) L	W	D	ODOR +/-	DRAINAGE COLOR	AMOUNT	TUNNELS +/-	UNDER-MINING +/-

SKIN INTEGRITY RISK ASSESSMENT SCALE

CLINICAL SUBSCALES	SCORE	CLINICAL SUBSCALES	SCORE
SENSORY PERCEPTION: LEVEL OF CONSCIOUSNESS		**MOBILITY***	
ALERT AND CLEAR, RESPONDS READILY	4	FULL ACTIVE RANGE, INDEPENDENTLY	4
LETHARGIC; CONFUSED; SLOW TO RESPOND; ALERT BUT NOT VERBAL	3	RESTRICTED MOVEMENT (LIMITED ASSISTANCE)	3
SEMI-COMATOSE; RESPONDS ONLY TO VERBAL OR PAINFUL STIMULI	2	MOVES ONLY WITH ASSISTANCE	2
COMATOSE; NO RESPONSE TO STIMULI	1	IMMOBILE/CONTRACTED**	1
		*A SCORE OF 3 OR LESS, REQUEST MD TO ORDER PT EVALUATION. EXCEPTION:	
		**ONLY IF NEW ONSET	
MOISTURE (INCONTINENCE, DRAINAGE, SKIN FOLDS...)		**NUTRITIONAL STATUS***	
NONE, SKIN CLEAR AND DRY	4	NEVER REFUSES A MEAL; NEGATIVE WGT. LOSS OR GAIN	4
ADDITIONAL SHEET OR GOWN CHANGE EVERY 24 HOURS	3	RECENT APPETITE CHANGES; GREATER OR LESS THAN 20% UBW*	3
ADDITIONAL SHEET OR GOWN CHANGE EVERY SHIFT	2	WEIGHT LOSS ≥ 10 LBS IN PAST 3 MONTHS; ALBUMIN 3.0 OR LESS; PERSISTENT NAUSEA, VOMITING, OR DIARRHEA; TPN/PPN; RECEIVING TUBE FEEDING**	2
SKIN MOIST ALMOST CONSTANTLY	1	NPO OR ON CLEAR LIQUID DIET > 3 DAYS	1
		*USUAL BODY WEIGHT.	
		**A SCORE OF 2 OR LESS, CONSULT DIETICIAN. ☐ CONSULT PLACED DATE____	
PHYSICAL ACTIVITY*		**FRICTION & SHEAR/GENERAL SKIN CONDITION**	
AMBULATES WITHOUT ASSISTANCE	4	NO PROBLEM, CLEAN AND DRY	3
AMBULATES WITH ASSISTANCE (OF PERSON OR DEVICE)	3	POTENTIAL PROBLEM; POOR TURGOR AREAS RED; RECEIVING TUBE FEED WITH HEAD OF BED ELEVATED	2
CHAIRFAST*	2	PROBLEM; EXISTING LESION(S), FREQUENTLY SLIDES DOWN IN BED OR CHAIR	1
BEDFAST*	1		
*A SCORE OF 3 OR LESS, REQUEST MD TO ORDER PT EVALUATION IF THIS IS A NEW ONSET OR RECENT CHANGE.			

PATIENTS WITH A TOTAL SCORE OF 16 OR LESS ARE CONSIDERED TO BE AT HIGH RISK FOR ALTERATION IN SKIN INTEGRITY,   TOTAL _____

SUMMATION QUESTIONS

IF YES RESPONSE:

1. IS PATIENT AT HIGH RISK FOR INFECTION AND/OR TRANSMISSION?	☐ YES	☐ NO	☐ INITIATED PRACTICE GUIDELINES - INFECTION	
2. IS PATIENT AT HIGH RISK OF FALLING OR OF INJURY?	☐ YES	☐ NO	☐ INITIATED PRACTICE GUIDELINES - SAFETY	
3. IS PATIENT AT RISK FOR THE DEVELOPMENT OF PRESSURE ULCERS?	☐ YES	☐ NO	☐ INITIATED PRACTICE GUIDELINES- SKIN INTEGRITY	
4. POTENTIAL FOR SELF-CARE DEFICIT AT DISCHARGE?	☐ YES	☐ NO	☐ CONSULTED: ☐ SOCIAL WORK ☐ HOME CARE	
5. IS THE PATIENT A SUSPECTED VICTIM OF ABUSE?	☐ YES	☐ NO	☐ SOCIAL WORK CONSULTED	
6. LEARNING NEEDS IDENTIFIED?	☐ YES	☐ NO	☐ PATIENT TEACHING FLOWSHEET, PIE NOTE, CRITICAL PATH (CIRCLE ALL THAT APPLY)	

■ ORIENTED TO UNIT   ■ ID BAND IN PLACE

NAME: _____ MR # _____

INITIAL DIAGNOSTIC DATA BASE (LABS, ECG, X-RAYS, ETC.):

CSC:	LAB SCAN:		ABG:	ECG:

CSC:
WBC
  MYELO _____
  BAND _____
  SEG _____
  LYMPH _____
  MONO _____
  EOS _____
  BASO _____
  SED RATE _____
  _____
HGB _____
HCT _____
MCV _____
MCH _____
MCHC _____
PLT _____
_____

COAGULATION:
PT _____
PTT _____
INR _____
_____

LAB SCAN:
  BUN _____
  NA _____
  K _____
  CL _____
  CO2 _____
  GLU _____
  CRE _____
  AN GAP _____
  ALT _____
  AST _____
  ALK PHOS _____
  T. BILI _____
  D. BILI _____
  LDH _____
  GTT _____
  AMYLASE _____
  LIPASE _____
  CALCIUM _____
  MAG _____
  PHOS _____
  URIC ACID _____
  ALBUMIN _____

CHOL _____
TRIGLY _____
HDL _____
LDL _____
_____
T4 _____
TSH _____

URINALYSIS:
  GLU _____
  OC BLD _____
  PROTEIN _____
  NIT _____
  BILI _____
  SP GR _____
  pH _____
  LEU _____
  WBC _____
  RBC _____
  SO EPI _____
  BACT _____
  _____

ABG:
  pH _____
  PaO2 _____
  PaCO2 _____
  HCO3 _____
  SaO2 _____
  THERAPY _____
SaO2 _____
THERAPY _____

X-RAYS: _____
_____
_____
_____
_____
_____
_____
_____

BACTERIOLOGY/SEROLOGY: _____
_____
_____

ECG:
_____
_____
_____
_____
_____
_____
_____
_____

SUMMARY: _____
_____
_____
_____
_____
_____
_____
_____

ADMITTING DIAGNOSIS: _____
_____
_____
_____
_____

TREATMENT PLAN: _____
_____
_____
_____
_____
_____
_____
_____
_____
_____

_____ MD/DO

_____	_____	_____
DATE	TIME	PRINT NAME

_____	_____
PAGER	MD/DO SIGNATURE

_____ RN/LPN

_____	_____	_____
DATE	TIME	NURSES SIGNATURE

_____ RN/LPN

_____	_____	_____
DATE	TIME	NURSES SIGNATURE

PHYSICIANS MUST COMPLETE SHADED AREAS

Health History

The health history is one of the main components of a clinical database. The following may be included in a health history:

- Basic demographic data
- Reason for seeking health care
- Medical history
- Medication and substance use history
- Health status information

Data Collection

Data for the health history may be obtained from primary or secondary sources. The health assessment interview is conducted to obtain primary source data.

Purpose of the Health Assessment Interview

The purpose of the health assessment interview is to obtain information about the individual, their health perceptions, functional status, and other factors relevant to health, healing, and illness.

The Interview Process

The interview process has three phases: introduction, working, and summary. Certain tasks and objectives characterize each phase.

Therapeutic Communication

Therapeutic communication is purposeful, goal-directed, and always focused on the person being interviewed. The nurse's knowledge of effective communication techniques as well as communication patterns to avoid can be applied to the conduct of the health assessment interview.

Interview Challenges

The most commonly encountered interview challenges are likely to occur with cultural variations, children, elders, cognitive limitations, anger, anxiety, depression, manipulation, seductive behavior, discussions about sexuality, and discussions about terminal illness.

Assessment Guidelines

Guidelines that are useful in the development of a health history include the following:

- The Initial Health Assessment Interview
- The Medical History (Past Health History and Review of Systems)
- The Medication and Substance Use History

Documentation

Two approaches may be used to document the health history:

- Narrative style documentation
- Standardized form completion

 Critical Thinking

You are admitting a 45-year-old female with metastatic breast cancer to the medicine service of a general acute care hospital. She has developed pneumonia. She is oriented but depressed and experiencing a great deal of pain.

1. Explain how you would initiate the interview with this person. Create a script of the first few sentences you might say.

2. Identify and describe an approach that could block therapeutic communication in this situation. Explain what is wrong with this approach.

3. If you could ask this person only three questions, decide what they would be and specify how you would ask them. Create a script for each question.

4. The patient states that she does not want to participate in the admission interview. How would you respond?

5. The patient starts to cry when you ask her how she has been managing at home. How would you respond?

BIBLIOGRAPHY

Bernstein, L., & Bernstein, R.S. (1985). *Interviewing: A guide for health professionals* (4th ed.). Norwalk, CT: Appleton-Century-Crofts.

Braverman, B.G. (1990). Eliciting data from the patient who is difficult to interview. *Nursing Clinics of North America, 25* (4), 743–750.

Dirckx, J.H. (1985). Talking with patients: The art of history taking. *Clinical Nurse Practitioner, 3,* 13–14.

Giger, J., & Davidhizar, R. (1995). *Transcultural nursing*. St. Louis: Mosby-Year Book, Inc.

Gordon, M. (1987). *Nursing diagnosis: Process and application* (2nd ed.). New York: McGraw-Hill.

Helms, J. (1985) Active listening. In G.M. Bulechek & J.C. McCloskey (Eds.). *Nursing interventions: Treatments for nursing diagnoses*. Philadelphia: W.B. Saunders.

Kasch, C. (1986). Toward a theory of nursing action: Skills and competency in nurse-patient interactions. *Nursing Research, 35* (4), 226–230.

Lee, M. (1996). Drugs and the elderly: Do you know the risks? *American Journal of Nursing, 96* (7), 25–31.

Leininger, M. (Ed.) (1988). *Transcultural nursing: Concepts, theories, and practice* (2nd ed.). New York: John Wiley & Sons.

Robinson, C.A. (1996). Health care relationships revisited. *Journal of Family Nursing, 2,* 152–173.

Santora, A. (1986). Communicating better with the elderly: How to break down barriers. *Nursing Life, 6* (4), 24–27.

Seversten, B.M. (1990). Therapeutic communication demystified. *Journal of Nursing Education, 29* (4), 190–192.

Smith, S. (1992). *Communication in nursing* (2nd ed.). St. Louis: Mosby-Year Book, Inc.

Travelbee, J. (1971). *Interpersonal aspects of nursing*. Philadelphia: F.A. Davis.

Whall, A. (1988). Therapeutic use of self. *Journal of Gerontological Nursing, 14* (2), 38–39, 46–47.

Williams, G.D. (1997). Preoperative assessment and health history interview. *Nursing Clinics of North America, 32* (2), 395–416.

Wong, D.L. (1995). *Whaley & Wong's essentials of pediatric nursing* (3rd ed.). St. Louis: C.V. Mosby.

The Physical Examination

ASSESSMENT GUIDELINES

- The Complete Physical Examination
- The General Survey

CHAPTER ORGANIZATION

Introductory Overview

Knowledge Base for Assessment
- Purpose of the Physical Examination
- Frameworks for the Interpretation of the Physical Examination

- Physical Examination Techniques
- Physical Examination Equipment and Instruments

Documentation: The Physical Examination

INTRODUCTORY OVERVIEW

In previous chapters, the primary data collection methods used by the nurse to conduct a health assessment of individuals were identified as the following:

Data Collection Methods for Health Assessment

- Assessment Interview
- Physical Examination
- Review of Records

In Chapter 2, you learned that the data obtained by interviewing and reviewing records is usually compiled into the component of the clinical database known as the health history. The other component of the clinical database consists of a record of the physical examination conducted by the clinician. The techniques and concepts presented in this chapter provide the foundation for conducting a comprehensive physical examination.

A *physical examination* is the observation of an individual in which the nurse uses the senses of sight, hearing, touch, and smell and the observation techniques of inspection, palpation, percussion, and auscultation. The nurse's perceptions during the physical examination are interpreted in light of the nurse's knowledge of normal and abnormal anatomy and physiology, nursing diagnoses, and clinical problems. The physical examination usually takes place after you have interviewed the person.

Before you conduct the physical examination, you should understand various frameworks for the conduct of the examination as well as how to interpret physical examination findings for relevance to a particular functional health pattern or body system. In addition, you should develop the basic technical skills that will serve as your tools for collecting data. The required technical skills include inspection, palpation, percussion, and auscultation and the correct use of examining instruments such as the stethoscope and ophthalmoscope.

The physical examination is conducted in a manner that will logically and systematically coordinate all the separate steps. Most clinicians will use a similar approach to conduct a physical examination. The two most common approaches for the conduct of the physical examination are the following:

Two Approaches to Physical Examination

- Head-to-Toe
- Body Systems

Although different clinicians use similar techniques and methods for conducting the physical examination, there may be different reasons for collecting data, and the data may be interpreted differently depending on your goals. Different clinical disciplines, for example, nursing or medicine, will have different ways to organize or interpret physical examination findings that may be obtained through a common process. In this book, functional health patterns serve as the organizational framework for interpreting physical findings to emphasize how your findings can serve as indicators of functional status and health problems managed by nurses. The detailed steps required to examine a particular area or system of the body are presented in Unit II. Physical examination is presented as a method of evaluating the various functional health patterns.

KNOWLEDGE BASE FOR ASSESSMENT

Basic knowledge and skills are required to successfully conduct the physical examination. The nurse's knowledge base should include an understanding of the purpose of the physical examination, the frameworks that may be used to choreograph the sequence of the physical examination and interpret findings, and the basic techniques, instruments, and equipment that are used to collect data during the physical examination.

Purpose of the Physical Examination

The observations you make by conducting a physical examination serve a number of purposes. First, thorough examination of body parts and systems provides an indication of the person's overall health status, including information about growth and development. Second, an examination can provide additional information about the clinical significance of any symptoms that were reported by the person during the interview. And, finally, physical status can provide an indication of how an individual is responding to various aspects of their health care, including responses to medication use or a person's response to special procedures.

The data and information obtained by conducting a physical examination, along with the information from the health history, provides the foundation for clinical judgment and diagnostic reasoning. A number of indicators for various nursing diagnoses and clinical problems can be identified and validated during the physical examination.

The Examination Sequence: Head-to-Toe Approach

Perhaps the most widely used sequence of conducting a comprehensive physical examination is the head-to-toe approach, in which the practitioner systematically examines every part of the body, beginning at the head and progressing down the body to the toes (Display 3-1). A detailed head-to-toe examination sequence for an adult, ambulatory person is outlined in the Guideline presented elsewhere in this chapter. This sequence can and should be modified according to the examiner's preferences, the setting, or because of the health status or age of the person you are examining.

Some practitioners prefer to use a body systems approach to organize and sequence the physical examination. The body systems approach focuses on examining each of the body systems, one at a time, including the neurologic, cardiovascular, respiratory, gastrointestinal, genitourinary, musculoskeletal, and integumentary systems. This approach is used most frequently when the purpose of the examination is to determine the function of a particular system. For example, for a person who has had acute myocardial infarction, the nurse may choose to examine the cardiovascular system to make judg-

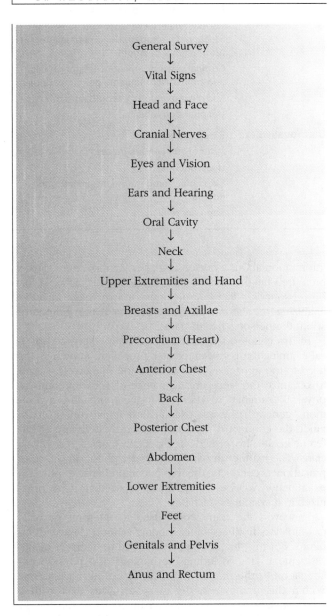

Head-to-Toe Examination Sequence for an Ambulatory Adult

General Survey
↓
Vital Signs
↓
Head and Face
↓
Cranial Nerves
↓
Eyes and Vision
↓
Ears and Hearing
↓
Oral Cavity
↓
Neck
↓
Upper Extremities and Hand
↓
Breasts and Axillae
↓
Precordium (Heart)
↓
Anterior Chest
↓
Back
↓
Posterior Chest
↓
Abdomen
↓
Lower Extremities
↓
Feet
↓
Genitals and Pelvis
↓
Anus and Rectum

ments about cardiovascular function. Physical examination components for four major body systems are shown in Table 3-1.

Frameworks for the Interpretation of the Physical Examination

As you learned in Chapter 1, there is a difference between data collection and the interpretation of data. Whereas data collection is the process of obtaining uninterpreted

TABLE 3.1 Body Systems Examination Focus for Four Major Body Systems

Body System	Examination Focus	Body System	Examination Focus
Neurologic	Mental status	**Respiratory**	Airway
	Cranial nerves		Breathing pattern
	Proprioception and cerebellar function		Chest—thoracic configuration, breath sounds, percussion tones, thoracic expansion, fremitus
	Peripheral nerve sensory functions (light touch, pain, temperature and pressure, vibration, joint position)		Skin color
	Cortical sensory functions (stereognosis, two-point discrimination; point location)	**Renal**	Skin—pigmentation, edema, uremic frost
	Muscle movement, strength, and tone		Abdomen—kidneys
	Deep tendon reflexes		Genitalia
Cardiovascular	Blood pressure		Rectum
	Arterial and venous pulses		Pelvic structures (females) or prostate (males)
	Heart sounds		
	Skin color, temperature, moisture, and edema		
	Capillary refill		

information about a person (*e.g.,* body temperature, blood pressure, height and weight, lung sounds, skin color, bowel sounds), data interpretation or assessment includes analyzing the information and data to make judgments about the person's health status.

In this chapter, the conduct of a comprehensive physical examination is presented as a procedure known as the head-to-toe approach. The head-to-toe framework serves to organize the steps and sequence of a comprehensive physical examination. The head-to-toe approach is a common "generic" physical examination framework used to guide the conduct of the examination by a variety of different healthcare providers, especially nurses and physicians. The manner in which a nurse, a physician, or other practitioner conducts the basic comprehensive physical examination will be a very similar proceeding in an organized and systematic fashion.

However, the frameworks used to interpret physical examination findings differ among various clinical disciplines. For this text, the approach used to interpret health assessment data, including the findings of a physical examination, is the framework of functional health patterns. Within this framework, the nurse analyzes data with a focus on how well an individual functions within the 11 functional health patterns: health perception and health management; nutrition and metabolism; elimination activity and exercise; cognition and perception; sleep and rest; self-concept; roles and relationships; sexuality and reproduction; coping and stress; and values and beliefs. This approach was chosen because it is pertinent to how nurses today must integrate and use the data they collect to focus on nursing diagnoses, level of health and wellness, individual strengths, and physiologic alterations as manifestations of human functioning. Nurses should conceptually organize data to arrive at nursing diagnoses, just as physicians organize data to arrive at medical diagnoses.

There are other frameworks for interpreting physical examination findings, including the medical model, with its focus on body systems findings that may indicate medical problems. Physicians traditionally analyze physical examination findings according to body systems, including the neurologic, cardiovascular, respiratory, gastrointestinal, genitourinary, endocrine, musculoskeletal, and integumentary systems. Nurses also may use this framework, especially when the nurse is assessing an ill or injured patient to evaluate the individual's response to medical intervention.

Functional health patterns can be easily and comfortably used as the framework for interpreting physical examination findings. Information presented in the context of body systems also has relevance to functional status. Tables 3-2, 3-3, and 3-4 show relationships among the various frameworks—head-to-toe physical examination, body systems, and functional health patterns.

Physical Examination Techniques

The four basic techniques of physical examination are *inspection, palpation, percussion,* and *auscultation,* together referred to as *observation.* These techniques enable you to collect data systematically using the senses of sight, touch, hearing, and smell. Physical appearance, behavior, communication patterns, and activity abilities can all be observed, as can a person's environment and events that effect him or her. Observing facial expression for signs of discomfort, detecting odors that indicate infection, listening to chest sounds to determine airway patency, and touching the skin to determine body temperature are all examples of observation.

Inspection

Inspection is the systematic and deliberate observation of the person using the senses of vision, smell, and hearing

TABLE 3.2   Correlating Data Associated with Functional Health Areas with Body Systems

The following table lists the functional health areas and the corresponding body systems that are assessed to elicit data about the patient's functional status.

Functional Health Area	Body Systems
Health perception and health management	Examination of all body systems is pertinent. Inferences about a person's health management practices can be derived from assessment of all body systems.
Nutrition and metabolism	*Integumentary system:* Alterations in appearance of the skin, hair, and nails may indicate actual or potential alterations in nutrition.
	Gastrointestinal system: Physical or functional alterations of the oral cavity may interfere with the ingestion of nutrients or indicate nutritional problems; physical or functional alterations of the gastrointestinal tract may interfere with the ingestion of nutrients or indicate nutritional problems.
	Endocrine system: Thyroid gland alterations and disruption of hypothalamic temperature regulation may alter basal metabolism.
Elimination	*Gastrointestinal system:* Alterations in the lower gastrointestinal tract (anus and rectum) may contribute to problems with elimination.
	Neurologic system: Neurologic alterations may disrupt neural control of bowel or bladder elimination.
	Musculoskeletal system: Musculoskeletal alterations may interfere with bowel or bladder control.
	Reproductive and genitourinary system: Alterations in pelvic or genitourinary structures may interfere with bladder elimination or control.
	Integumentary system: Skin integrity may be threatened with bowel or bladder incontinence.
Activity and exercise	*Cardiovascular system:* The cardiovascular system assists with meeting oxygen requirements during activity and exercise.
	Pulmonary system: The pulmonary system assists with meeting oxygen requirements during activity and exercise.
	Musculoskeletal system: Alterations in the musculoskeletal system influence mobility and exercise.
	Neurologic system: Neurologic alterations may interfere with activity and exercise.
Cognition and perception	*Neurologic system:* Neurologic alterations may influence cognitive and perceptual functions.
	Sensory system: An intact and functioning sensory system, including the special senses and deep senses, is essential for perception.
Sleep and rest	Examination of all body systems is pertinent. Sleep disorders may be secondary to alterations in many body systems. Conversely, sleep disorders can result in body system alterations.
Self-concept	Body system alterations are evaluated to determine whether they are related to threats to personal identity or body image.
Roles and relationships	Body systems usually are not evaluated to provide data about roles and relationships. Body system alterations that result in changes in lifestyle or daily activities, however, can threaten or disrupt usual roles and relationships.
Sexuality and reproduction	*Reproductive system:* Alterations in the development and physical status of reproductive structures (breasts, internal and external genitals) may contribute to altered patterns of sexuality or reproductive problems.
	Genitourinary systems: Alterations in genitourinary structures may contribute to sexual dysfunction or reproductive problems.
Coping and stress tolerance	The physiologic effects of stress may be apparent by examining various body systems, especially the cardiovascular, respiratory, gastrointestinal, and integumentary systems. Alterations in the endocrine system may be associated with an altered response to stress.
Values and beliefs	Body systems usually are not evaluated to provide data about values and beliefs. Health beliefs can influence the way a person perceives body system functions, however.

TABLE 3.3   Correlating Data Associated with Functional Health Areas with a Head-to-Toe Physical Examination

The following table shows how data collected by functional health areas interrelate with a head-to-toe physical examination.

Head-to-Toe Physical Examination	Functional Health Area
General survey	General visual observation of a person may provide information about the level of functioning within each of the 11 functional health areas. Additionally, each component of the general survey may provide data specifically relevant to a particular pattern problem. *Health perception and health management:* The patient's general state of health and any obvious signs of distress will provide clues to his or her health perception and health management practices. *Nutrition and metabolism:* Survey height, weight, and general appearance as clues to nutritional status. Note the appearance of the skin, which may be altered with severe nutritional–metabolic problems. *Elimination:* Be alert for odors that may be associated with dysfunctional elimination patterns. Note impaired mobility or cognitive function that may contribute to elimination problems. *Activity and exercise:* Note any signs of distress related to activity and exercise. Observe the patient's posture, motor ability, and any physical deformities. *Cognition and perception:* Survey mental status, level of awareness, and the ability to communicate, which provide data about cognition and perception. *Sleep and rest:* Note facial expressions, affect, and behaviors that may be associated with sleep deprivation. *Self-concept and coping and stress tolerance:* Body language and behavior may provide clues to patient's self-concept and level of anxiety.
Anthropometric measurements	*Health perception and health management:* Body composition may reflect health management practices in relation to nutrition and exercise. *Nutrition and metabolism:* Anthropometric measurements are used to evaluate nutritional status and provide information about body tissues (viscera, skeletal muscle, and subcutaneous fat stores), which are altered during starvation or obesity.
Vital signs	*Health perception and health management:* Note whether the patient participates in blood pressure screening, a health management practice. *Nutrition and metabolism:* Alterations in the basal metabolic rate may be related to body temperature changes. *Activity and exercise:* Alterations in vital signs may suggest activity intolerance.
Hair, scalp, and cranium	*Nutrition and metabolism:* The appearance of the hair may be altered with severe nutritional–metabolic patterns.
Eyes, and vision	*Cognition and perception:* Alterations in the eyes and visual acuity may interfere with visual sensation, perception, and cognition.
Ears and hearing	*Cognition and perception:* Alterations in the ears and hearing acuity may interfere with hearing sensation, perception, and cognitive functions.
Oral cavity	*Nutrition and metabolism:* Physical or functional alterations in the oral cavity may interfere with ingestion; alterations in the oral mucosa may be indicators of nutritional–metabolic patterns.
Cranial nerves	*Cognition and perception:* Intact cranial nerve function is essential for a number of sensory–perceptual functions, including eyesight, hearing, smell, touch, and taste.
Thyroid gland	*Nutrition and metabolism:* Thyroid alterations may affect basal metabolism.
Neck veins	*Activity and exercise:* The appearance of the neck veins may provide data about the cardiovascular system, whose function is essential for meeting oxygen requirements during activity.
Upper extremities	*Activity and exercise:* Observe the mobility of upper extremities and evaluate pulses to judge cardiovascular status.
Nails	*Nutrition and metabolism:* The appearance of the nails may be altered with severe nutritional–metabolic problems.
Breasts	*Health perception and health management:* Note whether the patient practices breast self-examination, a health screening practice.
Precordium and anterior thorax	*Activity and exercise:* The precordial examination provides data about the cardiovascular system; the anterior thorax examination provides data about the pulmonary system. Both systems are essential for meeting oxygen requirements during activity.
Posterior thorax	*Activity and exercise:* The posterior thorax examination provides data about the pulmonary system.

(continued)

TABLE 3.3   Correlating Data Associated with Functional Health Areas with a Head-to-Toe Physical Examination (continued)

Head-to-Toe Physical Examination	Functional Health Area
Abdomen	*Nutrition and metabolism:* Physical or functional alterations in abdominal organs may interfere with digestion, absorption, or metabolism. The appearance of the abdomen may be altered by nutritional problems. *Elimination:* Some abdominal examination alterations indicate elimination problems such as abdominal and bladder distention or bowel sound alterations.
Lower extremities	*Activity and exercise:* Examination of the lower extremities may indicate the status of tissue oxygenation and level of motor function. Evaluate lower extremity pulses to judge cardiovascular status.
Genitals and pelvis	*Health perception and health management:* Note whether the patient participates in testicular self-examination, a health screening practice. Note whether the patient has routine pelvic examinations and Pap smears, health management screening examinations. *Elimination:* Pelvic structure alterations may contribute to problems with elimination.
Anus and rectum	*Health perception and health management:* The digital rectal examination is a health management screening practice for the detection of colorectal cancer. *Elimination:* Anal–rectal alterations may contribute to problems with elimination.

to determine any normal or abnormal findings. Some parts of the body can only be effectively inspected by using special instruments. For example, an otoscope is required to inspect the ear; an ophthalmoscope is used to inspect parts of the eye; and a speculum is used to inspect the vagina. You should observe the following characteristics as you inspect: color, size, location, symmetry, movement, behavior, odors, and sounds.

The physical examination always begins with inspection—first, of the individual as a whole, and then proceeding to the careful inspection of each body area or body system as you conduct the head-to-toe examination.

The initial inspection of the individual as a whole is referred to as *the general survey.* Specific observations to consider in the conduct of the general survey are presented in an assessment guideline elsewhere in this chapter. Specific observations that should be made of body areas or systems are presented in the corresponding assessment guidelines presented throughout Unit II chapters.

Inspection always precedes the other basic techniques of physical examination. The usual sequence of examination of a particular body area occurs in the following order: inspection, palpation, percussion, and auscultation.

TABLE 3.4   Correlating a Body Systems Physical Examination with Functional Health Areas

Each body system can be affected by many areas of functional health. The following table lists the body systems along with the most important functional health areas that are assessed to elicit data about that body system.

Body System	Functional Health Areas	Body System	Functional Health Areas
Cardiovascular system	Activity and exercise Coping and stress tolerance	Musculoskeletal system	Elimination Activity and exercise
Endocrine system	Nutrition and metabolism Coping and stress tolerance	Neurologic system	Sleep and rest Elimination
Gastrointestinal system	Nutrition and metabolism Elimination Coping and stress tolerance	Pulmonary system	Activity and exercise Cognition and perception Sleep and rest
Genitourinary system	Elimination Sexuality and reproduction Coping and stress tolerance Sleep and rest	Reproductive system	Activity and exercise Sleep and rest Coping and stress tolerance Elimination
Integumentary system	Nutrition and metabolism Elimination Coping and stress tolerance	Sensory system	Sexuality and reproduction Cognition and perception

Inspection Guidelines

Focus on observation. Inspection can be a powerful data collection tool, provided you take your time and train yourself to concentrate and observe. You may feel awkward about "staring" at the person without "doing something," but with practice, this technique will seem more natural and comfortable. Do not proceed immediately to touching the area being examined. Effective inspection requires taking the time to look.

Use good lighting. Sunlight is the optimal type of lighting for inspection, especially when inspecting the skin. Fluorescent lighting can alter true skin color, and dim lighting will generally inhibit your inspection and may even result in missing certain conditions.

Expose body parts. As each body area is inspected, it should be completely exposed. For example, when examining the anterior chest, you would inspect the chest with the person's clothing removed to the waist. You should only expose the body area being examined and cover the person as soon as possible after exposure.

Make comparisons. Use the person as his or her own control by comparing your observations of the right and left sides of the body. Look for similarities and differences between symmetric body parts such as arms, legs, eyes, and ears.

Palpation

Palpation is the use of touch during the physical examination to make judgments about the following characteristics:

- Size (small, medium, large)
- Shape (well-defined, irregular)
- Texture (rough, smooth)
- Mobility (fixed, movable, still, vibrating)
- Quality of pulses (strong, weak, thready, bounding)
- Condition of bones and joints (tender, crepitus, rigid, fixed)
- Presence of tenderness or pain
- Temperature (warm, hot, cold)
- Moisture (dry, wet)
- Fluid accumulation (swelling, edema)
- Chest wall vibrations

Palpation occurs after inspection and often provides more information about your initial visual observations.

Palpation Guidelines

Warm your hands. Before you start, warm your hands by rubbing them together or holding them under warm water. Cold hands may startle the person and cause muscle tensing, which will inhibit your ability to feel underlying structures and features.

Minimize discomfort. Use a calm, gentle approach and explain to the person what you are doing to minimize anxiety. Identify any painful areas and palpate these areas last. You should start with light palpation

movements and monitor the person's facial expression as you proceed. Any expression of distress or discomfort should prompt you to use a lighter touch or stop.

Use the correct part of your hand. Different parts of the hand are used to palpate different types of structures. Use the fingertips for fine tactile discrimination such as that required for the palpation of skin texture, swelling, pulses, and to determine the presence of lumps, especially in the breasts or lymph nodes. Grasp, using the thumb and the fingertips, to detect the position, shape, and consistency of structures or masses. Use the back (dorsal surface) of the hand to evaluate the person's skin temperature. Temperature sensory nerves are concentrated in this area of your hand and the skin is very thin, which contributes to your sensitivity to temperature. To detect vibrations, use the palm of your hand, especially at the surface of the metacarpal joints at the base of the fingers.

Start light. Start with light palpation to evaluate surface features and accustom the person to your touch. Then you can proceed to deep palpation, if necessary, depending on the part of the body being palpated. For example, deep palpation is indicated during the examination of the abdomen to feel the abdominal contents.

Light palpation. Light palpation, the safest and least uncomfortable, involves exerting gentle pressure with the fingertips of your dominant hand and moving them in a circular motion (Fig. 3-1). Place your

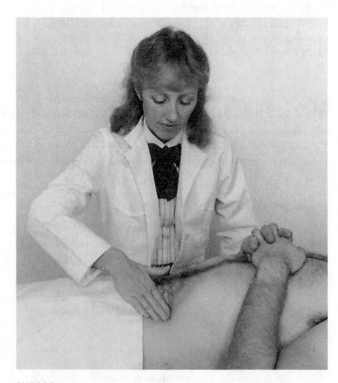

FIGURE 3.1 Light palpation. The fingertips are moved in a circular motion, depressing the body surface 0.5 to 0.75 inch (1 to 2 cm).

hand lightly on the body surface being examined and use your fingertips to depress the skin surface approximately 1 to 2 cm (0.5–0.75 inches). Exert and release fingertip pressure several times over an area. This press and release method is important for the best results. Exerting continuous pressure would tend to dull the examiner's tactile discrimination senses.

Deep palpation. Deep palpation follows light palpation and is usually conducted to detect abdominal masses. You will seldom use deep palpation for examining other areas of the body. The technique is similar to light palpation, except the skin is depressed about 2.5 to 5 cm (1–2 inches). A variation of this technique involves placing the fingertips of one hand over the fingertips of the palpating hand (Fig. 3-2). The top hand should press and guide the bottom hand to detect underlying masses.

Bimanual palpation. Bimanual palpation involves using both hands to trap a structure between them. One hand is used to apply pressure, and the other hand is used to feel the structure. This technique can be used to evaluate the spleen, kidneys, breast, uterus, and ovaries (Fig. 3-3).

Percussion

Percussion involves tapping the body parts with short, sharp strokes to create sound waves. Using percussion, you can determine the position, size, and density of underlying structures, as well as the presence of fluid or air

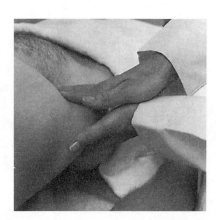

FIGURE 3.3   Bimanual palpation.

in a cavity. Tapping the body creates a sound wave that travels toward underlying areas. Sound reverberations assume different characteristics, depending on the features of the underlying structures. Percussing the right upper abdominal quadrant, for example, will usually elicit dull sounds, indicating the presence of the liver; tapping over the lungs should reveal resonant sounds associated with air-filled spaces. Percussion should be performed after an area has been palpated.

Three percussion methods can be used: mediate or indirect, immediate, and fist percussion (Fig. 3-4). The method chosen depends on the area to be percussed. *Mediate or indirect percussion* should be used to percuss the abdomen and thorax and can be performed by using the finger of one hand as a plexor (striking finger) and the middle finger of the other hand as a pleximeter (the finger being struck). *Immediate* percussion, used mainly to evaluate the sinuses or an infant's thorax, involves striking the surface directly with the fingers of one hand only. *Fist percussion*, used to evaluate the back and kidneys for tenderness, involves placing one hand flat against the body surface and striking the back of the hand with a clenched fist of the other hand.

Mediate (Indirect) Percussion Guidelines

Technique. Mediate or indirect percussion is the basic technique of two-handed percussion and is performed in the following manner:

1. Place the index or middle finger of your nondominant hand firmly against the surface being percussed. The other fingers, as well as the heel of this hand, should be raised to avoid contact with the body surface. Hold the finger firmly against the body surface throughout percussion, even when the other hand is not tapping it.
2. Use the middle finger of your dominant hand as the plexor. Hold the forearm horizontal to the surface being percussed. Keep the forearm stationary and use wrist motion to make striking movements.
3. Quickly strike the distal phalanx of the finger that is positioned on the body surface with the tip of the

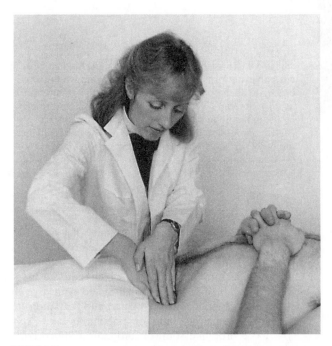

FIGURE 3.2   Deep palpation. The fingers are held at a greater angle to the body surface than in light palpation, and the skin is depressed 1.5 to 2 inches (4 to 5 cm). Deep palpation also may be done with only one hand.

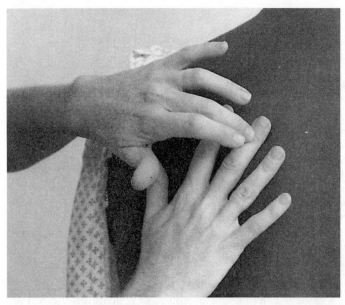

A

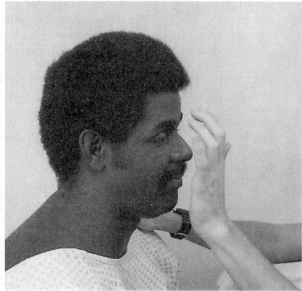

B

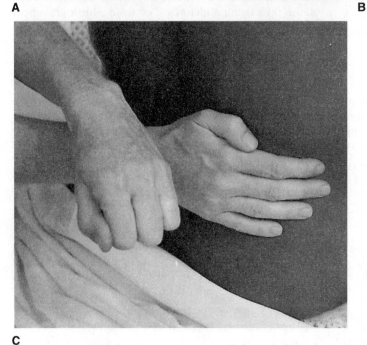

C

FIGURE 3.4 Three percussion methods. (**A**) Mediate percussion is performed with two hands, using the finger of one hand as the plexor and the finger of the other hand as a pleximeter. (**B**) Immediate percussion is performed by using the fingers of one hand to strike the surface. (**C**) Fist percussion involves placing one hand flat against the body surface and striking the back of the hand with the other hand.

finger of the other hand. Use only the wrist to generate motion, and quickly remove the striking hand after percussing to avoid muffling the percussion sound. You may percuss a single area two or three times before moving to the next area. Light tapping is more effective than heavy tapping.

4. Identify the percussion sound. Skillful percussion reveals one of five percussion sounds, depending on the density of underlying structures: flatness, dullness, resonance, hyperresonance, and tympany (Table 3-5). A *flat sound* is elicited by percussing over solid masses such as bone or muscle. A *dull sound,* which has a lower pitch than a flat sound, is elicited when the high-density structures, such as the liver, are percussed. *Resonance* is a hollow sound heard, for example, by percussing the lung. *Hyperresonance* is an abnormal sound with a pitch between resonance and tympany, and may indicate an emphysematous lung or pneumothorax. *Tympany* is a drumlike sound heard over air-filled parts such as the bowel or stomach.

5. Proceed to the next percussion area. Move from more resonant to less resonant areas, because detecting a change from resonance to dullness is eas-

TABLE 3.5 Percussion Sounds

Sound	Underlying Structure	Intensity	Pitch	Quality	Example
Flatness	Very dense tissue	Soft	High	Extreme dullness; a dead stop of sound	Normal: Muscle (thigh), bone (sternum) Abnormal: Collapsed lung, tumor
Dullness	Relatively solid tissue or organ	Medium	High	Thud-like	Normal: Liver, diaphragm Abnormal: Pleural effusion
Resonance	Part air and part solid	Loud	Low	Clear and hollow	Normal: Adult lung
Hyperresonance	Mostly air	Very loud	Lower than resonance	Booming	Normal: Child lung Abnormal: Emphysematous lung
Tympany	Air	Loud	High	Musical and drum-like	Normal: Gastric air bubble, puffed out cheek, intestine Abnormal: Air-distended abdomen

ier than detecting a change from dullness to resonance.

Common Errors in Percussing. The most common errors in performing mediate percussion are as follows:

- *Moving the forearm of the dominant hand.* Remember, all motion should be generated from the wrist.
- *Pressing the striking finger into the positioned finger.* Remove the striking finger immediately after tapping.
- *Causing injury to oneself or the client* by inadvertently striking the client or your own hand with a long fingernail. The fingernail of the plexor hand should be kept short.
- *Failing to hear the percussion note.* Eliminate environmental noise, including noise caused by bracelets or loose-fitting watches. If the note is still difficult to hear, check your technique.

Practice. You can practice mediate percussion on yourself as well as various surfaces to work on technique and the identification of sounds. Percuss over your abdomen while lying flat and listen for sound changes as you move across the abdominal surface. You should be able to detect dullness over the liver and tympany over an air-filled colon. Percuss your thigh to detect flatness and your puffed-out check to detect tympany. You may also percuss various other surfaces such as a tabletop.

Auscultation

Auscultation is the technique of listening to body sounds created in the lungs, heart, blood vessels, and abdominal viscera. Auscultation is usually the last technique used during the examination. The sequence usually progresses from inspection to palpation, percussion, and auscultation, except during the abdominal examination, when auscultation is the second step (after inspection). The reason for altering the sequence with the abdominal examination is that bowel sounds may be altered by the techniques of palpation and percussion so auscultation of bowel sounds is performed first to establish an appropriate baseline.

Immediate auscultation involves placing one's ear directly on the skin, such as over the lung. This method is rarely used because environmental noise frequently interferes with hearing. The usual method is *mediate auscultation,* or using a stethoscope to detect sounds. The best results are gained using a good-quality stethoscope. You should eliminate extraneous noise such as televisions, voices, and equipment sounds before performing auscultation. Do not create noise by moving the stethoscope over body hair or clothing or by touching the stethoscope tubing.

Auscultated sounds are described in terms of pitch, intensity, duration, and quality. *Pitch* is determined by the frequency of sound vibrations and should be classified as high or low. *Intensity* refers to the loudness of the sound. *Duration* refers to how long the sound lasts or how long it takes to occur in relation to a physiologic event such as systole. *Quality* of sound must be described using subjective terms such as tinkling, harsh, or blowing. Specific auscultatory guidelines are discussed throughout the text.

Physical Examination Equipment and Instruments

A comprehensive physical examination is conducted with the aid of various types of equipment and special instruments. Some equipment is simple, such as safety pins and cotton wisps used to evaluate sensory function. Special instruments may be more complex, such as stethoscopes, which are used to evaluate various body sounds. Some of the more complex, commonly used physical examination instruments are discussed in this section. More detailed descriptions of these and other instruments are also provided in Unit II chapter assessment guidelines.

Before starting the physical examination, you should assemble and organize all the equipment you expect to use so it is within easy reach (Fig. 3-5). You want to avoid

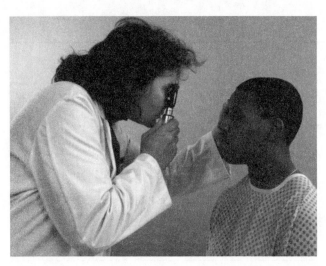 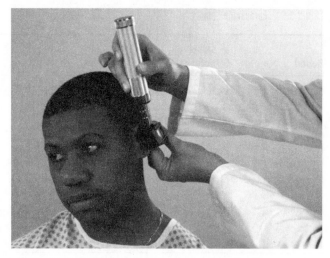

FIGURE 3.5 Various pieces of equipment used for physical examination. (Photos © B. Proud)

TABLE 3.6 Equipment Used for the Physical Examination

Equipment	Use
Paper, pencil, pen, recording forms	Documentation
Pillows, drapes	Positioning, privacy, and comfort
Gloves	Protection of examiner from body fluids
Cotton-tipped applicators	Specimen collection
Slides/specimen container	Specimen collection
Stethoscope	Vital signs, breath sounds, heart sounds, bowel sounds, vascular sounds
Sphygmomanometer	Vital signs
Thermometer	Vital signs
Watch with a second hand	Vital signs
Ophthalmoscope	Eye examination
Snellen chart	Vision testing
Otoscope	Ear examination, internal nose inspection
Tongue blades	Oral cavity
Penlight	Eye examination, oral cavity, sinuses
Dental mirror	Oral cavity
Gauze squares (4 x 4s)	Oral cavity
Cotton balls/wisps	Neurologic examination
Reflex hammer	Neurologic examination
Tuning fork	Ear examination
	Neurologic examination
Vaginal speculum	Pelvic examination
Water-soluble lubricant	Pelvic examination, anus and rectum examination
Flexible tape measure	Anthropometric measurements, extremities, organ size
Skinfold calipers	Anthropometric measurements
Safety pins	Neurologic examination
Platform scale with height attachment	Anthropometric measurements
Ruler with centimeter markings	Skin lesion examination, organ measurement, venous pressure measurement
Cover card	Eye examination
Doppler probe	Peripheral vascular examination
Goniometer	Musculoskeletal examination
Soap, coffee	Neurologic examination (smell)
Salt, sugar, lemon	Neurologic examination (taste)
Coin or key	Neurologic examination (stereognosis)

leaving the room to search for a piece of equipment once the examination has started. The types of equipment typically needed to conduct the physical examination are identified in Table 3-6.

Stethoscope

A stethoscope is used to evaluate sounds that are difficult to hear with the human ear, such as heart, bowel, vascular, and lung sounds. The stethoscope transmits sound to the ears while blocking out environmental noise (Fig. 3-6).

The chestpiece of the stethoscope is designed to detect high- or low-frequency sounds and consists of two main parts: the diaphragm and the bell. The flat, closed diaphragm filters out low-pitched sounds and is used to detect high-pitched sounds such as lung sounds. Best results are obtained by placing the diaphragm evenly and firmly over the person's exposed skin. Because the diaphragm has a relatively large surface, it transmits acute sounds over a wide area. The diaphragm should be at least 1.5 inches in diameter. Smaller diaphragm pieces are available for examining children.

The open bell portion of the chestpiece is used to detect low-frequency sounds such as diastolic heart murmurs. The bell should be at least 1 inch in diameter. The bell is placed gently on the person's skin. If too much pressure is applied, the bell will function as a diaphragm.

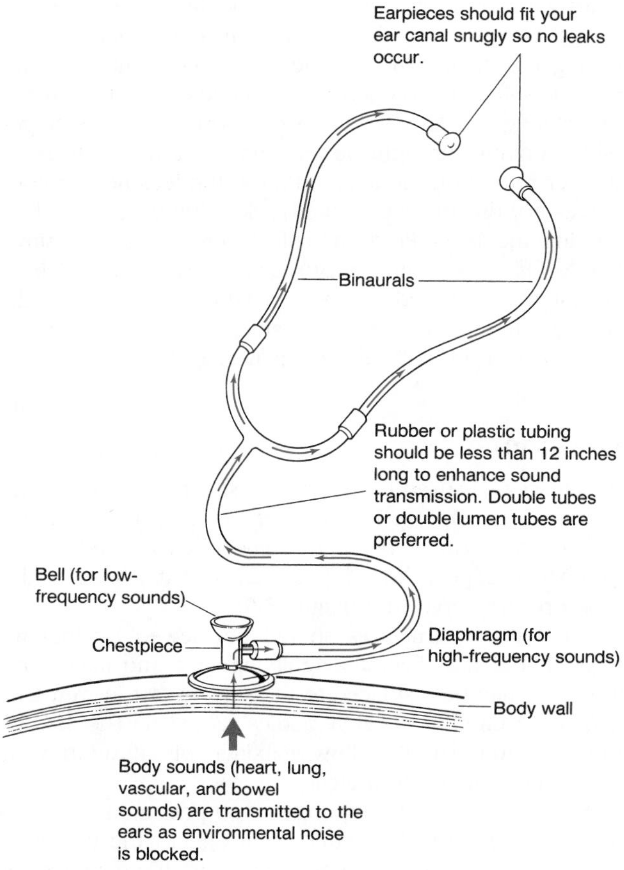

Faint sounds may be difficult to detect with the bell because of its relatively small size.

The stethoscope tubing is made of flexible rubber or plastic that is thick enough to block environmental sounds. Double tubes that are less than 12 inches long further enhance sound transmission.

The binaurals are placed in the ears and are positioned to project sound toward the tympanic membrane. The tips of the earpieces approximate the angle of the ear canal, and should fit snugly and comfortably. Manufacturers usually supply several earpieces so that a comfortable pair can be selected.

Doppler Probe

The Doppler probe is used to evaluate blood flow, especially when traditional methods such as pulse palpation or auscultation are inappropriate or ineffective. Common clinical applications include evaluating fetal heart sounds and peripheral pulses such as brachial, radial, femoral, popliteal, dorsalis pedis, and posterior tibial pulses (see Chap. 8). The Doppler probe, or transducer, is placed on the skin to send a low-energy, high-frequency sound beam (ultrasound beam) toward underlying red blood cells. Ultrasound waves are reflected off moving objects, in this case the red blood cells, and return to the Doppler transducer, which also functions as a receiver. The Doppler probe detects the change in sound frequency as sound is returned and converts the sound into an audible signal (Fig. 3-7). When blood is flowing through the vessel that is being evaluated, a pulsatile sound can be heard.

Doppler probes are available as pencil-shaped probes, flat discs, or stethoscope-like units. Each device usually has an on/off switch and a volume control dial. A small amount of gel can be applied between the end of the Doppler transducer and the client's skin to eliminate air interference. The probe is then placed gently on the skin over the vessel at approximately a 60-degree angle to the

Earpieces should fit your ear canal snugly so no leaks occur.

Binaurals

Rubber or plastic tubing should be less than 12 inches long to enhance sound transmission. Double tubes or double lumen tubes are preferred.

Bell (for low-frequency sounds)

Chestpiece

Diaphragm (for high-frequency sounds)

Body wall

Body sounds (heart, lung, vascular, and bowel sounds) are transmitted to the ears as environmental noise is blocked.

FIGURE 3.6   The stethoscope.

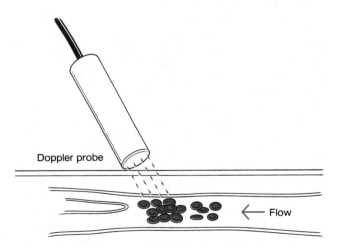

FIGURE 3.7   Doppler sound generation. The transmitting crystal emits an ultrasound beam through the skin to a vessel and moving red blood cells. The red cells reflect the ultrasound beam to the receiving crystal.

Doppler probe

Flow

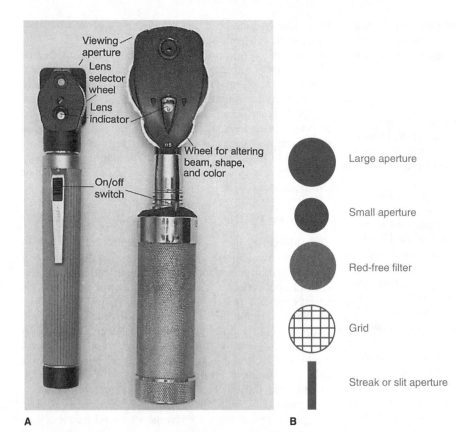

Large aperture

Small aperture

Red-free filter

Grid

Streak or slit aperture

FIGURE 3.8   **(A)** Front views of two different ophthalmoscopes. **(B)** Five apertures contained within the viewing aperture.

flow within the vessel. Excessive pressure applied to the skin may occlude the vessel.

Ophthalmoscope

An ophthalmoscope is used to inspect internal eye structures (see Chap. 9). The head of the ophthalmoscope is placed on a battery base and may be exchanged for an otoscope head. To understand the effective use of this instrument, it is important to become familiar with the structures of the ophthalmoscope head (Fig. 3-8A).

Internal eye structures can be viewed by directing a light source toward the person's pupil and looking through the viewing aperture. Light is directed away from the headpiece by a front mirror window. The viewing aperture may be adjusted by turning the aperture selection dial. To see the different apertures available on the ophthalmoscope model (Fig. 3-8B), shine the light toward a piece of paper and adjust the aperture selection dial. Usually, the large aperture is selected if pupils are dilated, and the small aperture is chosen if pupils are constricted. The slit aperture may be used to examine the anterior portion of the eye and evaluate fundal lesion levels. The grid aperture may be used to characterize, locate, and measure fundal lesions. The red-free filter or green beam may be used to evaluate the retina and disc, especially for any hemorrhaging, which appears black with this filter, whereas melanin pigments usually appear gray.

The ophthalmoscope lens can be adjusted to bring the internal eye structures into sharp focus, compensating for nearsightedness or farsightedness of the client or examiner. If necessary, you may wear contact lenses or glasses during the examination if the lens adjustment does not provide sufficient compensation. The lens can be adjusted by rotating the lens selection dial with the index finger while looking through the viewing aperture. At the zero diopter setting on the lens indicator, the lens neither converges nor diverges light. The black numbers, obtained by moving the lens selection dial clockwise, have positive values (+1 to +40) and improve visualization if the client is farsighted. The red numbers, obtained by counterclockwise rotation, have negative values (-1 to -20) and improve visualization if the client is nearsighted.

Otoscope

An otoscope is used to inspect the structures of the internal ear (see Chap. 9). The head of the otoscope should be placed on a battery base and may be exchanged for an ophthalmoscope head. The structures of the head of the otoscope are depicted in Figure 3-9.

Internal ear structures should be viewed by looking through the illuminated magnifying lens and speculum. The lens may be displaced to the side so that instruments can be inserted or foreign bodies removed. The size of the speculum should allow maximal visualization with minimal discomfort to the client.

Some otoscopes are equipped with pneumonic devices to introduce a small amount of air against the tympanic membrane, and may be used to evaluate the flexibility of the tympanic membrane.

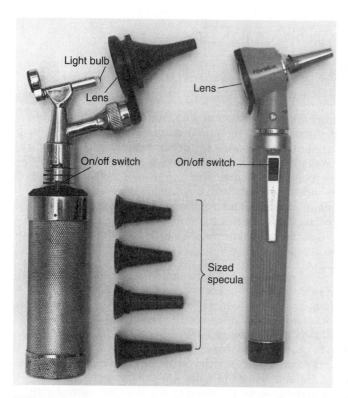

Light bulb

Lens

Lens

On/off switch

On/off switch

Sized specula

FIGURE 3.9   The otoscope.

Physical Examination   The Complete Physical Examination

GENERAL APPROACH

The physical examination usually takes place after the examiner has interviewed the individual. It is customary in an ambulatory setting, such as an outpatient clinic or physician's office, to conduct the interview with the client still wearing street clothes. The client changes into an examining gown after completion of the interview in preparation for the physical examination. The examiner, before the start of the interview, makes other preparations for the physical examination.

Prepare the Physical Examination Setting. The physical examination may be performed in a number of settings, including an outpatient clinic, a hospital room, or the client's home. In any case, common steps may be taken to optimize the examination setting. The examination should be conducted in privacy, preferably in a room where the door may be closed. In hospital rooms, privacy curtains should be drawn during the examination. Schedule the examination at a time when you can anticipate no interruptions. The room should be warm, quiet, and well lit. If you are unable to adequately raise the room temperature to acceptable levels, provide warm blankets for additional comfort during the examination. Eliminate any unnecessary noise such as sounds from TVs, radios, or nonessential equipment that might distract you as you try to listen to body sounds. Natural lighting, such as sunlight, is best for viewing the skin. Artificial lighting also can be used. A portable gooseneck lamp can provide additional high-intensity lighting as needed during parts of the examination. Position the examining surface (examination table or bed) in a manner that allows you to freely walk around it for easy access. Adjust the height so that you will not have to bend or stoop excessively as you conduct the examination. A roll-up stool should be available to use in parts of the examination for which

(continued)

you will be sitting. Finally, you will need a surface for holding all of your equipment such as a bedside table or Mayo stand.

Prepare Equipment, Forms for Documentation, and Prompts for the Examination Steps. Assemble all the necessary equipment and place it on a table so that it is easy to reach. You should also organize any documentation materials you may use during the examination. Many agencies have printed forms for recording the results of the examination. You may want to record a few findings during the examination but should conduct most of your documentation at the completion of the examination to avoid interrupting the flow of the examination. It is acceptable to prepare some notes that will help you remember all the steps of the examination, or the printed forms used for documentation may provide adequate cues as you proceed.

Prepare the Client. The client is informed of the purpose of the examination and asked to change into an examining gown. For example, you may say, "I'm going to examine you to evaluate your general health and follow-up on some of the symptoms you reported during our previous discussion," or "I am going to listen to your heart and lungs to see how you are responding to your treatments." Ask the person to change into the examining gown, removing all of their clothing except for the underwear, which will be removed during the genital examination. Then you should leave the room while the person changes. Provide adequate time and then return, knocking on the door before you enter.

Unless you require a urine specimen, the person should empty their bladder before you start the examination. If you require a specimen, provide the specimen container and give the person instructions for providing the specimen.

Explain the Steps of the Examination. Throughout the examination, explain what you are doing and why. You do not have to explain every step but instead focus on the more invasive procedures and give clear instructions during position changes. For example, during the eye examination with the ophthalmoscope, you may explain why you are darkening the room and how the person can assist you as you visualize eye structures by looking at a point on the ceiling and keeping the eyes wide open. You also should inform the person that you will be shining a bright light in their eyes.

Use Standard Precautions to Prevent the Transmission of Infectious Agents. During the physical examination, you should take precautions to prevent the transmission of infectious agents. Standard Precautions, established by the Centers for Disease Control and Prevention and the Hospital Infection Control Practices Advisory Committee in 1996, should be followed during the physical examination.

The following practices are recommended:

• Wash your hands thoroughly before initiating the examination. It is a good idea to wash your hands in the person's presence, which gives the message that you are genuinely concerned for his or her safety.
• Wash your hands again after contact with any contaminated surfaces or body fluids. Finally, wash your hands again at the completion of the examination.
• If you have an open cut or skin abrasion on your hands, wear gloves to protect the person being examined.
• Routinely wear gloves when contact with body fluids is likely. For example, wear gloves during the oral examination, the rectal examination, and the vaginal examination. Also, wear gloves when contact with soiled linens is likely.

(continued)

- Wear gloves when examining open skin lesions or if the person has a weeping dermatitis.
- Wear gloves to handle and clean soiled equipment such as vaginal speculums.
- Clean contaminated equipment using proper procedures and disinfectant agents.
- Wear gloves when collecting specimens (stool, urine, sputum, and wound drainage).
- If safety pins or other sharp objects are used during sensory testing, use a new pin for each person and discard each sharp object carefully to prevent injury.
- Wear a mask and protective goggles if you are performing a procedure in which there is a likelihood of being splashed by blood or other body fluids (*e.g.,* obtaining a sputum specimen).

Establish Appropriate Positioning. By convention, physical examination procedures are performed with the examiner positioned on the right side of the person, who is positioned in bed or on an examining table. Probably the most important reason for encouraging the examiner to stand on the right side is to minimize the examiner's movements from one side of the person to the other during the examination, which would be awkward. Moreover, most examination maneuvers are performed with the right hand, even in left-handed examiners making this position more convenient.

The position of the person being examined will be changed several times during a comprehensive examination. The examination should be organized to minimize the number of times position changes are required, because this can be tiring. Whenever a position is changed, the examiner should be attentive to any support that is needed as well as proper body alignment. For example, when the person is lying supine, a small pillow under the head will increase comfort. Also, prolonged sitting should not occur without proper back support. Some individuals will need assistance in moving from one position to another. Certain individuals will poorly tolerate some positions, and you will need to make appropriate modifications. For example, the person who has difficulty breathing because of respiratory or cardiac problems may not tolerate lying completely flat in the supine position. You may have to elevate the head of the bed or the examining table.

Make Appropriate Modifications for Infants and Children. When examining infants and children (Display 3-2), the head-to-toe examination sequence is commonly modified such that the least distressing aspects of the examination are conducted first (*e.g.,* listening to heart and lung sounds), whereas the most invasive procedures are postponed to the end of the exam (*e.g.,* examining the ears with the otoscope). You want to listen to the heart and lungs with the child quiet. If the child is asleep, take advantage of this quiet state and listen to heart and lung sounds. Infants and very young children may sit on the lap of the parent or guardian during the examination. Equipment should be presented in a nonthreatening manner and the child allowed to touch and play as appropriate when introducing equipment. More extensive guidelines for examining infants and children are presented in Chapter 16.

Make Appropriate Modifications for Elders. Some older persons will have difficulty making the usual position changes during the physical examination and require your assistance. In addition, some positions will be difficult if not impossible for the elder to assume. In general, you should keep position changes at a minimum if the person appears to have difficulty.

A lengthy physical examination can be tiring for elders. Allow for rest breaks as appropriate or conduct the examination over several visits if possible. More extensive guidelines for evaluating elders are presented in Chapter 17.

(continued)

Physical Examination   The Complete Physical Examination (continued)

Conduct the Preliminary Aspects of the Examination. At the beginning of the examination, before the person is positioned on the examining table, either before or after he or she changes into an examining gown, you may evaluate the following:

- Vital signs (temperature, pulse, respirations, and blood pressure)
- Height and weight
- Posture and gait
- Snellen visual acuity
- Cerebellar functions

These procedures are easy and nonthreatening and help you and the individual become more comfortable with each other. In addition, it helps the individual become accustomed to the examination. When the person is positioned on the examining table, you may start the examination by picking up the person's hands and examining nails, skin color, and joints. Most people do not perceive hand touching as too threatening, so this is a good way to establish your initial physical contact with the person.

DISPLAY 3.2

Examination Sequence
for Infants and Children

INFANTS

First   →   If baby is sleeping or being held and quiet, listen to heart sounds, lung sounds, abdomen

Next   →   Least distressing procedures, especially inspection and noninvasive palpation. Use general head-to-toe sequence.

Last   →   Invasive steps of the examination, including examination of the eyes, ears, and oral cavity; elicit the Moro reflex at the end of the examination.

TODDLERS

First   →   Make general survey observations of musculoskeletal functions and motor skills while child plays as you interview parent or caregiver

Next   →   Play "games"—for example, the Denver Development Screening Test or Cranial Nerve Testing

Next   →   Use the general head-to-toe sequence to conduct the least distressing procedures

Last   →   Invasive steps of the examination, including examination of the eyes, ears, and oral cavity.

PRE-SCHOOLERS

Similar to toddlers

SCHOOL-AGE CHILDREN

Similar to adult sequence

▼ ▼ ▼
GUIDELINES

Assessment Guidelines   The Complete Physical Examination

Procedure

What To Observe and Record

1. **Initiate the general survey.**
   a. The general survey begins when you first meet the client, in the waiting room or examination room, or while delivering bedside care.

   - General state of health
   - Signs of distress such as breathing difficulty, pain
   - Awareness, behavior, facial expression, mood (Chap. 9)

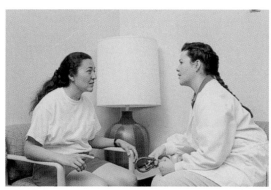

General survey

   b. Survey mobility and gait as the person walks into the room.

   - Height, weight, nutritional status (Chap. 6)

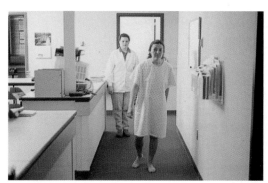

Surveying mobility and gait

   c. Continue the general survey as you examine each body region.

   - Hygiene, grooming, clothes
   - Skin condition (Chap. 6)
   - Odors
   - Posture, motor activity, physical deformities (Chap. 8)
   - Speech pattern (Chap. 9)
   - Apparent age vs. actual age

▼ ▼ ▼

GUIDELINES *continued*   The Complete Physical Examination

Procedure

With the client seated on the examination table, bed, or chair,

2. **Measure vital signs (Chap. 4).**

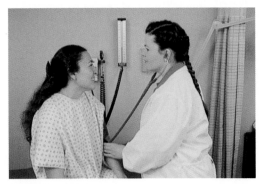

Measuring vital signs

3. **Examine the head.**
   a. Inspect and palpate the cranium.

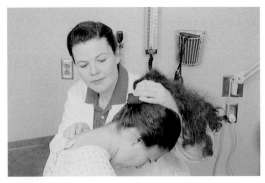

Inspecting the hair and scalp

   b. Palpate and auscultate the temporal arteries.

What To Observe and Record

- Blood pressure
- Pulse
- Respiratory rate
- Body temperature

- Hair (Chap. 6)
- Size, shape, and symmetry
- Tenderness
- Scalp smoothness

- Thickening
- Tenderness
- Bruits

Procedure

c. Inspect and palpate the face.

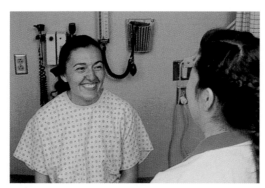

Inspecting the face

What To Observe and Record

- Symmetry
- Movements
- Tenderness
- Nodules
- Sinus tenderness (Chap. 6)

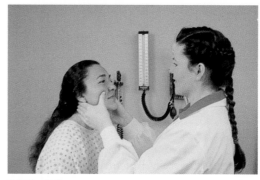

Palpating the face

d. Test cranial nerves V and VII (Chap. 9).

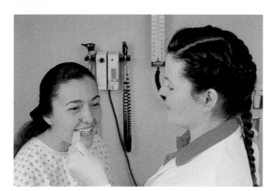

Testing motor function of cranial nerve V (trigeminal)

- Motor and sensory responses

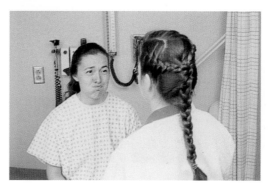

Testing motor function of cranial nerve VII (facial)

e. Inspect the nose and test cranial nerve I.

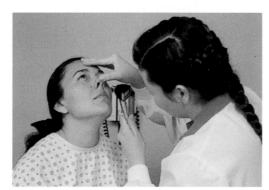

Inspecting the nose

- Patency
- Septum
- Mucosa
- Sense of smell

▼ ▼ ▼

GUIDELINES *continued*   The Complete Physical Examination

Procedure

4. **Examine the eyes and test vision** (Chap. 9).
   a. Inspect and palpate to evaluate external eye structures.

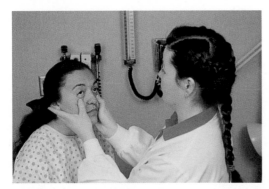

Inspecting the lower conjunctiva

   b. Evaluate visual acuity. Perform Jaeger chart testing of near vision now, or Snellen chart testing of far vision at the beginning of the examination.

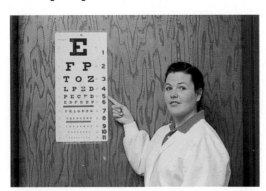

Testing visual acuity

   c. Test extraocular muscle function (cranial nerves III, IV, and VI).

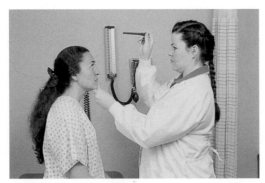

Testing extraocular eye movements

What To Observe and Record

- Shape and symmetry
- Eyelids and eyelashes
- Lacrimal glands, puncta, and lacrimal functions
- Upper and lower conjunctiva
- Lens, cornea, iris, and pupil

- Eye chart readings
- Peripheral vision

- Extraocular eye movements
- Eye movement during cover–uncover test
- Eye alignment and symmetry

▼ ▼ ▼

Procedure	**What To Observe and Record**

Procedure

   d. Test pupillary reflexes.

What To Observe and Record

- Reaction to light
- Accommodation

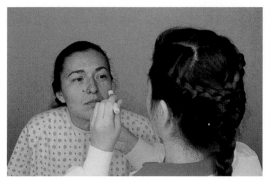

Testing pupillary light reflex

   e. Inspect internal eye structures with the ophthalmo-scope; darken the room if possible.

- Retina
- Retinal vessels
- Optic disc
- Macula

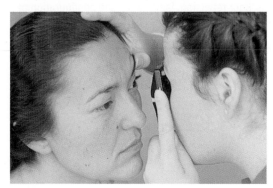

Inspecting the internal eye with the ophthalmoscope

5. **Examine the ears and test hearing** (Chap. 9).
   a. Inspect and palpate the external ear.

- Skin integrity
- Structure, alignment, and symmetry
- Tenderness

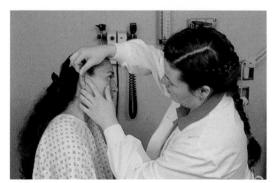

Palpating the external ear

▼ ▼ ▼

G U I D E L I N E S *continued*   The Complete Physical Examination

Procedure

b. Evaluate hearing.

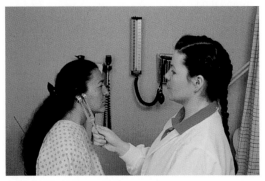

Testing hearing acuity

c. Inspect the ear canal and tympanic membrane with the otoscope.

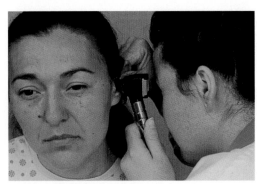

Inspecting the internal ear with the otoscope

6. **Examine the oral cavity** (Chap. 6).

a. Inspect and palpate the outer structures of the oral cavity.

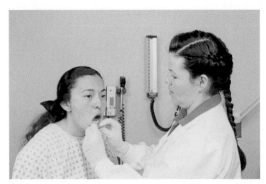

Palpating the lips

What To Observe and Record

- Ability to distinguish sounds varying in pitch and intensity
- Sound lateralization
- Perception of air conduction of sound vs. bone conduction

- Skin integrity
- Obstructions, foreign bodies
- Color, light reflection, landmarks, and configuration of the tympanic membrane

- Lips
- Jaw
- Temporomandibular joint
- Parotid glands

▼ ▼ ▼

G U I D E L I N E S   *continued*   The Complete Physical Examination

---

Procedure

b. Inspect and palpate the inner structures of the oral cavity.

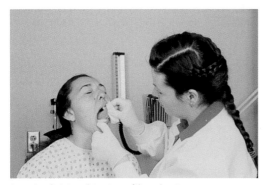

Inspecting the internal structures of the oral cavity

c. Test cranial nerves V, IX, and XII (Chap. 11).

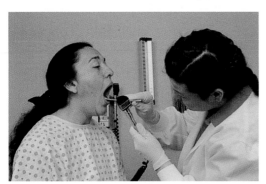

Testing cranial nerve IX (glossopharyngeal) by eliciting a gag reflex

What To Observe and Record

- Oral mucosa
- Tongue
- Inner cheek
- Hard and soft palates
- Oropharynx
- Uvula

- Motor responses

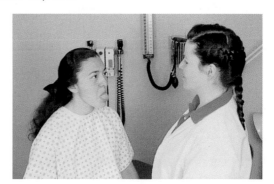

Testing cranial nerve XII (hypoglossal) by observing the tongue for symmetry and movement

7. **Examine the neck.**
   a. Inspect musculoskeletal structures.

   b. Palpate the lymph nodes (Chap. 6).

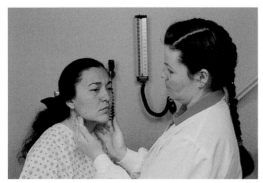

Palpating the cervical lymph nodes

- Alignment
- Symmetry
- Consistency
- Enlargement
- Nodules
- Tenderness

▼ ▼ ▼

G U I D E L I N E S   *continued*   The Complete Physical Examination

---

Procedure

c. Inspect and palpate the thyroid gland (Chap. 6)

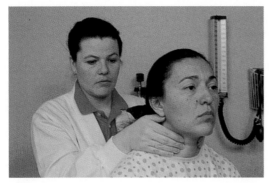

Palpating the thyroid gland

d. Test neck musculoskeletal function and cranial nerve XI.

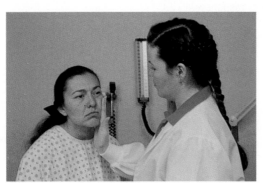

Testing motor function of cranial nerve XI (spinal accessory)

e. Palpate and auscultate the carotid arteries.

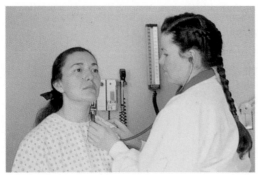

Auscultating the carotid artery

8. **Examine the upper extremities.**
   a. Inspect musculoskeletal structures, skin, and nails.

What To Observe and Record

- Consistency
- Enlargement
- Nodules
- Tenderness

- Muscle strength and tone
- Range of motion

- Pulsations
- Vascular sounds

- Skin integrity
- Muscle mass
- Alignment and symmetry

▼ ▼ ▼

Procedure	What To Observe and Record

Procedure

b. Test musculoskeletal function.

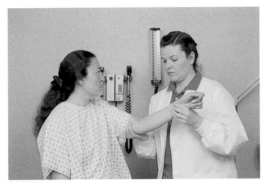

Testing range of motion of the upper extremity

c. Palpate brachial and radial arteries.

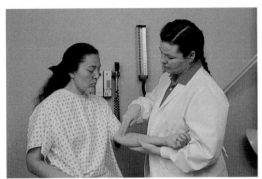

Palpating the brachial artery

d. Test deep tendon reflexes.

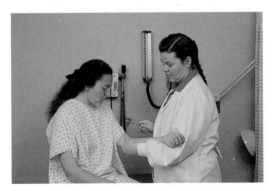

Testing the biceps deep tendon reflex

What To Observe and Record

- Muscle strength and tone
- Range of motion

- Pulsations

- Motor response

▼ ▼ ▼

G U I D E L I N E S *continued*   The Complete Physical Examination

Procedure

9. **Examine the anterior chest.**
   a. Inspect and palpate the breasts and axillae (Chap. 13)

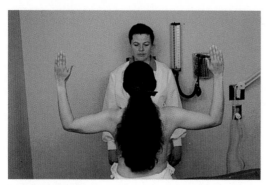

Inspecting the breasts

   b. Inspect, palpate, percuss, and auscultate the thorax (Chap. 8).

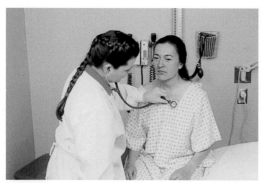

Auscultating the anterior chest

   c. Inspect, palpate, and auscultate the precordium (Chap. 8).

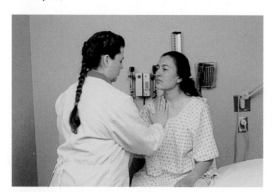

Palpating precordial landmarks

10. **Examine the back.**
    a. Inspect and test musculoskeletal structures.

What To Observe and Record

- Skin integrity
- Size, shape, and symmetry
- Consistency

- Skin integrity
- Ventilatory pattern
- Shape and symmetry
- Chest excursion
- Vibrations
- Percussion tones
- Breath sounds

- Pulsations
- Vibrations
- Heart sounds

- Spinal alignment
- Muscle tone
- Range of motion

▼ ▼ ▼

Procedure

b. Perform fist percussion over the spine and kidneys.

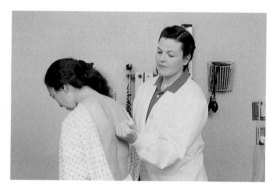

Percussing the spine

c. Inspect, palpate, percuss, and auscultate the posterior thorax.

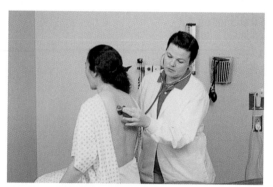

Auscultating the posterior thorax

What To Observe and Record

- Tenderness

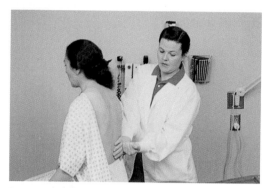

Percussing the kidney

- Same as anterior thorax

Position client supine on the examining table or bed. Elevate the head 30 degrees to 60 degrees to inspect the neck veins. The examiner stands on the right side.

11. **Inspect the neck veins** (Chap. 8).

- Jugular venous pulsations
- Central venous pressure

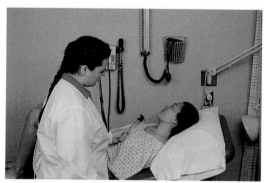

Inspecting neck veins

Procedure

12. **Examine the anterior chest** (as above, adding palpation of glandular breast tissue and precordial auscultation in the left lateral position.)

What To Observe and Record

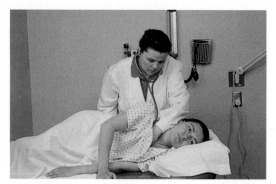

Auscultating precordial landmarks in the left lateral position

13. **Examine the abdomen.**
    a. Inspect, auscultate, palpate, and percuss the four abdominal quadrants (Chap. 6).

- Contour and symmetry
- Skin integrity
- Bulges
- Bowel sounds
- Vascular sounds
- Muscle tone
- Masses
- Organ characteristics
- Percussion tones
- Tenderness

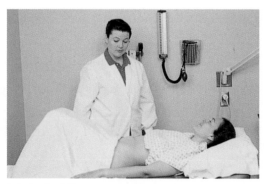

Inspecting the abdomen

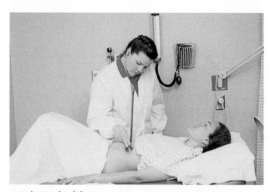

Auscultating the abdomen

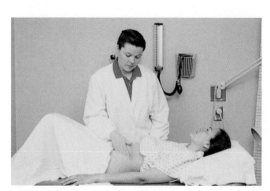

Palpating the abdomen

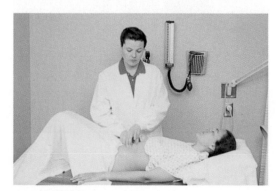

Percussing the abdomen

▼ ▼ ▼
GUIDELINES *continued*   The Complete Physical Examination

Procedure	What To Observe and Record
b. Palpate and percuss specific organs (liver, spleen, kidneys).	• Size • Consistency • Tenderness

14. Examine the lower extremities.
a. Inspect musculoskeletal structures, skin, and toenails.

b. Test musculoskeletal function.

c. Palpate popliteal, posterior tibial, and pedal arteries.

What To Observe and Record
- Skin integrity
- Muscle mass
- Alignment and symmetry
- Muscle strength and tone
- Range of motion
- Pulsations

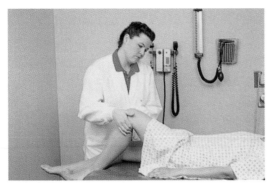

Palpating the popliteal pulse

d. Test deep tendon reflexes and plantar reflex.

- Motor response

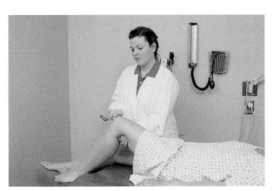

Testing the patellar deep tendon reflex

▼ ▼ ▼

G U I D E L I N E S   *continued*   The Complete Physical Examination

---

Procedure

Position the female client in the lithotomy position with stir-rups.

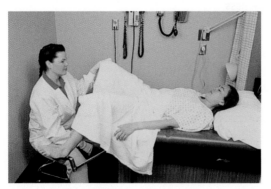

Positioning the client in the lithotomy position

15. **Examine the genitals and pelvis** (Chap. 13).
    a. Inspect the external genitals.

    b. Inspect the vagina and cervix.

    c. Palpate the vagina, uterus, and adnexa.

16. **Examine the rectum** (Chap. 7).

Assist the male client to a standing position.

17. **Examine the external genitals** (Chap. 13).
    a. Inspect and palpate the penis.

    b. Inspect and palpate the scrotum.

    c. Inspect and palpate for hernias.

18. **Examine the rectum.** (For male patients, different positions may be used and special attention is given to prostate pal-pation.)

What To Observe and Record

- Skin integrity
- Contour and symmetry
- Discharge
- Skin integrity
- Masses
- Discharge
- Muscle tone
- Position
- Size
- Consistency and masses
- Muscle tone
- Stool
- Tenderness
- Masses
- Bleeding, discharge

- Skin integrity
- Masses
- Discharge
- Skin integrity
- Size and shape
- Testicular descent and mobility
- Masses
- Tenderness
- Bulges

Physical Examination   The General Survey

GENERAL APPROACH

The general survey provides an indication of the person's overall health and outstanding physical features. The general survey is initiated on meeting the person and is usually the first step of a comprehensive physical examination. A number of judgments can be made about the person based on the general survey, including judgments about the following:

- General state of health
- Signs of distress
- Mental status
- Nutritional status
- Growth and development status

You should conduct the general survey by observing the following about the person:

- Age and general physical appearance
- Dress and grooming
- Body habitus
- Mobility
- Speech and behavior

▼ ▼ ▼

G U I D E L I N E S

Assessment Guidelines   The General Survey

Procedure

1. **Observe age and general physical appearance.**
   Determine whether the person looks his or her stated age.

   Note level of growth and development, including whether level of sexual development appears appropriate for gender and age.

   Observe general state of health. Determine whether the person appears well, chronically ill, or acutely ill.

   Observe general nutritional status and body weight.

   Observe the general appearance of the skin.

   Note the facial features.

Clinical Significance

- Appearance **older than stated age** associated with chronic disease, manual labor, chronic alcoholism, chronic smoking.
- The development of **secondary sex characteristics** (*e.g.*, facial hair, breast development in women) may be inhibited in **delayed puberty** and appear early with **precocious puberty**.

- **Cachexia:** Poor nutritional status is usually associated with chronic illness, such as cancer or advanced pulmonary disorders, and manifested by wasted, "walking skeleton" appearance, sunken eyes, temporal muscle wasting, and loose skin.
- Obesity of **Cushing's syndrome:** Endocrine disorder characterized by abnormal deposits of fat in the trunk, face (moon facies), and posterior neck area (buffalo hump).

Abnormal Findings (see Skin Assessment Guidelines in Chap. 6):
Pallor, cyanosis, jaundice, lesions

Normal
Facial features are symmetric with movement; appropriate smiling and frowning

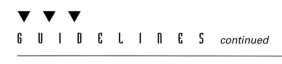

▼ ▼ ▼

G U I D E L I N E S *continued*   The General Survey

Procedure	Clinical Significance

Clinical Significance

Abnormal
Asymmetry of facial movements; poor eye contact may indicate depression/cultural variation; inappropriate smiling may indicate mental illness.

2. Observe speech and behavior.
Note the quality of the person's speech pattern, especially articulation and speech content.
Note general mental status, especially level of orientation to time, place, and person.

Note mood and affect.

Abnormal Speech Patterns
Slurred speech may indicate neurologic disorders; Inappropriate use of words needs to be more fully evaluated during the mental status examination; Slow, hoarse speech may be associated with hypothyroidism.

Normal
Pleasant affect, cooperative, level of eye contact appropriate for culture, smiles appropriately.

Variations
Poor eye contact and flat affect may occur with depression; hostile, distrustful, suspicious, angry behavior should be further evaluated.

Identify signs of distress that should receive immediate attention:

Acute illness

May be accompanied by pallor, diaphoresis, an increased ventilatory rate or effort, and guarding of painful areas.

Abnormal ventilatory patterns

Shortness of breath (dyspnea), labored breathing and use of accessory muscles, stridor (crowing sounds on inspiration or expiration), wheezing, and rapid breathing (tachypnea).

Cyanosis

Bluish discoloration of the skin and mucous membranes indicates poor cardiopulmonary status.

Acute anxiety

Some anxiety during the physical examination is to be expected. **Acute anxiety** may be characterized by fidgety movements; restlessness; cold, moist palms; and tense facial expressions.

Pain

Indicators of Acute Pain
Guarding or protecting the painful area; wincing; crying; moaning; diaphoresis.

Indicators of Chronic Pain (chronic mask of pain)
Flat or fixed facial expression; lackluster eyes; appearance of fatigue.

Trauma

Bleeding, inflammation, or other signs of physical injury should be evaluated further before proceeding with an interview or physical examination. Signs of physical abuse include multiple bruises at different stages of healing and excessive bruises above the knees or above the elbows.

3. Observe dress and hygiene.
Evaluate dress and hygiene in light of cultural norms, age, and socioeconomic status. Determine whether the person's dress is appropriate to the climate, looks well kept, and fits appropriately.

Significant Dress Observations
Clothing that is inappropriate for the climate may be noted in persons who are mentally ill, depressed, grieving, or poor. Also may be observed in persons with heat/cold intolerance. If clothes fit loosely, suspect recent weight loss.

▼ ▼ ▼
G U I D E L I N E S   *continued*   The General Survey

Procedure

Compare dress and hygiene on both sides of the body.

Note any general odors such as body odor and the odor of urine or feces. Observe for breath odors, including alcohol, acetone, urine, and ammonia.

4. **Examine body habitus (build) and determine body type.**

5. **Note posture, gait, and general mobility.**
   Watch the person walk, sit, and change positions.

Clinical Significance

Variations
Some cultures may not include the use of a deodorant, a clean-shaven look for men, or women shaving their legs; women's makeup may vary depending on culture; children who make their own choices regarding what to wear may choose clothes that do not match; and people of lower socioeconomic status may wear outdated clothing.

Poor Hygiene
Consider depression, dementia, schizophrenia.

One-Sided Neglect
A condition associated with lesions to the cerebral cortex manifested by inattention to grooming on one side of the body.

Alcohol on the breath may indicate acute intoxication; acetone is associated with diabetic emergencies; Urinous breath (uremic fetor) is a manifestation of chronic renal failure; an ammonia odor indicates advanced liver disease.

Three Basic Body Types
   Asthenics (ectomorphs)—appear thin and tall with long necks, chests, and abdomens. May have poorly developed musculature.
   Sthenics (mesomorphs)—Have an athletic appearance with average height, large bone structure, and good muscle development.
   Hypersthenics (endomorphs)—Have a short, round appearance and good muscle development. Tendency toward obesity.

Abnormal Posture
May be associated with disorders of the muscles, bones, or neurologic system. May observe curvatures of the spine—**lordosis, scoliosis,** or **kyphosis.** Typical postures may be observed in persons with chronic obstructive pulmonary disease (forward-leaning, tripod posture); depression (slumped shoulders) sciatica (deviation of the spine toward the affected side); and arthritis (rigid spine, stiff, moves as one unit).

Abnormal Gait
Exceptionally wide base; staggering and stumbling; shuffling or dragging nonfunctional leg; limping with injury; propulsion or difficulty stopping forward motion.

Types of Abnormal Gaits
Ataxic, hemiplegic, Parkinsonism, scissors, spastic, steppage, or waddling (see descriptions in Chapter 8).

Normal General Mobility
Full mobility for all joints; movement is voluntary, smooth, coordinated, accurate. No tics, tremor, or seizure activity.

DOCUMENTATION: THE PHYSICAL EXAMINATION

The approach for documenting physical examination findings varies depending on such factors as the examiner's preferences and policies and procedures stipulated by an agency for recording findings. General principles for documentation were discussed in Chapter 1.

Display 3-3 illustrates documentation of the physical examination using a narrative approach. The use of abbreviations is acceptable, but it has been kept to a minimum in this example.

Some agencies use a "charting by exception" method to document physical examination findings. This is usually applied to summarize the examiner's evaluation of each major body system. The underlying premise in the "charting by exception" method is that the examiner uses a standardized definition of what constitutes normal findings for each body system. If the examination findings correspond to the normal criteria, no additional documentation is required. Only the variations from the normal criteria are recorded. The example shown on Display 3-4 illustrates the "charting by exception" method used by nurses on a Medical-Surgical unit in an acute care hospital. Until you have developed your own abilities to fully describe normal findings in a narrative account, you should avoid the "charting by exception" method unless fulfilling an agency requirement. In this case, you may still want to develop your skills by describing normal findings in a separate recording.

DISPLAY 3.3

Documentation of the Physical Examination

Patient Name:	Jane Doe
General Survey:	The patient is a 61-year-old female who appears 5 to 10 years older than her stated age. She is seated on the examining table, constantly shifting position and picking at the paper covering the table. There are no signs of respiratory distress or pain. She is alert but disoriented to time, person, and place and requires frequent orientation to the examination process. She is cooperative when given simple instructions, but her attention span is short. She is thin and well groomed but wears no cosmetics. Eye contact is minimal. She talks throughout the examination, with some phrases being unintelligible.
Vital Signs:	BP 144/88 left arm seated; 142/88 left arm standing; 140/84 right arm seated; heart rate 90 and regular; respirations 16; otoscopic temperature 37.1
Skin:	Skin pink and dry; poor turgor; scattered lentigines over dorsal surfaces of the hands. Hair on head thick with some graying. Hair present on lower extremities.
Head:	Normocephalic without evidence of trauma. Nontender to palpation; scalp smooth; facial features symmetric.
Eyes:	Wears glasses; visual acuity with Snellen chart not assessed because patient unable to follow instructions. Able to read single words printed in phone book; unable to test peripheral vision due to lack of cooperation. EOMs intact; PERLA; eyelids symmetrical and without lesions; conjunctiva moist and pink; not injected. No discharge on palpation of lacrimal glands. Small opacity present on right lens. Fundoscopic exam reveals sharp discs bilaterally. A-V ratio 2:3 OU; fundus without lesions.
Ears:	External ears not tender to palpation. Otoscopic exam reveals left ear impacted with dark brown cerumen. Unable to see left tympanic membrane. Right ear has small amount of soft yellow cerumen. Right tympanic membrane pearly gray and scarred. Landmarks visible. Rinne, BC > AC on left; AC > BC on right. Weber, lateralization to the left side.
Nose:	Straight; no masses or drainage; patent bilaterally.
Sinuses:	Facial and maxillary sinuses nontender.
Oral Cavity:	Edentulous; no TMJ tenderness; oral mucosa pink, moist, and intact. No lesions seen or palpated on mucosa or tongue or beneath tongue. Tongue midline without fasiculations; gag reflex intact.

(continued)

Documentation of the Physical Examination (continued)

Neck:
Full range of motion; trachea midline; no visible jugular pulsations when seated upright; carotids negative for bruits. Thyroid borders easily palpable with no palpable thyroid masses. Thyroid not enlarged. Old, well-healed linear scar from surgical incision noted on anterior neck beneath thyroid. No adenopathy.

Chest:
Symmetric and effortless ventilatory pattern. Increased AP to lateral chest diameter. No visible or palpable masses. Breath sounds diminished at bases bilaterally with slight expiratory wheeze bilaterally. Upper lung fields auscultated for fine vesicular breath sounds. Fremitus not evaluated.

Breasts:
Breasts symmetric, atrophic, skin intact. No visible masses or changes in breast shape with movement. No palpable masses; no nipple discharge; no palpable axillary or supraclavicular nodes.

Heart:
No visible precordial pulsations. PMI not palpable. Auscultation reveals S1, S2, and Grade III/VI midsystolic murmur over Erb's point that does not radiate.

Vascular:
No bruits heard over carotid, renal, femoral, or abdominal arteries. Peripheral pulses all 3+ with the exception of pedal pulses—1+ bilaterally. Mild varicosities noted in lower extremities; Homans' sign negative bilaterally.

Back:
Marked kyphosis. No spinal tenderness.

Abdomen:
Abdomen flat with slight pulsation noted over abdominal aorta. No visible or palpable masses. Well-healed linear surgical scar noted over right upper quadrant. Active bowel sounds in all quadrants. Percussion note is tympanic over all quadrants. Liver span 10 cm by percussion. Abdomen not tender to palpation.

Rectal:
Atrophic skin tags present; anal sphincter tone intact. Hard stool in rectum—negative for occult blood. No masses palpable along rectal walls.

Genitals:
Wartlike lesion 1–2 cm noted on left vulvar surface. Parous cervix midline without discharge. Bimanual exam reveals no tenderness or palpable masses. Uterus midline and mobile.

Lymphatics:
No palpable or tender nodes in cervical, axillary, supraclavicular, epitrochlear, or inguinal chains.

Musculoskeletal:
Full range of motion to all extremities. Marked kyphosis; finger joints enlarged on both hands—nontender.

Neurologic:
Orientation as previously noted. Long-term memory intact more than short-term memory. Cranial nerves intact. Gross sensory function intact. Gait unsteady. Unable to cooperate with cerebellar testing. DTRS symmetrical—2–3+.

Documentation of the Physical Examination: Charting by Exception

PHYSICAL EXAMINATION FINDINGS

(Note: Record abnormal findings only; a blank space indicates normal exam)

Skin ☐ Normal ☑ Exceptions	Lentigines on dorsal surfaces of both hands
HEENT ☐ Normal ☑ Exceptions	Glasses; small opacity on right lens Right ear impacted with cerumen; AC>BC on right; Weber lateralize to left side
Respiratory ☐ Normal ☑ Exceptions	Diminished at bases and slight expiratory wheeze bilaterally
Cardiovascular ☐ Normal ☑ Exceptions	Grade III/VI midsystolic murmur over Erb's point that does not radiate
Peripheral Vascular ☐ Normal ☑ Exceptions	Pedal pulses 1+ bilaterally; mild varicosities in lower extremities
Gastrointestinal ☑ Normal ☐ Exceptions	
Lymphatic ☑ Normal ☐ Exceptions	
Neurologic ☐ Normal ☑ Exceptions	Disoriented to time, person, place; unable to concentrate and follow instructions; constant talking—not always intelligible. Short-term memory poor—some ability to recall distant past events; gait unsteady.
Musculoskeletal ☐ Normal ☑ Exceptions	Marked kyphosis. Finger joints enlarged both hands; nontender.
Genitalia ☐ Normal ☑ Exceptions	Wartlike lesion 1–2 cm noted on left vulvar surface
Rectal ☐ Normal ☑ Exceptions	Atrophic skin tags; hard stool in rectum

CHAPTER 3 SUMMARY

Physical Examination

The record of the physical examination, along with the health history, make up a clinical database. The physical examination is the observation of an individual in which the examiner uses the senses of sight, hearing, touch, and smell and the observation techniques of inspection, palpation, percussion, and auscultation.

Purpose of the Physical Examination

The purpose of the physical examination includes the following:

- To provide an indication of overall health status, including growth and development
- To provide additional information about the signifi-

cance and meaning of any symptoms reported during the interview
- To provide indicators of the person's response to various aspects of their health care

The Examination Sequence

The comprehensive physical examination is conducted in an organized manner that will ensure a complete, systematic, and efficient process. Two sequences for the conduct of the physical examination include the following:
- Head-to-toe
- Body systems

Interpreting Data

Nurses should use the functional health pattern framework to interpret the findings of the physical examination to facilitate diagnostic reasoning and the identification of problems and responses that concern nurses. A body system framework may be useful when the nurse is monitoring and treating responses to medical intervention.

Physical Examination Techniques

The four basic techniques of physical examination are:
- Inspection
- Palpation
- Percussion
- Auscultation

Physical Examination Equipment and Instruments

The comprehensive physical examination requires the use of various types of equipment and instruments. Before the examination, the equipment is assembled and organized. The examiner is familiar with the use and operation of all instruments.

Assessment Guidelines

Guidelines that are useful in the conduct of the comprehensive physical examination include the following:
- The Head-to-Toe Physical Examination
- The General Survey

Documentation

Two approaches may be used to document the physical examination:
- Narrative-style documentation of normal and abnormal findings
- Charting by exception–style of documentation of abnormal findings

---

 Critical Thinking

A 23-year-old woman presents to the hospital emergency room with severe abdominal pain. In addition to obtaining a brief history, a physical examination is required to adequately assess her and make the appropriate diagnosis.

1. Describe the primary observations you would make during the general survey of this patient.

2. Explain how the general survey would help you prioritize and organize the physical examination.

3. As you percuss the patient's abdomen, she asks you what you are doing. Demonstrate how you would explain your actions.

4. Defend the advantages of using a systematic approach as you examine each area of the body (*e.g.,* for each body area, you proceed by inspection, followed by palpation, auscultation, and finally, percussion).

Physical examination is a process involving skill and analysis. Skill is required to conduct the examination and requires attention to technique, timing, and sequence. Analysis is required to make judgments about examination findings and requires knowledge, problem solving, and creativity.

5. Specify how you would modify a head-to-toe examination sequence for an elderly woman confined to a wheelchair, who will remain seated in the wheelchair during most of the examination. The woman is hard of hearing and has left-sided weakness.

6. Plan and describe a sequence for examining the cardiovascular system for a healthy, ambulatory adult.

7. Review the physical examination results documented in Display 3-3 in this chapter. Using the data included in this example, identify indicators for each of the functional health patterns listed below:

Health Perception and Health Management
Nutrition and Metabolism
Elimination
Activity and Exercise
Cognition and Perception
Sleep and Rest
Self-Concept

BIBLIOGRAPHY

Baker, J.D. (1991). Assessment of peripheral arterial occlusive disease. *Critical Care Nursing Clinics of North America, 3*(3), 493–498.

Byers, V.B. (1973). *Nursing observation* (2nd ed.). St. Louis: C.V. Mosby.

Centers for Disease Control. (1991). Recommendations for preventing transmission of human immunodeficiency virus and hepatitis B virus to patients during exposure-prone invasive procedures. *Morbidity and Mortality Weekly Report, 40.*

Centers for Disease Control and Prevention and the Hospital Infection Control Practices Advisory Committee. (1996). *Guideline for isolation precautions in hospitals: Category 1B.* Atlanta: CDC.

Durbin, N. (1983). The application of Doppler techniques in critical care. *Focus on Critical Care, 10* (3), 44–46.

Fitzgerald, M.A. (1991). The physical exam. *RN, 54*(11), 34–39.

Gordon, M. (1987). *Nursing diagnosis: Process and application* (2nd ed.). New York: McGraw-Hill.

Holbrook, J., & Schneiderman, H. (1990). Honing physical diagnostic skills. *Patient Care, 24*(7), 123–141.

Hronek, C. (1995). Redesigning documentation: Clinical pathways, flowsheets, and variance notes. *Medical Surgical Nursing, 4.*

Littman, D. (1972). Stethoscopes and auscultation. *American Journal of Nursing, 72* (7), 1238–1241.

McConnell, W.E. (1990). Orderly assessment. *Emergency, 22* (10), 34–38.

Assessing Vital Signs

ASSESSMENT GUIDELINES

Body Temperature

Arterial Pulse

Respiratory Rate and Pattern

Blood Pressure Measurement

CHAPTER ORGANIZATION

Introductory Overview
- Interpretation of Vital Signs
- General Guidelines for Vital Sign Assessment

Body Temperature
- Anatomy and Physiology Review

Arterial Pulse
- Anatomy and Physiology Review

Respiratory Rate and Pattern
- Anatomy and Physiology Review
- Documentation

Blood Pressure
- Anatomy and Physiology Review

ＩＮＴＲＯＤＵＣＴＯＲＹ ＯＶＥＲＶＩＥＷ

Vital signs, also called *cardinal signs,* include body temperature, pulse, respiration, and blood pressure. Assessing vital signs provides a quick overview of a person's physiologic status. Vital signs also provide an indication of the intensity of other human responses such as pain, anxiety, fear, and activity tolerance.

INTERPRETATION OF VITAL SIGNS

Nurses routinely evaluate vital signs to monitor a person's physical status. Vital sign data should be interpreted in light of the person's baseline values, medical diagnoses, and medical history, medication history, and laboratory results. If deviations from normal or baseline values are detected, the nurse must determine whether additional assessment or intervention is indicated. Standard ranges for the various vital sign values in different age-groups are presented in Table 4-1.

If deviations from standard ranges are observed, you should proceed in the following manner. First, you should evaluate any deviations from "normal" in light of the person's own baseline vital signs. For example, a blood pressure of 90/60 mm Hg may deviate from the normal range for systolic blood pressure observed in published standards, but this value may represent the person's usual blood pressure and therefore be considered normal for that individual. Second, you should evaluate any deviations from normal in light of the person's overall physical status. For example, a blood pressure of 90/60 accompanied by cold, clammy skin, rapid heart rate, and decreased level of consciousness is significant and may indicate a state of shock. In this case, a life-threatening situation exists, and immediate additional assessment and intervention is required.

If deviations from normal pulse, respirations, and blood pressure are noted and if such deviations do not represent the person's baseline vital signs, additional assessment of the person should focus on the status of the following body systems: the cardiovascular system, the respiratory system, and neurologic system. Altered vital signs may be the first indication of life-threatening pathologic conditions involving these systems.

Deviations in body temperature, although significant and potentially life-threatening, do not usually indicate critical situations requiring immediate action. However,

---

TABLE 4.1 Vital Signs: Normal Range According to Age

| Age | Resting Pulse Rate* (beats/minute) | Ventilatory Rate (breaths/minute) | Blood Pressure | | Body Temperature† |
			Systolic‡ (mm Hg)	Diastolic (mm Hg)	
Newborn	120–170 Mean: 145	30–50	80±16 30–60 flush	46±16	35.9°–36.7°C (96.6°F–98.0°F) axillary
1 year	80–160 Mean: 120	20–40	96±30	66±25	36.2°–37.8°C (97.2°F–100.0°F) rectal
3 years	80–130 Mean: 106	20–30	100±25	67±23	>37.2°C (99.0°F) rectal
6 years	75–115	16–22	100±15	56±8	>37.0°C (98.6°F) oral
8 years	70–110	16–22	105±16	57±9	>37.0°C (98.6°F)
10 years	70–110	16–20	111±17	58±10	>37.0°C (98.6°F)
16 years	60–100	14–20	118±20	65±10	>36.7°C (98.1°F) oral
Adult	60–100	16–20	100–140	60–90	>36.7°C (98.1°F)
Elderly	60–100	16–20	Maximum 160	Same as adult	>36.0°C (96.8°F) oral

*After age 12, a boy's average pulse is 5 beats/minute slower than a girl's.
†Temperatures are subject to circadian rhythms in all age-groups.
‡Boys age 12 to 17 have slightly systolic blood pressure than do girls.

additional assessment is still indicated to make this type of determination.

General Guidelines for Vital Sign Assessment

When and how frequently vital signs are assessed is determined by standards of practice and the client's physical status. For example, for a postoperative patient in the first hour of recovering from general anesthesia, vital signs should be obtained frequently, every 5 to 15 minutes, until the patient's physical status meets certain recovery criteria. Hours later, when the person is fully ambulatory, vital signs may be assessed on a regular schedule or when a change occurs in the person's overall appearance or responses. Patients in acute care settings, including hospitals, are often subjected to routine monitoring of vital signs, such as once every hour, every 4 hours, or every 8 hours, depending on their health status. Vital signs are typically measured before conducting a physical examination.

Pulse, respirations, and blood pressure are influenced by diverse factors such as emotion and exercise. Therefore, every attempt should be made to measure vitals signs when the person is calm and at rest. A person who presents to a setting for blood pressure screening after climbing several flights of stairs should be seated and rested before blood pressure is taken. Vital sign values that are inconsistent with the person's baseline values should be double-checked and interpreted relative to overall physical status before therapeutic decisions are made.

BODY TEMPERATURE

Anatomy and Physiology Review

Each species has a genetically determined "set point" that represents the optimal core body temperature for maintaining normal physiologic activities. In humans, this set point is approximately 37° Centigrade (98.6° Fahrenheit), with slight variations in response to circadian rhythms, the menstrual cycle, activity, and age. The normal range of oral temperature in a resting person is 35.8°C to 37.3°C (96.4°F–99.1°F).

Body Temperature Is Influenced by the Following

- *Circadian Rhythms.* In a 24-hour period, body temperature will cycle to a low point in the early morning hours and reach a high point in the late afternoon or early evening (Fig. 4-1).
- *The Menstrual Cycle.* The basal body temperature fluctuates in women according to the phase of the menstrual cycle. After ovulation, there is a rise in the basal body temperature lasting until the beginning of the menses. If conception follows ovulation, the temperature rise will persist (Fig. 4-1).
- *Activity.* As basal metabolic activities increase, such

as occurs through the activity of skeletal muscle during exercise, the body heat increases. Internal regulating mechanisms restore the body heat to normal.
- *Age.* Infants and children may experience greater body temperature fluctuations than adults because the hypothalamus temperature-regulating mechanisms are immature. Because infants are unable to shiver, they are especially susceptible to lowered core temperatures and should be kept warm when exposed. Elders adapt slowly to changes in external temperature. An elder may feel cold when the environmental temperature is adequate because blood supply to the skin is diminished. Elders tend to have a lower body temperature than other age-groups, the average being 36.2°C (97.2° F).

Hypothalamic Regulation

The body's temperature set point is maintained through a thermostat process regulated by the hypothalamus in the brain. The thermostat maintains a balance between the effects of heat production and heat loss to maintain a relatively constant core body temperature with only minor fluctuations (±0.5°C). Heat production accompanies many activities, including food digestion, routine activities, strong emotions, and exercise. Heat loss occurs through radiation of heat away from the body, evaporation of sweat, convection, and conduction.

The hypothalamus can stimulate mechanisms to restore body heat to normal, including the following:

- *Sweating.* Sweating allows heat to escape from the body through evaporation.
- *Vasodilation.* Heat can escape the body by conduction and radiation when the blood vessels dilate.
- *Vasoconstriction.* Blood vessels can constrict and shunt blood to the body core, preserving body heat.
- *Hormone production.* An increase in thyroid hormone will increase body heat.

The hypothalamic thermostat is reset under certain conditions, such as infection. Substances released from leukocytes, called *pyrogens,* may cause an increase in body temperature to as high as 40°C (104°F) by interfering with temperature-lowering mechanisms in the hypothalamus. Controversy exists about the physiologic significance of such temperature elevation. It may represent an increase in the basal metabolic rate, which is essential for the body to fight invading organisms. Conversely, an increased temperature and basal metabolic rate lead to increased oxygen consumption in the body, which may be detrimental. Oxygen requirements increase 10% for every 1°C temperature increase. Fever may cause convulsions in young children, and tissue in the brain and other organs may be damaged as enzyme activity and transport processes are adversely affected by high temperatures. For these reasons, high temperatures associated with infections are generally considered pathologic.

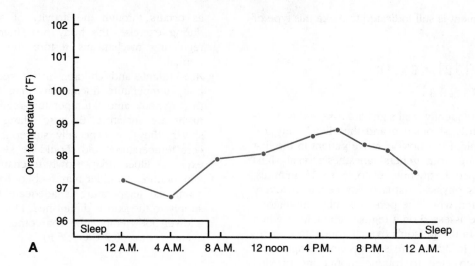

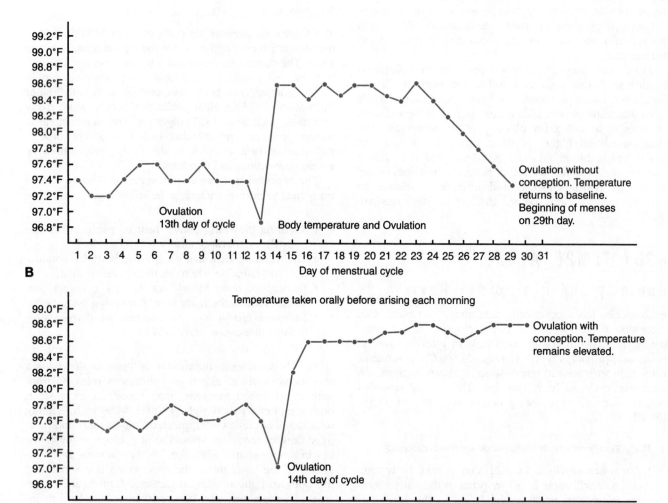

FIGURE 4.1 Body temperature variations. (**A**) Circadian variations. Note body temperature lowering during sleep. (**B** and **C**) Menstrual cycle and variations. Body temperature drops before ovulation and increases above the woman's baseline after ovulation.

Physical Examination   Body Temperature Assessment

GENERAL APPROACH

The body temperature is usually the first vital sign measured. By taking the person's temperature, you are putting the person at rest before measuring pulse, respiration, and blood pressure.

EQUIPMENT

Body temperature is determined by reading the measurement registered on a glass thermometer or an electronic thermometer, or on a monitor associated with a thermistor, such as on the tip of a thermodilution pulmonary artery catheter or Foley catheter. For an accurate reading, these instruments must be used and read correctly.

Electronic thermometers are more accurate and are preferred over glass thermometers. Electronic thermometers also afford less chance of cross-contamination because of the disposable probe covers.

SITE SELECTION AND INTERPRETATION

Body temperature may be measured at different sites, such as the mouth, the rectum, the tympanic membrane, and the axillae. Rectal and tympanic membrane measurements are considered most accurate and most closely related to core body temperature. The rectal site or tympanic membrane should be used in children under the age of 6 or for anyone who is confused, prone to seizure activity, comatose, or intubated (*e.g.,* endotracheally, nasogastrically). Some authorities recommend that rectal thermometers not be inserted in children younger than 2 years of age because of the risk of rectal perforation. The rectal method is also contraindicated after abdominoperineal resection or hemorrhoidectomy, and in persons with cardiac illness because rectal stimulation could lead to Valsalva maneuvers.

The oral method can be used in clients who are alert, cooperative, and older than 6 years of age. The client should be able to breathe through the nose and should be without oral pathology or recent oral surgery.

The axillary method is considered least accurate but is preferred for infants because it is safer than other methods.

Temperatures differ depending on measurement site. For example, rectal temperatures are usually 0.4°C (0.7°F) higher than oral temperatures, whereas axillary temperatures are 0.6°C (1°F) lower than oral temperatures. You should take into account the person's physiologic status as well as the time of day when interpreting temperatures.

ACCURACY

For accurate temperature measurement, the thermometer must be inserted properly and left in place for the required length of time. Numberous studies confirm that the optimal time for keeping oral glass thermometers in place is 8 minutes. However, this time should be increased (or the temperature reading postponed) if a hot or cold beverage was ingested immediately before the thermometer was placed in the mouth. Contrary to popular belief, oxygen administration by mask should not affect the accuracy of the reading. Electronic thermometer readings require much less time, often less than 10 seconds. Rectal glass thermometers may be left in place for 3 minutes.

EXAMINATION AND DOCUMENTATION FOCUS

Body temperature value

▼ ▼ ▼

G U I D E L I N E S

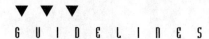

Assessment Guidelines Body Temperature

Measuring Temperature with Mercury Thermometer

Procedure

Clinical Significance

1. **Preparation:**

   a. Choose the type of thermometer to use. Use an "oral" thermometer for oral or axillary measurements and a "rectal" thermometer for rectal measurements.

   The mercury thermometer may be used for any site, but the distinctions are made to prevent cross-use and cross-contamination. Rectal thermometers are often designated with red on the blunt end.

   b. If you are taking the temperature orally, ask the person about recent ingestion of hot or cold beverages. Wait about 10 minutes before taking the temperature if hot or cold beverages were ingested.

   Hot or cold substances can alter the temperature of mouth tissues.

   c. Cleanse the thermometer. If the thermometer is stored in disinfectant solution, wipe off the disinfectant with a tissue or rinse under cold water. Wipe from the distal end to the bulb end holding the thermometer by the distal end.

   Unpleasant-tasting solutions should be removed before inserting.

   d. Shake down the thermometer to 35°C (95°F) or below. Hold the thermometer between your thumb and first finger at the distal end and shake downward by snapping the wrist.

   Be careful not to break the thermometer by shaking it too close to a hard surface (desk, tabletop).

2. **Measurement: oral temperature:**

   a. Ask the person to open his or her mouth. Place the thermometer bulb in the right or left sublingual pocket (on either side of the frenulum), and instruct the person to close the mouth and hold the thermometer in place between the lips.

   The large blood vessels in this area reflect core body heat.

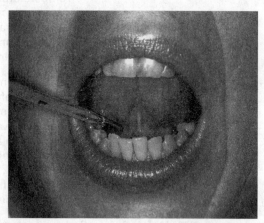

Oral temperature measurement: thermometer placement

▼ ▼ ▼

G U I D E L I N E S   *continued*   Body Temperature

Procedure

   b. Leave the thermometer in place for 4 to 11 minutes. Use this time to measure other vital signs.

   c. Remove the thermometer and wipe away any secretions with tissue from end to bulb. Hold the thermometer at eye level and read at the end of the mercury column.

   d. Wash in soapy water, then rinse and return to disinfectant solution or protective case after shaking down again.

3. **Measurement: axillary temperature:**

   a. Remove the person's clothing, exposing the arm and shoulder. Dry the axilla with a towel.

   b. Place the bulb in the center of the axilla. Fold the arm across the person's chest to keep the thermometer in place.

   c. Leave the thermometer in place for 10 minutes.

   d. Read and cleanse as you would an oral thermometer.

   e. Axillary temperatures usually register one degree lower than oral temperatures.

4. **Measurement: rectal temperature:**

   a. Lubricate the thermometer before inserting.

   b. Apply clean gloves.

   c. Place the person on the side with the knees slightly flexed. Expose the anus by lifting the buttocks. Insert the thermometer into the rectum. Point the thermometer toward the person's umbilicus, guiding it along the rectal wall. Insert the thermometer approximately 1 inch into the rectum.

   d. Hold the thermometer in place for 3 minutes.

   e. Read and cleanse the rectal thermometer as you would an oral thermometer.

   f. Rectal temperatures usually read 1 degree higher than oral temperatures.

Clinical Significance

The optimal placement time is 8 minutes (see Research Highlight at the end of this chapter), but often the peak temperature registers after 4 or 5 minutes.

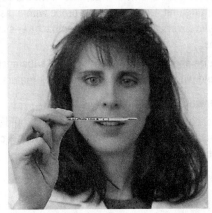

Reading the glass thermometer

Moisture should be removed from the skin to prevent a lower temperature reading through evaporation.

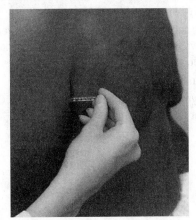

Axillary temperature measurement: thermometer placement

Never force or insert the thermometer into feces. Injury may result from improper placement.

▼ ▼ ▼

G U I D E L I N E S *continued*   Body Temperature

Measuring Temperature with Electronic Thermometers

Procedure

Clinical Significance

1. **Preparation:**
   a. Obtain the electronic thermometer from the battery-charging unit. Cover the metal probe with a disposable plastic cover according to the manufacturer's instructions.
   b. Inquire about ingestion of hot or cold substances as you would when using oral mercury thermometers.

2. **Temperature measurement:**
   a. Proceed to take the temperature as you would using a mercury thermometer by inserting the plastic-covered probe into the appropriate body area.

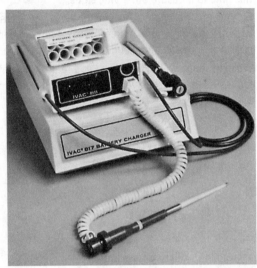

Electronic thermometer

   b. *Tympanic temperature:* Place tympanic probe in the ear canal so as to seal the opening.
   c. At the sound of the tone, note temperature reading, remove probe, and discard probe cover in the waste basket.
   d. Return thermometer to base unit.
   e. The tympanic membrane temperature is 0.8°C (1.4°F) higher than the normal oral temperature.

The blood vessels in the tympanic membrane reflect core body temperature.

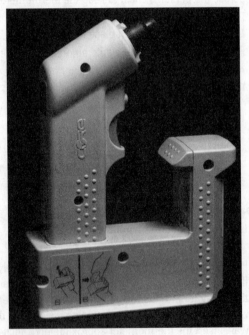

Tympanic thermometer

Documentation

Record the temperature in centigrade. You can convert between centigrade and fahrenheit with the following formulas:

- Degrees C = 5/9 (degrees F − 32)
- Degrees F = 9/5 (degrees C + 32)

Record the body temperature indicating the site used for temperature measurement. For example, (O) indicates oral, (AX) indicates axillary, and (R) indicates rectal. Temperature and other vital signs are typically recorded on flowsheets or presented graphically in the record so that trends are easily identified.

Nursing Diagnoses Related to Body Temperature Assessment

Hypothermia

Hypothermia occurs when body temperature registers between 25°C and 35°C (77°F to 95°F). In severe hypothermia, the temperature may not even register on the thermometer. Hypothermia occurs secondary to prolonged exposure to cold or administration of large volumes of unwarmed blood products. It may be induced for therapeutic purposes, such as total body cooling during heart surgery.

Physical signs of severe hypothermia include changes in the skin and cardiovascular system that are induced by cold injury. Prolonged cold causes damage to the capillary endothelium, resulting in "leaky" capillaries. When the patient is rewarmed, edema may occur as the plasma moves from the capillaries into the interstitial space. Such edema may occur in early postoperative periods following cardiopulmonary bypass surgery, during which the body temperature was lowered. The skin is usually cool to the touch, and excessive fluid shifts contribute to hypotension. The heart and respiratory rates may be severely decreased, and the person may be lethargic or unconscious. Severe hypothermia may not result in shivering, because in such cases this compensatory mechanism fails.

Frostbite is localized hypothermia, usually affecting exposed skin such as ears, fingers, or toes. Vascular injury caused by the cold may be so intense that vessel occlusion may be followed by ischemia. The initial vascular damage usually causes the affected part to appear red, changing to white as vessel occlusion progresses.

Hyperthermia

Hyperthermia, or hyperpyrexia, is an excessively high core body temperature, exceeding 39°C (102.2°F). Hyper-

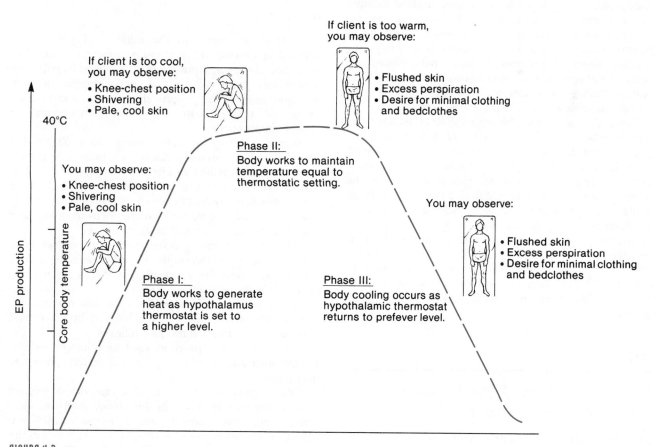

FIGURE 4.2 Three phases of fever.

thermia occurs secondary to hypothalamus damage, which may be caused by intracranial surgery, stroke, or traumatic head injury, or by the release of endogenous pyrogens from cells associated with inflammation and bacteria. Endogenous pyrogens reset the thermostat in the hypothalamus to a higher level. Consequently, higher body temperatures will be perceived as normal by the hypothalamus. In other words, a new equilibrium, defined as *fever,* will occur.

Fever Levels

Three phases of fever related to thermostat alteration have been identified. Each phase involves different assessment findings (Fig. 4-2).

Phase I occurs when the hypothalamic thermostat has been reset to a higher level. The body responds with heat-generating mechanisms as the core temperature rises from 37°C (98.6°F) to 40°C (104°F). The patient may assume a knee–chest position in an attempt to conserve body heat. Shivering may occur as the body attempts to generate necessary heat. The skin may be pale and cool to the touch, secondary to the conserving vasoconstriction.

Phase II occurs when the core temperature reaches the new thermostatic level. The body acts to protect this temperature with the usual hypothalamic mechanisms. Excessive cooling will cause shivering, and excessive temperature increases will result in cutaneous vasodilation and sweat gland secretion.

Phase III is often referred to as "breaking" the fever. Endogenous pyrogen production ceases, and the stimulus for a higher thermostat setting is removed. As the hypothalamic set point returns to its pre-fever level, hypothalamic-mediated cooling mechanisms lower body temperature. Severe diaphoresis, or diffuse perspiration, may occur as the sweat glands work to cool the body by evaporation. Placing the patient in a cooler environment or removing clothing will also help cool the body.

Some diseases show characteristic fever patterns that may be related to different patterns of endogenous pyrogen production. A sustained fever may accompany infectious diseases such as typhoid, for instance. In hyperthermia, relapsing fever alternates with periods of normal temperatures. Such a pattern may also be observed in patients with syphilis and malaria. A single daily fever spike, or remittent fever, is common in septicemic patients, whose temperatures rarely return to normal. An intermittent fever is usually characterized by diurnal variations of peaks and troughs. The patient's temperature may be high in the late afternoon and subnormal in the early morning. This pattern may occur with certain pyrogenic infections.

Clinical Problems Related to Body Temperature Assessment

Body temperature alterations may be noted with a number of pathologic conditions. Hypothermia may be ob-

served in persons with acute illnesses, including congestive heart failure, uremia, diabetes mellitus, drug overdose, respiratory failure, and hypoglycemia. The mechanism appears to be a failure of thermoregulation. Hyperthermia may be observed in persons with infectious diseases, central nervous system pathology, and heat stroke. Malignant hyperthermia is an inherited disorder characterized by a rapid increase in temperature following the administration of inhaled anesthetic agents or muscle relaxants. Malignant hyperthermia is life-threatening and represents a medical emergency.

ARTERIAL PULSE
Anatomy and Physiology Review

The arteries are strong, compliant vessels that carry oxygenated blood away from the heart to peripheral tissues. The elastic properties of the arterial walls cause the arteries to stretch during systole and recoil during diastole. The result is a palpable arterial pulse. The arterial pulse not only reflects the status of the arterial vasculature, it also provides an index of heart function. When vital signs are assessed, the pulse is evaluated primarily to determine heart rate and rhythm. However, the pulse may also be evaluated to determine vessel patency, the state of the arterial wall, and the contour and amplitude of the pulse. Related examination techniques are discussed in Chapter 8.

Pulse Rate

The pulse rate refers to the number of pulse beats counted in 1 minute. In most cases, pulse rate is equal to heart rate. However, if pulse rate is evaluated by palpating a peripheral pulse site, and the arterial pressure wave is not propagated to the peripheral site because of vascular disease or impaired heart contractility, heart rate may be faster than pulse rate.

Normal adult pulse rate ranges from 60 to 100 beats/minute. *Tachycardia* refers to a pulse rate greater than 100 beats/minute; *bradycardia* is a pulse rate less than 60 beats/minute. Children and infants generally have faster rates than adults (Table 4-1). Women have slightly faster rates than men, and elderly persons may have slightly faster rates than middle-aged adults.

Pulse rate is primarily determined by the automaticity rate of the sinoatrial (SA) node. The SA node is the normal cardiac pacemaker that spontaneously discharges at a rate of 60 to 100 times/minute.

Pulse rate is also influenced by autonomic nervous system activity, which, in turn, is influenced by the central nervous system and baroreceptor reflexes.

In the presence of psychophysiologic stressors, such as trauma, infection, fever, fear, pain, and anxiety, pulse rate may increase.

Other factors that influence pulse rate include oxygen and carbon dioxide levels in the blood, fluid and electrolyte status, drugs, exercise, and acid–base status. If you detect an alteration in pulse rate, you should investigate possible causes.

Physical Examination   Arterial Pulse Assessment

GENERAL APPROACH

For purposes of vital sign assessment, an arterial pulse is examined by auscultation or palpation to determine pulse rate and rhythm. Arterial pulses may also be examined to evaluate blood flow, arterial wall elasticity, and vessel patency. An examination of this nature is not required when eliciting vital signs but would be indicated during a comprehensive evaluation of the cardiovascular system (see Chap. 8, "Cardiovascular System").

PULSE SITES

Peripheral pulses can be palpated at areas where large arteries are close to the skin surface. Palpable pulses include the carotid, brachial, radial, femoral, popliteal, posterior tibial, and dorsalis pedis. The apical pulse may be palpated or ausculated over the heart apex as the left ventricle distends and recoils during systole and diastole. Because the radial or apical pulse sites are so accessible, they are most commonly used during vital sign assessment. An apical pulse, usually evaluated by listening with the stethoscope, is considered more accurate than a radial pulse if conditions exist that interfere with the transmission of the pulse to the periphery (*e.g.,* low cardiac output, atherosclerosis).

EQUIPMENT

Watch or clock with a second hand
Stethoscope (if pulse rate and rhythm are determined by auscultation)

EXAMINATION AND DOCUMENTATION FOCUS

Pulse rate
Pulse rhythm

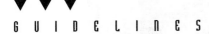

▼ ▼ ▼

G U I D E L I N E S

Assessment Guidelines   Arterial Pulse

Procedure

1. **Locate the radial pulse.**
   a. Place the pads of your first, second, and third fingers over the radial artery pulse point on the inner wrist surface over the radius.
   b. Press your fingers firmly against the artery and slowly release pressure until the pulse is palpable.

Clinical Significance

The thumb should not be used to locate the client's pulse because it has its own pulse.

Pressing too hard obliterates the pulse.

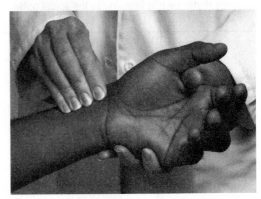

Radial pulse palpation

▼ ▼ ▼

G U I D E L I N E S *continued*   Arterial Pulse

2. **Count the pulse rate.**

   Use a watch with a second hand to count the pulse rate. If the pulse is regular, count for 30 seconds and multiply by 2. If irregular, count for a full minute and then evaluate the apical pulse, which may be more accurate.

Normal Findings

Pulse rate 60–100 beats/minute in adults (see also Table 4-1).

Deviations from Normal

A resting pulse rate less than 60 beats/minute may be considered normal in persons who participate in regular aerobic exercise.

A pulse rate greater than 100 beats/minute may be considered a normal response to exercise.

3. **Evaluate pulse rhythm.**

   Note the pulse rhythm while palpating the radial pulse.

Normal Findings

Regular rhythm

Deviations from Normal

Irregular rhythm; indicates cardiac dysrhythmias

4. **Locate the apical pulse.**

   In adults, the apical pulse is normally found at the fifth left intercostal space just medial to the midclavicular line. Palpate or auscultate the pulse with the stethoscope. Place the diaphragm of the stethoscope over the pulse site.

5. **Count the apical pulse rate.**

   Use a watch with a second hand and count the pulse for 1 full minute.

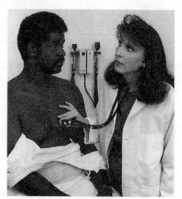

Apical pulse auscultation

6. **Identify a pulse deficit** (optional).

   a. Listen to the apical pulse while simultaneously palpating the radial pulse.

   b. Two nurses may simultaneously count the apical and radial pulses and record the difference to quantify the pulse deficit.

7. **Evaluate the pulse rhythm.**

   Note pulse rhythm while listening to the apical pulse.

A pulse deficit exists if the apical rate is greater than the radial rate. Pulse deficits may occur with dysrhythmias such as atrial fibrillation, or in severe heart failure when some heart contractions are too weak to propagate the arterial pressure wave to peripheral pulse sites. A pulse deficit also may indicate vascular disease.

Documentation

Record the pulse rate and rhythm, indicating which pulse site was used. Pulse rate and other vital signs are typically recorded on flowsheets or presented graphically in the record so that trends are easily identified. If the pulse rhythm is irregular, describe your findings in greater detail. Note also whether the pulse felt thready (weak) or strong.

Nursing Diagnoses Related to Pulse Assessment

A person with deviations from normal pulse rate, rhythm, and quality should be further evaluated for signs and symptoms of the following nursing diagnoses: Decreased cardiac output, Fluid volume deficit or excess, Altered tissue perfusion, and Activity intolerance. An increased pulse rate may also be an indicator of pain or anxiety.

Clinical Problems Related to Pulse Assessment

Pulse rate and rhythm alterations can indicate a number of pathologic conditions, including some that may be life-threatening. Pathology of the cardiovascular, respiratory, and neurologic systems can all affect the quality of the arterial pulse.

RESPIRATORY RATE AND PATTERN

Anatomy and Physiology Review

Respiration is the exchange of oxygen and carbon dioxide between the atmosphere and the cells of the body. The process of respiration includes *ventilation,* or air movement in and out of the lungs. *Breathing,* the alternate inspiration and expiration of air into and out of the lungs, is controlled by the respiratory center in the brain stem. The pons regulates respiratory rhythm, and the medulla controls respiratory rate and depth, which are affected by the carbon dioxide, hydrogen ion, and oxygen concentrations in the blood and body tissues.

Inspiration and expiration occur because of pressure changes within the lungs. Inspiratory pressure changes result primarily from muscle contraction, involving the diaphragm and external intercostal muscles. Expiration occurs passively as the muscles relax. Lung expansion is also influenced by lung and thoracic compliance (see Chap. 8). Evaluation of the respiratory system is further discussed in Chapter 8.

Physical Examination	Respiratory Rate and Pattern Assessment
GENERAL APPROACH	The respiratory rate and pattern may be observed visually by watching the person's chest rise and fall during inspiration and expiration. The examiner may also feel the chest movements by placing his or her hand over the chest.
EQUIPMENT	Watch or clock with a second hand
EXAMINATION AND DOCUMENTATION FOCUS	Respiratory (ventilatory) rate Respiratory (ventilatory) pattern

▼ ▼ ▼

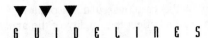

Assessment Guidelines   Respiratory Rate and Pattern

Procedure

1. **Minimize interference.**
   a. Evaluate respiratory rate while keeping your fingers on the radial pulse site, as if you are still evaluating the pulse.
   b. Alternatively, if the client is sleeping, you may count respiratory rate before assessing other vital signs.
   c. If the person appears to be holding his or her breath, a slight tap on the leg or shoulder may stimulate normal breathing.

2. **Observe the ventilatory movements.**
   a. You may either visualize or feel the person's respiratory movements. Visual observation involves watching the chest rise and fall. Tactile observation involves placing a hand on the chest to feel it rise and fall.
   b. Note also the work of breathing and the use of accessory muscles.

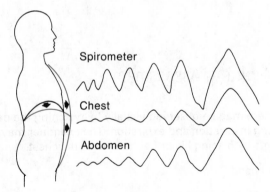

Normal breathing pattern: Inspiration is associated with downward movement of the diaphragm and outward movement of the chest and abdomen.

3. **Count the ventilatory (respiratory) rate.**
   Using a watch with a second hand, count the number of times the chest rises and falls in 30 seconds, and multiply by 2. If the respiratory rate is very slow or irregular, count for 1 full minute instead of 30 seconds.

4. **Describe the ventilatory pattern.**
   Note the rhythm, depth, and pattern of the respirations.

Clinical Significance

If the person is aware that you are counting the respiratory rate, the ventilatory pattern may be altered.

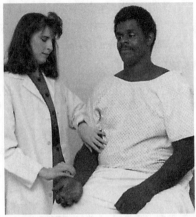

Tactile observation of the ventilatory rate

Respirations should be quiet and appear effortless. The chest and abdomen should move in a synchronous pattern.

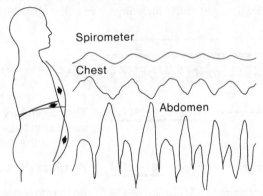

Ineffective breathing pattern: Asynchronous movement of the chest and abdomen. On inspiration, the abdomen moves inward while the chest moves outward.

Normal adult ventilatory rate: 12 to 20 breaths/minute at rest.

See "Ventilatory Patterns," Display 4-1.

Documentation

Record the respiratory rate, indicating the number of breaths per minute. Respiratory rate and other vital signs are typically recorded on flowsheets or presented graphically in the record so that trends are easily identified. The descriptive terms shown in Display 4-1 may be used to document various ventilatory patterns.

Nursing Diagnoses Related to Respiratory Rate and Pattern Assessment

A person with deviations from normal respiratory rates and patterns should be further evaluated for signs and symptoms associated with the following nursing diagnoses: Ineffective airway clearance, Ineffective breathing pattern, and Activity intolerance. An increased ventilatory rate may also be an indicator of pain or anxiety.

Clinical Problems Related to Respiratory Rate and Pattern Assessment

Alterations in respiratory rate and pattern can indicate a number of pathologic conditions, including some that may be life-threatening. Altered respiratory rates and patterns may be noted in patients with brain stem disorders, respiratory muscle dysfunction, or altered lung compliance.

BLOOD PRESSURE

Anatomy and Physiology Review

Physiologically, blood pressure is the product of cardiac output and peripheral vascular resistance. Blood pressure changes may indicate variations in cardiac output, peripheral arteriolar resistance, artery distensibility, amount of blood in the system, and blood viscosity.

Elastic properties of the arterial walls allow the arteries to stretch during systole and recoil during diastole. In addition to providing a palpable arterial pulse, this arterial activity accounts for the physiologic principle behind blood pressure measurement. Systolic blood pressure represents the maximum arterial pressure at the peak of systole, and diastolic blood pressure represents the lowest level of arterial pressure at the end of diastole. The difference between the systolic and diastolic blood pressures is the pulse pressure.

Blood pressure may be measured directly, with invasive arterial catheters connected to pressure-transducer systems, or indirectly, with a sphygmomanometer. Only the indirect method is discussed here.

Korotkoff Sounds. During indirect blood pressure measurement, a stethoscope is used to auscultate *Korotkoff sounds.* Korotkoff sounds reflect changes in blood flow through the artery as sphygmomanometer cuff pressure is released and the artery goes from a state of complete occlusion to maximum patency. Korotkoff sounds are generated as normal laminar blood flow is disrupted by cuff pressure, and resulting turbulent flow creates vessel wall vibrations. There are five distinct sound phases (Fig. 4-3).

Phase I sounds are the first sounds heard as the sphygmomanometer cuff pressure is released. The point at which sounds are first audible represents the systolic blood pressure. The sounds can be heard as clear tapping that gradually increases in intensity for a brief period, generated by rapid distension of the artery wall as the blood suddenly rushes into the previously collapsed artery. Sound intensity is related to the force of the blood flow.

Phase II sounds have a murmur-like or swishing quality. Murmurs represent turbulent blood flow and subsequent vessel wall vibration, created as blood flows from the relatively narrowed artery, caused by cuff inflation, to the wider artery lumen distal to the cuff.

Phase III sounds are clear, tapping sounds similar to phase I sounds, but more intense. Increased sound pitch and volume distinguish phase II from phase III sounds. During phase III, blood flow occurs during systole, but cuff pressure remains high enough to collapse the vessel during diastole.

Phase IV sounds are different from the previous sounds

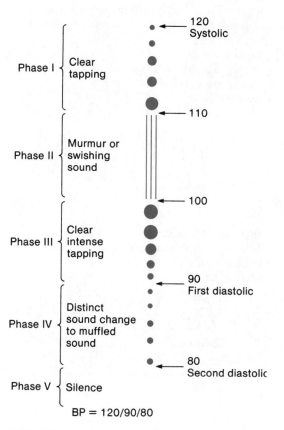

FIGURE 4.3 Korotkoff sounds: five phases.

DISPLAY 4.1

Ventilatory Patterns

NORMAL VENTILATORY PATTERN

- 12 to 20 breaths per minute
- Average tidal volume 350–500 mL (adults)
- Regular, occasional sigh breath
- Inspiration to expiration (I:E) ratio 1:2

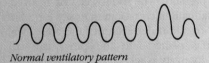

Normal ventilatory pattern

TACHYPNEA

- Rapid rate (>20 breaths per minute)
- Shallow—small tidal volume with each breath
- May be associated with CO_2 retention
- Regular rhythm
- I:E ratio approaches 1:1

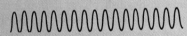

Tachypnea

HYPERVENTILATION

(Also called *central neurogenic hyperventilation* if secondary to lower midbrain or upper pons lesions, or *Kussmaul's breathing* when secondary to diabetic coma.)

- Rapid rate
- Deep—large tidal volumes
- May be associated with CO_2 loss
- Usually regular
- I:E ratio approaches 1:1

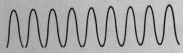

Hyperventilation

BRADYPNEA

- Slow rate (<12 breaths per minute)
- Tidal volumes vary depending on the cause
- Regular
- I:E ratio 1:2

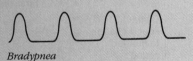

Bradypnea

CHEYNE-STOKES RESPIRATION

- Variable rate
- Apneic periods alternate with hyperventilation
- Depth of each breath varies in a cyclical pattern: shallow before and after apnea, deep with hyperventilation
- Regular-irregular—crescendo-decrescendo pattern

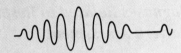

Cheyne-Stokes breathing

APNEA

- Complete cessation of breathing
- May be of a temporary nature

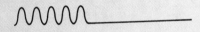

Apnea

BIOT'S BREATHING (ATAXIA)

- Variable rate
- Apnea alternates with breathing periods
- Depth variable—predominantly shallow
- Unpredictable irregularity

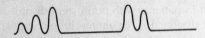

Biot's breathing (ataxia)

OBSTRUCTIVE BREATHING

- Noted with obstructive pulmonary disease
- Rate increases as air trapping occurs
- Becomes shallower with air trapping
- Longer expiratory phase

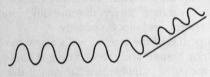

Obstructive breathing

in their muffled quality. The first diastolic sound occurs when the sound changes from a tapping to a muffled sound, and represents the diastolic blood pressure.

Phase V occurs when the sounds cannot be heard because normal laminar blood flow has been restored. The second diastolic sound occurs at the reading when the muffled sound first disappears.

Auscultatory Gap. Occasionally, if the person is hypertensive, no sounds will be heard between the systolic and diastolic pressures. This silence is called the auscultatory gap and may last for 10 to 20 mm Hg. The auscultatory gap, if not detected, represents a possible source of error in blood pressure measurement because phase III sounds may be mistaken for phase I sounds.

Blood Pressure Ranges. Normal blood pressure ranges for adults are 100 to 140 mm Hg systolic and 60 to 90 mm Hg diastolic (see Table 4-1). Blood pressure readings consis-

tently greater than 140/90 in adults may indicate hypertension. Few guidelines are available for the lower limits of hypertension in children.

Factors Affecting Arterial Blood Pressure. An abnormal blood pressure should be investigated to determine contributing factors. Arterial blood pressure is affected by the following factors:

- Cardiac output
- Heart rate
- Systemic vascular resistance
- Arterial elasticity
- Blood volume
- Blood viscosity
- Age
- Body surface area
- Exercise
- Emotions

Physical Examination   Blood Pressure Assessment

GENERAL APPROACH

Blood pressure may be measured by a number of methods: indirectly, by palpating an arterial pulse distal to a blood pressure cuff; indirectly, by auscultating Korotkoff sounds distal to a blood pressure cuff; or directly, by means of a catheter placed in an artery. A complete cardiovascular examination requires blood pressure evaluation on both arms.

EQUIPMENT

Stethoscope and Doppler Probe

Korotkoff sounds can be detected by listening over a pulse site distal to the blood pressure cuff. Usually, the sounds can be heard by placing the diaphragm of the stethoscope over the pulse site. If it is difficult to hear the sounds, use the bell (Kototkoff sounds are low frequency). If you still cannot hear the Korotkoff sounds, place a Doppler probe over the artery. You can also palpate the artery in the same manner as taking a pulse. Inflate the cuff, and record the point at which the first beat is palpated during cuff deflation as the systolic blood pressure. The diastolic pressure cannot be determined by palpation.

Sphygmomanometer

The term sphygmomanometer refers to the blood pressure cuff, connecting tubes, air pump, and pressure manometer (Fig. 4-4).

Blood Pressure Cuff.   Korotkoff sounds are generated when arterial flow properties are altered by inflation of the blood pressure cuff. The cuff has an air-distensible bladder and is covered with cloth. A rubber tube connects the air bladder to a hand-held rubber air pump used to inflate the cuff. Another rubber tube attaches to the manometer and indicates air pressure within the cuff. The entire cuff can be wrapped around the extremity and secured with Velcro or hooks.

For accurate measurement, the cuff should be wide enough to cover two thirds of the upper arm or upper thigh and long enough to completely encircle the extremity. For the average adult arm, a 12- to 14-cm-wide cuff should be sufficient. For the arm of the obese adult or when the pressure is taken at the thigh, use an 18- to 20-cm-wide cuff. Small cuffs are available for children. If the cuff is too small, an abnormally high blood pressure reading may result. Similarly, if the cuff is too large, the blood pressure may be underestimated.

(continued)

Physical Examination   Blood Pressure Assessment (continued)

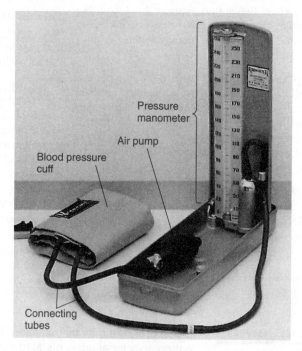

FIGURE 4.4   Sphygmomanometer.

Pressure Manometer.   The pressure manometer is the instrument that displays cuff pressure in millimeters of mercury (mm Hg), an indirect reading of the person's blood pressure. There are two types of pressure manometers: the aneroid instrument, which uses a needle that points to numbers on a calibrated dial, and the mercury manometer, which uses the height of a mercury column in a glass tube to indicate the pressure. The mercury manometer is read by looking at the mercury column meniscus at eye level and reading the corresponding number. Mercury manometers are more accurate simply because they do not require calibration. Aneroid manometers are calibrated against mercury manometers by using a Y connector between the two manometers.

POSITIONING

The person may be standing, seated, or supine during blood pressure measurement. An orthostatic or standing blood pressure should be evaluated by first measuring the pressure while the person is supine and then while he or she is sitting and standing. If the orthostatic value is significantly lower (>30 mm Hg), orthostatic hypotension is indicated and may point to excessive volume depletion, prolonged immobility, or neurologic disease.

The extremity that is being used for blood pressure measurement should be positioned at a level equal to or lower than the heart to avoid a false low reading. If the arm is used for measuring blood pressure, the forearm should be in a relaxed position (*e.g.,* resting on a tabletop). Alternatively, the person's forearm can be placed over your forearm.

REPEATING THE PROCEDURE

Occasionally, you may deflate the cuff too rapidly, or there may be another reason to question the accuracy of the blood pressure reading. In such a case you should repeat the blood pressure measurement. Before rechecking the pressure, completely deflate the cuff and wait for 1 minute, allowing for normal blood flow to return and ensuring that Korotkoff sounds are generated from a baseline flow state.

NONINVASIVE ELECTRONIC MEASUREMENT

Electronic devices are available for continuous noninvasive indirect blood pressure monitoring. A blood pressure cuff is applied to the person's arm, but the rubber connecting tubes attach to an electronic monitoring and inflation device rather than to a hand-held pump and manometer.

▼ ▼ ▼
GUIDELINES

Procedure

1. **Apply the blood pressure cuff.**

   Caution: Never apply a blood pressure cuff to an extremity where a hemodialysis access device such as a shunt or AV fistula is in place.

   a. *Upper arm:* Wrap the completely deflated blood pressure cuff snugly and smoothly around the client's bare upper arm. The bottom of the cuff should be approximately 1 inch above the antecubital space (closer in infants), and the center of the air bladder should be directly above the brachial artery.

   b. *Leg:* Wrap the blood pressure cuff around the thigh with the bottom of the cuff 1 inch above the knee. The remainder of the procedure for blood pressure measurement in the leg is similar to that for arm blood pressure measurement except that Korotkoff sounds should be auscultated over the popliteal artery.

2. **Estimate the systolic blood pressure by palpation** (optional after baseline established).

   a. Palpate the radial artery with the fingertips of your nondominant hand.

   b. Inflate the cuff while simultaneously palpating the artery. Close the valve on the air pump by turning it clockwise between the thumb and first finger of your dominant hand, and then squeeze the bulb.

   c. Note the point on the manometer at which the radial artery pulsation is no longer palpable.

   d. Inflate the cuff 20 mm Hg above this point when measuring the auscultated blood pressure.

Clinical Significance

Repeated occlusion of the device may contribute to clotting and limit the life-span of the device.

Inaccurate cuff placement may result in inaccurate BP measurement.

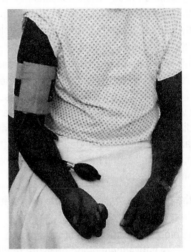

Blood pressure cuff placement

The systolic blood pressure values read 10 to 20 mm Hg higher in the leg than in the arm.

This method prevents measurement errors that might occur by not inflating the cuff high enough, or errors caused by the presence of an auscultatory gap. This step may be omitted if you are familiar with the client's usual blood pressure.

This provides a rough estimate of the systolic pressure.

▼ ▼ ▼

G U I D E L I N E S *continued*   Blood Pressure Measurement

Procedure	**Clinical Significance**

Procedure

3. **Auscultate the blood pressure.**

   a. Find the brachial artery by palpation. Place the diaphragm or the bell of the stethoscope over the brachial artery site.

   b. Inflate the cuff. Close the valve on the air pump by turning it clockwise between the thumb and first finger of your dominant hand, and then squeeze the bulb.

   c. Slowly deflate the cuff while auscultating the brachial artery. Deflate the cuff at a rate of 2 to 3 mm Hg per second by turning the air pump valve counterclockwise.

   d. Note the Korotkoff sounds and manometer readings. As the cuff is deflated, note the manometer reading when the first Korotkoff sound is heard. This is the systolic blood pressure. Read the first diastolic pressure at the point when the sounds become muffled. Read the second diastolic pressure at the point when the sound disappears completely. Finish deflating the cuff and remove, unless a second measurement is necessary. Wait 1 minute before reinflating.

4. **Repeat the procedure on the opposite extremity** (initial examination only).

   Check the blood pressure in the other arm and note any differences. Take subsequent blood pressure readings on the arm with the higher pressure.

Clinical Significance

Inflate the cuff until the manometer reading is 20 mm Hg above the client's usual systolic value.

Rapid deflation results in inaccurate readings.

Read the manometer at eye level to avoid error.

A 5- to 10-mm Hg difference is normal.

Greater pressure differences may indicate coarctation of the aorta, aortic aneurysm, or impaired blood flow to the upper arm arteries.

Documentation

The American Heart Association recommends that three blood pressure readings be recorded: the systolic, first diastolic, and second diastolic pressures. The recording would appear as follows: 130/82/26. Despite this recommendation, many health care providers record only the systolic and first diastolic readings, such as 112/70.

Record the blood pressure, indicating the extremity used and the client's position in order to make accurate comparisons. For example, "RA sit" indicates the use of the right arm with the person in the sitting position. Blood pressure, as well as other vital signs, is typically recorded on flowsheets or presented graphically in the record so that trends are easily identified.

Nursing Diagnoses Related to Blood Pressure Measurement

A person with deviations from normal blood pressure should be further evaluated for signs and symptoms associated wih the following nursing diagnoses: Decreased cardiac output, Fluid volume deficit or excess, Altered tissue perfusion, and Activity intolerance. An increased blood pressure may also be an indicator of pain or anxiety.

If a person has a medical diagnosis of hypertension, those nursing diagnoses that are associated with management of a complex and chronic disease should also be considered, including Noncompliance and Altered health maintenance.

ND_x

Clinical Problems Related to Blood Pressure Measurement

Hypertension

Hypertension is an intermittent or sustained elevation of systolic or diastolic blood pressure. Adults are diagnosed as having hypertension when the diastolic blood pressure is observed to be greater than 90 mm Hg or higher on at least two consecutive clinical assessments, or when the systolic blood pressure is greater than 140 mm Hg on at least two consecutive visits. Persons with hypertensive disease may have combined systolic and diastolic hypertension or isolated systolic hypertension.

Primary (essential) hypertension affects about 90% of all hypertensive individuals and occurs when there is no known cause for the elevated blood pressure. Secondary hypertension refers to elevated blood pressure that is related to some other underlying disease, such as renal failure or arteriosclerosis.

Risk factors for the development of primary hypertension include the following: family history of hypertension, advancing age, male gender, black race, obesity, high sodium intake, diabetes mellitus, cigarette smoking, and excessive alcohol intake.

Orthostatic (Postural) Hypotension

Orthostatic (postural) hypotension is a drop in both systolic and diastolic blood pressure when a person moves to an upright or standing position. For example, if the person has his or her blood pressure recorded as 138/88 while in a seated position and the value is recorded as 100/60 after standing, orthostatic hypotension exists. Additional observations may be noted as the person assumes an upright position, including dizziness, blurring or loss of vision, and fainting.

Orthostatic hypotension is associated with dehydration or volume depletion, antihypertensive medications, and prolonged immobility.

CHAPTER 4 S U M M A R Y

Vital Signs
The vital signs are typically measured at the beginning of the physical examination and include the following:
- Body Temperature
- Pulse
- Respiration
- Blood Pressure

Vital signs are interpreted against standard normal ranges and in light of the person's overall physical status, age, and activity level. The frequency of vital sign measurement and evaluation is determined by the clinical situation and setting.

Knowledge Base for Assessment
Knowledge of the anatomy and physiology of body temperature control and regulation, arterial pulse, respiration, and blood pressure provides a foundation for the evaluation of the vital signs.

Assessment Guidelines
Guidelines for the measurement and evaluation of vital signs include the following:

- Body Temperature
- Arterial Pulse
- Respiration
- Blood Pressure

Diagnostic Reasoning
Nursing diagnoses associated with vital sign variations include the following:
- Hypothermia
- Hyperthermia
- Ineffective thermoregulation
- Decreased cardiac output
- Fluid volume deficit (or excess)
- Altered tissue perfusion
- Activity intolerance
- Ineffective airway clearance
- Ineffective breathing pattern
- Pain
- Anxiety

Critical Thinking

You are conducting a routine physical examination of a 40-year-old man who is obese and in poor cardiovascular condition. He has just been seated in the examination room and appears out of breath and perspiring. The physical examination begins with the measurement of his vital signs.

1. Determine and discuss any additional background information about this person that would be useful as you evaluate his vital signs.

2. Propose and discuss several alternative explanations for an elevated blood pressure in this person.

3. Specify how you would minimize error when measuring this person's blood pressure.

4. Explain how you would further evaluate hyperventilation in this person.

5. You are unable to locate the radial pulse. Identify and explain your next actions.

BIBLIOGRAPHY

American Heart Association. (1987). *Recommendations for measuring human blood pressure determination by sphygmomanometer.* Publication No. 7001005. Dallas: AHA.

American Heart Association. (1980). *Recommendations for human blood pressure determination by sphygmomanometer.* Publication No. 70-019B, 80-100M. Dallas: AHA.

Cooper, K.M. (1992). Measuring blood pressure the right way. *Nursing 92, 22*(4), 75.

Erikson, R. (1980). Oral temperature differences in relation to thermometer and technique. *Nursing Research, 29,* 157–164.

Guyton, A.C. (1991). *Textbook of medical physiology* (8th ed.). Philadelphia: W.B. Saunders.

Hahn, W.K., et al. (1989). Blood pressure norms for healthy young adults: Relation to sex, age, and reported parental hypertension. *Research in Nursing and Health, 12,* 53–56.

Henneman, E.A., & Henneman, P.L. (1989). Intricacies of blood pressure measurement. Reexamining the rituals. *Heart and Lung, 18*(3), 263–273.

Hill, M.N. (1980). Hypertension: What can go wrong when you measure blood pressure. *American Journal of Nursing, 80*(5), 942–945.

Hollerbach, A., & Sneed, N. (1990). Accuracy of radial pulse assessment by length of counting interval. *Heart and Lung, 19*(3), 258–264.

US Department of Health and Human Services Report of the Second Task Force on Blood Pressure Control in Children. (1987). Bethesda, MD: National Institutes of Health.

US Department of Health and Human Services Report of the Joint National Committee on Detection, Evaluation, and Treatment of High Blood Pressure. (1988). Bethesda, MD: National Institutes of Health.

US Department of Health and Human Services (1993). The fifth report of the Joint National Committee on Detection, Evaluation, and Treatment of High Blood Pressure. *Archives of Internal Medicine, 153,* 154–183.

UNIT TWO

Health Assessment of Human Function

5. Assessing Health Perception and Health Management

6. Assessing Nutrition and Metabolism

7. Assessing Elimination

8. Assessing Activity and Exercise

9. Assessing Cognition and Perception

10. Assessing Sleep and Rest

11. Assessing Self-Concept

12. Assessing Roles and Relationships

13. Assessing Sexuality and Reproductive Patterns

14. Assessing Stress and Coping

15. Assessing Values and Beliefs

Assessing Health Perception and Health Management

ASSESSMENT GUIDELINES

Health Perception Interview (Health History)

Health Maintenance–Health Perception: Physical Assessment

CHAPTER ORGANIZATION

Introductory Overview

Assessment Focus
- Data Collection Methods
- Nursing Diagnoses

Knowledge Base for Assessment
- Health Maintenance
- Promoting Health

- Preventing Diseases
- Health Behaviors
- Risks to Health
- Environmental Safety

Health Perception–Health Management Pattern Assessment

INTRODUCTORY OVERVIEW

Health maintenance is based on the concept of health and an individual's ability to maintain a desired health status. A change in any body system can have a profound effect on health maintenance. Health maintenance is the foundation for planning short- and long-term objectives for individual health care. For example, the diagnosis of diabetes mellitus results in the individual learning new knowledge/behaviors about a health care regimen, dietary guidelines, and lifestyle changes. How the individual manages these changes will directly affect his or her health. Additionally, the new diagnosis impacts on the family's ability to manage the health of all of its members.

Health has been an evolving and elusive concept to define. The World Health Organization in 1986 defined health as a "state of complete physical, mental, and social well-being and not merely the absence of disease and infirmity" (p. 1). Different nursing theorists have proposed different definitions of health. For example, Florence Nightingale in 1860 (1969) defined health as "not only to be well, but to use well every power that we have"; Jean Watson (1985): "health refers to unity and harmony within the mind, body, and soul. Health is also associated with the degree of congruence between the self as perceived and the self as experienced" (p. 48); Betty Neuman (1989): health "is reflected in the level of wellness. When system needs are met, a state of optimal wellness exists; conversely, unmet needs reduce the wellness state" (p. 71); and Callista Roy (1984): "health is defined as a state and a process of being and becoming an integrated and whole person" (p. 39). Nola Pender (1995), a nurse and health promotion theorist, defines health as

> the actualization of inherent and acquired human potential through goal-directed behavior, competent self-care, and satisfying relationships with others while adjustments are made as needed to maintain structural integrity and harmony with relevant environments (p. 22)

Finally, in 1986, the Ottawa Charter for Health Promotion stated that

> Health is created and lived by people within the settings of their everyday life; where they learn, work, play and love. Health is created by caring for oneself and others, by being able to make decisions and have control over one's life circumstances, and by ensuring that the society one lives in creates conditions that allow the attainment of health by all members. (World Health Organization, 1986b)

Just as health professionals and organizations have different definitions of health, people and families the nurse interact with have different perceptions of the meaning of health. Individual and family meanings of health can be influenced by cultural and religious beliefs, learning/knowledge, and past experiences. These factors do influence interventions that nurses use to assist people in attaining and maintaining health. Traditionally, professional nurses have recognized the responsibility to promote and protect health rather than merely to treat illnesses. Florence Nightingale identified two types of nursing: health nursing and illness nursing. The speciality of community health nursing is dedicated to promoting and protecting the health of populations. In its 1980 Social Policy Statement, the American Nurses' Association states that nurses are responsible for maintaining and managing clients' routine health practices during wellness as well as during illness. However, health promotion and protection depend on how people perceive health and their ability to manage health activities within their environment. To assist people in maintaining optimal health, it is important to identify their health perceptions, health practices, promotion and preventive practices, and barriers to achieving or maintaining a desired health state.

ASSESSMENT FOCUS

Assessing an individual's health perceptions and health management abilities involves conducting a general inspection of the person's appearance, evaluating health habits, self-care abilities, health risks, self-examination techniques, and comparing data in the health history with observations. It also includes identifying safety hazards or health threats in the person's home and immediate environment. With a comprehensive assessment of health maintenance, the nurse will meet the following objectives:

- Identifying the individual's definition of health and perceptions of health status
- Evaluating biological, lifestyle, and environmental risk factors that may negatively impact health status
- Evaluating barriers and enhancements to maintaining/improving health status
- Evaluating ability to perform self-care and self-examination skills for health management
- Identifying new health behaviors/knowledge the individual desires

Data Collection Methods

Data collection is accomplished by the following methods:

Interview or Review of Records

Health Perception Focus

- The individual's definition of health
- The value the client places on health

Health Management Focus

- Factors influencing health management
- Risk factors that might disrupt health
- The client's ability to manage health, including performance of self-care and self-examination skills

Laboratory/X-ray Evaluation

- Focus is on promoting health
- Laboratory tests recommended by US Preventive Services Task Force for adults younger than 65 years of age (also see the following chapters for pregnancy and other age-group recommendations: sexuality and reproduction [Chapter 12], children and adolescents [Chapter 16], and elders [Chapter 17]):
  - Total blood cholesterol
  - Papanicolaou (Pap) test (women)
  - Mammogram
  - Fecal occult blood test or sigmoidoscopy

Physical Examination/Observations

- Observe for indicators of overall health status
- Signs of health maintenance capabilities
- Observation of risk factors
- Observation of self-care and self-examination techniques
- Preventive health screening activities
- Observation of the environment

The data that the nurse obtains should be analyzed in connection with cultural, psychosocial, developmental, and physiologic influences on health and related preventive practices. Thorough assessment of health perception and health management behavior will help identify and understand the client's strengths and risks and enable the nurse to plan with the individual or family appropriate nursing services. The components of the assessment for this pattern is a synthesis of all the other patterns. Gordon (1994) states that health perception-health management pattern is the "umbrella pattern": that all other patterns can be viewed as specific areas of health management. The goal of this pattern is to identify health strengths, health beliefs, health risks, and health deficits for which improvements are possible to maximize health status.

Nursing Diagnoses

Primary Nursing Diagnoses

Assessment of health perception and health management may result in the identification of one or more of the following NANDA nursing diagnoses:

High risk for aspiration
High risk for infection
High risk for injury
High risk for poisoning
High risk for suffocation
High risk for trauma
Altered growth and development
Altered health maintenance
Ineffective management of therapeutic regimen: individual
Ineffective management of therapeutic regimen: family
Effective management of therapeutic regimen
Altered protection
Health-seeking behaviors
Noncompliance (specify)

Secondary Nursing Diagnoses

Additional factors may contribute to health maintenance problems. These may include but are not limited to the nursing diagnoses of

Impaired adjustment
Altered family processes
Impaired home maintenance/management
Impaired mobility
Ineffective individual or family coping
Fatigue
Impaired memory
Knowledge deficit (specify)
Self-care deficit (specify)
Spiritual distress
Altered thought process

Stolte, in her text *Wellness: Nursing Diagnosis for Health Promotion* (1996), also suggests that nurses should use wellness nursing diagnoses as well as problem-oriented NANDA diagnoses. The use of wellness diagnoses acknowledges that healthy client responses are within the nursing domain. Additionally, wellness diagnoses recognize individual strengths and provide a more holistic picture of the client and nursing practice. Some nurses in the attempt to use NANDA taxonomy for wellness have changed existing NANDA diagnoses modifiers from negative to positive, such as *adequate, effective,* or *healthy* in place of *inadequate, ineffective,* and *impaired.* In the Health Perception and Health Management Pattern, there are two approved NANDA nursing diagnoses that are wellness focused: effective management of therapeutic regimen and health-seeking behavior. Possible wellness diagnoses for health management identified by Stolte and others include

Positive self-care strategies
Increasing compliance with prescribed treatment
Adequate immunization status
Assuming responsibility for health
Adequate health maintenance
Correct breast-self examination technique

KNOWLEDGE BASE FOR ASSESSMENT

Assessment of health perception and health management is based on understanding such concepts as health maintenance, promoting health, disease prevention, health behaviors, and health risks.

Health Maintenance

Health maintenance refers to activities people engage in to maintain a satisfactory level of health and includes responsible behavior such as exercising regularly, managing stress, receiving scheduled immunizations, and eating a balanced diet. Without responsible management, health cannot be maintained for an extended time.

Promoting Health

In 1990, the US Department of Health and Human Services put forth a set of objectives for the health of the US population (*Healthy People 2000*). The emphases of those objectives were on health promotion, health protection, and preventive services. Three specific overall goals were established: increasing the span of health life; reducing health disparity among Americans; and access to preventives services for all Americans. Nurses can and do have a major role in achieving these national goals through traditional and advanced practice activities. The health perception and health management functional health pattern is closely associated with *Healthy People 2000* objectives and outcomes. Health promotion includes activities that assist a person to develop internal and external resources to maintain or enhance physical, psychological, and social well-being. Such activities are not usually directed at any particular disease or condition but seek to enhance general well-being. Health promotion involves self-assessment, professional assessment, and health screening. Self-

assessments can be performed by any individual at home (*e.g.,* breast self-examination for women and testicular self-examination for men to detect for signs of cancer). Many self-assessment tools are available to instruct individuals on how to conduct self-examinations; these are often available in brochures distributed by hospitals and clinics or in books available at a general book store or library. For example, brochures published by the American Cancer Society ("Breast Self-Examination" and "Testicular Self-Examination"); *The New Our Bodies Our Selves* (The Boston Women's Health Book Collective, 1992); *50 Simple Things You Can Do To Save Your Life* (Faculty of the UCLA School of Public Health, 1991); and *Readers Digest: The Good Health Fact Book* (Shuher, 1992). Numerous hospitals and other health agencies provide information to the public via telephone call-in programs. Additionally, people are getting information via the World Wide Web on the Internet. The American Cancer Society, the American Heart Association, and similar organizations maintain websites. Numerous other health-related web pages are available on the Internet.

Professional health assessment and health screenings are conducted by health professionals, usually in a local clinic, hospitals, or schools. Occasionally, organizations or corporations may sponsor special health screenings (*i.e.,* blood pressure measurement, blood cholesterol levels, glaucoma testing) at various convenient locations such as a shopping mall or community center or in a special mobile unit. These special promotional screenings are usually announced by the local media and are a good opportunity for people to obtain a health screening either free or at a minimal charge at a convenient location.

Health promotion has two levels of intention: individual and populations. Individual health promotion is associated with personal lifestyle choices within the social setting, such as physical activity and fitness, tobacco/drug alcohol use, and family planning. Promoting health at the population level (known as health protection) is associated with environmental and regulatory measures designed to protect large population groups. Examples of health protection interventions are occupational safety and health regulations, fluoridation of public water, and safe playground designs. Nurses in settings other than public health departments have been involved in health promotion and protection activities such as tobacco cessation programs, lobbying for automobile restraint laws, parenting and childbirth preparation classes, and stress-management programs.

Preventing Diseases

Health care providers have traditionally advocated the prevention of diseases or illnesses by screening presumably healthy people. The concept of the annual physical examination was initially endorsed by the American Medical Association in the 1920s. In 1903 Lillian Wald demonstrated in the first school nurse project that nurses were effective in reducing the number of sick school days through early detection and treatment of health problems, control of contagious diseases, and health teaching. With the entry of school nurses, school records document that

98% of children previously excluded from school for health reasons were attending classes (Stanhope & Lancaster, 1996). Today, preventive health screening activities are divided into three levels: primary, secondary, and tertiary prevention.

Primary prevention refers to practices that prevent disease and injury from occurring. The focus is prevention before any pathology. Examples of strategies include immunizations, carseat restraints, and proper dental hygiene. Individual lifestyle behaviors also can be in this category; for example, reducing risk of developing hypertension by diet management, weight control, exercise program, and avoiding tobacco products. Clearly, primary prevention is the most cost-efficient approach to health management.

Secondary prevention includes measures to detect possible health problems at an early stage of development. The focus is early detection of health problems at the subclinical level so that early treatment will either rid the person of the condition or minimize or control the effects and prevent further problems. All screening programs in which the target population does not have the specific health problem are examples of secondary prevention. Examples include screenings for hypertension, scoliosis, colorectal cancer, developmental problems of children (Denver Development Screening Tests), breast cancer (mammography and self breast examination), diabetes (blood glucose tests), and cystic fibrosis and amniocentesis (chromosomal testing). When establishing screening clinics, tests or measurements should be appropriate for the target group. Screening for sickle cell anemia, which usually affects people of African heritage, would not be appropriate in a neighborhood of Vietnam immigrants. Similarly, if a target population worked from 8 AM to 5 PM weekdays, a screening clinic would be most efficient in the evenings or weekends. The availability of appropriate referrals and counseling for individuals with positive (abnormal) findings is essential and ethically mandated.

The early detection of diseases through screenings is linked with substantial reduction in morbidity (occurrence of a disease) and mortality (death of a disease). For example, the mortality rate for strokes has decreases 50% since 1972, primarily through early detection and treatment of hypertension (US Preventive Services Task Force, 1996). Screening tests are not diagnostic in nature but serve to identify individuals who need further diagnostic procedures. Screening tests should be accurate to detect those with a condition even when only a small indicator of the condition is present. However, the test needs to be specific enough that false positives rarely occur.

Tertiary prevention includes activities that promote maximum health *after* disability has occurred. Such activities may be carried out through self-help groups such as Alcoholics Anonymous and Reach for Recovery (a program to help postmastectomy patients). Nurses direct or co-direct programs such as cardiac rehabilitation, diabetic self-care programs, and rehabilitation programs for children with developmental disabilities. Tertiary prevention also includes monitoring of health problems through clinics such as a hypertension clinic where blood pressure is measured and referral to appropriate health provider when readings are beyond expected limits. People with hypertension may be monitored in a hypertension screening clinic, so that two levels of prevention occur simultaneously.

Health Behaviors

Self-Directed Behavior

An individual's level of health should be the result of individual choice based on genetic predisposition, knowledge, capabilities, and the amount of energy he or she is willing to expend on health behaviors. The ability of the person to choose a lifestyle and maintain that lifestyle is dependent on the person's internal and external resources. The individual's choice may not always be consistent with health knowledge and health professional values. For example, some people continue to use tobacco products in spite of information about hazards to health. However, if a person who uses tobacco is willing to eat properly, exercise regularly, and limit the amount of tobacco, then that person's health, although compromised by tobacco use, is enhanced by other conscious health-promoting behaviors.

Adherence Behavior

People have always based decisions about their health and health care on beliefs, perceived capabilities, knowledge, and resources. People determine when and to what extent a health professional should be consulted for health issues. Today, there is also a strong emphasis on containing health care costs, and individuals are encouraged to assume more responsibility to contain costs and maintain their health. Concurrently, people are changing their attitudes about health care, the relationship with healthcare providers, and participation in movements for consumer rights and self-care. More information about health, health options, and alternative health practices is available to the public via many avenues, including the Internet.

Adherence to prescribed health regimens is believed to help contain health costs. Conditions that increase the likelihood of people adhering to prescribed health regimens include the following:

- Participation in formulating the health regimen
- Informed agreement to the health regimen
- Knowledge of the problem or risk factor(s)
- Knowledge of available options and consequences
- Motivation
- History of success with health regimens
- Practical and noncomplex health regimen

Setting goals with healthcare providers assists clients in adhering to healthcare regimens. Short- and long-term goals are established, and target dates are set for evaluating how close the person has come to achieving goals. In addition, when people make agreements with themselves, they have a vested interest in achievement. Because experiences affect motivation, a person who has been unable to adhere to previous healthcare regimens is at greater risk for failure. Examine possible causes of failures, such as noninvolvement in setting the healthcare regimen, low expectation of success, and the cost of following the regimen. Success increases motivation and improves beliefs of self-efficacy. Small, easily achievable goals in the early stages of a complex healthcare regimen may prove to be very useful.

To increase adherence, healthcare regimens must be practical and as simple as possible. In numerous studies about medication adherence, researchers have overwhelmingly found that the more complex the regimen, the greater number of different medications, and the greater number of doses a day, the less adherence to the regimen. Because of lifestyle or certain limitations (physical, cognitive, or environmental), adherence to some regimens is improbable and inappropriate. When presenting options, consider the person's lifestyle and ability to follow through.

Risks to Health

Risk Factors

Risk factors are attributes that intensify a person's probability of developing a particular disease or condition. Identifying risk factors that may compromise a person's health or life is essential for health maintenance. Additionally, it is assumed that knowledge of risk factors before development of a disease or condition will motivate people to change their lifestyle to forestall or prevent illness or disability (Pender, 1995). Some risk factors pose health risks for everyone (such as poor air and water quality), whereas other risk factors may affect only certain ethnic, occupational, or familial groups. The following features are characteristic of risk factors: they vary in intensity (some risks pose greater threat than others, such as drinking alcohol and driving); the possibility of jeopardizing health increases as the strength of the risk factor increases; and multiple risk factors may present a greater risk through risk factor interaction (Pender, 1987).

Risk factors are identified through analysis of health history, laboratory tests, lifestyle, and physical and nutritional assessment. Computer programs have been developed to identify health risks and health promotion activities of individuals; these programs are available to health professionals and the public. Two of the many computer health risk appraisals available are the "Personal Wellness Profile" (available from Wellsource Inc., Clackamus, OR 1987) and "The Healthier People Health Risk Appraisal" (available from The Carter Center of Emory University, 1989).

Risk factors may be classified according to genetics, age, biologic characteristics, personal habits, lifestyle, and environment (Display 5-1). Risk for some genetic/biologic illnesses can easily be identified through the use of a three- to four-generation genogram. A genogram illustrates morbidity and mortality factors in a family (Fig. 5-1). Evaluating risk factors may show a person's vulnerability to disease or injury before the condition develops and enables the nurse to devise a health regimen with the client to reduce risks. Low socioeconomic status is a powerful risk factor; with poverty, the risk of developing and dying of chronic or preventable acute health problems increases dramatically. The nurse should evaluate each identified risk factor to determine the degree to which the factor can be controlled through modification of health behaviors and referral to social agencies.

DISPLAY 5.1

Risk Factor Classification

GENETIC

- Chromosomal abnormalities such as Down syndrome (trisomy 21)
- Family incidence of genetically transmissible conditions/diseases, such as cystic fibrosis, Huntington's chorea, hemophilia, diabetes, breast cancer, Duchenne's muscular dystrophy, phenylketonuria, sickle cell trait, and sickle cell anemia

AGE-RELATED

- Sensory deficits in elders
- Acute illnesses in children
- Homicide in young adults
- Development of chronic diseases in middle age

BIOLOGIC

- Elevated cholesterol level
- Elevated blood glucose level
- Altered immune status

PERSONAL HABITS

- Alcohol or drug abuse
- Tobacco use

LIFESTYLE

- Sedentary lifestyle
- Sunbathing
- Multiple sexual partners
- Low socioeconomic status

ENVIRONMENTAL

- Proximity to exposure to toxic substances (at home or work)
- Hazardous working conditions (fireman, farm worker)
- Excessive noise exposure
- Substandard housing

Risk factors associated with common dysfunctions or problems are identified in Display 5-2.

Potential for Injury

When assessing health and planning nursing care, consider the client's potential risk for injury. Injuries occur when a conflict exists between the individual and the external environment and may be influenced by the internal environment. Different age-groups are at risk for different types of injuries (see Chaps. 16 and 17). Potential injuries include not only lacerations, abrasions, and frac-

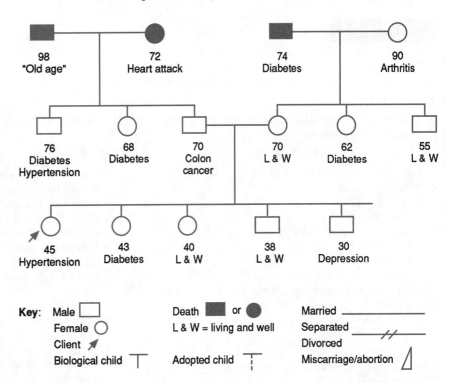

Key:

Male □		Death ■ or ●		Married ———	
Female ○		L & W = living and well		Separated —–//—	
Client ➚				Divorced	
Biological child ⊤		Adopted child ⊤ (dashed)		Miscarriage/abortion △	

FIGURE 5.1 Genogram, three generations.

---

tures, but also poisoning, infection, emotional distress, and disability.

Assessing the external environment involves evaluating hazards that may exist in the home, school, or play area, at work, and in other surroundings. Assessment also should include identifying potential contaminants such as polluted water or air, or the presence of allergens, poisons, and toxic substances.

The internal environment refers to biologic, genetic, and personality features of the individual. Certain disease processes and conditions compromise the body's ability to protect itself from injury. Diabetes mellitus, for example, complicates the body's attempt to recover from breaks in the skin's integrity. Human immunodeficiency virus (HIV) disease (acquired immune deficiency syndrome [AIDS]) interferes with the body's ability to prevent and fight infections. Immature taste buds and curiosity limit children's ability to protect themselves from bad-tasting poisons. Finally, lack of sight hinders a blind person from avoiding harmful obstacles.

Environmental Safety

Most accidents and many illnesses are preventable through protective measures. Assessing the external environment can show hazards and target environmental improvements that will prevent accidental injury. In addition, minimizing contamination of the environment is a primary prevention approach to acute and chronic illnesses and conditions.

The Home Environment

People of different ages are at risk for different hazards, even in the same environment. From infancy on, a person's environment enlarges to a peak size at some point in adulthood, and then with increasing age and infirmity, the size of the environment may contract. The internal environment influences the potential for injury or illness associated with environmental hazards. For example, a person with airborne allergies is more susceptible to environmental factors such as plant pollens and animal dander than persons without allergies.

Environmental risks in or around the home may include improperly stored household cleaning products, a nearby toxic waste disposal site, busy streets, a location near a high-traffic area such as an interstate highway (potential for lead poisoning), nearby smokestack industries, polluted or stagnant water, substandard housing, overcrowding, insects, rodents, lack of play areas, and poor food storage facilities.

When assessing a home, anticipating possible hazards is important. For example, medications on the kitchen table may be safe for the 70-year-old grandmother but not for her 2-year-old great-grandson. Assessment of the home environment for health promotion and injury prevention is focused on the following:

- The sanitation of the home and water supply
- Appropriate storage for food, perishable and nonperishable
- Safety features, such as working smoke and carbon monoxide alarms and safety catches on cupboards
- Potential outdoor hazards, such as unfenced yards near busy streets, unfenced swimming pools, and uneven sidewalks
- Potential indoor hazards, such as poor lighting, use of space heaters, drug storage in bathroom, and scatter rugs
- Neighborhood crime rate and crime precautions

DISPLAY 5.2

Risk Factors Associated with Common Dysfunctions and Problems

Some risk factors may be modified, whereas others, such as age, gender, and ethnicity, cannot. The former may be the focus of nursing interventions.

ATHEROSCLEROTIC HEART DISEASE

- Positive family history
- Increasing age
- Male gender
- Hypertension
- Elevated serum lipid levels
- Postmenopause
- Tobacco use
- Carbohydrate intolerance
- Diet high in calories, fats, cholesterol, refined sugars
- Obesity
- Type A personality

HYPERTENSION

- Positive family history
- Increasing age
- African heritage
- Pregnancy
- Oral contraceptive use
- Obesity
- Diabetes mellitus
- Tobacco use
- Heavy alcohol consumption

ABUSE OR VIOLENCE

- Crisis situations
- Dysfunctional family relationships
- Drug or alcohol abuse
- Threatened self-esteem
- Poor communication patterns
- Family history of abuse
- Gang membership

INFECTION

- Chronic disease status
- Altered immune status or function
- Altered skin or mucous membrane integrity
- Medications: antibiotics, antifungals, antivirals, steroids, immunosuppressants
- Therapeutic modalities: surgery, radiation, hyperalimentation, dialysis, invasive lines or procedures
- Contact with nosocomial agents
- Trauma
- Malnutrition
- Stress
- Prolonged immobility
- Thermal injuries
- Warm, dark, moist environments (skinfolds, under dressings)
- Age: children and elders

TRAUMA

- Physical alterations affecting judgment, coordination, sensory function, mobility, or level of consciousness
- Medications causing sedation or hypotension
- Use of alcohol or drugs
- Lack of use of automobile restraints, hard hats, motorcycle or bicycle helmets
- Unsafe household
- Stress
- Fire hazards
- Improper footwear
- Guns or other firearms in the home

Tools for Environmental Assessment

Evaluation tools, in the form of questionnaires or checklists, have been developed to assist nurses with environmental assessment. An age-related tool for evaluating the environment of children, known as Home Observation for Measurement of the Environment (HOME), has been used extensively by public health nurses (Caldwell, 1976). The following assessment areas for children from birth to 3 years are incorporated:

- Emotional and verbal responsibility of the parent
- Avoidance of restriction and punishment
- Organization of the physical and temporal environment
- Provision of appropriate play materials
- Parental involvement with the child
- Opportunities for variety in daily stimulation

Home safety assessment tools have also been developed for people with disabilities (Stanhope & Knollmueller, 1995), families (Keating & Kilmer, 1988),and elders (Burnside, 1988;). Hill and Smith (1989) have developed an assessment tool to evaluate the air, water, energy, safety, noise, light, and space in a person's environment. Bomar (1996) has developed an environmental health self-assessment tool that examines primary, secondary, and tertiary levels of prevention in the work place and home.

Individuals who have exposure to toxic substances in their work or home environment should have an exposure history to assess risks and to develop prevention interventions. Typically exposure histories are collected by occupational health nurses and others involved with care to individuals exposed to toxic substances such as farmers, mineral smelter employees, and anyone working with or near chemicals.

Health Care Environment

Nurses and other employees in health care agencies are responsible for providing a safe environment for clients, visitors, and employees. Many hospitals employ individuals, such as infection control nurses, to monitor safety conditions. Obvious hazards, such as frayed electrical cords, water spills, and malfunctioning equipment, place both the nurse and the client at risk for injury. In health care settings, nurses are more frequently injured than any other employee group; housekeeping personnel are also at high risk.

When assessing safety, note the condition of all equipment before use. Electrical equipment is especially hazardous if a short exists in the system. However, safety means more than safe equipment. Safety includes protection from nosocomial infections, hazardous or infectious wastes, excessive noise levels, unnecessary radiation exposure, invasion of personal space, and proper disposal of needles and other sharp instruments.

Safety assessment should consider the age, level of consciousness, functional capabilities, and level of cognitive of the individual. For example, a patient using oxygen should not be exposed to an open flame or tobacco smoking. A patient with a radium implant or infectious disease should be isolated to protect others, and a person with a suppressed immune system should be isolated to protect himself or herself from others. A confused person should not be left unsupervised. If a young child who can climb is left unattended in a crib, a safety net should be placed over the crib.

HEALTH PERCEPTION– HEALTH MANAGEMENT PATTERN ASSESSMENT

Nurses assess individuals and families in a variety of settings including hospitals, clinics, physician offices, nursing centers, community screenings, and over the telephone. In most situations, the nurse is able to see and touch the client to validate what is heard in making clinical judgments. However, with call-in programs such as "Call-a-Nurse," the nurse must assess the situation based on only what information is readily provided, questions asked, and information heard. There is a concern that information provided may be incorrect and place the nurse at risk legally. A few basic principles of telephone assessment or triage can reduce that risk and enhance quality service to callers. These principles are provided in Display 5-3.

DISPLAY 5.3

Principles of Telephone Assessment

The telephone has become an important link in today's health care. People leave the hospital sooner, with more demanding care needs, than a decade ago. Nurses are making discharge follow-up phone calls to assess the client's transition to home care and to identify problems. Consumers of health are using opportunities such as "Call a Nurse" to determine what to do before seeking in-office health care or to determine whether an emergency really exists. Nurses who work in telephone triage need to be able to assess the caller and the caller's problem and make critical decisions regarding treatment. Nurses working in this capacity should use approved protocols to guide assessment and decision making. According to Briggs (1997), all telephone triage protocols should contain **Key Questions** to ask, **Assessment** areas, and **Actions** the caller should take such as to call 9-1-1 or to call back if there is no improvement. Using approved protocols ensures providing the caller with correct information and reduces liability risks.

PRINCIPLES

- Listen carefully and do not make premature conclusions. Remember that callers may be embarrassed, confused, or afraid.
- Try to talk directly to the person with the problem or a responsible care provider (second-hand information can be incorrect).
- Carefully assess the problem; the caller may exaggerate or downplay symptoms.
- Note the level of anxiety of the caller.
- Provide the caller with the option to call back or seek medical attention if the problem continues or worsens.

- Use medically approved protocols to establish standards of care.
- Document all calls and advice given.
- Establish a helping relationship at the beginning of the call; skillful communication is a must.
- Get a brief description of the problem with the duration, onset, location, medical history, medications, allergies, and age of the person.
- Do not use medical jargon.
- Review and update protocols on a regular basis.

(Adapted from Briggs, J. [1997]. *Telephone triage protocols for nurses.* Philadelphia: Lippincott.)

Physical Examination — Health Perceptions and Health Management Assessment

GENERAL APPROACH

Evaluating Health Benefits, Behavior, and Risks

There is no universally accepted tool for measuring health perception–health management.

Data collected from other patterns are used in analysis for health perception–health management.

Promoting health should be a consideration with every nurse–client contact.

People of different ages and ethnic heritage are at risk for different problems, although some risks may be universal.

The health perception–health maintenance pattern tends to be abstract.

SCREENING

Screenings are secondary prevention activities to identify potential health problems.

Screenings are performed on people who, because of age, ethnicity, lifestyle, or genetics, are at risk for specific health problems.

Screening in other patterns such as nutrition may identify nursing diagnoses in health perception–health management pattern.

Specific screening for age and pregnancy have been identified by the US Preventive Services Task Force. Preventive services and screening identified by the US Preventive Services Task Force for people 24 to 65 years are illustrated in Display 5-4.

If a positive result is obtained in screening, additional diagnostic tests are needed; one elevated blood pressure reading does not make a person hypertensive.

Referral to appropriate healthcare providers is necessary for a comprehensive diagnosis. For example, positive scoliosis screening leads to referral to an orthopedist.

COMPREHENSIVE HEALTH PERCEPTION–HEALTH MAINTENANCE ASSESSMENT

A comprehensive health perception—health maintenance assessment should include the following components:
  Interview (health history)
  Laboratory analysis
  Physical assessment

ASSESSMENT AIDS

No specific equipment is needed for the assessment of health perception–health management pattern. If the client is using a piece of equipment for self-examination at home, for example, a monitor for blood glucose, the nurse should access the accuracy of the equipment if possible and the client's skill in using the equipment correctly.

An interview guide to suggest questions and record data is shown in Display 5-5.

DISPLAY 5.4

Preventive Health Recommendations for Ages 24–65 Years

SCREENING	FREQUENCY
Blood pressure	1–2 years
Height and weight	Annual
Total blood cholesterol	
Men 35–64	Annual
Women 45–64	Annual
Pap test (women)	Annual × 3, if normal then every 3 years
Fecal occult blood (50+)	Annual
Mammogram (women) 50–64	1–2 years
Clinical breast examination (women 40+)	1–2 years
Assess for problem drinking	Annual
Rubella serology or immunization history (women)	Once

COUNSELING	FREQUENCY
Tobacco cessation	Annual
Avoid alcohol when need to be alert (driving, etc.)	Annual
Dietary—limit fat and cholesterol, calorie intake	Annual
Balanced diet	Annual
Exercise program	Annual

Car seat restraint use	Annual
Bicycle/motorbike helmet	Annual
Smoke/carbon monoxide Detector	Annual
Unintended pregnancy	Annual
STD protection	Annual
Dental health	Annual

IMMUNIZATIONS	FREQUENCY
Tetanus–diphtheria booster	Every 10 years

CHEMOPROPHYLAXIS

Hormone replacement therapy Postmenopausal women	Annual

HIGH-RISK ONLY: TARGET GROUPS

TB screening:

Drug/alcohol abuse, low income, immigrants, HIV/AIDS

STD screening:

More than 1 sexual partner in 1 year, drug/alcohol abuse

Hepatitis vaccine:

High-risk sexual behavior, drug/alcohol abuse, health care workers, institutionalized person

(Adapted from Report of the US Preventive Services Task Force [1996].)

DISPLAY 5.5

Interview Guide: Health Perception—Health Maintenance

A structured interview guide may be used to facilitate data collection. The headings provided on this screening interview form correlate with major interview areas discussed in the text and may be copied when creating forms to record data in practice settings. If you are assessing the individual for more than just health perception–health maintenance, some of these data may be a duplication.

HEALTH PERCEPTION

Description of Health Now and in Last Year

How is your general health? _____

How has your health been in the last year? _____

What does it mean to you to be healthy? _____

Compared with others your age, how do you rate your health? _____

(When appropriate) What do you think caused this problem? _____

_____

(continued)

DISPLAY 5.5

Interview Guide: Health Perception—Health Maintenance *(continued)*

INFLUENCING FACTORS

Value: How important is health to you? _____

Control: Who makes decisions about your health care? _____

SOURCES OF HEALTH ADVICE

When you have a health question, whom do you contact? _____

RISK FACTORS

Does anyone in your family have   Who?
  • Cardiovascular disease _____
  • Hypertension _____
  • Cancer (type) _____
  • Diabetes mellitus _____
  • Drug or alcohol abuse _____
  • Genetic disorders (specify) _____
  • Depression _____
Do you use tobacco? (type and amount) _____
Have you ever tried to quit? _____ Would you like to quit now? _____
Do you use alcohol? (number of drinks per day/week/month) _____
  Do you ever believe you have had too much to drink? _____
Do you use car seat restraints? _____ How frequently? _____
Do you have a regular exercise program? _____
Are you currently sexually active? _____ Do you use any form of protection? (type) _____
What type of work do you do? (activities) _____
Do you have a smoke/fire and carbon monoxide detector in your home? _____

ABILITY TO PERFORM SELF-CARE

What do you do to stay healthy? _____
Are there any behaviors you would like to change? _____
In the past, have you had any difficulty following suggestions of health care providers? _____
What self-examinations do you perform? (BSE, TSE, blood pressure, blood glucose, skin; frequency) _____

_____

How comfortable are you with your self-examination skills? _____

HEALTH PROFESSIONAL SCREENING

Women: last Pap and mammogram and results _____
Last dental examination _____
Last cholesterol level _____
Last blood pressure measurement _____
Weight (recent gain or loss?) _____ Height _____
Immunizations: date   date
  • Tetanus–diphtheria _____   Hepatitis _____
  • Rubella (women) _____   Pneumonia _____
  • Influenza _____   Other _____
Prescription medications _____
Over-the-counter medications_____

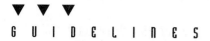

GUIDELINES

Assessment Guidelines   Health Perception Interview (Health History)

Procedure

1. Perception of health

Inquire about the person's perception of health by asking question such as:

"How is your general health?"

"How has your health been during the last year?"
or
"Have you missed any days from work or school because of illness?"

"What does it mean to you to be healthy?"

"How do you describe good health?"

"Compared with others your age, how is your health?"

When appropriate—

"What do you think caused this illness?"
and
"What have you done to treat this problem?"

2. Influencing factors

A. Value of Health

Inquire into the value the client places on health by asking questions such as, "How important is your health to you?" "On a scale of 1 to 10, with 10 being the highest, how important is it to you to stay healthy?"

Perceived Control

Determine the individual's locus of control regarding health status by asking:

"Who makes decisions about your health and health care?"

"Some people believe that they are 100% responsible for their own health status; what do you think of that?"
or
"Some people believe that good health is a matter of fate or God's will; what do you think?"

Clinical Significance

How a person describes his or her health influences health practices and related decision making. Remember how the individual describes health status and compare this with the nurse's findings. This will assist in determining the congruence between the nurse's perception and the client's perception and will influence decisions regarding interventions.

Note frequency of illnesses. Listen to descriptions of illnesses and how illnesses were managed. Are any themes present, such as delay in seeking health care, for example, "I had bronchitis for a month before I saw a doctor"?

This defines what the person means by *health*. Perceptions of health vary not only individually but also by age. As people age, there is an expectation of chronic illnesses such as arthritis. A person aged 70 with diabetes and arthritis may consider himself or herself to be healthy, whereas a person aged 20 with the same conditions may not rate health as good. For some people, being healthy means being able to go to work or work in the garden.

Listen for cues regarding a desire to be competent in health care activities and awareness of healthy practices.

Information provides the nurse with a cue to the individual's belief system regarding causes of illness (these may be influenced by culture and knowledge). Of the numerous herbal and folk remedies available, some may be helpful, such as chicken soup for colds, and others may be dangerous, such as *Azarcon* (a folk remedy for children that has recently been discovered to contain toxic levels of lead). The nurse also may discover the client has used another's prescription medication or used an antibiotic saved from the last illness.

People who place a high value on health generally are more active in their health management than people who place a lower value on health or believe that good health is one's fate.

Internal and external locus of control is a measurable concept that pertains to the individual's belief regarding who is in control. Individuals with an external locus of control believe that health status is dominated by chance or by other forces, such as God. People who believe that health is self-determined have an internal locus of control. Few people have an entirely internal or external locus of control. Knowing a person's locus of control traits can assist the nurse in identifying appropriate interventions and reinforcers. With health care reform and managed care, many people may believe that they have less control over health care decisions than in the past.

▼ ▼ ▼

Health Perception Interview (Health History)

Procedure

B. Sources of Health Advice
Interview the person to determine from whom he or she seeks advice about health.
> "When you have a question about health, whom do you contact?"
> "When you have a health question, what do you do?"
> "When you first become ill and don't know what to do, whom do you consult?"

3. Risk factors
Interview the individual to determine possible risk factors that could affect health.

Biologic and Genetic Risk Factors
- Review the record or ask whether there is a family history of any conditions such as cancer, heart disease, diabetes, or a genetic risk factor such as cystic fibrosis and premenopausal breast/ovarian cancer. Ask, for example,
> "Does anyone in your family have diabetes, cancer, or are there any other conditions that occur in your family?"
- Alternatively, complete a genogram.

Personal Habits
- Inquire into the individual's drug, alcohol, and tobacco use. If the person uses any of the above, the nurse may ask:
> "Have you ever tried or considered quitting the use of cigarettes?"
> "Have you ever regretted the amount of alcohol you drank after an event?"
> "Have you ever thought you drank too much?"
- Ask about car safety restraint use or helmet use with bicycle and motorcycles.

Lifestyle
- Inquire into regular exercise activities, for example:
> "Do you have a regular exercise routine?"
> "How frequently do you take the opportunity to engage in physical activity such as walking for 20 minutes or more?"

- When appropriate, inquire into the individual's sexual practices, for example:
> "Are you currently sexually active?"
> "Do you have more than one sexual partner?"
> "How many sexual partners have you had in the last 6–12 months?"
> "When engaging in sexual activity, what type of protection do you use?"

Clinical Significance

Women tend to be the "health care brokers" of the family; 70% of the time women determine when family members should seek health care (Triolo, 1987).

Sources of health advice may be family members, friends, friends/family in the health field, books, magazine articles, television programs, the Internet, and nontraditional health healers. Nontraditional healers in the United States include *Curanderos* and *Yerbero* (use of herbal remedies) (Hispanics), medicine men and women (Native Americans), lay midwives, folkhealers/practitioners, acupuncturists, and spiritual healers, among others.

A positive response for any risk factor may necessitate a more comprehensive assessment in another pattern. For example, a lifestyle that includes other than monogamous sexual encounters would cue the nurse to do a more extensive assessment of the sexuality pattern.

Knowledge of specific risk factors for the individual will allow the nurse to select appropriate screening tests. Risk factors associated with specific conditions/illnesses are identified in Display 5-2.

According to the Centers for Disease Control (CDC), tobacco accounts for 20% of deaths of all causes. Problem alcohol drinking with and without signs of dependency places individuals at high risk for future health and social problems. Nondependent heavy drinkers account for most alcohol-related mortality and morbidity in the general population, for example, automobile accidents (*Report of the US Preventive Services Task Force,* 1996).

Mandatory safety belt laws are in effect in most states, and restraints are required for all children. Helmets are also required in many states.

Over 50% of the people in the United States do not exercise on a regular basis. Physical activity could reduce mortality and morbidity for the following conditions: coronary heart disease, hypertension, obesity, diabetes, osteoporosis, and mental health disorders (*Report of the US Preventive Services Task Force,* 1996).

The CDC estimates that 12 million new cases of STDs (sexually transmitted diseases) occur in the United States each year. High-risk practices, including multiple sexual partners and nonuse of condoms, is a major problem in the United States. This is especially a problem in adolescents and young adults. (*Report of the US Preventive Services Task Force,* 1996).

Procedure

Environment

- Discover from the record or ask the person where he or she works, attends school, or lives. Ask:
  "What type of work do you do?"
  "What are your activities at work?"

- Ask whether there is a smoke/fire detector and carbon monoxide detector in the house.

4. Ability to perform self-care

A. Staying Healthy

Inquire what the person does to remain healthy. Ask questions such as:

- "What do you do to stay healthy?"
- "Are there any behaviors you would like to change?"
- "In the past, has it been easy or difficult to follow doctors' or nurses' suggestions?"
- "Do you have any goals to improve your health status?"
- "In the past, what has helped in meeting health goals?"
- "What makes it difficult to follow health advice?"
- "What makes it easier to follow health advice?"
- "Are there any behaviors you would like to change or behaviors you think you should change?"

B. Self-Examinations Performed

Inquire into self-examinations performed and level of competence in completing these examinations.

- For women, ask, "Do you perform a self-breast exam?" If yes, then "How often do you do a BSE and how comfortable are you with what you feel?"
- For men, ask, "Do you perform a self-testicular exam (TSE)?" If yes, then "How often do you do a TSE and how comfortable are you with what you feel?"
- Other self-examinations include:
  Skin for skin cancer
  Oral for dental caries and oral cancer
  Blood pressure for hypertension
  Blood glucose for diabetes
  Temperature for ovulation and fever

Clinical Significance

Some occupations, such as construction trades, fire fighting, and farm work, place workers at risk for environmental hazards, including trauma and exposure to toxic substances. If there has been an exposure to toxins, special assessments are recommended.

Housing or schools near busy highways and interstates can have ground contaminated with lead. Also, living in houses built before 1970 places children at risk for lead poisoning from lead-based paint.

Many fire deaths are associated with a nonworking smoke/fire detector. Be sure to ask how often batteries are replaced on battery-operated detectors.

Identifying what the person does to stay healthy provides a cue to the nurse regarding the number of activities a person deliberately engages in to stay healthy and the knowledge base the person has about health. This also provides an opportunity for the person to discuss the use of vitamins, minerals, and herbs used to maintain health status and to identify desired changes in current health behavior.

Additionally, it provides the nurse with information on what is a successful motivator/intervention for past experiences and difficulties encountered.

Situations such as limited transportation, the inability to read because of either illiteracy or visual acuity, and inability to open medication containers because of arthritis may interfere with a person's ability to engage in healthy behaviors.

Most breast and testicular tumors are first identified by the individual. Because early detection is important, it is important to discover whether the individual is practicing this self-examination procedure. If individuals assume responsibility for health care and detecting health problems, then they must have the knowledge, skill, and belief that what they are doing is correct.

▼ ▼ ▼

G U I D E L I N E S *continued*   Health Perception Interview (Health History)

Procedure

C. Frequency of Professional Screening Activities, Immunizations, and Medications

From the person's record or through interview, determine:

- The date of last Pap smear and frequency of screening for women
- The date of last mammogram for women older than 40.
- Last dental examination and frequency of dental evaluation
- Appropriate laboratory tests such as blood glucose and cholesterol
- Immunization status
- Medications, both prescription and over-the-counter medications taken; ask:
    "What medications are you now taking?"
    "Can you tell me what each one of these is for?"
    "Do you ever take vitamins, aspirin, or other medications you pick out yourself?"

Assessment Guidelines

A complete health perception and health management assessment includes consideration of laboratory values, x-rays, and test results, including cholesterol level, blood glucose, Pap smear, fecal occult blood, mammogram, prostate-specific antigen, tuberculosis skin test. The type of screening test used for any complete assessment is dependent on age (developmental tests are performed on children), gender (mammograms for women), and ethnic origin (blood glucose screening with ethnic high-risk groups such as Native Americans and people of Mexican heritage).

Laboratory Test

- Total blood cholesterol (see Chap. 8 for further discussion of cholesterol)

- Fecal occult blood test (stool guaiac) or sigmoidoscopy (see Chap. 9 for further discussion of colorectal diagnostic examinations)

Clinical Significance

This information is important for determining interventions for disease prevention. For example, if the person has not had a tetanus immunization in 15 years, the nurse could recommend receiving this immunization. Also, the nurse can observe for congruence between what the individual says and actual behaviors. Some people have phobias to dental care, and asking about this activity may make it easier for the person to discuss.

When asking about medications, ask specifically about over-the-counter medications such as aspirin and vitamins; people often forget these. Some over-the-counter medications are contraindicated if taking specific prescription medications such as warfarin sodium (Coumadin) and aspirin.

Laboratory/X-Ray Evaluations

Many of the diagnostic studies performed for health maintenance are not for diagnosing illnesses or conditions but to alert the health provider to potential problems and the need for a diagnostic workup. (See Display 5-4 for schedule for screening tests for adults; see Chaps. 13, 16, and 17 for the schedule for pregnant women, children, and elders). Most laboratory and x-ray tests used for this pattern are also used in other patterns, for example, blood and plasma glucose and cholesterol for nutritional and metabolic assessments.

Clinical Significance

Elevated blood cholesterol is a major modifiable risk factor for coronary heart disease, the leading cause of death in the United States (*Report of the US Preventive Services Task Force*, 1996).

For the identification of colorectal cancer and other anomalies such as polyps and hemorrhoids. Colorectal cancer has the second highest morbidity and mortality in the United States. When detected early as a localized problem, the 5-year survival rate is 91% (Wingo, Tong, & Bolden, 1995). Colorectal cancer risk doubles every 7 years after age 50.

▼ ▼ ▼

G U I D E L I N E S   *continued*   Health Perception Interview (Health History)

Laboratory Test	Clinical Significance
• Papanicoalaou (Pap) test (see Chap. 13 for further discussion)	The incidence of cervical cancer is increasing, and the risk increases with certain types of human papilloma virus (HPV). Treatment of localized cervical cancer has a 90% 5-year survival rate (Wingo, Tong, & Bolden, 1995).
• Blood or plasma glucose measurement	This test is only performed on adults at high risk for diabetes or those who have symptoms such as polyuria and polydipsia (excessive urination and thirst). Routine screening of people not at risk has not proved to be cost-effective.
• Prostate-specific antigen (men)	This screening is controversial and must be decided on an individual basis. As a routine screening for prostate cancer, it is recommended by the American Cancer Society and the American Urologic Association, but not recommended by the National Cancer Institute and the US Preventive Services Task Force.
X-Rays • Mammogram (women)	A soft-tissue x-ray of the breasts that is used to detect abnormalities such as cysts and cancerous tumors. These can be detected through mammography at sizes too small to palpate. Breast cancer is the second leading cause of cancer death in women.
Other • Tuberculosis skin test, PPD (tuberculin purified protein derivative serum)	For asymptomatic high-risk person. High-risk groups include close contacts of people with the disease, individuals with HIV, immigrants from countries with high rates of tuberculosis, low-income populations, injection drug users, and residents and employees of high-risk facilities such as healthcare facilities and prisons (*Report of the US Preventive Services Task Force*, 1996).

▼ ▼ ▼

G U I D E L I N E S

Assessment Guidelines   Health Maintenance–Health Perception: Physical Assessment

Procedure

The primary goals of the physical assessment related to health perception and health management are to

1. Identify visible evidence of the client's health perceptions and health management behavior.

2. Validate data obtained during the interview.

3. Identify problems with health management. The physical examination for this pattern can be organized around the following:

Clinical Significance

This information is analyzed to formulate nursing diagnoses and to identify possible problems of health management and ways health can be promoted through better management. The individual's health perception and health management skills impact all other functional abilities and health status. Therefore, information from other assessment areas can provide cues to health misinformation, conflict between health beliefs and traditional health practices, and problems or potential problems in health management.

▼ ▼ ▼

GUIDELINES *continued*

Health Maintenance–Health Perception:
Physical Assessment

Procedure

- Indicators of overall health status
- Health management skills
- Obvious risk factors
- Self-examination techniques
- Preventive health screening
- The environment

1. Indicators of overall health status:

A. Initial observation
- Does the person appear healthy or sick?
- Does your opinion of the client's health status—from poor to excellent—agree with the client's perception?

2. Assess for health management skills.

A. Observe general appearance
- General appearance includes overall appearance, hygiene, body odor, fit of clothes, and condition of nails and hair. Are there obvious dental caries and missing teeth?

B. Body structure

Measure height and weight, noting whether weight is appropriate for height.

Are body parts in proportion to body size and age?

Note any gross deformities or missing extremities.

Does muscle tone correlate with reported activity?

C. Mental status

Can the individual carry on a logical conversation?

Does health history seem accurate?

Do judgments about health or health care sound rational?

Are there signs of distress: crying, unable to sit in one position, wringing hands, not talkative, or overly talkative?

How easy is it for the nurse to establish a relationship with the client?

Clinical Significance

Verifying the client's perception with the nurse's provides valuable information (i.e., whether the client minimizes or exaggerates health problems or is fairly accurate). Many clients rate their health status as comparable with the rating by the health professional.

Proper dress and grooming can provide insight into the client's self-esteem, occupation (is the client wearing a uniform?), and ability to manage basic self-care needs.

Deviations from Normal
Any deviations should be followed up with the appropriate assessment. For example, an adult with an ammonia smell should alert the nurse to possible urinary incontinence, fruity breath may indicate diabetes mellitus.

Clinical observations should validate the client's health history.

Avoid making quick judgments or assumptions with initial impressions. Verify your judgments by confirming with the client. Individuals may not have enough time to clean up after work before a health appointment.

Deviations from Normal
Any unusual findings should be evaluated further in the appropriate pattern. For example, a client with a missing limb should be evaluated for mobility and risk for injury related to falls. Problems with obesity should be followed-up in the Nutrition–Metabolism pattern. Obesity places the individual at risk for cardiovascular problems, diabetes mellitus, and hypertension.

Deviations from Normal
Any unusual or unexpected finding should alert the nurse for a more extensive mental status assessment in the Self-Concept and Cognition Perception patterns.

If it is difficult to establish a helping relationship, the nurse may be ineffective in working with the client to initiate lifestyle change interventions.

An alert, logical mental status is helpful in managing health care. The mental status of a person is important in determining the amount of assistance needed to assume independence in health care. Some people are totally independent, others are totally dependent on others for health care, but most people fall somewhere between those two extremes.

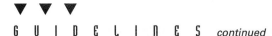

Health Maintenance–Health Perception:
Physical Assessment

Procedure

D. Observe gross mobility

Note any indications of potential interference with health maintenance activities, such as:

Mobility

Joint range of motion

Any obvious signs of arthritis of the hands

Ability to bend over

3. **Observe for obvious risk factors, including the following:**
   - Obesity
   - Racial/ethnic heritage that places the person at risk for specific conditions
   - Risky occupations
   - Socioeconomic status
   - Education

   Be careful not to make premature judgments without validation from client.

4. **Observe self-examination techniques.**

   For any self-examination performed (ie, blood pressure, blood glucose, testicular self-examination, and breast self-examination), observe the individual's techniques.

   See Display 5-6, "Breast Self-Examination" and Display 5-7, "Testicular Self-Examination"

5. **Preventive health screening**

   Health screenings are suggested for numerous conditions; a few of the more common ones are listed here.

   - Breast cancer (women)
     Risk factors:
     Never pregnant or first pregnancy after 35
     Early menarche (before 12)
     Late menopause (after 50)
     History of benign breast disease

Clinical Significance

The ability to perform such tasks as going to a store to purchase food and other necessities, preparing food, opening medication containers, going to the toilet to avoid incontinence, and bathing and dressing greatly impact the person's ability to effectively carry out health maintenance.

Deviations from Normal
Any deviation should alert the nurse to focus physical assessment in the Activity–Exercise pattern.

The identification of risks is of primary importance if health is to be maintained and risk minimized. People of certain heritage are at higher risk for certain disease or conditions, although changes in lifestyle or eating habits can reduce these risks. Type of clothing can often indicate whether a person engages in an occupation or activity that poses a health risk (i.e., someone working with toxic substances or construction worker). Educational level often can influence how well an individual can read and comprehend health care instructions or medication instructions. Educational level has a strong positive correlation with socioeconomic status.

If a person takes the time and energy to perform self-examinations, it is important that he or she does them properly and is assured that the conclusions are accurate. The vertical strip pattern of breast self-examination has been found to be more effective in covering more breast tissue than other methods (Murali & Crabtree, 1992). See Chapter 13 for discussion of health professional assessment of breasts and testicles.

Common Improper Techniques
Blood pressure cuff may be inappropriately placed, be the wrong size, or deflated too quickly.

Breast Self-Examination: Using insufficient finger pressure, using fingertips and not pads, neglecting to cover the entire breast tissue, especially near axilla.

Testicular Self-Examination: Performing examination while scrotum is not relaxed, neglecting to assess proximal area, not using enough pressure.

Health professional assessment of breasts every 3 years until age 40 and then yearly.

Other assessments: Mammography every 1–2 years for women age 50–69, beginning at 40 if at high risk. Breast self-examination monthly.

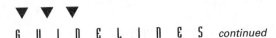

GUIDELINES *continued*

Health Maintenance–Health Perception:
Physical Assessment

Procedure

Family history of breast cancer, especially if before age 35

- Testicular cancer (men)
  Risk factors:
  Between ages 15 and 34
  Partially to totally undescended testicle
  History of maternal use of diethylstilbestrol or oral contraceptives during first trimester
  History of cryptorchidism, inguinal hernia, Klinefelter's syndrome (XXY), atrophy of testes, and hermaphroditism

- Colorectal cancer
  Risk factors:
  Family history of hereditary syndromes associated with colon cancer (familial polyposis)
  Ulcerative colitis
  High risk for adenomatous polyps

- Cervical cancer
  Risk factors:
  Multiple sexual partners
  History of human papilloma virus (HPV)

- Prostate cancer
  Risk factors:
  Advanced age
  Family history of early prostate cancer (before age 70)

- Heart disease/coronary artery disease
  Risk factors:
  Family history
  Hypertension
  Diabetes
  Obesity
  Hypercholesterolemia
  Tobacco use
  Sedentary lifestyle

- Diabetes mellitus (non–insulin-dependent diabetes mellitus [NIDDM]
  Risk factors:
  Obesity
  Family history of diabetes
  Member of following ethnic groups: Native Americans, Hispanics, African Americans

- Sexually transmitted diseases
  Numerous diseases can be transmitted sexually, including gonorrhea, syphilis, chlamydia, genital herpes, genital warts, human immunodeficiency virus (HIV/AIDS), and hepatitis.
  Risk factors:

Clinical Significance

Testicular examination by health professional annually, beginning with puberty.

Other assessment: Testicular self-examination, monthly

Digital rectal examination by health professional annually, beginning at age 40.

Other assessments: Sigmoidoscopy, fecal occult blood, barium enema, and colonoscopy. See Chapter 9 for discussion of these tests.

Pap test, beginning at age 18 or sexual activity. Schedule: 3 negative smears for 3 years and then once every 3 years if results remain negative.

Other assessments if positive Pap smear: cervicography and colposcopy (see Chapter 13).

Yearly digital rectal examination, beginning at age 40

Other assessments: Prostate-specific antigen (see discussion above) and fine-needle biopsy with positive tests

Blood pressure: Every 2 years if diastolic pressure under 85 and annually if between 85 and 89

Cholesterol screen: men aged 35–65 and women aged 45–65 annually

Weight annually

Other assessments: Triglycerides (see Chap. 6), electrocardiography with and without exercise (stress test; see Chap. 8)

Only people at risk are screened

Blood or plasma glucose

Other Assessments: 1-hour glucose challenge, Glucose tolerance test (GTT)

See Chapter 6 for further discussion

Only people at risk are screened on a regular basis; some screening routinely occurs with assessment for prenatal care.

Most screenings are cultures or blood tests.

See Chapter 13 for the discussion of these laboratory tests.

▼ ▼ ▼

G U I D E L I N E S *continued*   Health Maintenance–Health Perception:
Physical Assessment

Procedure

Multiple sexual partners
Unprotected sexual contact (nonuse or condoms)
Intravenous drug user (for HIV and hepatitis)

- Other screenings include skin, oral and thyroid cancer, vision, glaucoma, hearing, scoliosis, depression, dementia, and drug abuse.

6. Assess the environment.

- When possible, assess the environment for hazards. Consider the person's capabilities and how the environment enhances or detracts from managing health. For example, does a person with mobility problems only have access to a toilet on the second floor of a house? Is the confused patient in the room furthest from the nurses' station?

Clinical Significance

See Chapter 8 for vision, glaucoma, and hearing screening; Chapter 6 for skin, oral, and thyroid cancer; and Chapters 11 and 14 for depression, dementia, and drug use.

Environmental concern will vary depending on the age of the person and the person's specific capabilities; for example, side rails may not pose a problem for an alert hospitalized person, but a confused person may try to crawl over the rails and fall.

Potential Hospital Hazards
Fluid spills, frayed electrical cords, smoking in bed, loose "sharp" instruments, damaged equipment, inadequate lighting, inadequate hand washing

Potential Home Hazards
Children: toxic substances within the child's reach and access, peeling lead-based paint, windows not secured, uncovered electrical outlets, inappropriate toys, nonsecured play areas, swimming pools, matches, stairs, high water temperature, malfunctioning or absent fire and carbon monoxide detectors

Elders: frayed electrical cords, space heaters, smoking in bed or on overstuffed furniture, scatter rugs, poor lighting, lack of smoke/fire and carbon monoxide detectors, unlevel sidewalk, unstable furniture, slippery bathing area, cluttered walkways and stairs

DISPLAY 5.6

Breast Self-Examination

SCREENING RECOMMENDATIONS

The American Cancer Society recommends monthly BSE for women over age 20. About 90% of all breast lumps are found by women or their significant others.

Procedure

1. Examine the breasts in the tub or shower when skin is wet and hands move easily over breast tissue (*A, B*). Use the right hand to examine the left breast as you raise the left arm over the head to expose more breast tissue.

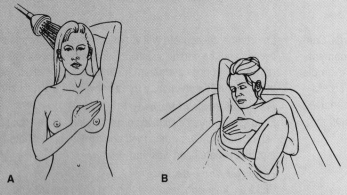

2. Examine the breasts in front of a mirror to detect unusual contours or changes in the skin appearance, such as puckering, dimpling, or retraction of the nipple. Note the appearance of the breasts in three different positions: arms at the sides (*C*), arms over the head (*D*), and hands on the hips while flexing the chest muscle (*E*).

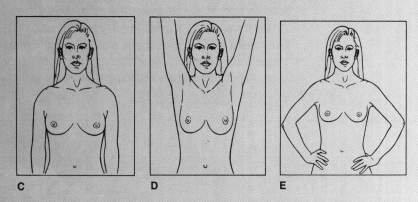

3. Examine the breasts lying down. Place a small pillow or blanket under your shoulder on the side being examined, to expose more breast tissue (*F*). Use the right hand to examine the left breast. Be thorough, proceeding in a circular pattern from the center of the breast outward. Feel the breast tissues that extend to the armpit. Squeeze the nipple to detect any discharge. (*G*). Any hard lumps, clear or bloody nipple discharge, or skin changes should be reported to a health professional.

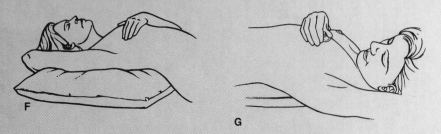

DISPLAY 5.7

Testicular Self-Examination

SCREENING RECOMMENDATIONS

Monthly testicular self-examination (TSE) is recommended by the American Cancer Society for early detection and cure of testicular cancer.

CHARACTERISTICS OF TESTICULAR TUMORS

An established testicular tumor is palpable as an irregular, nontender, fixed mass. A dragging sensation or heaviness may be reported. Nearby lymph node enlargement is rarely noted because the scrotal lymphatics drain deep within the abdominal cavity.

Procedure

1. TSE is performed as a 3-minute examination, preferably after a warm bath or shower when the scrotal skin is relaxed and easy to manipulate.
2. Examine each testicle along a horizontal plane by rolling the skin between the thumb and forefinger of each hand (A).
3. Repeat the procedure by feeling for lumps or other abnormalities along the vertical plane (B). Perform this examination on each testis. It is normal to find one testis larger than the other. Any hard lumps or nodules should be reported to a health professional. See Chapter 14 for examination guidelines for health professionals.

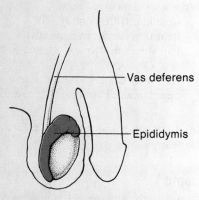

Normal anatomy

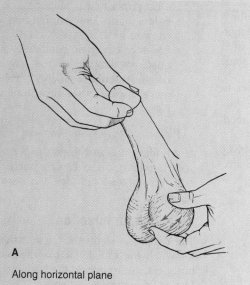

A

Along horizontal plane

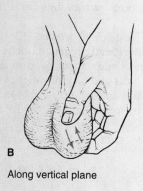

B

Along vertical plane

ND_x

Documentation

A normal examination finding may be documented as follows:

S: 50 year old African-American woman. No current health problems—believes health is "OK, but could be better"; 10-year history of hypertension (both parents had hypertension and diabetes—mother living, father dead 3 years—stroke); takes Cozaar 50 mg daily for blood pressure and motrin 400 mg three times per day for hip and knee joint discomfort. Walks 30 minutes 4–6 times per week, has a balanced diet but "has too many fried foods." Immunizations: tetanus 2 years ago, influenza last October. Performs BSE monthly, no lumps noted. Mammogram 2 years ago—normal, Pap smear 1 year ago—normal. Wears glasses for reading. Saw dentist 6 months ago, no problems. No specific questions or concerns, needs medications renewed.

O: Height 5′6″, weight 132, BP 116/74, P 72. Hygiene adequate. Dress appropriate. BSE—correct technique, normal findings confirmed. ROM in lower extremities within normal limits. Logical flow of conversation.

A. Health maintenance appropriate, at risk for diabetes (family history and ethnicity)

P. Schedule for mammogram and plasma glucose level (diabetes screening) now

Continue with monthly BSE

Return to dentist in 6 months

Pap smear in 2 years, tetanus in 8 years, influenza next October

Call with laboratory results and schedule for next appointment based on those results.

An abnormal examination finding may be documented as follows:

Example 1

S. Mr. Q, a 35-year-old white male seen at blood pressure clinic. Ran out of blood pressure medication (can't remember name) 5 days ago. Having "terrible headaches that make me want to cry" in the afternoons. Has had high blood pressure for 5 years. Talked with sister and plans to go to pharmacy to get medication filled this afternoon after cashing check. Doctor wants him to lose some weight.

O. BP 180/96, P 84. Height 5′9″, weight 230.

A. Management of therapeutic regimen, ineffective, related to lack of knowledge about need to take medication on a daily basis and lack of weight loss

P. Purchase medication and take dose this AM. (Mr. Q) Return tomorrow to screening clinic for BP measurement

Discuss need to take medication regularly and risks

Assess for weight loss and jointly make plan

Example 2

S: Cassandra, 23 years old, recently became sexually active. Never had pelvic examination and does not do routine breast self-examination. Here for oral contraceptives. Has had 1 sexual partner, using condoms for protection. Last menstrual period 9-12 (1 week ago)

O: Ht. 5′5″, weight 110. BP 110/72, P 70. Breast examination—no abnormalities

A: Health-seeking behavior: Contraception

P: To see Women's Health Nurse Practitioner for pelvic examination and to get prescription today

Instructed on BSE and return demonstration—done

After examination, review how to take oral contraceptives and possible side effects

Return to clinic in 3 months—call if any problems

Nursing Diagnoses Related to Health Perception and Health Maintenance

High Risk for Aspiration

The diagnosis High risk for aspiration is used for the individual who is at risk for secretions, fluids, or solid objects entering the tracheobronchial passages. This diagnosis is useful for people with altered consciousness, structural defects (such as cleft palate), and neurologic (such as cerebral palsy) and gastrointestinal disorders. Individuals with swallowing disorders also may be at risk for aspiration; however, if the goal is to improve swallowing, then the primary diagnosis is Impaired swallowing (see Chap. 6). With swallowing disorders, there is always a risk for aspiration.

History

The risk for aspiration may be increased in the following circumstances:

- Infants: Prematurity or cleft palate
- Children: Ages 1–3, especially when eating nuts, hard candy, popcorn, whole beans; toys with small pieces (for children under 3 a toy should not fit through a toilet paper tube), balloons
- Elders: Poor dentition that may cause food not to be chewed well
- Presence of certain conditions that interfere with adequate swallowing or the gag reflex, Parkinsonism, cerebrovascular accidents (stroke), dementia (Alzheimer's disease), post–head trauma, tracheoesophageal fistula

Physical Examination Findings

Any finding that documents a poor or absent gag reflex, poor dentition, presence of a tracheotomy, or prematurity in a newborn should alert the nurse to the potential for aspiration.

High Risk for Infection

The diagnosis High risk for infection involves a situation in which the individual has the potential for an opportunistic agent to invade the body and cause a localized infection of generalized illness.

History

Situations or condition that place the individual at risk would include:

- Reports of altered immune response related to an altered production of leukocytes, altered T-cell production, and altered circulation. Illnesses and conditions related to one or more of the above include HIV/AIDS, cancer, diabetes mellitus, hematologic disorders
- A severe nutritional deficit
- Incomplete immunization status
- Infants and elders
- Situational factors such as exposure to secondhand

smoke (especially children), trauma, unsafe sexual intercourse, hospitalization, exposure to infectious agents

Physical Examination Findings

As with other diagnoses in this pattern, physical examination findings from other patterns are used to confirm the diagnosis High risk for infection. For example, any break in the integumentary system increases the risk for infection. Any laboratory findings that document altered immune system, such as low white cell count, also place the individual at risk. Finding the presence of any infectious process in the body increases the risk for additional infections.

High Risk for Injury

The diagnosis High risk for injury is employed when the person is at risk for harm because of factors such as age, lack of knowledge of hazards, or perceptual/physiologic defect. This diagnosis is used to provide on-site protection, but not teaching about protection. The need for teaching about injury risk may be more appropriate under the nursing diagnosis Altered health maintenance or Health-seeking behavior. The diagnosis High risk for injury has subcategories of poisoning, suffocation, and trauma. These subcategories can be isolated so the nurse can focus only on that aspect of potential harm.

History

- History of accidents, especially those requiring medical attention
- Environmental hazards such as busy streets, substandard housing, unsafe sidewalks, gas leaks, absent or nonfunctioning smoke/fire and carbon monoxide alarms
- Any factor that can impair mobility such as syncope, arthritis, paralysis, multiple sclerosis, and seizures
- Age is a significant factor for specific risks. Infants are at risk for suffocation, poisoning, and burns. Elders are at risk for drug toxicity, bone fractures, burns, and falls.

Physical Examination Findings

Findings from other functional patterns are used to confirm the diagnosis High Risk for Injury. The presence of scars and bruises indicates a history of injury. Findings such as orthostatic hypotension, syncope, impaired vision, hearing loss, poor memory, confusion, tissue hypoxia, or neurosensory deficit should alert the nurse to the need to implement interventions to prevent potential injuries.

Altered Growth and Development

This nursing diagnosis is specifically for children who are at risk for impaired ability to perform age-appropriate developmental tasks. The inability to perform one or more of the skills in motor, personal, social, language, and cognition places the child at risk. This diagnosis is discussed in Chapter 16.

Altered Health Maintenance

Altered health maintenance is the potential interruption in health because of an unhealthy lifestyle that the person desires to change. A disease/illness is not present.

History

The ability to maintain health may be compromised under the following circumstances:

- Reports of unhealthy lifestyle or habits such as tobacco use, excessive caloric intake, substance abuse, excessive exposure to the sun, and unprotected nonmonogamous sexual intercourse
- Frequent use of potentially unsafe over-the-counter products
- Psychosocial disorders
- Situational factors such as lack of health knowledge, lack of access to health care, or inability to read or understand advice
- Any new diagnosis or skill required of an individual. The individual may not process sufficient knowledge or skill to manage a new healthcare regimen.

Physical Examination

The physical examination may show cues to Altered health maintenance such as poor hygiene, early tooth loss or teeth in poor repair, nonhealing wounds, obesity, and blood pressure or blood glucose level remaining elevated despite prescribed regimen.

Physical examination findings to support the diagnosis Altered health maintenance often come from other examination areas such as the integumentary and cardiovascular systems and cognitive status. The nurse should consider this any time the individual is not responding as expected or is given a new diagnosis, prescription, or activity to perform.

Ineffective Management of Therapeutic Regimen

The individual or family is at risk or is experiencing difficulty in incorporating a healthcare regimen into daily living to meet specific goals or to maintain health. The individual or family is having difficulty reaching positive/desired outcomes.

History

- A complex healthcare regimen, possibly including numerous medications (polypharmacy)
- Reports of difficulty managing healthcare regimen
- Financial cost of following regimen
- Exacerbation or nonimprovement of condition
- Previous unsuccessful experiences

Physical Examination

Listen closely to people describe their healthcare regimens—confusion, misconceptions, and lack of confidence in the regimen reduce the individual's ability to correctly follow recommendations. Sometimes the regimen is so complex or costly it is not possible for the individual to comply. Difficulty with memory, untoward effects, visual or hearing impairments, inability to open medication containers, lack of motivation, and health belief conflicts can create barriers to effectively managing a therapeutic regimen.

Management of Therapeutic Regimen, Effective

This is a positive nursing diagnosis that notes when the individual is meeting healthcare goals and is successful in managing care needs. Nursing interventions for this diagnosis would be anticipatory guidance to alert the individual to a potential problem to reduce negative impacts.

History

- Appropriate lifestyle choices
- Appropriate management of healthcare regimen
- Diseases/conditions remain within an expected range

Physical Examination Findings

Laboratory readings and other findings are within an expected range. For example, blood pressure readings remain below 140/90 and the blood glucose reading remain below 140 or the target range agreed on by the individual and the healthcare provider, or the individual may be meeting goals such as weight loss or lack of weight loss (individuals with anorexia).

Altered Protection

The diagnosis Altered protection is used to describe the situation in which the individual has a decreased ability, or is unable, to protect himself from harm. The goal of this diagnosis is to protect the person from threats. Similar diagnoses one may consider are High risk for infection and High risk for injury.

History

- An impaired immune system, impaired healing, altered blood clotting, maladaptive stress, neurosensory alterations, and autoimmune disorders
- Weakness, fatigue, immobility, skin breakdown, confusion, inadequate nutrition, substance abuse
- Being very young, very old, or having a debilitating disease such as Parkinsonism or HIV/AIDS

Physical Examination Findings

Examination findings for this diagnosis come from other examination areas such as the integumentary and lymphatic systems. The presence of reddened areas on the skin in an immobile patient should alert the nurse that the patient's skin needs to be protected. Laboratory findings that indicate an altered immune system or prolonged bleeding time also are evidence for added precautionary protection.

Health-Seeking Behaviors

The diagnosis Health-seeking behaviors is closely related to Health maintenance. With the diagnosis Health-seeking behaviors, however, the individual is actively seeking to improve his or her level of wellness through a change in health habits or the environment. This diagnosis is wellness-focused, whereas Altered health maintenance is illness/condition-focused.

History

The desire to enhance one's level of wellness is evidenced in the history by the following:

- Expressing a desire for health promotion
- Voicing a desire to gain greater control of own health, concern of environmental effects on health,

and unfamiliarity with health promotion resources in community
- Anticipated role change, for example, becoming a parent or retirement

Physical Examination Findings

Generally, there are no physical examination findings for this diagnosis; however, be alert while doing examination of other areas to the patient's voicing any concerns about health promotion.

Noncompliance (Specify)

Noncompliance occurs when the individual desires to adhere to a health regimen or health advice but is prevented from doing so by factors that impede adherence. To be noncompliant, the individual must have agreed through informed consent to follow the regimen or advice. Strategies used by the nurse aim to reduce or eliminate the barriers the client has encountered in attempting to comply. There are other reasons people may not follow health-related advice; in such cases, the nursing diagnosis of Noncompliance does not apply. If the person lacks the knowledge for compliance, the diagnosis should be Knowledge deficit. If the individual has made an informed, autonomous decision *not* to adhere to the regimen or health advice, a more appropriate diagnosis might be Altered health maintenance or Ineffective management of therapeutic regimen. For example, if a person knows that smoking is hazardous to one's health and refuses to quit, the diagnosis of Noncompliance would not apply because that person has never agreed to try to stop smoking. Noncompliance assumes that the person desires to comply but is prevented from doing so by other factors.

History

Factors that influence an individual's ability to comply with health advice or health regimen include the following:

- Socioeconomic status influences the ability to purchase medications and foods for special diets.
- Individuals with a history of noncompliance are more likely to be noncompliant than others who have complied. The person has insufficient knowledge regarding the advice, regimen, or health problem or inability to read directions.
- Complex, long-term regimens make it more difficult to maintain compliance.
- Lack of resources such as transportation, nearby pharmacy, and family support hinder compliance.

Physical Examination Findings

Findings from other patterns are used to support the diagnosis of Noncompliance (*i.e.,* the persistence or progression of symptoms that should have been controlled or eliminated with the treatment prescribed, or the occurrence of undesired outcomes, such as pregnancy, in a person with a prescription for contraceptives). Other findings such as confusion, impaired vision, or decreased hand dexterity, or laboratory findings of drug toxicity can alert the nurse to problems the individual may have in attempting to follow the advice of healthcare providers.

Clinical Problems Related to Health Perception and Health Maintenance

The focus of this health pattern is to prevent problems from occurring by identifying potential risks and barriers to the maintenance and promotion of health. The goal of the nurse is to assist the individual and the family to reduce risks, maintain or promote health, and protect the client from harm. Therefore, clinical problems in other areas create clinical problems in the health perception–health maintenance pattern.

Case Study

Susan, age 45, a single mother of two children, comes into a community clinic for health care. She has health insurance for herself but cannot afford premiums for her children. She is waiting to see whether the children will be covered under a new program specifically for children. Her children, Alexis, age 6 (1st grade), and Teresa, age 17 (12th grade), attend the clinic on a sliding scale fee. This is Susan's second visit to the clinic and her children's first.

Susan believes that her family has been healthy except for a few ear infections for Alexis. Teresa had problems with asthma when younger but has not missed any school in the past few years. Susan remains sexually active and has had the same partner for the past 7 years; she uses oral contraceptives to prevent pregnancy. She is concerned that she may need to use some other form of contraceptive as suggested at her last clinic appointment. She does not know whether Teresa is sexually active.

Susan desires to maintain the health of her family. If Alexis becomes ill, either she or Teresa stays home. Teresa stays home by herself when not feeling well. On nonschool days, Teresa must watch Alexis. Susan thinks her children get enough exercise but also worries about the amount of television they watch. Teresa may be a little overweight. Susan uses tobacco, about 1 pack per day. She denies the use of alcohol. Except for contraceptives, no one in the family takes any medication regularly. Teresa and Susan occasionally use aspirin, and Alexis uses Tylenol for minor aches and discomforts. Both of Susan's parents have diabetes, and her father has hypertension. Susan is unaware of health problems of either of her children's fathers or their families.

The family lives in a subsidized two-bedroom apartment. To give Teresa some space, Alexis and Susan share a room and have separate beds. Susan tries to have her family eat meals together, but often Teresa is out. Both children eat breakfast and lunch at school on a reduced-cost meal plan. Susan skips breakfast and sometimes has lunch at work. She works at a garment factory, sewing pieces of fabric together. Susan views maintaining health as important because she cannot afford to miss work, and she does not want the children to miss school.

The nurse notes that all three members of the family appear overweight but otherwise healthy, and they are all well groomed. Susan is attentive to all her children and allows Teresa to respond to questions about her own health. While talking to Teresa alone, the nurse discovers that Teresa smokes a pack of cigarettes every couple of days and is sexually active, but she doesn't want her mother to know about either activity. Teresa "sometimes uses a condom" but not regularly. She does not desire to become pregnant like her best friend.

Analysis

This profile illustrates the type of information you can collect by paying close attention to health-maintenance behaviors and using observation skills. Important factors to consider are: Who is responsible for managing the health of the family? What cultural factors influence health-related behaviors? What biologic factors, such a genetic background, influence health? Are there environmental conditions that influence health and safety? The assessment of this family's health maintenance indicated an essentially healthy family engaged in some healthy behaviors and some risky behaviors. Even though the nurse's first impression was that this was a healthy family, she conducted the assessment process in a thorough and systematic manner. She additionally discovered that Teresa and Susan needed immunizations and information about breast self-examinations. Also, no one in the family had a regular exercise routine.

Assessment Focus

The nurse recognized many cues reflecting the family's health perceptions and health management practices. The cues were organized in strength and risk factors.

Strengths

- Susan views the maintenance and improvement of health as important.
- The children eat three meals per day.
- Immunizations were up to date at the end of this visit.
- Susan has a single sexual partner and uses contraception.
- The three members talk comfortably together during the visit.
- Teresa is willing to share at risk behaviors with nurse.
- Susan would like to stop using tobacco.

Risks

- All are slightly overweight.
- No one follows a regular exercise routine.
- Susan does not do BSE.
- Teresa has unprotected sexual intercourse.
- Teresa has not discussed sexual activity and tobacco use with Susan.
- All are at risk for diabetes owing to family history, ethnicity (Mexican-American), and overweight.

Possible Nursing Diagnoses

Based on the nursing assessment, the possible diagnoses include Altered health maintenance related to tobacco use by Susan and Teresa and unprotected sexual intercourse by Teresa. Also, all family members have Altered health maintenance related to diet, inactivity, and family history that increases family's risk for diabetes.

The nurse talks with Susan, Teresa, and Alexis together to see what they would like to do about their diabetes risks. She individually talks with Susan about tobacco use and Teresa about tobacco and sexual activity. She refers Susan to a new tobacco cessation program at the clinic that is covered by her insurance. She encourages Teresa to talk to Susan, but also refers Teresa to the Women's Health Clinic for contraception and education about safe sex. Teresa is not interested to quitting her tobacco use at this time. Additionally, the nurse refers Susan to the social work department to determine whether the children are eligible for the new children's health insurance program.

CHAPTER 5 SUMMARY

Health perception and health management are evaluated to determine the following:
- The person's ability to maintain or improve health status
- Risk factors that may negatively affect health status
- The person's or family's knowledge base and ability to relate to health promotion and disease prevention

When assessing health perception–health management activities, the nurse should consider the following:
- Cultural influences on health status
- The level of responsibility for health maintenance the person is capable of assuming
- The person's cognitive ability and knowledge of health-related activities
- The value the person places on health
- Presence of any knowledge deficits and the person's willingness or ability to be compliant
- The complexity of the proposed healthcare regimen and the person's capabilities

The following information sources are used during assessment:
- 1. Interview and/or Review of Records
  - Focus
    - The individual's definition of health
    - The value the client places on health
    - Factors influencing health management
    - Risk factors that might disrupt health
    - The client's ability to manage health, including performance of self-care and self-examination skills
- 2. Laboratory/X-ray Evaluation
  - Focus
  - Laboratory tests recommended by US Preventive Services Task Force for adults younger than 65 years of age (also see children and adolescents, sexuality, and elder chapters for other age-group and pregnancy recommendations). Adults: total blood cholesterol
    - Papanicolaou (Pap) test (women)
    - Mammogram
    - Fecal occult blood test or sigmoidoscopy
- 3. Physical Examination/Observations
  - Observation of indicators of overall health status

- Signs of health maintenance capabilities
- Observation of risk factors
- Observation of self-care and self examination techniques
- Preventive health screening activities
- Observation of the environment

Health Maintenance–Health Perception assessment based on these principles and methods assists the nurse to identify defining characteristics and risk factors for the following nursing diagnoses:
High risk for aspiration
High risk for infection
High risk for injury
High risk for poisoning
High risk for suffocation
High risk for trauma
Altered growth and development
Altered health maintenance
Ineffective management of therapeutic regimen: individual
Ineffective management of therapeutic regimen: family
Effective management of therapeutic regimen
Altered protection
Health-seeking behaviors
Noncompliance (specify)

Related nursing diagnoses may be detected during health perception-health maintenance assessment, including problems that contribute to the management of health:
Impaired adjustment
Altered family processes
Impaired home maintenance/management
Impaired mobility
Ineffective individual or family coping
Fatigue
Impaired memory
Knowledge deficit (specify)
Self-care deficit (specify)
Spiritual distress
Altered thought process

Critical Thinking

Your agency has contracted to provide multi-phasic screening at a meat processing plant company picnic. Screening includes PSA for men older than age 40; glucose, cholesterol, and liver enzyme blood test; blood pressure; fecal occult blood; and providing health education on a variety of topics. Most employees do not have regular health care; although employees have free health insurance, it costs the employee to insure dependents. Health screening is being provided free to all who have company insurance.

1. How would you explain to an employee the purpose of the screening and possible benefits?

2. The second person you screen for blood pressure has a reading of 210/115. He denies he is at risk for anything. You explain the immediate risks. Others have told him that his blood pressure is a little high. What would your next action be?

3. Before you take a 40-year-old woman's blood pressure, she tells you that she has been on medication in the past but stopped it because it made her feel bad. She now takes garlic and grapefruit to control her blood pressure. Describe how you would show acceptance of her belief.

4. When the final results come in, you find that 20% of the population screened has untreated high blood pressure and 40% have very high cholesterol levels. What action would you take?

BIBLIOGRAPHY

American Nurses' Association (1980). *Nursing: A social policy statement*. Kansas City, MO: American Nurses' Association.

Bomar, P. (1996). *Nurses and family health promotion* (2nd ed.). Philadelphia: Lippincott.

Boston Women's Health Book Collective (1992). *The new our bodies our selves*. New York: Simon and Schuster.

Burnside, I. (1988). *Nursing and the aged* (3rd ed.). St. Louis: Mosby.

Caldwell, B. (1976). *Home observation measurement of the environment*. Little Rock, AR: University of Arkansas Center for Child Development and Education.

Caprenito, L. (1997). *Handbook of nursing diagnosis* (7th ed.). Philadelphia: Lippincott.

Gordon, M. (1994). *Nursing diagnosis: Process and application* (3rd ed.). St. Louis: Mosby.

Hill, J., & Smith., N. (1989). *Self care nursing* (2nd ed.). Norwalk, CT: Appleton-Century Crofts.

Horgan, P. (1987). Health status perceptions affect health-related behaviors. *Journal of Gerontological Nursing, 13*(12), 30–35.

Keating, S., & Kilmer, G. (1988). *Home health care nursing concepts and practices*. Philadelphia: Lippincott.

Murali, M., & Crabtree, K. (1992). Comparison of two breast self-examination techniques. *Cancer Nursing, 15*(4), 276–282.

Neuman, B. (1989). *The Newman systems model*. East Norwalk, CT: Appleton-Century Crofts.

Nightingale, F. (1969). *Notes on nursing*. New York: Dover Publications (original work published 1860).

North American Nursing Diagnosis Association (1996). *Nursing diagnosis: Definitions and classifications 1997–1998*. Philadelphia: NANDA.

Pender, N. (1995). *Health promotion in nursing practice* (3rd ed). Stamford, CT: Appleton & Lange.

Pender, N. (1987). *Health promotion in nursing practice* (2nd ed.). Norwalk, CT: Appleton & Lange.

Roy, C. (1984). *Introduction to nursing: An adaptation model* (2nd ed.). Englewood Cliffs, NJ: Prentice Hall.

School of Public Health (1991). *50 simple things you can do to save your life*. Los Angeles: UCLA Press.

Shuher, J. (1992). *Reader's Digest: The good health fact book*. New York: Reader's Digest.

Stanhope, M., & Knollmueller, R. (1995). *Public and community health nurse's consultant: A health promotion guide* (2nd ed.). St Louis: Mosby.

Stanhope, M., & Lancaster, J. (1995). *Community health nursing: Process and practice for promoting health* (4th ed.). St. Louis: Mosby.

Stolte, K. (1996). *Wellness: Nursing diagnosis for health promotion*. Philadelphia: Lippincott.

Triolo, P. (1987). Marketing women's health care. *Journal of Nursing Administration 17*(11), 9–14.

US Department of Health and Human Services (1990). *Healthy people 2000: New objectives to promote health, prevent disease*. Washington DC: Office of Disease Prevention and Health Promotion.

US Preventive Services Task Force (1996). *Guide to clinical preventive services* (2nd ed.). Baltimore: Williams & Wilkins.

Watson, J. (1985). *Nursing: Human science and human care*. East Norwalk, CT: Appleton-Century Crofts.

Wingo, P., Tong, T., & Bolden, S. (1995). Cancer statistics. *CA: Cancer Journal for Clinicians, 45*(1), 8–30.

World Health Organization (1986a). *Leadership for health for all: The challenge to nursing*. Geneva: World Health Organization.

World Health Organization (1986b). *Ottawa charter for health promotion*. Geneva: World Health Organization.

ASSESSMENT GUIDELINES

- Nutrition Interview (Health History)
- Diet Evaluation
- Diagnostic Studies of Nutrition Status
- Anthropometric Assessment
- Interpreting Physical Examination Findings Related to Nutrition
- Skin
- Wound Assessment
- Hair
- Nails
- Jaw and Oral Cavity
- Abdomen
- Evaluating Abdominal Fluid
- Thyroid Gland
- Lymphatic System

CHAPTER ORGANIZATION

PART 1: ASSESSING THE PATTERN

Introductory Overview
- Assessment Focus
- Nursing Diagnoses

Knowledge Base for Assessment
- Nutritional Processes
- Nutritional Requirements: RDA Analysis
- The Dietary Guidelines for Americans
- Eating Disorders

PART 2: PHYSICAL EXAMINATION TECHNIQUES

Integumentary System: Skin, Hair, and Nails
- Anatomy and Physiology Review

The Jaw and Oral Cavity
- Anatomy and Physiology Review

The Abdomen
- Anatomy and Physiology Review

The Thyroid Gland
- Anatomy and Physiology Review

The Lymphatic System
- Anatomy and Physiology Review

PART 1

ASSESSING THE PATTERN

INTRODUCTORY OVERVIEW

Comprehensive assessment of a person's nutritional and metabolic status can be a considerable undertaking. *Nutritional processes* (including *ingestion, digestion, absorption,* and *transport*), metabolic status, and the impact of dietary practices should all be thoroughly evaluated to adequately characterize nutritional and metabolic functions.

Nutrition status is influenced by multiple factors, including the balance between a person's nutrient intake (supply) and the body's energy requirements or metabolic needs (demand). To underscore the importance of these supply and demand relationships, the assessment of nutrition and metabolism is integrated. For example, the observation that a person's nutrient intake amounts to 2200 kilocalories (kcal) per day does not provide adequate information about nutrition status unless considered in relation to the person's metabolic needs. In a sedentary person without any conditions causing high metabolic demands, a 2200 daily kilocalorie intake may be excessive. Conversely, a 2200 daily kilocalorie intake may be inadequate if the person has high metabolic demands such as those associated with major wound healing.

Signs and symptoms of altered nutrition may be noted by observation of a person's general appearance and the condition of the skin, hair, and nails. Indicators of altered metabolism also should be considered during assessment of nutrition and metabolism. For example, signs and symptoms of infection, such as fever and lymphatic system alterations, are significant because metabolic needs generally increase with infection. Thyroid alterations are also significant because thyroid hormones play a major role in regulating metabolism.

Nutrition status is also evaluated by analysis of the person's diet. An adequate diet is one that supplies all essential nutrients in appropriate amounts and avoids excesses that predispose individuals to chronic diseases. Dietary practices are subject to many influences, including personal beliefs and culture, socioeconomic status, functional abilities, and the development of eating disorders. The indicators of a healthy diet must be familiar to health care providers conducting a nutrition assessment. The *1995 Dietary Guidelines for Americans* are presented in this chapter to illustrate the essential components of a healthy diet.

ASSESSMENT FOCUS

Nutrition assessment is the process of collecting and interpreting data for the purpose of identifying healthy nutrition practices, nutrition risks, altered nutrition status, and the effects of altered nutrition. With a comprehensive nutrition assessment, the nurse will meet the following objectives:

- Evaluating dietary practices in relation to recommended nutritional and weight standards
- Identifying the impact of various factors that may influence food and fluid consumption
- Evaluating indicators of nutrition risk

- Determining the status of the nutrition processes including ingestion, digestion, absorption, and metabolism
- Identifying specific nutrition alterations or problems

Data collection is accomplished by the following methods:

1. Interview or Review of Records Focus
   Patterns of weight gain or loss
   Dietary practices
   Functional status
   Socioeconomic variables
   Medical history
   Medication history

2. Diet Evaluation Focus
    Diet (food intake) history
    24-hour food recall
    Food frequency record
    Food diary
    Calorie count
3. Diagnostic Studies Focus
    Serum albumin
    Serum transferrin
    Total lymphocyte count
    Urinary urea nitrogen, state of nitrogen balance
    Hemoglobin, hematocrit, and transferrin
    Cholesterol
    Lipid profile
4. Physical Examination Focus
    Anthropometric measurement: height, weight, triceps skinfold, mid-arm circumference, mid-arm muscle circumference
    Signs and symptoms of nutritional or metabolic alterations detected during examination of general appearance, the integumentary system, oral cavity, abdomen, thyroid gland, or lymphatic system
    Skin lesions, wounds, and wound healing

Nursing Diagnoses

Assessment of the nutrition and metabolic pattern may result in the identification of one or more of the following primary nursing diagnoses:

Adequate nutrition
Altered nutrition: More than body requirements
Altered nutrition: Less than body requirements
Altered nutrition: Potential for more than body requirements

Secondary nursing diagnoses related to nutrition and metabolic status include the following:

Feeding self-care deficit
Ineffective breast-feeding
Altered growth and development
Impaired tissue integrity
Altered oral mucous membrane
Impaired skin integrity
Risk for impaired skin integrity
Constipation
Diarrhea
Fluid volume excess
Fluid volume deficit
Risk for fluid volume deficit
Risk for infection
Impaired swallowing (dysphagia)
Risk for aspiration
Knowledge deficit
Altered health maintenance
Ineffective management of therapeutic regimen
Noncompliance
Health-seeking behaviors

KNOWLEDGE BASE FOR ASSESSMENT

Important knowledge to guide you in the assessment of nutrition status includes an understanding of the nutritional processes—ingestion, digestion, absorption, transport, and metabolism. Knowledge of nutritional requirements, including the characteristics of a healthy diet, is also essential knowledge for the assessment process.

Nutritional Processes

Nutritional status is influenced by all of the processes involved in nutrient intake and use: ingestion, digestion, absorption, transport, and metabolism. Each process requires integrated anatomic and physiologic function. Physical examination techniques provide cues to functional status.

Ingestion involves the process of taking nutrients into the gastrointestinal tract. Under normal conditions, this process involves all activities that lead to placing food in the mouth. Significant influences include habits, culture, socioeconomic status, ability to prepare food, and satiety.

Digestion refers to breakdown of ingested nutrients in the gastrointestinal tract to forms that can be absorbed by the body. It involves a number of mechanical acts and chemical reactions occurring in the mouth, esophagus, and intestine.

Absorption involves the passage of digested food substances from the gastrointestinal tract to the blood or lymphatic circulation. The blood is then channeled to the liver, where metabolic processes occur.

Transport refers to the movement of nutrients across cell membranes. Transport problems are usually detected by laboratory screening. In a person with diabetes mellitus, for example, glucose is prevented from entering the cells, and serum blood sugar levels may be characteristically high.

Metabolism is the final process of nutrition. Metabolism consists of the processes that produce and use energy within body cells. The production and use of energy in the cell is a complex process that begins when the cell is fueled by nutrients. Ultimately, however, energy use must be matched by energy production to achieve optimal health.

In the human body, energy is used in two major ways: to maintain essential life processes, such as breathing, nervous system function, and blood circulation, and to support "nonessential" life activities such as running, working, thinking, and dealing with stress. Additionally, some energy is expended for nutritional processes such as digestion and absorption.

The amount of energy required for essential life processes is referred to as the basal metabolism or basal metabolic rate (BMR). The BMR is measured when the body is physically, metabolically, and emotionally at rest and is usually expressed in kilocalories per hour (kcal/hour). Surprisingly, a large number of kilocalories are required to maintain basal metabolic activities. For example, someone whose total energy needs are 2000 kcal/day may use as many as 1400 of these kilocalories for basal metabolism.

Metabolic processes are referred to as anabolic or catabolic. *Anabolism* is a constructive metabolic state in which ingested raw materials are converted to cell-building substances. *Catabolism* is a destructive metabolic process in that tissues or other substances such as glycogen are broken down to generate energy or heat.

Optimal metabolic function is characterized by a balance between anabolic and catabolic processes. Factors other than the amount and type of nutrients ingested daily may affect this balance and should be considered when assessing nutritional–metabolic status. Activity levels, hormonal imbalances, environmental temperature, stress, and illness may significantly influence the metabolic state.

Nutritional Requirements: RDA Analysis

In the United States, the federal government has published various nutritional guidelines to assist people in adhering to a healthy diet. The most well known of these guidelines are the *Recommended Dietary Allowances (RDAs)*, first published in the 1940s, and the *Dietary Guidelines for Americans,* most recently revised and published in 1995.

The RDAs focus on the prevention of dietary deficiencies that were more common in American society in the postwar years of the 1940s. To make judgments about diet using the RDA system, the following steps are taken:

1. *Data Collection.* An accurate food intake history is recorded for a 24-hour period (See *Diet Evaluation* elsewhere in this chapter).
2. *Nutrient Analysis.* For each food item consumed in the 24-hour period, the amount of kilocalories, proteins, fats, carbohydrates, vitamins, and minerals contained in the food is determined by consulting a food composition table.
3. *Identification of Nutrient Deficiencies.* The amounts of nutrients in the diet being analyzed are compared with a table of RDA values representing ideal daily nutrient intakes (see Appendix B).

The RDA diet analysis methodology has several shortcomings. First, nutrition disorders caused by deficiencies in vitamins and minerals are relatively rare in the American diet, with the exception of iron and calcium deficiencies in some high-risk groups. Second, the RDA system is complex and requires special skills and accurate analysis for good results, which limits reliable use by the general public. Third, RDAs have been established for healthy persons only and may not appropriately reflect the nutrition needs of people with acute or chronic illnesses. Finally, RDA standards have not been established for elders.

The Dietary Guidelines for Americans

The Dietary Guidelines for Americans (Display 6-1) call for moderation in the consumption of various food groups, and in so doing speak to the excesses common in most American diets, especially excesses in calories and fats. The guidelines serve as the basis for federal nutrition policy and provide research-based nutritional guidance in easily understood terms. Health care providers should become familiar with the guidelines to assist people in the evaluation and modification of their diets. It is essential to know what each guideline means and how it is important to health as well as how the guideline may be used for nutrition education. Seven dietary guidelines were issued by the US Departments of Agriculture (USDA) and Health and Human Services (HHS) in 1995.

Guideline #1: Eat a Variety of Foods

The variety guideline serves as the foundation for a healthy diet. At least 40 different nutrients are required to promote good health. It is preferable to obtain these nutrients through the consumption of a variety of foods rather than from the ingestion of a few highly fortified foods or supplements. In fact, some supplements may provide nutrients in excess of the recommended daily allowances, and this practice in itself may be harmful.

One way to assure variety in the diet is to choose foods daily from the *Food Pyramid* (Display 6-2). The Food Pyramid is an educational tool developed by the US Department of Agriculture to illustrate the message of dietary variety. The Food Pyramid replaces the Four Food Group classification system previously used by the federal government for nutrition education. The Food Pyramid may be used as a guideline for vegetarian diets and can accommodate different cultures, lifestyles, and religious perspectives.

Five major food groups and a sixth group—the "empty calorie" group—are included on the Food Pyramid. The Food Pyramid emphasizes choosing from among the following major food groups in the daily diet:

1. Breads, cereals, rice, and pasta
2. Vegetables
3. Fruits
4. Meat, poultry, fish, dry beans and peas, eggs, and nuts
5. Milk, yogurt, cheese

DISPLAY 6.1

Dietary Guidelines for Americans

☑ Eat a variety of foods
☑ Maintain or improve your weight
☑ Choose a diet with plenty of grain products, vegetables, and fruits
☑ Choose a diet low in fat, saturated fat, and cholesterol
☑ Use sugars only in moderation
☑ Use salt and sodium only in moderation
☑ If you drink alcoholic beverages, do so in moderation

DISPLAY 6.2

Food Guide Pyramid

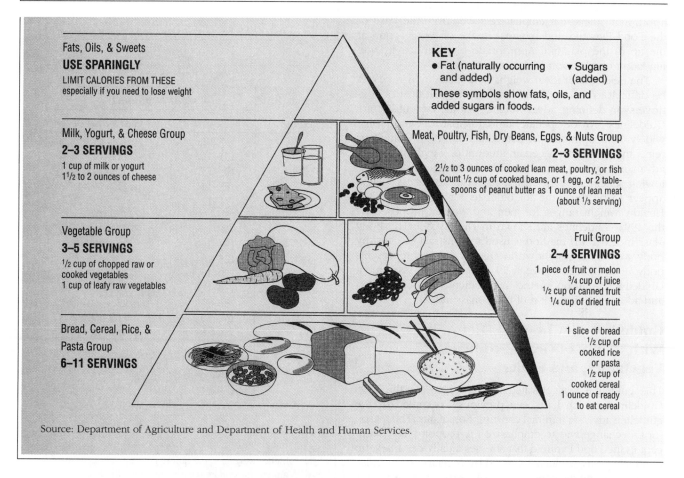

Fats, Oils, & Sweets
USE SPARINGLY
LIMIT CALORIES FROM THESE
especially if you need to lose weight

KEY
● Fat (naturally occurring   ▼ Sugars
and added)   (added)
These symbols show fats, oils, and
added sugars in foods.

Milk, Yogurt, & Cheese Group
2–3 SERVINGS
1 cup of milk or yogurt
1½ to 2 ounces of cheese

Meat, Poultry, Fish, Dry Beans, Eggs, & Nuts Group
2–3 SERVINGS
2½ to 3 ounces of cooked lean meat, poultry, or fish
Count ½ cup of cooked beans, or 1 egg, or 2 table-
spoons of peanut butter as 1 ounce of lean meat
(about ⅓ serving)

Vegetable Group
3–5 SERVINGS
½ cup of chopped raw or
cooked vegetables
1 cup of leafy raw vegetables

Fruit Group
2–4 SERVINGS
1 piece of fruit or melon
¾ cup of juice
½ cup of canned fruit
¼ cup of dried fruit

Bread, Cereal, Rice, &
Pasta Group
6–11 SERVINGS

1 slice of bread
½ cup of
cooked rice
or pasta
½ cup of
cooked cereal
1 ounce of ready
to eat cereal

Source: Department of Agriculture and Department of Health and Human Services.

At the top of the pyramid are fats, oils, and sweets sometimes referred to as "empty calories," to illustrate the minimal nutritional value of such foods. Consumption of these foods, which include salad dressing and oils, soft drinks, candy, and sweet desserts, should be limited. The circle (fat) and triangle (sweet) shapes concentrated at the top of the pyramid represent highly concentrated or added fats and sugars. The circle and triangle shapes scattered through the rest of the pyramid represent added and naturally occurring fats and sugars found in foods occurring in the major food groups.

The Food Pyramid suggests minimum daily servings for each food group. In addition, it illustrates proportionality by showing the relative amounts of each food that should be consumed daily. At a glance, the consumer can see that breads, cereal, rice and pasta should make up the largest amount of the daily dietary intake and that fats, oils, and sweets should be used sparingly.

Certain individuals need to make food choices to ensure adequate intake of calcium and iron. Many women and adolescent girls need to eat more calcium-rich foods, such as milk and milk products, to ingest enough calcium for healthy bone metabolism. Young children, adolescent girls, and women of childbearing age must take care to eat enough iron-rich foods such as lean meats, dry beans, and whole grain and iron-enriched breads or cereals.

Guideline #2: Balance the Food You Eat With Physical Activity—Maintain or Improve Your Weight

This guideline emphasizes the importance of considering both diet and physical activity (supply and demand) in relationship to weight maintenance, weight gain, and weight loss. Weighing either too much or too little can contribute to health problems. Obesity is far more common among Americans than being too thin and is associated with hypertension, heart disease, diabetes, and certain types of cancer. Generally, accumulation of fat in the abdominal area is considered more detrimental to health than fat accumulation in the hips and thighs.

Because many Americans may be overweight, this guideline stresses the message of preventing further weight gain by emphasizing weight maintenance. Ideally, 30 minutes per day of moderate physical activity will maintain weight or burn fat to reduce weight, provided dietary intake is controlled. By building muscle mass, exercise also will help prevent the weight loss that may occur with aging primarily because of muscle tissue loss or atrophy. Care must be taken when making weight loss recommendations for children, who still require adequate energy intake to maintain healthy growth and development. Overweight children should be encouraged to develop appropriate diets that emphasize foods from the base of the Food Pyramid and minimal intake of foods found at the tip of the pyramid. Appropriate physical activity and limitation of television is also important.

The desirable or ideal weight for a given individual can be difficult to define. There has been a great deal of controversy in defining "ideal weight," but the current Dietary Guidelines provide specific standards that renounce some widely held opinions. In particular, the 1995 Guidelines reject the belief that a certain amount of weight gain with advancing age is acceptable. The Guidelines make the following statement: "The health risks due to excess weight appear to be the same for older as for younger adults." Healthy weight ranges for men and women proposed by the 1995 Guidelines are shown in Display 6-3. The Body Mass Index (BMI) method is used to construct the healthy body weight ranges shown in Display 6-3 and represents body mass indices between 19 and 25. (See Assessment Guideline: Anthropometric Assessment, for calculation and additional discussion of body mass index).

Guideline #3: Choose a Diet With Plenty of Grain Products, Vegetables, and Fruits

This guideline was elevated to third place in the 1995 Guidelines, which had been previously occupied by the guideline advising minimal consumption of fats. The reason for this change was to emphasize the proportionality concept in the Food Pyramid that stresses a daily diet made up of mostly grain products followed by vegetables and fruits. By emphasizing the consumption of foods at the base of the pyramid in the appropriate proportions, there is less daily consumption of unhealthy fats. At a minimum, a person's daily diet should include six servings of grains, three servings of vegetables, and two servings of fruits. Foods from these groups provide complex carbohydrates needed to meet the body's energy needs, dietary fiber, and essential vitamins and minerals. These foods are also generally low in fats unless such substances are added in the course of food preparation. Dietary fiber is considered essential to proper bowel function and the prevention of chronic constipation, diverticular disease, and hemorrhoid formation. Fiber is best obtained from food sources rather than supplements because other components in fiber-containing foods provide nutritional benefits.

Guideline #4: Choose a Diet Low in Fat, Saturated Fat, and Cholesterol

The intent of this guideline is to encourage limited consumption of fats and cholesterol in the American diet because the health effects can be detrimental. High-fat diets are associated with atherosclerotic heart disease, certain forms of cancer, obesity, and non–insulin-dependent diabetes.

DISPLAY 6.3

Suggested Weights for Adults (Dietary Guidelines for Americans)

	SUGGESTED WEIGHTS FOR ADULTS	
	Weight in pounds[†]	
Height*	**19–34 years**	**35 years and older**
5'0"	97–128[‡]	108–138
5'1"	101–132	111–143
5'2"	104–137	115–148
5'3"	107–141	119–152
5'4"	111–146	122–157
5'5"	114–150	126–162
5'6"	118–155	130–167
5'7"	121–160	134–172
5'8"	125–164	138–178
5'9"	129–169	142–183
5'10"	132–174	146–188
5'11"	136–179	151–194
6'0"	140–184	155–199
6'1"	144–189	159–205
6'2"	148–195	164–210
6'3"	152–200	168–216
6'4"	156–205	173–222
6'5"	160–211	177–228
6'6"	164–216	182–234

*Without shoes.

[†]Without clothes.

[‡]The higher weights in the ranges generally apply to men, who tend to have more muscle and bone; the lower weights more often apply to women, who have less muscle and bone.

(Nutrition and your health: Dietary guidelines for Americans [3rd ed]. [Home and Garden Bulletin 232]. Washington, DC: U.S. Department of Agriculture and U.S. Department of Health and Human Services, 1990; 9.)

These recommendations should be applied to the amount of fat intake averaged over several days rather than applied to a single meal or daily intake. In other words, an occasional indulgence in a high-fat food may be acceptable if, on the average, fat intake is controlled. A practical and consumer-oriented method for evaluating fat intake is to refer to *Nutrition Facts Labels* displayed on many food items (Display 6-4). The label will indicate fat grams contained in a particular food.

Total fat intake should not exceed 30% of calories consumed per day. For a 2000-calorie diet, the upper limit would be 600 calories obtained from fat (2000 × .30). This is equal to 67 g fat (600 divided by 9, the number of calories provided by each gram of fat). The primary sources of

DISPLAY 6.4

Nutrition Facts Label

THE NEW [SIMPLE FORMAT] FOOD LABEL AT A GLANCE

The new food label will carry an up-to-date, easier-to-use nutrition information guide, to be required on almost all packaged foods (compared with about 60% of products up until now). The guide will serve as a key to help in planning a healthy diet.*

Serving sizes are now more consistant across product lines, stated in both household and metric measures, and reflect the amounts people actually eat.

The list of nutrients covers those most important to the health of today's consumers, most of whom need to worry about getting too much of certain items (fat, for example), rather than too few vitamins or minerals, as in the past.

The label will now tell the number of calories per gram of fat, carbohydrates, and protein.

Nutrition Facts

Serving Size 1/2 cup (114g)
Servings per Container 4

Amount Per Serving

Calories 90 Calories from Fat 30

	% Daily Value*
Total Fat 3g	5%
Saturated Fat 0g	0%
Cholesterol 0mg	0%
Sodium 300mg	13%
Total Carbohydrate 13g	4%
Dietary Fiber 3g	12%
Sugars 3g	
Protein 3g	

Vitamin A—80%	Vitamin C—60%
Calcium—4%	Iron—4%

*Percent Daily Values are based on a 2,000 calorie diet. Your daily values may be higher or lower depending on your calorie needs:

	Calories	2,000	2,500
Total Fat	Less than	65g	80g
Sat Fat	Less than	20g	25g
Cholesterol	Less than	300mg	300mg
Sodium	Less than	2,400mg	2,400mg
Total Carbohydrates		300g	375g
Fiber		25g	30g

Calories per gram:
Fat 9—Cholesterol 4—Protein 4

New title signals that the label contains the newly required information.

Calories from fat are now shown on the label to help consumers meet dietary guidelines that recommend people get no more than 30% of their calories from fat.

% Daily Value shows how a food fits into the overall daily diet.

Daily values are also something new. Some are maximums, as with fat (65 grams or less); others are minimums, as with carbohydrates (300 grams or more). The daily values on the label are based on a daily diet of 2,000 and 2,500 calories. Individuals should adjust the values to fit their own calorie intake.

*This label is only a sample. Exact specifications are in the final rules. Source: Food and Drug Administration, 1992.

saturated fat are from animal products and tropical oils (coconut, palm). Saturated fat intake should not exceed 10% of total calorie intake. This amounts to no more than 22 g saturated fat in a 2000 calorie per day diet.

Animal products are the source of all dietary cholesterol, and cholesterol levels can be effectively lowered, in most cases, by consuming less fat from animals. The daily dietary intake of cholesterol should not exceed 300 mg.

The 1995 Guidelines provide new fat recommendations for children over the age of 2 years. Children between 2 and 5 years of age should gradually decrease their dietary intakes of fat so that, by school age, no more than 30% of the calories in their diets are derived from fat.

Guideline #5: Choose a Diet Moderate in Sugars

Sugars, along with starch and fibers, are carbohydrates. All carbohydrates break down into sugars with digestion. Sugars supply calories but are limited in nutrients. High-sugar diets have not been correlated with the development of diabetes or hyperactivity. However, there is a positive correlation between high sugar intake and the development of obesity and tooth decay. Therefore sugars should be avoided to maintain weight and appropriate oral hygiene practices developed to prevent tooth decay.

Guideline #6: Choose a Diet Moderate in Salt and Sodium

Table salt contains sodium and chloride, and both are essential nutrients. Most people easily exceed the daily minimal requirements of these minerals. One reason may be that dietary salt is not just added at the table but is also added during the commercial processing of many foods and beverages. Sodium, along with heredity, obesity, and excessive alcohol consumption, has been implicated in the development of hypertension. Consumers are advised to limit daily sodium intake to less than 2400 mg. This can be evaluated by reading Nutrition Fact Labels on food products (see Display 6-4).

Guideline #7: If You Drink Alcoholic Beverages, Do So in Moderation

Alcohol is classified as a food and contains calories but little or no other nutritional value. Excess consumption of alcohol is associated with detrimental effects including dependency, impaired function and judgment, and, over the long term, additional serious health effects. In moderation, beneficial effects of alcohol are recognized, including positive effects on digestion and some protection from coronary artery disease. Coronary artery disease may be effectively prevented through proper diet and exercise, so alcohol ingestion should not be adopted primarily for this purpose.

Moderate alcohol intake is defined for women as no more than one drink per day and for men, no more than two drinks. A drink is defined as 12 ounces of regular beer or 5 ounces of wine or 1½ ounces of distilled spirits (80 proof).

The Guidelines identify those who should not drink alcoholic beverages, including children and adolescents; women who are pregnant or who are trying to conceive; individuals who plan to drive or engage in other activities that require attention or skill; individuals using medications, including over-the-counter; and individuals who cannot drink in moderation.

Pattern Assessment   Nutrition Assessment Guidelines

GENERAL APPROACH

There is no single, universally accepted tool for evaluating nutrition status. A combination of methods is often used to assess nutrition status. The specific focus or emphasis of nutrition assessment may vary across practice settings, institutions, and patient populations. Screening for nutrition problems should be a routine health assessment activity, even in ambulatory settings with healthy populations. Persons at high risk for nutritional problems include elders, people scheduled for surgery, people with cancer or chronic diseases, and people living in deprived environments.

NUTRITION SCREENING

Nutrition screening is an abbreviated assessment method that identifies people at moderate to high risk for nutrition problems. Screening involves taking a few critical measurements strongly associated with nutrition problems. Screening should be simple, straightforward, and easy to conduct by trained providers who may not have advanced expertise in nutrition assessment. Typical information used for screening nutrition status includes the following: height, weight, unintentional weight loss, change in appetite, special diet order, medical diagnosis, serum albumin level, hemoglobin, hematocrit, total lymphocyte count.

Nutrition screening is a common activity in hospitals. This type of screening is often conducted by nurses. Patients identified at risk for nutritional problems through the screening process are further evaluated. A sample hospital screening tool is shown in Display 6-5.

(continued)

DISPLAY 6.5

Nutrition Screening Report

MEDICAL CENTER REHABILITATION HOSPITAL

University of North Dakota
Grand Forks, North Dakota
Clinical Nutrition Services

NAME: _____
NUMBER: _____
ROOM/BED NO:_____

S:_____

_____

_____

O:

Age	Sex	Height	Weight

% Wt. Change	Usual Weight	IBW	%IBW

Score

_____

Dx: _____

Hx: _____   _____

_____

Diet Order: _____   _____

_____

Lab Data: (Date)   _____   _____   _____

                          _____   _____   _____

Decubiti Stage: I   II   III   IV

Diet Hx: _____

1. Appetite   Adequate   Poor < 10 Days   Poor > 10 Days   _____

2. N/V   Dysphagia   Diarrhea   _____

Total Points

A: Nutritional Status:

☐ High Risk   ☐ Moderate Risk   ☐ Low Risk
   (5+ pts)   (3–4 pts)   (<3 pts)

Requires further L.R.D. intervention   ☐ Yes   ☐ No

P:_____

_____

_____

_____

_____   _____
Signature   Date

DISPLAY 6.5

Nutrition Screening Report (continued)

NUTRITION SCREENING REPORT CRITERIA

Points will be accumulated in the following manner to determine the risk level of the patient upon admission and provide a basis for the type of nutritional care to be instituted.

A. Weight Status—Evaluation of previous weight/height ratio; recent weight loss or gain; % of the suggested Ideal Body Weight range (> 120% or < 90%).
> Number of Points Possible = 1

B. Admitting Diagnosis/History—Evaluation of presence of high risk diagnosis/history (ex: CVA, TBI, SCI, Dysphagia, etc.).
> Number of Points Possible = 1

C. Type of Diet Order—Diets other than regular will be evaluated in light of the patient's diagnosis.
> Number of Points Possible = 1

D. Laboratory Data—Review of recent (within 5 days) laboratory data that reflect compromised nutritional status (ex: serum albumin, CBC, etc.).
> Number of Points Possible = 1+; point will be assigned for each significantly abnormal laboratory value.

E. Skin Integrity—Evaluation for the presence of decubitus ulcers.
> Number of Points Possible = 1+; 1 point will be assigned for each stage (1–4).

F. Diet History—Evaluation of patient's appetite status.
> Number of Points Possible = 1+ (1 = <10 days, 2 = >10 days)

G. Diet History—Evaluation for the presence of factors affecting overall nutritional status.
> Number of Points Possible = 1+; 1 point assigned for each factor.

The points are then totaled to determine risk category based on the following:

> High risk (5+ points)
> Moderate risk (3–4 points)
> Low risk (1–2 points)

This will determine whether the patient warrants any further action by the licensed registered dietitian. A plan of action will be noted if appropriate.

(Courtesy of Medical Center Rehabilitation Hospital, Grand Forks, ND.)

Pattern Assessment — Nutrition Assessment Guidelines (continued)

NUTRITION RISK SCREENING IN ELDERS

The Nutrition Screening Initiative has developed a tool for nutrition screening of elders (Display 6-6). This screen is used to identify persons who may be candidates for home meal delivery, assistance with shopping or cooking, congregate meal programs, or nutrition intervention and education.

COMPREHENSIVE NUTRITION ASSESSMENT

A comprehensive nutrition assessment includes the following components:

Interview (health history)
Diet evaluation
Laboratory analysis
Physical assessment
Anthropometric assessment

EQUIPMENT FOR ANTHROPOMETRIC ASSESSMENT

Metric tape measure
Beam balance scale
Calipers

ASSESSMENT AIDS

Interview Guide to suggest questions and record data (Display 6-7)

DISPLAY 6.6

Nutrition Screening Initiative—Elder Screening

DETERMINE YOUR NUTRITIONAL HEALTH

The warning signs of poor nutritional health are often overlooked. Use this checklist to find out if you or someone you know is at nutritional risk.

Read the statements below. Circle the number in the yes column for those that apply to you or someone you know. For each yes answer, score the number in the box. Total your nutritional score.

	Yes
I have an illness or condition that made me change the kind or amount of food I eat.	2
I eat fewer than 2 meals per day.	3
I eat few fruits or vegetables, or milk products.	2
I have 3 or more drinks of beer, liquor, or wine almost every day.	2
I have tooth or mouth problems that make it hard for me to eat.	2
I don't always have enough money to buy the food I need.	4
I eat alone most of the time.	1
I take 3 or more different prescribed or over-the-counter drugs a day.	1
Without wanting to, I have lost or gained 10 pounds in the last 6 months.	2
I am not always physically able to shop, cook, or feed myself.	2
Total	

TOTAL YOUR NUTRITIONAL SCORE. IF IT'S—

0–2 **Good!** Recheck your nutritional score in 6 months.

3–5 **You are at moderate nutritional risk.** See what can be done to improve your eating habits and lifestyle. Your office on aging, senior nutrition program, senior citizen center or health department can help. Recheck your nutritional score in 3 months.

6 or more **You are at high nutritional risk.** Bring this checklist the next time you see your doctor, dietitian, or other qualified health or social service professional. Talk with them about any problems you may have. Ask for help to improve your nutritional health.

American Academy of Family Physicians
The American Dietetic Association
National Council on the Aging, Inc.
Remember that warning signs suggest risk but do not represent diagnosis of any condition.

(Developed by The Nutritional Screening Initiative [American Academy of Family Physicians; The American Dietetic Association; National Council on Aging, Inc.])

Pattern Assessment   Nutrition Assessment Guidelines (continued)

Screening Tools (Displays 6-5 and 6-6)
Institution-specific forms for recording data
Forms for recording dietary intake such as the 24-hour diet recall, food frequency record, or food diary

REFERENCE MATERIALS

Height and weight tables
Food composition tables
Recommended Daily Allowance (RDA) tables
Computer software programs for diet analysis

DISPLAY 6.7

Interview Guide: Nutrition

NUTRITION AND METABOLIC PATTERN

Height/Weight/Changes in Appetite

Height _____   Weight _____

Weight Fluctuations ❑ None   ❑ Gain   ❑ Loss (>10 pounds in last 3 months)*

Appetite   ❑ Normal   ❑ Increased   ❑ Decreased   ❑ Decreased taste

❑ Nausea   ❑ Vomiting (>3 days)*   ❑ Stomatitis

❑ Minimal PO intake (>5 days)*

Diet

Meals/Snacks (#/day) _____   Special Diet/Supplement _____

Compliance ❑ Yes   ❑ No   ❑ Previous dietary instruction/Typical daily diet:

  Breakfast _____

  Lunch _____

  Dinner _____

  Snacks _____

Fluid Intake: (8-oz glasses/day) ❑ Restricted   ❑ 0–5 glasses   ❑ 5–10 glasses   ❑ >10 glasses

Food Allergies: _____   Food Dislikes: _____

Nutrition Knowledge

Name basic foods groups _____

Name food high in calories; in fats: _____

Name foods with low nutritional value: _____

Learning needs: ❑ No   ❑ Yes   Explain: _____

FUNCTIONAL STATUS

Problem obtaining/preparing food: ❑ No   ❑ Yes*   Explain: _____

Swallowing difficulty: ❑ None   ❑ Solids*   ❑ Liquids*

Chewing difficulty: ❑ None   ❑ Meat   ❑ Fruits/Vegetables

Dentures: ❑ None   ❑ Upper   ❑ Lower   ❑ Partial   ❑ Full

MEDICAL HISTORY

Conditions related to nutritional risk: ❑ No   ❑ Yes   Explain/List: _____

Any changes in skin, hair, nails: _____

MEDICATION HISTORY

Potential food/drug interactions: ❑ No   ❑ Yes   Explain: _____

_____

*Consider consult with clinical dietician.

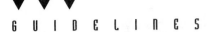

Assessment Guidelines Nutrition Interview (Health History)

Procedure	Clinical Significance

Procedure

1. Weight

Note: Measurement of weight is discussed elsewhere—See "Anthropometric Measurement"

Inquire about the person's weight, asking questions such as the following:

- "Is your weight today your usual weight?"
- "Have you had any recent weight change?"
- "Describe how your weight has changed."
- "Are you trying to lose (or gain) weight?"
- "How do you feel about your present weight?"
- "How would you describe your appetite?"

Reports of trying to lose weight should be evaluated in relation to whether an actual need for weight reduction is indicated.

People of normal weight trying to lose weight may be at risk for nutritional problems, weight cycling, development of eating disorders, and self-esteem problems, especially if they fail to lose weight.

2. Dietary practices

Interview the person to determine special dietary requirements and preferences, dislikes, eating habits, and food allergies.

Promote an atmosphere of interest, respect, and open-mindedness, especially when you ask about eating habits. Accept information about eating habits without passing judgment, recognizing that there are many individual variations.

Ask questions such as the following:

- "Do you require a special diet?"
- "Do you know the name of your diet?"
- "Do you have any special dietary needs?"

- "Do you have allergies to any food?"

Clinical Significance

Reports of sudden changes in weight may indicate serious health problems as well as nutritional problems and should be further investigated.

A report of unintentional weight loss may indicate a serious undiagnosed illness such as cancer.

Severe weight loss: Loss of 10% or more of body weight within 6 months or unintentional loss of more than 2 pounds per week. Associated with increased risk of disease development and premature death.

Weight cycling: Repeated weight loss and regain. Weight cycling is associated with an increased risk of disease development and premature death.

Eating disorders: Unusual eating patterns that are potentially life-threatening. Common eating disorders include *anorexia nervosa* and *bulimia nervosa.*

A report of sudden weight gain may indicate fluid retention, electrolyte imbalance, and medication side effects.

Assessment of a person's eating habits involves information that may be very personal and requires interpersonal skills for developing trust and rapport. Eating habits are personal because they reflect ethnic background, family customs, religious beliefs, philosophy, and other aspects of a person's lifestyle.

A special or therapeutic diet may be prescribed to meet a person's specific nutritional needs.

Asking about special needs also provides an opportunity for the person to identify dietary practices related to individual lifestyle, for example, vegetarian or kosher diets. Attention to special needs shows cultural sensitivity and respect for an individual's values and beliefs.

Therapeutic diet: A modified diet or meal plan that is specifically ordered for an individual in the treatment of symptoms or disease conditions. Specific terminology should be used to describe various therapeutic diets. For example, "1200 kcal/day diet" is more descriptive than "low-calorie diet" and "1500 mg/day sodium" is better than saying "low-sodium diet."

Food allergies are usually caused by proteins in foods such as the protein components of milk, eggs, nuts, and wheat.

▼ ▼ ▼

Procedure

- "Describe how you reacted when eating foods you are allergic to."

- "Can you name foods you dislike or wish to avoid?"
- "What types of fruits and vegetables do you like/dislike?"
- "How many meals do you eat a day?"
- "Do you snack between meals? Before bedtime?"

3. **Nutrition knowledge**

Ask the person whether they are familiar with the Food Guide Pyramid (see Display 6-2). Ask them to name the food groups on the pyramid and describe how many daily servings they should consume from each food group.

If the person is unfamiliar with the food guide pyramid, alternative questions may be asked to evaluate nutrition knowledge, such as:

- "Name some foods high in calories."
- "Name some foods with limited nutritional value."
- "If there was one thing you would do to improve your diet, what would it be?"

Determine whether the person can read food labels. The most reliable way to assess understanding of food labels is to display a label and ask the person questions about its content, such as:

- "Is this food high or low in fat (cholesterol, sodium)?"
- "How many fat grams will you consume with this food?"
- "How many fat grams could you consume in a day without exceeding recommended levels?"

4. **Functional status**

A combination of interviewing and direct observation can provide information about a person's functional status and level of independence with eating abilities. If the individual cannot participate in an interview, you may interview a significant other who is familiar with the person's eating abilities, or you may directly observe the person's eating abilities.

Interview Questions:

- "Do you have any difficulties with meal preparation?"
- "Do you have any problems with eating?"
- "Do you have any difficulty chewing? Swallowing? Choking during eating?"

Clinical Significance

Allergic reactions may follow different patterns:
- *Immediate* (within 1 hour)
- *Delayed* (within 24–48 hours)
- *Cyclical* (not always occurring)
- *Fixed* (always occurring after eating the item)

Allergic reactions may result in skin, gastrointestinal, respiratory, or central nervous system symptoms.

Determining food likes, dislikes, and meal patterns is helpful for menu planning.

Knowledge of the Food Pyramid and its application indicates basic understanding of healthy diet principles.

The responses to these questions may identify teaching/learning needs as well as obvious misconceptions about nutrition.

Food labels, called "Nutrition Facts," are required on approximately 90% of processed foods.

The ability to interpret food labels represents more sophisticated consumer knowledge of nutrition and may be most helpful for people adhering to therapeutic diets. (See Display 6-4.)

A decline in functional abilities increases the risk of developing nutritional problems.

If the person reports chewing problems, evaluate the oral cavity, especially the condition of the teeth and fit of dentures (if applicable).

If the person reports difficulty with swallowing or choking during eating, additional evaluation should be conducted.

▼ ▼ ▼
G U I D E L I N E S *continued*   Nutrition Interview (Health History)

Procedure	Clinical Significance

Procedure

5. Socioeconomic variables

Income
Determine whether economic factors play a role in the types of foods purchased. Ascertain whether the person can afford to purchase milk products or fresh fruit and vegetables.

Education
Evaluate educational level of the client or persons with primary responsibility for shopping and food preparation.

Mealtime Setting
Determine whether meals are eaten at home, with others, or alone.

6. Medical history
Screen the person for pathology that may place a person at nutritional risk

High-Risk Diagnoses
Cancer: head, neck, GI
Dehydration < age 4
Diabetes, new onset
Diabetic ketoacidosis
Dysphagia
Eating disorder
Failure to thrive
Malnutrition
Pressure ulcer
Renal failure
Traumatic brain injury/head injury

Moderate-Risk Diagnoses
Alcoholism/chemical dependency
Amputation (new)
Bowel obstruction
Bronchopulmonary dysplasia
Cancer (other than head, neck, GI) with metastasis
Cirrhosis
Crohn's disease
Dehydration > age 70
Diabetes, established
Fistula/abscess
Fractured hip
General debility
GI bleed
Hepatitis
Malabsorption
Pancreatitis
Pneumothorax
Sepsis
Short bowel syndrome
Spinal cord injury
Stroke/CVA/TIA
Subdural hematoma

Clinical Significance

Higher income does not necessarily mean better nutritional status, but higher income is more frequently associated with adequate diet than lower income.

Higher educational levels have been associated with better quality diets. Educational level has been found to be inversely related to the use of convenience foods.

At all socioeconomic levels in America, fewer meals are being eaten at home or in a family setting, which may adversely affect family stability. Elderly people who eat alone are at risk for nutritional problems and social isolation.

Various states of illness or pathology may have a significant impact on nutritional status by causing a primary nutrient deficiency related to inadequate intake or by contributing to a secondary deficiency related to altered digestion, absorption, or metabolism. If a medical problem is identified that has potential to alter nutritional status, additional evaluation is required to determine impact.

▼ ▼ ▼

Procedure

7. Medication history

Determine whether the person is taking any medications that may affect nutrition status by taking a medication history.

A medication history may be obtained at some other point in the sequence of the overall health assessment. The results of the medication history should always be analyzed for implications related to nutrition status.

Components of a Medication History Used in the Evaluation of Nutrition Status

Vitamin and mineral use

Prescription and nonprescription drug use

For each drug identified, determine:

- Purpose
- Dosage
- Whether it is taken with meals or between meals
- Duration of use
- Side effects perceived by individual

Drugs Influencing Appetite/Food Intake

Antipsychotic and sedatives

Cancer chemotherapies

Digoxin

Drugs Affecting Nutrient Availability

Aluminum or magnesium antacids

Anticoagulants

Cholestyramine

Vitamin B_{12} and fat-soluble vitamins

Corticosteroids

H_2 receptor blockers

Isoniazid, hydralazine, L-dopa

Salicylate

Drugs Affecting Nutrient Loss

Furosemide (Lasix)

Spironolactone

Thiazides

Clinical Significance

Drugs can alter both nutritional and metabolic states. Some drugs may interfere with nutritional processes; some foods may interfere with responses to a particular drug. Collectively, these relationships are referred to as food and drug interactions.

At highest risk for food and drug interactions:

Elders

People taking drugs for long duration

People taking more than two medications

People who are not eating well

Self-medication with vitamins and minerals is common, especially in elders. When taken in doses exceeding Recommended Daily Allowances (RDAs), vitamins and minerals may act as drugs and interact adversely with nutrients and nutritional processes.

Some drugs, especially some antibiotics, are less effective if taken with meals. Other drugs, such as iron preparations, are best taken with meals to minimize gastrointestinal irritation.

Nutritional Side Effects

Somnolence; disinterest in food

Nausea, vomiting, aversion to food

Anorexia, nausea, vomiting, weakness

Nutritional Side Effects

Phosphate depletion

Vitamin K antagonists

Decreased absorption of lipids, folate, iron

Gastrointestinal side effects

Decreased vitamin D activity

Vitamin B_{12} malabsorption

Vitamin B_6 antagonists

Iron loss secondary to gastrointestinal bleeding

Nutritional Side Effects

Loss of potassium, magnesium, chloride sodium, and water

Potassium sparing—hyperkalemia; fluid and electrolyte changes

Loss of potassium, sodium, magnesium, and zinc

▼ ▼ ▼
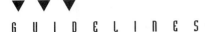

Assessment Guidelines   Diet Evaluation

Procedure

1. Diet (food intake) history

A number of methods can be used to determine dietary intake, including an interview, 24-hour food recall, food frequency recording, food diary recording, and a calorie count.

For any method, the examiner compares the information about the types and amounts of food ingested with established standards of sound nutrition, such as the Recommended Daily Allowances or Dietary Guidelines, to make judgments about the adequacy or inadequacy of the diet.

Simple Interview:

Ask the person to describe a typical day's diet and record their response. To get more detailed responses, related to the Dietary Guidelines, ask the person for the following types of information:

- "How many servings of breads, pasta, cereals, and rice do you consume each day?"
- "How many servings of fruits and vegetables do you consume each day?"
- "How many servings of dairy products, meats, beans, and nuts do you consume each day?"
- "How many servings of fats and sweets do you consume daily?"

2. 24-Hour food recall

The 24-hour food recall asks the person to report all food and beverages consumed during one 24-hour period.

Use a form, such as the one shown in Display 6-8 and ask the person to record the food and beverages consumed the previous day or during another, more representative, 24-hour period.

Use food models to help the person define portion sizes.

Review the results of the completed form with the person.

Evaluate the results using the Food Guide Pyramid.

Clinical Significance

A diet history is obtained to determine the characteristics of the person's typical daily diet. The purpose of evaluating the diet is to determine whether it supplies all the essential nutrients in appropriate amounts and avoids excesses that predispose individuals to chronic disease.

It may be difficult to obtain an accurate depiction of the diet with this approach, because 1 day may not be representative of the typical diet. In addition, people may forget the types and amounts of foods eaten, or they may be reluctant to reveal their eating patterns.

The underlying assumption in the use of the 24-hour recall method of diet evaluation is that a 24-hour period will be representative of the typical diet. Studies have indicated this is not the case. Therefore, this is considered one of the least reliable ways to evaluate diet. However, it is an easy and quick method of assessment.

A form can be completed by the person or used as an interview guide by the clinician.

Accurate interpretation of portion size is a major source of measurement error in the use of a 24-hour recall.

Reviewing the results provides an opportunity for additional clarification, recall, and discussion of dietary practices.

The Food Guide Pyramid can be used to assess the adequacy of the recorded diet.

DISPLAY 6.8

Forms Used to Assess Food Intake

DIET RECALL

What foods do you choose for your usual meals and snacks?

Morning _____

Noon _____

Night _____

Snacks _____

What specific foods have you eaten in the past 24 hours?

Morning _____

Noon _____

Night_____

Snacks _____

FOOD FREQUENCY CHECKLIST

How Often Have You Eaten the Following Foods?	Never; Less Than 1 Time per Week	1–2 Times per Week	More Than 3–7 Times per Week	Once a Day
Milk (8 oz)				
Whole				
2% fat				
1% fat				
Skim				
Chocolate				
Juices (4 oz)				
Citrus (orange, grapefruit)				

FOOD DIARY

Time B—Begin F—Finish	Food	Amount	Kcal	Place	Activity (TV, reading, etc.)	Position S—Sitting ST—Standing R—Reclining	Mood*	Degree of Hunger, 0–5

*A, angry; B, bored; D, depressed; H, happy; N, neutral; Ner, nervous; T, tired.

▼ ▼ ▼

G U I D E L I N E S *continued*   Diet Evaluation

Procedure

3. Food frequency record

The Food Frequency method of evaluating diet asks the person to indicate how often certain foods are ingested over a defined period, such as a week or a month.

Alternatively, the person may be asked to indicate how frequently certain foods are consumed, using the categories "frequently, seldom, or never."

Use a form, such as the one shown in Display 6-8, and ask the person to complete the tool for the specified timeframe (week, month).

Review the results with a recognized dietary standard to determine deficiencies or excesses.

4. Food diary

The Food Diary method for diet evaluation requires the person to record every food and beverage consumed over a certain period, usually 3 to 7 days. Instruct the person to record the food or beverage as soon as possible to assure accurate recording.

Use a form, such as the one shown in Display 6-8, to record food intake and associated eating behaviors.

Use food models to help the person define portion sizes.

Evaluate the nutrient content of the diet using standard references—RDA Tables or the Dietary Guidelines.

5. Calorie count

A calorie count is usually initiated by a clinical dietician to determine the exact number of calories ingested.

The clinical dietician will evaluate the results and make diet recommendations.

Clinical Significance

The Food Frequency record provides information about the types of foods consumed, but not the quantities.

A selective Food Frequency questionnaire may focus on food groups suspected of being deficient or excessive in the diet.

Food-frequency questionnaires are easier to complete than 24-hour recalls, because estimating portion size is not required.

When a Food Frequency evaluation is used in addition to the results from a 24-hour recall, a more complete dietary profile is obtained than by using either method alone.

The Food Diary may provide the most accurate record of dietary intake, provided the person is motivated to keep the diary. Accuracy of recording tends to decline after several days. Recording may influence people to alter their usual diet patterns.

Accurate interpretation of portion size is a major source of measurement error in the use of a food diary.

The average daily intake of various nutrients can be calculated by totaling the nutrients that were consumed during the entire period and dividing by the total number of days.

The primary use of a calorie count is to prescribe diets and supplements containing adequate calories for persons with nutritional deficits.

The calorie count is usually conducted in a health care facility, and data are recorded by a variety of caregivers on a form. The following information is recorded: all food and beverages consumed at meals and between meals, including dietary supplements; any foods obtained from visitors; nutrients obtained from intravenous fluids.

▼ ▼ ▼

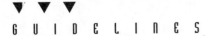

G U I D E L I N E S

Assessment Guidelines   Diagnostic Studies of Nutrition Status

Procedure

Laboratory data may be reviewed when assessing nutrition status to accomplish the following:

- Screen persons for nutritional problems
- Quantify the extent of protein-calorie malnutrition
- Identify specific deficiencies in essential nutrients

1. **Serum albumin transferrin and lymphocytes**

   Monitor albumin levels in persons at risk for protein-calorie malnutrition. Measurement of albumin is common in hospitalized patients, because it is a component of chemistry screening routinely ordered and monitored in acute care populations. Serum transferrin analysis may or may not be readily available and is more costly to measure.

   Total lymphocyte count is readily available in hospitalized patients who have had the laboratory analysis called a complete blood count (CBC).

Clinical Significance

Abnormal results of laboratory tests reviewed in this section are not always diet or nutritionally related. Furthermore, test results do not indicate whether the cause is malnutrition, related to an outcome of a disease, or related to treatment. Therefore, laboratory data must be carefully evaluated and interpreted.

Albumin, transferrin, and lymphocytes are serum proteins. Decreased serum levels indicate protein deficiencies.

A decrease in albumin (**hypoalbuminemia**) causes serum osmotic pressure to decrease so that fluid escapes the vascular space and causes edema. A person with severe protein malnutrition may develop an enlarged abdomen as fluid moves into the abdominal space.

Ascites: Fluid accumulation in the abdomen and subcutaneous compartments caused by relative lack of protein in the vascular space. Ascites occurs in the protein starvation disease *kwashiorkor.* The resulting fluid shifts give the victim a protuberant abdomen.

Many other conditions may lower lymphocyte count in addition to malnutrition. Lymphocytes are essential for immune function, and lower levels are associated with greater risk for infection.

Measures of Protein Status

Indicator	Normal Range	Moderately Malnourished	Severely Malnourished
Albumin (g/dL)	3.5–5.0	3.0–3.5	<3.0
Transferrin (mg/dL)	150–250	160–180	<160
Total lymphocyte count (cells/mm^3)	>1500	1000–1500	<1000

2. **Nitrogen balance**

   Evaluate nitrogen balance by comparing the 24-hour nitrogen intake (grams of protein ingested divided by 6.25) to nitrogen output over a 24-hour period. Nitrogen output equals the measured value for a 24-hour urine urea nitrogen (UUN) in grams plus 4 g nitrogen lost through feces.

   Nitrogen balance = Nitrogen in – Nitrogen out
   = (Protein intake/6.25) – (24-hour UUN + 4)

3. **Hemoglobin, hematocrit, and transferrin**

   Hemoglobin, hematocrit, and transferrin levels are decreased in persons with iron-deficiency anemias.

Nitrogen balance is an indicator of protein nutritional status and provides an indicator of metabolic status. Optimal nutritional status is associated with a positive nitrogen balance of +2 to +4 g. A positive nitrogen balance (**anabolism**) exists when input exceeds nitrogen output. A negative nitrogen balance (**catabolism**) occurs when intake is less than output. In a catabolic state, protein is being lost from muscle, and metabolic demands are not being met.

Iron deficiencies are among the most common nutrient deficiencies in the United States.

Procedure

Review these laboratory tests for abnormal values and determine risk for iron deficiency

Risk categories for iron-deficiency anemia:

- Infants
- Adolescent girls
- Menstruating women
- Pregnant women
- Elders
- People in low income groups

Clinical Significance

Iron-deficiency anemia: A condition characterized by an inadequate iron supply to support optimal formation of various red blood cells. As a result, tissue oxygenation needs are not met.

Normal Hemoglobin

Adult males 13–18 g/dL

Adult females 12–16 g/dL

Infants 9–14 g/dL

Children 11.5–15.5 g/dL

Normal Hematocrit

Adult males 42%–50%

Adult females 40%–48%

Infants 28%–42%

Children 35%–45%

Normal Transferrin

150–250 mg/dL

4. **Potassium and sodium**

Evaluate serum potassium levels to determine whether a potassium deficiency or potassium excess is present

Evaluate serum sodium levels to determine whether a sodium deficiency or sodium excess is present.

Normal serum potassium: 3.5–5.0 mEq/L

Hypokalemia (deficit): <3.5 mEq/L

Hyperkalemia (excess): >5.0 mEq/L

Normal sodium levels: 135–145 mEq/L

5. **Cholesterol and lipids**

If available, note values reported for total serum cholesterol and HDL cholesterol.

Refer persons with the following results for additional lipoprotein analysis:

Total cholesterol > 240 mg/dL

HDL levels < 35 mg/dL

Cholesterol and lipid evaluation is used to screen people at risk for cardiovascular disease.

People meeting criteria for additional screening will have lipoprotein analysis, including measurement of LDL cholesterol. Additionally, dietary modifications may be recommended.

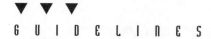

Assessment Guidelines   Anthropometric Assessment

Procedure	**Clinical Significance**

Procedure

Anthropometric assessment requires the measurement of several body dimensions, including height, weight, skinfold thicknesses, and various body circumferences.

Anthropometric measurements are obtained as a part of a comprehensive nutritional assessment and compared with established standards such as weight tables and other standard references to make judgments about nutritional status.

1. **Measure height**

   a. Instruct the person to stand erect, without shoes, against a wall to which a measuring tape has been affixed. Be sure the feet are together and the heels, buttocks, shoulders, and head are touching the wall.

   b. Record the height in centimeters.

   c. If the person cannot stand, measure the height in the supine position with body fully extended. Measure height from the heels to the top of the head with a tape measure.

2. **Measure and evaluate weight**

   a. Obtain weight using a beam balance scale after the person has voided. Bed scales may be used for immobile persons.

   b. Standardize the procedure as much as possible. Serial weights, such as daily weights in institutional settings, are obtained at the same time each day, with the person wearing the same amount of clothing.

   c. Record the weight in kilograms.

   d. Evaluate the body weight.

   Several methods may be used to evaluate body weight, including:
   - Ideal Body Weight (IBW) standards
   - Healthy Weight Range Tables
   - Body Mass Index (BMI) evaluation
   - Life Insurance Tables

Ideal Body Weight (IBW)
Adult Women:

100 lb for 5 feet of height plus 5 lb for each additional inch over 5 feet

Clinical Significance

Measuring these body dimensions provides information about three body tissues altered during starvation or obesity: visceral proteins, skeletal muscle, and subcutaneous fat.

In children younger than 3 years of age, head circumference and height are often measured as well. Growth retardation, indicated by these measurements, may be a sign of poor nutritional status.

Height is used to evaluate body weight and normal growth patterns in children.

Using the rod on a balance scale to measure height is less accurate than the method described here but more accurate than asking the person.

Metric measurements are used to determine other values derived from height, such as the body mass index and body surface area.

Beam balance scales are more accurate than bathroom scales.

A consistent method of weighing increases accuracy, especially in a setting with multiple caregivers.

Metric weight values (kilograms instead of pounds) are used in other calculations such as body mass index, drug dosages, and body surface area.

Experts disagree about the best way to define ideal or normal body weight. The methods described here are most commonly used in clinical practice.

The body weight ranges suggested by this method are criticized for being too narrow

▼ ▼ ▼

G U I D E L I N E S *continued*   Anthropometric Assessment

Procedure

Adult Men:

106 lb for 5 feet of height plus 6 lb for each additional inch over 5 feet

Ideal body weight may be adjusted up or down by 10%, depending on frame size.

To evaluate body weight using the IBW method, calculate %IBW of the person's actual body weight, using the following formula:

$$\%IBW = (\text{actual weight/IBW}) \times 100$$

Healthy Weight Range Tables

Acceptable weight ranges for adults were shown earlier in this chapter in Display 6-3.

The weight ranges in Display 6-3 apply to men and women of all ages. Weights at the higher end of each range represent people with more muscle and bone; the higher weights in any given range are not intended to encourage people to gain weight.

Body Mass Index (BMI) Evaluation

Body mass index is derived in the following way:

$$BMI = \frac{\text{weight in kilograms}}{\text{height in meters squared}}$$

or,

Using pounds and inches, calculate as follows:

$$BMI = \frac{\text{weight in pounds}}{\text{height in inches squared}} \times 705$$

Note: 1 kg = 2.2 lb. To convert pounds to kilograms, divide by 2.2

1 m = 39.37 inches. To convert inches to meters, divide by 39.37

Life Insurance Tables

Life insurance tables show average ideal weights based on mortality statistics. The tables provide different weight ranges for men and women based on height and body frame.

3. **Measure midarm circumference (MAC; in cm)**

   a. To measure MAC, determine the midpoint on the person's nondominant arm. With the arm in a relaxed position, palpate the acromial process at the top of the humerus. Sliding your fingers across the clavicle helps locate this landmark. Place a tape measure between the acrominal process and the olecranon process or elbow and mark the midpoint on the arm.

Clinical Significance

Interpretation

>120% of IBW	Obese
110–120% of IBW	Overweight
90–110% of IBW	IBW
80–90% of IBW	Mildly underweight
70–80% of IBW	Moderate underweight
<70% of IBW	Severely underweight

The weight ranges shown in Display 8-4 are included in the Dietary Guidelines for Americans and are intended for general screening and teaching.

The advisory committee that established the 1995 Dietary Guidelines for Americans rejected the concept that people can gain additional weight as they grow older without an adverse effect on health. Therefore, the suggested weight ranges for adults adopted for the dietary guidelines do not show different weight ranges for different adult age-groups, gender, or body frame size.

Body Mass Index is considered one of the best methods of quantifying obesity.

Assessment of Body Weight Using BMI

Category	BMI
Normal	19–27
Overweight	28–30
Obese	30–40
Morbidly obese	>40

Many authorities do not regard weights presented on Life Insurance tables as either ideal or desirable, and other methods are preferred in current clinical practice.

MAC reflects both muscle mass and fat. MAC is used to calculate midarm muscle circumference.

▼ ▼ ▼

G U I D E L I N E S   *continued*   Anthropometric Assessment

Procedure

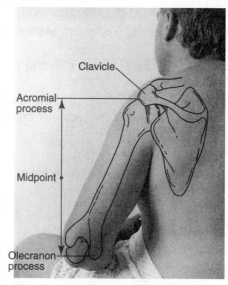

Finding the midpoint

b. Next, instruct the person to let the arm hang loosely at the side. Place a tape measure around the person's arm at the midpoint and record the measurement in centimeters.

Clinical Significance

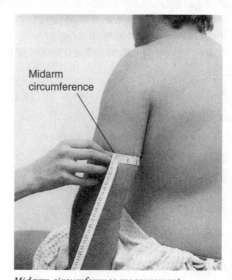

Midarm circumference measurement

c. Interpret the MAC. MAC decreases with undernutrition and increases with an increase in fat (obesity) or muscle (hypertrophy). Undernutrition may be indicated by a measurement below the 90% reference:

Adult MAC (cm)	Standard Reference	90% of Standard Reference Moderately Malnourished	60% of Standard Reference Severely Malnourished
Men	29.3	26.3	17.6
Women	28.5	25.7	17.1

d. Record the measured value as well as the number being used as the standard reference as follows:

MAC (cm) = 23 cm; 81% of standard

standard = 28.5 cm

▼ ▼ ▼
G U I D E L I N E S *continued*   Anthropometric Assessment

Procedure

4. Triceps skinfold (TSF; in mm)

a. Obtain the measurement on the nondominant arm, using plastic or precision metal calipers.

b. Find the midpoint of the arm, using the method described for MAC measurement.

c. With the arm hanging loosely at the side, grasp a fold of skin at the midpoint on the posterior aspect of the arm. Apply the caliper and take a reading after waiting for 3 seconds. Repeat the procedure three times.

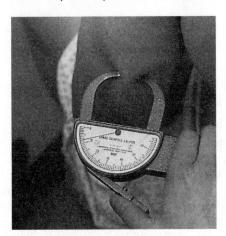

Measurement of triceps skinfold

Clinical Significance

Because at least half of body fat is directly below the skin, this measurement indicates total body fat.

Metal calipers can be calibrated, making them more accurate.

TSF is measured at the midpoint mark.

Measuring triceps skinfold requires practice. A common error is measuring underlying muscle as well as fat. To avoid such an error, grasp the fold of skin and ask the person to flex the arm muscle. If you feel the contraction, you have probably grasped muscle as well as fat. In this case, release the skin and try again.

d. Interpret the TSF. Fat stores decrease because of long-term undernutrition and successful weight loss. Obesity increases fat stores. Standard values are used to make clinical judgments:

Adult TSF (mm)	Standard Reference	90% of Standard Reference—Moderately Malnourished	60% of Standard Reference—Severely Malnourished
Men	12.5	11.3	7.5
Women	16.5	14.9	9.9

e. Record the measured value as well as the number being used as the standard reference as follows:

TSF (mm) = 12.87 mm; 78% of standard
Standard = 16.5 mm

5. Midarm muscle circumference (MAMC; in cm).

a. Calculate MAMC by using the following equation:

$$MAMC = MAC \text{ (cm)} - [0.314 \times TSF \text{ (mm)}]$$

b. Interpret the MAMC. MAMC decreases with undernutrition and increases with obesity and muscle hypertrophy. The severe muscle wasting of protein-calorie malnutrition is indicated by a MAMC of less than 15.2 cm in men and less than 13.9 cm in women:

Reflects skeletal muscle mass status.

MAC and TSF must be measured to derive the MAMC.

▼ ▼ ▼

Anthropometric Assessment

Procedure

Adult MAMC (cm)	Standard Reference	90% of Standard Reference Moderately Malnourished	60% of Standard Reference Severely Malnourished
Men	25.3	22.8	15.2
Women	23.2	20.9	13.9

c. Record the measured value as well as the number being used as the standard reference as follows:

    MAMC (cm) = 18.96; 81% of standard

    standard = 23.2

Clinical Significance

▼ ▼ ▼

G U I D E L I N E S

Assessment Guidelines   Interpreting Physical Examination Findings Related to Nutrition

Procedure

1. **Integrate physical examination findings into the overall assessment of nutrition and metabolism with special attention to the following:**
   a. General appearance
   b. The integumentary system
   c. Oral cavity
   d. Abdomen
   e. Thyroid gland
   f. Lymphatic system
   g. Cardiovascular system
   h. Respiratory system
   i. Neurologic system

2. **General appearance**
   - As you conduct a general survey at the beginning of the physical examination, note the general appearance of the person and whether he or she appears overweight or underweight.

   - Look for signs of muscle wasting.

   - Note and record patterns of fat distribution.

3. **Integumentary system**
   Observe the skin, hair, and nails for signs of malnutrition.

Clinical Significance

Some observations made during the head-to-toe physical examination may help you with nutritional assessment by indicating the status of nutritional processes—ingestion, digestion, absorption, transport, and metabolism. Physical assessment may also indicate general physical signs of altered nutrition status.

(Note: Complete assessment guidelines are presented elsewhere in this chapter for the integumentary system, oral cavity, abdomen, thyroid gland, and lymphatic system.)

Cachexia: A syndrome of weight loss, muscle wasting, subcutaneous fat depletion, and anemia due to calorie starvation. A cachexic person has a "walking skeleton" appearance.

Ascites: Abdominal enlargement caused by fluid shifts associated with protein malnutrition (kwashiorkor).

Atrophy: Muscle wasting associated with protein malnutrition or disuse. Muscle wasting in starvation states is most noticeable in the temporal area, the dorsum of the hands and along the spine.

Obesity is characterized by fat accumulation in the abdomen, hips, and thighs.

Starvation depletes subcutaneous fat in the abdomen, arms, and legs.

Signs of Malnutrition

Skin—Dryness; flakiness; sandpaper feel; red, swollen pigmentation of exposed areas; excessive bruising; pinpoint hemorrhages

▼ ▼ ▼
G U I D E L I N E S *continued*

Interpreting Physical Examination Findings
Related to Nutrition

Procedure

Clinical Significance

Flaky paint dermatosis: Generalized dryness of the skin that occurs with severe protein deficiencies (kwashiorkor). The skin may flake off like old paint.

Hair—Lusterless; dry, thin, sparse; easily plucked; bands of pigmentation

Flag sign: Alternating bands of light and dark hair that may indicate a protein or copper deficiency

Nails—spoon-shaped with iron deficiencies; brittle; transverse ridges across the nail plate; pale

4. **Oral cavity**

Observe the lips, tongue, oral mucosa, and condition of the teeth.

Signs of Malnutrition

Lips—Puffy, swollen, fissures at corner of the mouth

Cheilosis: Reddening and cracking at the corners of the mouth associated with Vitamin B_6 and riboflavin deficiencies

Tongue—pale or raw; scarlet red or purplish; lesions; smooth appearance

Oral mucosa—swollen; dryness; redness

Teeth—mottled; cavities; poor dentition

5. **Abdomen**

Observe the abdominal contour and condition of abdominal organs.

Note general indicators of GI dysfunction, including indigestion, diarrhea or constipation, poor appetite, and nausea.

Signs of Malnutrition

Ascites; liver enlargement

6. **Glands and immune system**

Palpate the thyroid and lymphatic glands.

Signs of Malnutrition

Enlarged thyroid; enlarged lymphatics; signs of frequent infections such as colds, poor wound healing, slow convalescence

7. **Cardiovascular and respiratory systems**

Observe heart rate and rhythm, blood pressure, and activity tolerance.

Obesity is associated with an elevated diastolic blood pressure and activity intolerance.

Starvation states are associated with low blood pressure, low energy levels, and weakness.

Note ventilatory patterns.

Pickwickian syndrome: A syndrome of respiratory compromise secondary to extreme obesity characterized by somnolence and hypoventilation. Fat accumulation around the chest restricts chest movement and impairs ventilation.

8. **Neurologic system**

A number of changes in neurologic function may be noted with vitamin B deficiencies, including the following:

Clinical Finding	*Possible Deficiency*
Confabulation, disorientation	Thiamine
Decreased position and vibratory sense; ataxia	Vitamin B_{12}; thiamine
Diminished deep tendon reflexes	Thiamine
Weakness, paresthesias, diminished tactile sensation	Vitamin B_{12}, pyridoxine, thiamine

Documenting Nutrition Assessment Findings

Data collected in the course of conducting a comprehensive nutritional assessment or nutritional screening come from many diverse sources, including interviews, anthropometric evaluations, medication histories, laboratory analyses, and observations. It is now common in clinical practice to record nutritional status data on a form specifically created to organize such a complex array of data into meaningful information about nutrition status. Forms used in the documentation of nutritional screening data should be created to guide the clinician toward an assessment of level of nutritional risk. A sample of a nutritional assessment screening form is found earlier in this chapter in Display 6-5.

Nursing Diagnoses Related to Nutrition Assessment

Altered Nutrition: Less Than Body Requirements

Altered nutrition: Less than body requirements is the diagnosis for a person who is experiencing or is at risk of experiencing weight loss and nutritional deficiencies because of either inadequate nutrient intake or excessive metabolic demands. The diagnosis of poor nutritional status is based on meeting one or more of the following criteria:

Anthropometric Data

- BMI < 19
- Weight less than 90% of ideal body weight
- Unintentional weight loss greater than 10% of weight within last 6 months
- Triceps skinfold (TSF), midarm circumference (MAC), and midarm muscle circumference (MAMC) less than 85% of the standard measurement

Nutrient Intake

- Inadequate food intake, fad dieting, numerous food intolerances or allergies
- Use of inadequate modified diet (i.e., clear liquid) for more than 3 days without adequate supplementation
- NPO for more than 3 days without adequate supplementation
- Difficulty chewing or swallowing
- Changes in taste, smell, or appetite

Laboratory Data

- Serum albumin less than 3.5 g/dL
- Low hemoglobin and hematocrit
- Total lymphocyte count < 1500 cell/m^3
- Decreased serum cholesterol level

Medical-Socioeconomic Factors

- Illness or other pathophysiologic process that interferes with nutrient intake or nutrient requirements processes
- High fever (>37°C) for more than 2 days
- Long-term use of medications that affect nutritional processes
- Alcohol abuse
- Inadequate food budget

Altered Nutrition: More Than Body Requirements

Altered nutrition: More than body requirements is the diagnosis for a person who is experiencing or is at risk of experiencing weight gain and the chronic diseases associated with obesity. The diagnosis is based on meeting one or more of the following criteria:

Anthropometric Data

- BMI > 27
- Overweight: Weight 10% over ideal body weight
- Obese: Weight 20% over ideal body weight
- TSF > 15 mm in men and >25 mm in women

Nutrient Intake

- Undesirable eating patterns
- Intake in excess of metabolic requirements

Lifestyle

- Sedentary activity patterns

Laboratory Data

- Total cholesterol > 240 mg/dL
- HDL Levels < 35 mg/dL
- LDL Levels > 130 mg/dL

Eating Disorders

Among the most common, and life-threatening, eating disorders are those that may affect adolescent and young adult women—anorexia nervosa, bulimia nervosa, and binge eating. Women in this age group are particularly vulnerable because of their tendency to go on strict diets to achieve an "ideal" figure. Most people with eating disorders share the following personality traits: low self-esteem, feelings of helplessness, and a fear of becoming fat. Dysfunctional eating behaviors may develop as a way to handle stress and anxiety and to gain a sense of control.

Anorexia nervosa occurs in 1% of American adolescent girls. It is characterized by intentional starvation and involves extreme weight loss—at least 15% below the person's usual body weight. The skin, hair, and nails take on characteristics of protein-calorie malnutrition. The skin becomes dry and flaky and covered with soft hair called lanugo. There is decreased tolerance to cold secondary to fat loss. Laboratory analysis indicates significant protein, iron, and calcium deficiencies.

Bulimia nervosa occurs in 2% to 3% of young women. It is characterized by a pattern of excessive overeating following by self-induced vomiting or other purging behavior such as abusing laxatives or diuretics, taking enemas, or excessive exercise. Because the binging and purging may occur in secret and body weight may be maintained, the disease may be well hidden from others. Repeated vomiting, with the high acid content, may wear down tooth enamel and can cause scarring on the backs of hands when the fingers are pushed down the throat to induce vomiting.

Binge eating disorder resembles bulimia with respect to a pattern of uncontrolled binge eating. However, unlike bulimia, the binge eater does not engage in purging behaviors. Usually these people develop serious weight problems and weight cycling. Binge eating disorder occurs in about 30% of people participating in medically supervised weight control programs.

PART 2
PHYSICAL EXAMINATION TECHNIQUES

INTEGUMENTARY SYSTEM: SKIN, HAIR, AND NAILS

Anatomy and Physiology Review

The skin is composed of three layers: the epidermis, the dermis, and the subcutaneous tissue. Hair, nails, sweat glands, and sebaceous glands are considered appendages of the skin. Figure 6-1 depicts a cross-sectional view of the skin.

Epidermis

The first layer of the skin, the epidermis, is thin and avascular. It provides protection from foreign invasion and prevention of fluid and electrolyte loss. The outermost epidermal layer (stratum corneum) consists of a horny layer of keratinized cells that are constantly being sloughed and replaced. If these cells are being sloughed at a rate exceeding replacement, the skin may appear thin and become chapped because the keratinized cells quickly lose water content when exposed to the outside environment.

The other layers of the epidermis contain living cells. The deepest layer (stratum germinativum) includes cells that contain the pigment melanin, which is responsible for skin color. The production and accumulation of melanin varies with race, age, heredity, and sun exposure. Aging is associated with lower levels of melanin production and local accumulations of melanin, especially on the backs of the hands.

Dermis

The middle skin layer, the dermis, is made up of connective tissue and blood vessels. Connective tissue in the dermis is largely made up of the proteins collagen and elastin, which give the skin its strength, structure, and flexibility. Skin wrinkling is associated with elastin degeneration and loss of subcutaneous fat. Pressure ulcers occur when the blood vessels in the dermal layer of skin are occluded. Constriction or dilation of the blood vessels in the dermis can affect skin color and temperature.

Subcutaneous Tissue

The innermost layer of skin, the subcutaneous layer, stores fat and connective tissue containing blood and lymph vessels, nerves, and glands. The subcutaneous level acts as an insulator, calorie reserve, heat source, and shock absorber. This layer varies in thickness mainly because of variations in fat accumulation.

Appendages

Hair is composed of keratin and consists of the visible portion, called the hair shaft, which is embedded in the hair follicle beneath the skin surface. Sebaceous glands secret oil into hair follicles and lubricate the skin. Hair is

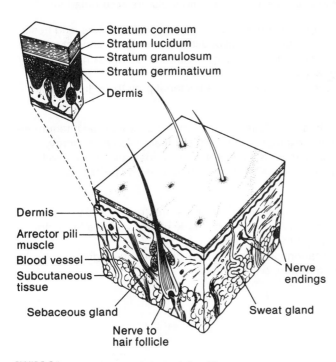

FIGURE 6.1 Cross-sectional view of the skin.

constantly being formed and shed; the scalp loses from 20 to 100 hairs per day.

The nails are composed of keratin. Low water content and sulfur contribute to nail hardness. The nail surface is called the plate. The lunula is the half-moon–shaped portion at the nail base. A rich capillary network is beneath the nail plate, making it possible to blanch the nail when pressure is applied. The skin surrounding the nail is susceptible to bacterial and fungal infections. Under normal conditions, a fingernail can completely regenerate within 170 days.

Two types of sweat glands are located in the skin: eccrine and apocrine. The eccrine glands are widely distributed over the body and secrete sweat in response to temperature elevations and nervous system stimulation. The apocrine glands are located in the axillary and genital areas and produce secretions that decompose in the presence of bacteria, causing the characteristic body odor.

Physical Examination Skin, Hair, and Nails

GENERAL APPROACH

Assess the skin, hair, and nails by inspection and palpation. Assess any abnormalities by asking the person how long the abnormality has been present; whether any associated pain or discomfort is present; what has made the skin condition worse or better; if there is a history of skin or drug allergies; and finally, what they have done to care for the skin problem.

EQUIPMENT

Metric ruler for measuring skin lesions
Gloves for skin palpation if body fluid precautions are indicated

EXPOSURE AND LIGHTING

Expose skin crevices and pressure points where lesions such as pressure ulcers may be in early stages of formation. Uncover wounds to assess healing and observe drainage. A good source of lighting will ensure thorough and effective skin examination and accurate assessment of skin color.

THOROUGHNESS

Examine the skin and hair thoroughly from the head to the toes with special attention to areas vulnerable to pressure ulcers and moisture accumulation:

- Bony prominences: occiput, scapulae, sacrum, greater trochanters, and heels
- Contact points: nares in contact with nasogastric tubes; lips in contact with endotracheal tubes; ears in contact with oxygen cannula tubing; skin covered by tape; skin covered by restraints
- Skinfolds that trap moisture and encourage bacterial growth, including skin under the breasts

COMPARISONS

Compare the left and right sides of the body whenever an abnormal integumentary finding is detected. For example, if the left foot feels cold and clammy, check the right foot for similar signs. Is an abnormal appearance in one nail plate evident in all of the nail plates? Does a rash appear on one arm but not the other?

EXAMINATION AND DOCUMENTATION FOCUS

- *Skin:* Color and pigmentation, moisture, temperature, texture and thickness, turgor and mobility, hygiene, lesions (particularly pressure ulcers for bedridden persons), and healing of any wounds
- *Hair:* Color and pigmentation, quantity, texture, distribution, hygiene
- *Nails:* Shape and configuration, color, lesions

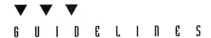

Assessment Guidelines   Skin

Procedure

1. **Inspect the skin to evaluate color and pigmentation**

Clinical Significance

Normal Findings

Lighter-pigmented races: Skin color will appear ivory to pink with possible olive or yellow overtones. Exposed areas are usually darker than nonexposed areas.

Darker-pigmented races: Skin color will appear tan to dark brown. The lips may have a bluish hue in people of Mediterranean descent. Blacks may have a blue or reddish hue to lips and mucous membranes.

Hyperpigmentation such as freckles on face and arms is common in light-skinned people.

Yellow skin may be associated with callusing or, when confined to a specific area, pigment retention.

Deviations from Normal Skin

Skin color deviations suggest compromises in metabolism, circulation, or oxygenation.

Pallor: Paleness; may be secondary to vasoconstriction or anemia.

Jaundice: Yellow cast; usually generalized if abnormal; secondary to impaired bilirubin metabolism. In a black person, jaundice is difficult to observe on the skin but can be detected by inspecting the sclera of the eyes for yellow discoloration. However, it is important to distinguish sclera yellowing from pigment accumulation in the sclera, which appears more concentrated.

Cyanosis: Bluish cast. Observe the distribution of cyanosis. Cyanosis of the mucous membranes and around the mouth (circumoral) is called central cyanosis and indicates hypoxemia. Cyanosis that involves the extremities and lips is called peripheral cyanosis and indicates reduced peripheral blood flow.

Erythema: Redness; when confined, reflects a local inflammatory response. Widespread erythema is associated with systemic vasodilation or polycythemia.

2. **Inspect and palpate the skin to evaluate moisture**

Normal Findings

Normal skin is dry, but moisture may accumulate in skin folds. A slightly warm, moist feeling is noted if the person is in a warm environment or is exercising and perspiring to cool the body. Anxiety may cause sweaty palms and perspiration in the axillae and on the forehead and scalp.

Deviations from Normal

Dryness, sweating, or oiliness may be abnormal but are not always clinically significant. Determine whether these conditions are widespread or confined to certain areas. Diaphoresis (profuse sweating) can occur in shock states in which case the skin also feels cold (cold and clammy). Abnormally dry skin may indicate dehydration.

▼ ▼ ▼

GUIDELINES *continued*   Skin

Procedure

3. **Palpate the skin to determine temperature**

4. **Inspect and palpate the skin to evaluate texture and thickness**

5. **Evaluate skin turgor by lifting a fold of skin between your thumb and forefinger**

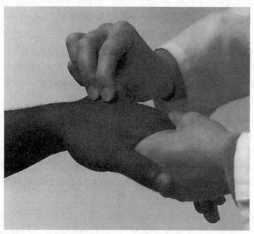

Evaluating skin turgor

6. **Survey general hygiene of the skin**

   Make note of infestations, irritating body secretions, or secretions with potential for disrupting skin integrity.

7. **Examine the skin for the presence of edema (swelling)**

   a. Survey dependent body parts. In bedridden persons, survey the lower extremities or sacrum.

Clinical Significance

Normal Findings

The skin should feel warm. Cool skin temperatures may also be normal if coolness is accompanied by a dry skin surface. Cold and clammy skin is a sign of shock.

Deviations from Normal

Local increases in skin temperature accompany acute inflammation. Cool skin temperature is noted with vasoconstriction or arterial insufficiency.

Normal Findings

Unexposed skin is smooth, whereas exposed skin may be rough, especially on the feet and hands. Skin thickness varies; the epidermis covering the eyelids and ears may be 1/50 inch thick, whereas the epidermis over the soles of the feet may be as thick as 1/4 inch.

Deviations from Normal

Note very thin skin that may be friable, easily broken, or disrupted in integrity. Very rough skin also may be abnormal.

Normal Findings

Skin is elastic and rapidly returns to original shape when grasped between thumb and forefinger.

Deviations from Normal

Poor skin turgor is demonstrated if the skin is slow to resume its original shape when pinched. Loss of turgor occurs with dehydration or as a normal aging process.

Normal Findings

Hygienic practices associated with the skin, such as frequency of bathing, vary widely depending on the individual's cultural and social practices and physiologic needs. Healthy skin usually is clean.

Deviations from Normal

Edema or swelling occurs as a result of excess fluid in the tissues. Causes include increased capillary hydrostatic pressure, which occurs from renal disease or congestive heart failure, and decreased capillary oncotic pressure, which occurs from protein deficits. In addition, edema may result from tumors or injuries that obstruct lymphatic drainage channels.

Edema in dependent body parts can be a sign of heart failure or may be a gravity-related distribution of excess fluid.

▼ ▼ ▼
GUIDELINES *continued*   Skin

Procedure

b. Press on edematous skin with your thumb or forefinger.

c. Quantify the extent of edema (grading edema) by gently pressing the edematous area with your thumb or fingers for up to 5 seconds. Note: The method of grading edema is somewhat subjective, and reported findings may vary between examiners. Nevertheless, grading edema is a common clinical practice. Serial examinations by the same examiner are most reliable. (See display, Grading Edema.)

8. Examine the skin for presence of lesions

a. Note any distinguishing characteristics of the lesion: color, texture, and general appearance.

b. Note size of lesion(s). You may want to measure the diameter with a metric ruler.

c. Note patterns of distribution for lesions.

Clinical Significance

For detailed descriptions of the types of skin lesions, see displays: Primary and Secondary Skin Lesions and Vascular Skin Lesions.

Some skin disorders are recognized according to distribution patterns over the body as well as on the basis of primary lesions. (See display, Distribution Patterns for Skin Disorders.)

Grading Edema

1+ Pitting Edema
- Slight indentation (2 mm)
- Normal contours
- Associated with interstitial fluid volume 30% above normal

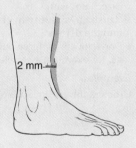
2 mm

2+ Pitting Edema
- Deeper pit after pressing (4 mm)
- Lasts longer than 1+
- Fairly normal contour

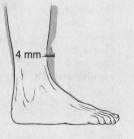
4 mm

3+ Pitting Edema
- Deep it (6 mm)
- Remains several seconds after pressing
- Skin swelling obvious by general inspection

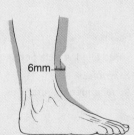
6mm

4+ Pitting Edema
- Deep pit (8 mm)
- Remains for a prolonged time after pressing, possibly minutes
- Frank swelling

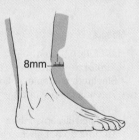
8mm

Brawny Edema
- Fluid can no longer be displaced secondary to excessive interstitial fluid accumulation
- No pitting
- Tissue palpates as firm or hard
- Skin surface shiny, warm, moist

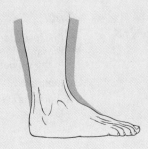

▼ ▼ ▼

G U I D E L I N E S *continued*   Skin

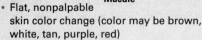

Primary Skin Lesions

Primary skin lesions are original lesions arising from previously normal skin. Secondary lesions can originate from primary lesions.

Macule, Patch

- *Macule:* <1 cm, circumscribed border
- *Patch:* >1 cm, may have irregular border
- Flat, nonpalpable skin color change (color may be brown, white, tan, purple, red)

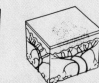

Macule

Patch

Examples:

Freckles, flat moles, petechia, rubella, vitiligo, port wine stains, ecchymosis

Vesicle, Bulla

- *Vesicle:* <0.5 cm
- *Bulla:* >0.5 cm
- Circumscribed, elevated, palpable mass containing serous fluid

Bulla

Vesicle

Examples:

Vesicles: Herpes simplex/zoster, chickenpox, poison ivy, second-degree burn (blister)

Bulla: Pemphigus, contact dermatitis, large burn blisters, poison ivy, bullous impetigo

Papule, Plaque

- *Papule:* <0.5 cm
- *Plaque:* >0.5 cm
- Elevated, palpable, solid mass
- Circumscribed border
- Plaque may be coalesced papules with flat top

Papule

Plaque

Examples:

Papules: Elevated nevi, warts, lichen planus

Plaques: Psoriasis, actinic keratosis

Wheal

- Elevated mass with transient borders
- Often irregular
- Size, color varies
- Caused by movement of serous fluid into the dermis
- Does not contain free fluid in a cavity as, for example, a vesicle

Wheal

Examples:

Urticaria (hives), insect bites

Nodule, Tumor

- *Nodule:* 0.5–2 cm
- *Tumor:* >1–2 cm
- Elevated, palpable, solid mass
- Extends deeper into the dermis than a papule
- Nodules circumscribed
- Tumors do not always have sharp borders

Tumor

Examples:

Nodules: Lipoma, squamous cell carcinoma, poorly absorbed injection, dermatofibroma

Tumors: Larger lipoma, carcinoma

Pustule

- Pus-filled vesicle or bulla

Examples:

Acne, impetigo, furuncles, carbuncles

Pustule

Cyst

- Encapsulated fluid-filled or semisolid mass
- In the subcutaneous tissue or dermis

Examples:

Sebaceous cyst, epidermoid cyst

Cyst

▼ ▼ ▼
GUIDELINES   *continued*   Skin

Secondary Skin Lesions

Secondary skin lesions result from changes in primary lesions.

Erosion

- Loss of superficial epidermis
- Does not extend to dermis
- Depressed, moist area

Examples:

Ruptured vesicles, scratch marks

Erosion

Ulcer

- Skin loss extending past epidermis
- Necrotic tissue loss
- Bleeding and scarring possible

Examples:

Stasis ulcer of venous insufficiency, decubitus ulcer

Ulcer

Fissure

- Linear crack in the skin
- May extend to dermis

Examples:

Chapped lips or hands, athlete's foot

Fissure

Scales

- Flakes secondary to desquamated, dead epithelium
- Flakes may adhere to skin surface
- Color varies (silvery, white)
- Texture varies (thick, fine)

Examples:

Dandruff, psoriasis, dry skin, pityriasis rosea

Scales

Crust

- Dried residue of serum, blood or pus on skin surface
- Large adherent crust is a scab

Examples:

Residue left after vesicle rupture: impetigo, herpes, eczema

Crust

Scar (Cicatrix)

- Skin mark left after healing of a wound or lesion
- Represents replacement by connective tissue of the injured tissue
- Young scars: red or purple
- Mature scars: white or glistening

Examples:

Healed wound or surgical incision

Scar

Keloid

- Hypertrophied scar tissue
- Secondary to excessive collagen formation during healing
- Elevated, irregular, red
- Greater incidence in blacks

Example:

Keloid of ear piercing or surgical incision

Keloid

Atrophy

- Thin, dry, transparent appearance of epidermis
- Loss of surface markings
- Secondary to loss of collagen and elastin
- Underlying vessels may be visible

Example:

Aged skin, arterial insufficiency

Atrophy

Lichenification

- Thickening and roughening of the skin
- Accentuated skin markings
- May be secondary to repeated rubbing, irritation, scratching

Example:

Contact dermatitis

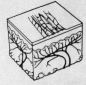

Lichenification

▼ ▼ ▼

G U I D E L I N E S *continued* Skin

Vascular Skin Lesions

Petechia (*pl.* petechiae)

- Round red or purple macule
- Small: 1–2 mm
- Secondary to blood extravasation
- Associated with bleeding tendencies or emboli to skin

Petechiae

Ecchymosis (*pl.* ecchymoses)

- Round or irregular macular lesion
- Larger than petechia
- Color varies and changes: black, yellow, and green hues
- Secondary to blood extravasation
- Associated with trauma, bleeding tendencies

Ecchymoses

Cherry Angioma

- Papular and round
- Red or purple
- Noted on trunk, extremities
- May blanch with pressure
- Normal age-related skin alteration
- Usually not clinically significant

Cherry angioma

Spider Angioma

- Red, arteriole lesion
- Central body with radiating branches
- Noted on face, neck, arms, trunk
- Rare below the waist
- May blanch with pressure
- Associated with liver disease, pregnancy, vitamin B deficiency

Spider angioma

Telangiectasis (Venous Star)

- Shape varies: spider-like or linear
- Color bluish or red
- Does not blanch when pressure is applied
- Noted on legs, anterior chest
- Secondary to superficial dilation of venous vessels and capillaries
- Associated with increased venous pressure states (varicosities)

Telangiectasis

▼ ▼ ▼
▼ ▼ ▼

G U I D E L I N E S   *continued*   Skin

Distribution Patterns for Skin Disorders

A number of skin disorders are recognized according to distribution patterns over the body as well as on the basis of the primary lesion.

Adult Atopic Eczema

Lesions noted especially on the flexor surfaces of the body.
Lesions: Erythema, papules, vesicles, pustules, crusts

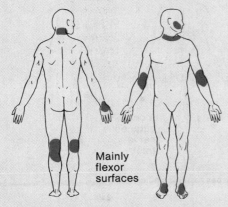

Mainly flexor surfaces

Adult atopic eczema

Psoriasis

Lesions noted especially on the extensor surfaces of the body.
Lesions: Pink or red based, topped with silvery scales; may be confluent (merged together)

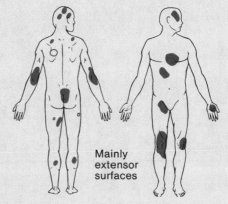

Mainly extensor surfaces

Psoriasis

Seborrheic Dermatitis

Lesions noted especially on the scalp, nasolabial folds, and axillary, interscapular, sternal, and genitocrural regions.
Lesions: Rounded, irregular, or circular, covered with yellowish or brownish gray greasy scales

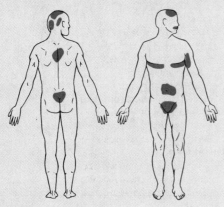

Seborrheic dermatitis

Contact Dermatitis

Affects surfaces in contact with the irritating agent. Diagram depicts contact dermatitis from contact with cosmetics, lotions, earrings.
Lesions: Erythema, papules, vesicles, pustules, crusts

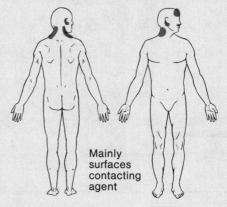

Mainly surfaces contacting agent

Contact dermatitis

(continued)

▼ ▼ ▼

G U I D E L I N E S *continued*   Skin

Distribution Patterns for Skin Disorders (continued)

Acne Vulgaris

Noted especially on face, neck, chest, and back.
Lesions: Papules, comedones, pustules

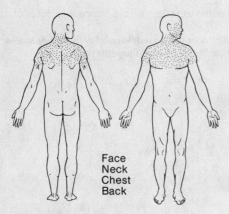

Face
Neck
Chest
Back

Acne vulgaris

Lichen Planus

Found primarily on extremities.
Lesions: Papules and scaly patches; associated with severe itching

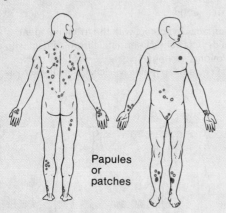

Papules
or
patches

Lichen planus

Herpes Zoster (Shingles)

Distribution is along cutaneous nerve tracts, almost always unilateral.
Lesions: Painful vesicles

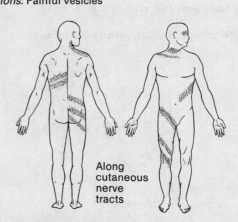

Along
cutaneous
nerve
tracts

Herpes zoster (shingles)

Pityriasis Rosea

Distributed mainly over the trunk; rare on the face.
Lesions: Macular lesions covered with scales; centers eventually clear, leaving elevated reddish rings with pale centers (ringworm-like)

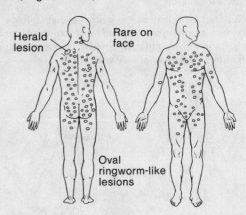

Herald
lesion

Rare on
face

Oval
ringworm-like
lesions

Pityriasis rosea

▼ ▼ ▼
GUIDELINES

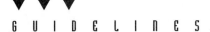
Assessment Guidelines Wound Assessment

Procedure	Clinical Significance

Procedure

1. **Inspect and evaluate the condition of wounds, noting the following:**

   a. Location and Size

   Observe and record the location of the wound.

   Measure the wound's length and width in centimeters.

   Measure the depth of the wound by inserting a sterile swab into the deepest part of the wound and measuring the extent the swab can be inserted in centimeters.

   b. Undermining or Tunneling

   If you suspect tunneling, slide a sterile swab into the tunnel until you meet resistance and measure its depth with a ruler.

   Record your findings to indicate the direction of the undermining or tunneling as well as the depth.

   c. Color of the Wound Bed

   Observe the color of the wound bed, and note how much of the wound bed is covered by either necrotic or granulation tissue.

   d. Wound Drainage

   Note any drainage in the wound bed as well as drainage adhering to old dressings.

   e. Wound Odor

   Observe the odor of the wound. If the wound is covered by a dressing, the wound should be cleaned before evaluating odor. Document the quality of the odor. If there is no odor, this observation should also be documented.

2. **Stage the wound as part of the initial evaluation.**

   Use staging only for the initial evaluation of the wound. Do not restage a wound as a method to denote healing.

   Use the staging guidelines of the National Pressure Ulcer Advisory Panel (see below).

   Based on inspection of the wound, assign one of the following stages:

   Stage I

   Nonblanchable erythema of intact skin

   The skin surface appears red and will remain red with light palpation, indicating underlying tissue damage.

Clinical Significance

Wounds should be carefully assessed and assessment findings documented to stage a wound (see below) and follow the wound healing progress.

Wound size is monitored to evaluate healing. One indicator of wound healing progress is progressive contraction (shrinking) of the wound surface area.

Undermining or *tunneling* in a wound refers to the development of a space or pocket between two layers of skin

Red or pink color: Indicates healing and the presence of granulation tissue.

Granulation tissue: Bright, shiny, "beefy-red" tissue in a wound bed consisting of new capillary buds, fibroblasts that synthesize collagen, and an extracellular matrix. Granulation tissue replaces lost or destroyed tissue in a wound.

Green, yellow, or *black color:* Indicates infection and the presence of necrotic (dead) tissue.

Clear or *serous drainage:* Normal in a healing wound

Green or *yellow (purulent) drainage:* Indicates infection

Sweet smell: May indicate decay

Foul smell: May indicate fecal contamination or a fistula.

Wound Staging: The initial evaluation of pressure ulcers and other types of wounds to quantify the extent of tissue loss. Wound staging is not used to evaluate progress or lack of progress toward wound healing, because healing does not always result in replacement of tissues that were destroyed in the original wound.

The use of standardized definitions helps ensure accuracy of wound staging.

▼ ▼ ▼

G U I D E L I N E S *continued*   Wound Assessment

Procedure

Stage II
Partial-thickness skin loss involving the epidermis or dermis. May present clinically as an abrasion, blister, or shallow crater.

Stage III
Full-thickness skin loss involving damage or necrosis of subcutaneous tissue that may extend down to, but not through, the underlying fascia. Undermining may or may not be present.

Stage IV
Full-thickness skin loss with extensive destruction, tissue necrosis, or damage to muscle, bone, or supporting structures. Undermining and sinus tracts may be present.

Clinical Significance

Partial-thickness skin loss (superficial tissue destruction): Refers to loss of epidermis or dermis. Occurs with a stage II wound. The mechanism of healing for partial-thickness wounds is relatively simple because there is no damage to blood vessels or loss of connective tissue.

Full-thickness skin loss (deep tissue destruction): Refers to loss of tissue from all three skin layers—epidermis, dermis, and subcutaneous tissue. The mechanism of healing full-thickness wounds is complex and involves replacement of connective tissue with granulation tissue.

Stages of Decubitus Ulcers

Stage I
- Blood stasis in underlying tissues (hyperemia)
- Not relieved by massage or pressure relief
- Reddened skin color
- Warm to touch

Stage II
- Epidermal tissue loss
- May be damage to the dermis
- Moist and depressed skin erosion

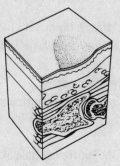

Stage I

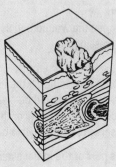

Stage II

(continued)

▼ ▼ ▼
G U I D E L I N E S *continued*   Wound Assessment

Stages of Decubitus Ulcers (continued)

Stage III

- Full-thickness skin loss
- Dermal ulceration may extend to the subcutaneous layer
- Serosanguineous or purulent drainage common

Stage IV

- Full-thickness skin destruction
- Ulceration into deeper tissue structures (fascia, connective tissue, muscle, bone)

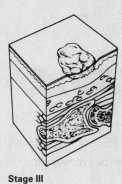

Stage III

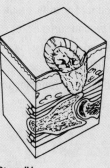

Stage IV

3. **Evaluate wound healing.**

   a. Conduct serial assessments of the wound and carefully document your findings to reliably note any changes in the appearance of the wound. Full-thickness wounds should be thoroughly assessed on a weekly basis.

   b. Observe the wound, noting surface area, wound bed color and drainage, and wound odor (See #1).

   c. Evaluate your findings with respect to the healing process expected for a particular type of wound.

   Note the amount of time it takes for the wound to heal.

Indicators of healing for a superficial wound (complete healing normally takes 10 to 14 days after wound resurfacing):

- Progressive decrease in wound surface area
- Decrease in surrounding tissue redness and swelling
- Blending of the wound area into the surrounding undamaged epidermis

Wound Healing Processes
Superficial Wounds (Stage II wounds)

- Only the epidermis is damaged
- No blood vessels are interrupted
- No need to synthesize connective tissue
- Mechanism of healing is tissue regeneration (resurfacing or re-epithelialization)
- Regeneration: damaged tissue heals by replacement with tissue identical to the original tissue
- Requires short timeframe
- Three phases of healing:
  - Epithelial migration
  - Cell division (mitosis) to supply new cells
  - Differentiation of new epidermis

▼ ▼ ▼

G U I D E L I N E S *continued*

Wound Assessment

Procedure

Indicators of healing for a full-thickness wound (complete wound healing may take months, depending on volume and surface area of the wound):

- Removal of eschar (scab)
- Decrease in surrounding tissue redness and swelling
- Appearance of granulation tissue
- Reduction in the amount of necrotic tissue and debris
- Gradual reduction in wound surface area
- Reduction in exudate and change from purulent to serous
- Appearance of epithelial tissue
- Blending of the wound into surrounding undamaged epidermis

Clinical Significance

Full-Thickness Wounds (Stage III or IV wounds)

- Tissue destruction involves all three skin layers
- Mechanisms of healing is tissue repair and tissue regeneration
- The new tissue that is formed is referred to as granulation tissue
- Three phases of healing
  - Inflammation
  - Granulation tissue production
  - Matrix formation and remodeling

Signs of Impaired Wound Healing

- Increased redness and swelling
- Suppuration (pus formation)
- Dehisence (disruption of wound layers)
- Change in wound bed color from pink or red to white, yellow, black
- Decrease in the amount of granulation tissue

▼ ▼ ▼

G U I D E L I N E S

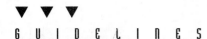

Assessment Guidelines   Hair

Procedure

1. **Inspect the hair to evaluate color and pigmentation.**

2. **Note the quantity of hair. Pull gently at a few strands to determine whether It comes out easily.**

Clinical Significance

Normal Findings

Normal hair color is largely influenced by genetic makeup and age. Natural hair colors include black, brown, red, and yellow. Pigment distribution is uniform in the hair shaft. Gray hair occurs secondary to loss of melanocytes and represents normal aging. Cosmetic alteration of healthy hair is a common practice in many cultures.

Deviations from Normal

Alterations in color and pigmentation may indicate nutrition alterations. Flag sign: Transverse depigmentation of the hair indicating nutrient deficiency, especially of copper and protein.

Normal Findings

Hair quantity generally increases after puberty in both males and females and decreases with age. Body hair quantity may vary greatly among healthy persons of both sexes.

Male balding that occurs as anterior regression of the hairline is a genetic tendency and is considered normal.

Deviations from Normal

Easy pluckability and sparse hair may be noted with protein deficiencies. Loss of hair may also occur with anemia, heavy metal poisoning, and hypopituitarism.

▼ ▼ ▼

G U I D E L I N E S   *continued*

Hair

Procedure

3. **Move a few strands of hair between your thumb and forefinger to evaluate texture.**

4. **Survey general hygiene of the hair and scalp.**
   Grasp handfuls of hair and pull it gently away from the scalp to better visualize the hair shaft and skin. Inspect carefully at the back of the head and neck.

Clinical Significance

Normal Findings
Normal hair texture may be coarse or silky. Dark-skinned people tend to have coarser hair, whereas light-skinned people will probably have fine or silky hair.

Deviations from Normal
Very coarse hair is associated with hypothyroidism. Very fine hair is associated with hyperthyroidism.

Normal Findings
Healthy hair and scalp will have a shiny appearance and will be free of lice infestations and nits (louse eggs).

Deviations from Normal
Flakiness, sores, and infestations are considered abnormal. Lice infestations may be more readily observed at the surface of the scalp.

▼ ▼ ▼

G U I D E L I N E S

Assessment Guidelines   Nails

Procedure

1. **Observe the shape and configuration of the nail.**

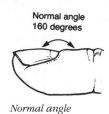

Normal angle
160 degrees

Normal angle

Clinical Significance

Normal Findings
Dorsal nail surface: slightly convex. Nail thickness: 0.3 to 0.65 mm. Angle at the nail base, at the skin–nail interface, is normally 160 degrees.

Deviations from Normal
Abnormal nail shape may indicate malnutrition.

Spooning: Concave nail plates; associated with iron-deficiency anemia.

Spooning

▼ ▼ ▼

G U I D E L I N E S   *continued*   Nails

Procedure

Estimate the angle at the base of the nail where the skin and nail interface.

Clinical Significnce

Clubbing: The angle at the base of the nail where the skin and nail interface is greater than 160 degrees. Clubbing is associated with congenital heart disease and pulmonary pathology. See the display, Nail Abnormalities, for other abnormalities and possible causes.

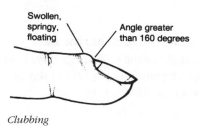

Swollen, springy, floating

Angle greater than 160 degrees

Clubbing

Nail Abnormalities

Onychorrhexis

- Brittle, fragile, uneven nail edge
- Associated with malnutrition, overhydration, thyrotoxicosis, chemical damage, radiation, aging

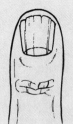

Onychorrhexis

Onychauxis

- Nail hypertrophy
- Associated with trauma, aging, fungal infections

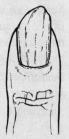

Onychauxis

Beau's Lines

- Transverse furrows in nail plate
- Associated with malnutrition, severe illness

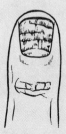

Beau's lines

Splinter Hemorrhages

- Blood streaks
- Associated with heart disease, hypertension, rheumatoid arthritis, neoplasms, trauma

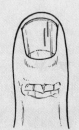

Splinter hemorrhage

Subungual Hematoma

- Blood clot
- Associated with trauma

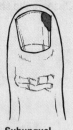

Subungual hematoma

▼ ▼ ▼

G U I D E L I N E S   *continued*   Nails

| Procedure | Clinical Significance |

Procedure

2. **Note the color of the nails.**

Clinical Significance

Normal Findings

Uniform with the exception of color difference between lunula and the rest of the nail. Nails appear pink in whites and may have a bluish hue in dark-skinned people.

Deviations from Normal

Nail lesions may alter the color of the nail plate.

Cyanosis: Bluish discoloration of the nail bed; associated with pulmonary pathology.

3. **Squeeze the nail between the thumb and the forefinger to determine capillary refill time.**

   When pressure is released, the nail will appear white (blanching). The number of seconds that elapse before the nail bed returns to its baseline color is the capillary refill time.

Normal Findings

Normal capillary refill time is less than 3 seconds.

Deviations from Normal

Capillary refill time greater than 3 seconds indicates poor tissue perfusion.

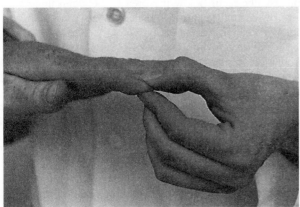

Determining capillary refill time

4. **Examine the nails for presence of lesions or other abnormalities.**

See display, Nail Abnormalities.

Documenting Integumentary Examination Findings

Describe the characteristics of any skin or nail lesions. Document the size of any lesions in the patient's record so that any changes may be monitored. It may be helpful to draw simple diagrams of any significant lesions and place them in the patient's record with accompanying dimensions.

Example 1: Normal Skin

Ms. J, aged 67, was recovering from a concussion after a motor vehicle accident. The patient was lethargic but arousable, and she had remained in bed for the 24 hours since hospital admission. Skin examination was conducted as part of a routine head-to-toe examination. Examination results were normal and recorded in the progress notes as follows:

> Skin pale flesh color, warm, and dry without lesions; no erythema over pressure points; no prolonged tenting when pinched, and no sacral or other types of dependent edema observed.

Example 2: Decubitus Ulcer

Mr. B, aged 88, was confined to bed after a massive cerebral vascular accident 6 months ago. He had developed a sacral decubitus ulcer that the nurses examined daily. Examination findings were charted as follows:

> Sacral ulcer 5 × 6 cm; epidermal surface disrupted and dermis exposed. Wound bed reddened without drainage; small yellow patch (0.5 × 0.5 cm) noted in center of ulcer.

Example 3: Normal Hair

A.J., aged 6, was examined by the school nurse during a pediculosis (lice) screening program. Special attention was given to the condition of the scalp and hair. Examination findings were recorded as follows:

> Hair thick, shiny, and clean. Scalp and hair shafts show no signs of flaking, redness, or infestation.

Example 4: Severe Malnutrition

G.H., aged 17, was hospitalized for treatment of severe anorexia nervosa. She was 60% below her ideal body weight. Her physical appearance had been altered as a result of malnutrition. The appearance of her hair was documented as follows:

> Hair is thin and coarse. Areas of depigmentation noted in transverse distribution. Hair pulls out easily with minimal tugging. Scalp skin flaky but without redness.

Example 5: Healthy Nails

The appearance of the nails is described with attention to shape and configuration, color, and lesions. Consider the following, for example:

> Nail plates smooth, uniform pinkish color, convex, and without lesions. Nail bed–skin angle 160 degrees. Capillary refill less than 3 seconds.

Example 6: Clubbing

Mr. K.K., aged 68, had a long history of chronic obstructive pulmonary disease secondary to a 40–pack-year history of cigarette smoking. Manifestations of chronic hypoxia were evident during the examination of the nails, and findings were recorded as follows:

> Nail beds dusky-cyanotic color. Capillary refill 3 seconds. All nails have increased nail bed–skin angle of approximately 190 degrees.

Nursing Diagnoses Related to Integumentary Assessment

Impaired Skin Integrity

The nursing diagnosis of Impaired skin integrity may be applied to a person whose skin is adversely altered. The indicators of impaired skin integrity include disruption of skin surface, destruction of skin layers, and invasion of body structures.

To identify persons at risk for impaired skin integrity, you also should determine the presence of any of the following risk factors:

- Incontinence
- Inactivity
- Immobility
- Poor nutritional status
- Mechanical factors such as friction/shear

Risk assessment tools are often used in clinical practice to determine at-risk status and initiate early preventive measures. Common risk assessment tools include the Norton Assessment Scale (Norton, McLaren, & Exton-Smith, 1962); the Braden Scale (Bergstrom, et al. 1986); and the Waterlow Scale (Standing, 1985)

Clinical Problems Related to Integumentary Assessment

Clinical Syndromes With Integumentary Manifestations

A number of clinical syndromes or disease states are characterized by alterations in the appearance or function of the integumentary system.

Diabetes Mellitus. People with diabetes mellitus are prone to chronic skin infections with skin ulceration, especially if the disease is poorly controlled. Such infections may occur because diabetes alters immunity and peripheral circulation. Candidal (yeast) infections are common and usually occur below the breasts, between fingers and toes, in the axilla, and in female genitals, producing erythema, swelling, pain, and itching.

Ulceration and infection may occur in the feet, where circulation is often impaired. The nurse should carefully inspect the feet for redness, swelling, and pain and report such signs of inflammation to a physician.

Shin spots (brownish, rounded, painless atrophic lesions) may be observed on the pretibial area of the adult with diabetes. Diabetics also may develop xanthomas, small round lesions resembling slightly elevated, soft plaques, on the lower legs or ankles.

Liver Disease. Many types of pathologic processes can affect the liver, and skin alterations may vary depending on the specific pathologic condition. Jaundice is a common finding in most types of liver disease. Edema also may occur and may be generalized or limited to the abdomen as protein metabolism and fluid dynamics of the liver are impaired.

Chronic and excessive alcohol consumption is a common cause of liver pathology. The skin examination may show palmar erythema, spider nevi over the upper chest, and skin changes associated with vitamin deficiencies. (Spider nevi are vascular skin lesions caused by capillary dilation and congestion.)

Renal Disease. Skin alterations observed with renal failure may be secondary to hematologic alterations caused by renal dysfunction. Pallor may be observed secondary to anemia. Purpura, a sign associated with platelet dysfunction, is caused by hemorrhage into the skin. The hemorrhage appears as a dark purple to brownish yellow macular lesion.

Some skin changes occur because the kidney can no longer metabolize or excrete certain substances. A yellow skin discoloration may occur secondary to pigment retention; it differs from jaundice in that the discoloration is not always generalized and does not affect the appearance of mucous membranes. Pigment retention may occur in the sclera and should not be confused with jaundice. Impaired metabolism may cause urate crystals to precipitate through the skin, causing a frosted appearance (uremic frost). Generalized edema may occur secondary to impaired protein metabolism and fluid retention.

Protein-Calorie Malnutrition. Changes in the hair are indicative of protein-calorie deficiencies. If the nurse can easily pull strands of hair from the scalp (easy pluckability), the person may have a protein deficiency. Alternating bands of dark and light hair (flag sign) may indicate a protein or copper deficiency. In general, protein-calorie malnutrition causes a dull, dry, sparse hair condition. Nail changes associated with protein-calorie malnutrition include a dull, lackluster appearance and transverse ridging across the nail plate.

With a protein deficiency such as kwashiorkor, the person's entire body may become dry, with the skin flaking off like old paint (flaky paint dermatosis). Flaky skin may be noted around the nose of clients with less severe protein malnutrition.

Vitamin-Mineral Deficiencies. In severe niacin deficiency (pellagra), the person's skin also flakes, but unlike flaky paint dermatosis, the condition is limited to sun-exposed areas. Flaking skin areas usually appear darker in color. Vitamin B_6 and riboflavin deficiencies cause cheilosis, a condition in which reddening and cracking occurs at the corners of the mouth. Vascular skin lesions may be noted with vitamin C and K deficiencies. Petechiae, especially around the hair follicles, are associated with vitamin C deficiency, whereas purpura occurs with a lack of vitamin K. Vitamin A deficiency is associated with hyperkeratosis, a condition in which hair follicles become plugged with excess keratin, causing rough skin.

Iron deficiencies may cause spooning of the fingernail plates, and copper and zinc deficiencies may cause hair thinning and pigmentation changes.

Cardiovascular Disease. Skin alterations observed in persons with cardiovascular disease are usually associated with impaired oxygenation and fluid volume alterations. Integumentary manifestations of impaired oxygenation include pallor and cyanosis. A person in cardiogenic shock will display cold, clammy, pale skin and prolonged capillary refill time (greater than 3 seconds). Persons with cardiovascular disease may have edematous-appearing skin secondary to fluid volume excesses that may occur with heart failure.

Peripheral Vascular Disease. Disease in the peripheral vascular system may occur in the venous or arterial vessels. It may be either chronic or acute; it will influence skin appearance accordingly.

Acute arterial occlusion may cause the skin to feel cold and to appear mottled or pale. Skin changes may progress to bleb formation, skin necrosis, cyanosis, and gangrene. *Any such finding, in addition to loss of peripheral pulses, signals a medical emergency.*

Chronic arterial occlusion, which occurs with atherosclerosis, may result in atrophic skin changes, including hair loss in the involved area (usually a lower extremity) and skin thinning. Rubor is noted when the extremity is dependent, and blanching occurs with elevation. The affected extremity may be cool on palpation.

Chronic venous insufficiency usually affects the lower extremities, and ankle edema is common. Stasis ulcers may form as a result of fluid pressure on surface capillaries. Scar tissue from previously healed stasis ulcers is common. The skin surface appears thin, shiny, and atrophic. Skin color may be cyanotic, and brownish pigment may accumulate.

Skin Cancers. Different types of skin cancer have characteristic abnormal lesions. The American Academy of Dermatology developed the "ABCD" formula as a guide to determine which lesions warrant further investigation. The "ABCD" rules are as follows:

- *Asymmetry.* Half of the skin lesion does not match the other half.
- *Border irregularity.* The edges of the skin lesion are scalloped, notched, or ragged.
- *Color.* Pigmentation varies throughout the lesion. Shades of tan, brown, and black are present. Red, white, and blue may add to a mottled appearance.
- *Diameter.* The lesion has increased in size, or the diameter of the lesion is greater than 6 mm (roughly that of a pencil eraser).

Actinic keratosis is a premalignant skin lesion found on areas that have been exposed to the sun. Usually, the lesion appears as a small, scaly papule with underlying erythema; scales return if the lesion is scraped off. In most cases, the borders of the lesion are well circumscribed but may become indistinct when undergoing malignant transformation. Lesions commonly occur in fair-skinned, light-haired people.

Basal cell carcinoma is a malignant skin lesion that may occur in a fair-skinned person who has been chronically exposed to sunlight. The small papular lesion grows very slowly, reaching only 1 to 2 cm in diameter after 1 year. Lesion borders usually appear semitranslucent and waxy. Telangiectatic vessels may appear, and the center of the lesion may ulcerate and invade the underlying tissue.

Squamous cell carcinoma may develop from actinic keratoses. The lesion appears as a small, hard, conical nodule that rapidly grows and invades surrounding tissues. Ulcers with poorly defined, irregular borders accompany such rapid growth.

Malignant melanoma, the most lethal type of skin cancer, arises from a malignant transformation in the melanocytes and may, in the precancerous state, exist as a mole that develops into a lesion with more elevation, more pigmentation, and a tendency to bleed easily. Lesion borders become irregular, and pigmentation may be blue, purple, red, or black.

Infection and Infestations

Skin infections or infestations are identified according to the characteristics and distribution of the lesions. It is important to question the patient about how the lesion developed and any associated symptoms that might help to establish the diagnosis.

Bacterial Skin Infections. Impetigo, a common bacterial skin infection, is caused by staphylococci, streptococci, or both. The bacteria are transmitted by touch, and the infection commonly occurs on the face or other exposed body areas. The lesions may appear as macules, vesicles, or pustules that become crusted and rupture. A red base is found beneath denuded lesions. The patient should be questioned about symptoms of intense itching.

Folliculitis is an inflammation of the hair follicles caused by staphylococci. Pustules may be present at the surface of the hair follicle, and the hair shaft may be observed at the center of the pustule. This infection occurs most commonly on skin that has been shaved, on the buttocks, and on areas with hair follicles. Itching may accompany the infection.

Furuncles, boils, and carbuncles are deep-seated staphylococcal infections of hair follicles. A carbuncle is the coalescence of several furuncles. The lesion is pustular with a rounded, raised core that eventually opens, releasing necrotic tissue and pus. Furuncles and boils commonly occur on the back of the neck and the buttocks.

Viral Skin Infections. Herpes is responsible for many common viral skin infections. Two types of herpes simplex viruses, HSV-1 and HSV-2, have been identified. The HSV-1 virus infects the oral mucosa, labia, eyes, and the skin overlying sensory nerve segments. The HSV-2 virus infects the genitals, anus, and oral mucosa by sexual transmission. Lesions associated with both virus types are small vesicles that eventually rupture and form crusts. Erythema and itching may precede vesicle formation.

Fungal Skin Infections. Monilial or candidal infections are caused by yeast-like fungi that are part of the normal skin flora. The most common sites where this normal flora may become pathogenic are the genital, anal, and axillary areas as well as beneath breasts and between fingers and toes. The lesions appear as bright red, eroded patches. Satellite vesicopustules may or may not be present. Whitish, curd-like secretions may be observed in the affected areas, especially on oral or vaginal mucous membranes. The person may report severe itching.

Tinea (ringworm) is a fungal infection that usually occurs on the groin, scalp, feet, or trunk. The lesions vary slightly in appearance, depending on site. Tinea capitis (scalp ringworm) appears as round, scaly gray patches that cause hair breakage and lead to small bald areas. Tinea corporis (body ringworm) appears as a group of lesions surrounded by a ring. Within the ring, scaling with central clearing occurs. Small vesicles may be noted at the border of the ring. Tinea cruris (groin ringworm), also known as "jock itch," appears as erythematous macules with sharp margins. The center of the macule is clear, but vesicles appear at the borders. Tinea pedis (foot ringworm), also known as "athlete's foot," occurs in the interdigital webs and soles of the feet. In the acute phase, a reddened macular rash appears and may be followed by fissuring and tissue maceration.

Common Infestations. Scabies is a parasitic infestation of the skin caused by *Sarcoptes scabiei,* or itch mite, which usually affects the hands, wrists, axillae, genitalia, and inner aspect of the thighs. The skin of the head and neck is rarely affected. Associated lesions include small papules, vesicles, and burrows that result after the mite enters the skin to lay eggs. Burrows appear as short, irregular marks that look like they were made by a sharp pencil.

Pediculosis (lice infestation) affects the scalp, body, and pubic hairs. The eggs (nits) are visible small, white particles. The skin underlying the infested area usually appears excoriated.

Noninfectious Inflammatory Processes

Contact dermatitis, a form of eczema, is an inflammatory skin condition caused by exposure to external factors (primary irritant contact dermatitis) or specific allergens in a sensitized person (allergic contact dermatitis). Causal agents include plant oils and pollens, soaps, detergents, industrial chemicals, and rubber. Lesions appear as erythematous macules that may form vesicles and crusts. The lesions are easily infected and then discharge a purulent exudate. Distribution depends on the location of the skin that contacts the causative agent. For example, the hands may be affected if the agent is a dishwashing detergent. Similarly, the face may be affected if a cosmetic is the causative agent.

THE JAW AND ORAL CAVITY
Anatomy and Physiology Review

The oral cavity includes the lips, salivary glands, tongue and taste buds, gingiva, teeth, hard and soft palates, uvula, tonsils, and pharynx. Except for the teeth, the visible structures of the oral cavity are covered by a mucous membrane referred to as the oral mucosa.

Oral Mucosa

The oral mucosa is composed of three layers: the epithelium, the lamina propria, and the submucosa (Fig. 6-2). The oral mucosa keeps the mouth hydrated, aids in digestion, and serves as both a mechanical and a chemical barrier to trauma and infectious organisms.

The epithelial cells undergo rapid and continuous cell

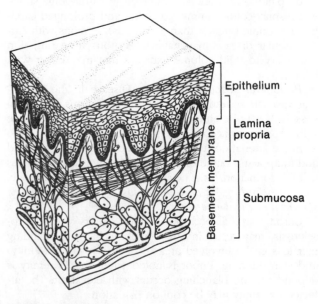

FIGURE 6.2 Cross section of the oral mucosa.

growth and differentiation. The epithelial surface is renewed every 7 to 14 days. Epithelial cell differentiation varies throughout the oral cavity. For example, epithelial cells in the tongue evolve to form the papillae that contain the taste buds, and lip and cheek epithelia differentiate into cells that secrete saliva.

Blood flow through the lamina propria and submucosa accounts for the pink color of the oral mucosa. Cyanosis may occur with hypoxemia. Erythema is common with inflammation. The submucosa is thin and tough over the roof of the mouth or palate, providing the ability to withstand mechanical stress. It is thicker in the lips, cheeks, and tongue, giving a softer appearance.

Salivary Glands

A number of glands secrete saliva, including the parotid glands located beneath each ear, the submandibular and sublingual glands in the floor of the mouth, and the buc-

cal glands in the epithelium of the lips and the cheeks (Fig. 6-3). The opening of the parotid gland is marked by a small papillae called Stensen's duct. The submandibular gland openings, called Wharton's ducts, are located under the tongue at the base of the frenulum. Each sublingual gland has approximately 20 ducts that open at the base of the mouth.

Normally, 1500 mL of saliva is produced in a 24-hour period. Saliva production is regulated by the salivary nuclei located in the brain stem, which are stimulated by certain tastes, odors, and tactile stimulations and even by food thoughts. Excessive salivation may be observed during nausea because the salivary nuclei and vomiting center are in close proximity in the brain.

Saliva hydrates and cleanses the oral mucosa and provides protection from bacterial infections. The normal pH of the saliva (6.0 to 7.0) contributes to the maintenance and growth of the normal bacterial flora. If this pH balance is disrupted, the risk of infection increases.

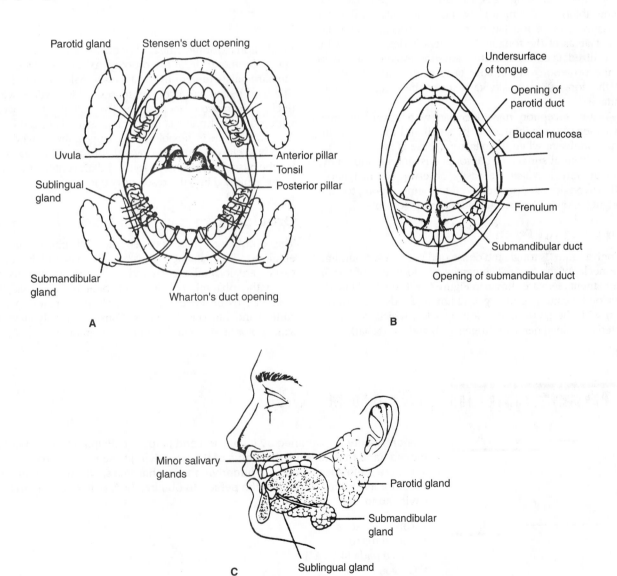

FIGURE 6.3 Salivary glands. (**A** and **B**) Gland openings into the oral cavity. (**C**) Anatomic location of the salivary glands.

Substances within saliva such as lytic enzymes and the immunoglobulin secretory IgA further inhibit bacterial growth. Saliva also has an important digestion function because it contains enzymes that initiate starch breakdown.

Tongue and Taste Buds

The tongue is a muscular organ infiltrated with fat and mucous and serous glands. The tongue functions in speech, food mixing, and swallowing.

The dorsal surface of the tongue is covered by papillae, which give the tongue a rough appearance. Taste buds, composed of epithelial cells, are located on the papillae surfaces. Taste sensations are conducted to the cerebral cortex by sensory divisions of cranial nerves VII (facial) and IX (glossopharyngeal). Epithelial taste cells undergo rapid synthesis and differentiation and are highly vulnerable to radiation and chemotherapeutic agents, which destroy rapidly dividing cells. Although all taste buds have some ability to distinguish sweet, sour, salty, and bitter sensations, these four sensations are associated with different areas of the tongue. Sweetness is detected best by specialized taste buds at the anterior tongue; bitterness at the posterior tongue; sour taste at the lateral surfaces of the tongue; and salty taste over the tongue's entire surface.

Taste perception may decrease with advancing age. Taste sensation is influenced by smell and may be diminished or absent when the olfactory sense is impaired.

The ventral surface of the tongue is smooth and shiny, and underlying veins are easily observed. Cranial nerve XII (hypoglossal) provides motor innervation to the tongue, allowing numerous muscular movements.

Gingiva and Teeth

Gingiva (gum) is tough and dense oral mucosa surrounding the necks of the teeth. The names and locations of the 32 permanent teeth are shown in Figure 6-4. Teeth facilitate digestion by cutting, grinding, and mixing foods in coordination with the jaw's mastication muscles, which are innervated by cranial nerves V (trigeminal) and VII (facial).

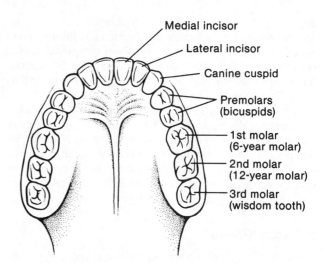

FIGURE 6.4   The permanent teeth.

Palate

In addition to forming the roof of the mouth, the palate separates the mouth from the oropharynx and is divided into the hard palate (anteriorly) and the soft palate (posteriorly). The hard palate has a convex shape and is covered with a thick, pale mucous membrane. The soft palate, covered with a thin, red mucous membrane, extends to the uvula. The soft palate is flexible and changes shape when the mouth is relaxed. It moves upward during swallowing, closing the nasopharynx and pharynx and preventing food from being aspirated into the respiratory tract.

Oropharynx

The oropharynx lies between the soft palate and the epiglottis. The palatine tonsils, small masses of lymphoid tissue, are located on each side of the oropharynx beneath the pharyngopalatine arch behind the uvula. The epithelial tissue covering the tonsils invaginates to form surface indentations or crypts. Tonsils normally have the same color as surrounding mucous membranes.

Physical Examination   Jaw and Oral Cavity

GENERAL APPROACH   The oral cavity is examined by inspection and palpation. Palpate lesions with a gloved hand to determine the status of the underlying tissues. Cancerous lesions are often associated with underlying tissue hardness, which is secondary to tumor infiltration. Interview the person to obtain a history if you note oral cavity abnormalities.

EQUIPMENT
- Tongue blades
- Dental mirror
- Gauze pads (4" × 4")
- Gloves
- Penlight or flashlight

(continued)

Physical Examination Jaw and Oral Cavity (continued)

EXPOSURE AND LIGHTING

Use a flashlight or penlight to inspect the oral mucosa. Before the examination, ask the person to remove any dental prostheses. To facilitate inspection, displace the person's tongue with gauze or tongue blades and use a dental mirror.

EXAMINATON AND
DOCUMENTATION FOCUS

- *Mucous membranes:* Color and pigmentation, moisture, texture, hygiene, lesions
- *Structural integrity:* Structural symmetry, tooth alignment, deformities
- *Functional ability:* Cranial nerves (IX [glossopharyngeal], X [vagus], XII [hypoglossal]); taste sensation; chewing: swallowing; speech

EXAMINING THE ORAL CAVITY
OF THE UNCONSCIOUS
OR SEMICONSCIOUS PATIENT

An oral examination is relatively easy to perform when the person is fully alert and cooperative. The person with a decreased level of consciousness, however, presents a special challenge. Because the risk for oral mucosa alterations is high in persons with decreased level of consciousness, frequent reassessment is warranted.

Often, semiconscious and unconscious people clench their jaws and resist opening their mouths, especially after tactile stimulation of the lips or oral mucosa. Attempting to force the jaw open may be unsuccessful or harmful. The best approach is to wait until the person spontaneously opens the jaw and inspect as much of the oral mucosa as possible by shining a penlight into the mouth without touching the person.

If spontaneous jaw opening does not occur, the mouth may be opened by using a chin-lift maneuver such as that used for opening an obstructed airway. Place the fingers of one hand under the lower jaw while lifting the chin forward to open the mouth. To perform a thorough inspection, place a hard plastic bite block between the upper and lower teeth. Never place your fingers in the mouth. When using a block, take precautions against unnecessary tissue trauma. Remove the block quickly, not forcefully, after the spontaneous release of the jaw pressure. A block should never compromise the airway.

Be sure to assess for tissue trauma from tubes passing through the oral cavity, such as an endotracheal tube.

▼ ▼ ▼

G U I D E L I N E S

Assessment Guidelines   Jaw and Oral Cavity

Procedure

1. **Inspect and palpate the outer structures of the oral cavity.**

   a. Assess for malocclusion by asking the person to open and shut the jaw and expose the teeth. While the mouth is opened and closed, palpate the temporomandibular joint for tenderness and deviation.

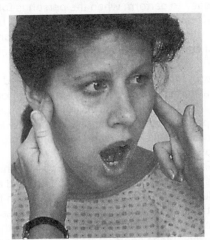

Temporomandibular joint palpation

   b. Inspect and palpate the skin over the parotid glands (anterior to the ear lobes) for symmetry and swelling.

   c. Inspect and palpate the lips.

2. **Examine the dorsal surface of the tongue while evaluating cranial nerves XII (hypoglossal) and X (vagus).**

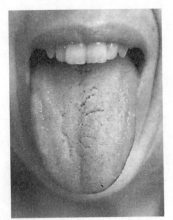

Dorsal surface of the tongue

Clinical Significance

Normal Findings

Upper and lower front teeth should align when the jaw is clenched.

Full range of voluntary motion to the mandibular joints exists; that is, the jaw can open and shut completely, and the upper and lower jaws can move from side to side.

Deviations from Normal

Teeth may be missing or may deviate from normal alignment. The significance of such findings is determined by assessing functions such as chewing and talking. Missing teeth often are replaced by partial or complete dentures, which should align with the surrounding teeth or jaw.

Deviation from Normal

Parotid gland enlargement, unilateral or bilateral.

Normal Finding

Lips are symmetric, although asymmetry is common and considered normal unless functional interference occurs.

▼ ▼ ▼

G U I D E L I N E S *continued*   Jaw and Oral Cavity

Procedure

a. To inspect the dorsal tongue surface, ask the person to extend the tongue and say "ah."

b. Note symmetry of the tongue and uvula when the tongue is protruded.

c. Observe the motion of the soft palate when the person says "ah."

3. **Inspect the hard and soft palates.**

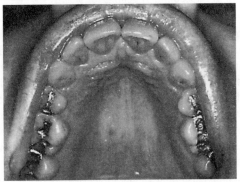

Palate inspection

Ask the person to tilt the head back with mouth open, and examine the palate with a light or dental mirror.

4. **Examine the oropharynx, posterior tongue, and uvula.**

a. If the person has difficulty holding the tongue flat, gently depress it with a tongue blade. Be careful not to initiate a gag reflex; to relax and reassure the person, explain the procedure.

Clinical Significance

Normal Finding

Taste buds give the posterior tongue a slightly rough texture.

Deviations from Normal

The appearance of the tongue mucosa is altered with malnutrition, inflammation, infection, and inflammatory states. During inflammatory states, the tongue forms a protective coating of a whitish cast; however, such a coating should not be confused with the white plaques that may adhere to the tongue as exudate from certain infections.

Deviations from Normal

Loss of symmetry may indicate pathologic processes involving the nervous system. Tongue deviation as well as tremors indicate a problem with cranial nerve XII (hypoglossal).

Cranial nerve X (vagus) has one branch that innervates the soft palate.

Normal Finding

Normal nerve function is indicated by the soft palate's rising when the client says "ah."

Normal Findings

The anterior surface of the hard palate is corrugated. The palate is symmetric with no midline openings.

Structural abnormalities of the palate are often genetic.

Normal Finding

The oral mucosa of the tonsils is pink and moist and may be characterized by crypts and indentations.

Deviation from Normal

Erythema restricted to the oropharynx usually represents a localized infection of that structure.

▼ ▼ ▼

G U I D E L I N E S *continued*   Jaw and Oral Cavity

Procedure

b. Use a dental mirror to inspect the posterior pharynx and uvula.

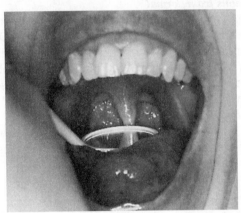

Inspection of posterior pharynx and uvula

c. Elicit a gag reflex by touching the posterior wall of the pharynx with the tongue blade or dental mirror.

5. **Examine the lip and cheek (buccal) oral mucosa.**

a. Examine the underside of the lips and anterior surface of the gums by displacing the lips with fingers or gauze.

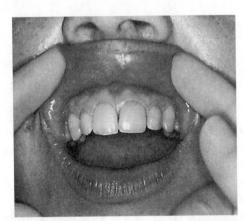

Lip displacement

Clinical Significance

A gray oropharynx is a sign of diphtheria.

Normal Finding

Gagging with this maneuver indicates normal function of cranial nerve IX (glossopharyngeal).

Normal Findings

Oral mucosa color inside the cheek (buccal mucosa) and lips may vary according to race. Blacks may have a slight blue undertone, and whites may have a pink or red undertone. In all races, the remaining oral mucosa appears pink, but variations in shade are normal depending on the thickness of mucosa layers. Although rare, hyperpigmentation may occur in dark- and light-skinned people as freckle-like macules inside the buccal mucosa.

The oral mucosa should appear moist secondary to saliva secretion, smooth, and free of lesions and exudates.

Deviations from Normal

Abnormal color changes include pallor (paleness or lack of color), cyanosis (bluish cast), erythema (redness), and gray mucous membranes. Any color changes are recorded in terms of location and distribution. Cyanosis usually indicates systemic hypoxemia and is distributed throughout the oral mucosa. Pallor reflects vasoconstriction of the vessels in the mucosa, which may occur with shock or before acute inflammatory states such as stomatitis. Stomatitis erythema is characterized by a sharp line of demarcation at the mucocutaneous border of the lips. Intensified pigmentation of the oral mucosa may be noted with Addison's disease.

▼ ▼ ▼

G U I D E L I N E S *continued*   Jaw and Oral Cavity

Procedure

b. Examine the inner cheek by using a tongue blade or gloved finger to displace the cheek laterally and expose the surface.

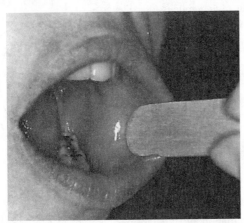

Inner cheek inspection: Using the tongue blade to expose the buccal mucosa

Clinical Significance

Excessive dryness of the oral mucosa (xerostomia) occurs when salivary gland activity is arrested. Excessive moisture may be observed in early stages of inflammation.

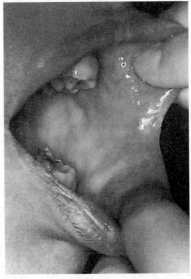

Inner cheek inspection: Using the fingers to expose the buccal mucosa

6. **Examine the lateral and ventral tongue surfaces.**

   a. Inspect the mucosa by displacing the tongue laterally.

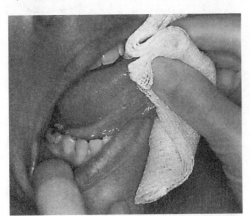

Lateral displacement of the tongue

   b. Then, ask the person to touch the hard palate with tongue tip, and examine the ventral surface. Palpate oral mucosa of the mouth floor with a gloved finger.

Oral lesions, including malignancies, may be hidden beneath the tongue. Accumulation of food and debris may indicate poor hygiene or impaired chewing or swallowing.

▼ ▼ ▼

G U I D E L I N E S   *continued*   Jaw and Oral Cavity

Oral Lesions and Conditions

Lip Vesicles

- Small lesions
- Occur singularly or in clusters
- Serous, fluid-filled masses

Example:

Herpes simplex

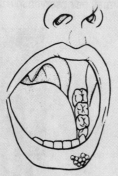

Lip vesicules

Lip Ulcers

- Necrotic loss of lip tissue

Examples:

The chancre that is the primary lesion of syphilis. A chancre ulcerates in the center and leaves a crusty residue. Pressure ulcer, such as those resulting from prolonged contact with tubes.

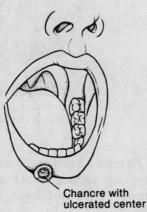

Chancre with ulcerated center

Lip ulcer

Squamous Cell Carcinoma

- May appear as plaque, warty papule, or ulcer
- Nonhealing lesion
- Appears on lips or underside of tongue
- Most common form of oral cancer
- If not healed within 2 to 3 weeks, should be evaluated to rule out malignancy

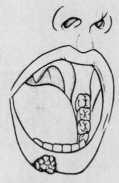

Squamous cell carcinoma

Mucocele

- Small, bluish, mucus-filled cyst
- Benign
- May be removed for cosmetic purposes

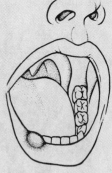

Mucocele

Cheilitis

- Inflammation and crust formation
- Lower lip most often affected
- May be chronic
- Cause often unknown

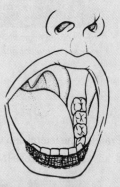

Cheilitis

Torus Palatinus

- Nodular mass midline on the hard palate
- Benign
- Masses away from the midline may represent malignancies
- May not develop until adulthood

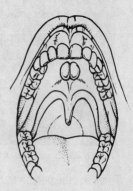

Torus palatinus

(continued)

▼ ▼ ▼

G U I D E L I N E S   *continued*   Jaw and Oral Cavity

Oral Lesions and Conditions (continued)

Fordyce Spots (Granules)

- Small yellow papules on oral mucosa
- Represent sebaceous glands
- Common benign lesion

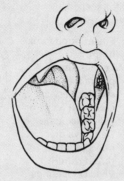

Fordyce spots

Glossitis

- Tongue becomes bright red, edematous, and smooth as papillae are lost
- Associated with stomatitis, malnutrition, chronic illness

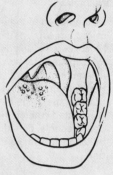

Glossitis

Aphthous Stomatitis (Canker Sore)

- Ulcerated lesion of oral mucosa
- Surrounded by white halo
- Tender
- Heals and recurs spontaneously
- May occur in groups

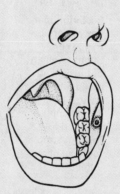

Canker sore

Hairy Tongue

- Hairy appearance secondary to papillae elongation
- Papillae dark brown or black
- Benign
- Associated with antibiotic therapy

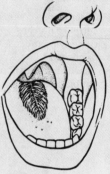

Hairy tongue

Leukoplakia

- Smooth, white, paint-like patch on the oral mucosa
- May represent a premalignant transformation of oral mucosa
- Associated with oral tobacco usage

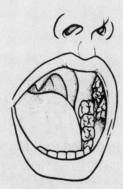

Leukoplakia

Pseudomonas Infection

- Necrotic ulcers
- Dark brown central eschar (scar)
- Surrounded by erythematous ring

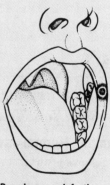

Pseudomonas infection

(continued)

▼ ▼ ▼

G U I D E L I N E S *continued*   Jaw and Oral Cavity

Oral Lesions and Conditions (continued)

Stomatitis

- Inflammation of the oral cavity
- Mucosa, red, dry, edematous
- Predisposes oral mucosa to ulceration
- Red demarcation line may be noted at the vermilion border
- Associated with chemotherapeutic agents, dehydration, infectious agents, and radiation

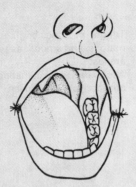

Stomatitis

Candida albicans (Yeast, Thrush, Moniliasis)

- Oral mucosa covered by white, curd-like patches
- Underlying mucosa may be bright red
- Associated with chronic illness, antibiotic therapy

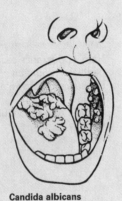

Candida albicans

Streptococcal Pharyngitis

- Posterior pharynx bright red
- Tonsils, uvula, pillars may be swollen and covered with white or yellow exudate
- Definitive diagnosis requires throat culture
- Physical findings may vary

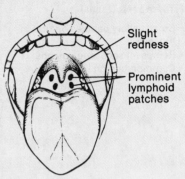

Slight redness

Prominent lymphoid patches

Streptococcal pharyngitis

Viral Pharyngitis

- Posterior pharynx red or normal in color
- Slight swelling of tonsils and uvula may occur
- Throat culture required to rule out streptococcal pharyngitis

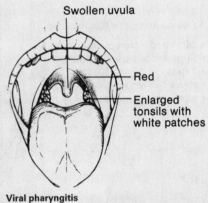

Swollen uvula

Red

Enlarged tonsils with white patches

Viral pharyngitis

Documenting Jaw and Oral Cavity Examination Findings

Example: Normal Jaw and Oral Cavity

The following was recorded after examining a 30-year-old woman:

Temporomandibular joint palpated with jaw movement—no clicks, tenderness, or restricted range of motion. Parotids nonpalpable. Slight overbite but no associated impairment of chewing or talking. Tongue moist and shiny, and midline without tremor during protrusion. Gag reflex intact. Uvula and soft palate rises with "ah." Tonsils missing. No lesions seen or palpated on tongue, oral mucosa, or palate.

Nursing Diagnoses Related to Oral Cavity Assessment

Impaired Oral Mucous Membrane

Impaired oral mucous membrane is a state in which a person experiences disruptions in the oral cavity. During examination, you may recognize alterations as well as determine contributing factors.

Poor Hygiene. Oral hygiene practices vary among individuals and are influenced by personal preference, sociocultural factors, and health status. Poor oral hygiene is reflected by the presence of both food debris and excessive plaque accumulation. Halitosis (bad breath) may not always indicate poor hygiene and may occur with systemic diseases.

Poor oral hygiene can contribute to or exacerbate most pathology to the oral cavity. Food debris may accumulate in the crevices between teeth. Excessive plaque buildup may be observed as a yellow or brown cast. Inadequate hygiene is a common cause of dental caries and periodontal disease. Both conditions may occur when excessive plaque accumulates on teeth and gingiva, destroying surfaces.

Periodontal disease (pyorrhea) is associated with plaque accumulation in dental pockets between gums and teeth. Such dental pockets enlarge as debris continues to accumulate. An inflammatory response is usually initiated; the gingiva appears swollen and red, and pus may be noted. Eventually, the gingiva recesses from the neck of the teeth, and teeth may loosen. Gingival tissue may become inflamed, and abscesses may form secondary to dental caries. Although you should screen the person for these oral mucosa lesions, regular dental examinations are essential.

Nutritional Impairment. Alterations in lip and oral mucosa may be caused by severe vitamin B and C deficiencies. For example, lack of B vitamins may result in reddened vermilion and cracks at the corners of the mouth (cheilosis). Vertical fissures may appear across the entire outer lip surface. In addition, the tongue may become swollen, bright red, and painful. Taste bud papillae may atrophy, and a smooth tongue surface also may occur. Painful ulcers (glossitis) may develop. In severe vitamin C deficiency (scurvy), the gingiva becomes spongy, bleeds easily, and recedes. The teeth may loosen and fall out.

Fluid Imbalance. The most common type of fluid imbalance that alters the oral mucosa is dehydration. Dehydration causes redness and dryness of the oral mucosa. Saliva production decreases, and saliva becomes more viscous.

Factors contributing to oral mucosa dehydration include inadequate hydration and actions of certain drugs, such as cholinergic blocking agents and antihistamines. A pattern of mouth breathing may decrease intravascular pressures, resulting in diminished blood flow to the oral mucosa that may contribute to dryness. Rapid respiratory rates lead to dehydration as the saliva is used to humidify inspired gases faster than saliva is produced. Oxygen administration, even with humidification devices, may cause additional oral cavity dryness.

Mechanical Trauma. Common sources of mechanical trauma include poorly fitting dentures, braces, endotracheal or nasogastric tubes, and oral cavity surgery. Improper suctioning and oral hygiene also can affect the oral mucosa. Assessing the surface of the oral mucosa that contacts prostheses or tubes is extremely important. The classic signs of inflammation—redness, swelling, pain, heat, and functional impairment—are usually observed with traumatic injury to the oral mucosa.

Chemotherapeutic Agents. Anticholinergic agents and antihistamines may contribute to oral mucosa dehydration, whereas antibiotics may upset microbial flora in the mouth. Chemotherapeutic agents used in cancer treatment are among the most damaging to the oral mucosa and cause generalized stomatitis or oral cavity inflammation secondary to a lethal effect on rapidly dividing oral mucosal epithelial cells. The surface of the mucosa appears erythematous, dry, and edematous, and may be prone to ulceration. A bright red inflammatory demarcation line may be observed at the vermilion border.

Impaired Swallowing

Swallowing is a complex physiologic maneuver that occurs in four phases: oral preparatory, oral, pharyngeal, and esophageal. In general, swallowing problems are assessed by taking a history, checking cranial nerve functions, observing the placement and control of food in the oral cavity, inspecting the oral cavity, and palpating for a normal swallowing movement over the throat.

The oral preparatory phase involves placing the food in the mouth and preparing the food for the next phase with the teeth and the tongue. The phase ends with the tongue placing the bolus of chewed food between the tongue and the palate in preparation for the oral phase. Problems with the oral preparatory phase result from injury to cranial nerves V, VII, and XII and the resulting dysfunction of the facial, oral, and tongue muscles. Dysfunction is indicated by drooling and food being pocketed in the mouth. Mumbled speech and asymmetry of mouth movements or the smile may be additional indicators of neuromuscular dysfunction.

The oral phase involves placing the tongue against the hard palate, elevating the larynx, and propelling food into the pharynx. Problems result from injury to cranial nerve XII, which innervates the tongue. The person with this problem may cough or choke when trying to swallow. Because the tongue is paralyzed, food falls into the airway.

The pharyngeal phase of swallowing propels food from the mouth to the esophagus and is accomplished by constriction of pharyngeal muscles that are innervated by cranial nerves IX, X, and XI. Normal function of these muscles is associated with a gag reflex. The person with this problem may complain of food stuck in the throat or may experience nasal regurgitation, coughing, or choking associated with swallowing. They also may experience hoarseness.

During the esophageal phase of swallowing, the upper esophagus sphincter closes, preventing regurgitation of food into the respiratory tract. Swallowing difficulties associated with this phase are rare.

NDₓ

Clinical Problems Related to Oral Cavity Assessment

Diabetes Mellitus. Similar to the skin, the oral mucosa of patients with diabetes mellitus is susceptible to infection and ulceration because the disease alters circulation and immunity. After 10 to 15 years, a significant thickening of the vessels in the oral mucosa occurs. Impaired circulation may lead to ischemic ulcer formation in the mouth. Such lesions often heal slowly, and secondary infection is common.

Renal Disease. Severe renal disease, characterized by retention of ammonia in the body, can lead to oral mucosa impairment. Ammonia, secreted into the oral cavity through the saliva, is caustic and may cause gingival bleeding and buccal mucosa ulceration. The mouth may become dry (xerostomia), which further threatens the oral mucosa. The breath may have an ammonia odor (uremic breath), and the person may report a metallic taste.

Cancer. Oral tumors may disrupt the patient's oral mucosa. Some systemic cancers, especially leukemia, also affect the oral cavity. Cancer treatments, including surgery, radiation, and chemotherapy, can further disrupt the oral mucosa.

Depending on the procedure, cancer surgery may disrupt the person's oral mucosa by affecting self-care abilities or nutritional status, or by causing physical trauma.

Radiation therapy for head and neck cancers is related to death of rapidly dividing epithelial cells. The effects may be noted within 1 to 2 weeks after treatments have begun and include inflamed mucosa, decreased saliva production, and diminished taste sensation.

THE ABDOMEN
Anatomy and Physiology Review

Because the abdomen extends from the diaphragm to the pelvis, physical examination provides cues to the status of the gastrointestinal system and related processes such as digestion, secretion, absorption, and metabolism, as well as to the status of the genitourinary system. Certain vascular anomalies and inflammatory processes also may be detected during the abdominal examination. Although many abdominal organs are difficult to examine, some examination techniques provide indirect information about organ function. In the case of abnormal findings, abdominal examination should be augmented with diagnostic studies such as x-rays, ultrasound, endoscopic procedures, and laboratory tests.

Abdominal Assessment Landmarks

Generally, the structures of the abdomen are not visible, but occasionally outlines of organs or structures may be observed in very thin clients. Likewise, abdominal structures are not easily palpated. The only structures that are normally palpable include the right edge of the liver at the right costal margin, the lower pole of the right kidney (in thin persons), the colon in the lower left quadrant, and rectus abdominal muscles in the midline, and aortic pulsations (in thin clients, especially women). A full and distended bladder is also palpable.

Because anatomic structures are not visible, a reference map of the abdomen is helpful. The four- and the nine-region maps are widely used (Fig. 6-5). These maps may be used to describe the location of abnormal physical examination findings and symptoms such as pain.

The four-region map divides the abdomen into four quadrants. An imaginary line extending from the xiphoid process to the symphysis pubis is crossed at the umbilicus by another line. The four regions are referred to as right and left upper quadrants and right and left lower quadrants. A knowledge of which abdominal organs are located in which quadrants is necessary for assessment findings to be meaningful.

The nine-region map is more specific. The numbers assigned to each of the nine regions are standard but may be confusing (see Fig. 6-5B). Midline regions are numbered first, and then numbers are assigned in a systematic

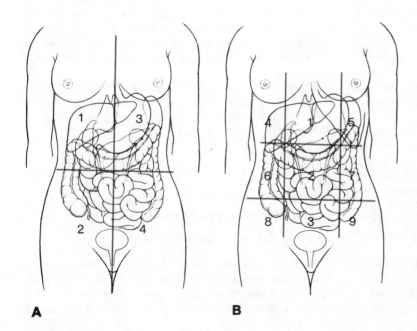

A **B**

FIGURE 6.5 **(A)** Four-region abdominal map: (1) right upper quadrant, (2) right lower quadrant, (3) left upper quadrant, (4) left lower quadrant. **(B)** Nine-region abdominal map: (1) epigastric, (2) umbilical, (3) hypogastric (pubic), (4) right hypochondriac, (5) left hypochondriac, (6) right lumbar, (7) left lumbar, (8) right inguinal, (9) left inguinal.

manner to right and left areas, starting at the costal area and extending downward, as follows:

1: Epigastric
2: Umbilical
3: Suprapubic
4 & 5: Right and left hypochondriac
6 & 7: Right and left lumbar
8 & 9: Right and left inguinal

Gastrointestinal Motility

The esophagus, stomach, and small and large intestines are capable of peristalsis, a wave-like involuntary movement caused by contractions of the longitudinal and circular smooth muscles in the organ walls. Peristalsis depends on a functioning myoelectric complex and is influenced by the presence of food, diet composition, drugs, irritating substances such as bacteria and bile salts, and various hormones. Gastrointestinal tract distension, such as occurs from a food bolus, initiates a reflex muscular contraction of the area above and distal to the distension. Such contractions result in a progressive movement of food and fluids through the gastrointestinal tract. Although the mechanism is not clearly understood, peristalsis also occurs in fasting states to clear the gastrointestinal tract.

Peristaltic movements of the small intestine are more readily evaluated by a physical examination. A peristaltic "rush," or rapidly moving peristaltic wave, may be observed in a thin person by watching the surface of the abdomen. Peristaltic movements also may be evaluated by auscultating the abdomen. Created by peristaltic movements of fluid and air, bowel sounds are tinkling or gurgling sounds with a relatively high pitch and should be evaluated based on pattern and quality. Occasionally, such sounds can be heard without a stethoscope.

Because peristalsis is continual, bowel sounds should always be present, even during fasting. Sound frequency and intensity depend on the stage of digestion. Bowel sounds usually occur every 5 to 15 seconds and are more frequent 4 to 8 hours after a meal when intestinal contents are propelled over the ileocecal valve (right lower quadrant). Hypoactive or decreased bowel sounds, such as one every 2 minutes, may reflect an improperly functioning small intestine. Decreased peristalsis is associated with extensive handling of the bowel during surgery, severe hypokalemia, peritonitis, paralysis of the intestinal wall (paralytic ileus), and advanced intestinal obstruction.

Hyperactive or increased bowel sounds, such as every 3 seconds, may occur with diarrhea as intestinal contents are rapidly moved through the system, or in the early stages of intestinal obstruction, which causes distention of the bowel proximal to the obstruction. Distention stimulates an increase in the rate and force of peristalsis, which produces more frequent and higher-pitched bowel sounds (borborygmi).

The Peritoneum

The peritoneum is the double membrane that lines the abdominal cavity; it contains many blood vessels, lymphatic ducts, and nerves. The two layers, the visceral peritoneum and the parietal peritoneum, are separated by serous fluid. This thick membrane supports the abdominal organs, transports water and electrolytes from the abdominal cavity to the vasculature, and protects abdominal organs from infection and inflammation.

Early detection of peritoneal injuries is important because they can be life-threatening if peritoneal functions are impaired. After peritoneal injury, the bowel may be initially hyperactive, manifested by increased bowel sounds, as impaired transport mechanisms across the peritoneum retain substances and distend the bowel. Abdominal distention and rigidity also occur secondary to fluid accumulation in the retroperitoneal space. Because the peritoneum contains many nerves, the person with peritoneal injury usually experiences severe pain. You may note rebound tenderness, which is pain elicited immediately after deep, quick palpation of the person's abdomen.

Vasculature

Arterial blood is supplied to the abdomen by arterial branches from the abdominal aorta. One branch, the celiac artery, further divides into five major branches that supply blood to the stomach, spleen, gallbladder, pancreas, and duodenum. Another major branch, the superior mesenteric artery, supplies the jejunum, ileum, cecum, and ascending colon, and part of the transverse colon. The inferior mesenteric artery branches off the aorta to supply the transverse, descending, and sigmoid colon and rectum.

You may evaluate the abdominal aorta by inspection and palpation because of pulsations that may be seen and felt. If the person has arterial obstructions affecting any of the abdominal vessels, you may find a bruit during auscultation.

The portal vein system collects blood from the entire gastrointestinal tract and delivers it to the liver. Portal vein hypertension, such as occurs with liver disease, may contribute to dramatic physical examination findings. Portal vein pressure is increased, causing congestion of blood. Consequently, collateral vessels develop to divert the flow from congested areas. The increased congestion often leads to spleen enlargement. In addition, increased pressures may force fluid out of the venous system. Ascites may be noted when fluid accumulates in the abdomen. Another consequence of portal hypertension is impaired delivery of important substances of digestion to the liver for further metabolism. Physical signs will depend on which metabolic process is affected. For example, vitamin K, a clotting factor, may not be optimally metabolized by the liver and may lead to a bleeding disorder.

Physical Examination Abdomen

GENERAL APPROACH

The abdomen is examined in the following sequence: Inspect, auscultate, percuss, lightly palpate, and deeply palpate. Always auscultate the abdomen first, because percussion and palpation may alter the character of bowel sounds. Use the diaphragm of the stethoscope to auscultate high-pitched bowel sounds and the bell of the stethoscope to detect lower-pitched vascular sounds such as bruits, venous hums, and friction rubs.

Perform light palpation before deep palpation. Percussion and palpation may be combined; preferably, you should assess an organ completely by both methods before continuing. For example, percuss the liver borders, then palpate the liver.

EQUIPMENT

• Stethoscope
• Metric ruler or tape measure

POSITIONING, PREPARATION, AND EXPOSURE

Ask the person to assume a supine position with knees slightly flexed to help relax the abdominal muscles. Place a pillow beneath the head and knees for complete relaxation. Instruct the person to place arms at the sides or across the chest. If the arms are over the head, the abdomen may tighten, making examination difficult. The person's bladder should be empty. Stand at the person's right side because many special examination techniques involve the liver and other right-side structures.

Because there may be apprehension about the examination, provide appropriate explanations and drape the chest and groin to ensure modesty. If the person is ticklish or extremely anxious about the procedure, begin palpating the abdomen with the person's hand under your hand.

Before initiating the examination, ask if any abdominal areas are especially tender or painful. Such areas should be examined last, and care should be taken not to aggravate any existing discomfort.

Keep the examining room, your hands, the stethoscope and the person warm during the examination to avoid abdominal tensing.

MEASUREMENTS

Measure skin lesions on the abdomen with a metric ruler, and measure abdominal distention to monitor changes. Wrap a tape measure around the abdomen at the umbilicus or highest point, and then mark the exact area where the tape measure was placed on the skin for accurate successive measurements. Special techniques are available for measuring abdominal enlargement during pregnancy, and are discussed in Chapter 13. Measure the width of aortic pulsations if you suspect an aneurysm and if pulsations are visible.

OTHER CUES

Monitor facial expression and body language during the examination. Be especially sensitive to facial expressions of pain, tenderness, and anxiety. Try to determine what action precipitated a change in expression.

EXAMINATION AND DOCUMENTATION FOCUS

• *Inspection:* Contour, symmetry, masses, pulsations, peristalsis, skin integrity, respiratory movements
• *Auscultation:* Bowel sounds, vascular sounds
• *Percussion:* Tone, outline of abdominal organs
• *Palpation:* Muscle tone, organ characteristics, tenderness, masses, pulsations, fluid accumulation

▼ ▼ ▼

G U I D E L I N E S

Assessment Guidelines   Abdomen

Procedure

1. Inspect the outer abdominal surface.

   a. Stand at the person's right side with his or her abdomen exposed and note symmetry, masses, pulsations, skin integrity, and respiratory pattern. Ask the person to cough to elicit previously unseen masses.

   b. Sit or stoop and view the abdomen tangentially to evaluate contour and peristaltic rushes.

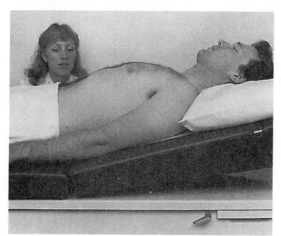

Tangential inspection of the abdomen

Clinical Significance

Normal Findings

Abdomen symmetric around the midline. No visible masses. Pulsation of the abdominal aorta at the midline and peristaltic rushes may be seen in thin people.

Deviations from Normal

No lesions should be present other than secondary lesions in the form of surgical scars. Although scars usually are not considered abnormal, the procedure that caused the scar and the related sequelae of abdominal adhesions should be considered.

Striae (stretchmarks) may be present if the skin has been stretched, as in pregnancy, obesity, abdominal tumors, and Cushing's disease.

Respirations are abdominal in men (the abdomen rises and falls with breathing).

Deviations from Normal

Visible abdominal masses: A mass that appears as a bulge when the person coughs or raises the head and shoulders may represent a hernia, an abnormal projection through the abdominal wall. Abdominal wall defects allow structures such as peritoneum, fat, bowel, or bladder to protrude. If the bulging is intermittent and appears only with coughing, the hernia is *reducible. Incarcerated hernias* always contain some abdominal contents. *Strangulated hernias* are so tightly constricted that the blood supply is cut off. Gangrene may result without surgical intervention.

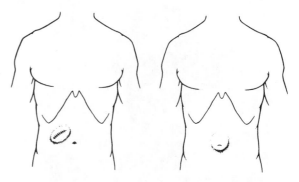

Incisional hernia   *Umbilical hernia*

▼ ▼ ▼

G U I D E L I N E S *continued*   Abdomen

Procedure

c. Identify altered abdominal contours.

Clinical Significance

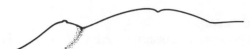

Generalized enlargement with umbilicus inverted

Gas distention, obesity

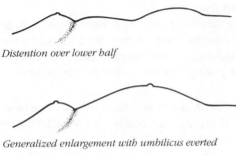

Distention over lower half

Ovarian mass, pregnancy, bladder distention

Ascites, tumor, umbilical hernia

Generalized enlargement with umbilicus everted

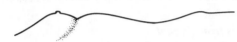

Starvation, replacement of subcutaneous fat with muscle

Scaphoid abdomen

2. **Auscultate the abdomen.**

a. Listen for bowel sounds using the diaphragm of the stethoscope. Listening to each quadrant is not necessary if pitch and frequency are normal. If bowel sounds are hypoactive or absent, listen for 1 or 2 minutes in each quadrant.

Normal bowel sounds: High-pitched, "gurgling" sounds. Irregular frequency; range from 5 to 35/minute.

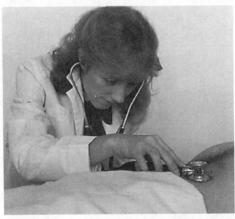

Abdominal auscultation: Listening for bowel sounds

▼ ▼ ▼

G U I D E L I N E S *continued*   Abdomen

Procedure

b. Use the bell of the stethoscope to auscultate vascular sounds and friction rubs over the abdomen.

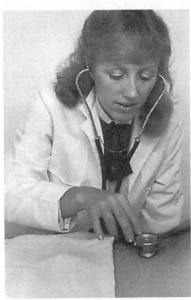

Abdominal auscultation: Listening for vascular sounds

3. **Percuss the four abdominal quadrants.**

Systematically percuss the four quadrants of the abdomen to evaluate abnormal sounds.

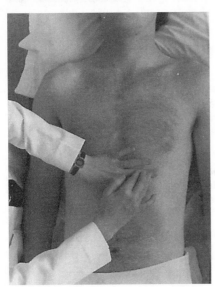

Abdominal percussion

Clinical Significance

Deviations from Normal

Vascular sounds (bruits and venous hums) are not normal findings. A friction rub indicates an inflammatory process.

A venous hum is a systolic bruit often heard when the liver is cirrhotic. Atherosclerosis of the renal and iliac arteries, and partial occlusion may cause bruits. Friction rubs may be heard over a damaged liver or spleen.

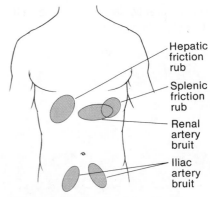

Auscultatory landmarks of the abdomen

Normal Findings

Tympany predominates, with dullness heard over solid organs and masses.

Deviations from Normal

Abdominal masses and fluid percuss as dull. For example, epigastric, ovarian, and uterine tumors that displace hollow, tympanic-sounding bowel cause a dull percussion note.

▼ ▼ ▼

G U I D E L I N E S *continued*   Abdomen

Procedure

4. Percuss the liver.

a. Percuss to find the upper and lower liver borders at the midclavicular line, starting at a level below the umbilicus. A tympanic note should be heard at this point, indicating gas in the underlying bowel. As you percuss along the midclavicular line toward the heard, the sound will change to dull near the lower costal margin. This change in percussion note quality indicates the location of the lower liver border. Mark or visualize this reference point for use in your measurement.

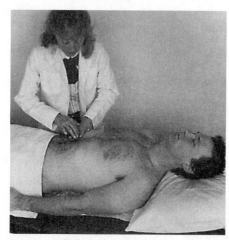

Percussing the lower liver border

Clinical Significance

Liver size can be estimated by identifying the upper and lower borders of the liver and measuring the distance between the borders (the liver span) in centimeters. Percussion is used to identify the location of each border.

Normal liver span: 6 to 12 cm at the midclavicular line; 4 to 8 cm at the midsternal line.

Because liver span is related to lean body mass, men and taller people usually have greater spans than women and shorter people.

Deviations from Normal

The liver may be displaced downward if the diaphragm is low, which may occur in obstructive pulmonary diseases. However, liver span should not be affected.

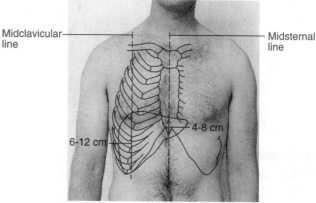

Normal liver span

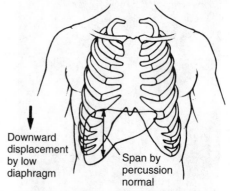

Liver displacement

▼ ▼ ▼

G U I D E L I N E S   *continued*   Abdomen

Procedure

To locate the upper liver border, percuss downward along the midclavicular line starting at the upper thorax. Be sure that you percuss between the ribs. A resonant percussion note indicates underlying lung tissue. The sound change to dull at the location of the upper liver border.

Mark or visualize this reference point. Measure the distance between the two reference points to determine the liver span at the midclavicular line.

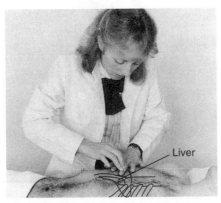

Abdominal percussion: Locating the upper liver border

A number of conditions can alter percussion findings and interfere with the accurate identification of liver border locations. For example, pleural effusions, pneumonia consolidation, or lung masses in the upper thorax or excessive abdominal gas at the lower border may alter normally expected percussion findings. These conditions need to be considered as potential errors in measurement.

Clinical Significance

Deviations from Normal

Liver enlargement: The liver is usually enlarged in cases of cirrhosis, hepatitis, and venous congestion such as occurs with right heart failure.

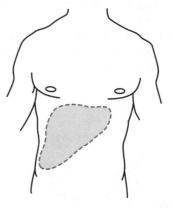

Liver enlargement

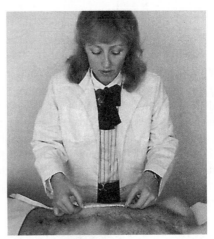

Measuring the liver span

▼ ▼ ▼

G U I D E L I N E S *continued*   Abdomen

Procedure

5. **Percuss the stomach and spleen.**

   a. The gastric air bubble in the stomach produces a tympanic percussion sound, which you can note by percussing at the left lower rib cage.

   b. Percuss splenic dullness at the area of the left 10th rib, posterior to the midaxillary line. This may be difficult to hear with the person supine, but it may be easier with the person lying midway between the supine and right lateral positions.

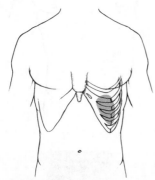

Location of the spleen

6. **Lightly palpate the four abdominal quadrants.**

   Lightly palpate by indenting the abdomen about 1 cm. Use smooth, circular movements with your finger pads, holding the fingers together. Systematically palpate each quadrant, noting any masses, muscle tenderness, or guarding. Monitor facial expression. If the person is not relaxed, the entire abdomen may feel tense. Encourage the person to take slow, deep breaths and exhale with the mouth open. The abdomen should feel relaxed on exhalation.

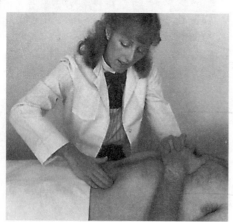

Light abdominal palpation

Clinical Significance

Stomach and spleen percussion is conducted to locate landmarks and to locate and note the size of the spleen.

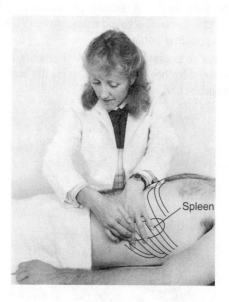

Abdominal palpation is conducted to identify painful areas, masses, abdominal distention, and abdominal rigidity.

Normal Findings

Abdominal muscles may be palpable. They should feel relaxed on light palpation rather than tightly contracted or spastic. Muscle contraction may be noted with anxiety.

Rectus abdominis muscle: This muscle includes two large, midline muscles that extend from the xiphoid process to the symphysis pubis, tightly approximated at the abdominal midline. Occasionally, a separation of the rectus abdominal muscle can be observed, especially in obese or pregnant persons, by palpating the midline as the person raises the head. A midline ridge may occur with this maneuver, but it does not represent a significant problem.

▼ ▼ ▼

Procedure

7. **Deeply palpate the four abdominal quadrants.**

   a. Using the same hand position, deeply palpate the abdominal quadrants, but avoid jabbing movements. If depressing the abdomen is difficult, again try placing one hand over the other.

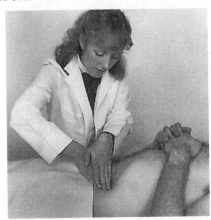

Deep abdominal palpation

   b. Check for rebound tenderness by depressing the abdomen and then quickly withdrawing your fingers. If the person indicates this maneuver is painful, then rebound tenderness is present.

8. **Palpate the liver, spleen, and kidney.**

   a. Either of two techniques may be used to palpate the liver. First, place your left hand beneath the 11th and 12th ribs and pull the person slightly upward.

   Next, place your right hand lateral to the rectus muscle with your fingers pointing toward the ribs. Ask the person to take in a big breath and hold it. Then, apply downward pressure and move your right hand under the rib cage. Ask the person to exhale while you attempt to palpate the liver edge, which should project toward your hand with this maneuver.

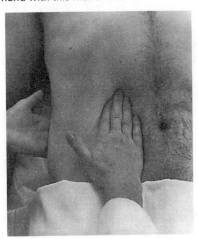

Liver palpation: Bimanual technique

Clinical Significance

Palpable masses: Masses should be further evaluated to determine size, shape, consistency, and mobility. Location should be described in reference to the abdominal wall. A mass may be inside the abdominal wall or deep within the abdominal cavity. While palpating the mass, ask the person to raise the head and shoulders. If the mass is still palpable, it is inside the abdominal wall. Muscle tenseness caused by raising the head will prevent you from palpating deep abdominal masses.

Abdominal structures commonly mistaken for masses include the aorta, rectus abdominus muscle, uterus, feces, filled colon, and sacral promontory (felt by deep palpation in very thin people). Stool is usually palpable as a tubular structure, as opposed to the rounded structure of an abnormal mass.

Tenderness: Although the abdomen is not normally tender to palpation, some people may complain of tenderness on deep palpation, especially over the abdominal aorta, the cecum (lower right quadrant), and the sigmoid colon (lower left quadrant).

Rebound tenderness may indicate inflammation of the peritoneum.

Liver, spleen and kidney palpation is conducted to note size, location, irregularities, and tenderness of these organs.

The liver may be impossible to feel by either method. Palpation is more easily performed on a very thin client or a client with an enlarged liver (hepatomegaly).

Normal Finding
Firm, smooth, nontender liver edge at or above the costal margin.

Deviations from Normal
Enlargement, irregular or nodular edges; tenderness on palpation is associated with heart failure and hepatitis.

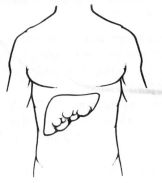

Nodular liver

▼ ▼ ▼

G U I D E L I N E S *continued* Abdomen

Procedure

b. Alternatively, you may use the hooking technique to palpate the lower liver border. Stand at the person's right side, facing the feet. Place both hands side by side at the lower liver border (previously determined by percussion). As the person inhales, press inward and pull upward toward the costal margin, feeling for the lower liver border.

Clinical Significance

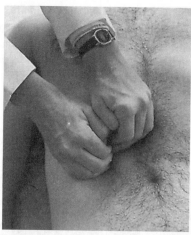
Liver palpation: Hooking technique

c. Palpate the spleen in the left upper quadrant. Remain on the person's right side and reach over the person, placing your left hand under the left costal margin. Gently pull the person upward with your right hand below the costal margin, and push upward to palpate. Ask the person to take in a deep breath and hold it, which may bring the spleen into line with your fingers.

Usually, the spleen must be enlarged to three times its normal size before it is palpable. Remember that palpation may further damage the spleen, especially if it is enlarged. Palpating the spleen is therefore not usually indicated, or is done very carefully by an experienced examiner.

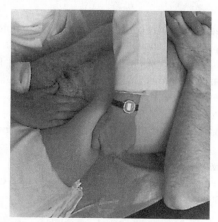
Palpating the spleen

An alternative technique is to repeat these movements with the person lying on the right side with knees flexed. This position moves the spleen slightly forward, making palpation easier.

d. The pole of the right kidney may be palpated in very thin people. The left kidney is difficult to detect on palpation. Place your upper hand at the costal margin with fingertips at the midclavicular line. Place your lower hand beneath the person. As the person inhales deeply, exert pressure to try to palpate the lower pole of the kidney. Palpation technique is identical for the left and right sides.

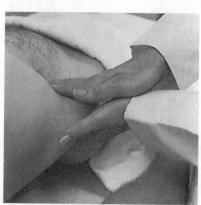
Palpating the right kidney

▼ ▼ ▼

Assessment Guidelines   Evaluating Abdominal Fluid

A distended abdomen may be further evaluated to differentiate fluid accumulation in the abdominal wall (interstitial fluid) from fluid accumulation in the abdominal cavity. Ascites is the accumulation of fluid in the abdominal cavity resulting from fluid lost from the vascular space. In starvation states, decreased intravascular protein will reduce plasma oncotic pressure, causing an outpouring of fluid into the abdominal cavity. In portal vein hypertension, increased hydrostatic pressure pushes fluid from the vessels into the abdominal cavity.

Procedure

1. **Percussion.**

   a. Percuss the abdomen to detect fluid.

   b. Percuss for shifting dullness. Place the person in a lateral position and percuss the abdomen. Note any changes in the percussion notes with position changes. As ascites fluid gravitates to the dependent side, the area where you have percussed dullness also shifts. Shifting dullness is not usually observed with interstitial edema.

2. **Palpation.**

   a. Palpate for a fluid wave. With the person lying supine, either the person being examined or another person should place the lateral edge of his or her hand firmly along the abdominal midline to prevent impulse transmission through the subcutaneous fat. Then, tap one side of the abdomen, and feel and observe any movement to the opposite side of the abdomen. A positive fluid wave indicates ascites.

Clinical Significance

Fluid in the abdominal cavity or abdominal wall percusses as dullness.

Distinguishes ascites fluid, which is free-floating in the abdominal cavity and therefore gravity-dependent, from interstitial edema, which is more evenly distributed and less affected by gravity.

A large accumulation of free fluid within the abdominal cavity is associated with a fluid wave.

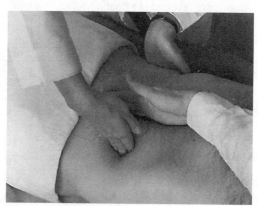

Evaluating abdominal fluid

▼ ▼ ▼

GUIDELINES *continued*   Evaluating Abdominal Fluid

Procedure

b. *Ballottement* is a special palpatory technique used to identify a floating object in the abdomen.

Place your fingers at a right angle to the person's abdomen and slightly depress the abdominal wall. While holding the abdomen in this position, note the rebound of a floating part against your fingers.

Ballottement may also be done bimanually. Place one hand on the anterior surface of the lateral abdomen and the other hand under the client's back. Use your top hand to push the abdomen toward your lower hand. Again, note rebound of a floating object, this time with your lower hand.

Clinical Significance

With ascites, a person's abdominal organs are actually floating in the abdomen. The pregnant uterus also represents a floating abdominal structure.

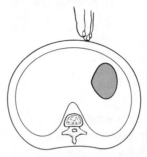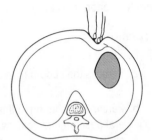

Single-handed ballottement

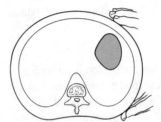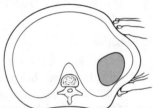

Bimanual ballottement

NDₓ

Documenting Abdominal Examination Findings

Example 1: Normal Abdomen

Mr. K, aged 55, had an abdominal examination as part of his routine annual health assessment. The examination results were normal and recorded as follows:

Abdomen flat, symmetric, with well-developed musculature. No visible masses or pulsations; skin intact without lesions. Active bowel sounds heard over all quadrants. Liver span percussed 10 cm at midclavicular line. Nontender to light and deep palpation. No palpable masses.

Example 2: Abdominal Pain

Mr. H, aged 38, has been experiencing chronic, crampy abdominal pain. The abdominal examination findings are abnormal and recorded as follows:

Abdominal inspection reveals no masses, skin lesions, pulsations; abdomen flat. Light palpation reveals diffuse tenderness, poorly localized but most pronounced in lower quadrant; no involuntary guarding, muscle rigidity, or rebound or referred pain.

NDₓ

Nursing Diagnoses Related to Abdominal Assessment

Indicators for the following elimination problems may be noted during the abdominal examination:

- Constipation
- Diarrhea
- Urinary retention

Although such diagnoses are thoroughly explored in Chapter 7, significant abdominal findings are included here because of the interrelationships of body systems.

Constipation

Constipation commonly causes gaseous distention of the abdomen. Gas accumulates and stretches the bowel walls, resulting in a tympanic abdomen. The contour becomes more rounded as distention progresses. The person may feel abdominal fullness and cramping. Peristaltic movements may decrease with constipation. Bowel sounds may be hypoactive.

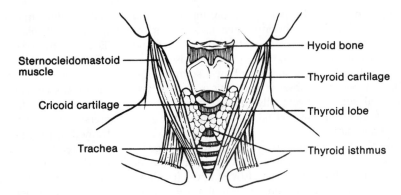

FIGURE 6.6 The thyroid gland.

Diarrhea

Diarrhea involves rapid movement of watery contents through the intestinal tract. Peristalsis increases, leading to two significant findings during the abdominal examination: the person may report cramping and abdominal pain, and the bowel sounds are usually more intense and frequent.

Urinary Retention

Urine retention in the bladder changes the normal abdominal contour. The area above the symphysis pubis may be distended. On palpation, bladder outlines may be evident, and the person may report tenderness. Percussion of a distended bladder results in dullness rather than tympany.

Clinical Problems Related to Abdominal Assessment

Inflammatory Processes

Although abdominal assessment can provide clues to the nature of inflammatory processes, a definitive diagnosis usually relies on additional information from endoscopic tests, radiographic examinations, and laboratory analyses. Nevertheless, nurses need a basis for evaluating signs and symptoms of inflammatory processes in the continual surveillance of the patient.

Stomach. Stomach inflammation occurs with gastritis and gastric ulcers. You may note epigastric tenderness and guarding to both light and deep palpation. Often, the person will report feelings of fullness and pressure in this area. Epigastric tenderness related to a gastric ulcer occurs more often when the stomach is empty and is relieved by food or antacids. Gastric ulcer pain may be referred to the person's left subcostal region.

Epigastric tenderness and guarding may occur on palpation when the person has a duodenal ulcer. The pain is most intense 45 to 60 minutes after food ingestion or during the night. Such pain may radiate below the costal margins to the back. Occasionally, a unilateral spasm of the rectus abdominis muscle may be palpated over the duo-

denal bulb in the right upper quadrant. Antacids may help relieve the intensity of this pain.

Perforation of a gastrointestinal ulcer represents a life-threatening emergency. Initially, the person may experience an acute onset of abdominal pain often accompanied by nausea and vomiting. Several hours later, abdominal rigidity may occur as the abdominal muscles become spastic. Generalized rebound tenderness may occur, and bowel sounds may be absent because peritoneal inflammation inhibits intestinal motility.

Gallbladder. An inflamed gallbladder (cholecystitis) may cause pain in the epigastric or right upper quadrant area, usually precipitated by a large, fatty meal. The pain may be accompanied by nausea and vomiting. Guarding, rebound tenderness, and jaundice may be noted. A positive Murphy's sign, a sharp increase in pain with inspiration, may be elicited with acute cholecystitis: place your thumb below the right costal margin and ask the person to inhale deeply.

Appendix. Acute appendicitis may cause pain and tenderness in the right lower quadrant, which is aggravated by activity and coughing. The person can usually identify the area of maximal tenderness. You may note signs of peritoneal irritation, including muscle rigidity, rebound tenderness, and decreased bowel sounds. Psoas and obturator signs may be positive. The psoas sign is related to contact irritation of the iliopsoas muscle. Ask the person to assume a supine position and raise the right leg at the hip. Exert pressure on the person's thigh. Right lower abdominal pain with this maneuver constitutes a positive psoas sign. The obturator muscle may also be irritated by acute appendicitis. The obturator sign is positive when lower quadrant pain results from the following maneuver: Ask the person to flex the right leg at the hip and knee. Then, internally and externally, rotate the patient's leg at the ankle.

Diverticulum. Acute diverticulitis may cause tenderness in the lower left quadrant of the abdomen. The person may report cramping pain in this area, which is occasionally relieved by a bowel movement.

Obstructive Processes

Organic. An organic bowel obstruction may be caused by hernias, postoperative adhesions, neoplasms, foreign bodies, and intussusceptions.

Organic obstruction is associated with colicky abdominal pain and tenderness that becomes more intense as the obstruction develops. The abdomen becomes distended. Initially, peristalsis is increased as the muscles of the bowel contract in reaction to the increasing distension. You may note high-pitched, splashing bowel sounds (borborygmi), and you may observe peristaltic rushes across the abdominal surface. Eventually, bowel sounds cease, and the abdomen is silent. Vomiting, constipation, and a shock-like state may occur.

Functional. A functional obstruction, also called paralytic ileus or adynamic ileus, is a neurogenic impairment of peristalsis. It may be precipitated by surgical handling of the bowel, peritoneal irritation, or acute illnesses. Functional obstruction causes continuous rather than colicky pain. The abdomen is usually distended, with minimal abdominal tenderness. Borborygmus is absent. Bowel sounds are hypoactive or absent, and vomiting is common.

THE THYROID GLAND

Anatomy and Physiology Review

The thyroid gland, the largest endocrine gland in the body, is located in the anterior neck between the larynx and the trachea (Fig. 6-6). Two lobes are separated by a narrow band of tissue, or isthmus, which lies below the cricoid cartilage. The thyroid gland is a highly vascularized tissue and has a rubbery texture on palpation.

Histologically, there are two distinct cell types in the thyroid gland that produce different hormones: the follicular cells produce triiodothyronine (T_3) and thyroxine (T_4), and the parafollicular cells (C cells) produce thyrocalcitonin. Two parathyroid glands are located on the posterior surface of each lobe of the thyroid gland and are not palpable.

The primary function of the thyroid gland is to control the metabolic rate with the hormones T_3 and T_4. Thyrocalcitonin has an effect on calcium metabolism. Hormone secretion is influenced by a negative feedback mechanism formed by the interrelationships among the hypothalamus, the anterior pituitary, and the thyroid gland. Iodine, derived from bread, iodized salt, seafood, milk, and eggs, must enter the thyroid for the synthesis of T_3 and T_4. Daily iodine requirements range from 100 to 200 μg.

Triiodothyronine is the thyroid hormone responsible for most of the physiologic body activities. Although the thyroid secretes a greater amount of T_4, it is readily converted to T_3 in the periphery. Triiodothyronine affects most cells. It increases the basal metabolic rate, which results in increased oxygen consumption; increases chemical reaction rates; and increases heat production. In addition, T_3 stimulates the metabolism of essential nutrients, including carbohydrates, fats, and proteins, and promotes human growth by acting synergistically with insulin and growth hormone. Because of the wide range of effects of this hormone, many body systems may be influenced by pathologic conditions of the thyroid gland. Therefore, in persons with thyroid disorders, assessment should include attention to cardiovascular, gastrointestinal, neurologic, and integumentary (including hair and nails) systems. Thyroid gland dysfunction may be present even if physical examination of the thyroid gland indicates normal findings.

Physical Examination Thyroid Gland

GENERAL APPROACH

The thyroid gland is examined by inspection and palpation. Auscultation is indicated if the gland is enlarged or if other findings, such as laboratory results or other physical examination findings, indicate altered thyroid function. Auscultate with the stethoscope bell to screen for a lower-pitched vascular bruit, an abnormal vascular sound indicative of vascular congestion.

EXPOSURE AND LIGHTING

For easier thyroid gland inspection, ask the person to swallow from a glass of water during the examination. As the person tilts the head back slightly and swallows, observe the anterior neck for any unusual bulges. Using tangential lighting may help you note any subtle changes in contour or symmetry.

EXAMINATION AND DOCUMENTATION FOCUS

- Size and shape
- Consistency
- Tenderness
- Occurrence of vascular sounds

▼ ▼ ▼

GUIDELINES

Assessment Guidelines   Thyroid Gland

Procedure

1. **Inspect the area of the anterior neck containing the thyroid gland.**

   a. Ask the person to hold the head and neck in a normal, relaxed position. Note any deviation or bulges in the area of the trachea, as well as outlines of the thyroid and cricoid cartilages.

   b. As the person extends the neck slightly and swallows water, note the upward, symmetrical movement of the trachea and other cartilage.

2. **Palpate the thyroid (anterior approach).**

   a. Stand facing the person, whose neck should be relaxed but held in slight extension to expose the underlying gland.

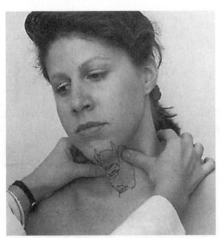

Lateral displacement of the thyroid: Anterior approach

   b. Use the pads of your first and second fingers to locate the area of the thyroid isthmus directly below the cricoid cartilage. Ask the person to swallow, which causes the isthmus to rise. You will note a rubbery texture on palpation.

   c. Next, move your hands laterally to palpate the thyroid lobes.

Clinical Significance

Normal Finding

The thyroid is usually too small to be observed as a change in the shape of the neck.

Deviations from Normal

Goiter. Thyroid gland enlargement (goiter), caused by generalized hyperplasia of the thyroid gland, may be apparent on inspection. Goiters may be diffuse or slightly asymmetric, and may be softer in texture when palpated. Goiters indicate an iodine deficiency, goiterogenic substance ingestion, or thyroid inflammation.

The thyroid gland is attached to the trachea and rises with swallowing. Goiters may rise with swallowing.

Use either the anterior or posterior approach to palpate the thyroid. (The posterior approach may be easier to use.)

Overextension may tense the surrounding muscles, making palpation difficult.

Normal Findings

Size and shape: The thyroid gland weighs between 20 and 25 g. The two lobes, which are connected by a central isthmus, give the gland a butterfly shape. The right lobe is slightly larger than the left. Each lobe is approximately 5 cm in length and 2 cm thick. Enlargement is associated with goiter.

▼ ▼ ▼

G U I D E L I N E S   *continued*   Thyroid Gland

Procedure

d. Then, place your fingers anterior to the large sternoclei-domastoid muscle of the neck. Ask the person to swallow while you feel for any masses or bulges on the lateral lobes.

e. Palpate the left lobe of the thyroid. Ask the person to tilt the head slightly forward and to the right. Use your left thumb to displace the thyroid gland in a lateral left position while you palpate the left lobe with the thumb and fingers of your right hand. The lobe will be more palpable if you ask the person to swallow. Repeat the procedure for the right lobe.

3. **Palpate the thyroid (posterior approach).**

a. Stand behind the person, who should be seated with the neck slightly flexed to relax the neck muscles.

b. Rest your thumbs on the back of the person's neck and lightly place your fingers below the cricoid cartilage. Then palpate the middle isthmus as the person swallows some water.

c. Ask the person to turn the head slightly to the side, and palpate the lobes. Use your fingers on the opposite side to displace the gland in a lateral direction so that the fingers over the side being palpated can more readily feel the lobe. Ask the person to swallow as you examine the lobe. Repeat the procedure for the opposite side.

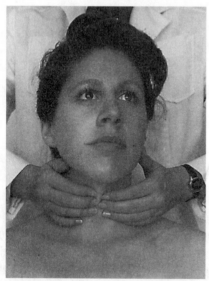

Posterior approach to the thyroid gland

4. **Auscultate the thyroid (optional).**

Auscultate for bruits over each lobe, using the bell of the stethoscope.

Clinical Significance

Consistency: Lobe edges are slightly irregular and give the thyroid gland a rubbery texture on palpation. Hardened nodules or masses are not normal and can be easily distinguished from the usual texture. A single firm nodule may represent a benign cyst or a malignancy. Malignant nodules are often painless on palpation. Multiple nodules are found in some types of goiter. Conditions such as Hashimoto's disease and carcinoma cause the gland to become firm.

Tenderness: Palpation does not usually elicit tenderness, although the person may experience mild discomfort. Palpation tenderness reflects various forms of thyroiditis. Often, the pain will radiate to the ears.

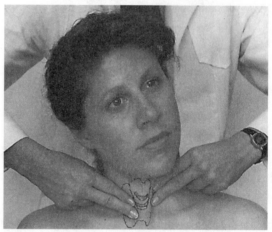

Lateral displacement of the thyroid: Posterior approach

Deviations from Normal

Vascular sounds may be auscultated in persons with hyperthyroidism. Blood flow through the vascular gland is accelerated, and increased turbulence generates a bruit. Occasionally, a bruit is accompanied by a palpable thrill.

Documenting Thyroid Examination Findings

Normal results of a thyroid examination may be documented as follows:

Thyroid palpated as symmetric without enlargement. Texture consistent with no masses, nodules, or tenderness.

An abnormal examination may be documented as follows:

Thyroid palpated as symmetric without enlargement Small, hard nodule observed on right lobe. No tenderness.

Nursing Diagnoses Related to Thyroid Assessment

Thyroid problems may contribute to a number of health problems treated by nurses. Persons with hypothyroidism are at increased risk for the following: Decreased cardiac output related to decreased metabolic rate, decreased cardiac conduction, and atherosclerosis; Activity intolerance related to lethargy, fatigue, and depressed neuromuscular status; and Altered nutrition: Less than body requirements related to decreased metabolic rate, poor appetite, and depressed gastrointestinal function.

Persons with hyperthyroidism are at increased risk for the following: Altered nutrition: Less than body requirements related to hypermetabolic state, increased fluid and calorie requirement, and fluid loss through diaphoresis; Impaired skin integrity related to extreme diaphoresis, fever, excessive restlessness, movement, tremor, and rapid weight loss; Altered thought processes related to insomnia, decreased attention span, and irritability; and Anxiety related to concern about disease and related treatments.

Clinical Problems Related to Thyroid Assessment

Thyroid dysfunction such as hypo- or hyperthyroidism may result in systemic clinical manifestations. Signs of *hypothyroidism* include the following:

Fatigue and lethargy
Weight gain
Cold hands and feet, cold intolerance
Memory impairment
Decreased peristalsis and constipation
Coarse, dry, scaling skin; dry, brittle hair
Menorrhagia or amenorrhea
Neurologic signs—polyneuropathy, cerebellar ataxia
Hypercholesterolemia

Enlarged heart
Hypotension
Slow speech; deep, hoarse voice

Signs of *hyperthyroidism* may include the following:

Nervousness, emotional lability, irritability, apprehension
Restlessness
Rapid pulse and palpitations
Hypertension
Heat intolerance, profuse perspiration, flushed skin
Fine tremor of hands
Constipation or diarrhea
Bulging eyes (exophthalmos)
Weight loss and emaciation
Goiter (in some cases)

THE LYMPHATIC SYSTEM
Anatomy and Physiology Review

The lymphatic system is examined to detect abnormalities such as enlarged or tender lymph nodes, lymphedema, and lymphangitis. Lymph nodes consist of encapsulated lymphoid tissues that function as filters for lymphatic fluid. Superficial lymph nodes are located in the head, neck, supraclavicular areas, breasts, axillae, epitrochlear areas, inguinal regions, and popliteal fossae (Fig. 6-7). They can be examined by palpation. Enlargement of the

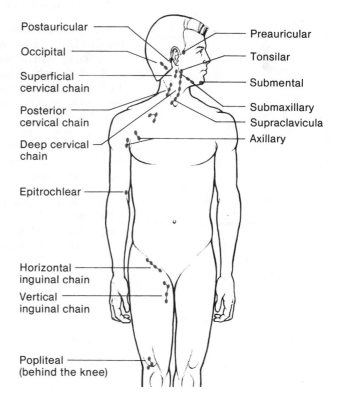

FIGURE 6.7 Distribution of lymph nodes.

superficial lymph nodes may represent a benign deviation from normal, local infection, or neoplasm. Lymph nodes may be painful in association with acute inflammatory processes. *Lymphadenitis* refers to inflammation of the lymph nodes.

Lymphatic channels drain fluid from the body tissues to lymphatic vessels that empty into the bloodstream through the lymphatic ducts in the thorax. Obstruction of flow through lymphatic vessels results in movement of fluid from lymphatic vessels to the interstitial space. The tissue swelling is referred to as *lymphedema*.

Lymphangitis is an inflammatory process along the course of lymphatic vessel that is manifested by a red streak on the skin. It is caused by the spread of bacteria through the lymphatic vessel to the lymph node.

Physical Examination   Lymphatic System

GENERAL APPROACH

The superficial lymph nodes are dispersed throughout the body. Therefore, examination of the lymphatic system may be incorporated into the head-to-toe physical examination. For example, lymph nodes of the neck are examined after the head; lymph nodes of the breast are evaluated during the breast examination. If abnormalities of the lymph nodes or lymphatic vessels are suspected, you should examine carefully the body area that drains toward the affected lymph node or vessel for signs of inflammation, infection, swelling, or injury.

The superficial lymphatic system is examined by inspection and palpation. Enlarged lymph nodes are detected more easily by light palpation than by deep palpation. Some variability is found among individuals in the number and location of lymph nodes in a particular area. Therefore, you should palpate the entire area where a lymphatic chain may be located. Encourage the person to report any tenderness experienced during palpation.

PALPABLE LYMPH NODES

Palpable lymph nodes should be distinguished from underlying tissue such as muscle. Unlike other surrounding tissue, an enlarged lymph node usually can be rolled up and down and side to side between the examiner's fingers.

Small palpable lymph nodes are common. Palpable nodes that are less than 1 cm wide, mobile, nontender, and discrete often are considered benign, but such findings still should be documented. You may detect a shotty node associated with frequent or chronic inflammation. A shotty node is enlarged over 1 cm, mobile, nontender, hard, and nodular. Malignancies may result in palpable lymph nodes that characteristically are nontender, nonmobile (fixed to underlying tissues), irregularly shaped, and firm, rubbery, or nodular. Such findings warrant further evaluation.

EXAMINATION AND DOCUMENTATION FOCUS

- *Inspection:* Location of any visible nodes, presence of swelling or red streaks
- *Palpation:* Palpable nodes are described in terms of location, size (millimeters or centimeters), consistency, discreteness, mobility, and tenderness. Determine when the palpable node was first noticed by the patient.

▼ ▼ ▼

Assessment Guidelines   Lymphatic System

Procedure

1. **Inspect and palpate the lymphatics of the head and neck.**

   a. Inspect the skin overlying the head and neck lymphatic chains for swelling, redness, or red streaks.

   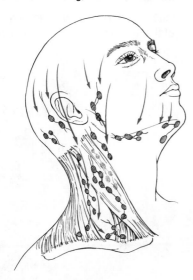

   b. Palpate the lymphatics of the head and neck.

   Right and left sides may be examined simultaneously as you palpate the lymphatic areas of the head and neck. Slight flexion of the head and turning the head away from the area being examined may be helpful. Systematically palpate the nodes of the head and neck, using a sequence such as the following:

   (1) Preauricular (in front of the tragus of the ear)

   (2) Postauricular or mastoid (overlying the mastoid process)

   (3) Occipital or suboccipital (at the base of the skull)

   (4) Tonsilar (at the angle of the lower jaw)

   (5) Submaxillary (midway between the angle of the lower jaw and chin)

   (6) Submental (midline behind the tip of the chin)

   (7) Superficial cervical chain (over the sternocleidomastoid muscle)

   (8) Posterior cervical chain (anterior to the trapezius muscle)

   (9) Deep cervical chain (embedded in the sternocleidomastoid muscle). The deep cervical chain is difficult to palpate. Hook thumb and fingers around the sternocleidomastoid muscle and then palpate.

   (10) Supraclavicular (within the angle formed by the sternocleidomastoid muscle and clavicle)

Clinical Significance

Normal Findings

Superficial nodes are not palpable and not tender on palpation.

Deviations from Normal

Superficial nodes, less than 1 cm in diameter, may be normal in adults. Lymph nodes may be up to 3 cm in healthy children.

Infection: Lymph nodes may become enlarged, warm, and tender in head and throat infections. Enlarged postauricular lymph nodes may be noted in otitis media.

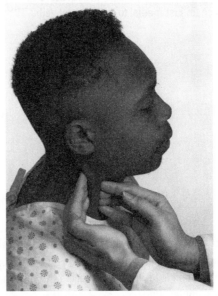

Palpation: Deep cervical chain

▼ ▼ ▼

Assessment Guidelines   Lymphatic System

Procedure

2. **Inspect and palpate the lymphatics of the breast, axillae, and supraclavicular area.**

3. **Inspect and palpate the lymphatics of the epitrochlear area.**

   The epitrochlear nodes are located just above the medial epicondyle of the humerus. To palpate for epitrochlear nodes, flex the patient's elbow 90 degrees, and palpate above the epicondyle in the groove created by the biceps and triceps muscles.

Clinical Significance

This is part of the routine breast and axillae examination. See Chapter 13.

Deviations from Normal

Enlargement and tenderness may be associated with infection of the ulnar aspect of the forearm and the fourth and fifth fingers.

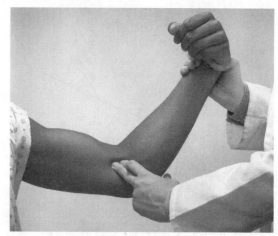

Palpation: Epitrochlear nodes

4. **Inspect and palpate the lymphatics of the inguinal region.**

   The superficial inguinal lymph nodes may be palpated with the patient lying supine with the knees slightly flexed. Palpate for the horizontal superficial inguinal chain along the inguinal ligament. Palpate for the vertical superficial inguinal chain just medial to the femoral vein.

Enlargement and tenderness may be associated with infection of the lower abdominal and pelvic regions and lower extremities.

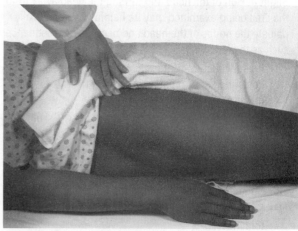

Palpation: Superficial inguinal lymph nodes

5. **Inspect and palpate the lymphatics of the popliteal fossa.**

   Palpate for the popliteal nodes in the posterior fossa of the knee. Palpation is facilitated by placing the knee in a position of slight flexion.

Enlargement and tenderness may be associated with infection of the heel and foot.

Documenting Lymphatic Examination Findings

Example 1: Normal Superficial Lymphatics

Lymph nodes generally are not visible or palpable. In this case, the results of the examination may be documented in the following manner:

> No visible or palpable lymph nodes in the [specify body area or lymphatic chain]. No tenderness on palpation; no edema or skin color changes.

Example 2: Benign Palpable Lymph Node

Mary, aged 14, had a physical examination before participating in school sports. The examination of the superficial lymphatic chains of the neck was recorded as follows:

> No palpable neck nodes except right tonsillar node, 1.5 × 1.0 cm. Node is nontender, soft, and mobile with well-defined borders. Node has been palpable for several years and unchanged in size. History of frequent sore throat before age 8 years.

Example 3: Generalized Lymphadenitis

Max, aged 24, has been tired lately and experiencing tenderness under his arms and in the groin area. He is a recovering intravenous drug user. The examination of the superficial lymphatic system was recorded as follows:

> Axillary lymph nodes palpable bilaterally. Nodes are tender, matted, nondiscrete, warm, soft, mobile, and irregularly shaped. Inguinal lymph nodes palpable bilaterally. Nodes are tender, matted, and warm. No other palpable lymph nodes.

Nursing Diagnoses Related to Lymphatic Assessment

A person with enlarged and painful lymph nodes (lymphadenitis) should be evaluated further for signs and symptoms of the following nursing diagnosis: Pain related to swelling and inflammation. Consider also the nursing diagnoses of Anxiety and Fear for persons undergoing evaluation.

Clinical Problems Related to Lymphatic Assessment

An enlarged or tender lymph node can be associated with a number of disease entities. Localized lymphadenopathy may suggest a bacterial infection in an area draining into that lymphatic chain. Generalized lymphadenopathy is the presence of palpable lymph nodes in three or more lymph node chains. This condition may be associated with systemic infectious processes, lymphoma, leukemia, or collagen vascular disorders. Additional diagnostic evaluation is usually indicated and may include lymphatic biopsy.

CASE STUDY

Anna Olsen was an 80-year-old widow who lived alone in her own home. She was a participant in a Meals-on-Wheels program that delivered nutritional noonday meals, Monday through Friday. The Medicare HMO that Mrs. Olsen belonged to had contracted with a home health agency to conduct nutritional screening assessments on all of its participants enrolled in Meals-on-Wheels programs. The nurse conducting the home visit and nutrition screening observed the following during the preliminary evaluation. Mrs. Olsen was 5'4", weighed 104 pounds, and appeared emaciated. Mrs. Olsen stated that she relied on the Meals-on-Wheels program because she could no longer drive to the grocery store or prepare meals because of failing eyesight. Mrs. Olsen often would save a portion of the noonday meal and reheat it for her evening meal. On weekends, she would prepare canned soups and apple juice. Her daughter-in-law regularly brought groceries to her home. Although she reported her appetite was good, she thought she did not eat as she had 5 years earlier and had noticed that her clothes were looser. Mrs. Olsen wore her upper and lower dentures only to eat. The physical examination showed loose dentures with inflamed gingiva from denture contact. The oral mucosa was dry.

On the basis of the initial nutrition screening, the nurse conducted a more in-depth assessment of Mrs. Olsen. The additional assessment was conducted to further evaluate overall nutritional status as well as contributing factors that placed Mrs. Olsen at risk for poor nutritional status. Health-promoting factors were also identified. The additional assessment information could be used in planning interventions to improve Mrs. Olsen's health status.

Profile Analysis

This chapter presents the concepts and skills used to conduct a comprehensive assessment of nutrition status. Nutrition screening is based on the identification of key physiologic indicators of impaired nutritional status, and comprehensive assessment takes into account many diverse aspects of nutritional processes as well as the individual's overall health history. Nutrition screening is especially important in elders. Some published studies have indicated that as many as 50% of independent living elders do not meet their recommended energy or protein intakes. Furthermore, many older people and their

CASE STUDY (continued)

caregivers or families may not report or recognize nutrition-related problems because they are erroneously believed to part of the normal aging process. Elders in meals-on-wheels programs are considered a population at risk for poor nutritional status in spite of their participation. The additional assessment of elders, such as Mrs. Olsen, can be used to determine whether additional nutritional or other interventions will be helpful to maximize health, nutritional status, and functional independence.

Assessment Focus

In addition to evaluating the indicators of nutritional status, the nurse focused the assessment on Mrs. Olsen's abilities to manage tasks of daily living, especially in relation to safety, food preparation, self-administration of any medications, and maintaining the home.

The nurse's general knowledge about independent living elders further influenced her approach to nutritional assessment. For example, the nurse knew that elderly people living alone were at greater risk for malnutrition even if adequate food was available and there were no problems with ingesting or metabolizing nutrients. Possible factors contributing to the risk of poor nutritional status in this population included:

- Loss of appetite secondary to inadequate social stimuli for preparing or enjoying meals
- Chronic illness or depression
- Unbalanced dietary intake
- Excessive calorie intake
- Mechanical eating problems

Based on this understanding of nutritional risks, the nurse recommended additional interventions as well as ongoing evaluation and analysis of nutritional status over the next few weeks until some improvement was observed.

Preliminary Nursing Diagnoses

Based on visual observation, the nurse judged Mrs. Olsen's body weight to be more than 10% below the ideal for her height and frame. This single observation suggested the nursing diagnosis of Altered nutrition: Less than body requirements. The nurse's next task was to consider possible contributing factors and to conduct additional assessment to either support or rule out each possibility. The following observations were made:

- Mrs. Olsen did not eat all of the food made available through the noonday meal service. Even though her daughter-in-law delivered groceries, weekend meals were not balanced.

- Mrs. Olsen reported ill-fitting dentures and displayed evidence of oral trauma from her dentures.

Additional Assessment

In addition to the most obvious factors already identified, the nurse also investigated additional factors that might be contributing to a compromised nutritional status. For example, Mrs. Olsen's medical history was further evaluated to determine whether there might be an underlying pathologic process that further impaired her appetite and ability to absorb nutrients. Even though Mrs. Olsen reported a good appetite and had adequate food supplies in her home, the nurse wondered why she did not finish her prepared meal portions. She also wondered how well Mrs. Olsen understood the principles of a balanced diet or whether she suffered from depression. Although she believed that poor dentition was the most probable contributing factor to her poor appetite, the nurse decided to follow-up on all such possibilities.

A more thorough interview about food and fluid intake, emotional status, and knowledge about nutrition was conducted. Additionally, the nurse examined the oral cavity and measured height and weight.

Final Nursing Diagnoses

Further evaluation showed that mealtime had been viewed by Mrs. Olsen as an important time for social interaction in the past when other people were in the home. Living alone, Mrs. Olsen felt isolated at mealtime and had less interest in preparing balanced meals. Her failing eyesight did not appear to interfere with her ability to use the stove or prepare meals. Mrs. Olsen's ill-fitting denture caused painful chewing that often prevented her from finishing her meals. She did not seek professional care, believing that her dentures would never fit well. Mrs. Olsen expressed that she was even more apathetic about weekend meals that she had to prepare and eat alone. The resulting nursing diagnosis was Altered nutrition: Less than body requirements related to social isolation and ill-fitting dentures.

Finally, the nurse identified the strengths that would be important for promoting an optimal state of health. The following observations were indicators of strengths:

- Remains alert and mobile
- Receives some nutritional meals
- Receives groceries from a family member
- Able to prepare basic meals
- No debilitating chronic illnesses

These strengths were considered when planning additional interventions to improve nutritional status.

The assessment of nutrition and metabolism focuses on analyzing
- The quality of the diet in relation to metabolic needs
- The degree to which the body demonstrates that the ingested nutrients are adequately used

Comprehensive nutritional assessment addresses the following:
- Dietary practices
- Factors influencing food and fluid consumption
- Nutritional risk factors
- Status of the nutritional processes
- Nutritional alterations or problems

Data Collection Methods

1. Interview and Review of Records
   - Patterns of weight gain or loss
   - Dietary practices
   - Functional status
   - Socioeconomic status
   - Socioeconomic variables
   - Medical history
   - Medication history
2. Diet Evaluation
   - Diet (food intake) history
   - 24-hour food recall
   - Food frequency record
   - Food diary
   - Calorie count
3. Diagnostic Studies Review
   - Serum albumin, transferrin, and lymphocytes
   - Nitrogen balance
   - Hemoglobin, hematocrit, and transferrin
   - Potassium and sodium
   - Cholesterol and lipids
4. Physical Examination
   - Anthropometric measurement
   - Integumentary system
   - Jaw and oral cavity
   - Abdomen
   - Thyroid gland
   - Lymphatic system

Primary Nursing Diagnoses
- Adequate nutrition
- Altered nutrition: More than body requirements
- Altered nutrition: Less than body requirements
- Altered nutrition: Potential for more than body requirements

Clinical Problems Related to Nutritional and Metabolic Dysfunctions

Metastatic processes involving the skin, oral cavity, and lymphatic system

Inflammatory gastrointestinal processes

Gastrointestinal obstruction

Critical Thinking

You are the nurse counseling a 65-year-old man who is receiving radiation therapy for rectal cancer on an outpatient basis. Nutritional problems are likely over the 6-week course of therapy. This is the patient's first week of therapy. A primary treatment goal is to design a plan to meet the patient's nutritional needs.

Learning Exercises

1. Select and describe the approach you would use to establish a useful database pertaining to this patient's nutritional status. Explain how you would proceed if you had only 30 minutes to spend with the patient, and approximately one third of that time would be used to answer questions and teach him about the overall treatment plan.

2. Specify how your nutrition database would help you establish realistic treatment goals for this patient.

3. The patient is unable to maintain a food diary. Identify and describe alternative approaches for assessing his diet.

4. Explain how you would use laboratory values to evaluate the patient's nutritional status.

BIBLIOGRAPHY

Academy of Science—National Research Council, Food and Nutrition Board. (1989). *Recommended dietary allowances, selected standard heights in adults.* Washington, DC.

Berecek, K. (1975). The etiology of decubitus ulcers. *Nursing Clinics of North America, 10,* 157.

Bergstrom, N., Braden, B., Laguzza, A., & Holman, A. (1987). The Braden Scale for predicting pressure sore risk. *Nursing Research, 36,* 205–210.

Bishop, C.W., Bowen, P.E., & Ritchey, S.J. (1981). Reference data (percentiles) for midarm circumference, triceps skinfold, and midarm muscle circumference. *American Journal of Clinical Nutrition, 34,* 25–30.

Bruce, B., & Wilfley, D. (1996). Binge eating among the overweight population: A serious and prevalent problem. *Journal of the American Dietetic Association, 96*(1), 58–61.

Bryant, R. (1987). Wound repair: A review. *Enterostomal Therapy, 14*(6), 262–266, 268.

Bryant, R.A. (1992). *Acute and chronic wounds: Nursing management.* St. Louis: C.V. Mosby.

Carter, R.L., Sharbaugh, C.O., & Stapell, C.A. (1981). Reliability and validity of the 24-hour recall. *Journal of the American Dietetic Association, 79,* 542–547.

Coulston, A.M., Craig, L., & Voss, A.C. (1996). Meals-on-wheels applicants are a population at risk for poor nutritional status. *Journal of the American Dietetic Association, 96*(6), 570–573.

Curtas, S. (1989). Evaluation of nutritional status. *Nursing Clinics of North America, 24*(2), 301–303.

Dose, A.M. (1995). The symptom experience of mucositis, stomatitis, and xerostomia. *Seminars in Oncology Nursing, 11*(4), 248–255.

Food and Nutrition Board. (1989). *Recommended dietary allowances* (10th ed.). Washington, D.C: National Academy Press.

Flory, C. (1992). Perfecting the art: Skin assessment. *RN, 55*(6), 22–27.

Frisancho, A.R. (1981). New norms of upper limb fat and muscle areas for assessment of nutritional status, *American Journal of Clinical Nutrition, 30,* 2540–2548.

Gallagher, J. (1995). Management of cutaneous symptoms. *Seminars in Oncology Nursing, 11*(4), 239–247.

Gauwitz, D.F. (1995). How to protect the dysphagic stroke patient. *American Journal of Nursing, 95*(8), 34–38.

Gee, C.F. (1990). Nutrition and wound healing. *Nursing: The Journal of Clinical Practice, Education, and Management, 4*(18), 26–28.

Grant, J.P. (1986). Nutritional assessment in clinical practice, *Nutrition Clinical Practice, 1*(1), 3–11.

Grant, M.M., & Rivera, L.M. (1995). Anorexia, cachexia, and dysphagia: The symptom experience. *Seminars in Oncology Nursing, 11*(4), 266–271.

Gray, D.P., & Smith, P. (1983). Nutritional assessment of the surgical patient: A nursing perspective. *Nutritional Support Services, 3*(9), 64–66.

Harrison, M. (1995). Pressure sores: Assessing the risk. *Nursing Standard, 9*(23), 32–34.

Home and Garden Bulletin No. 232. (1995). *Nutrition and your health: Dietary guidelines for Americans* (4th ed.). Washington, D.C.: US Departments of Agriculture and Health and Human Services.

Home and Garden Bulletin No. 252. (1992). *Food Pyramid Guide: A guide to daily food choices.* Washington, D.C.: US Department of Agriculture.

Institute of Medicine, Food and Nutrition Board. (1994). *How should the recommended dietary allowances be revised?* Washington, D.C: National Academy Press.

Jacobs, B.B., & Jacobs, L.M. (1988). Anatomy of the abdomen. *Emergency Care Quarterly, 3*(4), 1–11.

Jacobs. B.B., & Jacobs, L.M. (1988). Assessment of the abdomen. *Emergency Care Quarterly, 3*(4), 12–21.

Keithley, J.K. (1985). Nutritional assessment of the patient undergoing surgery, *Heart and Lung, 14*(5), 449–456.

Kennedy, E., Meyers, L., & Layden, W. (1996). The 1995 Dietary Guidelines for Americans: An overview. *Journal of the American Dietetic Association, 96*(3), 234–237.

Kohlmeier, L., Mendez, M., McDuffie. J., & Miller, M. (1997). Computer-assisted self interviewing: A multimedia approach to dietary assessment. *American Journal of Clinical Nutrition, 65*(4; suppl): 1275S–1281S.

Lachance, P., & Langseth, L. (1994). The RDA concept: Time for a change? *Nutrition Review, 52*:266–270.

Lazarus, G.J., Cooper, D.M., Knighton, D.R., et al. (1994). Definitions and guidelines for assessment of wounds and evaluation of healing. *Wound Repair and Regeneration, 2,* 165–170.

Leininger, M.M. (1988). Transcultural eating patterns and nutrition: Transcultural nursing and anthropological perspectives. *Holistic Nursing Practice, 3*(1), 16–25.

Levine, J.M., & Totolos, E. (1995). Pressure ulcers: A strategic plan to prevent and heal them. *Geriatrics, 50*(1), 32–37.

Loogman, E.A. (1992). Nutritional assessment in nursing. *Gastrointestinal Nursing, 14*(4), 189–194.

Makelbust, J., & Margolis, D. (1995). Pressure ulcers: Definition and assessment parameters. *Advances in Wound Care, 8*(4), 6–7.

Marius, E. (1992). An appetite for life: Assessing and meeting nutritional needs. *Professional Nursing, 7*(11), 732–737.

Neilly, L.K., & Darr Ellis, R.A. (1984). Nailing down a diagnosis. *Nurse Practice, 9*(5), 26–34.

Norton, D., McLaren, R., Exton-Smith, A.N. (1962). An investigation of geriatric nursing problems in hospitals. *National Corporation for the Care of Old People,* London.

O'Hanlon-Nichols, T. (1995). Commonly asked questions about wound healing. *American Journal of Nursing, 95*(4), 22–24.

O'Toole, M.T. (1990). Advanced assessment of the abdomen and gastrointestinal problems. *Nursing Clinics of North America, 25*(4), 771–776.

Panel for the Prediction and the Prevention of Pressure Ulcers in Adults. (1992). *Pressure ulcers in adults: Prediction and prevention.* Clinical Practice Guideline Number 3. AHCRR Publication No. 92-0047. Rockville MD: Agency for Health Care Policy and Research, Public Health Service, U.S. Department of Health and Human Services.

Rice, R. (1995). Wound assessment and documentation. *Home Healthcare Nurse, 13*(2), 75–76.

Rhodes, V.A., Johnson, M.H., & McDaniel, R.W. (1995). Nausea, vomiting, and retching: The management of the symptom experience. *Seminars in Oncology Nursing, 11*(4), 256–265.

Schakel, S.F., Sievert, Y.A., & Buzzard, I.M. (1988). Sources of data for developing and maintaining a nutrient database. *Journal of the American Dietetic Association, 88,* 1268–1271.

Sims, L.S. (1996). Uses of the recommended dietary allowances: A commentary. *Journal of the American Dietetic Association, 96*(7), 659–662.

Standing, J. (1985). *Somerset Health Authority pressure sore survey.* Taunton: Somerset Health Authority.

Young, M. (1988). Malnutrition and wound healing. *Heart and Lung, 17*(1), 60–69.

Assessing Elimination

ASSESSMENT GUIDELINES

- Bowel Elimination Interview (Health History)
- Bladder Elimination Interview (Health History)
- Diagnostic Studies of Elimination
- Stool
- Urine
- Interpreting Physical Examination Findings Related to Elimination
- Anus and Rectum

CHAPTER ORGANIZATION

PART 1: ASSESSING THE PATTERN

Introductory Overview
- Assessment Focus
- Nursing Diagnoses

Knowledge Base for Assessment
- Physiology of Bowel Elimination

- Anatomy and Physiology of Bladder Elimination

PART 2: PHYSICAL EXAMINATION TECHNIQUES

Anus and Rectum
- Anatomy and Physiology Review

PART 1

ASSESSING THE PATTERN

INTRODUCTORY OVERVIEW

Eliminating body waste is a complex process influenced by physiologic, pathologic, nutritional, environmental, and cultural factors. Assessment involves more than analyzing and quantifying urine and stool specimens. It also includes evaluation of the structures involved in elimination, risk factors and contributing factors for elimination problems, and the person's responses to problems with elimination.

Bowel and bladder elimination problems—especially constipation and urinary incontinence—are common health problems that are often underreported, undetected, and, as a result, left untreated. The overall impact of untreated elimination problems on quality of life is staggering, affecting self-esteem, social and sexual activity, and physical health. The economic consequences are also significant. Incontinence management is often considered to be a nursing issue. Your assessment of the person with elimination problems may often identify basic problems that may be readily responsive to independent nursing management or be the basis for referral to other clinical providers.

ASSESSMENT FOCUS

Elimination includes bowel and urinary elimination. The assessment of elimination focuses on the evaluation of bowel and urinary elimination functions and patterns to determine optimal health promotion practices, prevent elimination problems, and identify appropriate interventional strategies for persons with elimination problems. With a comprehensive assessment of elimination, the nurse will meet the following objectives:

- Describing the person's bowel and bladder elimination patterns in terms of frequency, amount, and usual habits
- Identifying self-care practices and knowledge about elimination
- Identifying risk factors and causative factors associated with altered elimination
- Evaluating the effects of elimination problems on physical, social, and psychological health
- Differentiating between various elimination problems

Data collection is accomplished by the following methods:

1. Interview and/or Review of Records
   - Bowel elimination focus
     - Usual bowel movement pattern
     - Altered bowel movement pattern
     - Self-care practices
     - Functional status
     - Medical history
     - Medication history
   - Bladder elimination focus
     - Usual voiding pattern
     - Altered urinary elimination patterns
     - Self-care practices
     - Functional status
     - Medical history
     - Medication history
2. Diagnostic Studies Focus
   - Radiographic studies of the bowel and urinary system
   - Urodynamic testing—cystometrogram; electromyography; pressure–flow studies
   - Postvoid residual volumes
3. Specimen Analysis Focus
   - Stool
   - Urine
4. Physical Examination Focus
   - General survey
   - Abdominal examination
   - Genitourinary structures (pelvic examination in women)
   - Anus and rectum

Nursing Diagnoses

Assessment of elimination patterns may result in the identification of one or more of the following primary nursing diagnoses:

Constipation
Perceived constipation
Colonic constipation

Diarrhea
Bowel incontinence
Altered urinary elimination
Stress incontinence
Reflex incontinence
Urge incontinence
Functional incontinence
Total incontinence
Urinary retention

Secondary nursing diagnoses related to bowel and bladder elimination problems include the following:

Body image disturbance
Fluid volume deficit
Risk for fluid volume deficit
Hopelessness
Ineffective coping
Self-care deficit
Self-esteem disturbance
Altered sexuality patterns
Impaired skin integrity
Risk for impaired skin integrity

KNOWLEDGE BASE FOR ASSESSMENT

Assessing elimination requires an understanding of the processes of bowel and bladder elimination. Each process has a physiologic basis that may be influenced by many factors, such as diet, age, activity, exercise, stress, drugs, and pathologic condition.

Physiology of Bowel Elimination

The amount of stool or feces evacuated from the bowel is related to the amount and composition of ingested food. Food intake, however, is not essential for producing a bowel movement. Stool can form from the cellular residues desquamated from the intestinal tract lining, as well as from intestinal gland secretions, bacteria, blood, and other substances. Under normal, nonfasting conditions, food residue (chyme) that passes through the ileocecal valve (the junction between the small and large intestines) contributes to total stool weight. At this point, most nutrients have been absorbed from the chyme; the bolus of food is further processed, with the semiliquid chyme being converted into solid stool that can be evacuated from the rectum. The formation and evacuation of stool is the result of the following normal colonic functions: fluid and electrolyte absorption, peristaltic contractions, and defecation (Fig 7-1).

Absorption

Fluid and electrolyte absorption, a process of converting semiliquid chyme into formed stool, occurs across the mucosal surfaces of the colon. Normally, the colon can absorb 90% of the water received from the small intestine. Absorption occurs passively and is enhanced when segments of the colon contract. Circular muscles in the colon constrict around the lumen and divide the colon into segments, holding the chyme in contact with the absorptive surface. If the chyme remains in prolonged contact with the mucosal surface of the colon, too much water is absorbed, and the stool may become hard and dry. Conversely, if muscle tone is decreased and segmenting con-

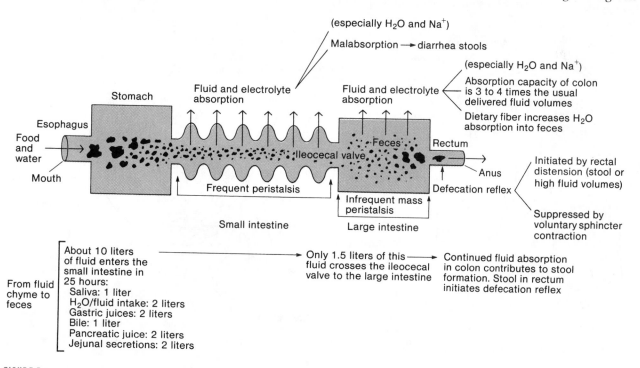

FIGURE 7.1 Summary of normal colonic functions contributing to feces formation and evacuation: fluid and electrolyte absorption, peristalsis, and defecation.

tractions do not occur, the chyme may trickle through the colon with little water being absorbed, resulting in liquid stools. Dietary fiber is an efficient water absorber. High intake of dietary fiber, therefore, may cause stools to be softer secondary to increased water retention.

Peristalsis

Wavelike peristaltic movements propel the stool toward the sigmoid colon and rectum. Unlike the frequent peristaltic activity in the small intestine, peristalsis of the large intestine is relatively infrequent, with mass peristaltic movements occurring only two to four times daily. Mass peristalsis in the colon can be initiated by the gastronomic reflex that occurs when food reaches the stomach, by bulk-forming agents such as fiber in the intestinal lumen, and by the stool in the rectum. Adding bulk to the diet causes the lumen of the colon to distend, which results in increased peristaltic activity to move feces through the colon. Usually parasympathetic nervous system discharge stimulates peristalsis in the colon, whereas sympathetic nervous system stimulation inhibits peristalsis. Prolonged stress may affect the autonomic nervous system and may result in bowel elimination problems, with alternating constipation and diarrhea.

Defecation

Defecation is the movement of stool out of the rectum. The defecation reflex is initiated when stool enters the rectum. Secondary to the defecation reflex, the internal and external anal sphincter relax, which allows the stool to be evacuated. The defecation reflex may be suppressed by voluntarily contracting the external anal sphincter. The ability to suppress the defecation reflex is essential for bowel control, but continued suppression may have adverse effects, contributing to constipation and fecal impaction.

Anatomy and Physiology of Bladder Elimination

The structures of the urinary tract include the kidneys, renal pelvis, ureter, bladder, urethra, and urinary meatus (Fig. 7-2). From the major calices of the kidney, urine drains into the renal pelvis and then into the ureter. The ureter from each kidney attaches to the bladder wall.

The urinary bladder is a hollow, muscular organ that stores and expels urine. The bladder muscle is called the detrusor muscle. The size and shape of the bladder vary. When the bladder is empty, it is triangular and lies entirely within the pelvic structure. When the bladder is full, it is more spherical and extends upward and anteriorly in the abdominal cavity. This causes the lower abdomen to appear distended.

The urethra extends from the urinary bladder to the urinary meatus. The male urethra traverses the prostate gland, and urinary alterations, such as retention, hesitancy, and narrow stream may be noted if the prostate gland is enlarged. The female urethra is relatively short compared with the male urethra. In women, good pelvic muscle tone is required to maintain voluntary control of the urethral sphincter.

Bladder elimination occurs when urine is excreted through the external urinary sphincter. Urine production occurs in the nephrons of the kidneys. If no urine is produced, as in renal failure, a problem exists with urine production, not bladder elimination.

The process of emptying the bladder may be called

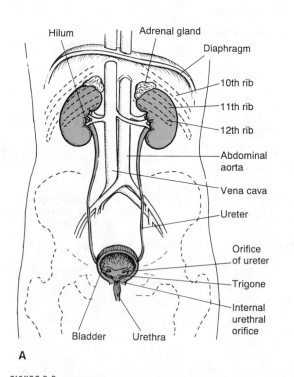

A

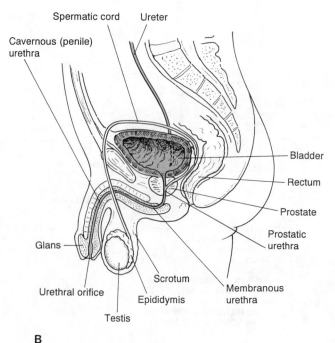

B

FIGURE 7.2 (**A**) Anatomic structures of the urinary tract. (**B**) The male urinary tract.

micturition, voiding, or urination, and it is a reflex children learn to control voluntarily between ages 2 and 4 years. In adults, the urge to void is felt when the bladder fills with approximately 200 mL of urine. When the bladder fills with 350 to 400 mL of urine, pressure from the urine volume stimulates specialized nerve endings in the bladder detrusor called stretch receptors, which in turn stimulate a reflex arc at the second to fourth sacral segments of the spinal cord. Eventually, in response to volume, the detrusor muscle contracts, strengthening the urge to void (Fig. 7-3). Without conscious control, urine would enter the urethra, the external sphincter would relax, and voiding would occur. Voiding remains under voluntary control until bladder volume approaches 700 mL, when most people lose the ability to delay voiding.

Neural Voiding Mechanisms

Messages are sent along neural pathways between the cerebral cortex and the sacral segments of the spinal cord as the bladder fills with urine and during the act of voiding (see Fig. 7-3). If environmental conditions are not suitable for voiding, messages from the brain will inhibit the reflex arc and lead to voluntary contraction of the external bladder sphincter. If conditions are favorable, the brain will send a message encouraging the external sphincter to relax, and urine will be voided. Brain messages also direct the detrusor muscle to contract until all urine has been expelled from the bladder.

Neural Pathway Disruptions

Disease and injuries may cause lesions along the central neurogenic pathways involved in voiding (see Fig. 7-3). If the pathway from the frontal cortex to the pontine-mesencephalic reticular formation is disrupted, voluntary voiding may be affected. Brain tumors, organic brain syndrome, cerebrovascular accident, and head injuries can cause such disruptions. Consequently, the bladder may empty secondary to involuntary reflex contraction of the detrusor and involuntary relaxation of the urethral sphincter, or voiding may occur at inappropriate times because of scrambled brain messages, a condition known as *upper motor neuron bladder* or *reflex bladder*.

Injury to the neural pathway from the pontine-mesencephalic reticular formation to the parasympathetic nucleus in the S2–S4 area of the spinal cord (reticulospinal

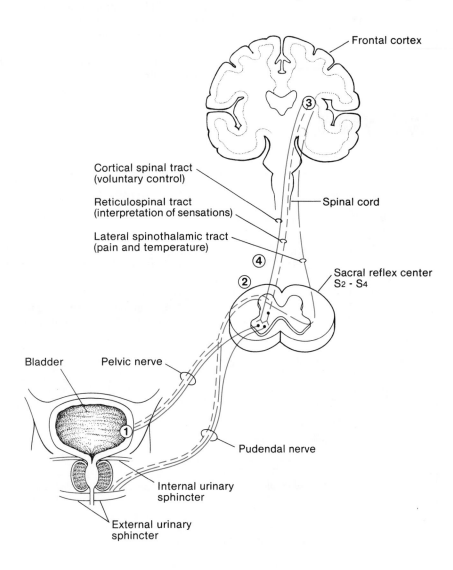

FIGURE 7.3 Urine elimination: Neuromuscular mechanisms. (1) Bladder stretch receptors send messages to the brain signaling bladder fullness. (2) Spinal (sacral) reflex causes sphincter relaxation and detrusor contraction when bladder is full. (3) Voluntary controls inhibit the spinal reflex until the person is ready to void. (4) Motor impulses are sent to the detrusor and sphincters so that voiding occurs.

Labels in figure:
Frontal cortex
Cortical spinal tract (voluntary control)
Reticulospinal tract (interpretation of sensations)
Lateral spinothalamic tract (pain and temperature)
Spinal cord
Sacral reflex center S2 - S4
Bladder
Pelvic nerve
Pudendal nerve
Internal urinary sphincter
External urinary sphincter

tract) may affect voiding coordination. Normally, the detrusor contracts as the external urethral sphincter relaxes. If these actions are not coordinated and the bladder involuntarily contracts, the flow may be partially obstructed by a contracted sphincter. Incontinence accompanied by urine retention in the bladder results.

The corticospinal tract houses the neural connections between the brain and the pudendal nucleus. Injury to this pathway may affect the ability to voluntarily interrupt the urinary stream.

Damage to the pelvic nerve, which leaves the spinal cord to innervate the bladder, may cause areflexia, or the inability of the detrusor to contract. Consequently, urine is retained in the bladder, a condition also referred to as *lower motor neuron bladder, hypotonic bladder,* or *atonic bladder.*

The hypogastric nerve and the pudendal nerve are needed to stimulate external sphincter contraction. If these nerves are damaged, stress incontinence and decreased sphincter tone may result.

Pattern Assessment Elimination

GENERAL APPROACH

An accurate description of a person's usual bowel and bladder elimination patterns is the basis for clinical judgments about elimination status and functions. Some people may be reluctant to discuss details of elimination because they find the discussion embarrassing. A straightforward and nonjudgmental approach is required. If the person is cognitively impaired, it may be difficult to conduct a meaningful interview. In this case, other approaches should be used to develop the elimination history, including reviewing medical records, interviewing family members or care providers, and directly observing elimination patterns. Special attention should be given to the assessment of persons at high risk for bowel elimination problems. Risk factors include inadequate diets, immobility, chronic use of medications affecting the bowel, neurologic dysfunctions, and chronic illnesses.

ASSESSMENT AIDS

Interview guide to suggest questions and record data (Display 7-1)
Voiding/incontinence records

DISPLAY 7.1

Interview Guide: Elimination

ELIMINATION PATTERN

Bowel

No. of Bowel Movements/day _____ Date of Last BM _____
Bowel Pattern: ❑ Normal ❑ Constipation ❑ Diarrhea > 3 days ❑ Incontinent
Pattern Change: ❑ No ❑ Yes Explain: _____
Use of Laxatives/Enemas: ❑ No ❑ Yes Explain/List: _____
Any of the following: ❑ Rectal pain ❑ Abdominal cramping ❑ Straining for BM
　　　　　　　　　　 ❑ Hard stools ❑ Blood in stools ❑ Excessive flatulence

Bladder

Voiding Pattern: ❑ Normal ❑ Frequency ❑ Urgency ❑ Dysuria
Pattern Change: ❑ No ❑ Yes Explain: _____
Incontinence: ❑ N/A ❑ Total ❑ Daytime ❑ Nighttime ❑ Occasional
　　　　　　　 ❑ Inability to perceive bladder cues ❑ Difficulty delaying voiding

Elimination Devices

❑ N/A ❑ Intermittent catheterization
❑ Ostomy: Type:_____ Appliance: _____
❑ Indwelling Catheter—Date inserted _____ ❑ Incontinent briefs
❑ External catheter ❑ Penile implant—Type _____

(continued)

DISPLAY 7.1

Interview Guide: Elimination (continued)

Elimination Function Knowledge

Self-Care for Constipation: _____

Self-Care for Incontinence: _____

Self-Care for Urinary Tract Infections: _____

Learning Needs ❑ No ❑ Yes Explain: _____

Functional Status

Problems Getting to Bathroom in Time ❑ No   ❑ Yes

Mobility Problems ❑ No   ❑ Yes Explain: _____

Medical History

Conditions Related to Problems with Bowel Elimination: ❑ No   ❑ Yes Explain: _____

_____

Conditions Related to Problems with Bladder Elimination: ❑ No   ❑ Yes Explain: _____

_____

Medication History

Medications Influencing Bowel Function: ❑ No   ❑ Yes Explain/List: _____

_____

Medications Influencing Bladder Function: ❑ No   ❑ Yes Explain/List: _____

_____

▼ ▼ ▼

GUIDELINES

Assessment Guidelines Bowel Elimination Interview (Health History)

Procedure

1. Usual bowel movement pattern

Determine the individual's perception of his or her usual bowel elimination pattern and whether he or she views this pattern as normal or abnormal.

Ask questions such as the following:

- "On the average, how many bowel movements do you have each day?"

- "What time of day do you usually have a bowel movement?"

- "Have you noticed any changes in the frequency of your bowel movements?"

- "How would you define constipation?"

Clinical Significance

So-called "normal" bowel elimination patterns can vary extensively among individuals. The individual's perception of a "normal" pattern can be used as a baseline to determine whether significant changes in bowel elimination have occurred.

Asking the person about the usual time of day for bowel movements helps characterize an individual's typical pattern. Many people have bowel movements at the same time every day, such as after a meal, in response to the gastrocolic reflex. Habitually ignoring this reflex may contribute to constipation.

Any recent changes in bowel patterns should be thoroughly evaluated. Changes in bowel patterns may be an indicator of more serious problems such as colon cancer.

Constipation should be evaluated in relation to the person's definition of constipation. A person who typically has a bowel movement every other day may not experience constipation. Similarly, a pattern of several bowel movements a day may be typical rather than abnormal.

▼ ▼ ▼

G U I D E L I N E S   *continued*   Bowel Elimination History (Health History)

Procedure

- "How is your usual bowel pattern affected by changes in routine, such as travel, different surroundings, or schedule changes?"

2. **Altered bowel movement patterns—constipation and diarrhea**

Further evaluate any reports of constipation by determining whether there are additional signs and symptoms, including the following:

- Rectal pain
- Feeling of fullness or pressure in the rectum
- Straining with bowel movements
- Abdominal pain or cramping
- Abdominal distention (bloating)
- Hard stools that are smaller in size and volume than usual
- Bloody stools
- Urinary incontinence

Further evaluate any reports of diarrhea by determining whether there are additional signs and symptoms, including the following:

- Abdominal pain or cramping
- Loose, liquid stools
- Urgency
- Changes in stool color

3. **Self-care practices**

Determine whether the person engages in any self-care practices to treat or prevent problems with bowel elimination.

   a. *Diet and Fluid Intake:* Determine the person's daily fluid intake. Quantify the amount of fluid ingested on an average day as well as the type of fluids being consumed.

Evaluate the person's intake of dietary fiber. Foods high in dietary fiber include the following:

- Whole-grain breads
- Cereals
- Raw fruits
- Raw vegetables

Clinical Significance

Changes in routine commonly contribute to bowel elimination changes by disrupting daily patterns, imposing time constraints, or interfering with privacy. In these circumstances, the defecation reflex may be suppressed, either voluntarily or involuntarily. Unnatural positioning, such as having to use a bedpan in a supine position, also may inhibit bowel movements.

Constipation: A change in normal bowel habits characterized by a decrease in frequency or passage of hard, dry stools.

The presence of any of these associated signs and symptoms will further support a diagnosis of constipation and may indicate contributing factors such as dehydration, hemorrhoids, or colon dysfunction.

Rectal pain is usually caused by stool being retained in the rectum.

Tenesmus is rectal pain associated with the urge to defecate and a sensation of incomplete emptying after defecation. Tenesmus can be a symptom of constipation, rectal tumors, or colon inflammation.

Urinary incontinence may be an indicator of fecal impaction.

Diarrhea: A change in normal bowel habits characterized by the frequent passage of loose, fluid, unformed stools.

Self-care practices involving diet, fluid intake, exercise, and self-administration of over-the-counter preparations influence bowel elimination patterns.

Adequate hydration is necessary to add weight, bulk, and softness to stools. Dehydration, from either inadequate intake or increased fluid losses, results in excessive water reabsorption from the intestinal chyme. This contributes to hard stools and constipation.

Optimal daily fluid intake to promote normal bowel function: six 8-ounce servings of water.

Coffee, tea, and grapefruit juice may have a diuretic effect, in which case less fluid is retained in the stool.

Dietary fiber contributes to stool bulk by promoting water retention in stool. Two to four grams of fiber daily helps prevent constipation and hemorrhoid formation. Low-fiber diets have been associated with colon diseases, including diverticulosis, irritable bowel syndrome, appendicitis, and colon cancer.

▼ ▼ ▼

Procedure

Determine whether specific foods known to affect bowel function are regularly ingested, such as the following:

Food

Prunes

Diary products in persons with lactase deficiency

Tube feedings

b. *Activity and Exercise:* Evaluate the individual's pattern of activity and exercise. Determine level of mobility and type and frequency of exercise.

c. *Laxatives, Enemas, and Suppositories:* Ask the person whether he or she uses laxatives, enemas, or suppositories to initiate bowel movements.

If the answer is "yes," determine how often this occurs and under what circumstances. Determine whether the person has an expectation of a daily bowel movement.

Determine the type of laxative being used.

Types of Laxatives

Lubricants

Bulk forming

Saline cathartics

Stimulants

4. **Functional status**

A combination of interviewing and direct observation can provide information about a person's functional status and level of independence with toileting.

Interview Questions

- "Do you have any difficulty getting to bathroom facilities in time?"
- "Do you have any problems with dressing or adjusting clothing?"

Observe levels of mobility and ability to dress independently. Determine the availability of toileting facilities. Are the facilities visible and easily accessible?

Also note the use of physical restraints—posey vests, wrist restraints.

Clinical Significance

Note: For a more comprehensive diet assessment, a 24-hour diet recall may be recommended (see Chap. 6).

Effect on Bowel Function

Laxative effect

Bowel irritation secondary to malabsorption of diary products—abdominal cramping, pain, and diarrhea

Diarrhea complications: Complications may be prevented by avoiding formula contamination, hypertonic formulas, and inadequate protein replacement.

Bowel elimination is facilitated by good muscle tone in the abdominal and pelvic muscles, which are used during defecating to propel the stool. Good overall muscle tone also strengthens the muscles responsible for peristalsis. Immobility may cause muscle weakness and inhibit mass peristalsis needed for defecation.

Using prescribed or over-the-counter preparations to promote bowel elimination is a common and potentially harmful self-care practice. Forty percent of Americans older than age 60 years have reported using laxatives on a weekly basis for constipation.

People who have expectations of a daily bowel movement tend to engage in overuse of laxatives, enemas, and suppositories.

Excessive use of stimulant laxatives may aggravate constipation. Stimulant laxatives act on the nerve endings in the colon to stimulate peristalsis. If used excessively, colon nerve function is disrupted, resulting in a cycle of constipation followed by more laxative use.

A decline in functional abilities increases the risk for stool or urine incontinence. Functional deficits most strongly associated with incontinence include impaired mobility, inability to transfer, and loss of manual dexterity required to manipulate clothing.

Physical restraints limit mobility and may contribute to incontinence.

▼ ▼ ▼

G U I D E L I N E S *continued*   Bowel Elimination History (Health History)

Procedure

5. Medical history

Screen the person for medical explanations of bowel elimination problems.

Conditions Associated with Constipation

Spinal cord injury

Bowel obstruction

Hypothyroidism

Hypocalcemia

Cancer

Surgery

Conditions Associated with Diarrhea

Crohn's disease

Ulcerative colitis

Acute bowel infections

Diverticulitis

Bowel obstruction

Hyperthyroidism

Diabetes mellitus

Adrenal insufficiency

Hypercalcemia

Conditions Associated with Stool Incontinence

Head injury

Stroke/CVA

Spinal cord injury

Fecal impaction

6. Medication history

Determine whether the person is taking medications that may affect bowel function by taking medication history.

Medication

Laxatives, stool softeners, or enemas

Anticholinergics

Tricyclic antidepressants

Anti-parkinsonism drugs

Antihistamines

Major tranquilizers

Broad-Spectrum Antibiotics

Ampicillin

Clindamycin

Lincomycin

Tetracycline

Neomycin

Cephalosporins

Clinical Significance

Medical problems may be the primary cause of bowel elimination problems or a risk factor because of the impact the medical problem has on mobility, food and fluid intake, or cognitive and functional abilities.

Polypharmacy: The ingestion of multiple medications is associated with an increased risk of bowel elimination problems.

Effect on Bowel Function

May irritate bowel mucosa and contribute to diarrhea. Long-term use may have an adverse effect on colon muscle tone and aggravate constipation.

Constipating effect—reduce contractility of the smooth muscle of the bowel

Diarrheal effect—by altering the normal bowel flora

▼ ▼ ▼

G U I D E L I N E S   *continued*   Bowel Elimination History (Health History)

Procedure

Antacids
   Gelusil
   Maalox
   Riopan
   Amphogel
Narcotics (opiates)
   Codeine
   Morphine
   Meperidine (Demerol)

Ask additional questions about laxative use to determine the person's motivation and the effects of these products. If the person reports using over-the-counter laxatives, ask questions about usual bowel patterns, type of laxative used, and frequency of use.

Clinical Significance

Diarrhea effect

Constipating effect—reduce smooth muscle tone of the colon, resulting in less frequent mass peristaltic movements

The Food and Drug Administration has documented widespread overuse of over-the-counter laxatives. Laxative use may occur in persons who do not consider themselves constipated. Overuse may be influenced by advertising, lack of knowledge, or belief in the benefits of regular purging. Habitual overuse of laxatives may diminish the normal defecation reflex.

▼ ▼ ▼

G U I D E L I N E S

Assessment Guidelines   Bladder Elimination Interview (Health History)

Procedure

1. **Usual voiding pattern**

   Determine the person's usual voiding pattern by asking questions such as the following:
   - "How many times a day do you void (go to the bathroom; pass water)?"
   - "How many times do you void at night?"

   Determine whether there are symptoms of altered urinary patterns by asking questions such as the following:
   - Frequency—"Do you think you are voiding more often than usual?"

   - Urgency—"Do you ever lose urine before you can arrive at the bathroom?"
   - Nocturia—"Do you have to get up at night to go to the bathroom?"
   - Enuresis—"Do you have trouble holding your urine when you are sleeping?"

Clinical Significance

Asking a person about his or her usual voiding pattern will establish the individual's baseline or lead to a discussion about symptoms of altered voiding patterns.

Frequency: Voiding more often than usual may be a sign of urinary tract infection.
Normal Frequency: Once every 3 to 6 hours. Normal frequency fluctuates in relation to fluid, caffeine, and alcohol intake.
Urgency: A sudden need to void that may be associated with inflammation of the bladder or urinary tract.
Nocturia: Nighttime voiding. May occur in persons with congestive heart failure, who tend to diurese fluids at night.
Enuresis: Bed wetting or involuntary voiding during sleep. Normal in preschool-age children. May be associated with urinary tract infection in older children.

▼ ▼ ▼

GUIDELINES *continued*   Bladder Elimination Interview (Health History)

Procedure

- Dysuria—"Do you experience pain when you urinate?" Further evaluate pain by inquiring about location, character, duration, radiation, and aggravating or relieving factors.

- Hesitancy—"Do you have difficulty starting your urine flow?" "Are you taking any antihistamines (cold medicines; allergy medicines)?"

- Dribbling—"Do you lose urine when you don't want to?" "Do you wear a pad or other protective device to collect your urine?"

2. **Altered urinary elimination pattern—urinary incontinence**

   Question the person about urinary incontinence:
   - "Do you have trouble with bladder control?"
   - "Do you have trouble holding your urine (water)?"

   For persons reporting urinary incontinence, ask additional questions to determine the following:
   - How long they have experienced incontinence
   - Frequency, timing, and amount of continent and incontinent voids
   - Precipitating factors such as being unable to get to the bathroom in time; sneezing, laughing, or other factors associated with increased abdominal pressure; medical conditions affecting functional, cognitive, or fluid status
   - Other symptoms of lower urinary tract dysfunction—nocturia, dysuria, hesitancy, interrupted stream, hematuria, pain, frequency, urgency, increased leakage
   - Fluid intake pattern
   - Alterations in bowel habits or sexual functions
   - Use of pads, briefs, or other protective devices

3. **Self-care practices**

   Determine whether the person engages in any self-care practices to treat or prevent problems with urine elimination.

Clinical Significance

Dysuria: Pain associated with voiding that may be symptomatic of many conditions, including urinary tract infections, urethral stricture, prostate disease, prolapsed uterus, and cancer of the cervix. Pain over the bladder area may indicate a urinary tract infection or bladder distention. Flank (side or back) pain is associated with upper urinary tract infections and stones in the urinary tract.

Hesitancy: Difficulty starting the flow of urine. May be associated with neurologic dysfunction or lower urinary tract obstruction. Antihistamines stimulate muscle tone of the bladder sphincter, which may contribute to hesitancy.

Dribbling: Involuntary passage of urine that may be associated with weakened bladder sphincter tone, hypotonic bladder, reduced bladder capacity, or sagging of the structures that support the bladder.

Urinary Incontinence: Involuntary loss of urine sufficient to be a problem. Urinary incontinence (UI) affects approximately 10 million Americans. This prevalence could be reduced through appropriate diagnosis and treatment.

In addition to obtaining a more extensive history from a person reporting urinary incontinence, the assessment also should include the following (discussed in detail elsewhere):

- Abdominal examination to detect masses, fullness, tenderness, and to estimate the postvoid residual volume (see complete examination guideline in Chap. 6)
- Genital examination in men to detect abnormalities of the foreskin, glans penis, and perineal skin (see complete examination guideline in Chap. 13)
- Pelvic examination in women to note atrophy of the vaginal mucosa, uterine prolapse, tenderness, and overall muscle tone (see complete examination guideline in Chap. 13)
- Rectal examination to evaluate rectal sensation, tone, fecal impaction, masses, bimanual estimation of postvoid residual volume and to estimate prostate gland contour and consistency
- Urinalysis
- Voiding/incontinence record (see Examination Guideline for Bladder Retraining in Chap. 18)

▼ ▼ ▼

G U I D E L I N E S *continued*   Bladder Elimination Interview (Health History)

Procedure

a. *Fluid Intake:*
Determine the person's daily fluid intake. Determine the amounts and types of fluids ingested in a typical 24-hour period.

b. *Activity and Exercise:*
Evaluate overall degree of physical fitness. Determine whether the person is familiar with or regularly engaging in pelvic strengthening exercises (*e.g.,* Kegel's exercises).

c. *Urinary Tract Infections:*
Ask about self-care practices to prevent or treat urinary tract infections:

- "What do you do to prevent (or manage) urinary tract infections?"

d. *Self-Treatment of Urinary Retention:*
If the person has a problem with urinary retention, ask how he or she manages this problem:

- "What helps you start urination?"

e. *Urinary Incontinence:*
Ask the person how they prevent or manage urinary incontinence.

4. Functional status
Evaluate functional status and level of independence with toileting activities (see discussion of Functional Status assessment in previous section "Bowel Elimination Interview").

Clinical Significance

Some people may decrease their fluid intake in an attempt to control urinary incontinence. This practice may actually aggravate urinary incontinence, especially if concentrated urine in the bladder becomes infected. Also, a critical volume of urine in the bladder is needed to maintain optimal detrusor muscle tone.

Optimal daily fluid intake to stimulate the bladder's stretch receptors and keep the urine dilute is 48 to 64 ounces of fluid. Caffeine and alcohol have irritating effects on the bladder.

Normal bladder elimination is facilitated by good pelvic muscle tone. Pregnancy may weaken the muscles involved in voiding, including the overall tone of the bladder sphincter.

Optimal self-care practices for urinary tract infections:

- Increase fluid intake—dilutes the urine and creates a less favorable environment for bacterial growth.
- Acidify the urine (*e.g.,* by drinking cranberry juice)—inhibits bacterial growth.
- Practice good hygiene (especially important in women), including voiding after intercourse, wiping the perineum from from to back after a bowel movement, and showering rather than bathing—all of these practices prevent bacteria from entering the urethra.

Optimal self-care practices for urinary retention:

- Trigger point stimulation to initiate voiding. Different methods will work for different people, such as stroking the inner thighs, tapping the abdomen, pulling the pubic hair, massaging the sacrum, and manually stretching the anal sphincter.
- Credé maneuver—manual expression of urine from the bladder by applying pressure over the suprapubic area

Common self-care practices for urinary incontinence:

- Fluid restriction (note: may aggravate UI)
- Following a toilet schedule
- Wearing an incontinence pad or external catheter
- Intermittent self-catheterization to assure complete bladder emptying
- Exercising the pelvic floor to strengthen voiding muscles

A decline in functional abilities increases the risk for urine incontinence.

▼ ▼ ▼

Procedure	Clinical Significance

Procedure

5. Medical history

Screen the person for medical explanations of bladder elimination problems:

- Urinary tract (system) infections

- Urinary tract obstructions—fecal impaction, masses, urinary calculi, prostatic hypertrophy
- Restricted mobility—may have medical causes such as arthritis, poor eyesight, Parkinson's disease
- Excessive urine production (polyuria) with the following medical causes—hypercalcemia, hyperglycemia, diabetes insipidus, congestive heart failure, low albumin

6. Medication history

Determine whether the person is taking medications that may produce side effects affecting urine elimination.

Medication

Anticholinergics
   Antihistamines
   Antidepressants
   Antipsychotics
   Antispasmodics

Sedatives
   Flurazepam
   Diazepam
   Alcohol

Diuretics
   Furosemide
   Ethacrynic acid
   Bumetanide

Alpha-Adrenergic Agents
   Decongestants
   Sympatholytics (*e.g.,* prazosin, terazosin, doxazosin)
Calcium Channel Blockers

Clinical Significance

Urinary tract infections may be associated with dysuria and urgency, making it difficult to get to the bathroom on time.

Urinary tract obstructions contribute to the development of urine retention, which may result in overflow incontinence.

Limited mobility is an aggravating or precipitating cause of incontinence.

Polyuria can lead to incontinence.

Effect on Urinary System

Anticholinergic side effects include urinary retention with associated urinary frequency and overflow incontinence.

Long-acting sedative agents may accumulate, especially in elders, causing confusion and secondary incontinence.

Loop diuretics cause fast diuresis that may overwhelm bladder capacity and lead to polyuria, frequency, and urgency. This may precipitate incontinence.

Alpha-adrenergics may decrease sphincter tone in the proximal urethra, contributing to the development of stress incontinence.

Calcium channel blockers may reduce smooth muscle contractility in the bladder, contributing to urinary retention and overflow incontinence.

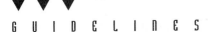

Assessment Guidelines   Diagnostic Studies of Elimination

Procedure

1. **Altered bowel elimination—common diagnostic studies**

   Note: A physician will usually determine the necessity for performing additional diagnostic studies of bowel function.

   - Plain abdominal radiograph (X-ray)—KUB

   - Barium enema—the instillation of barium, an x-ray contrast material, into the large intestine through the rectum, followed by the taking of x-ray images of the colon and rectum

   - Protosigmoidoscopy and colonoscopy—the examination of the anal canal, rectum, and colon through an endoscope inserted through the rectum, allowing visualization and biopsy of the colon mucosa and structures

2. **Tests of upper urinary tract function**

   Note: A physician will usually determine the necessity for performing additional diagnostic studies of the urinary system.

   Intravenous pyelogram (IVP)—The x-ray examination of the renal pelvis, ureters, and bladder. Dye is injected into the urinary system to make the structures opaque and visible on radiographic media.

3. **Tests of lower urinary tract function**

   a. Postvoid residual (PVR) volume

   Measurement of PVR volume is recommended for all persons with urinary incontinence.

   ### *Estimation Methods*

   Estimation of PVR volume can be made by abdominal palpation or percussion or bimanual evaluation. Bimanual evaluation requires palpation of the bladder by trapping the bladder between both of the examiner's hands. One hand is placed above the bladder on the abdominal surface, and the other hand is placed beneath the bladder, using a rectal approach.

Clinical Significance

Additional diagnostic studies may be performed for persons with altered bowel elimination to diagnose pathologic conditions contributing to bowel elimination changes.

A KUB may be obtained to determine the extent and distribution of feces throughout the colon in persons with constipation.

A barium enema may be obtained to determine the presence of various pathologic conditions of the bowel, including colorectal cancer, inflammatory bowel disease, polyps, and diverticula.

Endoscopic examination of the colon may be used to determine the presence of malignancies or inflammatory bowel disease, and to locate the source of lower gastrointestinal tract bleeding.

Abnormal dye retention in the bladder indicates bladder neck obstruction. Renal stones or calculi also may be visualized. Renal pathology also may be indicated by IVP studies.

Postvoid residual (PVR) volume: The amount of fluid remaining in the bladder immediately following the completion or urination. PVR volume is evaluated to determine the presence of urinary retention.

Clinical Interpretation of PVR Volumes

- Less than 50 mL—normal

- 50 to 199 mL—requires additional clinical interpretation of findings; additional clinical judgment is required to determine whether PVR volumes in this range are "normal" or "abnormal"

- Greater that 200 mL—abnormal

▼ ▼ ▼

Procedure

Specific Methods

Catheterization

Pelvic ultrasound

Radiographic studies

Radioisotope studies

Catheterization Method: A few minutes after voiding, a bladder catheterization is performed. The catheter is inserted, the bladder is drained of urine, and the catheter is removed (in-and-out catheterization). The amount of urine obtained by catheterization is measured and recorded as the PVR volume.

Portable Ultrasound Method: The bladder is scanned immediately after voiding with a portable ultrasound device to measure PVR volume. Specialized equipment and training is required for this method of measuring residual volumes.

b. Provocative Stress Testing

The person is instructed to cough vigorously while the examiner observes for urine loss from the urethra.

c. Cystometrogram

This test is performed by specially trained technicians. The person is instructed to void; the bladder is then catheterized and PVR volume measured. A special catheter that allows for pressure measurements is used for cystometric testing. The catheter is left in the bladder to complete the cystometrogram. Another catheter that measures abdominal pressure may be placed in the rectum or vagina.

During cystometric testing, sterile water may be instilled into the bladder via the catheter. A 50-mL, open-ended catheter-tip syringe is attached to the bladder catheter and held 15 cm above the pubic bone. Fifty-milliliter increments of sterile water are instilled into the bladder via gravity. The person is instructed to tell the technician when the first urge to urinate occurs, when the bladder feels full, and when it feels as though the bladder can hold no more. At this point, or after the instillation of 500 mL sterile water, the catheter may be removed, and the person may be asked to perform maneuvers causing increased pressure on the bladder and observed for urine leakage. The person is then asked to void, and the amount of fluid voided is measured. Various pressure/volume measurements are obtained throughout the procedure.

Clinical Significance

The catheterization method provides a specific quantitative measurement of PVR volume. In-and-out catheterization is an invasive procedure that may be uncomfortable and associated with infection risk. This method is not recommended in men with a history of prostatic obstruction because of the urethral trauma that might be caused by forcing a catheter through an obstructed urethra.

This method for assessing PVR volume is less invasive than catheterization. The initial cost of the ultrasound device may prohibit widespread use.

Provocative stress testing is a method of identifying stress incontinence by direct visualization of urine leakage from the urethra with maneuvers that will create pressure on the bladder, such as coughing. If leakage occurs with these maneuvers, a diagnosis of stress incontinence may be indicated.

The cystometrogram (cystometry) is a test used to assess bladder function by measuring the pressure/volume relationship of the bladder. The cystometrogram is used to evaluate detrusor activity, sensation, capacity, and compliance. There are different variations of the test, depending on the problem being investigated. However, the test always involves insertion of a catheter into the bladder.

Filling cystometrogram: Assesses pressure–volume relationships of the bladder during bladder filling and storage. Determines bladder capacity and the integrity of the urinary sphincters during physical stress. This test provides additional data to reveal mechanisms of stress incontinence.

Voiding cystometrogram: Provides assessment of detrusor contractility, voiding detrusor pressure, and the ability of the bladder to empty itself. Diminished voiding pressure indicates diminished detrusor contractility. Elevated voiding pressures may indicate an obstruction.

▼▼▼ ▼   ▼

Procedure

d. Electromyography

This test is performed simultaneously with the filling/voiding cystometrogram. Electrodes placed in the rectum or vagina measure the strength of muscle contraction during voiding.

e. Bulbocavernous Reflex

This test may be performed by simple physical examination methods. Prepare the person before performing this procedure by explaining what you are going to do. Many people find this procedure embarrassing, especially if there is no preparation. To perform the test, the examiner places a gloved finger in the person's rectum. With the finger in the rectum, the examiner then squeezes the glans penis of the male or the clitoris of the female. If the reflex is positive (present), the rectal sphincter will contract around the examiner's finger.

f. Pressure–Flow Study

The pressure flow study is performed immediately after the filling cystometrogram and simultaneously with the voiding cystometrogram. Multiple position changes may be required during this study (*e.g.,* standing, squatting, sitting).

Clinical Significance

Electromyography can be used to assess the electrical activity in the striated muscles of the pelvic floor involved in maintaining urinary continence and the electrical activity of the urinary sphincters. Elevated electromyographic activity of the urinary sphincter with voiding suggests inhibition of spontaneous voiding. This may explain a mechanism for urinary retention.

The bulbocavernous reflex is tested as part of a comprehensive evaluation of the lower urinary tract. The test is used to identify or rule out neurologic causes of urinary incontinence. A positive test indicates an intact sacral reflex arc and an intact voiding reflex.

A pressure–flow study involves simultaneous measurements of bladder pressure, electromyography, and urine flow. This study differentiates voiding problems due to an underactive detrusor muscle from those related to impaired innervation of urinary sphincters. It also can indicate whether an obstructive process is contributing to voiding problems.

Physical Examination   Stool Specimen Analysis

GENERAL APPROACH

Stool specimens may be observed in the patient care setting or further tested in the clinical laboratory by qualified technologists. In the patient care setting, stool is examined to describe general characteristics and volume. Testing stool for the presence of occult blood is also commonly conducted outside the clinical laboratory. Nurses should be cautioned that they may not have proper authorization to perform certain diagnostic testing of stool specimens at the bedside. Check with an agency's clinical laboratory before engaging in any diagnostic testing outside the clinical laboratory. Clinical laboratory analysis of stool is aimed at identifying and quantifying various substances such as fat, blood, organisms, and urobilinogen.

CLINICAL LABORATORY ANALYSIS OF STOOL

Fecal fat (normally < 7 g/24 h): Documents malabsorption of fat (steatorrhea). The principal site of fat absorption is the small intestine.

Occult blood (normally negative): Indicates hidden bleeding, especially in the bowel.

Ova and parasites (normally negative): Microscopic examination of the stool may show parasitic ova, cysts, larvae, or trophozites. A positive test indicates infestation of the intestinal tract.

(continued)

Physical Examination   Stool Specimen Analysis (continued)

Stool culture (usually shows normal flora): Indicates the nature of pathogenic organisms.

Fecal urobilinogen (normally 10 to 250 IU/100 g): Indicates hemolytic anemia (indicated by higher values) and biliary obstruction (indicated by lower values).

SPECIMEN COLLECTION

Stool collected for cultures must be delivered to the laboratory while still warm, usually within 30 minutes of collection, to avoid overgrowth of normal resident organisms and obscuring of abnormal organisms such as parasites.

If the stool is being cultured for organisms such as bacteria, parasites, or viruses, three consecutive stool samples may be evaluated, because organisms may not be passed with every stool.

Stool collected for chemical analysis should be refrigerated if immediate delivery to the laboratory is not possible.

Specimens should be placed in a clean container and covered. Wax-lined containers should not be used for stools being analyzed for fat content because wax can interfere with results.

The specimen container does not need to be filled unless the stool will undergo chemical analysis, in which case quantity is important. For example, fecal fat analysis involves determining the fat content of all stools excreted for a particular period, such as 24 hours.

BARIUM EFFECT

Barium is a radiopaque compound instilled into the lower bowel during certain x-ray studies and eventually excreted through the stool.

Barium in the stool will not interfere with most cultures, provided a relatively large stool sample is obtained.

Barium will interfere with cultures for parasites.

EXAMINATION AND DOCUMENTATION FOCUS

Color
Consistency and shape
Volume
Odor
Composition

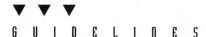

GUIDELINES

Assessment Guidelines   Stool

Procedure

1. **Observe the color of the stool.**

Clinical Significance

Normal Findings

Stool is light or dark brown as a result of the pigments stercobilin and urobilin, which are derived from the breakdown of bilirubin in the intestine. Certain foods and medications may alter normal color.

Dark brown to black: Indicates presence of iron pigments from large amounts of meat protein or iron-containing drugs.

Black: Indicates ingestion of licorice, anti-inflammatory drugs such as phenylbutazone and oxyphenbutazone, or bismuth compounds such as Pepto-Bismol.

▼ ▼ ▼

G U I D E L I N E S *continued*   Stool

Procedure

If food and drugs are ruled out as the reason for altered stool color, other causes should be investigated. Consultation with a physician may be indicated if any of the following colors are noted: black, maroon, gray, tan, clay, or yellow.

2. **Note the consistency and shape of stool.**

3. **Determine the volume of stool excreted with each bowel movement and in a 24-hour period.**

Clinical Significance

Green: Indicates ingestion of spinach or senna laxatives. In children and infants, green stools indicate rapid transit of food through the bowel.

White or gray: Indicates ingestion of barium or drugs containing aluminum hydroxide, such as Amphojel.

Red: Indicates ingestion of beets or cocoa.

Deviations from Normal

Black or maroon: May indicate bleeding in the gastrointestinal tract. Blackened stool may also be tarry (melena).

Gray, tan, or clay: May indicate that bile, which contains bilirubin, is not being adequately produced or distributed, perhaps due to biliary tract obstruction.

Yellow: May indicate excess fat in the stool, secondary to fat malabsorption syndromes.

Normal Findings

Stools are usually soft because they are 75% water, and are tubular in shape like the rectum.

Deviations from Normal

Hard, nodular stools, which may be excreted as small, rocklike masses, may be the result of constipation or spastic colon. Fluid or mushy stools usually occur with diarrhea and may appear greasy because the fat content is high, perhaps secondary to fat malabsorption syndromes. Fat-infiltrated stools often float in the toilet because fat is light and buoyant. Stools that are narrow, flat, or ribbon-like, rather than tubular, may indicate rectal obstruction or spastic colitis. Such obstructions may be secondary to tumors, strictures, or hemorrhoids.

Normal Findings

A person who eats a healthy diet usually excretes an average stool volume of 100 to 200 g/day. Not all people who ingest healthy diets defecate on a daily basis.

Deviations from Normal

Excessive volumes of watery stool may be noted with diarrhea. Low volumes are usually associated with constipation or prolonged fasting.

▼ ▼ ▼

G U I D E L I N E S *continued*   Stool

Procedure

4. **Note the odor of the stool.**

5. **Note the composition of the stool.**

Clinical Significance

Normal Findings

Stool odor varies and is influenced by diet. Odors occur secondary to bacterial action in the colon. A sour odor may be noted in the stool of infants.

Deviations from Normal

Distinct changes in fecal odor are noted when stools contain excessive fat or blood. Cancers that invade the rectum or colon may cause a putrid or decaying odor.

Normal Findings

Stool is normally composed of 75% water. The remaining dry matter consists of food residues, such as cellulose, fats, and proteins; bacteria (*E. coli*); inorganic salts; and residues from intestinal juices, such as pigments, and sloughed epithelial cells.

Deviations from Normal

Blood, mucus, parasites and foreign objects are not normal fecal constituents.

Bright red *blood* throughout the feces may indicate lower intestinal bleeding. Blood on the stool surface or on toilet paper may indicate rectal or anal canal bleeding, commonly caused by hemorrhoids and anal fissures. Occult blood is small quantities of blood in the stool that is not visible to the naked eye. Occult blood may be a sign of cancer or ulceration of the intestinal tract and requires further evaluation.

Mucus, although not always an abnormal finding, may be a sign of bowel inflammation. Mucus, diarrhea stools may be observed in ulcerative colitis, an inflammatory disease of the colon.

Parasites, including nematodes (roundworms) and tapeworms, may be visible on close examination of the stool. However, the ova and larvae of these organisms may be visible only with a microscope. Other microscopic organisms that may be excreted in the stool include protozoa and helminths.

Foreign objects, deliberately or accidentally ingested, may be found in the feces. This finding is most common in children.

▼ ▼ ▼

GUIDELINES *continued*   Stool

Procedure

6. **If indicated, test the stool for occult blood (guaiac test).**

   a. Properly prepare the patient.

   Diet Instructions: For testing conducted at home, instruct the person to alter diet 3 days before and during testing. Diet restrictions include all meat products, horseradish, and turnips. Before testing, the person should ingest high-residue foods such as raw vegetables, bran products, and nuts.

   Medication Instructions: Drugs may cause erroneous test results. If possible, anti-inflammatory preparations, steroids, or broad-spectrum antibiotics should not be taken before the stool is tested.

   Assess the patient's understanding of the procedures because this test often must be repeated several times at home.

   b. Assemble the necessary supplies. Presently, several commercial products are available. Stool is applied to specially prepared slides or filter paper and treated with a chemical solution that causes a color change.

   c. Apply a small stool specimen to slide or filter paper.

   d. Allow specimen to dry.

   e. Apply the required amount of developing solution to the slide or filter paper. Commercially prepared guaiac solution is commonly used.

   f. Wait the recommended time and read test results. The results should be read precisely 30 seconds after the solution is applied if commercially prepared guaiac slides are used.

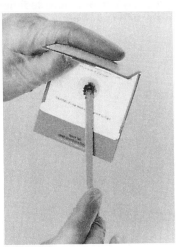

Stool application to guaiac slide

Clinical Significance

This test is an important screening procedure for detecting gastrointestinal bleeding, which may indicate colon cancer or ulcer disease.

This test is based on detecting peroxidase activity in the hemoglobin molecule. Peroxidases in these foods can result in false-positive results.

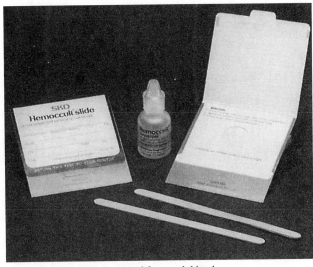

Commercial kit for testing stool for occult blood

Normal Findings

A negative result is indicated by no color change or a green color change, depending on the test.

Deviations from Normal

If occult blood is present, a blue ring will form around the stool specimen, indicating a positive result. A positive result should be followed by physician consultation. In addition, the test should be repeated several times to rule out a false-negative result or to detect intermittent bleeding.

Documenting Stool Examination Findings

Several descriptors may be used to document stool characteristics. The color, consistency and shape, and composition should be documented. The presence of occult blood revealed by guaiac testing is charted "guaiac positive." A sample documentation for a normal stool may be as follows: "Excreted soft, formed, brown stool on commode. Guaiac negative."

Descriptors for Documenting Stool Characteristics

	Normal Findings	Deviations from Normal
Color	Brown, tan, green-yellow	Black, maroon, bloody, white
Consistency and Shape	Soft, formed	Loose, liquid, hard, nodular, rocklike, stringy, greasy
Composition	No foreign particles	Blood, mucus, parasites, undigested food, guaiac positive

Physical Examination Urine Specimen Analysis

GENERAL APPROACH

Urine may be evaluated by inspection and smell or by clinical laboratory analysis. In the patient care setting, urine is observed for general appearance, odor, and volume, including voided volumes and residual volumes. Evaluation of urine volumes is especially relevant to the evaluation of urinary incontinence. Commercially prepared dipsticks may be used in the patient care setting to determine various urine constituents, pH, and specific gravity. Dipsticks are commercially prepared plastic sticks that register color changes when dipped into a fresh urine sample. The resulting color changes are compared with a standard reference to quantify various urine constituents. Nurses should be cautioned that they may not have proper authorization to perform certain urine tests (including dipstick tests) at the bedside. Check with an agency's clinical laboratory before engaging in any diagnostic testing outside the clinical laboratory. Clinical laboratory testing of urine is aimed at identifying and quantifying various substances, organisms, pH, and specific gravity.

SPECIMEN COLLECTION

Urine specimens to be used in analytic tests or cultures should be clean-catch, midstream specimens.

Urine that is sent to the clinical laboratory should be refrigerated to slow bacterial growth or decomposition and should be analyzed within 1 hour.

Urine for analysis should never be collected from the bottom of a catheter drainage bag, because the urine will probably contain more sediment and be contaminated with bacteria, thereby distorting test results.

EXAMINATION AND DOCUMENTATION FOCUS

Color
Transparency
Odor
Volume
Specific gravity
pH
Cells, casts, and crystals
Electrolytes

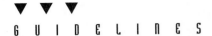

GUIDELINES

Assessment Guidelines Urine

Procedure	Clinical Significance

Procedure

1. **Observe the color of the urine.**

2. **Observe transparency of urine.**

3. **Note odor of the urine.**

Clinical Significance

Normal Findings
The normal color of urine ranges from pale to dark yellow because of the pigment urochrome. The variation in color reflects the urine concentration and the foods and drugs ingested. The normal color variations include pale yellow, colorless, bright yellow, yellow-orange, yellow-green, red, red-pink, and blue-green.

Pale yellow to colorless: Indicates urine is diluted because of increased fluid intake.

Bright yellow: May indicate ingestion of drugs such as acriflavine mepacrine, nitrofurantoin, and large doses of riboflavin.

Yellow-orange: Indicates ingestion of the drug phenazopyridine (Pyridium).

Yellow-green: Indicates ingestion of rhubarb.

Red: Indicates ingestion of beets or candies containing fuscin dye.

Red-pink: Indicates ingestion of phenolphthalein, a constituent of many over-the-counter laxatives.

Blue-green: Indicates ingestion of drugs containing the dye methylene blue.

Deviations from Normal
Colorless: Kidneys may not be concentrating the urine, as occurs in diabetes insipidus.

Yellow-orange: May indicate liver or gallbladder disease. Color changes are secondary to excess urobilin or bilirubin pigments.

Red, reddish brown, or brown-black: May indicate the presence of hemoglobin and be caused by trauma to urinary structures, reactions to blood transfusion, or lysis of red blood cells.

Brown to black: Indicates Addison's disease. The color change is due to urinary excretion of melanin.

Whitish cast: May represent bacteria or cell products of an inflammatory response (polymorphonuclear neutrophil leukocytes, or PMNs).

Normal Findings
Freshly voided urine is normally clear. Refrigerated urine or urine that is allowed to stand may become turbid as bacteria ferments. Urine contaminated with sperm or menstrual blood may appear cloudy.

Deviations from Normal
Cloudy urine (also called turbid urine) indicates the presence of abnormal cells or constituents such as excessive white blood cells (WBCs), calculi, pus, bacteria, or fats. In such cases, sediment may form at the bottom of the specimen container.

Normal Findings
Urine is normally aromatic. Ingestion of multivitamins or vitamin B may cause a strong, sharp odor. Eating asparagus may give the urine a grasslike odor.

▼ ▼ ▼

G U I D E L I N E S *continued*   Urine

Procedure

4. **Measure volume of urine using a container calibrated in milliliters.**

   a. Determine the postvoid residual (PVR) volume, if indicated. Encourage the person to void and record the voided volume, then catheterize the bladder immediately and record the amount of urine obtained. This is the postvoid residual volume. Amounts greater than 50 mL may be abnormal. The evaluation of PVR volume is discussed elsewhere (see "Diagnostic Studies of Elimination").

   b. Determine bladder capacity, if indicated.
      Bladder capacity is the volume determined by adding the voided volume to the PVR volume.

5. **Determine the urine specific gravity using a dipstick.**

Clinical Significance

Deviations from Normal

An acetone odor indicates ketosis resulting from diabetic ketoacidosis and other starvation states. If the urine has an ammonia scent, the probable cause is infection, especially by *Proteus,* a bacterium capable of splitting urea into ammonia by-products. A smell of decay indicates infection and results from bacterial cell death. A musty odor is associated with phenylketonuria (PKU). A fecal odor indicates the existence of a rectal fistula.

Normal Findings

Normally 1200 to 1500 mL of urine is voided per day. Greater amounts may be voided if there is excessive fluid intake. Normally, the bladder can store 300 to 600 mL of urine before voiding becomes essential. Usually urine is not retained in the bladder after voiding.

Deviations from Normal

Oliguria: In oliguria, less than 500 mL of urine is voided per day. The cause may be an elimination problem such as urine retention in the bladder or pathologic conditions related to urine production in the kidney. Determining PVR volume (urine drained from the bladder by a catheter immediately after voiding) may help differentiate these oliguric states. Oliguria secondary to renal pathology usually does not result in significant residual volumes. However, if bladder function is impaired, which can occur when infection interferes with normal muscular contraction of the bladder muscles or when the bladder outlet is obstructed, then high residual volumes may be noted. Residual volumes exceeding 50 mL are generally considered abnormal.

Polyuria: Polyuria refers to urine volumes of 2500 mL or greater per day, which may occur with diuretic therapy, endocrine dysfunction, or renal pathology. Cerebral pathology may undermine the influence of antidiuretic hormone (ADH), leading to increased urine production. The diuretic phase of renal failure also may be associated with large urine volumes.

Deviations from Normal

A bladder capacity greater than 1000 mL may indicate urinary retention.

Specific gravity is a measurement of urine density, a product of the volume of urine produced by the kidneys and the amount of particulate matter in the urine. Specific gravity indicates whether urine is diluted or concentrated.

Normal Findings

The normal adult range for specific gravity is 1.003 to 1.030, with the higher number representing more concentrated urine. The normal range for elderly people is between 1.016 and 1.022 because the ability to concentrate urine decreases with age.

▼ ▼ ▼
G U I D E L I N E S   *continued*   Urine
_____

Procedure

Clinical Significance

Deviations from Normal
Urine specific gravity may be lowered with excessive urine production after increased fluid intake or ingestion of diuretic medications.

Deviations from Normal
Increased urine specific gravity indicates decreased urine volume or an increased amount of particulate matter in the urine. The latter condition may be related to excessive glucose or protein, as in uncontrolled diabetes mellitus and nephrotic syndrome.

Decreased urine specific gravity occurs with diabetes insipidus, acute renal failure, water intoxication, and severe hypokalemia.

6. **Determine the urine pH using a dipstick.**

Normal Findings
Urine is slightly acid with a normal pH of 5 to 7. A high intake of meat protein or foods such as cranberry juice may acidify the urine further. Urine that is tested early in the morning may be more acidic because a mild respiratory acidosis occurs during sleep, and the kidneys compensate by excreting more hydrogen ions. A more alkaline pH is noted in urine that is allowed to stand before it is tested. The bacterial action and the loss of carbon dioxide cause the urine to lose its acidity. Vegetarian diets also may cause alkaline urine.

Deviations from Normal
Increased alkalinity is noted with bacterial infections that are caused by organisms that split urea, such as *Proteus* and *Pseudomonas*. A more alkaline urine also occurs with respiratory alkalosis, because the kidneys attempt to compensate by excreting more bicarbonate ions, and with renal diseases such as chronic glomerulonephritis and renal tubular acidosis.

Increased acidity results from metabolic or respiratory acidosis because the kidneys excrete more hydrogen ions from the body, and from electrolyte disturbances such as hypokalemia and hypochloremia.

7. **Examine the urine for cells, casts, and crystals.**
Cells, casts, and crystals are detected by microscopic urine examination in the clinical laboratory but may be visible on gross inspection when large quantities are present.

Normal Findings
Cells normally found in the urine include white blood cells (WBCs), red blood cells (RBCs), and epithelial cells from sloughing of dead cells in the urinary system. In normal urine, WBCs are more numerous than RBCs, with four or five WBCs and two or three RBCs per high-power field. WBCs are more abundant in the urine of females.

Casts are molded elements formed by cellular or fibrous accumulations in urinary structures. Although casts are usually considered pathologic, an occasional hyaline cast may appear in normal urine. For example, hyaline casts may be observed in urine after strenuous exercise or diuretic therapy as well as in pathologic states such as inflammatory renal disease, but are usually considered normal if few in number and in the absence of other casts.

▼ ▼ ▼

Procedure

8. **Determine the electrolyte composition of the urine, using a dipstick.**

Clinical Significance

Crystals are normally formed in the urine, and the type of crystal formed is pH dependent. In acid urine, calcium oxalate, uric acid, and urate crystals may be present; in alkaline urine, phosphate and carbonate crystals may be noted. Although considered a normal finding, crystals indicate urinary calculi (stones).

Deviations from Normal

Cells: An increased amount of epithelial cells indicates renal tubule disease and associated cell necrosis. An increased amount of RBCs is associated with systemic bleeding disorders such as overcoagulation; renal disease and renal trauma, including trauma from Foley catheters; and lower urinary tract pathology, including strictures, calculi, and bladder infections. An increased WBC count is found in most renal and urinary tract diseases. Bacteria are noted in urinary tract infections and in specimens contaminated by anal or vaginal excretions.

Abnormal casts are classified according to cell type and formation. Aside from the hyaline cast, the presence of casts in urine is abnormal and usually indicates renal pathology.

Crystals that contain cystine, tyrosine, or leucine are abnormal and may form large calculi that usually interfere with normal urinary elimination.

Normal Findings

Normal urine should not contain glucose, ketones, or proteins.

Deviations from Normal

Glucose, ketones, and proteins in the urine are always abnormal. Proteinuria indicates kidney glomeruli damage. Glucosuria usually occurs secondary to hyperglycemic conditions such as diabetes mellitus (uncontrolled), and endocrine and liver disorders. Additionally, renal disease may prevent proper glucose reabsorption in the renal tubules and may cause glucose to spill into the urine. Ketones usually appear in the urine when the body breaks down fats for energy, as in starvation states, diabetes mellitus, vomiting and diarrhea, and conditions that increase the basal metabolic rate.

NDx

Documenting Urine Examination Findings

To document urine characteristics, note the color, transparency, odor, and volume. Dipstick results are charted + or −, depending on whether a particular component is detected. Positive values are occasionally given a number to indicate magnitude, for example, "glucose, 4+."

Descriptors for Documenting Urine Characteristics

	Normal Findings	*Deviations from Normal*
Color	Straw, amber, yellow	Red, brown, orange, bloody
Transparency	Clear	Cloudy, sediment (specify color, *e.g.*, white, brown)
Odor	Aromatic	Ketosis, ammonia, fecal
Volume	1200–1500 mL/day	Anuria, oliguria, polyuria

▼ ▼ ▼
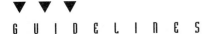
G U I D E L I N E S

Procedure

Integrate physical examination findings into the overall assessment of elimination, with special attention to the following:

- General appearance
- Abdomen
- Genitourinary structures
- Anus and rectum
- The neurologic system

(Note: Complete examination guidelines are presented elsewhere in this chapter for the anus and rectum.)

1. **General appearance**

    Observe the person's general appearance and note whether there are any indicators of elimination problems or related risk factors.

    Note signs of stool or urine incontinence.

    Determine the status of functional abilities, including mobility, transfer ability, manual dexterity, vision, and hearing.

    Evaluate the appearance of the skin, especially in the perineal area, for any person with bowel or bladder incontinence.

2. **Abdomen**

    (Note: Techniques for abdominal examination are discussed in Chap. 6.)

    Observe the abdomen for signs of bladder distention. An enlarged bladder may be observed by inspection, palpation, or percussion. An enlarged bladder may be tender with palpation.

    Note general indicators of constipation, including abdominal distention, diminished bowel sounds, or palpable stool in the colon.

3. **Genitourinary structures**

    (Note: Techniques for genitourinary structure examination are presented in Chap. 13.)

    Inspect and palpate genitourinary structures to determine the functional status of structures involved in voiding.

    Conduct a pelvic examination in women to assess perineal skin condition, genital atrophy, pelvic prolapse (cystocele, rectocele, uterine prolapse), and perivaginal muscle tone, and to estimate PVR volume using the bimanual approach.

Clinical Significance

Some observations made during the physical examination may indicate problems with elimination. A physical examination may also be conducted to further evaluate a known elimination problem, such as urinary incontinence or constipation.

Incontinence may be indicated by distinctive odors, the presence of incontinence pads, or appliances such as external catheters. The use of strong perfumes might indicate an attempt to mask offensive odors.

Independence in toileting self-care activities is evaluated by considering the status of functional abilities.

There is a high risk for impaired skin integrity with stool or urine incontinence.

Bladder distention indicates urine retention.

The abdomen may be palpated to provide a crude estimate of postvoid residual (PVR) volume.

Alterations in genitourinary structures may contribute to elimination problems.

A pelvic examination is indicated in women with stress incontinence of urine to evaluate the pelvic muscle tone.

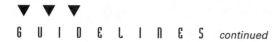

Procedure

Inspect the vaginal mucosa and note any dryness, redness, or thinning that would indicate atrophic vaginitis (hypo-estrogenic vaginitis).

Palpate the anterior vaginal wall and urethra and observe for any urethral discharge or tenderness.

4. Anus and rectum

Examine the rectum to test for perineal sensation, sphincter tone, bulbocavernous reflex, fecal impaction, and rectal mass, and to evaluate the consistency and contour of the prostate gland in males.

5. Neurologic system

Observe level of consciousness and cognitive status.

Test sacral reflexes and perineal sensation.

Clinical Significance

Abnormalities in urethral sphincter tone in women have been attributed to diminished levels of estrogen. The urethral sphincter cannot be directly visualized. However, the vaginal mucosa is also effected by estrogens and can be directly observed.

Discharge or tenderness of these structures may indicate infection or other inflammatory process.

These are the aspects of the rectal examination most relevant to diagnosing and managing elimination problems.

Impaired mental status is a risk factor for incontinence and potential problems with self-toileting.

Reflex testing provides an indication of the status of neurologic processes involved in elimination.

Nursing Diagnoses Related to Bowel Elimination Assessment

Constipation

Constipation is defined as "a state in which an individual experiences a change in normal bowel habits characterized by a decrease in frequency or passage of hard, dry stools." Causes include change in lifestyle, immobility, and painful defecation.

The defining characteristics for constipation include decreased activity level; less frequent defecation than usual; hard, formed stools; palpable mass; a reported feeling of rectal pressure; a reported feeling of rectal fullness; and straining to defecate. Additional defining characteristics include abdominal pain; appetite impairment; back pain; headache; interference with daily living; and laxative use.

Constipation may be classified as Perceived constipation or Colonic constipation. Perceived constipation occurs when the person makes a self-diagnosis of constipation and treats himself or herself with laxatives to assure a daily bowel movement. Colonic constipation refers to a bowel elimination pattern characterized by hard, dry stool.

Constipation Related to Change in Lifestyle

History. Changes in a person's lifestyle may impair the response to the normal defecation reflex. Significant

lifestyle changes include situations that cause or interfere with usual bowel elimination habits, such as travel or schedule changes, and the use of laxatives or drugs that decrease colonic motility. Inactivity also may contribute to constipation. In addition, many disease processes can alter lifestyle and bowel function. The person's chief complaint will often be infrequent stools rather than lifestyle changes. Consequently, you need to initiate a thorough nursing history.

Physical Examination. The rectal examination may indicate a palpable fecal impaction. Abdominal distension may be noted, and it may be accompanied by restlessness and an increase in flatulence.

Stool. The stool may be hard, dry, and formed. Stool size may vary.

Constipation Related to Immobility

History. A decrease in mobility is associated with decreased peristaltic activity and loss of muscle strength, both of which contribute to constipation. Hospitalization often limits mobility because of enforced bed rest and restricted activity resulting from the presence of tubes, intravenous lines, and other equipment used in therapy. The person may report infrequent, hard stools.

Physical Examination and Stool. See "Constipation Related to Change in Lifestyle," above.

Constipation Related to Painful Defecation

History. Painful defecation may lead to a pattern of ignoring the defecation reflex. Hemorrhoids may be the cause of this discomfort. Severe abdominal cramping may also make defecation painful. The person may report infrequent stools, rectal itching, and straining during defecation.

Physical Examination. The anorectal examination may show conditions that cause painful defecation. Anal fissures or hemorrhoids may be visible or indicated by extreme pain when the anal canal is palpated. Further assess the rectum for other causes of painful defecation, such as prostatic enlargement, abscesses, and fecal impactions. The perineum may be excoriated.

Stool. The stool is often hard and dry. If lesions such as hemorrhoids are present, the stool may be streaked with bright red blood. The stool may be narrow if rectal masses or colonic dysfunction exists. Stools should be assessed for occult blood.

Diarrhea

Diarrhea is defined as "a state in which an individual experiences a change in normal bowel habits characterized by the frequent passage of loose, fluid, unformed stools." Diarrhea may result from infectious processes affecting the gastrointestinal tract, nutritional and malabsorption disorders, changes in lifestyle, drug side effects, and bowel surgery.

The defining characteristics for diarrhea include abdominal pain; cramping; increased frequency; increased frequency of bowel sounds; loose, liquid stools; and urgency.

History. Diarrhea results from hyperperistalsis of the small intestine or colon. Because diarrhea is a manifestation of more than 100 clinical entities, determining the probable cause may be difficult. Investigate factors associated with infectious processes, obstructive neoplasms, ulcerative colitis, Crohn's disease, and malabsorption syndromes. The person may report frequent, loose, or watery stools, defecation usually more than three times per day, or pain and abdominal cramping with defecation. Loss of fluid and electrolytes accounts for complaints of weakness.

Physical Examination. Observable signs of dehydration include poor skin turgor, increased body temperature, hypotension, and weight loss. The rectal examination may show marked tenderness or a mass such as fecal impaction or tumor. Rectal examination with a proctoscope by a physician may show changes in the mucosal lining of the sigmoid colon that are characteristic of inflammatory diseases such as ulcerative colitis. Bowel sounds are usually hyperactive.

Stool. The stool may be liquid or mushy. Stool color, odor, and composition may indicate the probable cause.

Bowel Incontinence

Bowel incontinence is defined as the involuntary passage of stool. Causative factors include conditions that impair neuromuscular function of the colon, rectum, and anal sphincters. Cognitive and perceptual impairment also may be a contributing factor.

History. A person who is alert and oriented may not report fecal incontinence because of embarrassment. Therefore, you should ask questions during the interview

to elicit this information and to ascertain how frequently the incontinence occurs and to identify contributing factors such as neurologic lesions or mental confusion. Question the person about factors relating to constipation, because fecal impaction is one of the most common causes of fecal incontinence.

Physical Examination. The rectal examination can provide information about muscle tone and sphincter strength. A fecal impaction may be palpated. A prolapsed anus or other rectal masses may contribute to incontinence. General muscle strength also should be assessed, although a weak and debilitated person may not have the strength to contract anal sphincters. Skin excoriation may be noted around the anus and buttocks.

Stool. Stool consistency may range from formed to liquid. The appearance of the stool may help determine probable causes of incontinence.

NDx

Clinical Problems Related to Bowel Elimination Assessment

Inflammatory and Infectious Processes

Examination of the anus, rectum, and stool may indicate inflammatory or infectious bowel or rectal disease, in which case the patient should be referred to a physician. Additional assessment, including stool analysis and culture, x-ray, and proctoscopic examination, may be necessary. Understanding the signs and symptoms of certain pathologic conditions that affect bowel function will help you monitor the patient's response to the disease process and treatment.

Ulcerative Colitis. This inflammatory disease, of unknown cause, affects the colon and rectum. Bloody, mucoid diarrhea with as many as 30 stools per day usually indicates ulcerative colitis. Defecation may be painful and is often accompanied by abdominal cramping and rectal tenesmus. The rectal mucosa usually becomes inflamed and may bleed easily. Signs of fluid and electrolyte depletion, including weight loss, fever, weakness, and fatigability, also may be present. This disease may involve a series of remissions and exacerbations.

Crohn's Disease. Also called regional enteritis, this inflammatory bowel disease can be easily confused with ulcerative colitis because it is also characterized by remissions, exacerbations, abdominal cramping, and diarrhea. Crohn's disease may affect the small or large intestine. The lesion it causes on the intestinal wall differs from the lesion caused by ulcerative colitis. In the early stages, abdominal cramping occurs, usually aggravated by constipation and relieved by a bowel movement. In later stages, exacerbations are characterized by colicky pain in the right lower abdominal quadrant, fever, and abdominal tenderness. Diarrheal stools may occur. The disease invades the bowel mucosa, increasing the risk of fistula formation. Lesions of the anus, anal canal, and rectum are common.

Acute Gastroenteritis. This disease also may be characterized by diarrheal stools caused by pathogens that invade the intestinal tract. The pathogens may be viral, bacterial, or parasitic. Often the disease is self-limiting and will resolve spontaneously within 72 hours. Stool cultures may show the causative organism. The patient may appear ill; fever, signs of dehydration, and abdominal cramping often accompany attacks. Rectal examination results are usually normal, but diarrheal stools may cause skin excoriation.

Diverticulitis. This inflammatory process may occur when small pouches, called diverticula, form in the colon and are irritated by feces. The person's bowel elimination pattern may be characterized predominantly by constipation, occasionally alternating with diarrhea. Abdominal pain is usually relieved by a bowel movement. Stool testing will show occult blood in 20% of cases. Diverticula may bleed, resulting in massive gastrointestinal hemorrhage.

Malabsorption Syndromes

Malabsorption syndromes involve impaired absorption of fats, proteins, or carbohydrates across the intestinal wall. Malabsorption occurs to some extent with any condition causing rapid intestinal transit and diarrheal stools, as in Crohn's disease and acute gastroenteritis. Common malabsorption syndromes include celiac disease and nontropical sprue. People suffering from these diseases are unable to digest gluten and gliadin, proteins found mainly in wheat. Stools are high in fat content (steatorrhea), appear foamy, and may float. Diarrhea usually occurs as nonabsorbed substances pull excessive water into the bowel, causing distention and hyperperistalsis. The person may lose weight and become malnourished.

Hemorrhage

Gross or occult blood in stools is associated with gastrointestinal hemorrhage from diverse causes such as peptic ulcer disease, ulcerative colitis, diverticulosis, tumors, or hemorrhoids. Stools may become liquid if large amounts of blood enter the colon. Melena or black, tarry stools may be noted when bleeding originates in the small intestine. A maroon stool may indicate bleeding in the colon. Bright red blood within the stool or streaking on the outside surface is associated with bleeding in the lower sigmoid colon, rectum, and anal canal.

Irritable Bowel Syndrome

Irritable bowel syndrome (IBS), or spastic colon, is considered an elusive entity. It is characterized by recurrent abdominal pain and altered bowel elimination patterns. Although there appears to be intestinal motor dysfunction, no bowel pathology is found. Symptoms vary among people and in the same person from one time to another. Most people with this disorder have two or three of the six cardinal symptoms of IBS:

1. Relief of pain with defecation
2. Onset of pain associated with more frequent defecation
3. Onset of pain associated with looser stools
4. Distention of the abdomen
5. Rectal dissatisfaction (feeling of incomplete evacuation)
6. Passage of mucus with stools

Hyperplastic Growths

Colon and Rectum Cancer. The likelihood of developing colon or rectum cancer increases between the ages of 40 and 60 years. If the condition is detected early, 90% of patients respond favorably to treatment. Often the earliest sign is a change in the bowel elimination pattern, either diarrhea or constipation. At later stages, rectal bleeding, abdominal pain and distention, general malaise, and weight loss may be noted. Most rectosigmoid tumors are palpable during the rectal examination. The tumor is usually a hard, firmly embedded mass that may have an irregular border. Palpation of the mass rarely causes pain. The stool usually contains occult blood. Persons with a palpable rectal mass should be referred to a physician.

Prostate Cancer. Men older than age 60 are at highest risk for prostate cancer. Initially, the patient may notice prostatic hyperplasia symptoms, including hesitancy and straining with urination, dribbling, and a decreased caliber of the urinary stream. Urine retention may occur as the enlarging prostate obstructs the bladder outlet. Rectal examination may indicate a hard, fixed, enlarged prostate gland. Nodular masses may be palpable.

Nursing Diagnoses Related to Urinary Elimination Assessment

Altered Urinary Elimination

Altered urinary elimination is defined as a state in which the individual experiences a disturbance in urine elimination. The signs and symptoms include dysuria, frequency, hesitancy, incontinence, nocturia, retention, and urgency. Among the most common causes of altered urinary elimination is a lower urinary tract infection.

Stress Incontinence

Stress incontinence refers to the involuntary leakage of small amounts of urine (less then 50 mL) during momentary episodes of increased intraabdominal pressure. The following are contributing factors:

1. Loss of the normal urethrovesical angle or muscular support structures, such as from multiple births, pregnancy, pelvic tumors, or obesity
2. Weak sphincter tone due to childbirth or prolonged bladder catheterization

Assessment. Stress incontinence is more common in postmenopausal women and is associated with activities such as coughing, sneezing, lifting heavy objects, and climbing stairs. The amount of urine lost with each incontinent episode is variable. The pelvic examination may show cystocele or uterine prolapse.

Reflex Incontinence

Reflex incontinence refers to incontinence related to a permanent neurologic lesion that causes voiding to be controlled by spinal cord reflex. The incontinent episodes occur at relatively predictable intervals, when a specific bladder volume is reached. It may occur in the following conditions:

1. When messages between the spinal cord reflex arc and brain are interrupted, such as in spinal cord injury or multiple sclerosis
2. When the spinal cord reflex is inappropriately inhibited or not inhibited, as in cerebral pathology, including cerebrovascular accident (CVA), tumors, or organic brain syndrome

Assessment. Predictable voiding patterns are usually noted. Voiding may be initiated by maneuvers that stimulate the reflex arc, including tapping the abdomen above the symphysis pubis, stroking the inner thigh, and pulling the penis or pubic hair. Residual urine volumes may be high.

Urge Incontinence

Urge incontinence refers to involuntary urination that occurs immediately after a strong sensation to void. Urgency results from the following conditions:

1. Irritation of bladder stretch receptors, through infection, concentrated urine, or neuropathies
2. Severe reduction of bladder capacity, which may occur secondary to severe pelvic inflammatory disease or prolonged bladder drainage by an indwelling Foley catheter. The pressure of the uterus during pregnancy may also decrease bladder capacity.
3. Increased urine production, such as from diuretic therapy

Assessment. The urine elimination pattern is usually characterized by urgency, frequency, and bladder spasm. Continence may be maintained if the person is able to reach toilet facilities quickly. If infection is the contributing factor, dysuria may accompany voiding. Urine analysis and culture may indicate bacterial growth.

Functional Incontinence

Functional incontinence refers to the involuntary and unpredictable loss of urine. There is no warning sign such as urgency. This condition usually occurs because the person cannot reach bathroom facilities in time. People in unfamiliar environments and people with cognitive or motor deficits are at greatest risk.

Total Incontinence

Total incontinence, or uncontrolled incontinence, refers to an unpredictable or continuous urine loss. The following are contributing factors:

1. Loss of voluntary control mechanisms, such as occurs with cerebral pathologic conditions such as CVA, tumors, or organic brain syndrome
2. Loss of neuronal control in pathways to the bladder, such as with severance or destruction of motor and sensory neurons below the voiding reflex arc (surgery, trauma)
3. Fistula formation

Assessment. Constant bladder flow may accompany total incontinence. The elimination pattern also may be

characterized by urinary frequency, urgency, and nocturia. Incontinence is usually obvious unless a catheter or other appliance is used. Skin integrity is often impaired if urine comes in contact with the skin. Bladder capacity is usually decreased. Residual urine may not be observed.

Urinary Retention

Urinary retention refers to the inability to completely empty the bladder and may occur in the following conditions:

1. Hypotonic bladder (bladder muscle atrophy)
   a. Lesions affecting the motor roots of the S2–S4 spinal cord, such as occur with poliomyelitis, Guillain-Barré syndrome, trauma, or tumor
   b. Lesions affecting the sensory roots of the S2–S4 spinal cord, such as occur in diabetes mellitus
2. Strong sphincter tone, which is induced by drugs such as antihistamines and psychotropics
3. Urethral obstruction from prostatic hypertrophy, surgical swelling, fecal impaction, or vaginal and rectal packs

Assessment. When urine is retained in the bladder, the lower abdomen over the symphysis pubis may become distended. Urine output is significantly decreased or absent. Dribbling of urine or overflow incontinence may occur when the bladder fills to capacity. The person may experience a sensation of bladder fullness if the sensory fibers of the sacral spinal cord are intact and may strain in an attempt to empty the bladder. Bladder capacity eventually increases, and residual urine volumes are usually high. Because of urine stasis in the bladder, the risk of infection increases. Urinalysis may indicate high concentrations of white blood cells and bacteria.

Clinical Problems Related to Urinary Elimination Assessment

Many pathologic problems that contribute to urinary retention or incontinence are permanent alterations. In these cases, recognizing the pathologic condition helps you make the correct nursing diagnosis and implement appropriate treatment. Recognizing potentially reversible pathologic conditions will help identify persons who should be referred to a physician.

Inflammatory and Infectious Processes

Acute lower urinary tract infection is usually characterized by dysuria, frequency, and urgency. Urine may be cloudy and voided in small volumes. Urinalysis may indicate bacteria and increased white and red blood cell concentrations. A urine culture helps to identify specific bacterial organisms.

Upper urinary tract infection is characterized by lethargy, fever, chills, headache, and occasionally vomiting. Abdominal pain and tenderness over the costovertebral angle may be noted. The urine usually contains bacteria as well as elevated white and red blood cell counts and increased amounts of protein. The serum white blood cell count is also usually elevated.

Prostatitis, inflammation of the prostate gland, may cause a lower urinary tract infection or may mimic this condition. Dysuria, frequency, and urethral discharge may be noted. The prostate examination may show an enlarged, boggy, and tender gland. Palpating the prostate may result in purulent urethral discharge. Pus cells and bacteria may be noted in the urine sample obtained after the prostate is palpated. Other symptoms include perineal pain and low back pain, which may be intensified with ejaculation or a bowel movement.

Urinary Stones

Urinary stones, or calculi, occur secondary to numerous conditions, including metabolic disease, urinary tract infection, and necrotic kidney disease. The signs and symptoms of urinary stones depend on where the stones are located in the urinary system. Kidney stones are often asymptomatic.

Stones that become trapped in the ureters usually produce intense, colicky pain in the lower back or abdomen that may radiate to the sides or legs. Back or abdominal muscle spasms may be noted. The person may experience mild shock. Urine may contain increased white blood cells

and red blood cells and increased amounts of bacteria. Urine crystals may be present, providing information about stone type, such as uric acid or cystine.

Bladder stones irritate the bladder and may cause symptoms such as dysuria, urgency, and frequency. The stone may occlude the bladder neck, in which case the urinary stream may be interrupted. The bladder may become palpable as urine is retained. Urine may contain increased white and red blood cells and increased amounts of bacteria.

Renal Failure

Acute renal failure occurs when normal kidney function suddenly ceases. The ensuing fluid and electrolyte imbalances may produce a life-threatening condition. Immediate physician referral is crucial if you detect signs of acute renal failure during nursing assessment. The client may experience sudden oliguria. Urine examination reflects loss of kidney function. The urine may contain abnormal constituents such as protein and hemoglobin. Specific gravity is usually abnormally low (1.010–1.016). Systemic effects alter blood chemistry. For example, serum creatinine, blood urea nitrogen, potassium, and phosphate levels are usually increased. The person may experience anorexia, nausea and vomiting, hypertension, and fatigue.

PART 2

PHYSICAL EXAMINATION TECHNIQUES

ANUS AND RECTUM

Anatomy and Physiology Review

The terminal structures of the large intestine, beginning at the sigmoid colon, include the rectum, the anal canal, and the anus (Fig. 7-4). The physical examination of these structures is commonly referred to as the rectal examination. The integument around the sacrum, gluteal cleft, and perineum (the external area between the vulva and anus or the scrotum and anus) also should be inspected during the rectal examination because of the proximity of these structures.

Anus. The skin of the anus, the outlet of the anal canal, is hairless and darker and moister than the skin surrounding the perineum, because the anus is a mucocutaneous junction. The mucous lining of the anal canal is usually not visible because the anus is held tightly closed by external and internal sphincter muscles. The mucous lining may be examined by exerting slight pressure on each side of the anus. Normally, the anus appears as intact skin without lesions.

Anal Canal. The anal canal is located between the anus and the rectum and is an epithelium-lined structure, 2.5 to

4 cm long. It is important to consider the angle of the anal canal when examining and inserting devices such as thermometers or rectal tubes: The anal canal lies along a line extending anteriorly from anus to umbilicus (see Fig. 7-4).

The internal and external sphincter muscles surround the anal canal and keep the terminal end closed except during defecation. The external sphincter consists of striated muscle under voluntary control and is innervated by the somatic nervous system. The nerve endings are very sensitive to painful stimuli, such as careless digital examination. The levator ani muscles of the pelvic floor augment the contraction of the external sphincter. The internal sphincter consists of smooth muscle controlled by the autonomic nervous system.

The external hemorrhoidal plexus, a vascular structure, is located in the tissue surrounding the anal canal. Vessel enlargement in the plexus is related to venous swelling or thrombosis, resulting in external hemorrhoids. Venous enlargement may occur secondary to increased hydrostatic pressure in capillary vessels, caused by various conditions, including portal hypertension, pregnancy, habitual straining during defecation, and prolonged standing. The proximity of external hemorrhoids to somatic nerve endings causes this condition to be potentially painful, especially during defecation.

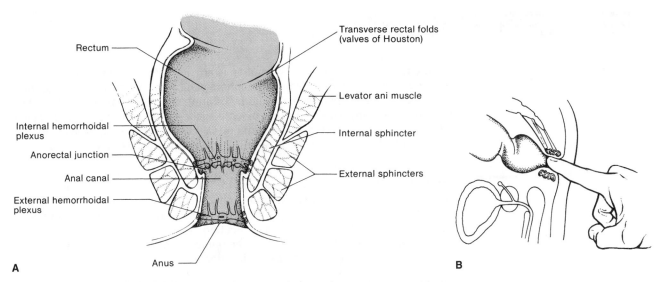

FIGURE 7.4 (**A**) Gross anatomy of the anus and rectum. (**B**) Orientation of the anus and rectum. Note the angle of the anal canal and how the examining finger should be inserted.

Rectum. The rectum is a mucosa-lined structure 12 cm in length. The entire length of the rectum cannot be palpated by digital examination. The boundary between the anal canal and the rectum, called the anorectal junction or pectinate or dentate line, is not palpable. However, the diameter of the bowel lumen usually enlarges at this point and is palpable. The rectum extends posteriorly toward the sacrum, with the posterior wall of the rectum being oriented almost 90 degrees from the anal canal. Normally, the mucosa overlying the posterior wall is smooth. The zona hemorrhoidalis surrounds the anorectal junction and is slightly superior to it. In the underlying tissue, veins anastomose and form a ring around the anorectal junction. Congestion, dilation, and thrombosis of these vessels may result in internal hemorrhoids.

In men, the posterior surface of the prostate gland is palpable through the anterior rectal wall. The prostate consists of two lateral lobes divided by a slight indentation called the median sulcus. The entire gland weighs approximately 20 g and is 4 cm wide and 2.5 cm long. The prostate gland may become enlarged and compress the urethra, which may affect bladder elimination. The prostate gland is also susceptible to malignant growth and should be examined to screen for cancer.

The upper portion of the rectum is surrounded by several transverse folds of mucosa called the valves of Houston. These folds are palpable as ridges and are often mistaken for masses during the rectal examination. The valves of Houston may function to hold feces in the rectum when flatus is passed.

Physical Examination   Anus and Rectum

GENERAL APPROACH

The main techniques used in the anorectal examination are inspection and palpation. The areas examined include the peripheral and gluteal skin, the anal canal and rectum, and the prostate gland in men and the cervix and uterus in women. The presence and characteristics of any stool accumulations are noted.

To lessen the person's physical discomfort, your nails should be well-trimmed and no rings should be worn. Extreme pain during palpation is associated with fissures and hemorrhoids. *Do not force the examination if pain persists.* In such a case, consult a physician to determine whether a lesion is present. A more extensive examination might require that the area be anesthetized. The physician may decide to inspect the anal canal and lower rectum with an anoscope, a speculum that allows epithelial and mucosal surfaces to be viewed.

EQUIPMENT

Gloves (nonsterile examination type)
Water-soluble lubricant (*e.g.,* KY Jelly, Lubrifax)

(continued)

Physical Examination   Anus and Rectum (continued)

MINIMIZING ANXIETY

For many people, the rectal examination is an uncomfortable and embarrassing procedure. A more comfortable atmosphere can be established by draping the person to lessen embarrassment and by offering simple explanations about the procedure and any sensations that may be elicited, such as the urge to defecate when the anal canal and distal rectum are palpated. Men should be warned that they may feel the urge to void when the prostate gland is palpated.

HYGIENIC MEASURES

Although you wear gloves during the examination, good handwashing is essential after the examination is completed. Take care not to contaminate the perineum with fecal material that may adhere to gloves. If the person has fecal impaction, liquid stool may ooze from the rectum during the digital examination. For people who are at risk for defecating during the examination, place a protective pad beneath the buttocks. The person's skin should be cleaned after the examination, either by you or by the client.

POSITIONING

The person may assume any of several positions during the rectal examination. Selecting a position depends on examination purpose and the person's mobility.

The left lateral position (Sims' position) requires the person to lie on the left side with the upper leg flexed in a manner that brings the knee to the chest (Fig. 7-5). Masses (including fecal impactions) in the lower rectum can be easily palpated with the person in this position. The upper rectum may be difficult to palpate because this position will displace it away from your finger. However, for a person who is confined to bed, this position is easiest to assume.

The knee–chest position (genupectoral position) requires the person to bend at the knees with the thighs upright and the head and shoulders resting on the examining table (Fig. 7-6). This position allows for optimal observation of the perineum and palpation of the prostate gland.

The standing position requires the person to stand at the end of the examining table and bend at the waist while supporting the upper body on the table (Fig. 7-7). Palpating the prostate gland is easier with the person in this position than in the knee–chest position.

The squatting position requires the person to bend at the hips and knees, while leaning slightly forward and supporting the body weight with the hands and forearms (Fig. 7-8). Rectal prolapse (protrusion of the rectal mucosa through the anus) is most easily observed with the person in this position. It also allows you to palpate a more extensive area of the rectum and detect possible rectal-sigmoid lesions of the pelvic floor.

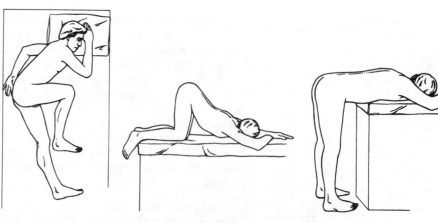

FIGURE 7.5   Left lateral (Sims') position.

FIGURE 7.6   Knee–chest (genupectoral) position.

FIGURE 7.7   Standing position.

Physical Examination   Anus and Rectum (continued)

The lithotomy position (dorsosacral position) requires the person to lie on his or her back with the thighs flexed toward the abdomen and the legs pulled up on the thighs (Fig. 7-9). This position also may be achieved by placing the heels in stirrups attached to the table. This method is used for women undergoing pelvic and rectal examination, because the rectal examination is often conducted as part of the pelvic assessment in women. For men, however, the lithotomy position is not ideal because it does not provide the best position for palpating the prostate.

EXAMINATION AND
DOCUMENTATION FOCUS

Perineal and gluteal skin: Color and pigmentation, secretions or excretions, lesions

Anal canal and rectum: Muscle tone, prostate gland or cervix and uterus, stool accumulation, tenderness, lesions, and masses

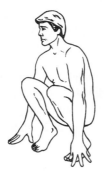

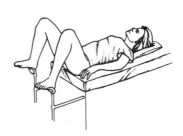

FIGURE 7.8   Squatting position.

FIGURE 7.9   Lithotomy (dorsosacral) position.

▼ ▼ ▼
GUIDELINES

Assessment Guidelines   Anus and Rectum

Procedure

1. **Inspect the integument of the sacrum, gluteal folds, and perineum.**

   a. Position the person in the standing or left lateral position. If the lateral position is used, displace the buttocks with your nondominant hand. If the standing position is used, spread the buttocks apart with your hand. Use a small penlight to assess more easily the condition of the skin.

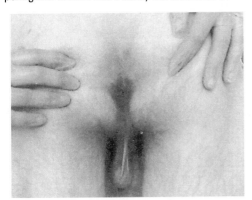

Inspection: Sacrum, gluteal folds, perineum

Clinical Significance

Deviations from Normal
A dimple or tuft of hair in this area may indicate a pilonidal cyst or sinus.

Pilonidal cyst (a cyst in the area of the sacrum or coccyx usually near the upper gluteal fold): This condition is congenital and forms when a small amount of epithelial tissue becomes trapped beneath the skin surface. Hair may grow from this tissue. The cyst is significant because it may trap debris, become infected, and lead to fistula formation.

▼ ▼ ▼

GUIDELINES *continued*   Anus and Rectum

Procedure

b. Inspect the perineum, noting any redness, excretions, or lesions including fissures, warts, hemorrhoids, and scars.

c. Inspect the perianal region and ask the person to perform a Valsalva maneuver (bear down as though having a bowel movement). Then note any bulges, fissures, hemorrhoids, or polyps revealed by this maneuver.

2. **Palpate the anal canal and rectum.**

a. Relax the external anal sphincter. Use your nondominant hand to spread the buttocks. Your dominant hand should be gloved, with the index finger lubricated. Using the pad of the index finger of your dominant hand, exert slight, even pressure against the anus. This will relax the sphincter, and facilitate inserting your examining finger into the anal canal. Using the tip of the finger, rather than the pad, will cause greater pain and sphincter tightening.

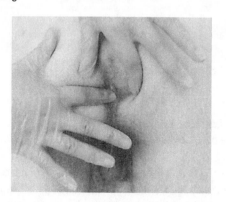

Clinical Significance

Normal Findings

Perineal skin color matches the color of the surrounding skin. Skin immediately surrounding the anus may be darker (reddish brown), especially in children. The surface of the skin should be clear of fecal material. The anal area should be free of lesions or signs of skin irritation such as erythema or rashes.

Deviations from Normal

Excretions of fecal material may indicate poor hygiene practices. Other excreted substances, such as blood or mucus, should not be present. Possible lesions include protrusions, bluish discolorations, and fissures in the anal area. Skin tags (irregular flaccid skin sacs) may be noted around the anus if the client has a history of external hemorrhoids. Skin tags are usually benign and painless, forming as hemorrhoids expand through skin connective tissue and becoming flaccid when hemorrhoids resolve.

The digital examination may be painful if the external sphincter is not relaxed before the examining finger is inserted.

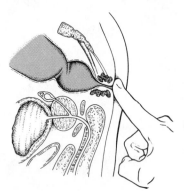

Relaxation of the external sphincter

▼ ▼ ▼
G U I D E L I N E S *continued*   Anus and Rectum

Procedure

b. Palpate the anal canal. Insert your gloved examining finger into the anal canal, moving the finger in the direction of the umbilicus. Ask the person to tighten the external sphincter by squeezing around your finger so that you can assess muscle tone. To palpate, rotate your finger, which will expose the entire lumen of the anal canal. Stop the examination if the person experiences extreme pain.

c. Palpate the levator ani muscles. Advance your examining finger through the anal canal. At the anorectal junction, palpate the levator ani muscles on the lateral-posterior surfaces of the rectal wall.

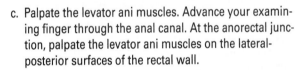
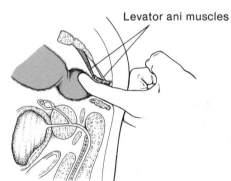

Palpation: Levator ani muscles

d. Palpate the lateral and posterior rectal walls. Advance your examining finger and systematically palpate the right lateral wall, posterior wall, and left lateral wall of the rectum, noting any tenderness or masses. The posterior wall may be difficult to palpate because it extends furthest from the anal opening. Ask the person to bear down while you palpate the posterior wall, to expose any palpable masses higher in the rectum.

Clinical Significance

Normal Findings

The external sphincter should remain closed until voluntary muscle contraction (as occurs during defecation) pulls it open. Good sphincter tone is present if the person can voluntarily contract the sphincter around the examiner's finger.

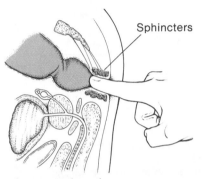

Palpation: Anal canal

The levator ani muscles play an important role in bowel control. The muscles may be difficult to palpate, but should be smooth and firm.

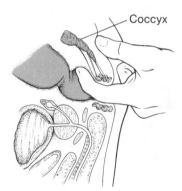

Palpation: Posterior rectal wall

Stool accumulation: Soft, formed stool may be palpable in the rectum; hard or putty-like stool may indicate fecal impaction.

Masses: Palpable masses are abnormal (see display "Anal and Rectal Masses"). Stool, tampons (felt through the anterior wall of the rectum), and the valves of Houston should not be mistaken for masses.

▼ ▼ ▼

Anal and Rectal Masses

Note: Discovering a mass during the rectal examination may warrant referral to a physician. Further examination, including tissue biopsy, may be indicated to rule out a malignancy.

External Hemorrhoid

- May be visible at the anal opening unless thrombosed
- Small, shiny, bluish nodules
- May appear only when the person performs a Valsalva maneuver
- Tender to palpation

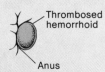

Thrombosed hemorrhoid

Anus

External hemorrhoid

Internal Hemorrhoid

- Located above the anorectal junction
- Not always palpable, unless thrombosed
- If palpable, should feel smooth and soft

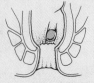

Internal hemorrhoid

Rectal Prolapse

- Red mucosa protruding through the anus
- May appear only when the person performs a Valsalva maneuver

Rectal prolapse

Rectal Tumor

- May be palpable anywhere along the anal canal or rectum
- Hard, nodular, irregular
- May or may not have a rolled edge
- Firmly embedded in surrounding tissue
- Nontender to palpation

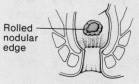

Rolled nodular edge

Rectal tumor

Rectal Polyps

- Small, rectal tumors
- Pedunculated polyps develop on a stalk and are freely moveable
- Sessile polyps lie close to rectal mucosa

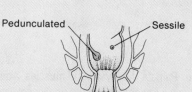

Pedunculated   Sessile

Rectal polyps

Procedure

e. *In men:* Palpate the prostate and anterior rectal wall. Rotate the examining finger to palpate the anterior wall. Identify the lateral lobes and median sulcus of the prostate gland, noting size, tenderness, consistency (firm or boggy), and nodules.

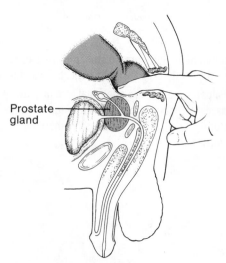

Prostate gland

Palpation: Prostate gland

Clinical Significance

Normal Findings

The prostate is round, 4 cm wide and 2.5 cm long, with a palpable median sulcus or groove separating the two lobes. It should feel firm and be free of nodules and masses. When palpated, it should not cause tenderness, although it may cause an urge to urinate (see display, "Prostate Conditions").

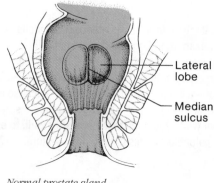

Lateral lobe

Median sulcus

Normal prostate gland

▼ ▼ ▼
G U I D E L I N E S *continued*   Anus and Rectum

Prostate Conditions

Benign Prostatic Hypertrophy

- Symmetric enlargement of the prostate
- Gland feels boggy
- Median sulcus may disappear
- Common after age 50
- May compress urethra and interfere with urination

Smooth, elastic, symmetrical

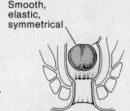

Benign prostatic hypertrophy

Prostate Malignancy

- Palpable mass on prostate
- Hard, irregular, fixed
- May be painless on palpation
- May cause prostate to feel asymmetric

Hard, irregular, fixed

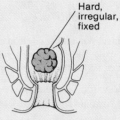

Carcinoma of the prostate: Advanced

Irregular, hard

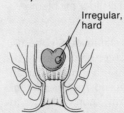

Carcinoma of the prostate: Single nodule

Acute Prostatitis

- Prostate enlarged (may be asymmetrical)
- Tender to palpation

Swollen, tender

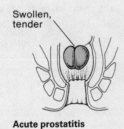

Acute prostatitis

Procedure

f. *In women:* Palpate the cervix. Examine the anterior rectal wall as part of the pelvic examination with the woman in the lithotomy position (this technique is described in greater detail in Chap. 15). Rotate the examining finger and palpate the anterior wall. Palpate the rounded tip of the cervix, noting any tenderness or nodules. Ask the woman to bear down in order to assess for uterine prolapse.

3. **Complete the examination.**

a. Slowly withdraw your examining finger from the rectum. Note the color of any stool adhering to the glove and check the stool for occult blood (see guaiac test, p. 257).

b. Give the person tissue to clean the anus, or clean the perineum yourself as you finish the examination.

Clinical Significance

Cervix: A firm, round, smooth mass felt through the anterior wall; not tender on palpation.

Uterus: Difficult to palpate by rectal examination unless prolapsed.

NDx

Documenting Anus and Rectum Examination Findings

Example 1

Hal, aged 44, had an anorectal examination as part of a routine health assessment. The results were normal and recorded as follows:

> Perineal skin and anus clean and intact. Small amount of soft stool in rectum; no masses or tenderness. Prostate smooth, firm, nontender, and without masses; size 4 by 2 cm.

The same results may be summarized in a problem-oriented format:

S: Reports no change in bowel elimination patterns; regular pattern—BM every am after breakfast.
O: Perineal skin and anus clean and intact. Small amount of soft stool in rectum; no masses or tenderness. Prostate smooth, firm, nontender, and without masses; size 4 by 2 cm.
A: Normal anorectal examination results.
P: Follow-up with routine exams.
   Test stool for occult blood.
   Teach significance of sudden change in bowel elimination pattern.

Example 2

Mr. G, aged 72, had an anorectal examination after reports of urinary hesitancy. The results were abnormal and recorded as follows:

> No masses, nodules, or stool palpable in rectum. Prostate enlarged and soft on palpation, unable to palpate median sulcus; no palpable prostate masses.

The same results may be summarized in a problem-oriented format:

S: Reports "can't get my water going"; reports occasional constipation.
O: No masses, nodules, or stool palpable in rectum. Prostate enlarged and soft on palpation; unable to palpate median sulcus; no palpable masses.
A: Prostate enlarged—possibly related to benign prostatic hypertrophy.
P: Refer to physician.

Example 3

Mrs. L, aged 55, had experienced intermittent constipation and noted bloody stools. The anorectal examination results were abnormal, and she was referred to her physician. The documentation was as follows:

> Firm, irregular, nonmobile mass palpated on posterior rectal wall 5 cm from anus; nontender to palpation, gross blood noted on examining glove.

CASE STUDY

Ricardo, aged 16, was being discharged from a rehabilitation center. Three weeks earlier he had been involved in a gang confrontation and shot in the back with a 9-mm assault weapon. The incident resulted in a complete transection of his spinal cord at the S2 level. His lower extremities were permanently paralyzed, confining him to a wheelchair. He had also lost voluntary control of bowel and bladder functions.

During the early phase of his recovery, Ricardo had been completely incontinent of stool and urine. The rehabilitation team developed a treatment plan for bowel and bladder control. Ricardo had early success with bowel retraining.

As a result of his spinal cord injury, Ricardo could not feel pressure as his bladder filled with urine, and he had no perception of an urge to urinate. His bladder would fill with urine, which eventually resulted in overflow dribbling without his knowledge. Eventually, he would become aware of the odor of urine or a caregiver would identify urine incontinence during routine monitoring. Ricardo's pattern of bladder elimination was characterized by overdistention of the bladder and eventual overflow incontinence. The rehabilitation team worked with Ricardo to teach him methods for complete bladder emptying. At regular intervals, Ricardo would be encouraged to void into a urinal and decompress the bladder by applying manual pressure over the lower abdomen. Occasional measurements of PVR volumes were obtained by in-and-out catheterization to evaluate the effectiveness of manual bladder decompression. With practice, Ricardo achieved complete daytime urinary continence with PVR volumes of less than 50 mL.

Three days before his scheduled discharge, Ricardo again began experiencing urinary incontinence. PVR volumes were greater than 250 mL. Urinalysis indicated signs of infection. His skin was becoming irritated from contact with urine. The rehabilitation team recommended adding nonsterile, clean intermittent self-catheterization to Ricardo's bladder training program to more effectively decompress the bladder. Ricardo was upset about having to perform this additional procedure and often refused to participate. He became angry and withdrawn, occasionally making statements about no longer having his manhood. He was verbally abusive to the rehabilitation team. His friends were caught supplying him with various street drugs that affected his ability to participate in treatment.

Profile Analysis

Ricardo had a permanently altered elimination pattern as a result of irreversible damage to his lower spinal cord. Although assessing the nature of his bladder elimination problem and his response to his bladder training program were important, evaluating factors that might interfere

CASE STUDY   *continued*

with Ricardo's successful ongoing management of elimination functions was also crucial.

Assessment Focus

The rehabilitation team initially focused their assessment efforts on thoroughly evaluating the bladder elimination pattern. People such as Ricardo who have had lower spinal cord injury most often have urinary incontinence for the following reasons:

- Message transmission between the brain and the spinal cord reflex arc is interrupted, in which case voiding occurs at predictable intervals after the bladder fills to a critical volume (reflex incontinence).
- The detrusor muscle no longer contracts effectively, the bladder fills with urine, and constant dribbling occurs from the overfilled bladder (urinary retention with overflow incontinence).

Reflex incontinence may be treated effectively with bladder training regimens emphasizing regular voiding schedules. Urinary retention is identified by confirming high PVR volumes. The success of bladder decompression methods used to eliminate urinary retention (*e.g.*, manual massage of the lower abdomen or intermittent catheterization) can also be evaluated by monitoring PVR volumes.

The initial assessment focus of the rehabilitation team caring for Ricardo was evaluation of his typical bladder elimination pattern, volume of urine spontaneously voided, PVR volumes, and bladder capacity. In addition, the team monitored urine specimens for signs of infection, his fluid intake, and skin integrity.

Preliminary Nursing Diagnoses

During the acute phase of Ricardo's rehabilitation, the following diagnoses were identified relative to elimination functions and prioritized for intervention:

Bowel incontinence
Risk for constipation
Altered urinary elimination pattern
Reflex incontinence
Urinary retention
Risk for impaired skin integrity
Risk for infection

As important to long-term success with bowel and bladder training as learning specific techniques to control elimination functions is the consideration of the ongoing challenges to self-esteem and coping. It is also important to evaluate the social support systems that may or may not be available to the person.

Additional Assessment

Now that Ricardo's elimination pattern was well characterized, the rehabilitation team began to focus their assessment efforts on the impact of Ricardo's condition on his self-esteem, his abilities to cope with disability, and his responses to his impending discharge from the rehabilitation center. Thoughts of discharge were frightening to Ricardo. He was fearful of managing without his caregivers and felt he could not reliably depend on his mother to help him. He lived with his mother and four younger siblings in a poor, inner-city neighborhood. His mother worked full-time and could be away from home up to 12 hours a day. He was also concerned about his status and image with his friends. He was despondent about his "lost freedom" and "lost manhood." He had not been abusing drugs before his injury but had found comfort in this activity during his recovery. He was feeling overwhelmed with these thoughts and expressed little desire to maintain behaviors that had helped him regain control over elimination functions. He was at great risk of losing this control without additional intervention.

The rehabilitation team believed that continued management of elimination functions would be crucial to the successful return of Ricardo to his home setting. Strengths and risk factors related to effective management were summarized as follows:

Strengths

- Maintains control over bowel elimination
- Has demonstrated ability to manage bladder elimination
- Considered ready for discharge

Risks

- Permanent altered elimination patterns secondary to lower spinal cord injury
- Threats to self-esteem and body image
- Threats to physical well-being: infection and risk for impaired skin integrity
- Lack of effective social support systems
- Return to environment characterized by street violence, poverty
- High risk for continued substance abuse

Revised Nursing Diagnoses

Ricardo's plan of care was revised to incorporate additional diagnoses that would be addressed to the extent possible before discharge from the rehabilitation center. Among the diagnoses added to Ricardo's active treatment plan were the following:

Body image disturbance
Self-esteem disturbance
Risk for ineffective management of therapeutic regimen

These additional diagnoses were incorporated into Ricardo's care plan, and additional intervention was initiated.

CHAPTER 7 S U M M A R Y

Assessment of Elimination

Elimination pattern assessment focuses on the following:
- The individual's perceptions of bowel and bladder elimination patterns
- Self-care practices and knowledge related to elimination functions
- Risk factors and causative factors associated with altered elimination
- The effects of elimination problems on physical, social, and psychological health
- Differentiation of various elimination problems to determine the most effective management and intervention

Important principles to remember when assessing bowel and bladder elimination include the following:
- People may avoid discussing problems with elimination because of feelings of embarrassment or hopelessness. You should convey empathy and acceptance.
- Elimination patterns cannot be adequately described by merely quantifying stool and urine. Many factors influence elimination, and the relative impact of diet, activity, medications, lifestyle, and pathologic conditions should be evaluated.
- People are often concerned about bowel regularity, but wide variations exist in "normal" patterns.
- Most people with bowel or urinary incontinence respond to bowel or bladder training, provided interventions are based on accurate assessment.
- Physical examination as a component of elimination assessment is aimed at determining bowel and bladder function in relation to elimination and identifying adverse effects of elimination problems. You should also examine body structures related to elimination to detect actual or potential pathologic conditions and make appropriate treatment referrals.

Data Collection Methods

1. Interview or Review of Records
   Usual bowel or bladder elimination patterns
   Altered bowel or bladder elimination patterns
   Self-care practices related to elimination
   Functional status
   Medical history relevant to elimination functions
   Medication history relevant to elimination functions
2. Diagnostic Studies Review
   Radiographic studies of the bowel and urinary systems
   Urodynamic tests (cystometrogram, electromyography, pressure–flow studies)
   Postvoid residual volumes

3. Specimen Analysis
   Stool
   Urine
4. Physical Examination
   General appearance
   Abdomen
   Genitourinary structures
   Anus and rectum
   The neurologic system

Primary Nursing Diagnoses

- Altered bowel elimination
  - Constipation
  - Perceived constipation
  - Colonic constipation
  - Diarrhea
  - Bowel incontinence
- Altered patterns of urinary elimination
  - Altered urinary elimination
  - Stress incontinence
  - Reflex incontinence
  - Urge incontinence
  - Functional incontinence
  - Total incontinence
  - Urinary retention

Clinical Problems Related to Elimination Dysfunctions

1. Inflammatory and infectious processes of the anus and rectum
   a. Ulcerative colitis
   b. Crohn's disease
   c. Acute gastroenteritis
   d. Diverticulitis
2. Hyperplastic growths
   a. Colon and rectal cancer
   b. Prostate cancer
3. Malabsorption syndromes
4. Hemorrhage
5. Irritable bowel syndrome
6. Inflammatory and infectious processes of the urinary tract
   a. Upper urinary tract infection
   b. Lower urinary tract infection
7. Urinary stones
8. Renal failure

Critical Thinking Exercises

You are the contract nurse for an assisted living facility. Most of the residents are elderly, ambulatory, and able to feed, dress, and toilet themselves. During your weekly visit, you are asked to evaluate an 82-year-old female resident who has suddenly become incontinent of urine. She is extremely hard of hearing but otherwise healthy, with a medical history of congestive heart failure and hypertension. If this resident remains incontinent, she will no longer be able to live at this facility. To intervene, you must first determine the nature of her incontinence.

Learning Exercises

1. Select and describe the approach you would use to determine the nature of this person's bladder elimination problem. How would you differentiate among the following: urinary retention, total incontinence, urge incontinence, stress incontinence, reflex incontinence, and functional incontinence?

2. Because of her hearing problem, you are unable to elicit a good history of this person's perception of her incontinence. Moreover, because she is not observed around the clock by care providers, you do not have data from other sources to help you understand her bladder elimination patterns. Given these limitations, plan and describe your strategy for ensuring a thorough and accurate assessment of this person.

3. Explain what you could learn about this person's problem from examining the physical surroundings.

BIBLIOGRAPHY

Abbott, D. (1992). Objective assessment ensures improved diagnosis: Principles and practice of urodynamics. *Professional Nurse, 7*(11), 740–742.

Agency for Health Care Policy and Research Urinary Incontinence Guideline Panel. (1992). *Urinary incontinence in adults: Clinical practice guideline* (AHCPR Pub. No. 92-0038). Rockville, MD: Agency for Health Care Policy and Research, Public Health Service, U.S. Department of Health and Human Services.

Beckman, N.J. (1995). An overview of urinary incontinence in adults: Assessment and behavioral interventions. *Clinical Nurse Specialist, 9*(5), 241–274.

Bisanz, A. (1997). Managing bowel elimination problems in patients with cancer. *Oncology Nursing Forum, 24*(4), 670–686.

Blaivas, J.G. (1985). Pathophysiology of lower urinary tract dysfunction. *Urologic Clinics of North America, 12,* 215–224.

Blaivas, J.G. (1990). Diagnostic evaluation of incontinence in patients with neurologic disorders. *Journal of the American Geriatrics Society, 38,* 306–310.

Brink, C.A., Sampsell, C.M., Wells, T.J., Diokno, A.C., & Gillis, G.L. (1989). A digital test for pelvic muscle strength in older women with urinary incontinence. *Nursing Research, 38*(4), 196–199.

Brooks, M.J. (1995). Assessment and nursing management of homebound clients with urinary incontinence. *Home Healthcare Nurse, 13*(3), 11–16.

Cheater, F. (1996). Promoting urinary continence. *Nursing Standard, 10*(42), 47–54.

Crooks, V.C., Schnelle, J.F., Ouslander, J.P., & McNees, M.P. (1995). Use of the minimum data set to rate incontinence severity. *Journal of the American Geriatrics Society, 43*(12), 1363–1369.

Diokno, A.C., Normolle, D.P., Brown, M.B., & Herzog, A.R. (1990). Urodynamic tests for female geriatric urinary incontinence. *Urology, 36*(5), 431–439.

Dowd, T.T., & Campbell, J.M. (1995). Urinary incontinence in an acute care setting. *Urologic Nursing, 15*(3), 82–85.

DuBeau, C.E., & Resnick, N.M. (1991). Evaluation of the causes and severity of geriatric incontinence: A critical appraisal. *Urology Clinics of North America, 18,* 243–256.

Fantl, J.A., Wyman, J.F., McClish, D.K., & Bump, R.C. (1990). Urinary incontinence in community-dwelling women: Clinical, urodynamic, and severity characteristics. *America Journal of Obstetrics and Gynecology, 162*(4), 946–951.

Gray, M., Rayome, R., & Moore, K. (1995). The urethral sphincter: An update. *Urologic Nursing, 15*(2), 40–53.

Hahn, K. (1987). Think twice about diarrhea. *Nursing '87, 17*(9), 78–90.

Hahn, K. (1988). Think twice about urinary incontinence. *Nursing '88, 18*(11), 65–67.

Harari, D., Gurwitz, J.H., & Minaker, K.L. (1993). Constipation in the elderly. *Journal of the American Geriatrics Society, 41*(10), 1130–1140.

Harari, D., Gurwitz, J.H., Avorn, J., Choodnovskiy, I., & Minaker, K.L. (1994). Constipation: Assessment and management in an institutionalized elderly population. *Journal of the American Geriatric Society, 42*(9), 947–952.

Ireton, R.C., Krieger, J.N., Cardenas, D.D., et al. (1990). Bladder volume determination using a dedicated, portable ultrasound scanner. *Journal of Urology, 143*(5), 909–911.

Maestri-Banks, A., et al. (1996). Assessing constipation. *Nursing Times,* May 22–28.

Mager-O'Connor, E. (1984). How to identify and remove fecal impaction. *Geriatric Nursing, 5,* 158–161.

McBride, R.E. (1996). Assessing and treating urinary incontinence. *Home Healthcare Nurse, 14*(1), 27–32.

McCormick, K.A. (1991). From clinical trial to health policy—research on urinary incontinence in the adult, Part I. *Journal of Professional Nursing, 7*(4), 147.

McCormick, K.A., Newman, D.K., Colling, J., & Pearson, B.D. (1992). Urinary incontinence in adults. *American Journal of Nursing, 92*(10), 75–92.

McLane, A.M., & McShane, R.E. (1986). Empirical validation of defining characteristics of constipation: A study of bowel elimination practices of healthy adults. In M.E. Hurly (Ed.). *Classification of nursing diagnoses: Proceedings of the sixth national conference.* St. Louis: C.V. Mosby.

McLane, A.M., McShane, R.E., & Sliefert, M. (1984). Constipation: Conceptual categories of diagnostic indicators. In M.J. Kim, G.K. McFarland, and A.M. McLane (Eds.). *Classification of nursing diagnoses: Proceedings of the fifth national conference.* St. Louis: C.V. Mosby.

McShane, R., & McLane, A.M. (1988). Constipation: Impact of etiological factors. *Journal of Gerontological Nursing, 14*(4), 31–34, 46–47.

Moore, T., Matyas, Y., & Boudreau, A. (1996). Describing and analyzing constipation in acute care. *Journal of Nursing Care Quality, 10*(3), 68–74.

North American Nursing Diagnosis Association (1996). *NANDA nursing diagnosis definitions and classification 1997–1998.* Philadelphia: NANDA.

Ouslander, J.G., Leach, G.E., & Staskin, D.R. (1989). Simplified tests of lower urinary tract function in the evaluation of geriatric urinary incontinence. *Journal of the American Geriatrics Society, 37*(8), 706–714.

Ouslander, J., Leach, G., Staskin, D., et al. (1989). Prospective evaluation of an assessment strategy for geriatric urinary incontinence. *Journal of the American Geriatrics Society, 37*(8), 715–724.

Ouslander, J.G., Simmons, S., Tuico, E., et al. (1994). Use of a portable ultrasound device to measure post-void residual volume among incontinent nursing home residents. *Journal of the American Geriatrics Society, 42*(11), 1189–1192.

Resnick, N.M. (1995). Urinary incontinence. *Lancet, 346,* 94–99.

Shaw, B. (1996). Primary care for women: Management and treatment of gastrointestinal disorders. *Journal of Nurse Midwifery,* Mar–Apr 1996.

Skelly, J., & Flint, A.J. (1995). Urinary incontinence associated with dementia. *Journal of the American Geriatrics Society, 43*(3), 286–294.

Tunink, P. (1988). Alteration in urinary elimination. *Journal of Gerontological Nursing, 14*(4), 25–30.

Voith, A.M. (1986). A conceptual framework for nursing diagnoses: Alterations in urinary elimination. *Rehabilitation Nursing, 11,* 18–21.

Voith, A.M., & Smith, D.A. (1985). Validation of the nursing diagnosis of urinary retention. *Nursing Clinics of North America, 20*(4), 723–729.

Williams, M.E., & Gaylord, S.A. (1990). Role of functional assessment in the evaluation of urinary incontinence: National Institutes of Health Consensus Development Conference on Urinary Incontinence in Adults, Bethesda, MD, USA, October 3–5, 1998. *Journal of the American Geriatrics Society, 38*(3), 296–299.

Woodtli, A. (1995). Stress incontinence: Clinical identification and validation of defining characteristics. *Nursing Diagnosis, 6*(3), 115–122.

Woodward, S. (1995). Assessment of urinary incontinence in neuroscience patients. *British Journal of Nursing, 4*(5), 254–258.

Wozniak-Petrofsky, J. (1996). Urodynamics for the primary care nurse. *Geriatric Nursing, 7*(3), 115–119.

Wyman, J. (1988). Nursing assessment of the incontinent geriatric outpatient population. *Nursing Clinics of North America, 23*(1), 169–187.

ASSESSMENT GUIDELINES

Activity and Exercise Interview (Health History)

Diagnostic Studies for Evaluation of Activity and Exercise Functions

Interpreting Physical Examination Findings Related to Activity and Exercise

Heart and Precordium

Arterial Pulses

Neck Veins

Nose and Sinuses

Lungs and Thorax

Bones, Joints, and Muscles

CHAPTER ORGANIZATION

PART 1: ASSESSING THE PATTERN

Introductory Overview
- Assessment Focus
- Data Collection Methods
- Nursing Diagnoses

Knowledge Base for Assessment
- Physiologic Basis for Activity and Exercise Assessment
- Activity Assessment Using Metabolic Equivalents (METs)

PART 2: PHYSICAL EXAMINATION TECHNIQUES

Cardiovascular System
- Anatomy and Physiology Review

Respiratory System
- Anatomy and Physiology Review

Musculoskeletal System
- Anatomy and Physiology Review

PART 1

ASSESSING THE PATTERN

INTRODUCTORY OVERVIEW

Routine daily activities require energy expenditure and the ability move freely in one's surroundings. Assessment of an individual's activity and exercise pattern will determine the person's tolerance for activity, degree of physical mobility, and abilities to perform self-care activities. In healthy persons interested in improving or maintaining levels of physical conditioning, the assessment of this pattern can reinforce the positive effects of exercise. Evaluating activity and exercise patterns in persons with cardiovascular or mobility deficits can provide the basis for planning nursing care such as modifying activities of daily living or prescribing safe and effective exercise programs to build endurance.

ASSESSMENT FOCUS

Cardiovascular and respiratory responses to activity are evaluated in both health and illness states. Activity and exercise assessment is a process of identifying typical activity and mobility patterns, self-care abilities and limitations, risk factors for activity intolerance, and physiologic responses to exertion. A comprehensive assessment of the pattern will meet the following objectives:

- Describing the person's typical activity pattern, including activities of daily living, leisure activities, and exercise habits
- Evaluating activity and exercise patterns for positive effects on cardiovascular function and stress management
- Determining whether current physical abilities are sufficient for meeting self-care needs
- Identifying risk factors or conditions associated with activity intolerance
- Identifying physiologic, behavioral, and psychological responses to normal and altered activity patterns

Data Collection Methods

Data collection is accomplished by the following methods:

1. Interview or Review of Records Focus
   - Typical daily activities, exercise pattern and leisure activities
   - Self-care abilities and use of assistive devices (if applicable)
   - Activity tolerance
   - Medical history
   - Medication history
2. Diagnostic Studies Review
   - Cardiovascular focus:
       - Complete blood count, lipid profile, serum enzymes
       - Noninvasive studies: Chest radiograph, electrocardiogram (ECG), Holter monitor, stress test, echocardiography, plethysmography
       - Nuclear medicine studies: positron emission tomography (PET), thallium scan
       - Invasive studies: cardiac catheterization, angiograms
   - Pulmonary focus:
       - Arterial blood gas measurement
       - Pulmonary function studies
       - Oximetry
   - Musculoskeletal focus
       - Radiographic studies
       - Electromyography
3. Physical Examination Focus
   - Vital signs
   - Skin temperature and moisture
   - Mental status changes
   - Signs and symptoms of activity intolerance detected during the examination of the cardiovascular and respiratory systems
   - Signs and symptoms of mobility problems and self-care deficits identified by general observation or examination of the musculoskeletal system

Nursing Diagnoses

Assessment of the activity and exercise pattern may result in the identification of one or more of the following primary nursing diagnoses:

Activity intolerance
Risk for activity intolerance
Diversional activity deficit

Impaired home maintenance management
Impaired physical mobility
Impaired walking
Impaired wheelchair mobility
Impaired wheelchair transfer ability
Impaired bed mobility
Bathing/hygiene self-care deficit
Dressing/grooming self-care deficit
Feeding self-care deficit
Toileting self-care deficit
Fatigue

Secondary nursing diagnoses may be identified as you examine major body systems supporting activity and exercise functions. Examination of the cardiovascular, respiratory, and musculoskeletal systems may indicate these secondary diagnoses:

Altered (specify type) tissue perfusion (renal, cerebral, cardiopulmonary, gastrointestinal, peripheral)
Fluid volume excess
Risk for fluid volume imbalance
Decreased cardiac output
Impaired gas exchange
Ineffective airway clearance
Ineffective breathing pattern
Inability to sustain spontaneous ventilation

KNOWLEDGE BASE FOR ASSESSMENT

Physiologic Basis for Activity and Exercise Assessment

Engaging in activity and exercise requires an adequate supply of energy for physical work (muscle contraction), functioning joints and limbs, and motivation. Energy for physical work is obtained through the body's anaerobic and aerobic metabolic pathways. Anaerobic metabolism does not require oxygen and is capable of providing energy for short-duration, high-intensity activity. Energy for prolonged activity is provided by aerobic pathways, which require a constant oxygen supply. Normal physical responses to exercise are related to the body's attempt to meet oxygen requirements. These responses include a slight increase in heart rate and blood pressure, dilation of the blood vessels, and increase in the rate and depth of ventilation. These changes occur to deliver an increased supply of blood, oxygen, and nutrients to tissues to meet increased metabolic demands during exercise.

Oxygen Delivery

The supply of oxygen to muscle tissues depends on oxygen being diffused into the blood through the lungs and transported by hemoglobin molecules. Oxygen enters the body by diffusion across alveolar–capillary membranes in the lungs. Usually this process is not a factor in limiting physical activity unless there is underlying pulmonary dysfunction (such as excessive pulmonary secretions or edema that interferes with gas diffusion, altered lung ventilation, or obstructive pulmonary disease). In other words, for most people, getting oxygen into the body is not a problem affecting activity tolerance. Similarly, most people have adequate hemoglobin molecules to transport the oxygen.

Conversely, transporting oxygen to muscle tissue, which may occur at different efficiency levels, can be a factor that limits activity tolerance. The delivery of oxygen to muscle cells, where it enters metabolic, energy-producing pathways, depends on effective cardiac output and aerobic capacity.

Cardiac Output

Cardiac output, the product of heart rate and stroke volume, is the amount of blood ejected from the left ventricle with each contraction. Resting cardiac outputs do not differ significantly among people; however, a person's maximally attainable cardiac output can be increased by regular exercise, thereby promoting activity tolerance. Exercise improves cardiac output by increasing stroke volume.

Assessing activity tolerance by physical examination is based on understanding the physical indicators of effective cardiac output. Normally, the heart rate increases as activity increases to raise the cardiac output and increase oxygen delivery to the tissues. The gradient for heart rate increase is greater in people who have had exercise training because they tend to have lower resting heart rates. Age-related norms have been established for exercise-induced maximal heart rates (Table 8-1). Exercise-induced maximal heart rates should be determined by taking the pulse 10 to 15 minutes after continuous aerobic exercise, such as jogging or cycling. Optimal physical fitness is associated with maximum heart rates 60% to 80% of age-related norms or 60% to 80% of the person's pretraining maximal heart rate. A maximal heart rate that is lower than the norm indicates that cardiac output has been in-

TABLE 8.1 Age-Related Norms for Exercise-Induced Maximal Heart Rates*

Age	Maximal Heart Rate*	80% Maximal	60% Maximal
20	200	160	120
25	195	156	115
30	190	152	114
35	185	148	111
40	180	144	108
45	175	140	105
50	170	136	102
55	165	132	99
60	160	128	96
65	155	124	93

*Optimal physical fitness is associated with maximal heart rates 60% to 80% of age-related norms or 60% to 80% of the person's pretraining maximal heart rate.

Pretraining maximal heart rate = 220 – age in years.

creased by stroke volume rather than heart rate, a positive adaptation to regular physical activity.

Using heart rate as an indicator of activity tolerance is most reliable when other aspects of cardiac function, such as contractility and left ventricular compliance, are normal. Failure of the heart rate to increase with activity or return to a resting level 5 minutes after the activity or exercise ends is considered abnormal. Also, a sustained high heart rate increases the heart's oxygen demands, which, if unmet, can tax the myocardium.

Aerobic Capacity

Aerobic capacity refers to the maximal rate at which oxygen can be used, and may be measured during exercise testing by determining the peak oxygen consumption rate (Vo_2 max), the maximum volume of oxygen the body extracts and uses from inspired air. A person's maximal oxygen consumption rate or aerobic capacity is a commonly used criterion for evaluating physical fitness. Genetic makeup largely determines aerobic capacity, but a number of other factors contribute and should be considered when assessing a person's activity tolerance.

Aerobic capacity can be increased by 20% in a person who engages in regular aerobic exercise. The following exercise pattern promotes aerobic capacity:

- *Type:* Continuous activity, such as running, cycling, stair climbing, swimming, or aerobic dancing
- *Frequency:* 3 to 5 days per week
- *Intensity:* 60% to 80% age-related maximum heart rate obtained and maintained during the exercise period
- *Duration:* 15 to 60 minutes, depending on intensity of the exercise

Diseases of the pulmonary, cardiovascular, or musculoskeletal systems may limit aerobic capacity. In such cases, oxygen debts may occur more readily and may be more difficult to compensate for, resulting in fatigue or, in extreme cases, cardiopulmonary compromise such as cardiac dysrhythmias, chest pain, or ineffective breathing patterns. However, people with such problems may improve aerobic capacity through individually prescribed activity and exercise programs. In addition, if a person's resting and maximum heart rates are lowered through exercise adaptation, myocardial oxygen consumption can be lowered, an accomplishment having significant implications for people with underlying cardiac disease.

Activity Assessment Using Metabolic Equivalents (METs)

Evaluating a person's activity and exercise capabilities in terms of maximum oxygen consumption rate may not always be practical because necessary data may not be available. In such cases, metabolic equivalents (METs) may be used to estimate oxygen costs for various activities. Table 8-2 presents METs for a variety of self-care, work, and leisure activities.

One MET is the average amount of oxygen a person consumes at rest, approximately 3.5 mL/kg body weight/min. When a person lies quietly at rest, the amount of oxygen consumed is 1 MET. A person who leads a sedentary life but who is not incapacitated by disease should be able to perform at least 10 METs of work with no adverse effects. Researchers continue to recommend activity levels in terms of METs for patients with disease limitations, such as acute myocardial infarction. The METs values may be used to evaluate activity and exercise capabilities.

Metabolic equivalents are often used in prescribing exercise rather than in estimating activity capability. One of the problems with prescribing activity based on METs is that the guidelines fail to account for individual differences. For example, an obese person who sits up for the first time after surgery may consume a different amount of oxygen than would a thin person. Similarly, a person with high stress may use more oxygen during a particular activity than the MET guideline indicates.

Pattern Assessment   Activity and Exercise Assessment Guidelines

GENERAL APPROACH

For healthy clients, the assessment of activity and exercise functions begins by obtaining a history of the individual's patterns of activity, exercise, leisure, and self-care activities. Going through a specific assessment of the person's activities communicates that the nurse believes that activity and exercise are very important to the person's health. This alone may lead the person to become more active in beneficial ways.

The interview also focuses on factors that interfere with usual or desired activities, such as disorders of the cardiovascular, respiratory, or musculoskeletal systems. Any symptoms of these disorders expressed during the interview should be noted. Most, but not all, of the history may be obtained by interviewing the person. Additionally, records may be reviewed.

EVALUATING A PERSON WITH CARDIAC IMPAIRMENT

Additional information is obtained if you are evaluating a person with a known cardiac disorder, for example, a person with coronary artery disease. This addi-

(continued)

TABLE 8.2   Metabolic Equivalents (METs) Associated with Various Activities

1 MET	1 to 2 METs	2 to 3 METs	3 to 4 METs	4 to 5 METs
Home Activities • Bed rest • Sitting • Eating • Reading • Sewing • Watching television **Occupational Activities** • No activity allowed **Exercise or Sports Activities** • No activity allowed	**Home Activities** • Dressing • Shaving • Brushing teeth • Washing at sink • Making bed • Desk work • Driving car • Playing cards • Knitting **Occupational Activities** • Typing (electric typewriter) **Exercise or Sports Activities** • Walking 1 mph on level ground	**Home Activities** • Tub bathing • Cooking • Waxing floors • Riding power lawn mower • Playing piano **Occupational Activities** • Driving small truck • Using hand tools • Typing (manual typewriter) • Repairing car **Exercise or Sports Activities** • Walking 2 mph on level ground • Bicycling 5 mph on level ground • Playing pool • Fishing • Bowling • Golfing (with motor cart) • Operating motorboat • Riding horseback (at walk)	**Home Activities** • General housework • Cleaning windows • Light gardening • Pushing light power mower • Sexual intercourse **Occupational Activities** • Assembly-line work • Driving large truck • Bricklaying • Plastering **Exercise or Sports Activities** • Walking 3 mph • Bicycling 6 mph • Sailing • Golfing (pulling hand cart) • Pitching horseshoes • Archery • Badminton (doubles) • Horseback riding (at slow trot) • Fly-fishing	**Home Activities** • Heavy housework • Heavy gardening • Home repairs, including painting, and light carpentry • Raking leaves **Occupational Activities** • Painting • Masonry • Paperhanging **Exercise or Sports Activities** • Calisthenics • Table tennis • Golfing (carrying bag) • Tennis (doubles) • Dancing • Slow swimming

5 to 6 METs	6 to 7 METs	7 to 8 METs	8 to 9 METs	10 or more METs
Home Activities • Sawing soft wood • Digging garden • Shoveling light loads **Occupational Activities** • Using heavy loads • Lifting 50 pounds **Exercise or Sports Activities** • Walking 4 mph • Bicycling 10 mph • Skating • Fishing with waders • Hiking • Hunting • Square dancing • Horseback riding (at brisk trot)	**Home Activities** • Shoveling snow • Splitting wood • Mowing lawn with hand mower **Occupational Activities** • All activities listed previously **Exercise or Sports Activities** • Walking or jogging 5 mph • Bicycling 11 mph • Tennis (singles) • Waterskiing • Light downhill skiing	**Home Activities** • Sawing hard wood **Occupational Activities** • Digging ditches • Lifting 80 pounds • Moving heavy furniture **Exercise or Sports Activities** • Touch football • Swimming (backstroke) • Basketball • Ice hockey	**Home Activities** • All activities listed previously **Occupational Activities** • Lifting 100 pounds **Exercise or Sports Activities** • Running 5.5 mph • Bicycling 13 mph • Swimming (breaststroke) • Cross-country skiing	**Home Activities** • All activities listed previously **Occupational Activities** • All activities listed previously **Exercise or Sports Activities** • Running 6 mph or faster • Gymnastics • Football (contact)

*One MET equals the average amount of oxygen a person consumes at rest, about 3.5 mL/kg of body weight/minute.
Actual energy requirements may vary depending on body size (e.g., obesity), physical condition, skill level, temperature and humidity, emotions, and intensity of the activity.

Pattern Assessment   Activity and Exercise Assessment Guidelines (continued)

tional information is especially helpful in a cardiac rehabilitation setting, where this level of assessment helps determine the person's risk for activity intolerance or other adverse events. This level of exercise assessment can be used for medical clearance for more strenuous activity. Information used for medical clearance assessment is often obtained through sophisticated, invasive diagnostic methods that are beyond the usual scope of the nurse's independent assessment. Look in the medical record for the following important indicators of activity tolerance in the person requiring medical clearance:

1. Measurement of functional capacity: A graded treadmill stress test provides this information.
2. Left ventricular function
   If the person has been subject to a cardiac catheterization procedure, look at the procedure note for the measured ejection fraction, an indicator of left ventricular function.
   Ejection fraction ≥ 50%: no significant left ventricular dysfunction
   Ejection fraction 31% to 49%: mild to moderately depressed left ventricular dysfunction
   Ejection fraction ≤ 30%: severely depressed left ventricular function
3. Presence and extent of myocardial ischemia: Indicated by ECG changes, catheterization reports of vessel blockage, and symptoms such as chest pain
4. Presence and extent of cardiac dysrhythmias: Indicated by ECG and telemetry recordings

SELF-EVALUATION OF PHYSIOLOGIC RESPONSES TO EXERCISE

Persons who have cardiac disease or even healthy persons in conditioning programs may need to self-evaluate their responses to various activities. It is important to know whether activity is being tolerated at appropriate levels. Activity instructions such as "Don't overdo" or "do what you think you can" are vague and uncertain. Three measures that may be used for self-evaluation:

- Heart rate
- Dyspnea index
- Ratings of perceived exertion

Teach the person to measure their heart rate by palpating the carotid artery pulse. Count for 15 seconds and multiply by 4. The counted value is then compared to a standard value such as a prescribed maximum heart rate to evaluate activity tolerance.

The dyspnea index (DI) measures how hard the person is breathing. Instruct the person to begin this measurement by taking a normal-sized breath and then counting out loud to 15, taking about 8 seconds. Tell the person to take a breath only when they feel the need to and continue counting. The number of breaths taken between the counts of 1 and 15 indicates how hard the person is breathing. If four or more breaths are needed, the person should slow down their activity level or stop and rest.

The Measure of Perceived Exertion Scale (Display 8-1) can be used to assign a grade to one's perception of exertion with different activity levels. In general, if a person with compromised cardiac function exceeds a score of 13, activity should decrease. The Perceived Exertion Scale is especially helpful for persons taking beta-blockers such as propranolol (Inderal; Wyeth-Ayerst, Philadelphia, PA) or metoprolol (Lopressor; Novartis Pharmaceuticals, East Hanover, NJ) because these medications will not allow a person to reach a target heart rate.

ASSESSMENT AIDS

- Interview guide to suggest questions and record data (Display 8-2)

DISPLAY 8.1

Perceived Exertion Scale

PERCEIVED EXERTION SCALE	DATE	ACTIVITY	SCORE	NOTES
6				
7 Very, very light				
8				
9 Very light				
10				
11 Fairly light				
12				
13 Somewhat hard				
14				
15 Hard				
16				
17 Very hard				
18				
19 Very, very hard				
20				

DISPLAY 8.2

Interview Guide: Activity and Exercise

ACTIVITY AND EXERCISE PATTERN

Activity Pattern

Typical daily activities:_____
Exercise Pattern: type _____ frequency _____· intensity _____ duration _____
Leisure activities:_____

Self-Care Activities

Self-Care Ability	0	1	2	3	4	5	
Eating/Drinking							
Bathing							0 = Independent
Dressing/Grooming							1 = Assistive device
Toileting							2 = Assistance from person
Bed Mobility							3 = Assistance from person
Transferring							and equipment
Ambulating							4 = Dependent/unable
Stair Climbing							5 = Change in last week
Shopping							
Cooking							
Home Maintenance							

Assistive Devices ❑ none ❑ cane ❑ walker ❑ wheelchair ❑ bedside commode
❑ trapeze ❑ Other: _____

Activity Tolerance

❑ No problems with activity ❑ Unsteady gait ❑ Weakness ❑ Dyspnea at rest
❑ Chest pain/angina ❑ Leg pain ❑ Joint/muscle/back pain
❑ Difficulty breathing (Specify: dyspnea, air hunger, wheezing, orthopnea) ❑ cough
❑ Vertigo/dizziness/lightheadedness
❑ Palpitations
❑ Other: _____

Medical History

Conditions related to problems with activity/exercise: ❑ No ❑ Yes
  ❑ family history of heart disease ❑ angina ❑ heart attack ❑ hypertension
  ❑ congestive heart failure ❑ rheumatic heart disease ❑ heart murmur
  ❑ heart/valve surgery ❑ abnormal ECG ❑ stroke ❑ emphysema
  ❑ bronchitis ❑ asthma ❑ pneumonia ❑ musculoskeletal trauma ❑ arthritis
  ❑ osteoporosis ❑ weight-bearing problems ❑ head trauma
  ❑ spinal cord injury ❑ multiple sclerosis ❑ sensory deficits
Comments: _____
Smoke: ❑ No ❑ Yes Estimated pack-years (Packs/day × # years smoking) _____

Medication History

Medications influencing activity/exercise functions or responses: ❑ no ❑ yes
Explain/List: _____

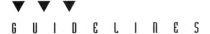

Assessment Guidelines   Activity and Exercise Interview (Health History)

Procedure	Clinical Significance

Procedure

1. Activity pattern—daily activities, exercise pattern, and leisure activities

Ask the person to describe a typical day's activities, including exercise and leisure activities. Occasionally, it may be helpful if the person keeps an activity diary that may be evaluated after several days.

- "Describe a typical day's activities."
- "How do you feel about your physical fitness?"
- "Are there any reasons you cannot participate in an exercise program?"
- "Do you follow a regular exercise routine?" (If so, describe: type, frequency, intensity, duration)
- Type—"What type of exercise activity do you engage in?"
- Frequency—"How many times a week do you exercise?"
- Intensity—"Do you know your pulse rate before, during, and after exercise? How would you describe the intensity of your exercise?"
- Duration—"How long does each exercise session last?"
- "What do you do for leisure/recreation?"

2. Self-care activities

Use observation and interviewing to evaluate self-care activities—feeding, dressing, toileting, bathing. Note the degree of independence the person experiences in relation to each of these activities.

Ask specific questions about abilities to eat, bathe, go to the bathroom, dress independently, and maintain a home. If the person reports any problems, you should further assess by observing functional abilities to conduct self-care activities.

Determine whether the person uses assistance devices (canes, walkers, splint/brace, commode, wheelchair, special tools) to carry out activities.

Review the person's health history to evaluate factors that can affect self-care abilities.

Grade self-care abilities using a zero to four scale.

    Level 0: Performs self-care activity independently

    Level 1: Requires assistive device

    Level 2: Requires assistance from person

    Level 3: Requires assistance from person and equipment

    Level 4: Dependent/unable

Clinical Significance

For some people, their everyday activities are their primary source of exercise. If there is minimal evidence of exercise and leisure activities, continue to probe for possible causes such as lack of time or motivation. Try to identify the person's leisure interests.

Exercise patterns promote physical fitness if they meet the following criteria:

Type: Continuous activity, *e.g.,* jogging, cycling, swimming, brisk walking

Frequency: 3–5 times per week

Intensity: 60–80% age-related heart rate obtained

Duration: 15–60 minutes, depending on the intensity of the exercise

Certain self-care deficits require additional clinical judgment for the diagnosis. For example, a person with diabetes may appear to have no self-care deficits, but on further questioning may show that bathing is a problem because she has difficulty differentiating water temperatures. Because a diabetic person is at risk for neuropathy and impaired circulation, there is also risk for associated self-care deficits.

Factors That Can Influence Self-Care Abilities

Age and developmental status; culture, values, and beliefs; socioeconomic status; cognitive abilities and knowledge base; motivation; medical history; activity restrictions.

Grading self-care abilities using a standardized scale improves consistency of observations among different examiners; it also helps in the identification of changes in self-care levels

▼ ▼ ▼

GUIDELINES *continued*   Activity and Exercise Interview (Health History)

Procedure

3. Activity tolerance

Ask questions to determine how the person tolerates activity:

- "Describe any problems you experience with usual activities and exercise."
- "How do you feel after walking two blocks?"
- Do you experience any of the following (with activity/exercise): chest pain, arm pain, leg pain, joint/muscle/back pain; breathing difficulty—shortness of breath, air hunger, wheezing, orthopnea, fatigue or weakness; lightheadedness, dizziness; clammy skin; frequent stopping/resting

4. Medical history

Review the person's medical history to identify conditions and risk factors that may contribute to activity intolerance.

Ask the person whether they smoke, and if so, number of packs per day and number of years smoking.

Determine whether there is a history of cardiovascular dysfunction: family history of cardiac disease, hypertension, angina, myocardial infarction, congestive heart failure, rheumatic heart disease, heart murmur, heart/valve surgery, abnormal ECG, stroke.

Determine whether there is a history of pulmonary dysfunction: emphysema, bronchitis, asthma, pneumonitis.

Determine whether there is a history of neurologic dysfunction: musculoskeletal trauma, arthritis, osteoporosis, weight-bearing problems, head trauma, spinal cord injury, multiple sclerosis, myasthenia gravis, sensory deficit.

5. Medication history

Medications that may be taken for cardiovascular dysfunctions:

  Beta-blockers
  Antihypertensives
  Digoxin
  Aspirin/anticoagulants
  Over-the-counter

Clinical Significance

Focus on reports of pain, discomfort, fatigue, dyspnea, and cough. The characteristics of these symptoms can often be a clue to underlying medical problems such as cardiovascular disease or pulmonary illness.

Angina: Chest pain that results from the inability of the heart's vascular supply to keep up with metabolic demand.

Intermittent Claudication: Leg pain that results from inadequate blood supply and oxygen to leg muscles and resolves with rest.

Dyspnea: Shortness of breath is a pulmonary symptom or may accompany cardiac disease.

Orthopnea: The need to assume a more upright position to breathe.

Persons taking beta-blockers such as propanolol (Inderal) or metoprolol (Lopressor) may not reach target heart rates during exercise.

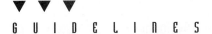

▼ ▼ ▼
G U I D E L I N E S

Procedure	Clinical Significance

Procedure

The major body systems that are considered during an assessment of activity and exercise functions include the cardiovascular, respiratory, and musculoskeletal systems. In addition to physical examination of these systems, a number of diagnostic tests may be performed to evaluate structures and functions.

1. **Diagnostic tests of cardiovascular function**

   Blood Tests:

   Complete blood count (CBC)

   Hematocrit

   Hemoglobin

   Anemia: Indicated by low hematocrit/hemoglobin. Cardiac output may increase to accommodate anemia.

   Lipid Profiles (serum cholesterol, triglyceride, and lipoprotein levels)

   Lipid abnormalities may indicate a risk for coronary artery disease, generalized atherosclerosis, and lipid disease.

   Serum enzymes (CPK, LDH, SGOT, HBD)

   Enzyme elevation occurs after cell death in the myocardium, for example, myocardial infarction.

   Noninvasive Cardiovascular Studies

   Chest x-ray

   The chest x-ray shows heart size, orientation, enlargement of individual chambers, calcification of valves.

   Electrocardiogram (ECG, EKG)

   Electrocardiogram: Graphic recording of electrical activity in the heart providing information about cardiac rhythm disturbances, conduction defects, cellular death or injury patterns, and electrolyte status.

   Holter monitoring

   Provides ECG recording over an extended period (24 hours); The person wears a compact monitor during all of their usual activities.

   Stress test or exercise tolerance test

   Monitors the ECG as the person performs prescribed exercises such as walking on a treadmill. Used in the evaluation of activity tolerance and the diagnosis of myocardial ischemia.

   Echocardiography

   Cardiac Ultrasound. Scanning to evaluate cardiac structures, especially the chambers and the valves.

   Plethysmography

   This procedure detects deep vein thrombosis in the lower extremities. Pressure cuffs are applied to the legs, inflated, and vessel pressure measured. If the pressure fails to immediately return to normal after cuff release, thrombosis should be suspected.

   Nuclear Medicine Studies

   Positron emission tomography (PET)

   PET Study: Radioactive tracers are injected and then evaluated to determine the metabolic status of myocardial tissue, including the location and exact size of a myocardial infarction, reversible versus irreversible myocardial tissue damage, and the effects of various treatments.

   Thallium scanning

   Thallium Scan: Used in the evaluation of coronary artery disease. Thallium, a radioactive tracer, is injected. Thallium accumulates in normal myocardium but not in areas that are not perfused. Ischemic areas show decreased radioactive activity or cold spots.

▼ ▼ ▼

GUIDELINES *continued*

Diagnostic Studies for Evaluation of Activity and Exercise Functions

Procedure	Clinical Significance
Invasive Cardiovascular Studies Cardiac catheterization Arteriograms	*Cardiac catheterization* can be performed on either the right or the left side of the heart. Pressures in the various cardiac chamber are determined, and blood samples may be obtained for blood gas analysis. This study can evaluate left ventricular function, measure cardiac output, and confirm pathologic conditions. *Angiograms* are radiographic studies of the heart chambers and vessels. Contrast medium is injected, and rapid-series x-ray films are obtained. Occlusive processes are readily identified.
2. **Diagnostic studies of pulmonary functions** Arterial blood gas (ABG) Components of the ABG: • Partial pressure of oxygen (PO_2) • Partial pressure of carbon dioxide (PCO_2) • Bicarbonate level • Percentage of oxygen saturation (SO_2) • pH Pulmonary function tests	The PO_2 value indicates how well the lungs are delivering oxygen to the blood. The PCO_2 indicates how well the lungs eliminate CO_2. The pH of the arterial blood indicates acid–base status. Abnormalities in blood gas values may indicate a respiratory disorder or a metabolic problem. Pulmonary function tests (PFTs) are used to measure lung capacity and lung volumes. Test results can differentiate obstructive or restrictive pulmonary diseases, determine surgical anesthesia risk, and monitor therapeutic responses. PFTs measurement involves use of a spirometer, a device that measures volumes of air that move in and out of the lungs during ventilation.

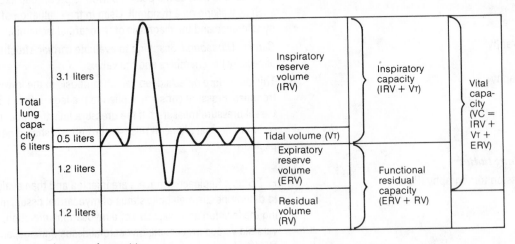

Lung volumes and capacities.

| Oximetry | *Oximetry* is a noninvasive method of monitoring oxygen and carbon dioxide levels in the blood. |

▼ ▼ ▼

G U I D E L I N E S *continued*

Diagnostic Studies for Evaluation of Activity and Exercise Functions

Procedure	Clinical Significance
3. **Diagnostic tests of musculoskeletal functions**	
Radiographic Studies	
The musculoskeletal system may be evaluated radiographically, using a number of different modalities:	
Diagnostic x-rays	Used to diagnose fractures, degenerative conditions, impingement, or tumors
Magnetic resonance imaging (MRI)	Used to identify musculoskeletal trauma, tumors, and spinal conditions
Computed tomography (CT scan)	Used to identify musculoskeletal trauma and other disorders
Bone scintigraphy (bone scan)	Used primarily to identify metastatic processes in the bone
Myelography (myelogram)	Involves injection of radiopaque solution along spinal canal to identify abnormalities, including herniated discs or tumors
Arthrography (arthrogram)	The radiographic study of joints after injection of a contrast material
Electromyography	The graphic reading of nerve and muscle responses to electrical stimulation. Indicates nerve status and muscle disorders

▼ ▼ ▼

G U I D E L I N E S

Assessment Guidelines Interpreting Physical Examination Findings Related to Activity and Exercise

Procedure

1. **Integrate physical examination findings with the assessment of activity and exercise with special attention to the following:**
   - General appearance
   - Vital signs
   - The neurologic system
   - The integumentary system
   - The cardiovascular system
   - The respiratory system
   - The musculoskeletal system

   (Note: Complete examination guidelines are presented elsewhere in this chapter for the cardiovascular, respiratory, and musculoskeletal systems).

2. **General appearance**

   During the general survey, note whether there are problems with movement by observing gait, posture, and obvious alterations such as missing limbs. Note the pattern of wear on the shoes, especially the heels, which could indicate altered walking movements. Note any prostheses. Survey muscle mass and muscle tone, noting any limb atrophy.

Clinical Significance

Physical examination related to activity and exercise focuses on identifying any limitations to physical movement, the status of the body systems essential for oxygenation, activity, and exercise, and physiologic responses to activity

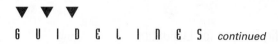

Interpreting Physical Examination Findings Related to Activity and Exercise

Procedure	Clinical Significance
Survey grooming.	Appearance and general hygiene may reflect a person's ability to meet self-care needs.
Look for general signs of activity intolerance by observing facial expression and mental status. Look for facial expressions of pain, anxiety, decreased level of consciousness. Note the general condition of the skin, especially color.	Pallor and cyanosis reflect oxygenation problems and may be associated with activity intolerance.
3. Vital signs Evaluate pulse at rest and with activity, ventilatory rate, and blood pressure.	Pulse rate should increase with increases in activity up to an age-defined level. Pulse rates should gradually return to normal after exercise.
4. The neurologic system *(Note: Techniques for the examination of the neurologic system are discussed in Chapter 9)* Review the medical history for neurologic problems and indications of neurologic dysfunction during the physical examination.	Numerous neurologic dysfunctions, including sensory deficits such as impaired vision of hearing, contribute to activity and exercise problems. Neurologic factors may contribute to self-care deficits, mobility problems, and respiratory disorders.
5. The integumentary system *(Note: Techniques of skin examination are discussed in Chapter 6)* Examine the skin, with special attention to the skin over the lower extremities.	Changes to skin appearance may be observed secondary to cardiovascular or function dysfunctions: *Edema:* swelling related to circulatory problems *Nail Clubbing:* Associated with chronic hypoxia *Loss of Normal Hair Distribution (legs):* effect of poor circulation

Nursing Diagnoses Related to Activity and Exercise Assessment

Activity Intolerance

Activity intolerance is the inability to endure or tolerate an increase in activity. However, you should also consider the diagnosis potential for activity intolerance, to identify persons at high risk and prescribe appropriate activity restrictions for this problem. Causes of activity intolerance include cardiovascular and pulmonary disease and cardiovascular deconditioning, as well as noncardiovascular factors such as depression, chronic illness, and prolonged immobility. People may be screened for this problem by considering various aspects of a person's health history and physical examination.

If the patient has heart disease, the four levels of the New York Heart Association's Functional and Therapeutic Classification may be used to help predict the appropriate activity tolerance level (see p. 295). The patient's condition can be classified according to the severity of symptoms elicited during activity and exercise.

The most feasible way in the clinical setting to assess a person's activity capabilities is to monitor continuously his or her response to activity. Assess vital signs before, immediately after, and 3 minutes after monitored activities to determine the person's tolerance level. Note other physical changes as well as any symptoms the patient reports.

Vital Signs. Vital signs indicate an ability to tolerate activity and a normal or abnormal response to activity.

Normal

- *Resting level:* Pulse 60–100 beats/min; blood pressure < 140/90; respirations < 20 breaths/min
- *Immediately after activity:* Pulse rate and strength increased; systolic blood pressure increased; respiratory rate and depth increased
- *Three minutes after activity:* Pulse rate within 6 beats/min of resting pulse

Abnormal

- *Resting level:* Pulse > 100 beats/min; blood pressure > 140/90; respirations > 20 breaths/min
- *Immediately after activity:* Pulse rate and strength decreased, irregular pulse; systolic blood pressure

decreased or unchanged; excessive increase or decrease in respiratory rate

- *Three minutes after activity:* Pulse rate greater than 7 beats/min over resting rate

Physical and Cognitive Changes. The following changes also may indicate poor activity tolerance: pallor, diaphoresis, cyanosis, incoordination, ECG changes, and confusion.

Symptoms. Activity intolerance may be associated with the following symptoms: fatigue, weakness, exertional pain, dyspnea, dizziness, and vertigo.

Clinical Problems Related to Activity and Exercise Assessment

Activity intolerance may be accompanied by symptoms of pain, discomfort, fatigue, dyspnea, or cough. The characteristics of these symptoms can often be a clue to underlying medical problems such as cardiovascular disease or pulmonary illness.

Cardiac Chest Pain. Cardiac chest pain occurs with angina, pericarditis, and aortic aneurysm. Angina occurs from an oxygen debt in the myocardium and may be precipitated by activity. The pain is often described as a squeezing, pressing, or tightening sensation; it is seldom described as sharp. The pain also may be precipitated by stress, hypoglycemia, or the ingestion of a heavy meal. Often, anginal pain radiates throughout the chest or to the arms or jaw and may be difficult to pinpoint.

Pericarditis pain occurs when the membranes or pericardium around the heart become inflamed. Unlike episodic anginal pain, pericardial pain is persistent, sharp, and usually aggravated by deep breathing.

A dissecting aortic aneurysm usually causes a constant, intense, searing pain that may radiate to the back, anterior chest, or abdomen. It requires immediate medical attention.

Activity Tolerance Classification. For persons with cardiac disease, activity tolerance may be characterized by using the New York Heart Association's Functional and Therapeutic Classification System as follows:

- *Class I:* Person with heart disease who is asymptomatic. Ordinary physical activity does not cause undue fatigue, palpitation, dyspnea, or angina.
- *Class II:* Slight limitation of physical activity. The person has no distress at rest, but ordinary physical activity results in fatigue, dyspnea, or angina.
- *Class III:* Significant limitation of physical activity. The person has no distress at rest, but even low-intensity self-care activities cause fatigue, palpitation, dyspnea, or angina.
- *Class IV:* Symptoms at rest. The person may have angina or dyspnea even at rest, and any physical activity aggravates symptoms.

Pulmonary Chest Pain. Pulmonary chest pain is often called pleuritic chest pain because the pain is secondary to inflammation of the pleural surfaces lining the lungs and inner thoracic cage. Inflammation may be caused by infection, tumors, trauma, or pneumothorax. Breathing aggravates pleuritic pain, which is usually sharp or knife-like. To avoid or lessen the discomfort, the person may take shallow breaths and splint the chest (lean toward or put pressure on the affected side to minimize chest excursion). A person with pleuritic pain usually feels short of breath because of poor lung ventilation and gas exchange. Activity may be poorly tolerated because of the altered breathing pattern.

Claudication. Intermittent claudication is a sharp, cramping, squeezing pain that occurs in the legs in response to activity or exercise. The pain may result from ischemia, or oxygen deficit, and it usually occurs in the presence of atherosclerosis in the major arteries supplying the leg. If the pain, which usually dissipates with rest, persists more than 10 minutes after rest, another cause may be indicated, such as arthritis. Intermittent claudication usually occurs in the calf muscles and is brought on by walking. The amount of walking that precipitates the pain indicates the severity of the arterial occlusion. Therefore, you should ask specific questions about the amount of walking that brings on the pain and the length of time the pain lasts.

Musculoskeletal Pain. Musculoskeletal pain is often associated with movement. It is important to determine whether the pain is attributable to alterations in the joints (articular pain) or in the surrounding structures such as muscles, tendons, or bones (periarticular pain). If you suspect musculoskeletal pain, follow the special physical examination procedures described in Physical Examination of the Musculoskeletal System. Often, musculoskeletal pain is localized, as in the case of degenerative joint disease, which may produce pain in the knees, hips, neck, fingers, or back. If the pain can be reproduced by direct palpation, ischemia can be ruled out as the cause. Specific movements also may reproduce the pain. Articular pain may be associated with stiffness and swelling of the affected joint.

Fatigue and Weakness. Fatigue may be expressed as a lack of energy or "pep." You should explore whether it is caused by physiologic factors or by psychological factors such as depression or boredom. The duration of the fatigue is also an important factor. Fatigue that is relatively rapid and recent in onset and that cannot be associated with physical work may represent infection, a fluid balance disturbance, anemia, or a cardiac or peripheral circulatory compromise. In such cases, even minimal activity may cause fatigue. Chronic fatigue, especially if accompanied by symptoms of psychological distress, may be secondary to depression or anxiety. In this case, ask the person about events that occurred when fatigue first became a problem.

Weakness, often erroneously confused with fatigue, is a symptom associated with decreased muscular strength. Rarely of psychological origin, weakness may result from muscle or nerve dysfunction and requires more elaborate diagnostic testing.

Shortness of Breath. Shortness of breath, or dyspnea, may reflect cardiac, pulmonary, or psychogenic problems. Hyperventilation, which occurs when an excessive accumulation of carbon dioxide is excreted, may occur during exercise or in other states of metabolic acidosis, and should not be confused with dyspnea.

You should ask whether the person has difficulty breathing when lying down (orthopnea), which may indicate severe congestive heart failure, asthma, pulmonary edema, chronic obstructive pulmonary disease (COPD), pneumothorax, or pneumonia. In persons with orthopnea, dyspnea can be relieved only in either a sitting or standing position.

Dyspnea during exertion may be related to impaired ventilation, which occurs with restrictive or obstructive pulmonary disease, diffusion defects, or ineffective breathing patterns. Dyspnea at rest usually occurs with severe cardiac disease rather than chronic pulmonary disorders. It is also associated, however, with acute pulmonary problems, such as asthma, pneumothorax, and pneumonia.

Cough.   Coughing may indicate pulmonary or cardiac problems and should be evaluated further. If the cough is productive, evaluate the amount, consistency, and color of any expectorated material, and note the presence of blood.

PART 2
PHYSICAL EXAMINATION TECHNIQUES

CARDIOVASCULAR SYSTEM
Anatomy and Physiology Review

The Heart and Great Vessels

The heart is a hollow, cone-shaped, muscular organ located beneath and to the left of the sternum. It is divided into a left and right side, each of which consists of an upper atrial chamber and a lower ventricular chamber. The chambers contract and relax in a syncopated rhythm that constitutes the beat of the heart. The atria are tilted slightly toward the back, whereas the ventricles extend to the left and toward the anterior chest wall.

The top of the heart is referred to as the *base,* whereas the conical bottom is called the *apex.* The apex is close enough to the chest wall to transmit a visible pulsation during ventricular contraction. The pulmonary artery, aorta, and right ventricle face the anterior chest wall (Fig. 8-1). Heart size varies according to the size of the person. The size and shape of a person's clenched fist closely approximate the size and shape of his or her heart. The great vessels attached to the heart include the aorta, the pulmonary artery, the superior and inferior venae cavae, and the pulmonary veins (see Fig. 8-1).

Blood Flow

Blood flows through the heart by way of a series of chambers and one-way valves (Fig. 8-2). The superior and inferior venae cavae return deoxygenated blood to the heart from peripheral veins. Blood enters the right atrium,

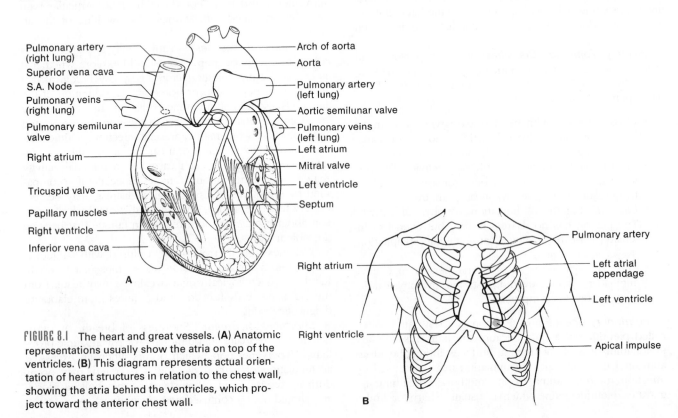

FIGURE 8.1   The heart and great vessels. (**A**) Anatomic representations usually show the atria on top of the ventricles. (**B**) This diagram represents actual orientation of heart structures in relation to the chest wall, showing the atria behind the ventricles, which project toward the anterior chest wall.

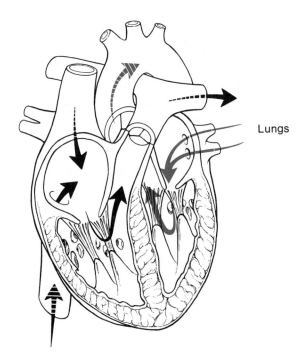

FIGURE 8.2   Blood flow through the heart.

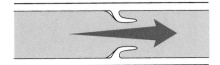

High flow

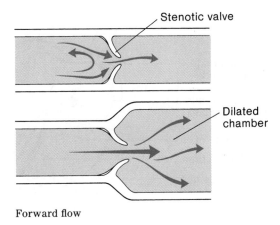

Stenotic valve

Dilated chamber

Forward flow

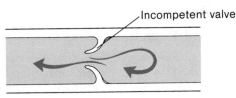

Incompetent valve

Backward flow

FIGURE 8.3   Origin of murmurs. **(Top)** High flow; **(middle)** forward flow through abnormal valves or chambers; **(bottom)** backward flow through abnormal valves or structures.

which is a thin-walled, low-pressure filling chamber, passes through the tricuspid valve, and enters the right ventricle, which is a higher-pressure pumping chamber. Blood is then ejected from the right ventricle through the pulmonary valve and into the pulmonary artery, which carries blood to the lungs. Blood becomes oxygenated while flowing through the extensive capillary network of the lungs, before returning to the left atrium by way of the four pulmonary veins. The blood then passes through the mitral valve and finally enters the left ventricle, which is a thick-walled, high-pressure pumping chamber. Ventricular contraction ejects the blood through the aortic valve into the aorta, which distributes blood throughout the body.

Altered Blood Flow: Murmurs

Murmurs are abnormal heart sounds or vibrations. They may occur at any point in the cardiac cycle and are caused by high rates of blood flow or turbulent blood flow over diseased valves.

Three main factors contribute to the intracardiac sounds called murmurs (Fig. 8-3):

1. High flow rates through normal or abnormal valves
2. Forward flow of blood through a constricted or irregular valve or into a dilated vessel or chamber
3. Backward or regurgitant flow through an incompetent valve, septal defect, or patent ductus arteriosus

The Conduction System

As electrical impulses cause heart muscle to depolarize, the heart's pumping chambers contract. This electrical impulse originates in the sinoatrial (SA) node near the right atrium and spreads through atrial conduction pathways to the atrioventricular (AV) node located at the interventricular septum (Fig. 8-4). This wave of atrial depolarization corresponds to the P wave on the ECG. The electrical impulse pauses at the AV node, allowing the ventricles to fill completely with blood before ventricular contraction. This phase of the cardiac cycle appears as the PR interval on the ECG. Next, the impulse travels rapidly through the bundle of His and down the left and right bundle branches to the terminal Purkinje fibers. The ECG configuration for this phase is called the QRS complex. Repolarization of the ventricles corresponds to the T wave on the ECG.

Arterial Blood Vessels

The arteries are strong, compliant vessels that carry oxygenated blood away from the heart to peripheral tissues. The elastic properties of the arterial walls cause the arteries to stretch during systole and recoil during diastole. This results in a palpable arterial pulse and is the physiologic principle behind blood pressure measurement (see Chap. 4).

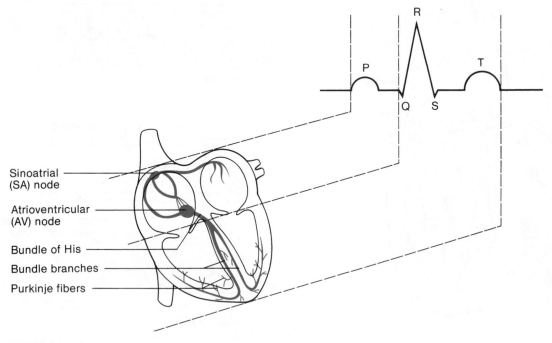

FIGURE 8.4 The cardiac conduction system in relation to the electrocardiogram.

Venous Blood Vessels

Veins are low-pressure vessels that carry deoxygenated blood to the heart. They have a larger capacity and thinner walls than arteries. Blood flow through the veins does not usually produce pulsations. However, pulsations may be noted in large central veins, such as the right internal jugular, and are caused by pressures generated in the right atrium during the cardiac cycle. Venous pulses have several distinct components, including the positive *a, c,* and *v* waves and negative descent waves, *x* and *y* (Fig. 8-5). Normally, only the *a* and *c* waves are readily detectable during the physical examination. The cardiac events generating these waves are discussed in the following section.

Veins distend when the intravascular volume increases; this may be noted in the great veins of the neck. See the section entitled Examination Guidelines: Neck Veins, later in this chapter.

The Cardiac Cycle

The cardiac cycle includes all events between ventricular contractions (see Fig. 8-5). Understanding the cardiac cycle is important for assessing cardiovascular function because changes in blood flow during the cycle cause tension and vibration, which affect the heart valves and other structures. The sounds that are generated may be auscultated with the stethoscope. Electrocardiogram waveforms, pulsations in great veins, and arterial waveforms also correspond to events in the cardiac cycle.

Ventricular systole and diastole are the two major phases of the cardiac cycle. During heart auscultation, these phases can be distinguished by noting the heart sounds as "lub-dub"; "lub," or the first heart sound (S_1), signals the beginning of systole, and "dub," or the second

heart sound (S_2), signals the beginning of diastole. When the heart rate is between 60 and 100 beats/min, the cardiac cycle lasts approximately 0.86 seconds. Systole, the time between S_1 and S_2, is shorter than diastole. When heart rates are greater than 100 beats/min, diastole shortens, and systole and diastole periods become almost equal. The cardiac cycle can be traced from the beginning of diastole as follows:

1. Rapid Inflow. Blood flows into the atria from the venae cavae and pulmonary veins. This movement increases the pressure in the atria over the pressure in the ventricles, which causes the AV valves to open and blood to flow rapidly into the ventricles.

Assessment Implications

- An abnormal heart sound, called the opening snap (OS), may occur during rapid inflow and is caused by the rapid opening motion of a diseased and stenotic mitral valve.
- The third heart sound, S_3, may be heard during rapid filling and results from sound vibrations generated when blood hits the ventricle walls. This heart sound is common in healthy young adults and children, and is called a physiologic S_3. In pathologic states, the vibrations may be generated by an increased volume load to the ventricles or by blood hitting a noncompliant ventricular wall. Third heart sounds are commonly noted with congestive heart failure.

2. Diastasis. During this phase, the inflow of blood from atria to ventricles continues, but at a much slower rate.

3. Atrial Systole. A wave of atrial depolarization spreads through the atria, initiating an atrial contraction, which

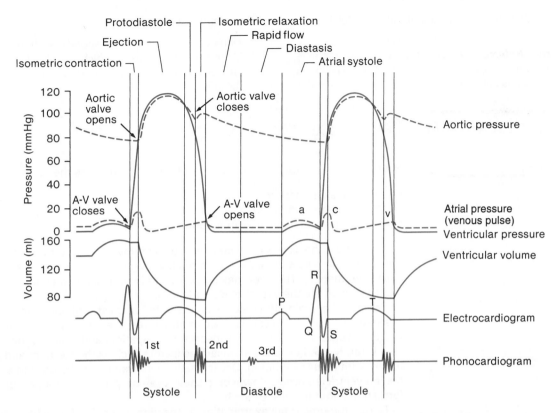

FIGURE 8.5 The cardiac cycle, showing changes in heart pressures and volumes, electrocardiogram, and phonocardiogram (graphic recording of heart sounds.)

forces the remaining 30% of blood into the ventricles, a process referred to as the "atrial kick."

Assessment Implications

- As pressure is transmitted to the venous system from atrial contraction, an *a* wave can be noted on the jugular venous pulsation (see Fig. 8-5).
- The P wave, PR interval, and beginning of the QRS complex can be noted on the ECG.
- An abnormal heart sound, called S_4, may be heard during atrial contraction. This sound is produced as blood rapidly enters the ventricles because of increased blood volume or decreased ventricular wall compliance.

4. Isometric Contraction. Systole begins as pressure increases in the ventricle walls, forcing the AV valves to shut. The increasing pressures cause the downstream pulmonic and aortic valves to open. No blood enters or leaves the ventricles.

Assessment Implications

- The first heart sound, S_1, results from vibrations related to AV valve closure. Because two valves are actually closing, S_1 may be split into mitral and tricuspid components.
- When the valve closures transmit pressure to the venous system, a *c* wave is produced. The *c* wave is difficult to see when inspecting the jugular venous pulsations but may be noted if the pressure is recorded as a waveform.
- An abnormal heart sound, or ejection click, is produced when the tricuspid valves open, either when one of the valves is diseased or when ejection is rapid through a normal valve.

5. Protodiastolic Ejection. After the aortic valve opens, blood flows rapidly from the left ventricle. At the same time, the right ventricle empties through the open pulmonic valve. When the blood flow ceases, the pressure in the ventricles becomes lower than the pressure in the great arteries. Subsequently, blood flows back toward the ventricles, forcing the aortic and pulmonic valves to close.

Assessment Implications

- When the aortic and pulmonic valves close, a second heart sound, S_2, is produced. During inspiration, S_2 may be heard as a split sound as increased blood volume is returned to the right side of the heart, causing pulmonic closure to occur slightly later than aortic closure.
- The T wave can be observed on the ECG.
- If hemodynamic monitoring is being performed, the dicrotic notch on the arterial waveform will correspond to aortic valve closure.
- A midsystolic click may be heard during the middle of protodiastolic ejection. This high-frequency, snapping noise is believed to be related to prolapsing or

backward motion of the mitral valve leaflets during systole.

6. Isometric Relaxation. After the aortic valve closes, ventricle pressure falls, and the ventricles relax while maintaining a constant volume.

Assessment Implication

- Isometric relaxation corresponds with the v wave in the venous pulse, which results from the increased atrial pressure caused by venous return to the heart.

Physical Examination   Cardiovascular System

GENERAL PRINCIPLES

Physical examination of the cardiovascular system involves the following:

- Precordial examination
- Arterial pulse examination
- Neck vein (venous pulse) examination

In addition, the skin is inspected during a cardiovascular examination to evaluate color changes, edema, and textures that might indicate cardiovascular disease (see Chap. 6). The liver may be evaluated in persons with congestive heart failure to evaluate the extent of pump failure.

Precordial examination focuses on the anterior chest wall and determining the status of underlying cardiovascular structures (the heart and great vessels). Precordial examination involves inspection, palpation, and auscultation. Percussion is rarely used because extracardiac factors such as the sternum and ribs interfere with heart evaluation. Occasionally, percussion may be used to evaluate the left ventricle border. However, a chest x-ray may provide more accurate information about the size of the heart.

During the precordial examination, inspection and palpation usually precede auscultation. However, it may sometimes be helpful to perform the two simultaneously, especially when abnormal findings are noted. For example, if an abnormal pulsation is detected by inspection and palpation, it is helpful to auscultate while palpating the pulse or inspecting neck veins to learn where the pulsation falls in the cardiac cycle.

It is also important to note whether findings occur during early, middle, or late systole or diastole, as well as whether they occur intermittently or continuously. Also, describe any variations with the breathing pattern.

Arterial pulses are generally assessed by palpating with the fingertips at points where an artery wall can be sufficiently compressed so that the artery's elastic recoil can be felt as pressure is transmitted from the aorta. Arterial pulses also may be detected by more sensitive equipment, such as Doppler ultrasound. Carotid and femoral arteries as well as the abdominal aorta should be auscultated with the bell and diaphragm of the stethoscope. Except for the carotids, pulses should be palpated bilaterally and simultaneously to make meaningful comparisons.

The neck veins are evaluated to determine the characteristics of the venous pulse to make judgments about the function of the right side of the heart. Jugular venous pulsations (JVP) and central venous pressure (CVP) can be determined by assessing the neck veins.

Jugular venous pulsations and CVP may be assessed by inspection as well as by invasive monitoring devices capable of producing a waveform or pressure scale reading. Inspection involves observing the column of venous blood in the internal jugular vein. Internal jugular vein pulsation can be distinguished from carotid artery pulsation by noting the difference in the type of stroke. The JVP is characterized by several low-amplitude and positive upstrokes, as opposed to one brisk upstroke in the arterial pulse. To make this distinction, palpate the carotid artery on the opposite side while viewing the JVP. An alternative method is to ask the person to lie flat, which causes visible jugular vein distension. When the person sits up, the jugular vein distension will disappear because the vein will collapse. Pulsation from the internal jugular vein also may be identified by placing pressure on the neck just above and parallel to the clavicle.

(continued)

Physical Examination   Cardiovascular System (continued)

In approximately 20 seconds, the vein will fill, and the distension will become exaggerated.

EQUIPMENT

Stethoscope with bell and diaphragm
Ruler for measuring neck vein distention
Light source to provide tangential lighting
Doppler for detecting arterial pulses (optional)

EXAMINING ROOM PREPARATION

To auscultate heart sounds accurately, the examination should take place in a quiet room. As with any procedure that requires the person to be exposed, privacy as well as comfort should be maintained. The examination should be conducted with the person sitting or lying on a table or bed that will allow for various position changes.

EXPOSURE AND LIGHTING

Tangential lighting, such as side lighting from a gooseneck lamp, is effective for casting shadows on the anterior chest or neck veins and thus making chest movements or venous pulsations more visible. The chest should be partially draped except during inspection, when the entire precordium must be surveyed. Listening to heart sounds through clothing is unreliable and inadvisable.

PRECORDIAL EXAMINATION POSITIONS

During the precordial examination, the examiner stands at the person's right side. If possible, the person's position is changed during the examination to bring underlying cardiac structures closer to the chest wall (Fig. 8-6).

The *supine position,* with the person's arms resting comfortably at the sides, will be adequate for most of the examination. The upper torso may be elevated to a 30-degree angle. The *forward-sitting position* will bring the base of the heart closer to the chest wall and is most effective for evaluating thrills and murmurs. The *left lateral decubitus position* will allow the apex of the heart to move closer to the chest wall and is best for detecting mitral valve murmurs.

PRECORDIAL LANDMARKS

Because the heart and great vessels are not visible, a system of precordial landmarks is used to guide the examination and provide locations for describing any sounds and pulsations observed during the examination. Heart sounds are created by valve movements and blood flow in the heart. Heart sounds are heard at the chest wall, but the area where you hear a sound may not be the area from which it originated. This is because blood flow transmits the sound away from

(continued)

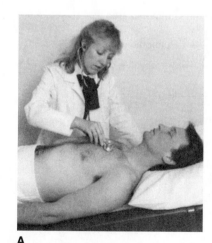

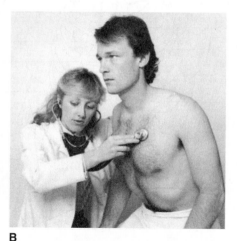

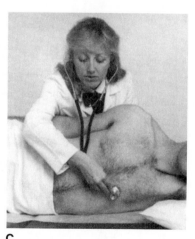

A   **B**   **C**

FIGURE 8.6   Precordial examination positions. (**A**) Supine position; (**B**) forward-sitting position; (**C**) left lateral decubitus position.

its point of origin. Heart sounds originating with the valves are detected in the direction of blood flow at one of the following landmarks (Fig. 8-7):

The *aortic area,* located to the right of the sternum at the second intercostal space, represents the direction of blood flow from the aortic valve and the direction of sound transmission after closure of the aortic valve. Auscultatory findings related to the aortic valve may be heard at this point.

The *pulmonic area,* located to the left of the sternum at the second intercostal space, represents the pulmonic valve, which is located slightly lower than the second intercostal space. This landmark correlates with the outflow tract of the pulmonic valve.

The *tricuspid area,* located to the left of the sternum at the fifth intercostal space, represents the tricuspid valve, which is actually more superior and to the right of the sternum. The tricuspid area represents the outflow tract of the tricuspid valve and the direction of sound transmission after valve closure.

The *mitral or apical area,* located at the fifth left intercostal space just medial to the midclavicular line, represents a valve and a cardiac chamber. Blood flows from the mitral valve, which is superior and to the right, into the mitral or apical area. The apex of the left ventricle also lies beneath this area, and a pulsation may be palpated as the ventricle contracts.

Additional precordial landmarks may be useful during the examination (Fig. 8-8):

The *sternoclavicular area* overlies the sternum and its junctions with both clavicles, as well as portions of the left and right intercostal spaces. These structures can serve as a landmark for assessing the aortic arch and pulmonary artery, which are located to the left of the first intercostal space.

The *right ventricular area* overlies the heart's right ventricle, which faces the anterior chest and extends from the third intercostal space to the distal end of the sternum. The right lateral border of the right ventricular area overlies the right atrium. The left ventricle is located under the left lateral border.

(continued)

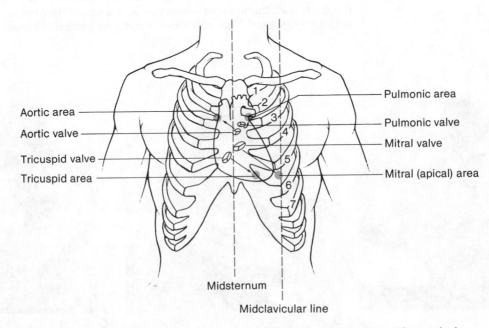

FIGURE 8.7   Heart sounds and precordial landmarks. Heart sounds are referred from valvular points of origin to the auscultatory or precordial landmarks. Sound travels in the direction of blood flow and may be heard at some distance from the valve.

Physical Examination Cardiovascular System (continued)

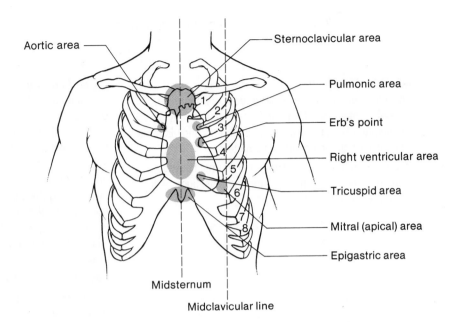

Aortic area — Sternoclavicular area

Pulmonic area

Erb's point

Right ventricular area

Tricuspid area

Mitral (apical) area

Epigastric area

Midsternum

Midclavicular line

FIGURE 8.8 Additional pre-cordial landmarks.

Erb's point, the third left interspace, is included in the right ventricular area. Aortic and pulmonic valve sounds may be transmitted to this point.

The *epigastric area* represents the same anatomic region for both abdominal and cardiac examinations. Aortic or right ventricular pulsations may be detected in this area.

The *ectopic area* represents a landmark where abnormal precordial pulsations can be palpated in persons with left ventricular wall disorders secondary to angina or diffuse myocardial disease. Usually, such pulsations may be detected in the left mid-precordium, just above the left ventricular apex. However, this location varies among people.

EXAMINATION AND DOCUMENTATION FOCUS [PRECORDIUM]

- *Inspection:* Pulsatile movements
- *Palpation:* Pulsatile movements, vibrations
- *Auscultation:* Heart rate and rhythm, heart sounds and murmurs

EXAMINATION AND DOCUMENTATION FOCUS [ARTERIAL PULSES]

- Ease of palpation
- Rate and rhythm of pulsation
- Character of the arterial wall
- Auscultatory findings
- Contour and amplitude

EXAMINATION AND DOCUMENTATION FOCUS [NECK VEINS]

- Pulse contour and amplitude
- Distention
- Height of venous pulsation

▼ ▼ ▼
G U I D E L I N E S

Assessment Guidelines   Heart and Precordium

Procedure

1. **Inspect the precordium.**

   a. With the person supine, observe from the right side. (Viewing the person from the foot of the bed may also be helpful.) Note the precordial landmarks and visualize the position of the underlying structures.

   b. Observe each precordial area for abnormal heaves, thrusts, paradoxical movements, and pulsations. Also note the breathing pattern.

2. **Palpate the major precordial landmarks.**

   a. With the person supine, palpate each precordial area, aortic, pulmonic, Erb's point, tricuspid, mitral with the ball of the hand. Palpate pulsations with the fingertips. You may place the stethoscope lightly on the chest as you palpate, to time findings with the cardiac cycle.

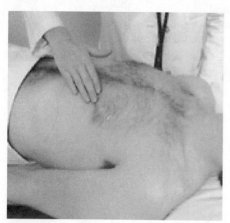

Precordial palpation with fingertips

   b. Note any pulsations, thrills, or rubs that must be further described in terms of location, amplitude, duration, and direction of impulse.

   c. You may palpate with the person in the forward-sitting position or left lateral decubitus position. However, changing to these positions at the end of the examination may be easier.

Clinical Significance

Normal Findings

Apical pulse or PMI: Pulsation known as the apical pulse or point of maximal impulse (PMI) may be seen at the mitral area. This pulsation represents the outward thrust of the left ventricle during early systole and is caused by the heart wall recoiling as blood is ejected. A normal PMI is observed in the mitral area and should be no larger in diameter than 2 or 3 cm. However, during the later stages of pregnancy, this pulse may be noted above the fifth intercostal space because the diaphragm is displaced upward. The apical impulse may not be visible in all people, especially those who are obese or who have large breasts.

Deviations from Normal

Pulsations in the epigastric area may be noted in thin people. However, such a finding may be abnormal and should be further evaluated.

A heave or lift is a sustained, forceful movement of the ventricle during systole associated with an increased workload. Right ventricular heave is best observed at the sternal border. Left ventricular heave is observed at the apex.

The ball of the hand is most sensitive to vibrations; fingertips are sensitive to pulsations.

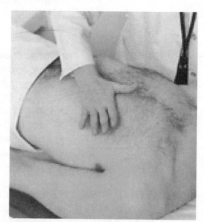

Precordial palpation with ball of hand

Normal Findings

Pulsatile movements: Normally, only pulsations over the mitral area corresponding to the PMI can be palpated.

Deviations from Normal

Vibrations: Palpable thrills, associated with murmurs, sound and feel like a purring cat and are not normal in any precordial area.

▼ ▼ ▼
G U I D E L I N E S *continued*   Heart and Precordium

Procedure	Clinical Significance

Procedure

3. **Auscultate the major precordial landmarks.**

   a. With the person supine, systematically proceed from one landmark to the next in this sequence: aortic, pulmonic, Erb's point, tricuspid, mitral.

      Listen for several cardiac cycles at each landmark.

      Listen to each sound and try to block out all other sounds.

      Auscultate each area using the diaphragm and the bell of the stethoscope.

      At each landmark identify S_1 and S_2, normal splitting of S_1 and/or S_2, extra heart sounds and murmurs (Display 8–3, "Abnormal Heart Sounds," and Display 8–4, "Murmurs")

4. **Identify S_1 and S_2.**

   The first heart sound, S_1, may be heard as a single sound and will be loudest at the apex when the diaphragm of the stethoscope is used.

   The second heart sound, S_2, may be heard as a single sound and will be loudest at the base of the heart. Note intensity and any sound splitting.

Clinical Significance

Heart rate: Normal resting heart rate is between 60 and 100 beats/minute but may be lower in people who are physically well-conditioned.

Rhythm: Usually rhythm will be regular, but it does vary in some persons, especially children and young adults. You may note an irregular rhythm that varies with respiration. During inspiration, venous return is greater and the heart rate may increase to compensate for the larger volume of blood. The rate will then decrease with expiration.

The diaphragm is used to detect higher-pitched sounds such as S_1, S_2, and aortic regurgitation murmurs. The bell is used to detect lower-pitched sounds such as S_3 and S_4.

S_1 represents the closing of the mitral and tricuspid valves.

S_2 represents the closing of the aortic and pulmonic valves.

Normal Findings

In a person with a normal heart rate and rhythm, the first and second heart sounds will be readily distinguished by the longer time between S_1 and S_2. Usually S_1 will be loudest at the mitral or apical area, and S_2 will be loudest at the pulmonic area. Also, S_1 may be heard almost simultaneously while palpating the upstroke of the carotid pulse.

Noting such variations may help when identifying S_1 and S_2 in persons with rapid heart rates.

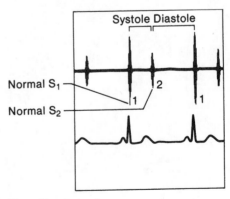

Normal heart sounds

DISPLAY 8.3

Abnormal Heart Sounds

ABNORMAL S₁ SPLITTING

Widely split first sound: S_1 may be abnormally split. Listen for a widely split S_1 with the diaphragm of the stethoscope.

This split may be secondary to electrical or mechanical causes, such as bundle-branch block and ventricular ectopy, that result in asynchronous ventricular contraction. A widely split first sound may be confused with other abnormal sounds, such as ejection clicks, that occur at this point in the cycle.

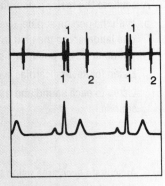

Widely split S₁

ABNORMAL S₂ SPLITTING

Second sound splitting: S_2 splitting during expiration is considered abnormal and may occur as either fixed splitting or splitting that is accentuated on inspiration. Use the diaphragm of the stethoscope at the base of the heart to detect this sound.

Splitting occurs because aortic and pulmonic valves close at least 0.03 seconds apart. Delayed pulmonic valve closure may be noted with right bundle-branch block or pulmonic stenosis.

Reserved second sound splitting (paradoxical split): Reversed or paradoxic S_2 splitting can be noted with expiration (unlike a normal or widely split second sound, which is detected on inspiration).

Paradoxical splitting occurs when the pulmonic valve closes first because of delays with left ventricular ejection related to left bundle-branch block or aortic stenosis.

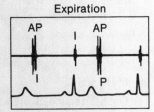

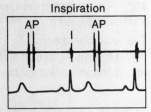

S₂ splitting

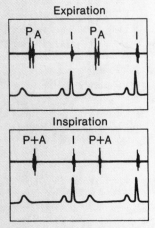

Reversed S₂ splitting

(continued)

DISPLAY 8.3

Abnormal Heart Sounds (continued)

THIRD HEART SOUND (S₃)

The third heart sound, S_3, also called the ventricular gallop, is a low-frequency sound best heard using the bell of the stethoscope at either the apical area (for S_3 of left ventricular origin) or lower right ventricular area (for S_3 of right ventricular origin). The sound may be accentuated during inspiration (sounds like "Ken-tuc-ky").

S_3 is usually pathologic but may occur normally in young children or in people with high cardiac outputs. However, it is rarely normal in people over age 40 years. S_3 is associated with congestive heart failure and tricuspid or mitral valve insufficiency. This early diastolic sound represents rapid ventricular filling and is related to vibrations caused by blood forcefully hitting the ventricular wall.

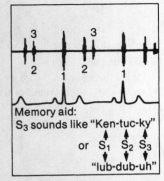

Third heart sound: S₃

OPENING SNAP (OS)

An opening snap (OS) is an abnormal early diastolic sound with a sharp quality, frequently mistaken for S_2 splitting or for an S_3. However, an OS will occur earlier than S_2 splitting or S_3. An OS will be detected at a higher pitch than S_3. This abnormal sound can be heard throughout the precordium and will not vary with respirations. Opening snaps occur secondary to the opening of a stenotic or stiff mitral valve.

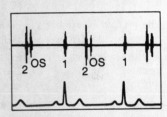

Opening snap

FOURTH HEART SOUND (S₄)

The fourth heart sound, S_4, also known as the atrial gallop, occurs near the end of diastole when the atria contract. Use the bell of the stethoscope to detect this low-frequency sound. Left ventricular S_4 sounds will be loudest at the apical area when the person assumes a supine or left lateral decubitus position. Right ventricular S_4 sounds will be loudest at the lower right ventricular area when the person assumes a supine position, and may increase in volume during inspiration (sounds like "Ten-nes-see").

S_4 occurs after atrial contraction and is caused by vibrations when blood flows rapidly into the ventricles. Vibrations result from the flow of a high blood volume or if the ventricle wall has low compliance. Associated conditions include coronary artery disease, hypertension, aortic and pulmonic stenosis, and acute myocardial infarction.

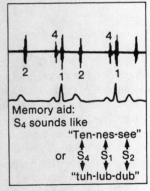

Fourth heart sound: S₄

SUMMATION GALLOP

When S_3 and S_4 occur simultaneously, the sound is called a *summation gallop*. Summation gallops are associated with severe congestive heart failure.

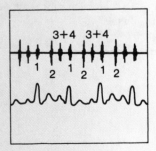

Summation gallop

(continued)

DISPLAY 8.3

Abnormal Heart Sounds (continued)

EJECTION CLICK

Heard just after the first heart sound, an *ejection click* is a high-frequency sound. This systolic sound can be heard widely throughout the precordium, unlike the more localized and lower-pitched S_4 sound.

Ejection clicks are produced by the opening of a diseased aortic or pulmonic valve or by rapid ejection through normal valves.

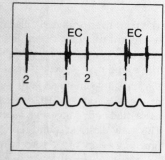

Ejection click

MIDSYSTOLIC CLICK

The *midsystolic click* is a high-frequency, snapping sound that can be heard in middle or late systole. Listen for this sound over the mitral or apical area.

A midsystolic click is attributed to mitral valve leaflet prolapse during left ventricular ejection.

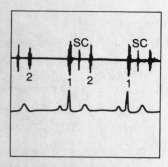

Midsystolic click

PERICARDIAL FRICTION RUBS

This extracardiac sound is a high-pitched, scratchy sound that can be simulated in the following manner: grasp the stethoscope in the left hand with the diaphragm facing the palm. Rub the thumb of the right hand back and fourth over the first and second finger metacarpal joints and listen to the simulated sound. Pericardial friction rubs are loudest at the left second, third, or fourth intercostal spaces and may be heard throughout the cardiac cycle, that is, throughout systole and diastole. There are three possible components of a pericardial friction rub: presystolic, systolic, and early diastolic. The rub is called *triphasic* if all three sounds are heard.

Pericardial friction rubs result from inflammation of the pericardial membrane.

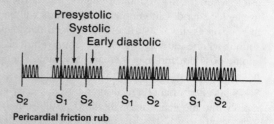

Pericardial friction rub

DISPLAY 8.4

Murmurs

CRITERIA FOR DESCRIBING MURMURS

All murmurs should be evaluated in terms of timing, intensity, quality, location, radiation, ventilation, and the effect of position changes.

1. TIMING

Does the murmur occur during systole or diastole? (Diastolic murmurs are usually pathological.) Describe the exact timing in relation to the cardiac cycle as follows:

a. A pansystolic (holosystolic) murmur is continuous throughout systole.

b. A midsystolic (ejection) murmur begins after S_1, peaks in midsystole, and ends before S_2.

c. A protodiastolic murmur occurs early in diastole.

d. A presystolic murmur occurs late in diastole.

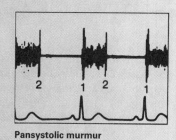

Pansystolic murmur

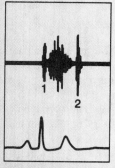

Midsystolic (ejection) murmur

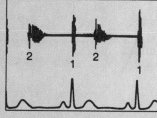

Protodiastolic murmur

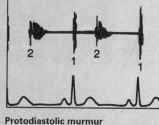

Presystolic murmur

2. INTENSITY.

How loud is the murmur? Use the following grading system to describe the murmur intensity:

I—Barely audible

II—Audible but quiet

III—Clearly heard

IV—Loud; may be associated with thrill

V—Very loud; palpable thrill; may hear with stethoscope partially off chest

VI—Very loud; palpable thrill; can hear without using stethoscope

3. QUALITY.

What is the quality, pitch, and pattern of the murmur? Describe pitch using terms such as *high* or *low* and quality with terms such as *blowing*, *harsh*, or *musical*. Pattern refers to changes in murmur intensity.

a. *Crescendo:* The murmur becomes progressively louder.

b. *Descrescendo:* The murmur becomes progressively softer.

c. *Crescendo-decresendo:* The murmur peaks in intensity.

4. LOCATION

Over which precordial landmark is the murmur loudest?

Murmurs are recorded as a fraction, with the grade as the numerator and "VI" (which indicates the grading scale used) as the denominator. Example: grade II/VI.

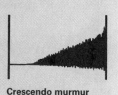

Crescendo murmur   **Decrescendo murmur**

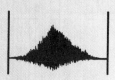

Crescendo-decrescendo murmur

(continued)

Murmurs (continued)

5. RADIATION.
Is the sound of the murmur transmitted to other areas of the precordium? Murmurs usually radiate in the direction of blood flow.

6. VENTILATION AND POSITION.
Is the murmur affected by inspiration, expiration, or position changes?

NURSING ROLE

Your role in evaluating murmurs is to detect new murmurs and changes in existing murmurs. You should make appropriate referrals based on your assessment. Describe the murmur(s) in relation to the criteria described below. Although specific murmur diagnosis is often the cardiologist's responsibility, you should be able to recognize life-threatening murmurs, such as a mitral regurgitation murmur in the patient who has recently had a myocardial infarction. Such a murmur, often having a sudden onset, may indicate papillary muscle rupture. The ensuing left-sided heart failure is a frequent cause of death.

COMMON MURMURS

Physiologic Murmurs

- Nonpathologic murmurs also called physiologic or innocent murmurs
- Can only be detected during systole
- Normal during late pregnancy and in children
- Also associated with increased cardiac output states such as anemia or hyperthyroidism

Mitral Regurgitation

- Pansystolic (holostolic)
- Grade varies from I to V
- High-pitched, blowing murmur
- Heard at the apex with the person in the left lateral decubitus position
- May radiate to the back and left axilla
- Caused by backward blood flow through a "leaky" mitral valve
- Associated findings: S_3, diminished S_1, S_2 splitting

Aortic Stenosis

- Midsystolic ejection murmur
- Grade varies
- Harsh with a crescendo-decrescendo pattern
- Heard clearly at the aortic area with the person in the forward-sitting position
- May radiate to the neck and back

- Caused by blood flow over a narrowed aortic valve
- May be accompanied by a thrill in the aortic area
- Other associated findings: left ventricular lift, ejection, click, and diminished aortic closing sound

Aortic Regurgitation

- Pandiastolic
- Difficult to hear—often graded I/VI
- Decrescendo, high-pitched, blowing
- Heard over the aortic area during exhalation (or holding breath) with the person in the forward-sitting position
- May radiate to the left sternal border
- Caused by backward blood flow from the aorta into the left ventricle
- S_3 and S_4 common; diastolic thrill may be palpable at the left sternal border

Mitral Sounds

- Usually middiastolic or presystolic
- Difficult to hear—less than grade III
- Low-pitched, rumbling quality
- Heard best at the apex with the person in the left lateral decubitus position
- Caused by blood flowing through a narrowed mitral valve during diastole
- Associated findings: Accentuated S_1, OS, diastolic thrill palpated of the apex

▼ ▼ ▼

Procedure

5. **Identify normal splitting of the first and second heart sounds.**

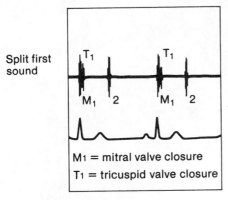

Split first sound

M1 = mitral valve closure
T1 = tricuspid valve closure

Split S_1: Normal variation

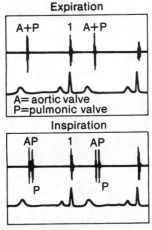

Expiration

A+P   1   A+P

A= aortic valve
P=pulmonic valve

Inspiration

AP   1   AP

P   P

Split S_2: Normal variation

6. **Identify extra heart sounds and murmurs.**

   a. Once S_1 and S_2 and any normal splitting patterns have been identified, concentrate on identifying any other extra sounds and murmurs that are timed in relation to the cardiac cycle and ventilatory pattern.

7. **Auscultate the precordium with the person assuming different positions (optional).**

   a. Auscultate with the person in the forward-sitting position.

   b. Auscultate with the person in the left-lateral decubitus position.

Clinical Significance

Because the left side of the heart normally contracts before the right side, two sounds are produced with S_1 (M_1 and T_1) and S_2 (A_2 and P_2). However, the interval may be too short to differentiate these sounds.

Normal Findings

Split first sound: A split S_1 may be heard close to the tricuspid area or lower left sternal border (LLSB). There is no respiratory variation with a split S_1.

The two components of this sound, M_1 and T_1, are related to mitral and tricuspid valve closure, and occur 0.2 to 0.4 seconds apart.

Split second sound: Normal S_2 splitting, also called a physiological split, may be heard on inspiration. On expiration, S_2 is again heard as a single sound.

Inspiration increases blood return to the right side of the heart. At the same time, the pulmonary vasculature capacity increases, causing more blood to pool, thereby decreasing the amount of blood entering the left side of the heart. As a result, the left ventricle is emptied more rapidly than the right ventricle and aortic valve closure precedes pulmonic valve closure by about 0.04 seconds.

Extra heart sounds and murmurs may be abnormal (See Display, "Extra Heart Sounds and Murmurs").

Forward-sitting position brings the base of the heart closer to the chest wall.

Left-lateral decubitus position brings the apex of the heart closer to the chest wall.

▼ ▼ ▼
G U I D E L I N E S

Procedure

1. **Palpate the central and peripheral arterial pulses.**

   a. Locate and palpate the following arterial pulses: carotid, brachial, femoral, popliteal, posterior tibialis, and dorsalis pedis.

   Carotid pulse: Locate the carotid pulse just medial to and below the angle of the jaw.

   Use light pressure and never palpate both carotid arteries at the same time to avoid compromising cerebral blood flow.

   Feel the contour and amplitude of the pulse.

   Avoid palpating the carotid sinus area above the carotid pulse

   Brachial pulse: Locate the brachial pulse just medial to the biceps tendon.

Clinical Significance

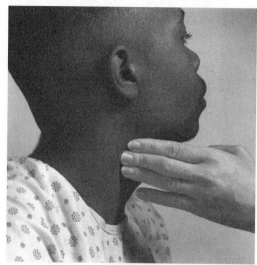

Palpation of the carotid pulse

Strong pressure stimulates the carotid sinus and may result in bradycardia, hypotension, or even cardiac arrest.

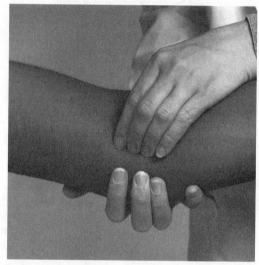

Palpation of the brachial pulse

▼ ▼ ▼
GUIDELINES *continued*   Arterial Pulses

Procedure

Clinical Significance

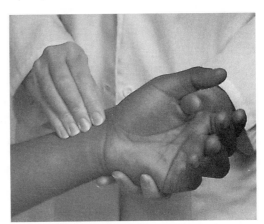

Palpation of the radial pulse

Radial pulse: Locate the radial pulse at the medial, inner wrist.

Femoral pulse: Locate the femoral pulse below the inguinal ligament.

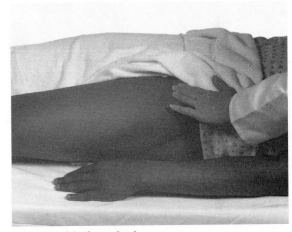

Palpation of the femoral pulse

Popliteal pulse: Locate the popliteal pulse. Place the thumbs on the patella and the remaining fingers of both hands in the popliteal space. Hold the leg slightly flexed at the knee. Use firm pressure. The popliteal pulse is difficult to palpate.

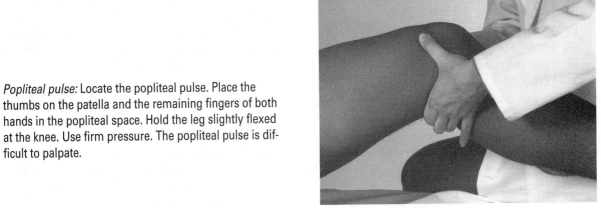

Palpation of the popliteal pulse

▼ ▼ ▼

G U I D E L I N E S *continued*   Arterial Pulses

Procedure   **Clinical Significance**

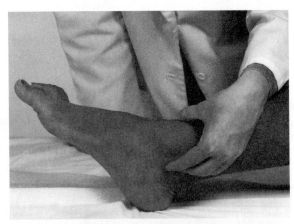

Palpation of the posterior tibial pulse

Posterior tibialis pulse: Locate the posterior tibialis pulse behind and slightly below the medial malleolus of the ankle.

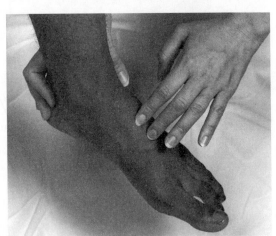

Palpation of the dorsalis pedis pulse

Dorsalis pedis pulse: Locate the dorsalis pedis pulse with the foot slightly dorsi-flexed on the top of the foot just lateral to the extensor tendon of the great toe.

b. Palpate, using the fingertips of the first and second fingers (or first, second, and third fingers).

c. Palpate left and right pulses individually as well as simultaneously.

   Exception: Never palpate both *carotid* pulses at the same time.

d. Palpate each pulse to determine ease of palpation, rate and rhythm, character of the arterial wall, and contour and amplitude.

   Ease of palpation: Note how easy or difficult is to feel each pulse and how much pressure it takes to obliterate the pulse.

Do not use your thumb. Because the thumb has a pulse, you may feel your pulse more readily than the patient's pulse.

Simultaneous palpation of pulses on right and left sides helps you make comparisons. Findings should be identical. Asymmetric pulses suggest arterial occlusion.

Normal Findings
Arterial pulses should be easy to palpate and should not be easily obliterated by pressure from your fingers.

Deviations from Normal
Nonpalpable pulses: A pulse may be difficult to palpate in cases of atherosclerosis, which causes vessel stiffness and diminished artery wall elasticity. Nonpalpable pulses may also be related to cessation of blood flow and should be further evaluated with Doppler ultrasound.

▼ ▼ ▼
G U I D E L I N E S *continued*   Arterial Pulses

Procedure

Rate and Rhythm: Observe the rate and rhythm of each pulse; compare with the apical (precordial) pulse.

Character of the arterial wall: Note how the arterial wall feels.

Contour and Amplitude: Note bounding of pulse, weakness, changes in upstroke and downstroke, and irregular patterns. Pulse contour and amplitude indicate volume and pressure relationships within the vessel and are difficult to assess by palpation. However, contour and amplitude may be assessed easily by examining pressure waveforms, obtained by intraarterial pressure monitoring.

2. **Auscultate the carotid and femoral arteries.**
   Auscultate for bruits, using the bell of the stethoscope.

Clinical Significance

Normal Findings
The pulse rate and rhythm should correlate with the rate and rhythm detected by precordial auscultation.

Deviations from Normal
Pulse deficit: A pulse deficit can be detected by simultaneously palpating a peripheral pulse and auscultating the precordial pulse. A pulse deficit exists if the peripheral pulse rate is slower than the precordial pulse rate. Pulse deficits indicate that myocardial contraction is not forceful enough to perfuse the extremities. This condition may be noted with cardiac dysrhythmias such as atrial fibrillation, atrial tachycardias, or premature ectopic depolarizations.

Normal Findings
The arterial wall will normally feel soft and pliable.

Deviations from Normal
The vessel wall may feel like a rope if atherosclerosis is present.

Normal Findings
Normal contour is characterized by a smooth upstroke. The dicrotic notch represents closure of the aortic valve.

Normal amplitude is represented by a pulse pressure (the difference between systolic and diastolic pressures) of approximately 30 to 40 mmHg. This pulse is recorded "3+" on a 0 to 4 scale.

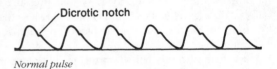

Normal pulse

Deviations from Normal
See Display 8-5, "Abnormal Pulse Patterns."

The bell detects low-pitched sounds—bruits are low-pitched.

Normal Findings
Silent on auscultation

Deviations from Normal
Bruits: A bruit, the vascular equivalent of a murmur, can be heard as a blowing sound caused by restrictive blood flow through vessels. Bruits may be auscultated over the carotid and femoral arteries and the abdominal aorta, indicating occlusive arterial disease.

DISPLAY 8.5

Abnormal Pulse Patterns

PULSUS MAGNUS

- Bounding pulse
- Increased pulse pressure
- Rapid upstroke and downstroke
- 4+ on a 0 to 4 scale
- Associated with atherosclerosis and hyperkinetic circulatory states as noted in hypertension, fear and anxiety, exercise, hyperthyroidism, anemia, patent ductus arteriosus, and aortic regurgitation

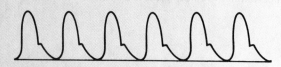

PULSUS PARVUS

- Small weak pulse
- Decreased pulse pressure
- Delayed upstroke and prolonged downstroke
- 1+ on a 0 to 4 scale
- Associated with low cardiac output states such as cardiogenic shock, cardiac tamponade, and severe cases of aortic and mitral stenosis

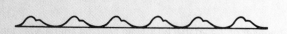

PULSUS ALTERNANS

- Heart rate is regular but the pulse alternates in size and intensity
- Difficult to assess by palpation; noted as the pulse is auscultated for blood pressure measurement
- Associated with a weakened myocardium and accompanying severe hypertension or left ventricular failure

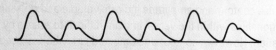

PULSUS PARADOXUS

- Exaggerated response to inspiration
- Normally, the pulse intensity or systolic pressure is lower during inspiration and is noted as a less than 10-mm Hg decrease in systolic blood pressure during inspiration
- A decrease of more than 10 mm Hg during inspiration indicates pulsus paradoxus
- Associated with severe heart failure, pericardial tamponade, severe lung disease, and constrictive pericarditis

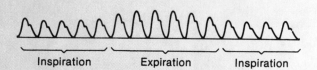

Inspiration   Expiration   Inspiration

PULSUS BISFERIENS ("DOUBLE-BEATING" PULSE)

- Two pulses can be palpated during systole
- Associated with premature cardiac contractions, pericardial effusion, and constrictive pericarditis

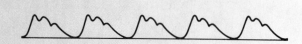

▼ ▼ ▼

G U I D E L I N E S   *continued*   Arterial Pulses

___

Procedure

3. **Perform the Allen test (optional).**

Occlude the radial artery with your fingers and ask the person to make a tight fist.

While you continue to hold pressure on the radial artery, ask the person to open the fist and note whether the color returns to the hand.

Clinical Significance

The Allen test is a method for determining the patency of the ulnar artery. The pulsation from the ulnar artery is difficult to palpate, yet in some clinical situations this artery must be assessed for patency. For example, when an intraarterial catheter is placed in the radial artery to monitor blood pressure, the ulnar artery must be patent to assure adequate collateral blood circulation to the hand.

This maneuver forces blood away from the hand and causes skin blanching.

Ulnar artery patency is indicted by color returning rapidly to the hand.

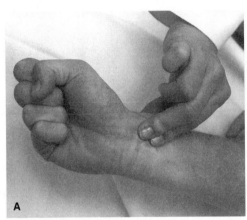
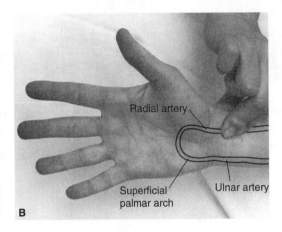

Allen test

▼ ▼ ▼
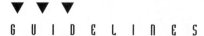

GUIDELINES

Assessment Guidelines   Neck Veins

Procedure

1. **Observe the jugular venous pulsation (JVP).**

   Observe the person from the right side.

   Position the patient with the torso elevated 30 to 45 degrees and inspect the venous pulse. Turn the person's head slightly to the left.

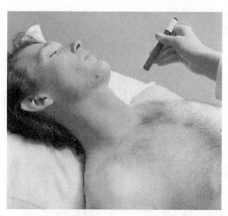

Neck vein inspection

   Provide tangential lighting to the neck area.

   Observe the jugular venous pulsation (JVP) for several cardiac cycles. Note distinct components of the venous pulse. Considerable skill is necessary to detect the distinct JVP components by inspection. However, such components are relatively easy to detect on a graphic waveform.

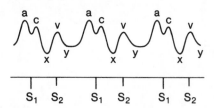

Jugular venous waveform in relation to S_1 and S_2

Clinical Significance

The jugular veins are assessed by inspection because palpation obliterates the vein.

The right internal jugular vein is more visible than the left because of the proximity to the right heart.

The venous pulse is normally not visible with the person sitting fully upright. A flat position is undesirable because the vein is fully distended and pulsations are indistinguishable.

Tangential lighting accentuates shadows and makes any pulsations more visible.

Normal Findings

Normal JVP: Several pulse waves may be noted in the JVP that reflect pressure changes in the right side of the heart. Three positive waveforms include *a, c,* and *v*. The *c* wave, reflecting atrial systole, may be a distinct wave, or appear as a notch on the *a* wave, or be absent. The *c* wave is the largest positive waveform and may increase in amplitude during inspiration. The *c* waveform represents tricuspid valve closure. The *v* waveform represents right atrial filling.

The negative waveforms include *x* and *y*. The x descent occurs with ventricular systole as the height of the venous blood column declines. The y descent occurs when blood from the right atrium flows rapidly into the right ventricle.

Deviations from Normal

Abnormal JVP: Conditions that increase resistance to right ventricular filling, such as tricuspid stenosis, right ventricular failure, pulmonary hypertension, and pulmonary stenosis, may cause the *a* wave amplitude to increase (*cannon* a *waves*). Decreased-amplitude *a* waves may be noted in clients with atrial fibrillation and ventricular pacemakers. Tricuspid regurgitation may increase *v* wave amplitude. Cardiac tamponade may cause an increase in both *a* and *v* waves.

▼ ▼ ▼
GUIDELINES *continued*   Neck Veins

Procedure

2. Estimate central venous pressure (CVP) by measuring the height of pulsation in the internal jugular vein.

a. Choose a standard reference point from which to measure the height of pulsation in the internal jugular vein. The zero reference point, at the level of the right atrium, may be difficult to determine with accuracy. Therefore, use the sternal angle, which is approximately 5 cm above the right atrium, as the reference point.

b. Measure the distance, in centimeters, from the sternal angle to the top of the distended jugular vein.

c. Add 5 cm to the value obtained, for a rough estimate of central venous pressure.

3. Check for hepatojugular reflux.

With the person raised 30 to 60 degrees, compress the right upper quadrant for 30 to 60 seconds with your palm.

The hepatojugular reflux is positive if the JVP level rises with this maneuver.

Clinical Significance

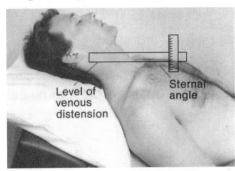

Estimating CVP

Normal central venous pressure is 3 to 5 cm above the sternal angle when the trunk is elevated 30 to 60 degrees.

CVP elevation may be attributed to right or left ventricular failure, pulmonary hypertension, pulmonary emboli, or cardiac tamponade.

Perform this maneuver if you suspect right ventricular failure.

The increased abdominal pressure increases venous return to the right side of the heart. If the right ventricle is impaired, pressure in the neck veins will increase.

ND$_x$

Documenting Cardiovascular Examination Findings

Precordial Examination Findings

Example 1: Normal Heart and Precordium

Mr. L, aged 20, was examined at the college health center as a prerequisite for playing college basketball. The precordial examination findings were normal and were recorded as follows:

> No visible pulsations on anterior chest. PMI palpable at left 5th ICS; 2 cm in diameter. Heart auscultation: Regular rhythm, rate 68 beats/min, S1 and S2 identified. No extra heart sounds, murmurs, or rubs.

The same findings may be summarized in a problem-oriented format:

S: Denies previous cardiovascular problems, including hypertension or rheumatic heart disease. No chest pain or dyspnea at rest or with activity.

O: No visible pulsations on anterior chest. PMI palpable at left 5th ICS; 2 cm in diameter. Heart auscultation: Regular rhythm, rate 68 beats/minute, S1 and S2 identified. No extra heart sounds, murmurs, or rubs.

A: No abnormalities detected on precordial examination.

P: Continue with routine follow-up examinations. Counsel about risk factors for cardiovascular disease; reinforce health benefits of present physical activities.

Example 2: Myocardial Infarction

Mr. H, aged 72 years, was a patient in the coronary care unit (CCU) after an acute anterior myocardial infarction 2 days ago. Heart sounds were auscultated several times a day. Examination findings were abnormal and were recorded as follows:

> Apical pulse regular, rate 80 beats/minute. S4 heard at LSB, 5th ICS. No murmurs. Pericardial friction rub heard over left precordium, loudest at LSB, 5th ICS.

The same findings may be summarized in a problem-oriented format:

S: Reports occasional sharp anterior chest pain with deep inspiration. Reports pain has no pressure-like or squeezing quality.

O: Apical pulse regular, rate 80 beats/minute. S4 heard at LSB, 5th ICS. No murmurs. Pericardial friction rub heard over left precordium, loudest at LSB, 5th ICS.

A: S_4 recorded on admission and not a new finding—probably indicates underlying heart disease. Pericardial rub is of new onset. Suspect post-MI (myocardial infarction) pericarditis.

P: Inform physician about rub. Reinforce need to report chest pain and inform about probable cause of current pain. Continue cardiac auscultation q4h and as condition changes.

Documenting the Quality of the Arterial Pulse

To establish consistency, arterial pulses are graded using the following criteria:

0 = Absent
1+ = Diminished; thready; easily obliterated
2+ = Normal; not easily obliterated
3+ = Increased; full volume
4+ = Bounding; hyperkinetic

Example 1: Normal Findings

If all peripheral pulses are noted as normal, you may record your findings as follows:

All peripheral pulses readily palpable and findings symmetric: 2+, regular rhythm, smooth contour, and brisk upstroke.

The results of examining normal carotid arteries may be recorded as follows:

Carotid pulse regular rhythm, rate 72, 2+ (bilaterally) with brisk upstroke. No bruits.

Example 2: Cardiogenic Shock (Pulsus Parvus)

All peripheral pulses diminished (1+). Delayed upstroke.

Neck Veins

Example 1: Normal Findings

The results of examining normal neck veins may be recorded as follows:

JVP noted 2 cm above sternal angle with upper body elevated 45 degrees (CVP estimated at 7 cm). Distinct *a* waves observed. Hepatojugular reflex negative.

Example 2: Right Ventricular Failure

Jugular veins distended in upright position. Hepatojugular reflex positive.

Nursing Diagnoses Related to Cardiovascular Assessment

Decreased Cardiac Output

Decreased cardiac output occurs when the amount of blood pumped from the heart has decreased, adversely peripheral tissue perfusion. The person also should be evaluated for conditions associated with a potential for decreased cardiac output, such as dehydration or dysrhythmias.

Symptoms. A number of reactions are associated with low cardiac output, including fatigue, weakness, dyspnea, syncope, vertigo, and coughing. Poor gastrointestinal tract perfusion may contribute to anorexia or nausea and result in constipation. Brain hypoxia usually results in dizziness and disorientation, and sometimes in loss of consciousness.

Physical Examination Findings. Decreased cardiac output may result in a lowered blood pressure, because the blood pressure is a product of cardiac output and peripheral resistance. Consequently, the sympathetic nervous system is stimulated, resulting in vasoconstriction, tachycardia, and decreased peripheral perfusion. You may note cool, diaphoretic, and possibly cyanotic skin. Urine output usually declines because kidney perfusion is compromised. Peripheral pulses may be difficult to palpate or may be diminished.

If cardiac output decreases because of poor left ventricular pump function, the blood in the left side of the heart will eventually back up to the lungs, right side of the heart, and venous system. You may note crackles on lung auscultation, an increase in CVP (jugular vein distention), a gallop rhythm, and peripheral edema.

Altered Tissue Perfusion

Inadequate tissue perfusion may be chronic or acute. Persons with chronic alteration in tissue perfusion should be evaluated by a physician for possible pharmacologic or surgical treatment. Chronic alteration in tissue perfusion is also considered a nursing diagnosis because nurses may treat associated functional deficits such as confusion, inability to ambulate safely, and impaired skin integrity. Acute alterations in tissue perfusion, such as acute arterial occlusion from a thrombus or embolus, are life-threatening clinical problems and are not usually considered nursing diagnoses.

Chronic Altered Cerebral Tissue Perfusion

A chronic decrease in the brain's arterial perfusion is most often associated with circulatory system dysfunction, for example:

- Low cardiac output states such as congestive heart failure; cardiac dysrhythmias; Stokes-Adams syndrome
- Vessel occlusion related to cerebral vessel atherosclerosis (especially at bifurcations of the vertebrals and carotids); subclavian steal syndrome (decreased brain blood supply secondary to left subclavian or innominate artery occlusion)
- Other hypotensive states such as orthostatic (postural) hypotension; carotid sinus syndrome

History. Vertigo (dizziness) is a common symptom indicating inadequate brain perfusion. The person may report "blacking out," episodes of confusion, memory or vision loss, or other neurologic deficits. Ask whether symptoms are associated with position changes or with other activities. Sudden head movements may aggravate symptoms in persons with carotid sinus syndrome; sudden changes in body positions are associated with ortho-static hypotension. Often a history of prolonged immobil-ity or bed rest contributes to orthostatic hypotension. Per-sons with subclavian steal syndrome may report that arm exercise precedes vertigo (or syncope).

Physical Examination Findings. Possible changes in function may be noted that are consistent with the per-son's history, such as restlessness, confusion, and altered mentation. Bruits may be auscultated over the vertebral or carotid arteries, indicating partial occlusion from athero-sclerotic plaque. The absence of bruits, however, does not always indicate normal vessels. Orthostatic hypotension is indicated by the following blood pressure changes when the person moves from sitting to standing or lying to sit-ting: a decrease in systolic blood pressure of greater than 20 mm Hg and a decrease in diastolic blood pressure of greater than 10 mm Hg. To compensate, the pulse rate may increase. A blood pressure difference of more than 10 mm Hg in both arms may indicate brachiocephalic artery atherosclerosis.

Chronic Altered Cardiopulmonary Tissue Perfusion

Cardiopulmonary tissue perfusion may be decreased in disease states such as congestive heart failure, myocardial infarction, angina pectoris, and pulmonary edema. Poor heart and lung perfusion is associated with dysrhythmias, especially tachycardia, cardiac chest pain, dyspnea, and tachypnea.

Chronic Altered Gastrointestinal Tissue Perfusion

Blood shunting from the gastrointestinal system may occur with prolonged stress or shock. Inadequate perfusion of gastrointestinal organs also may be associated with se-vere congestive heart failure. Gastrointestinal motility may be adversely affected, and the person may report related symptoms such as constipation, nausea, and vomiting.

Chronic Altered Renal Tissue Perfusion

A decrease in renal tissue perfusion may occur when the blood supply to renal arteries or arterioles is de-creased, as may occur with hypovolemia, congestive heart failure, shock, or thrombosis. The person may be oliguric, anuric, or edematous and may display other signs that in-dicate renal failure, such as azotemia.

Chronic Altered Peripheral Tissue Perfusion Related to Interruption of Arterial Flow

Arterial flow interruption may affect tissue perfusion in upper or lower extremities. The history, symptoms, and physical examination findings vary, depending on the exact arterial lesion site. During assessment, you may note the following common features:

Claudication. Intermittent claudication, a cramping, squeezing pain that occurs in the affected extremity dur-ing activity, may be the symptom that causes the person to seek health care.

Atrophic Skin Changes. Atrophic skin changes may be noted over the affected extremities, including a decrease in subcutaneous fat and muscle mass; thin, tight, shiny skin; lack of hair growth; and slow-growing, ridged, thick nails.

Such changes result from lack of oxygen. In people with unilateral vessel occlusion, atrophic skin changes can be noted easily by comparing one limb with the other.

Cool Skin Temperature. In patients with arterial oc-clusion, the skin may be cool or cold secondary to a de-creased blood supply to the skin.

Skin Color Changes. Evaluate skin color by having the person raise the affected extremity and noting any color changes. Extremities with arterial occlusion are usu-ally pale when elevated because gravity further reduces the blood supply. As the person lowers the limb, you may note dependent rubor (redness) as the capillaries refill. Cyanosis may occur in advanced stages as more oxygen is extracted from hemoglobin to compensate for the de-creased blood flow. Prolonged skin blanching (>3 sec) after pressure is applied and then released at the nail bed indicates slow capillary refill.

Skin Lesions. Skin lesions associated with severe ar-terial insufficiency include ulceration and necrosis (gan-grene). Such lesions are most often noted in areas of trauma such as shins, feet, and toes. Wound healing may be delayed.

Pulses Not Palpable. Pulses distal to the occlusion site may not be palpable.

Bruits. Bruits may be auscultated if vascular narrow-ing of major arteries causes turbulent blood flow. If you suspect arterial occlusion, listen over all major arteries where pulses are being palpated.

Chronic Altered Peripheral Tissue Perfusion Related to Interruption of Venous Flow

Chronic venous insufficiency most often affects the lower extremities. This condition develops slowly and oc-curs because the venous valves become incompetent and fail to close completely. As a result, venous pressure in-creases, leading to the following physiologic changes: ac-cumulation of edema fluid in surrounding tissues sec-ondary to high hydrostatic pressures; rupture of small venules; atrophy of skin and tissue from inability of oxy-gen to diffuse into high-pressure areas; and eventual necrosis from ischemia. Such alterations contribute to the following assessment findings:

Pain. Pain may or may not be present and may be less severe than arterial occlusion pain. The person may experience a dull, aching pain in the lower extremities after standing for prolonged periods, which contributes to higher venous pressures. Itching is a common symptom, especially around the ankles.

Skin Changes. The skin may be edematous, but edema may be somewhat relieved by leg elevation. At-rophic changes may accompany the edema. The temper-ature and color of the skin may be normal in affected extremities. However, skin color may reflect possible cyanosis when the extremity is maintained in a dependent position. A brownish color, resulting from stasis pigmenta-tion, may be noted over the lower extremities. This occurs as small vessels rupture and the red blood cell pigment hemosiderin, along with melanin, stains the tissues brown.

Painless ulcerations may form at the internal malleolus because the poorly perfused tissue is susceptible to injury.

Healed ulcers may appear as thin scars that easily break down again with minor trauma. Skin ulcers are easily infected. The limb also may be eczematous. Gangrene usually does not develop.

Obscured Pulses. Although often obscured by tissue edema, pulses are usually palpable.

ND_X

Clinical Problems Related to Cardiovascular Assessment

Cardiovascular examination may indicate many clinical problems such as heart murmurs, pericardial friction rubs, bruits, hypertension, and cardiac dysrhythmias. Some of these findings represent chronic conditions that you should monitor for changes. If you detect any abnormal findings, consult the physician.

Acute Arterial Occlusion

Acute arterial occlusion represents a medical-surgical emergency, requiring prompt assessment and diagnosis. Occlusion may occur secondary to embolism or thrombosis; the clinical signs depend on the site of occlusion. Although the signs are similar to those that occur with chronic alterations in tissue perfusion related to interruption of arterial flow, the onset is more sudden and irreversible. If the occlusion occurs in an extremity, the following signs may be noted: pain (sudden or gradual in onset), numbness, tingling, coldness, absence of pulses distal to the occlusion, pallor or mottling, superficial vein collapse, limb weakness, and paresthesias. Eventually, skin blebs and gangrenous necrosis may occur. Pain may not be present in all cases. The most reliable assessment finding is the absence of a previously palpated (or auscultated) pulse.

You should regularly check the peripheral pulses of patients at high risk, such as those with mitral valve stenosis, atrial fibrillation, and transmural myocardial infarction.

RESPIRATORY SYSTEM

Anatomy and Physiology Review

The pulmonary components of the respiratory system begin with the nose, mouth, and sinuses. Air is inhaled through the nose, where it is warmed and filtered before it enters the trachea and bronchial passages and passes into the lungs. The trachea is lined with mucus-producing cells that trap foreign material and with cilia (fine hair-like projections) that sweep mucus upward through the airway. Mucus is also moved upward by the cough reflex, which is especially strong at the bifurcation, or carina, where the trachea branches into the right and left mainstem bronchi. The right mainstem bronchus is shorter, wider, and more vertically aligned than the left mainstem bronchus. The bronchi divide into secondary branches

that enter the lungs at the hilum. The bronchi gradually narrow into bronchioles and lead into alveoli in the lungs.

The lungs are spongy, elastic structures that occupy the thorax. The outer lung surface is covered by the visceral pleura, which is separated from the parietal pleura lining the chest wall by a layer of fluid (the intrapleural space). The area between the right and left lungs is referred to as the mediastinum. A normally functioning respiratory system relies on intact neurologic and muscular systems.

The Nose and Sinuses

The nose and sinuses may be examined during the routine examination of the head or when a patient reports problems with these areas. Common problems associated with the nose include trauma, obstruction, and irritation or drainage secondary to colds and allergies. The primary symptom of sinus problems is pain that may result from inflammatory processes. Obstruction and dental disease are the most common causes of sinus inflammation.

The primary functions of the nose include olfaction and warming, moisturizing, and filtering inspired air. Olfaction is evaluated by testing the first cranial (olfactory) nerve (see Chap. 9).

Inspired air is warmed and humidified by passing through the three *turbinates* (Fig. 8-9). The turbinates consist of bony projections on the lateral walls of each nasal cavity. Only the middle and inferior turbinates are visible

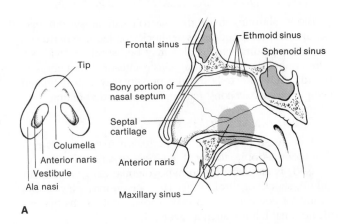

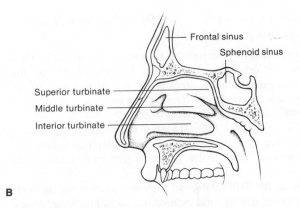

FIGURE 8.9 The nose and sinuses. **(A)** Cross-section of the nose. **(B)** Nasal turbinates.

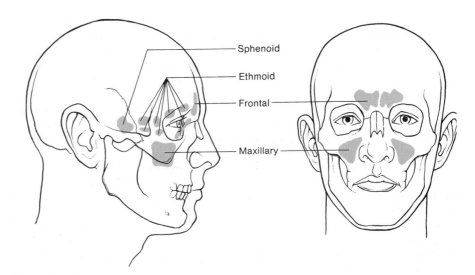

FIGURE 8.10 The four paranasal sinuses of the skull.

during physical examination. Turbinates are lined with ciliated epithelial cells, a large vascular supply, and mucus-secreting glands. The sinuses drain into the nose through small openings in the turbinates. When the turbinates are edematous, as might occur with a common cold, these openings may become obstructed. As a result, fluid may collect in the sinuses and provide a medium for bacterial growth. Pressure from fluid buildup contributes to the pain of acute sinusitis.

The four paranasal sinuses of the skull include the sphenoid, ethmoid, frontal, and maxillary sinuses (Fig. 8-10). Only the frontal and maxillary sinuses are accessible for physical examination. The sinuses normally are air filled and have no known function in humans; they are believed to be vestigial. The sinuses are lined with mucus-secreting cells and drain into the nose.

Thoracic Landmarks

The lungs are enclosed in the thorax and surrounded by the ribs. The sternum serves as the anterior thoracic border, whereas the thoracic spine borders the thorax posteriorly. The diaphragm forms the "floor" of the chest cavity and sits higher on the right side than on the left side. The right lung has three lobes and is larger than the left lung, which has two lobes. The lower lobe of the left lung curves slightly around and under the heart.

Chest landmarks for locating the underlying structures include the suprasternal notch at the top of the sternum between the clavicles; the sternal angle (angle of Louis), which is a palpable, slight outward projection of the sternum; 12 thoracic vertebrae; and 12 pairs of ribs (Fig. 8-11). The sternal angle is the starting point for counting ribs and intercostal spaces. The intercostal spaces have numbers that correspond to the overlying ribs. Identifying the ribs by palpation is usually easier along the midclavicular line, as opposed to the sternal border, where proximal sternal cartilages may interfere. Only the cartilages of the first seven ribs attach directly to the sternum. The costal margin refers to the proximal rib surface that slopes down and away from the sternum. The costal angle is formed by costal margin intersections.

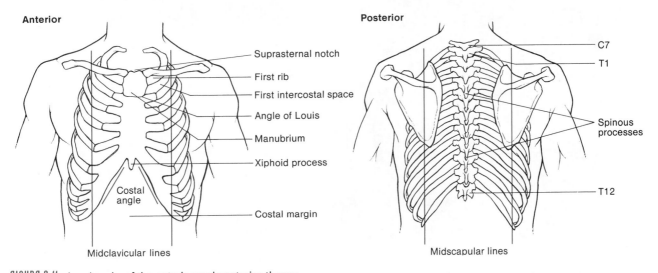

FIGURE 8.11 Landmarks of the anterior and posterior thorax.

Imaginary lines are also useful for determining lung field location and include the midsternal line, midspinal line, left and right midclavicular lines (vertical lines from the mid-point of each clavicle), left and right anterior axillary lines, left and right posterior axillary lines, and left and right mid-axillary lines that progress vertically from the left and right axillae apex (Fig. 8-12).

Anteriorly, the lung apices extend approximately 1.5 inches above the clavicles. Posteriorly, the apices extend to the first thoracic vertebra. The inferior lung borders extend from the sixth rib, midclavicular line, to the eighth rib, mid-axillary line. Posteriorly, the lower lung borders are located at the tenth thoracic vertebra (T10) on expiration and at T12 on deep inspiration.

The approximate location of the fissures that divide the lungs into lobes may be determined by noting the following landmarks. Posteriorly, the lungs divide into upper and lower lobes at an angle stretching from the spinous process of T3 obliquely down and laterally. On the anterior surface, the lower lobes are divided from the upper lobes on the left, and from the upper and middle lobes on the right by bilateral imaginary lines extending medially and inferiorly from the fifth rib, midaxillary line, to the sixth rib, mid-clavicular line. On the right lateral chest surface, the right upper and right middle lobe division is located by a line drawn medially from the fifth rib, midaxillary line, to the fourth rib, midclavicular line.

Ventilation Mechanics

Inspiration and expiration occur as a result of pressure changes within the lungs. The inward pull of the lungs and the outward pull of the chest wall create a negative pressure that prevents the lungs from collapsing. During expiration, when the lungs are at rest, lung pressure is equal to atmospheric pressure. During inspiration, the diaphragm contracts and moves downward. Then external intercostals pull the ribs up, and lung pressure becomes negative, allowing air to flow in. When the inspiratory muscles relax, lung pressure becomes positive, and air is expelled.

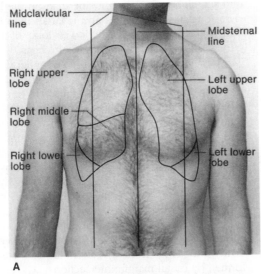

A

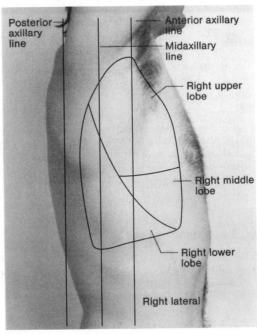

B

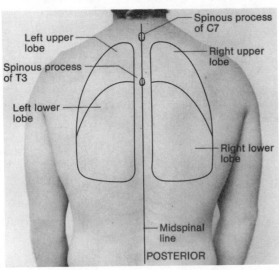

C

FIGURE 8.12 Reference lines for thoracic examination.

The diaphragm is the major muscle used during inspiration and is controlled by phrenic nerves from the third to the fifth cervical vertebrae. Accessory muscles, such as the trapezius muscles, scalenes, and sternocleoidmastoids, are used during extra inspiratory efforts; the abdominal muscles and internal intercostal muscles are used in extra expiratory efforts.

The compliance of the lungs and thorax also affects breathing and involves the ability of the lungs and thorax to expand and overcome their natural elastic recoil. Pressure is required to put a sufficient volume of air in the lungs to overcome elastic recoil. Compliance is considered to be high or low, depending on the pressure needed to expand the lungs. If the lung expands easily, for example, compliance is high, whereas if more pressure is needed to expand the lung, compliance is low, in which case the lung is called "stiff." Because of the surface tension in the fluid that lines the alveoli, these tiny air sacs tend to shrink. Surfactant, a phospholipid substance, is secreted by the alveoli to lower the surface tension. The decreased surface tension prevents alveolar collapse and reduces breathing efforts.

Respiratory muscle strength and compliance affect lung volumes, which vary with body size, age, and sex. The total lung capacity, or the amount of gas in the lungs after full inspiration, involves residual and tidal volumes and expiratory and inspiratory reserve volumes (see "Diagnostic Tests," Pulmonary Function Tests).

- *Residual volume* is the amount of air remaining in the lungs after a maximal expiration.
- *Tidal volume* is the amount of gas inspired or expired during normal ventilation.
- *Expiratory reserve volume* is the amount of air that can be exhaled after a normal expiration.
- *Inspiratory reserve volume* is the amount of air that can be inspired above maximal inspiration.

The neurons of the respiratory center are located in the brain stem. The pons regulates the respiratory rhythm, and the medulla controls respiration rate and depth, which are affected by the carbon dioxide, hydrogen ion, and oxygen concentrations in the blood and body tissues.

For tissues to be oxygenated, the oxygen within the alveoli must be transported into the blood. Carbon dioxide and oxygen are exchanged across the alveolar–capillary membrane through the process of diffusion. The membrane has a large, thin surface area, approximately 1 μm thick, which allows gas to be diffused rapidly. Almost all of the oxygen in blood combines with hemoglobin in red blood cells. An adequate amount of hemoglobin is essential for tissue oxygenation. Carbon dioxide moves from the capillaries to the alveoli to be removed through respiration. While in the blood, carbon dioxide is transported in the form of bicarbonate.

Within the circulatory system, the right and left pulmonary arteries transport deoxygenated blood to the lungs from the right side of the heart and then branch into arterioles that lead into the alveolar–capillary network. The pulmonary veins transport oxygenated blood to the left side of the heart. The oxygenated blood is distributed throughout the body.

Physical Examination   Respiratory System

GENERAL PRINCIPLES

The nose and sinuses are common sites for infection. Examine the nose and sinuses in persons with symptoms of upper respiratory infections, headaches, or breathing obstruction. The nose is inspected and palpated. The sinuses are inspected, using a light source for illumination, and palpated.

Inspection, palpation, percussion, and auscultation are used to assess the lungs and thorax. These techniques may be performed in the order cited, or they may be performed simultaneously, especially if abnormal findings are noted.

EQUIPMENT

Nasal speculum (optional)
Light source for transillumination of the sinuses
Stethoscope with diaphragm and bell

POSITIONING, PREPARATION, AND EXPOSURE

A quiet, warm room with adequate natural light is essential when examining the lungs and thorax. The person should assume a position that is comfortable and suitable and allows for easy examination of the anterior and posterior chest. If the person is short of breath, the head of the bed or examining table should be elevated. An equally comfortable position is to sit up and lean forward with arms supported on a table, especially if dyspnea is secondary to COPD. If such a position is impossible, the semi-Fowler's position can be used when the anterior chest is examined. This position allows the person to lean forward, supporting weight on the upper legs or on the siderails (if confined to bed) while the posterior chest is examined. If the person's condition does not allow for any of these maneuvers, a side-lying position can be used to examine the posterior chest, and the supine position can be used to examine the anterior chest.

(continued)

Physical Examination   Respiratory System (continued)

To reassure the person, explain the procedure as much as possible. Alleviating anxiety is important because apprehension could cause unnatural breathing. The person should undress to the waist; a woman should remove her bra. A loose-fitting examining gown may be used and a drape placed over the person to provide privacy.

CUES

Observing the person's general condition can provide important information about respiratory function. Alertness, level of consciousness, skin color, rate and depth of respirations, diaphoresis, nasal flaring, or breathing problems while speaking provide cues about respiratory function. Extreme agitation may indicate a low blood oxygen level. During the general inspection, ask specific questions about the person's usual state of health and any signs of respiratory problems such as a cough, sputum production, fever, edema, fatigue, or shortness of breath. Also note any external sounds associated with breathing, such as wheezing, grunting, or grasping.

EXAMINATION AND DOCUMENTATION FOCUS (NOSE)

- *Inspection:* Shape and configuration of external structures; position and integrity of nasal septum; color of the mucous membranes; color and swelling of the turbinates; discharge, lesions, masses, and foreign particles
- *Palpation:* Patency of the nares; displacement and tenderness along ridge and soft tissues

EXAMINATION AND DOCUMENTATION FOCUS (SINUSES)

- *Inspection:* Quality of transillumination
- *Palpation:* Tenderness

EXAMINATION AND DOCUMENTATION FOCUS (LUNGS AND THORAX)

- *Inspection:* Trachea position, thoracic configuration and symmetry, ventilatory pattern, muscle movements, masses or lesions
- *Palpation:* Symmetry of ventilatory movements, tactile fremitus, tenderness and masses, crepitus
- *Percussion:* Percussion tones, diaphragmatic excursion
- *Auscultation:* Quality of breath sounds, voice transmission

▼ ▼ ▼

GUIDELINES

Assessment Guidelines   Nose and Sinuses

Procedure	Clinical Significance
1. Inspect the external nose.	***Normal Findings***
a. Note shape and configuration.	The shape of the external nose varies greatly among people because of genetic differences and alterations secondary to trauma or cosmetic surgery.
	Deviations from Normal
	Deviations in the shape or configuration of the external nose generally are not significant unless indicative of recent trauma or associated with airway obstruction. Areas of recent swelling should be palpated for tenderness.
b. Observe nares during ventilation.	***Deviations from Normal***
	Flaring of the nares indicates respiratory distress.
c. If nasal discharge is present, note the character (watery, purulent, mucoid), color, amount, and whether it is unilateral or bilateral.	***Deviations from Normal***
	Nasal discharge (rhinitis): Rhinitis has many causes, including the following:

▼ ▼ ▼
GUIDELINES *continued* Nose and Sinuses

Procedure

2. Evaluate nasal patency.

Occlude the naris by placing your finger along one side of the nose. Ask the person to breathe in and out with the mouth closed. Repeat with the other naris.

3. Inspect the internal nose.

a. Tip the person's head back and look through the nares to view the vestibule, septum, and inferior and middle turbinates. To enhance visualization of internal structures, place your thumb against the tip of the nose to move it. Hold a penlight in your other hand to illuminate the internal structures. A nasal speculum may facilitate inspection by dilating the outer naris, but such instruments are rarely recommended because they are invasive and may irritate tender tissue. An otoscope with a short wide-tip attachment also may be used.

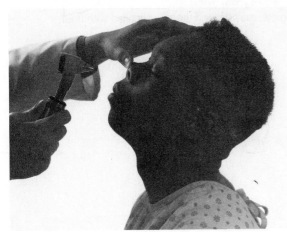

Inspecting the internal nose

b. Note the color and condition of the nasal mucosa, the appearance of the turbinates, and the appearance of the nasal septum.

Clinical Significance

1. Common cold—Clear, watery discharge of acute onset; associated findings include red, edematous nasal mucosa; purulent discharge may be noted after 3 to 5 days and represents secondary bacterial infection.

2. Allergies and hay fever—Clear, water discharge that may be acute (hay fever) or chronic (allergic rhinitis); the nasal mucosa appears pale and edematous; allergic rhinitis may be accompanied by nasal polyps.

3. Cerebrospinal fluid rhinnorrhea—Clear, water discharge noted after facial trauma or basilar skull fractures; glucose-positive.

4. Sinusitis—Purulent discharge; usually unilateral following a cold; chronic sinusitis may result in unilateral or bilateral purulent discharge.

5. Foreign body—Unilateral purulent discharge.

Normal Findings

The nares should be patent. Normal nasal breathing should be quiet.

Deviations from Normal

Masses or foreign particles may interfere with airway patency.

Normal Findings and Deviations from Normal

Nasal septum: Deviation of the nasal septum is common. Severe deviation may interfere with patency. The septum should not be perforated.

Nares: The nares should be patent. Masses or foreign particles may interfere with airway patency.

Mucous membranes: The nasal mucosa is pink or dull red. A small amount of clear, watery discharge may be noted.

Turbinates: The tubinates should be nonedematous, without masses, and pink or dull red.

Polyps: Polyps appear as small, peduncular masses and are associated with allergic rhinitis. Most polyps develop between the medial and inferior turbinates. Polyps may interfere with nasal patency and the sense of smell.

Epistaxis (nasal bleeding): The nasal turbinates and mucosa have high vascularity. Therefore, epistaxis secondary to trauma or spontaneous rupture of blood vessels may be profuse. Epistaxis may be associated with chronic sinusitis, nose picking, and cocaine abuse.

▼ ▼ ▼
G U I D E L I N E S   *continued*   Nose and Sinuses

Procedure

4. Palpate the sinuses.

a. Palpate the frontal sinuses. Press upwards from the eyebrows with your thumbs. Avoid pressing against the eye orbits.

b. Palpate the maxillary sinuses with your thumbs or fingertips by pressing upward under the zygomatic process (cheekbones).

Clinical Significance

Deviations from Normal

Tenderness in response to palpation is associated with inflammation.

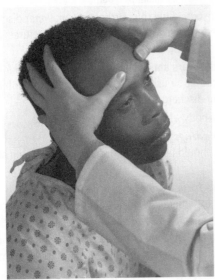

Palpating the frontal sinuses

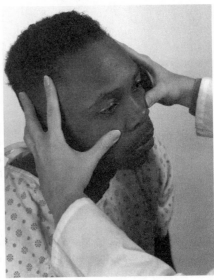

Palpating the maxillary sinuses

5. Transilluminate the sinuses.

If tenderness is elicited, transilluminate the sinuses to detect accumulation of fluid or masses.

a. Transilluminate the frontal sinuses by pressing a bright light source (may use the otoscope light) firmly against the medial supraorbital rim. This procedure should be done in a completely darkened room.

Normal Finding
A glow above the eye.

Deviation from Normal
No glow; may occur if the sinus is filled with fluid.

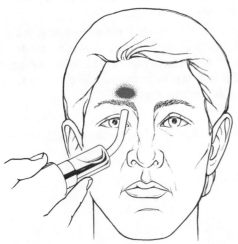

Transillumination of the frontal sinus

▼ ▼ ▼

Procedure

b. Transilluminate the maxillary sinus by asking the person to tilt the head back and open the mouth. Press the light against the skin just below the medial aspect of the eye.

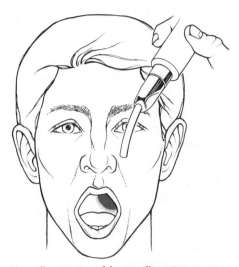

Transillumination of the maxillary sinus

Clinical Significance

Normal Findings

A glow should be noted in the area of the hard palate.

Deviations from Normal

No glow.

▼ ▼ ▼

G U I D E L I N E S

Assessment Guidelines   Lungs and Thorax

Procedure

1. **Inspect the thorax.**
   a. Inspect the thorax with the person sitting upright and uncovered to the waist. Note the symmetry of the thorax, muscles used for ventilation, the ventilatory pattern, and skin condition. Proceed systematically, inspecting the anterior thorax and noting landmarks. Some landmarks are readily visible, particularly in a person with little body fat. Palpate to locate landmarks that you cannot see.
   b. Inspect the posterior thorax when you have completed all aspects of the anterior examination.

Clinical Significance

Normal Findings

Position of the trachea: The trachea should be located midline, without deviating to the left or right.

Thoracic configuration: In adults, the normal ratio of antero-posterior chest diameter to lateral chest diameter is approximately 1:2.

Chest movements: Each side of the chest should have equal upward and outward movement with inspiration. A downward movement of the diaphragm and an outward movement of the chest and abdomen should occur with each effective inspiration. The reverse should occur with expiration. Generally, women breathe with thoracic movement, whereas men and children usually breathe from the diaphragm (abdominally). In effective, normal breathing, accessory muscle use should not occur.

▼ ▼ ▼

G U I D E L I N E S *continued*   Lungs and Thorax

Procedure

2. **Palpate the thorax.**

   a. Use your fingertips to palpate the chest and intercostal spaces for tenderness, alignment, bulging, or retraction. As you palpate, note the amount of muscle mass over the chest wall. Palpate any masses or sinus tracts (rare, blind, tube-like structures opening onto the skin). Examine any reported tender areas last.

   b. To assess for crepitus, palpate with the fingertips, especially around any wound site or any tube that invades the chest, such as chest tubes or intravenous lines.

   c. Evaluate tactile fremitus. Fremitus is vibration of the chest wall produced by vocalization. Ask the person to say "one, two, three" or "ninety-nine" while you palpate the thorax from left to right and then from right to left, using the heel or ulnar surface of your hand to detect vibrations. Usually, palpating with one hand works best to assess tactile fremitus, although both hands may be used to compare the left and right sides of the thorax. When evaluating the posterior chest, ask the person to fold the arms across the chest to move the scapulae partially out of the way.

Clinical Significance

Deviations from Normal

Thoracic configuration: With aging, the dorsal curve of the thoracic spine may increase, resulting in an increased anteroposterior chest diameter. This "barrel chest" is a normal variant in older persons. An abnormal barrel chest may be noted in persons with COPD.

Impaired chest movements may occur with pain or abdominal distension. A paradoxical movement of the chest wall may be the result of fractured ribs.

Abnormal ventilatory patterns: See Chapter 4, Display 4–1.

Masses and lesions: Masses or lesions in the neck or thorax are abnormal and require further investigation.

Normal Findings

The sternum, costal cartilages, ribs, intercostal spaces, and spine should not be tender on palpation. Muscles are palpable and should feel firm, smooth, and symmetrical.

Deviations from Normal

Palpable masses are abnormal.

Deviations from Normal

Crepitus, or crepitation, is a crackling sound produced when subcutaneous tissue containing air is palpated. Crepitus is an abnormal finding.

Always make comparisons between left and right sides.

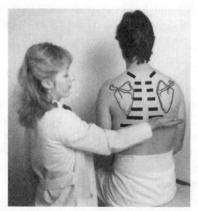

Evaluating tactile fremitus: Ulnar surface of hand

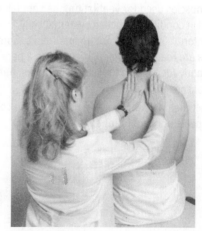

Evaluating tractile fremitus: Heel of hand

▼ ▼ ▼
G U I D E L I N E S   *continued*   Lungs and Thorax

Procedure

Clinical Significance

Normal Findings
Tactile fremitus: When the person speaks, tactile fremitus, a palpable vibration, should be felt on the chest wall. Fremitus is usually most noticeable where the trachea branches into the right and left mainstem bronchi in the upper chest near the sternal border. Fremitus is usually decreased or absent over the precordium.

Deviations from Normal
Increased tactile fremitus is associated with conditions favoring sound transmission in the chest, such as pneumonia with consolidation, atelectasis (with open bronchus), lung tumors, pulmonary infarction, and pulmonary fibrosis.

Decreased tactile fremitus is associated with conditions that interfere with sound transmission through the chest, such as pleural effusions, pleural thickening, pneumothorax with lung collapse, bronchial obstruction, tumors or masses in the pleural space, and emphysema.

3. **Evaluate the chest expansion.**
   a. *Anterior approach:* To evaluate chest expansion anteriorly, place your hands over the anterolateral chest with thumbs extended along the costal margin, pointing to the xiphoid process. Ask the person to breathe deeply and note the movement of your hands.

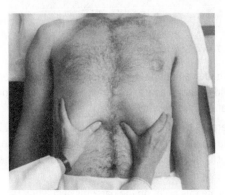

Evaluating chest expansion: Anterior approach

   b. *Posterior approach:* To evaluate chest expansion posteriorly, place your hands on the posterolateral chest with your thumbs at the level of the tenth rib. Ask the person to breathe deeply and note the movement of your hands.

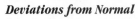

Normal Findings
Your thumbs should move an equal distance apart on each side as the person takes a deep breath.

Deviations from Normal
A lag in thoracic movement may indicate underlying lung or pleura disease.

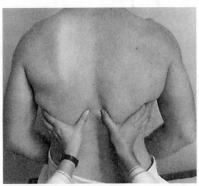

Evaluating chest expansion: Posterior approach

Procedure

4. **Percuss the thorax.**

   a. Evaluate percussion tone over lung fields.

   Percuss the thorax from the apices to the bases, moving from the anterior surface to the lateral areas, and then to the posterior surface.

   Always compare findings between right and left sides of the thorax.

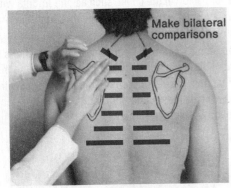

   Thoracic percussion

   When evaluating the posterior chest, ask the person to fold the arms across the chest to move the scapulae partially out of the way.

   b. Percuss to determine diaphragmatic excursion. Locate the upper edge of the diaphragm by noting where the normal lung resonance changes to dullness when percussing the posterior thorax.

   Locate this point on the person's skin when the person is holding a deep breath and mark it. Then, locate this point on the person's skin following a deep exhalation and mark it. The difference between marks is the diaphragmatic excursion.

5. **Auscultate the lungs.**

   a. Auscultate breath sounds.

   When auscultating the lungs, mentally picture the lung segment located beneath the thoracic landmarks. To locate the lobes of the lungs, palpate thoracic landmarks. With the person in a lateral position, palpate the free-floating ribs or costal margins, and count four intercostal spaces upward to locate lower lung borders. Remember that when the person is supine, organs are displaced and lung expansion is altered.

Clinical Significance

Use percussion to determine boundaries of organs and to detect the relative amounts of air, fluid, and solid material within the underlying lung.

Normal Findings

Normal percussion tone: In adults, the lungs emit a resonant tone when percussed. Children's lungs are normally hyperresonant.

Deviations from Normal

Hyperresonance: A hyperresonant or tympanic note is produced when air accumulates in the lungs or pleural cavity. Examples: emphysema, pneumothorax.

Dullness: A dull or flat percussion tone is produced by vibrations from solid masses or fluid in the lungs. Examples: pneumonia, atelectasis, masses, pleural effusion, and hemothorax.

Normal Findings

The diaphragmatic excursion is the distance between the levels of dullness with deep inspiration and full expiration, and normally ranges from 3 to 6 cm. The diaphragm should be slightly higher on the right side.

Auscultating the lungs helps to evaluate air flow as well as identify normal and abnormal breath sounds.

▼ ▼ ▼
G U I D E L I N E S *continued*   Lungs and Thorax

Procedure

Use the diaphragm of the stethoscope to auscultate the lungs. Ask the person to sit up, if possible, and to breathe slightly slower and deeper than normal, with the mouth open. Auscultate the anterior, posterior, and lateral lung fields. Listen to at least one full inspiration and expiration in each location that you auscultate.

Observe the client for dizziness and lightheadedness, which may indicate hyperventilation. If hyperventilation does occur, allow the client to rest.

Systematically listen to the chest, beginning with the apices and moving down to the bases in a zigzag, side-to-side manner. Compare one side with the other.

If the patient is unable to sit, auscultate the posterior and lateral lung fields while the person lies on first one side and then the other. Compare the findings from both sides.

Avoid misleading noises by placing the stethoscope firmly on uncovered skin. In addition, prevent the stethoscope or the person from moving during auscultation. To prevent extraneous sounds caused by the stethoscope moving over hair, dampen chest hair with a washcloth.

b. Note the quality of the breath sounds.

If you hear any abnormal breath sounds, note their location and where they occur in the ventilatory cycle. Ask the person to cough after the initial auscultation and note changes in adventitious sounds. If the person has complained of difficulty breathing, but you heard no abnormal sounds initially, check for adventitious sounds again after the person coughs.

Clinical Significance

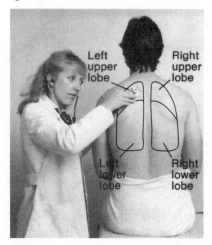

Lung auscultation

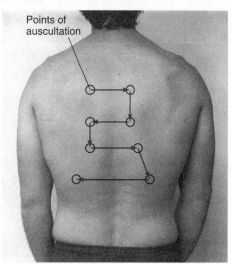

Pattern for lung auscultation

Normal Findings

Normal breath sounds: Normal breath sounds may vary according to the area auscultated. *Vesicular breath sounds* are low-pitched, soft, breezy sounds that can be heard over the lung fields of the anterior, posterior, and lateral chest. These sounds are usually longer and louder during inspiration than during expiration. *Bronchial breath sounds* are loud, high-pitched, and hollow and are a normal finding over the trachea. The inspiratory phase is shorter than the expiratory phase. *Bronchovesicular breath sounds* are found in the mainstem bronchi area and are heard anteriorly in the first and second intercostal spaces and between the scapulae posteriorly. The inspiratory and expiratory phases of bronchovesicular sounds are equal. They have a soft, breezy quality and are lower-pitched than bronchial sounds, but higher-pitched than vesicular sounds.

▼ ▼ ▼

GUIDELINES   *continued*   Lungs and Thorax

Procedure

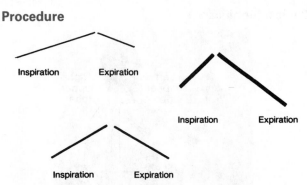

Bronchovesicular breath sounds

c. Auscultate for voice transmission.

Listening for voice transmission is an adjunctive technique used when abnormalities are found during inspection, palpation, percussion, or auscultation. Ask the person to say "one, two, three" or "ninety-nine," and
auscultate the lung fields. To assess for egophony, ask
the person to say "ee-ee-ee."

Clinical Significance

Deviations from Normal
See Display 8-6, "Abnormal (Adventitious) Breath Sounds."

Normal Findings and Deviations from Normal:
Normally, the sounds are muffled, but if the voice is transmitted loudly and clearly, lung tissue consolidation may be indicated. *Bronchophony* (loud, distinct voice transmission), *whispered pectoriloquy* (clear transmission of whispered sounds),
and *egophony* (/e/ to /a/ change in sound) are normally heard
over large airways (bronchi) and associated with abnormal
conditions, including consolidation and pleural effusions.

DISPLAY 8.6

Abnormal (Adventitious) Breath Sounds

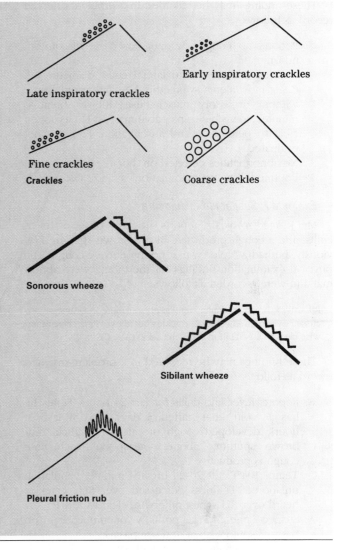

Late inspiratory crackles

Early inspiratory crackles

Fine crackles
Crackles

Coarse crackles

Sonorous wheeze

Sibilant wheeze

Pleural friction rub

CRACKLES

Crackles (formerly called rales) are soft, high-pitched, discontinuous popping sounds that occur during inspiration. The sounds are timed in relation to inspiration.

Crackles occur secondary to fluid in the airways or alveoli, or to opening of collapsed alveoli. Crackles in late inspiration are associated with restrictive pulmonary disease. Crackles in early inspiration are associated with obstructive pulmonary disease. *Fine crackles* in early inspiration are caused by small airway closure. *Coarse crackles* in early inspiration are associated with bronchitis or pneumonia.

WHEEZES

Sonorous wheezes (formerly called rhonchi) are deep, low-pitched, rumbling sounds that are heard primarily during expiration and caused by air moving through narrowed tracheobronchial passages. Narrowing may be caused by secretions or tumor.

Sibilant wheezes (formerly called wheezes) are continuous, musical, high-pitched, whistle-like sounds that are heard during inspiration and expiration. They are caused by narrowed bronchioles and are associated with bronchospasm, asthma, and buildup of secretions.

PLEURAL FRICTION RUB

A *pleural friction rub* is a harsh crackling sound like two pieces of leather being rubbed together, and may be heard during inspiration alone or during both inspiration and expiration. This sound may disappear when the breath is held.

Pleural friction rubs are secondary to inflammation and loss of lubricating pleural fluid.

Documenting Respiratory Examination Findings

Nose and Sinus Examination Findings

Example 1: Normal Nose and Sinus

Examination findings were normal and were recorded as follows:

External bony structures of the nose without deformity. Nares both patent. Nasal septum midline. Nasal mucosa and turbinates pink, moist, and without discharge or masses. Frontal and maxillary sinuses nontender.

Example 2: Upper Respiratory Infection

Examination findings were abnormal and were recorded as follows:

Nares not patent, mouth breathing required. Copious, bilateral white discharge from nares. Nasal mucosa and turbinates swollen and bright red. Frontal sinuses nontender. Maxillary sinuses tender bilaterally. Unable to transilluminate maxillary sinuses.

Lung and Thorax Examination Findings

Example 1: Normal Thorax

Ms. S, aged 22 years, had a thorax examination as part of a routine annual health assessment. The examination results were normal and were recorded as follows:

Trachea midline; AP to lateral chest diameter 1:2. Chest movements symmetric. Ventilation unlabored without accessory muscle use. RR 16 breaths/minute. No visible or palpable masses. Lungs sound clear to percussion and auscultation. Fremitus not evaluated.

These findings may be recorded in a problem-oriented record as follows:

S: Reports no cough, dyspnea, or chest discomfort; nonsmoker
O: Trachea midline; AP to lateral chest diameter 1:2. Chest movements symmetric. Ventilation unlabored without accessory muscle use. RR 16 breaths/minute. No visible or palpable masses. Lungs sound clear to percussion and auscultation. Fremitus not evaluated.
A: No abnormalities detected on thoracic exam
P: Routine follow-up examinations as indicated

Example 2: Suspected Pneumonia

Mr. J, aged 42 years, reports an acute onset of fever, chills, and a cough productive of red-brown sputum. Previously, he had a "cold" with a nonproductive cough. The physical examination findings for the thorax were abnormal and were recorded as follows.

RR 20–24 breaths/minute; ventilation unlabored. Dullness percussed over right lower lobe; crackles heard over RLL; chest otherwise clear to auscultation and percussion (A & P).

These findings may be recorded in a problem-oriented record as follows:

S: Reports fever and chills for last 24 hours. States he has a "cold" that started 3 days ago. In last 24 hours, developed cough productive of thick, red-brown sputum, "about a teaspoon" each time cough is productive.
O: Temp: 104°F. RR 20–24 breaths/minute; ventilation unlabored. Dullness percussed over RLL; crackles heard over RLL; chest otherwise clear to A & P.
A: Suspect pneumonia, possibly pneumococcal, on basis of sputum color and symptoms.
P: Refer to physician. Assist with ongoing diagnostic procedures: Obtain sputum sample for C & S; chest x-ray.

ND$_X$

Nursing Diagnoses Related to Respiratory Assessment

Impaired Gas Exchange

Impaired gas exchange (IGE) involves an actual or potential decrease in the passage of gases (oxygen and carbon dioxide) between the alveoli in the lungs and the vascular system. Impaired gas exchange is characterized by a decreased Po_2, decreased hemoglobin saturation, or an increased Pco_2, as determined by arterial blood gas testing.

Hypoxia, an inadequate tissue oxygen supply, and respiratory acidosis may accompany IGE.

History. Gas exchange across the alveolar–capillary membrane may be impaired under the following circumstances:

- Gas diffusion is blocked by secretions or fluid, such as those caused by mucus accumulation, inflammatory or infectious processes, or pulmonary edema.
- Loss of lung surface for gas diffusion, which occurs in cases of atelectasis, emphysema, tumor, and lobectomy
- Loss of lung elasticity and compliance, which occurs in cases of COPD and adult respiratory distress syndrome (ARDS)

In addition, extrapulmonary factors, such as pain, anxiety, and central nervous system depression, may affect pulmonary gas exchange.

To avoid inspiratory pain, which often occurs after chest or abdominal surgery, a patient may hypoventilate. As a result, secretions accumulate and atelectasis may occur. People with IGE may report feeling short of breath, fatigued, or disoriented.

Physical Examination Findings. Characteristic signs that indicate hypoxia, such as restlessness and dyspnea, may be noted with IGE. Initially, blood pressure, heart rate, and cardiac output may increase to compensate for the low Po_2. With increasing hypoxia, changes in mental status may occur, resulting in reduced responsiveness, drowsiness, and confusion as the pH drops and acidosis occurs. The respiratory rate increases initially, then becomes slow and shallow as the consciousness level decreases.

Hypoxia causes the skin to become diaphoretic and cooler as cardiac output decreases. Skin color and nail beds become dusky blue-gray to cyanotic (blue to purple). In people with dark skin, especially blacks, the mucous membranes in the mouth are a better indicator of tissue oxygenation. Observable signs that indicate dyspnea with IGE include an intolerance to lying flat. The person usually prefers to sit up with hands on the knees, or lean over a table. You will note an increased respiratory rate or increased respiratory effort with activity. Chronic IGE with carbon dioxide retention is associated with an increased anteroposterior chest diameter (barrel chest).

Ineffective Airway Clearance

The diagnosis of Ineffective airway clearance (IAC) is closely related to that of IGE because the former will eventually lead to the latter. Ineffective airway clearance occurs when partial or complete airway obstruction threatens to prevent air passing through the respiratory tract.

History. Ineffective airway clearance occurs in the same situations as IGE. Acute problems with airway clearance may be caused by improper positioning, edema of the upper airway structures, and mechanical obstruction such as choking.

Physical Examination Findings. Signs of ineffective airway clearance include a weak, ineffective cough; an abnormal respiratory rate, rhythm, or depth; dyspnea; wheezing; crackles; abnormal or decreased breath sounds; inability to remove secretions; and asymmetric chest expansion. A person with thick, sticky sputum, for example, may have difficulty removing the secretions because of an ineffective cough, resulting in increased breathing and changed respiratory rate or rhythm. Airway secretions also may produce adventitious breath sounds. The factors mentioned under IAC could also contribute to IGE.

Ineffective Breathing Pattern

Ineffective breathing patterns occur from impairment of ventilatory function. Either hypoventilation or hyperventilation may be accompanied by dyspnea. Hypoventilation decreases carbon dioxide exchange, which can cause respiratory acidosis. Hyperventilation increases carbon dioxide exchange, which can lead to respiratory alkalosis. Any chest pain that accompanies breathing difficulty will alter the breathing pattern. In turn, an ineffective breathing pattern may lead to IAC. Diagnosing Ineffective breathing pattern may be accomplished by observing any use of accessory muscles of respiration; shortness of breath, irregular respirations; hyperventilation; shallow, guarded, or rapid respirations; or difficulty breathing when not in an upright sitting or standing position.

Clinical Problems Related to Respiratory Assessment

Altered Elasticity and Compliance

Conditions that alter the lung's elasticity and compliance include COPD and ARDS. Chronic obstructive pulmonary diseases include asthma, chronic bronchitis, and emphysema. Wheezing, dyspnea, and a prolonged expiration phase are observable signs that indicate an asthmatic attack.

The patient with emphysema may appear as a "pink puffer," with a pink or flushed skin tone. The classic barrel chest is present, and the patient may be underweight and dyspneic. Emphysema involves decreased elastic recoil with increased lung compliance that causes air to be trapped in the alveoli.

Adult respiratory distress syndrome is diagnosed by chest radiograph and arterial blood gas analysis. Hypoxemia, which is refractory to oxygen therapy, indicates ARDS. Other signs include dyspnea, increased respiratory rate, tachycardia, and restlessness. A dry cough may be present. Rusty, frothy sputum that turns dark red may appear later in the disease process. Lung compliance is reduced in ARDS.

Inflammatory and Infectious Processes

Pneumonia is an inflammatory process, often having an infectious component. The patient may report chills, shortness of breath, pleuritic chest pain, fever, hemoptysis, and a cough that produces purulent sputum. Chest assessment may show crackles, wheezes, decreased breath sounds, and dullness on percussion. The diagnosis is confirmed through chest radiograph, blood cultures, sputum analysis, leukocyte counts, and arterial blood gas results.

Bronchitis may be acute or chronic. The person with chronic bronchitis is typically cyanotic and edematous, appearing as a "blue bloater." Dyspnea, wheezing, coarse crackles, and a chronic cough with sputum production are characteristics of chronic bronchitis.

Lung tuberculosis causes a cough that also produces purulent sputum, sometimes with traces of blood (hemoptysis). Fever and weight loss also may be noted. However, the patient also may be asymptomatic. The diagnosis is determined by chest x-ray findings, sputum culture, and a positive tuberculin test result.

A *lung abscess* may also cause fever and weight loss. Dyspnea, pleuritic chest pain, and a cough producing much bloody, purulent sputum also may occur.

Empyema (purulent material in a pleural space) may occur as a complication of respiratory infection, chest trauma, or surgery. Empyema produces shortness of breath, pleuritic chest pain, and fever.

Chest Trauma and Disease Alterations

Chest trauma or disease processes can cause anatomic and mechanical alterations in the lungs and thereby affect respiratory function. For example, blunt chest trauma may cause injuries, such as pneumothorax, tension pneumothorax, or flail chest. Penetrating trauma can cause a hemothorax (blood in the pleural space) or hemopneumothorax (blood and air in the pleural space).

Physical findings associated with a *pneumothorax* include limited respiratory excursion on the affected side and decreased or absent breath sounds. Crepitus may be present. Apprehension, dyspnea, and pleuritic chest pain may occur with a pneumothorax, which may be caused by a spontaneous or traumatic rupture of a lung bleb.

A *tension pneumothorax* may cause severe dyspnea and severe pleuritic chest pain. The trachea deviates toward the unaffected side, and the affected side shows limited respiratory excursion and absent breath sounds. Cyanosis and shock also may be present.

A *flail chest* results from multiple rib fractures. The chest wall becomes unstable, resulting in inadequate respiratory exchange. Paradoxic chest wall movement may be noted. When the uninjured chest areas expand, the injured portion depresses. The injured area "flails out" during expiration. Only minimal air movement will be noted. The person will probably be dyspneic and cyanotic.

A *bronchial tumor* typically causes a cough. Dyspnea or chest pain may occur, with either pleuritic or dull discomfort. Other signs include tracheal deviation toward the normal side, absent breath sounds, and a dull or flat percussion note over the tumor area if the tumor is large. The person may be asymptomatic until the tumor has advanced into the pleura and chest wall or until distant metastases appear.

Pulmonary emboli are caused by venous thrombi fragments detaching and migrating to the lungs, or they may be caused by fat emboli associated with long-bone fractures. Pulmonary alterations vary with the size of the embolus. When an embolus occludes a pulmonary artery, alveoli are ventilated but not perfused. Dyspnea is common. Tachypnea and tachycardia also may be present. Often the patient feels anxious and restless but does not know why. If partial lung infarction occurs, pleuritic chest pain and hemoptysis may result. A massive pulmonary embolus usually causes sudden shock, cyanosis, respiratory distress, and tachypnea, confusion, and anxiety. If the patient has a long-bone fracture or has had orthopedic surgery and then develops dyspnea, tachycardia, and a high fever, you should suspect a fat embolus. Petechiae usually appear over the thorax and upper extremities. Arterial blood gas analysis, chest radiograph, and ventilation-perfusion lung scan are commonly used to diagnose pulmonary emboli.

Pulmonary edema may occur gradually or suddenly. An initially dry cough usually progresses to a cough that produces pink, frothy sputum. Paroxysmal nocturnal dyspnea and orthopnea are present with gradual onset. Peripheral edema may be noted in the feet and ankles. Acute pulmonary edema causes dyspnea, tachypnea, and tachycardia. The patient's skin is cool, clammy, and cyanotic. Moreover, the person is usually apprehensive and must have the head elevated or sit up to breathe. Dry crackles may be heard first at the lung bases, progressing to wheezing, moist, bubbling adventitious sounds throughout the chest. Chest radiograph usually verifies pulmonary edema. Acute pulmonary edema is an emergency that requires immediate medical intervention.

Aspirating a solid object causes a cough, dyspnea, and wheezing. Respiratory distress, cyanosis, and the inability to speak indicate that an object is lodged in the airway. Aspirating materials such as water, gastric acid, or nasogastric tube feedings may cause an inflammatory reaction with decreased surfactant production and a resultant decreased lung compliance. Patients especially at risk for aspiration are those with a decreased level of consciousness and those without intact airway protective mechanisms.

Inhalation injuries result from smoke inhalation, thermal burns, or carbon monoxide poisoning. If the exposure is severe enough, mucous membrane edema and bronchospasms occur. Coughing, wheezing, dyspnea, and cyanosis are noted. Headache and depressed mentation also may be present, especially with carbon monoxide poisoning.

MUSCULOSKELETAL SYSTEM
Anatomy and Physiology Review

The musculoskeletal system includes bones, muscles, and joints as well as supporting structures such as tendons, ligaments, cartilage, bursae, and fasciae. Bones provide support and levers for movement; joints act as fulcrums for the levers; and muscles provide the force to move bones around the joints.

Bones

The human skeleton is composed of 206 bones, 80 of which make up the axial skeleton, including the skull bones, vertebral column, sternum, and ribs. The 126 bones of the appendicular skeleton include the bones of the upper and lower extremities. Bones are further classified according to shape at maturity:

- *Flat bones* function mainly to protect the body, and include skull bones, ribs, sternum, scapulae, and pelvis. Flat bones cannot function as levers and therefore do not directly contribute to body movement.
- *Long bones* function as levers during movement and include the femur, tibia, fibula, phalanges, humerus, ulna, and radius.
- *Short bones* provide strength during movement and include the carpals and tarsals.
- *Irregular bones* include all other bones. The bones of the vertebrae are classified as irregular and have important functions for protection and mobility. Irregular bones of the face contribute to movements necessary for eating and facial expressions.

Bones and associated processes (enlargements or protrusions) often serve as landmarks during physical assessment.

Bone Processes

- *Crest:* A ridge or linear process, such as the iliac crest
- *Condyle:* A rounded process forming a joint surface, such as the knuckle
- *Head:* A rounded end of a bone separated from the main body of the bone by a constricted neck, such as the femoral head
- *Spine:* A pointed, slender process, such as the vertebral spines
- *Trochanter:* A large, rounded process for muscle attachment, such as below the head of the femur
- *Tubercle:* A small, rounded process, such as the tubercle on the clavicle, where the deltoid muscle attaches
- *Tuberosity:* A large, rounded process, but smaller than a trochanter, such as the ulnar tuberosity

Bone Formation. Bone formation is a complex, ongoing physiologic phenomenon. Ideally, an equilibrium exists between bone formation (deposition) and bone loss (resorption). Numerous factors may disrupt this equilibrium in persons with bone deformities or histories of spontaneous pathologic fractures, which are associated with high rates of bone resorption (Display 8-7). People on long-term bed rest are at higher risk for disproportionate bone loss because they do not perform activities that use long bones. Bone deformities are also attributed to hereditary disorders.

Joints

The joints, or articulations, are composed of tissues associated with the articulating bone surfaces. Body movements are impossible without joints, which are classified according to the degree of mobility:

- *Synarthroses* are immoveable joints, such as the fused suture lines noted on mature skulls.
- *Amphiarthroses* are joints with restricted movement, such as the pubic symphysis.
- *Diarthroses,* or *synovial joints,* are freely moveable joints such as the shoulder, elbow, hip, and knee.

Physical examination should be focused on these joints.

Synovial Joints. In addition to the articulating bone surfaces, the joint is composed of a joint capsule, ligaments, muscle, and tendons (Fig. 8-13), and in some cases bursae or menisci. The *joint capsule* is a sac-like structure between bones bordered by the articular cartilage and surrounding ligaments. The outer layer of the joint capsule is fibrous; the inner, synovial layer secretes synovial fluid, which lubricates the joint and prevents friction during movement. *Ligaments, muscles,* and *tendons* provide joint stability. *Bursae,* pad-like structures that provide protection from friction, are located between moving surfaces such as bones, tendons, and ligaments. Bursae are associated with shoulder, elbow, hip, knee, and heel joints.

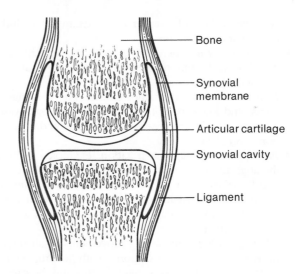

FIGURE 8.13 Synovial joint structure.

Menisci, crescent-shaped pieces of cartilage, may be found between articulating surfaces of some joints, such as the knee and shoulder.

Synovial joints are classified according to the degree of movement:

- *Ball and socket joints* are most freely moveable and are created when the head of one bone fits into the

---

DISPLAY 8.7

Factors That Influence Bone Deposition and Resorption

INCREASED BONE DEPOSITION

- Exercise, bone stress
- Growth hormone
- Fluoride*

INCREASED BONE RESORPTION

- Parathyroid hormone excess
- Vitamin D hormone†
- Adrenocortical steroid excess
- Calcium deficiency (dietary or malabsorption)
- Phosphorus deficiency (dietary, malabsorption, renal loss)
- Anabolic steroid deficiency (androgen, estrogen)
- Immobilization
- Acidosis
- Pregnancy and lactation
- Osteolytic neoplasms (including leukemia)
- Prostaglandins

DECREASED BONE DEPOSITION

- Immobilization, disuse, bed rest
- Growth hormone deficiency
- Adrenocortical steroid excess

DECREASED BONE RESORPTION

- Calcium
- Phosphorus
- Parathyroid hormone deficiency
- Calcitonin
- Magnesium deficiency
- Anabolic steroids
- Alkalosis
- Mithramycin
- Diphosphates

*Excessive fluoride causes uncalcified osteoid deposition and produces osteomalacia.

†Osteolytic effect of parathyroid hormone requires vitamin D hormone.

concave surface of another bone; examples include the hip and shoulder.

- *Condyloid joints,* such as the wrist, move freely except for axial rotation. They are created by oval and elliptical bone surface articulation.
- *Hinge joints,* such as the elbow, interphalangeal joints, and knee, permit only forward and backward movements and are created by concave and convex bone articulation.
- *Pivot joints* permit bone rotation; examples include the atlas and axis joints of the head and the elbow.
- *Saddle joints,* such as the carpometacarpal joint of the thumb, are created when two bones with concave and convex surfaces articulate, joining in a reciprocal manner.
- *Gliding joints* permit sliding movements in all directions and occur when two bones with flat articulating surfaces meet. The intervertebral joints and the carpal bones of the wrist are classified as gliding joints.

Intervertebral Joints. The moveable joints of the vertebral column do not have synovial fluid in the joint capsules between the articular surfaces as do other synovial joints. Intervertebral joints contain fibrocartilaginous discs with central, flexible cores (the nucleus pulposus) that function as shock absorbers between bones.

Joint Movements. Joints vary in the types of movement they can accommodate. During physical examination, joint movement or range of motion (ROM) is evaluated for a particular joint:

- *Abduction:* Movement away from the midline of the body, such as raising an arm to the side or spreading fingers apart
- *Adduction:* Movement toward the midline of the body, such as lowering an arm
- *Flexion:* Bending at a joint, such as the hip, to create a lesser angle between two bones (sitting)
- *Extension:* Straightening a joint, such as the hip, to create an angle at or near 180 degrees between two bones (standing)
- *Hyperextension:* Extending a body part beyond anatomic position, such as tipping the head backward
- *Eversion:* Turning a body part outward, such as moving the foot at the ankle joint so that the sole faces outward
- *Inversion:* Turning a body part inward, such as moving the foot at the ankle joint so that the sole faces inward
- *Pronation:* Rotating the forearm so that the palm faces downward
- *Supination:* Rotating the forearm so that the palm faces upward
- *Rotation:* Turning a bone around an axis, such as moving the head from side to side
- *Circumduction:* Moving a limb to create a cone shape, with the joint forming the apex of the cone and the distal part of the limb tracing a complete circle

- *Protraction:* Moving a bone forward on a plane parallel to the ground, such as moving the lower jaw forward
- *Retraction:* Moving a bone backward on a plane parallel to the ground

Processes that may restrict normal joint movement include pain, muscle spasm, intervertebral disc herniation, fibrosis (contracture), and bony fixation.

Muscles. The skeletal or striated muscles provide force to move bones around the joints. They can be easily assessed during physical examination because the person can control contractions and relaxations. You should inspect and palpate skeletal muscles during the physical examination.

The microscopic fibers in a single muscle together form a large, central muscle body and are attached to bones either directly, by tendons (cord-like connective tissue), or by aponeuroses, which are broad, flat sheets of connective tissue. The distal end of the muscle is called the insertion and attaches to the bone being moved by the muscle's contraction. The proximal end of the muscle is the origin and attaches to the bone that is held stationary during movement.

Muscle Action. In response to neurologic stimulus, the muscle shortens in length, or contracts. As the muscle relaxes, it elongates. Movement is based on bone movements created by muscle contraction across a joint. Muscles are named in a manner that describes some feature associated with the muscle, such as the movement that is produced by the muscle, the orientation of the muscle fibers, the location of the muscle, the number of origins at the proximal end of the muscle, the shape of the muscle, or the point of attachment:

- *Muscles named for joint movement created by the muscle contraction:* Flexor hallucis brevis (flexes great toe); extensor carpi ulnaris (extends wrist); abductor digiti (abduct fingers); adductor magnus (adducts thigh); rotatores spinae (rotate vertebral column)
- *Muscles named for orientation of the muscle fibers:* Transverse thoracic (narrows the chest); oblique external abdominal (contracts abdomen)
- *Muscles named for their location:* Intercostals (draw ribs together)
- *Muscles named for the number of origins at the proximal end:* Biceps (flexes arm); triceps (extends forearm)
- *Muscles named for shape:* Trapezius (draws head back and to the side)
- *Muscles named for the point of attachment:* Sternocleidomastoid (rotates the head)

Signs of Muscle Dysfunction. Muscle dysfunction can result from a number of factors, including fluid and electrolyte depletion, overuse or disuse, malnutrition, and altered innervation. Clinical signs and symptoms that indicate muscle dysfunction include cramps, muscle strain, muscle atrophy, fasciculations, and tetany.

Cramps are caused by spasms of muscle fiber groups, often caused by dehydration and sodium or potassium depletion. *Muscle strain*, manifested by pain, stiffness, and swelling, usually results from excessive muscle use. Pain is often worse near the joint or associated ligaments. *Muscle atrophy* or wasting may result from loss of muscle innervation, malnutrition, or disuse. *Fasciculations* are twitches of muscle fibers and are noted as rapid move-ments of overlying skin. Twitches may occur sponta-neously, indicating no muscle dysfunction, or may be associated with irritable muscle tissue. Degenerative nervous system disease is a common cause of fascicula-tion. *Tetany*, tonic muscle spasms, is most frequently noted in the extremities. Conditions causing hypocal-cemia, such as parathyroid or vitamin D deficiencies, may cause tetany.

Physical Examination   Musculoskeletal System

GENERAL PRINCIPLES

The musculoskeletal system varies significantly among different age-groups (see Chaps. 16 and 17). In general, musculoskeletal assessment focuses on eval-uating the extremities and the vertebral column. Evaluation of musculoskeletal function in relation to other body parts is integrated into the examination of other body systems. Part of the oral cavity assessment, for example, involves evaluating temporomandibular joint function; during the rectal or pelvic exami-nation the muscles involved in bowel or bladder elimination are evaluated; and during pulmonary assessment the muscles involved in ventilation are exam-ined. Muscles should be further evaluated to determine whether movement is coordinated. Muscle assessment also involves evaluating neurologic function; this aspect of the physical examination is discussed in Chapter 9.

Assess the musculoskeletal system by inspection and palpation. Ask the per-son to report any pain, tenderness, or other sensations when musculoskeletal structures are palpated. Use special maneuvers, such as ROM testing and mus-cle strength testing, to evaluate joints. Hold the palm of your hand over the person's joints during ROM maneuvers to detect crepitation (grating) and defor-mities.

You should judge whether certain maneuvers or procedures are appropriate. In cases of suspected trauma, such as bone fractures, for example, ROM maneu-vers could cause considerable pain and aggravate the injury. In general, if light or deep palpation of a musculoskeletal structure causes pain, and the cause of the pain is uncertain, ROM should not be evaluated until a cause for the pain can be determined. Similarly, if pain develops during ROM testing, take special care to prevent further injury. In the case of injury to an extremity, you should examine the unaffected side first to determine the person's usual musculoskele-tal function. Moving the neck and spine is strictly contraindicated if the person has had an accident that may have caused spinal injury.

EQUIPMENT

Metric tape measure
Goniometer (to measure joint angles)

THOROUGH ASSESSMENT VERSUS SCREENING ASSESSMENT

A thorough musculoskeletal examination is a lengthy procedure, involving eval-uation of joint ROM and skeletal muscle strength. A thorough examination may not be indicated for all persons or may not be tolerated because of fatigue or ac-tivity intolerance. If the person shows no overt signs of musculoskeletal dys-function, then a screening examination may be sufficient. To determine whether a screening examination is appropriate, ask the person the following questions:

Do you have any pain or tenderness in an extremity or when you move? Does this pain affect your daily activities?
Do you have a history of injuries to any muscles, bones, or joints?

In addition, note any deformities apparent on general inspection, such as ab-normal gait or stance and improper body alignment. To screen for muscu-loskeletal dysfunction, observe the manner in which the person walks, moves from a sitting to a standing position, shakes hands, and manipulates clothing. If

(continued)

Physical Examination   Musculoskeletal System (continued)

such simple screening techniques indicate no musculoskeletal problems, the following components may be eliminated from the musculoskeletal examination: comprehensive testing of ROM and muscle strength, and limb measurement.

Specific screening techniques, such as scoliosis screening in adolescents, may be used to detect musculoskeletal problems in certain high-risk groups.

EXPOSURE

The person can remain gowned or draped during much of the musculoskeletal examination, especially when you assess distal parts of the extremities. Underwear can be worn when body alignment and spinal configurations are assessed.

MEASUREMENTS AND COMPARISONS

In a comprehensive examination, measurements and comparisons are useful in describing joint ROM, muscle strength, and the length and circumference of the arms and legs.

Joint ROM can be measured in degrees with a protractor device called the goniometer (Fig. 8-14). The zero reference arm of this device should be aligned with the neutral position of the joint. The person should move the joint through a specific ROM and hold the final position while the other arm of the goniometer is moved to this position and the angle measured. This measurement may be compared with normal values. Record only values that deviate from normal by 10% to 20%. Differences in ROM may be noted by comparing joint movement between left and right sides.

The length or circumference of the limbs may be measured with a cloth tape measure if there appear to be any inequalities between the right and left sides. Accurate measurements are necessary for different health care providers to make meaningful comparisons over time. Serial measurements of limb circumference are most reliable when landmarks are specified or marks made on the person's skin with nontoxic markers to indicate tape measure placement. Measurement landmarks for the extremities may be designated as follows:

- *Entire arm:* Acromion process to the tip of the second finger
- *Upper arm:* Acromion process to olecranon process
- *Forearm:* Olecranon process to ulnar styloid process
- *Entire leg:* Anterosuperior iliac spine to tibial malleolus
- *Upper leg:* Anterosuperior iliac spine to medial condyle of the knee
- *Lower leg:* Medial condyle of the knee to tibial malleolus

MUSCULOSKELETAL PAIN

Although musculoskeletal pain is not considered normal, muscle pain, or *myalgia,* that results from overusing poorly conditioned muscles is usually benign. Crepitation (a grating sound) with joint movement is abnormal.

(continued)

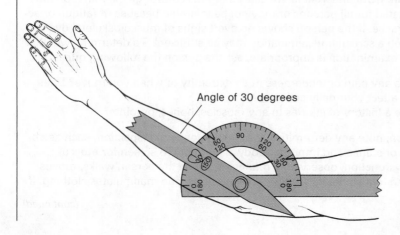

Angle of 30 degrees

FIGURE 8.14 The goniometer is used to measure degrees of joint motion. The zero point is placed at the extended anatomic position. This example shows 30 degrees of flexion at the elbow.

Physical Examination   Musculoskeletal System (continued)

Musculoskeletal pain should be distinguished from visceral pain during the examination. Unlike visceral pain, musculoskeletal pain can usually be elicited by palpation, is aggravated by movement of associated structures, and usually does not have a characteristic pattern such as those observed with the pain of angina or pleurisy.

EXAMINATION AND DOCUMENTATION FOCUS

- Structural symmetry and alignment
- Ease and ROM
- Muscle strength and tone
- Muscle mass
- Skin appearance over joints
- Deformities, pain, and crepitation

EVALUATING RANGE OF MOTION

Every joint in the body has a normal ROM, or maximum possible movement. Joint movements are described by range measured in degrees of a circle and by type of movement. When the range of movement is stated in degrees, the neutral joint position is 0 degrees. An example of ROM description for a simple hinge joint, such as the knee, is "flexion, 130 degrees." Motion may be possible in several directions, depending on joint type.

Differences in exercise levels, general health, and genetics account for normal differences among people. Generally, joint motion occurs with ease if the degree of movement is within 10% to 20% of the maximum possibility. ROM is normal if movement occurs without stiffness, pain, or crepitation. Joint movement past the normal maximum possibility may be abnormal, indicating ligament tears, abnormal connective tissues, or joint fracture.

EVALUATING MUSCLE STRENGTH AND TONE

Muscle strength is graded on a 0 to 5 scale:

0—No detectable muscle contraction
1—Barely detectable contraction
2—Complete ROM or active body part movement with gravity eliminated
3—Complete ROM or active movement against gravity
4—Complete ROM or active movement against gravity and some resistance
5—Complete ROM or active movement against gravity and full resistance

Normal muscle strength is between 3 and 5 on this scale, and differs among people. Although the dominant side may be slightly stronger, muscle strength is usually equal bilaterally. In general, muscles that act as flexors and abductors are stronger than extensors and adductors.

Muscle tone can be detected during partial contraction of muscles, even at rest. Partial contraction is attributable to continual neural stimuli and keeps muscles ready for action. The muscles should appear firm or well developed. Twitching of muscle fibers in the relaxed state is not typical. An occasional, isolated twitch, however, is considered normal.

▼ ▼ ▼

G U I D E L I N E S

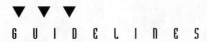

Assessment Guidelines   Bones, Joints, and Muscles

Procedure

1. **Survey gross motor movement and posture.**

   Ask the person to walk across the room, or note the person's movements and stance when he or she enters the examining room. Note gross motor movements (gait, posture, or stance) and range of motion of joints used for walking.

   In addition to noting the style of gait, note the patterns of wear on the shoes, especially the heels, which could indicate unequal pressures or abnormal walking movements. Prostheses such as walkers, canes, crutches, or artificial limbs that may modify gait should also be noted.

   Note posture (stance). Posture or stance refers to the body position the person assumes when standing or sitting.

2. **Evaluate trunk musculoskeletal, structures (vertebral column, paravertebral muscles, scapulae, pelvis).**

   a. Ask the person to stand, facing you; note the alignment and symmetry of the spine, scapulae, and iliac crests. Observe the muscles for tone and note any visible spasms.

Clinical Significance

Normal Findings

Normal gait is smooth and even and is usually accompanied by symmetrical arm swinging. In normal walking, the heel should gently strike the floor with the knee extended. Weight should then be smoothly transferred along the length of the foot toward the metatarsals. With the knee slightly flexed, the foot should lift off the floor. Walking movements should be coordinated.

Deviations from Normal

Abnormal gaits may be described as ataxic, hemiplegic, parkinsonian, scissors, spastic, steppage, or waddling. The different types of abnormal gait as well as the conditions associated with each are further described in Display 8–8, "Abnormal Gaits."

Good posture is characterized by proper alignment of body parts. Deviations from good posture, usually resulting from musculoskeletal or neurologic pathology, may provide cues about the person's activity and exercise abilities.

Normal Findings

Normal alignment: Normal alignment is present if an imaginary line can be drawn through the ear lobe, shoulder, hip, femoral tochanter, center of the knee, and front of the ankle. The elbow, finger, ankle, and knee joints should be slightly flexed. Viewed from the front, the following structures should be at an even level: right and left shoulders; right and left iliac crests; right and left knees.

Symmetry: The bones and muscles on each side of the body are symmetric with respect to size, shape, and function. Surface features, such as trochanters, crests, and other bony prominences, should also be symmetric. Measured length and circumference of matching structures should also be equal. A 1-cm difference in length between left and right extremities is usually considered clinically insignificant.

DISPLAY 8.8

Abnormal Gaits

ATAXIC GAIT

The foot is raised high and strikes the ground suddenly with the entire sole. The person may stagger or fall to one side. Occurs with cerebellar disorders; alcohol or barbiturate toxicity.

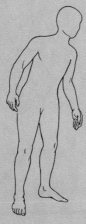

Ataxic gait

PARKINSONIAN GAIT (FESTINATING)

Body bends forward, rigid, with flexion of elbows, wrists, hips, and knees. Steps are short and shuffling with feet barely leaving the ground. May walk on toes as though pushed. Starts slowly and gradually accelerates Sudden forward movement (propulsion) may continue until person can grasp some object for support. Occurs with Parkinson's disease and other basal ganglia defects.

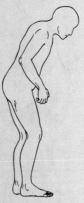

Parkinsonian gait

HEMIPLEGIC GAIT

One leg is paralyzed. The paralyzed leg is abducted and swung around so that the foot comes forward and to the front, or the paralyzed leg may be dragged forward in a semicircle. Occurs with unilateral upper motor neuron disorder, as in stroke.

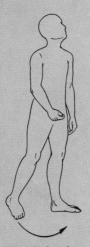

Hemiplegic gait

SCISSORS GAIT

Legs cross of the thighs or knees with each step. Takes short steps. Very slow and awkward leg movements. Occurs with upper motor neuron disorders, as in stroke.

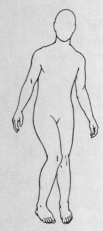

Scissors gait

DISPLAY 8.8

Abnormal Gaits (continued)

STEPPAGE GAIT

Foot and toes lifted high with knees flexed. Foot brought to ground suddenly, heel first, with slapping noise. Person watches ground to know where to place foot. Occurs with peripheral neuritis, late stages of diabetes, alcoholism, and chronic arsenic poisoning.

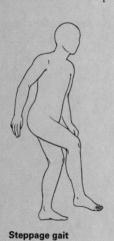

Steppage gait

WADDLING GAIT

Feet wide apart, and stride resembles that of a duck. Regular steps. Occurs with congenital hip displacement with lordosis, muscular dystrophy.

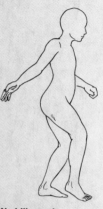

Waddling gait

▼ ▼ ▼

G U I D E L I N E S   *continued*   Bones, Joints, and Muscles

---

Procedure

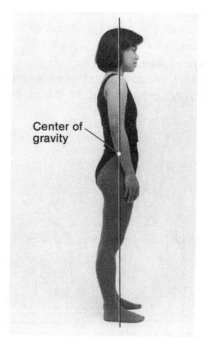

Normal musculoskeletal alignment:
Side view

b. View the person from the side, and note spinal curvatures. Also note abnormalities, such as exaggerated curvatures or straightening of the lumbar curve of the spine.

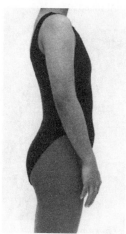

Normal vertebral
column alignment

Clinical Significance

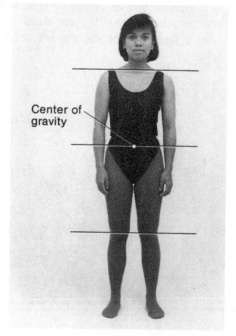

Normal musculoskeletal alignment: Front view

Normal Findings

Normal vertebral column alignment: Normally, when viewed from the side the vertebral column is characterized by concave curvature of the cervical spine, convex curvature of the thoracic spine, and concave curvature of the lumbar spine. The spine should be straight when viewed from behind the person. Exaggerated curvatures should be considered abnormal, even if oriented in a normal direction.

Deviations from Normal

Spinal deformities: Lordosis, abnormal concavity of the lumbar spine; *kyphosis,* abnormally increased rounding of the thoracic curve; *gibbus,* a projection along the vertebral column caused by a collapsed vertebra.

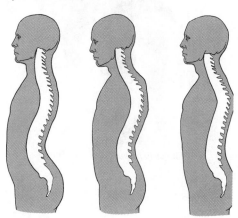

Spinal deformities: (left) *lordosis;* (center) *kyphosis;*
(right) *gibbus*

▼ ▼ ▼

GUIDELINES *continued*   Bones, Joints, and Muscles

Procedure

c. Ask the person to bend forward at the waist. Stand be-hind the person and note the ease of mobility, the orien-tation of the supine and scapulae, and curvature of the spine.

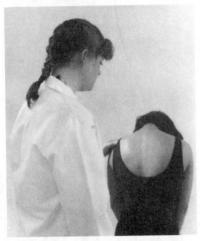

Spine inspection

d. With the person standing, sitting, or lying prone, pal-pate the vertebral column with the fingertips. Note any tenderness or bony deformities.

e. Lightly pound the length of the spine with the ulnar sur-face of your hand, and note any tenderness.

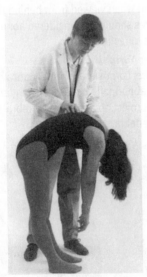

Fingertip palpation of the spine

Clinical Significance

Normal Findings

The entire spine should appear smooth and convex, and the vertebrae should remain midline.

Deviations from Normal

Scoliosis is lateral deviation of the thoracic spine best observed if the person bends at the waist from a standing position.

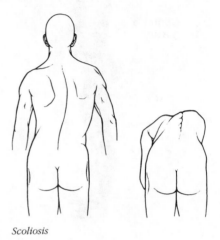

Scoliosis

Normal Findings

No tenderness elicited on palpation.

Deviations from Normal

Point tenderness (tenderness elicited on palpation); may indi-cate degenerative joint disease.

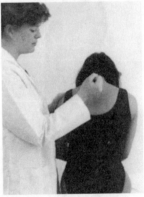

Fist palpation of the spine

▼ ▼ ▼

G U I D E L I N E S *continued* Bones, Joints, and Muscles

Procedure

3. **Test range of motion and muscle strength of the neck.**

    a. Check flexion and extension of the cervical spine by asking the person to touch the chin to the chest and then tip the head backward.

    b. To evaluate muscle strength, ask the person to repeat these movements while you press your hand against the person's forehead during flexion and against the occiput during extension.

    c. To evaluate cervical spine rotation, ask the person to turn the head toward the right and left shoulders while keeping the shoulders stationary.

    d. Then apply resistance to the temples and ask the person to repeat the movements, to assess muscle strength.

    e. Finally, to evaluate lateral bending of the cervical spine, ask the person to try and touch the ear to the shoulder while keeping the shoulders stationary.

    f. Then apply pressure to the person's right and left occiputs to evaluate muscle strength.

Clinical Significance

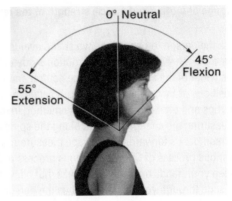

Neck range of motion: Flexion and extension

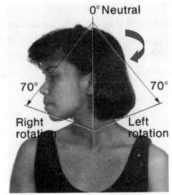

Neck range of motion: Rotation

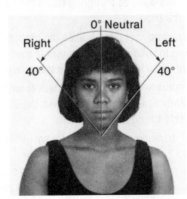

Neck range of motion: Lateral bending

▼ ▼ ▼

G U I D E L I N E S   *continued*   Bones, Joints, and Muscles

Procedure

4. **Test range of motion and muscle strength of the remaining spine.**

   a. Ask the person to bend at the waist and evaluate forward flexion. Measure range of motion by determining the width of the angle between the neutral and flexed positions or by measuring the length between the fingertips and the floor. An alternative method involves measuring the change in length along the spine as the person bends forward. Place a tape measure from the spinous process of C7 to the spinous process of S1. Keep your hands on these landmarks, but allow the tape to slide through your fingers at S1 as the person leans forward.

   b. To evaluate spinal extension, ask the person to lean backward.

   c. Extensor muscle strength is best evaluated with the person in the prone position. Instruct the person to try to lift the head and shoulders while you apply resistance by placing your hand between the scapulae.

   d. To evaluate lateral bending of the spine, ask the person to bend sideways as though to touch the hand to the side of the knee.

   e. Then evaluate spinal rotation as the person turns the head and the shoulders as one unit to the left and then the right while holding the pelvis stationary.

   f. Ask the person to repeat this maneuver while you place your hands against the right and left shoulders to evaluate muscle strength.

   g. *Special maneuvers.* Two special maneuvers, *Patrick's sign* and *Lasègue's sign,* are indicted for persons with back pain. Because the person should be supine, you may postpone these maneuvers until you are ready to evaluate the lower extremities.

   Lasègue's sign is elicited by asking the person to raise one leg at a time off the examining table.

Clinical Significance

Normal Findings

Normally, the length should increase about 4 inches in adults. If length does not increase, you should suspect conditions that limit vertebral joint mobility, which cause the back to remain straight with forward flexion.

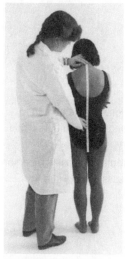 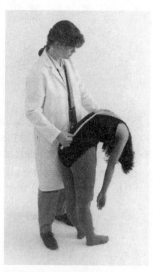

Evaluating spine range of motion: Upright

Evaluating spine range of motion: Bending over

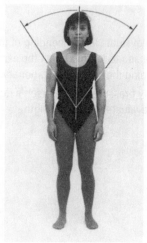

Spine range of motion: Lateral bending

Deviations from Normal

Positive Lasègue's sign is indicated by pain in the back with this maneuver, and indicates back injury.

▼ ▼ ▼
G U I D E L I N E S *continued*   Bones, Joints, and Muscles

Procedure

Patrick's sign is elicited by placing the heel of one foot on the opposite knee. Then, the hip of the flexed extremity is abducted.

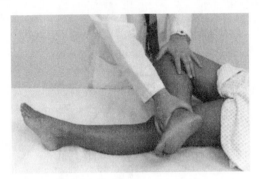

Assessing for Patrick's sign

5. **Evaluate shoulder musculoskeletal structures.**
   a. With the person standing, sitting, or supine, inspect the shoulders from the front, and note right- and left-side symmetry. Inspect the skin over the clavicles for bulges or protrusions. Note the shoulder posture (erect, slumped, hunched).

   b. With your fingertips, palpate along the clavicles outward to the shoulders and note any discomfort or deformities. Visualize sternoclavicular and acromioclavicular joint locations as you move your fingers along the clavicles. Locate the greater tubercle of the humerus by palpating the shoulder as the person abducts and adducts at the shoulder, allowing you to differentiate between scapula and humerus at the glenohumeral joint. Ask the person to rotate the shoulder externally, and palpate just medial to the greater tubercle to locate the long head of the biceps. Palpate along this cord-like tendon, and note any tenderness. Finally, palpate the deltoid muscle.

Clinical Significance

Positive Patrick's sign is indicated by pain with this maneuver, and indicates sacroiliac joint disease.

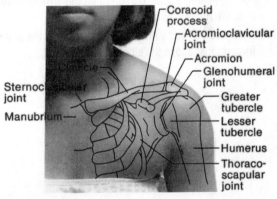

Shoulder musculoskeletal structures

Deviations from Normal

Skin bulges or protrusions are associated with clavicular fracture.

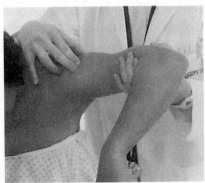

Shoulder palpation

Deviations from Normal

The deltoid muscle overlies the nonpalpable subdeltoid bursa; palpation may cause pain if *bursitis* is present.

▼ ▼ ▼

Procedure

6. **Test range of motion and muscle strength of the shoulder.**

   a. To evaluate flexion, ask the person to raise the arm anteriorly until pointing overhead.

   b. Apply resistance to the upper anterior arm just above the elbow. To test muscle strength, ask the person to repeat the shoulder flexion. Then apply pressure over the posterior surface of the upper arm just above the elbow to test muscle strength during shoulder extension.

   c. For abduction, ask the person to lift the arm laterally until the fingers point overhead.

   d. Apply resistance by placing your hand over the upper forearm just above the elbow.

   e. To test adduction, ask the person to bring the arm over the chest.

   f. Apply resistance over the medial aspect of the upper arm above the elbow to test muscle strength during adduction.

Clinical Significance

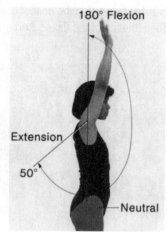

Shoulder range of motion: Flexion

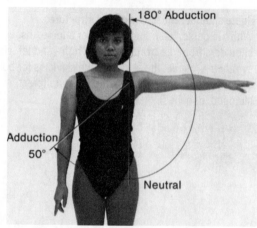

Shoulder range of motion: Abduction

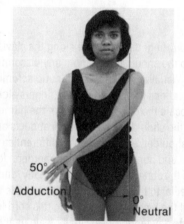

Shoulder range of motion: Adduction

▼ ▼ ▼
G U I D E L I N E S   *continued*   Bones, Joints, and Muscles

Procedure

g. Finally, to evaluate external and internal shoulder joint rotation, ask the person to flex the elbow and raise the arm to shoulder level, holding the hand with the fingers extended and palm facing the floor. Note external rotations as the person rotates the forearm posteriorly, back and forth. Note internal rotation as the person rotates the forearm anteriorly so that the fingertips point to the floor.

Clinical Significance

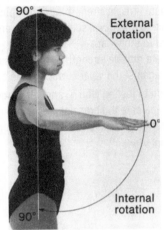

Shoulder range of motion: Rotation

7. **Evaluate elbow musculoskeletal structures.**

   Inspect and palpate the posterior elbow surface with your thumb and forefinger as the person bends the elbow at an angle of flexion just greater than 90 degrees while you support the forearm with your other hand. Note the medial and lateral condyles of the humerus and the olecranon process of the ulna. Note any bony deformities, and carefully compare opposite sides.

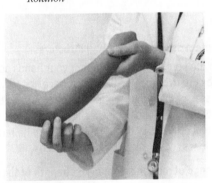

Elbow palpation

Deviations from Normal

The olecranon bursa lies between the condyles of the humerus and is not normally palpable but may be tender if inflamed. The ulnar nerve is palpable posteriorly between the olecranon process and medial epicondyle.

8. **Test range of motion and muscle strength of the elbow.**

   a. Instruct the person to hold the upper arm straight while bending at the elbow in a manner that allows the fingers to touch the shoulder. The opposite of this action is extension.

   b. To test muscle strength, ask the person to repeat the maneuvers, and apply your hand to the medial surface and then to the dorsal surface of the wrist during both flexion and extension.

   c. Finally, to test supination and pronation, ask the person to extend the forearm or rest the forearm on a flat surface with the palm facing down. Supination occurs when the person rotates the forearm so that the palm faces upward, and pronation occurs when the person rotates the forearm so that the palm faces downward.

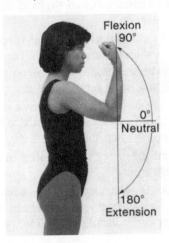

Elbow range of motion: Flexion and extension

▼ ▼ ▼

G U I D E L I N E S   *continued*   Bones, Joints, and Muscles

Procedure

d. To evaluate muscle strength during supination, apply resistance to the dorsal surface of the person's hand just distal to the wrist.

e. To evaluate muscle strength during pronation, apply resistance against the volar surface of the person's thumb

f. In addition to testing elbow range of motion and muscle strength, palpate the brachial pulse on the side opposite the olecranon process and check the bicep and tricep reflexes (see Chap. 9).

9. **Evaluate wrist musculoskeletal structures.**

   Grasp the person's wrist with both your hands so that both thumbs are over the dorsal wrist surface. Identify the bony processes of the radius (on the thumb side) and the ulna. Palpate the radiocarpal joint, a slight groove just distal to the radial process. With both thumbs, palpate remaining wrist bones.

10. **Test range of motion and muscle strength of the wrist.**

    a. To check flexion (palmarflexion) and extension (dorsiflexion), ask the person to bend the hand downward at the wrist and upward with fingers pointing up, respectively.

    b. To test muscle strength, place your hand against the volar surface of the person's hand during flexion and against the dorsal surface of the hand, over the carpals, during extension.

    c. To check radial wrists deviation, ask the person to hold the elbow aligned with the wrist and bend the wrist sideways toward the thumb side. Apply resistance by pressing against the person's thumb.

    d. Check ulnar deviation with the elbow and wrist in the same position, but instruct the person to bend the wrist sideways, away from the body.

    e. To test muscle strength, apply resistance along the person's little finger.

    f. In addition to evaluating the musculoskeletal structure of the wrist, palpate the radial pulse and check the supinator (brachioradialis) reflex (see Chap. 9).

Clinical Significance

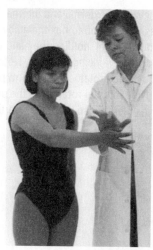

Evaluating muscle strength during elbow range of motion

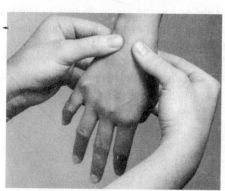

Wrist palpation

▼ ▼ ▼
G U I D E L I N E S *continued*   Bones, Joints, and Muscles

Procedure

11. Evaluate hand musculoskeletal structures.

Focus hand assessment on the finger joints, which are susceptible to degenerative joint disease.

With the person's fingers slightly flexed, use your thumb and forefinger to palpate the metacarpophalangeal joints, which feel like grooves just distal to the first knuckle. Then, palpate the interphalangeal joints.

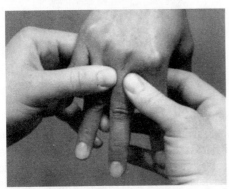

Metacarpophalangeal joint palpation

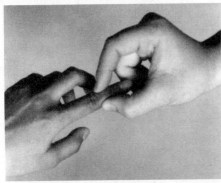

Interphalangeal joint palpation

12. Evaluate range of motion and muscle strength of the fingers.

a. To evaluate finger and thumb flexion and extension, ask the person to make a fist and then straighten the fingers.

b. Test resistance to extension by placing your hand over the person's clenched fist before the hand is opened.

Clinical Significance

Deviations from Normal

Finger deformities include mallet finger (position of permanent flexion due to loss of extensor ability), boutonnière and swan-neck deformities (associated with rheumatoid arthritis), claw fingers (associated with injury to ulnar and medial nerves), and nodules (associated with osteoarthritis).

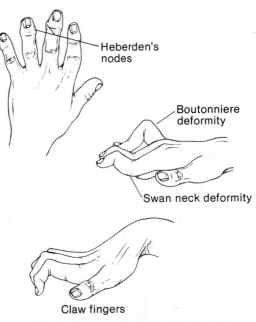

Finger deformities

▼ ▼ ▼

Procedure

c. Test finger abduction as the person spreads the fingers apart and adduction as the person holds the fingers tightly together.

d. To test adductor strength, place your thumb against the person's index finger and your other fingers against the person's little finger.

e. To test thumb abduction and adduction, ask the person to move the thumb up and outward from the palm and then return the thumb to the neutral position.

f. *Special maneuvers.* If the person reports pain and burning in the hand, special examination maneuvers should be performed to rule out carpal tunnel syndrome.

Test for *Phalen's sign* by holding the wrist in flexion position.

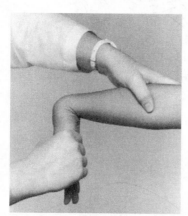

Testing for Phalen's sign

Test for *Tinel's* sign by tapping the palm of the hand (volar percussion).

Evaluate *opposition* by asking the person to touch the thumb to the fingertips of the same hand.

Clinical Significance

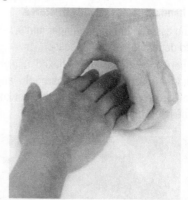

Evaluating muscle strength during finger range of motion

Deviations from Normal

Carpal tunnel syndrome results from pressure on the median nerve as it passes through the wrist. Signs include a positive Phalen's sign, a positive Tinel's sign, decreased sensation in the areas of the medial nerve distribution, atrophy of the thenar eminence, and weak opposition in the thumb of the affected hand.

Phalen's sign is positive if wrist burning is aggravated when the wrist is held in prolonged flexion, usually for 1 or 2 minutes.

Tinel's sign is positive if volar percussion produces tingling or shocklike pain.

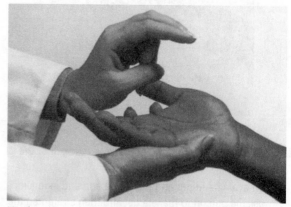

Tinel's sign

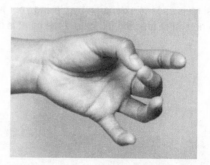

Evaluating finger-to-thumb opposition

▼ ▼ ▼
G U I D E L I N E S *continued*   Bones, Joints, and Muscles

Procedure

13. Evaluate hip musculoskeletal structures.

Because the hip joint is essential for walking movements, evaluate gait and stance during the general inspection. The hip may be assessed with the person standing or supine. Range of motion maneuvers are the same for both positions. However, the person needs greater strength and balance to perform such maneuvers while standing.

Palpate the hip joint and surrounding structures. Place your fingertips over the lateral aspect of the iliac crest with the palm of your hand over the lateral hip. The greater trochanter of the femur and the nonpalpable trochanteric bursa lie beneath the surface of your palm. Palpate around this process and note any joint tenderness or pain. Palpate the area surrounding the hip, thigh, and buttock muscles.

14. Evaluate range of motion and muscle strength of the hip.

a. To evaluate hip flexion, ask the person to lift the leg without bending at the knee.

b. Check muscle strength by placing your hand over the anterior surface of the upper leg as the person repeats hip flexion.

c. Note extension as the person returns the leg to the neutral position.

d. Test extensor muscle strength by placing your hand over the posterior surface of the upper leg during hip extension.

e. To check abduction, ask the person to move the entire leg away from the body. Check adduction by having the person move the leg across the midline so that one leg lies over the other.

f. Apply resistance over the lateral leg surface during abduction and the medial leg surface during adduction.

Clinical Significance

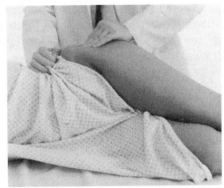

Hip palpation

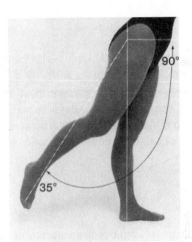

Hip range of motion: Flexion and extension

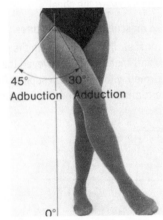

Hip range of motion: Abduction and adduction

▼ ▼ ▼

G U I D E L I N E S   *continued*   Bones, Joints, and Muscles

Procedure

g. Finally, to evaluate external rotation, ask the person to turn the foot outward while holding the leg straight. To evaluate internal rotation, ask the person to turn the foot inward.

Clinical Significance

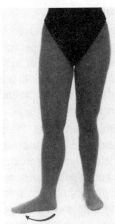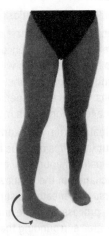

Hip range of motion: External rotation   *Hip range of motion: Internal rotation*

h. To test muscle strength, apply resistance against the lateral or medial aspects of the ankle.

i. *Special maneuvers.* The special maneuvers discussed with assessment of the trunk may be performed in conjunction with the hip examination because such assessments are based on hip range of motion maneuvers.

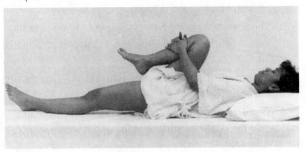

Thomas test

If you suspect a hip flexion contracture or note restricted range of motion, perform the Thomas test. Ask the person to assume a supine position and flex the knee, pulling it toward the chest.

Deviations from Normal

The Thomas test result is positive if the opposite leg flexes at the hip and knee with this maneuver. A positive result is abnormal and indicates a hip flexion contracture on that side.

15. **Evaluate knee musculoskeletal structures.**

The knee is most easily evaluated with the person seated, with the hips and knees flexed. However, the examination may be performed with the person supine. Apley's test should be performed with the person in a prone position (see p. 361).

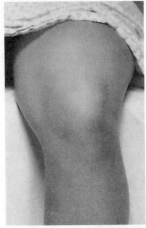

Knee musculoskeletal structure

▼ ▼ ▼

G U I D E L I N E S   *continued*   Bones, Joints, and Muscles

Procedure

a. Inspect the front of the knee and note alignment, deformity, and the contour of the quadricep muscle and any atrophy of this muscle.

b. Focus palpation on the suprapatellar pouch, a sac-like structure separating the patella from surrounding structures.

   To help make fluid more accessible to palpation, displace the pouch downward by placing one of your hands over the quadriceps at the top of the knee and exerting slight downward pressure.

   Use your other hand to palpate along each side of the patella and over the tibiofemoral joint space. Palpate with the fingertips and stabilize the opposite side of the knee with the thumb of your examining hand. Displace the pouch upward by placing one of your hands over the lower part of the knee and applying slight pressure upward and inward. Palpate the area from the quadriceps to the patella with your fingertips. Note any tenderness, bogginess, edema, or thickening. If you suspect fluid, patella ballottement and evaluation for a bulge sign are indicated (see 16c).

c. In addition to evaluating the musculoskeletal structures of the knee, palpate the popliteal pulse, located at the back of the knee in the popliteal fossa, slightly lateral to the midline. Then check the patellar reflex (see Chap. 11).

Clinical Significance

Normal Findings

Normal contour, which may be lost with swelling, is indicated by hollows on each side of the patella.

Deviations from Normal

Fluid accumulation following injury or disease may be easily detected at the suprapatellar pouch.

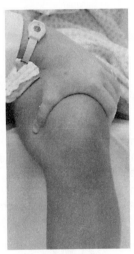
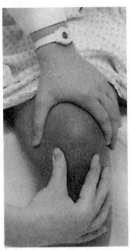

Displacing the suprapatellar pouch   *Palpating the suprapatellar pouch*

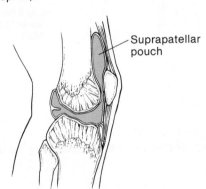

— Suprapatellar pouch

Internal knee structure

16. **Evaluate range of motion and muscle strength of the knee.**

    a. To evaluate flexion, ask the person to stand and bend the knee, bringing the heel toward the buttocks. If the person is supine, the hip must also be flexed to perform this action. Note extension as the person returns the knee to the neutral position.

    b. To test muscle strength of the knee during flexion, place your hand against the back of the ankle. During extension, move your hand to the front of the ankle.

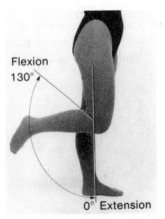

Flexion 130°

0° Extension

Knee range of motion: Flexion and extension

▼ ▼ ▼

Procedure

c. *Special maneuvers.* Two techniques may be used to check for fluid accumulation in the knee:

(1) To perform *patella ballottement,* place one of your hands over the quadriceps and apply downward pressure to distribute accumulated fluid in the suprapatellar pouch toward the patella. With the first and second fingers of your other hand, tap the patella against the femur and note the patella rebounding against your examining fingers.

(2) To elicit a *bulge sign,* milk any suprapatellar fluid away from the medial half of the knee by using the ball of your hand to apply firm upward pressure along the medial side. Repeat this motion several times. Briskly tap the lateral side of the knee several times. Note the medial area where you just displaced fluid.

McMurray's test is used to detect meniscus injuries. With the person supine or seated, place one of your hands against the medial side of the knee to stabilize it. With your other hand, grasp the person's ankle and rotate the lower leg and foot inward while trying to extend the leg.

Clinical Significance

Deviations from Normal

If the patella rebounds (ballots) against your fingers, fluid is present in the knee.

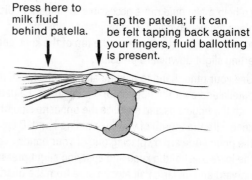

Press here to milk fluid behind patella.

Tap the patella; if it can be felt tapping back against your fingers, fluid ballotting is present.

Patella ballottment

Deviations from Normal

A medial bulge with lateral tapping indicates fluid movement in the joint. In such a case, the bulge sign is positive.

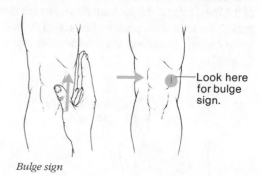

Look here for bulge sign.

Bulge sign

Deviations from Normal

The leg cannot be extended if a meniscus injury is present.

Procedure

Apley's test also detects meniscus injuries and foreign or floating objects in the joint. The person should be prone with the knee flexed at 90 degrees. Grasp the person's foot and apply pressure. Then rotate the foot externally and internally.

Clinical Significance

Deviations from Normal

Knee locking or clicking and popping sounds indicate loose objects and injury.

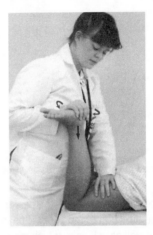

Apley's test

Knee stability is evaluated by attempting to move the knee in an abnormal manner. With the person supine, and the leg straight, grasp the thigh with one hand and the ankle with the other. Then, attempt to adduct and abduct the leg at the knee.

Evaluate the anterior and posterior cruciate ligaments by trying to elicit a *drawer sign.* With the person supine, flex the knee and grasp the lower leg firmly with both hands. Attempt to push the knee back and forth while stabilizing the person's foot by sitting on it.

Deviations from Normal

Movement with adduction indicates a tear of the medial collateral ligament, whereas movement with abduction indicates dysfunction of the lateral collateral ligament.

Deviations from Normal

Normally there is no movement. Forward movement indicates anterior cruciate tears, and backward movement indicates posterior cruciate tears.

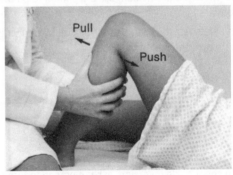

Testing knee stability

17. **Evaluate ankle musculoskeletal structures.**

    a. With the person seated or supine, inspect the ankle and note any swelling or deformity. Compare the contour of the left and right ankles.

    b. To palpate, stabilize the ankle by cupping one of your hand's behind the heel. Palpate with the fingers of your other hand.

▼ ▼ ▼

G U I D E L I N E S   *continued*   Bones, Joints, and Muscles

Procedure

   c. Palpate the posterior tibial pulse located slightly below the medial malleolus. Also test the Achilles reflex (see Chap. 9).

18. **Evaluate range of motion and muscle strength of the ankle.**

   a. To evaluate dorsiflexion, ask the person to bend the toes in the direction of the knee. Then, note range of motion as well as calf pain, which may indicate deep vein thrombosis in the lower leg (positive *Homans' sign*).

   b. Check resistance to dorsiflexion with your hand over the dorsal foot surface.

   c. To check plantar flexion, ask the person to point the toes.

   d. Evaluate resistance to plantar flexion by applying pressure over the ball of the foot.

   e. To check ankle inversion, ask the person to turn the sole of the foot inward at the ankle joint, and apply resistance to foot arches to check muscle strength.

Clinical Significance

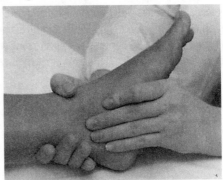

Ankle palpation

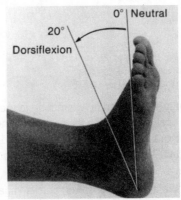

Ankle range of motion: Dorsiflexion

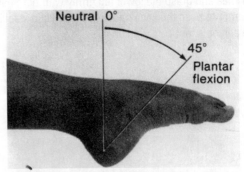

Ankle range of motion: Plantar flexion

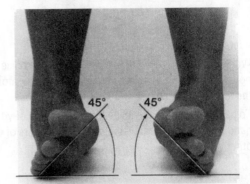

Ankle range of motion: Inversion

▼ ▼ ▼

G U I D E L I N E S   *continued*   Bones, Joints, and Muscles

---

Procedure

f. Check eversion as the person turns the soles of the feet outward at the ankle joint, and place your hands against the lateral aspect of the fifth metatarsal bones to check muscle strength.

Clinical Significance

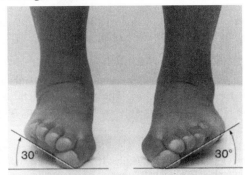

Ankle range of motion: Eversion

19. **Evaluate foot musculoskeletal structures.**

   a. Inspect the feet and note skin integrity, condition of the nails, and any deformities.

   b. Palpate the metatarsal bones and the metatarsal joints between the forefinger and thumb.

   c. The dorsalis pedis pulse is noted just lateral to the extensor tendon of the great toe.

Deviations from Normal

Foot deformities: Equinus and calcaneal deformities.

Toe deformities: Claw hammer toe.

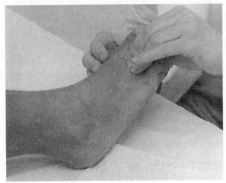

Metatarsal palpation

20. **Evaluate foot range of motion.**

   a. Stabilize the foot by cupping one of your hands around the heel. Ask the person to turn the foot inward (adduction) and then outward (abduction).

   b. To evaluate the toes for flexion and extension, ask the person to bend and straighten the toes.

   c. To check abduction of the toes, ask the person to fan the toes apart; for adduction, return the toes to the neutral position.

Documenting Musculoskeletal Examination Findings

Documentation of musculoskeletal examination findings may reflect the overall status of the musculoskeletal system or may focus on specific body parts.

Example 1: Normal Musculoskeletal Function

Mr. W, aged 30 years, had a routine annual health assessment at the industrial clinic. The musculoskeletal screening examination findings were normal and were recorded as follows:

Reports no previous musculoskeletal injuries or pain except for a sprained left ankle 3 years ago that healed without complications. Gait smooth and coordinated; extremities symmetric and posture upright. ROM required for general movement during examination intact; specific testing not done. Muscle strength 4 to 5; well-developed muscle mass. No visible musculoskeletal deformities.

These findings may be recorded in a problem-oriented format as follows:

S: Reports no musculoskeletal pain or movement limitations. Exercise program includes speed walking and using machine weights. Sprained left ankle 3 years ago that healed without sequelae.

O: Gait smooth and coordinated; extremities symmetric and posture upright. ROM required for general movement during examination intact; specific testing not done. Muscle strength 4 to 5; well-developed muscle mass. No visible musculoskeletal deformities.

A: No abnormalities detected by musculoskeletal screening examination.

P: Routine follow-up examinations as indicated. Evaluate exercise habits to see whether he uses warm-up and cool-down periods to prevent muscle strain and injury.

Example 2: Ankle Injury

Mr. T, aged 38 years, reported to the emergency clinic with left ankle pain after a fall during a softball game. The lower extremity examination findings were abnormal and were recorded as follows:

Left ankle edematous and ecchymotic compared with right ankle. Guards left ankle by not bearing weight. ROM impaired because of pain, but he is able to move ankle and toes. Left pedal pulse 3+.

These findings may be recorded in a problem-oriented format as follows:

S: "I twisted down on my ankle sliding into second base." Reports intense pain with weight bearing. Did not hear any snapping or cracking sounds when injured.

O: Left ankle edematous and ecchymotic compared with right. Guards left ankle by not bearing weight. ROM impaired because of pain, but he is able to move ankle and toes. Left pedal pulse 3+.

A: Possible soft tissue injury to left ankle; need to rule out bone injury.

P: Immobilize left ankle; apply ice packs; notify physician; obtain x-ray if advised by physician.

Nursing Diagnoses Related to Musculoskeletal Assessment

Impaired Physical Mobility

Impaired physical mobility is a state in which the person experiences limitation in the ability to engage in independent physical movement.

History. The person may describe limitations in movement or activities. Listen for reports of pain, tenderness, or soreness with movement. Consider underlying pathologic conditions such as trauma, inflammatory disease, or degenerative conditions. Determine what effect mobility problems are having on the person's capacity to perform activities of daily living.

Physical Examination Findings. In general, a person with impaired physical mobility will exhibit the following: inability to move purposefully within the environment; limited ROM; reluctance to attempt movement; decreased muscle strength. Impaired physical mobility caused by injury may be associated with the following physical examination findings: edema, bruising, or deformity at the injured area; guarding of injured part. When mobility is impaired because of inflammatory conditions of the musculoskeletal system, the following may be observed: edematous joints with enlargement and deformity; skin over affected areas that is warm and tender to palpation.

Clinical Problems Related to Musculoskeletal Assessment

Degenerative Joint Disease

Degenerative joint disease, also called osteoarthritis, is a disease manifested by degenerative changes in the articular cartilage, especially in the major weight-bearing joints (hip, knee, lower back) and hand joints.

History. Degenerative joint disease occurs more commonly in older people and is almost universal in people older than age 75 years. Overuse of the joints has been indicated as contributing to the problem. Degenerative joint disease may be a long-term sequela to joint trauma. Symptoms of the disease vary with severity. Early in the disease, the person may report pain when the involved joint is subjected to stress. Later, the pain may be felt even at rest. The person may also report joint stiffness. The joints may be asymmetrically involved.

Physical Examination. The joints become limited in ROM, and pain may be elicited with movement. Joint swelling or deformity may be present. There may be point tenderness over the affected joints. Occasionally, crepitations or crunching may be heard as the joint is moved.

Rheumatoid Arthritis

Rheumatoid arthritis is a systemic, autoimmune inflammatory disease of the body's connective tissue. Women are affected more often than men. The disease is most prevalent in the 30- to 50-year age-group.

History. The person will typically complain of joint pain or stiffness on arising in the morning. The joints are usually symmetrically involved. The joint pain may diminish throughout the day or it may stay the same. Painful episodes of the disease are cyclic. Remissions may be associated with decreased levels of activity. The small joints of the hands and the feet are usually the first joints to become affected.

Physical Examination. Examination of infected joints usually shows signs of inflammation (swelling, warmth, redness). Passive motions and pressure elicit pain. Rheumatoid nodules may develop at or near the affected joint.

Bursitis

A bursa is a sac that is filled with a small amount of synovial fluid and located over a bony prominence (elbow, knee, greater trochanter of the femur). Bursae facilitate movement of overlying tendons and muscles. Inflammation of the bursa, through trauma or repeated use, is referred to as bursitis.

History and Physical Examination. The person usually can report a mechanism of injury for the affected joint, such as one involving repeated flexion and extension of the elbow. Movement of the affected joint results in pain and tenderness. Over the affected bursa, the area may be red, hot, and edematous with pain that may or may not radiate to surrounding areas.

Herniated Disc Syndrome

This is an acute problem that can occur in persons of any age, typically after age 30 years. The intervertebral disc of the spinal cord ruptures, compressing the nearby spinal nerves.

History and Physical Examination. The onset of symptoms is abrupt, and a snap may be felt in the back just before the onset of pain. There is low back pain that frequently radiates into the lower extremity. Numbness may be felt in the distribution of the sciatic nerve. The person appears in obvious distress and may have difficulty bearing weight on the leg in pain. The person is most comfortable sitting or lying flexed in the fetal position. The paravertebral muscles may be tender and in spasm. Straight leg raising in the supine position is painful. The person may be unable to lie supine with the affected leg straightened out.

CASE STUDY

Enrico Garcia, aged 26 years, was a patient in the CCU with severe heart failure resulting from dilated cardiomyopathy. He had first experienced symptoms of heart dysfunction 4 years earlier after a viral illness. At that time, he was treated with digoxin, furosemide (Lasix), and warfarin sodium crystalline (Coumadin). Approximately 3 years later, hydrazine and captopril were added to the therapeutic regimen because of further deterioration. Five months before this hospital admission, Enrico had to leave his job because of increasing fatigue and dyspnea. While Enrico's condition was being evaluated to see whether he should undergo a heart transplantation, nursing efforts were directed toward maintaining cardiac function. Enrico's activities were restricted to prevent further cardiac decompensation. To evaluate the activity prescription, the nurses monitored Enrico's response to permitted activities. On bed rest he had no dyspnea; he felt well rested, with a pulse of 98 beats/minute, and his skin was warm and dry. While being transferred from bed to chair one day, however, Enrico became lightheaded and began to have trouble breathing. His pulse became weak and rapid at 160 beats/minute, and his skin was cool with cyanosis around the mouth. Enrico was returned to bed to rest. His symptoms persisted for 30 minutes.

For the patient with severe heart failure, even simple activities may further compromise physiologic function. Nurses monitor the patient's response to activity to prevent further deterioration, and to plan interventions that will improve activity tolerance by promoting rest, oxygenation, and cardiac function. Monitoring a patient's response to activity is complex and requires drawing conclusions more specific than statements such as "tolerated activity well" or "did not tolerate activity." Without more specific details about the person's response, planning appropriate interventions may be difficult.

Case Study Analysis

Enrico experienced potentially life-threatening cardiorespiratory compromise in response to activity. In this case, the nurse should focus on the assessment of activity tolerance so that timely interventions could be implemented.

Assessment Focus

For a person with impaired cardiovascular or respiratory functions, the nurse should make a judgment about his or her capabilities before permitting activity. If the nurse believes that the person is at risk for activity intolerance, before permitting activity he or she should make a decision about what types of data to collect and about what signs of activity intolerance to consider valid and reliable.

Before moving him to the chair, Enrico's nurse noted that despite the severity of his illness, the patient's cardiovascular parameters were stable. Based on this assessment, Enrico

CASE STUDY *continued*

was moved to the chair despite the risk of activity intolerance. Ongoing nursing evaluation of activity response focused on the following: watching the cardiac monitor for heart rate changes from baseline, resting levels, and cardiac dysrhythmias; noting signs of decreased cardiac output, such as changes in skin color, temperature, and moisture, all readily apparent by general observation; and evaluating blood pressure for cues to activity intolerance.

Nursing Diagnosis

Evaluating Enrico's response to activity revealed several important cues. First, his heart rate increased, which in itself is not sufficient to identify activity intolerance, be-

cause increased heart rate is a normal response to increased activity, contributing to the higher cardiac output needed to sustain activity. The nurse noted other cues, however, such as lightheadedness, weak pulse, and cool skin, indicating that cardiac output was not augmented. The nurse then made the appropriate decision to return Enrico to bed. Ongoing monitoring showed that 30 minutes elapsed before Enrico's condition stabilized. Normally, heart rate should return to preactivity levels within 3 to 5 minutes.

Based on the nursing assessment, the nurse established the diagnosis of Activity intolerance. Enrico's activity prescription was modified to prevent further cardiovascular deterioration.

CHAPTER 8 SUMMARY

Assessment of Activity and Exercise
The assessment of activity and exercise is focused on the following:
- Typical activity patterns, including activities of daily living, leisure activities, and exercise habits
- The positive effects on cardiovascular function and stress management
- Current physical abilities for meeting self-care needs
- Risk factors or conditions associated with activity intolerance
- Physiologic, behavioral, and psychological responses to normal and altered activity patterns

Data Collection Methods
1. Interview and Review of Records
   Typical daily activities, exercise pattern, and leisure activities
   Self-care abilities and use of assistive devices
   Activity tolerance
   Medical history
   Medication history
2. Diagnostic Studies Review
   Blood surveys
   Noninvasive cardiac studies
   Nuclear medicine studies
   Invasive cardiac studies
   Arterial blood gases (ABGs)
   Pulmonary function studies
   Oximetry
   X-rays
   Electromyography

3. Physical Examination
   Vital signs
   Integumentary system
   Mental status
   Signs and symptoms of activity intolerance during the examination of the cardiovascular and respiratory systems
   Signs and symptoms of mobility problems and self-care deficits identified by general observation or examination of the musculoskeletal system

Primary Nursing Diagnoses
Activity intolerance
Risk for activity intolerance
Diversional activity deficit
Impaired home maintenance management
Impaired physical mobility
Impaired walking
Impaired wheelchair mobility
Impaired wheelchair transfer ability
Impaired bed mobility
Bathing/hygiene self-care deficit
Dressing/grooming self-care deficit
Feeding self-care deficit
Toileting self-care deficit
Fatigue

Clinical Problems Related to Activity and Exercise Dysfunctions
Pathology of the cardiovascular and pulmonary systems

Critical Thinking

A local business is sponsoring a "Wellness Program" and developing a screening program to evaluate wellness and physical fitness levels. The employees range in age from 18 years to 70 years. The sponsor is planning to complete each individual screening session within 20 minutes. Screening techniques commonly used by health clubs are being considered, including measurement of resting and exercise-induced heart rates, anthropometrics, flexibility, and blood pressure.

Learning Exercises

1. Determine and describe the types of information needed to make judgments about physical fitness.

2. If you were to add an additional screening option to this program, describe what it would be and specify your rationale for the addition.

3. Develop a plan for evaluating physical fitness for persons with physical disabilities who could not participate in some of the exercises included in a typical screening program.

4. Select and describe the aspects of the musculoskeletal, cardiovascular, and respiratory examinations you believe would be most useful when making judgments about physical fitness.

BIBLIOGRAPHY

Ahrens, T. (1993). Respiratory monitoring in critical care. *AACN Clinical Issues in Critical Care Nursing, 4*(1), 56–65.

American Association of Cardiovascular and Pulmonary Rehabilitation. (1991). *Guidelines for cardiac rehabilitation programs.* Champaign, IL: Human Kinetics.

Bennett, A.F., & Sauer, H.C. (1991). Special considerations in cardiovascular assessment of the aged. *Nurse Practitioner Forum, 2*(1), 55–60.

Clark, J.R. (1993). Listen closely: Assessing heart sounds. *JEMS: Journal of Emergency Medical Services, 18*(10), 46–47.

Criscitiello, M.G. (1990). Fine-tuning the cardiovascular exam. *Patient Care, 24*(11), 51–74.

Dillon, P. (1994). Reviewing respiratory assessment skills. *Nursing, 24*(6), 68–70.

Dougherty, C.M. (1985). The nursing diagnosis of decreased cardiac output. *Nursing Clinics of North America, 20*(4), 787–799.

Eakin, P. (1989). Assessment of activities of daily living: A critical review, part 1. *British Journal of Occupational Therapy, 52*(1), 11–15.

Estok, P.J., & Rudy, E.B. (1986). Jogging: Cardiovascular benefits and risks. *Nurse Practitioner, 11*(5), 21–28.

Fabius, D.B. (1994). Understanding heart sounds: Solving the mystery of heart murmurs. *Nursing, 24*(7), 39–44.

Fabius, D.B., & Stunkard, J. (1994). Understanding heart sounds: Uncovering the secrets of snaps, rubs, and clicks. *Nursing, 24*(7), 45–50.

Franklin, B.A. (1995). Diagnostic and functional exercise testing: Test selection and interpretation. *Journal of Cardiovascular Nursing, 10*(1), 8–29.

Gehring, P.E. (1992). Vascular assessment. *RN, 55*(2), 22–30.

Gender, M. (1988). Development of a comprehensive nursing history and physical assessment program in a rehabilitation setting. *Rehabilitation Nursing, 8*(5), 17–21.

George, M. (1988). Neuromuscular respiratory failure: What the nurse knows may make a difference. *Journal of Neurosurgical Nursing, 20*(2), 110–117.

Gettman, L.R. (1993). Fitness testing. In Durstine, J.L., King, A.C., Painter, P.L., Roitman, J.L., Zwiren, L.D., Kenney, W.L. (Eds.). *American College of Sports Medicine's resource manual for guidelines for exercise testing and prescription* (2nd ed.). Philadelphia: Lea and Febiger.

Geyer, N., & Naude, S. (1996). Continuing education: Clinical diagnostic skills: Assessment of the chest and lungs. *Nursing News (South Africa), 20*(5), 42–44.

Gordon, M. (1979). Assessing activity tolerance. *American Journal of Nursing, 76,* 72–75.

Gordon, M. (1979). The concept of nursing diagnosis. *Nursing Clinics of North America, 14*(3), 487–496.

Grap, M.J., Glass, C., & Constantino, S. (1994). Accurate assessment of ventilations and oxygenation. *MEDSURG Nursing 3*(6), 435–442.

Guzzetta, C. E., & Dossey, B.M. (1983). Nursing diagnosis: Framework, process, and problems. *Heart and Lung, 12*(3), 281–291.

Herman, J.A. (1986). Nursing assessment and nursing diagnosis in patients with peripheral vascular disease. *Nursing Clinics of North America, 21*(2), 219–231.

Ishii, K. (1995). Physical capacity assessment of the acute cardiovascular patient. *Journal of Cardiovascular Nursing, 9*(4), 53–63.

Jones, A. (1995). A brief overview of the analysis of lung sounds. *Physiotherapy, 81*(1), 37–42.

Kim, M.J. (1984). Physiologic nursing diagnosis: Its role and place in nursing taxonomy. In M.J. Kim, G.K. McFarland, & A.M. McLane (Eds.). *Classification of nursing diagnoses: Proceedings of the fifth national conference.* St. Louis: C.V. Mosby.

Kirton, C.A. (1997). Assessing S3 and S4 heart sounds. *Nursing '97,* July 52–53.

Louden, R.G. (1987). The lung exam. *Clinical Chest Medicine, 8,* 265–272.

Massey, J.A. (1986). Diagnostic testing for peripheral vascular disease. *Nursing Clinics of North America, 21*(2), 207–281.

Milde, F. (1988). Impaired physical mobility. *Journal of Gerontological Nursing, 14*(3), 20–24, 38–40.

Pflieger, K.L., & Strong, W.B. (1992). Screening for heart murmurs:

What's normal and what's not. *Physician and Sportsmedicine, 20*(10), 71–74.

Questad, K.A., & Alquist, A. (1994). Exercise assessment in clinical practice. *Physical Medicine and Rehabilitation Clinics of North America, 5*(2), 243–253.

Rossi, L., & Leary, E. (1992). Evaluating the patient with coronary artery disease. *Nursing Clinics of North America, 27*(1), 177–188.

Rothenberg, M.H., & Graf, B.K. (1993). Evaluation of acute knee injuries. *Postgraduate Medicine, 93*(3), 75–82, 85–86, 149–151.

Saul, L. (1983). Heart sounds and common murmurs. *American Journal of Nursing, 83,* 1679–1689.

Striesmeyer, J. (1993). A four step approach to pulmonary assessment. *American Journal of Nursing, 93*(8), 22–31.

Treml, L.A. (1996). Assessing patient mobility: Mobility screening as part of a community-based geriatric assessment. *Home Care Provider, 1*(1), 26–29, 48.

Assessing Cognition and Perception

ASSESSMENT GUIDELINES

- Cognition and Perception Interview (Health History)
- Mental Status Evaluation
- Diagnostic Studies for Evaluation of Altered Mental Status
- Interpreting Physical Examination Findings Related to Cognition and Perception
- Pain
- Cranial Nerves
- Deep Tendon Reflexes
- Superficial Reflexes
- Sensory System and Cerebellar Functions
- Eyes
- Testing Visual Acuity
- Ears
- Hearing

CHAPTER ORGANIZATION

PART 1: ASSESSING THE PATTERN

Introductory Overview
- Assessment Focus
- Data Collection Methods
- Nursing Diagnoses

Knowledge Base for Assessment
- Dimensions of Cognition
- Dimensions of Perception

Pain
- Definitions of Pain
- Anatomy and Physiology Review
- Pain Theories

PART 2: PHYSICAL EXAMINATION TECHNIQUES

The Cranial Nerves
- Anatomy and Physiology Review

Motor System and Reflexes
- Anatomy and Physiology Review

Sensory System and Cerebellar Functions
- Anatomy and Physiology Review

The Eyes and Vision
- Anatomy and Physiology Review

The Ears and Hearing
- Anatomy and Physiology Review

PART 1

ASSESSING THE PATTERN

INTRODUCTORY OVERVIEW

Perception is the process of acquiring information about the environment through the senses and interpreting sensory input in a meaningful way. *Cognition* is the act or process of understanding and knowing. Cognition involves intellectual functions and associated operations such as memory, learning, motivation, reasoning, thinking, and following instructions. Perception and cognition are closely interrelated, and alterations in either process may affect the other one.

Communication, including communication through speech, involves sending and receiving messages. Alterations in cognitive and perceptual processes (such as those that result from damage to the language areas of the cerebral cortex) or alterations of the special senses may interfere with communication. Communication is also an interpersonal process and may be influenced by the type of relationship one person has with another. Therefore, communication problems should be evaluated from the perspective of roles and relationships as well as from the perspective of cognition and perception.

ASSESSMENT FOCUS

Cognitive and perceptual assessment is a broad domain encompassing many dimensions of human function. Cognitive assessment may be the basis for evaluating factors involved in health education teaching and learning processes commonly referred to by clinicians as *patient and family education.* In another situation, the nurse may be caring for a person with a neurologic problem and the assessment of cognitive and perceptual functions may be directed toward the evaluation of the central or peripheral nervous systems. The assessment of cognition and perception also may focus on the evaluation of the status of the sensory organs and structures required for vision, hearing, taste, touch, smell and position sense. Finally, sensory–perceptual experiences, such as pain, hallucinations, and altered thought processes may be the focus of the clinical assessment. Considering this comprehensive scope of cognitive and perceptual functions, a thorough assessment of cognition and perception will be conducted to meet the following objectives:

- Identifying factors relevant to health education teaching and learning processes
- Determining the status of neurologic functions
- Determining the status of the special senses: sight, hearing, smell, touch, and taste
- Determining the status of deep senses, including kinesthetic (position) and vestibular (balance) senses
- Identifying the person's perceptions of self and surroundings

- Identifying persons at risk for injury because of sensory and perceptual alterations
- Evaluating human responses to sensory and perceptual alterations

Data Collection Methods

Data collection is accomplished by the following methods:

1. Interview or Review of Records Focus
   Mental status
   Status of sensory structures and functions
   Teaching and learning evaluation
   Medical history
   Medication history
2. Pain Assessment (if applicable) Focus
   Perceptions and self-reports of pain
   Physiologic responses
   Behavioral responses
   Cognitive attempts to manage pain
3. Diagnostic Studies Review Focus (diagnostic approach to acute mental status changes)
   Complete blood count
   Electrolytes
   Liver and renal function tests
   Blood alcohol levels
   Toxicology screening
   Radiologic assessment
   Lumbar puncture (if indicated)
4. Physical Examination and Observation Focus
   Neurologic functions
   Mental status evaluation

Signs and symptoms of neurologic dysfunction detected during the examination of cranial nerves, reflexes, and motor and sensory systems

Physical examination of the eyes and ears

Nursing Diagnoses

Assessment of the health education teaching and learning process may result in the identification of the following primary nursing diagnosis:

Knowledge deficit (specify)

Assessment of neurologic and sensory functions may result in the identification of one or more of the following primary nursing diagnoses:

Altered thought process
Acute confusion
Chronic confusion
Impaired memory
Impaired environmental interpretation syndrome
Impaired verbal communication
Sensory–perceptual alterations (specify): Visual, auditory, kinesthetic, gustatory, tactile, olfactory
Unilateral neglect
Potential for injury
Risk for autonomic dysreflexia

Assessment of pain perception may result in one of the following diagnoses:

Pain
Chronic pain

KNOWLEDGE BASE FOR ASSESSMENT

Dimensions of Cognition

Cognitive functions include the ability to think and learn, understand, communicate, and interact with the environment. Thinking requires mental processes such as understanding and being aware. Learning encompasses both thinking and doing. Learning is used in connection with some aspect of behavior such as solving a problem or carrying out a skill. Assessment of cognition is based on observing the following: *level of consciousness, awareness, thought processes,* and *communication processes.*

Consciousness consists of two dimensions: arousal and content. *Level of consciousness* refers to degree of wakefulness or arousability and is regulated by the upper brain stem, the reticular activating system (RAS), and the interaction of these structures with the cerebral hemispheres.

The content or *awareness* dimension refers to a person's ability to integrate and organize thoughts, emotions, and mental processes. Awareness is dependent on the functions occurring within the cerebral cortex. The cerebral cortex is divided into four lobes: frontal, temporal, parietal, and occipital (Fig. 9-1). The frontal lobe is divided into three functional areas: the prefrontal area, the motor area, and Broca's area. Psychic and cognitive functions, including personality, judgment, attention span, moral and ethical behaviors, drive, and depth of feeling, originate in the prefrontal area. Motor speech originates in Broca's area. Speech functions are also controlled by Wernicke's area, located in the temporal lobe of the cerebral cortex.

Thought processes that are evaluated as part of the mental status evaluation include abstract thinking, problem solving, insight, memory, and judgment. These capacities are regulated by the frontal lobe of the cerebral cortex. Thought processes are evaluated by observing the person's ability to perform various cognitive tasks, such as interpreting statements, solving problems, memorizing, and making judgments.

Communication processes include a person's speech patterns and abilities to comprehend language. Specific areas of the cerebral cortex regulate speech and language functions. The motor aspects of speech, such as the movements of the lips, tongue, and vocal cords, are controlled by Broca's area in the cerebral cortex (see Fig. 9-1). Speech functions are also controlled by Wernicke's area,

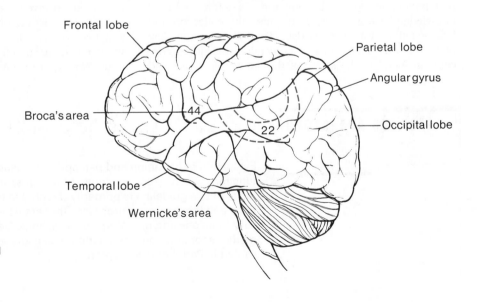

FIGURE 9.1 The cerebral cortex. Lateral view of the cerebral cortex showing speech areas.

located in the temporal lobe of the cerebral cortex. The left cerebral hemisphere is the dominant hemisphere for language function in over 90% of right-handed persons. Therefore, left hemisphere strokes are commonly associated with aphasia, whereas right hemisphere strokes are less likely to cause aphasia. In left-handed persons, the left hemisphere is dominant for language only 50% to 75% of the time.

Despite the concept of cerebral hemisphere dominance, it should be remembered that both hemispheres have some language function. The left hemisphere is responsible for propositional language such as word order, choice, and combinations to form phrases and sentences. The right hemisphere is responsible for affective language such as melody of speech, emotional tone, and intonation.

Wernicke's area (Brodmann's #22) is located in the temporal lobe of the dominant hemisphere and processes word symbols, which allows for understanding and interpretation. *Broca's area* (Brodmann's #44), located in the frontal lobe of the dominant hemisphere (see Fig. 9-1), functions in the propositional language aspects and involves converting messages in the brain into words, phrases, and sentences in a manner consistent with grammatical rules. Another major speech and language area is located at the angular gyrus of the parietal lobe, which receives all incoming sensory stimuli and relates stimuli to language.

Variations in cognitive functions may be age-related. For example, babies acquire knowledge through direct interaction with their surrounding environment, whereas older children are capable of logical thinking. A person's educational level, life experiences, and culture may influence cognitive functions. Cognitive functions may be temporarily or permanently impaired as a result of illness, stress, medications, or abuse of substances such as alcohol or drugs. Therefore, when you conduct a cognitive assessment, you should consider factors that might be influential in the person's background and environment.

Dimensions of Perception

Perception, the process of interpreting reality and events, is a multidimensional phenomenon. Therefore, a broad knowledge base is necessary to guide the collection and interpretation of assessment data. The following overview of the various dimensions of perception introduces concepts included in the scope of this knowledge base and suggests other areas of human function that should be considered during the assessment process.

Physiologic Dimension. The body houses mechanisms for receiving sensory stimuli from the environment, transmitting sensory impulses to the brain, discriminating the nature of stimuli received, and formulating and performing reaction responses. Basic knowledge about ascending and descending neural pathways and brain function is essential for understanding and assessing this aspect of perception. In this chapter, these structural and physiologic aspects are further discussed in Part II with the Anatomy and Physiology Reviews associated with the cranial nerves, motor, system and reflexes, sensory system and cerebellum, eyes, and ears.

Cognitive Dimension. Nerve impulses reaching the brain activate various cortical association areas in brain tissue. A person's responses are shaped by his or her previous experiences, age, and intellectual abilities, with storage areas of the brain becoming activated and memory triggered by the nerve impulses. As past experiences are remembered, learned behaviors or conditioned responses to these stimuli are initiated, and meaning becomes associated with the sensory experience. Without memory and experience, or the cognitive processing of nerve impulses, a person would perceive many sensory stimuli as undifferentiated environmental events.

Personal or Cultural Dimension. An individual's personality and cultural background can influence perceptions. Usually, personal and cultural experiences enhance perceptual functions. For example, culture gives meaning to the words used when communicating with others. Personal experiences, family experiences, cultural norms, and the expectations of other persons serve as frames of reference to validate a person's perceptions. At times, because of personal or cultural influences, an individual's perception of reality may not agree with society's standards. Such a person may be considered by others to be highly individualistic or unrealistic and unable to think clearly.

Behavioral Response Dimension. Everyone evaluates his or her own perceptions of reality. Reactions may be described positively as adaptive, goal-oriented, appropriate, or constructive, or negatively as inappropriate, nonadaptive, or destructive. Often negative reactions occur when incoming stimuli are perceived as unfamiliar, repetitious, boring, or meaningless.

Pattern Assessment   Cognition and Perception Assessment Guidelines

GENERAL APPROACH

Evaluation of cognition and perception focuses on the assessment of cognitive functions, sensory and perceptual functions, and neurologic functions. The focus of this guideline is primarily directed at the evaluation of cognitive functions and the screening processes that are used to make judgments about sensory functions and neurologic dysfunctions. Detailed physical examination methods for additional evaluation of sensory and neurologic functions are presented in Part II of this chapter.

(continued)

The assessment of cognition and perception begins by obtaining a history focused on the general status of cognitive processes, special senses, and general neurologic indicators. The history is compiled by interviewing the person or family members, reviewing records, and reviewing the medical history and medication history. The interview also provides an opportunity to further evaluate cognitive functions through the direct observation available to the examiner of the person's level of consciousness, awareness, thought processes, and communication abilities.

SCREENING COGNITIVE AND PERCEPTUAL STATUS

Screening is an abbreviated assessment method that identifies people at risk for cognitive and neurologic problems. A screening interview may be sufficient if the person appears to have no sensory–perceptual alterations, as would be the case if the person were fully alert, communicated easily, ambulated readily, and displayed no signs of pain, fatigue, or irritability. A screening interview is based on questions about the status of the special senses, especially vision and hearing. The person is asked about participation in recommended screening programs for detection of visual or hearing problems and about any other problems with the special senses.

EVALUATING A PERSON WITH COGNITIVE IMPAIRMENT

If the screening interview indicates potential or actual problems, or if the general survey indicates a problem with any cognitive functions, then a more comprehensive evaluation is indicated. In the presence of cognitive impairment, such as altered thought processes, it may be difficult to conduct an interview because of the person's inability to participate in a meaningful way. In this case, you should use techniques designed for mental status evaluation and testing. You also can obtain additional information from family members or caregivers.

COMPREHENSIVE NEUROLOGIC ASSESSMENT

A comprehensive neurologic assessment includes the following:

- Mental status evaluation
- Cranial nerve assessment
- Reflex testing
- Motor system assessment
- Sensory system assessment

MENTAL STATUS EVALUATION

Mental status evaluation is conducted to make judgments about the status of cognitive functions, including level of consciousness, awareness, thought processes, and communication abilities. Mental status evaluation may be conducted during a routine assessment process or it may be initiated to evaluate a sudden change in cognitive status. Serial measurements of mental status are indicated for acute mental status changes. A variety of methods may be used to assess mental status, including the following:

- Interview and observation
  During the interview, the examiner can observe the person's orientation, judgment, affect, speech, and language abilities (See "Mental Status Evaluation" for specific assessment procedures).
- Glasgow Coma Scale
  The Glasgow Coma Scale is a standardized assessment tool used to evaluate level of consciousness (see "Mental Status Evaluation" for a description of the use of the Glasgow Coma Scale).
- Cognitive screening instruments: "Mini-Mental State Examination"
  Cognitive screening instruments have been developed to aid in the assessment of mental status in clinical settings. One of the most common screening instruments, "The Mini-Mental State Examination," evaluates cognitive functions by administering and scoring a set of 11 questions (see Display 9-1). The

(continued)

DISPLAY 9.1

Mini-Mental State Examination

Patient _____ Examiner _____ Date _____

Maximum
Score   *Score*

ORIENTATION

5   ( )   What is the (year) (season) (date) (day) (month)?
5   ( )   Where are we: (state) (county) (town) (hospital) (floor).

REGISTRATION

3   ( )   Name 3 objects: 1 second to say each. Then ask the patient all 3 after you have said them.
                           Give 1 point for each correct answer. Then repeat them until he learns all 3.
                           Count trials and record.

                                                                                       Trials _____

ATTENTION AND CALCULATION

5   ( )   Serial 7's. 1 point for each correct. Stop after 5 answers. Alternatively spell "world" backwards.

RECALL

3   ( )   Ask for the 3 objects repeated above. Give 1 point for each correct.

LANGUAGE

9   ( )   Name a pencil, and watch (2 points)
                           Repeat the following "No ifs, ands, or buts." (1 point)
                           Follow a 3-stage command:
                              "Take a paper in your right hand, fold it in half, and put it on the floor." (3 points)
                           Read and obey the following:
                           Close your eyes (1 point)
                           Write a sentence (1 point)
                           Copy design (1 point)
_____   Total Score
                           ASSESS level of consciousness along a continuum _____

                                                             Alert   Drowsy   Stupor   Coma

                                                                                       (continued)

Pattern Assessment   Cognition and Perception Assessment Guidelines (continued)

maximum score possible on this test is 30. Scores that are 27 or higher are considered normal. The examination is easy to conduct and can be completed in approximately 10 minutes. This instrument is useful for the initial as well as serial evaluations of mental status. Serial evaluations enable the examiner to make judgments about improvement or deterioration of mental status. The Mini-Mental State Examination is designed to measure cognitive functions but not moods or thought processes. It is considered a good tool for identifying dementia or delirium states.

ASSESSMENT AIDS

• Interview Guide to suggest questions and record data (Display 9-2)
• Screening tools (see Display 9-1)
• Institution-specific forms for recording data

DISPLAY 9.1

Mini-Mental State Examination (continued)

INSTRUCTIONS FOR ADMINISTRATION OF MINI-MENTAL STATE EXAMINATION

Orientation

(1) Ask for the date. Then ask specifically for parts omitted, e.g., "Can you also tell me what season it is?" One point for each correct.

(2) Ask in turn, "Can you tell me the name of this hospital?" (town, country, etc.). One point for each correct.

Registration

Ask the patient if you may test his memory. Then say the names of three unrelated objects, clearly and slowly, about 1 second for each. After you have said all three, ask him to repeat them. This first repetition determines his score (0–3), but keep saying them until he can repeat all three up to six trials. If he does not eventually learn all three, recall cannot be meaningfully tested.

Attention and Calculation

Ask the patient to begin with 100 and count backwards by 7. Stop after 5 subtractions (93, 86, 79, 72, 65). Score the total number of correct answers.

If the patient cannot or will not perform this task, ask him to spell the word "world" backwards. The score is the number of letters in correct order. *e.g.,* dlrow = 5, dlorw = 3.

Recall

Ask the patient if he can recall the three words you previously asked him to remember. Score 0–3.

Language

Naming: Show the patient a wrist watch and ask him what it is. Repeat for pencil. Score 0–2.

Repetition: Ask the patient to repeat the sentence after you. Allow only one trial. Score 0 or 1.

3-Stage command: Give the patient a piece of plain blank paper and repeat the command. Score 1 point for each part correctly executed.

Reading: On a blank piece of paper, print the sentence "Close your eyes," in letters large enough for the patient to see clearly. Ask him to read it and do what it says. Score 1 point only if he actually closes his eyes.

Writing: Give the patient a blank piece of paper and ask him to write a sentence for you. Do not dictate a sentence; it is to be written spontaneously. It must contain a subject and verb and be sensible. Correct grammar and punctuation are not necessary.

Copying: On a clean piece of paper, draw intersecting pentagons, each side about 1 in., and ask him to copy it exactly as it is. All 10 angles must be present, and 2 must intersect to score 1 point. Tremor and rotation are ignored.

Estimate the patient's level of sensorium along a continuum, from alert on the left to coma on the right.

(From Folstein, M.F., Folstein, S.E., & McHugh, P.R. [1975]. Mini-mental state. *Journal of Psychiatric Research, 12,* 189–198. Reprinted with permission.)

DISPLAY 9.2

Interview Guide: Cognition and Perception

COGNITIVE AND PERCEPTUAL PATTERN

Mental Status

❏ Alert ❏ Unresponsive ❏ Lethargic ❏ Restless ❏ Combative
❏ Oriented × _____
Confusion: ❏ None ❏ Intermittent ❏ Nighttime ❏ Total

Vision

❏ Normal ❏ Impaired Explain:_____
Last eye examination: _____ Last glaucoma testing _____
❏ Eyeglasses ❏ Contact lenses ❏ Prosthesis ❏ Cataracts ❏ Blind spots ❏ Diplopia ❏ Eye infections
❏ Eye itching ❏ Photophobia ❏ Redness ❏ Pain ❏ Visual blurring ❏ Eyestrain ❏ Headaches

Hearing

❏ Normal ❏ Impaired Explain:_____
Hearing aid(s) ❏ No ❏ Yes ❏ Left ❏ Right
Last hearing examination: _____
Ear hygiene practices: _____
❏ Ear infections ❏ "Swimmer's" ear ❏ Ear ringing, buzzing ❏ Ear pain/fullness ❏ Tinnitus

Speech

❏ Normal ❏ Slurred ❏ Garbled ❏ Expressive Aphasia
Language barrier ❏ No ❏ Yes

Taste, Smell, Touch

Any problems with taste, smell, touch: ❏ No ❏ Yes Explain:_____
_____

Teaching and Learning

Learning needs: ❏ No ❏ Yes Explain: _____
Barriers to learning: ❏ None ❏ Communication ❏ Language ❏ Physical factors ❏ Motivation ❏ Anxiety
❏ Depression ❏ Cognitive impairment
Preferred method of learning: ❏ Written materials ❏ Video ❏ Demonstration and discussion

Pain/Discomfort

❏ None ❏ Acute ❏ Chronic
Description _____
Aggravating/relieving factors:_____
Pain management: _____
Personal definition of adequate pain control: _____

Medical History

Conditions related to problems with cognition and perception: ❏ No ❏ Yes
Explain/list:_____

Medication History

Medications influencing cognition and/or perception: ❏ No ❏ Yes
Explain/list:_____

▼ ▼ ▼
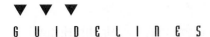
G U I D E L I N E S

Procedure	Clinical Significance

1. Mental status

Screen mental status by observing the person's level of consciousness, speech quality, orientation, and thought processes.

Often, you can form an initial judgment about mental status based on your general observations during the interview. If your initial observations indicate alterations in mental status, then you may want to ask more direct questions such as the questions presented below that elicit data about orientation.

Observe orientation to time, place, and person by noting responses to the following questions:

- (Time) Do you know today's date (day of week, year, season)?
- (Place) Where do you live? Where are we now? What city/state is this?
- (Person) What is your name? My name?

Evaluate thought processes as you interview the person. Listen to the person's responses to your questions and determine whether his or her ideas and thoughts make sense.

If normal findings are not observed, conduct a thorough assessment of mental status (See next section).

Normal Findings (Level of Consciousness)
The person is awake, alert, and aware of stimuli in the environment.

Normal Findings (speech)
The person can clearly articulate words and conduct an appropriate conversation.

Normal Findings (orientation)
The person demonstrates appropriate understanding of time, place, and person.

Normal Findings (thought processes)
The person demonstrates responses to questions that are appropriate to the context and conversation.

2. Special senses evaluation (vision, hearing, taste, smell, and touch)

Note: To evaluate the status of the special senses, ask questions that focus on the functional status of the eyes and ears, the ability to taste, smell, and touch, and any problems the person identifies with the sensory organs.

If sensory deficits are identified, evaluate the person's specific responses or adaptations to the deficits. For example, a problem with vision should lead you to ask about self-care abilities and the potential for injury; problems with hearing should prompt questions about the person's ability to communicate and interact with others; problems with positions sense and tactile abilities should prompt questions about measures taken to prevent injury; and problems with taste and smell should initiate discussion of any effects on nutritional status.

Eyes and Vision

Inquire about vision and any visual or eye changes.

- "Have you experienced any recent changes in your vision?"

A sudden loss of vision may be an emergency, and the person should be referred immediately to a physician. A gradual loss of vision may be related to aging, diabetes, or hypertension.

- "Do you see any spots (floaters) in front of your eyes?"

Floaters may be common in persons older than 40 years of age or nearsighted persons. They usually require no additional follow-up.

- "Do you have any blind spots?"

Scotoma: A blind spot in the visual field. Possible causes include glaucoma, pressure on the optic nerve, increased intracranial pressure, or retinal detachment. Refer to a physician.

- "Do you have any difficulties seeing at night?"

Night blindness is associated with optic atrophy, glaucoma, and vitamin A deficiency.

▼ ▼ ▼

Procedure

- "Do you experience double vision (diplopia)?"
- "Do you see halos or rainbows around objects?"
- "Do you have any discharge from the eyes?"
- "Do you have any eye pain?"

Ask about eye examination and self-care practices:

- "Have you ever had your vision tested? If so, when was your last eye exam?"
- "Do you wear glasses/contact lenses? How do they work for you?"
- "How do you care for contact lenses? How long do you wear them? What type of cleaning system do you use?"

- "Are you exposed to potential hazards that may affect your eyes?
- If so, do you wear protective goggles?"
- "Have you ever had a screening test for glaucoma? If so, when was your last screening examination?"

Ask about pathologic conditions that may affect the eyes and vision:

- "Do you have any history of injury or surgery to the eye(s)?"
- "Do you have a history of cataracts or glaucoma?"

Ask about the effects of any vision losses on ability to perform usual activities or work.

- "How has your loss of vision affected your ability to take care of yourself? To work?"

Ears and Hearing

Ask about hearing acuity and any hearing problems.

- "Do you have any trouble hearing?" If yes, describe onset—gradual or sudden; character—loss of all hearing or loss of ability to hear certain sounds.

- "Is there a family history of hearing loss?"

Clinical Significance

Diplopia is associated with increased intracranial pressure.

Halos are associated with narrow-angle glaucoma.

Discharge from the eyes indicates an infection.

Itching or burning: Associated with allergies, superficial irritation.

Stabbing or deep, aching pain: May indicate the presence of a foreign body.

Vision testing is a health promotion practice and an effective way to screen for vision impairments. A thorough eye and vision examination is recommended every 2 years (more often if problems are identified).

People who wear eyeglasses may be in need of a change in their current prescription, especially if they report eyestrain and frontal headaches after prolonged reading or other visual activities. Improper cleaning of contract lenses can lead to infection and irritation.

Industrial accidents can cause injury to the eye but are often preventable by protective eyewear.

Glaucoma is an eye disease characterized by increased intraocular pressure. Bifrontal headaches in a person older than age 40 years may be a symptom of glaucoma. The person should be referred for additional screening and testing.

Chronic illnesses associated with visual impairments include hypertension and diabetes.

Visual impairment may affect the person's ability to perform usual activities of daily living, the ability to drive, or work performance. The person may not be able to read patient education materials, medication instructions, or fill insulin syringes. Abilities to cook and maintain personal hygiene may be affected.

A person with a hearing problem may hesitate to disclose this problem. Look for other cues. For example, speaking with a distorted tone of voice, lip reading, paying special attention to gestures, listening with the head turned to one side, leaning toward the interviewer, or displaying a strained facial expression while listening to the interviewer speak.

Sudden Onset of Hearing Loss

Associated with trauma or upper respiratory infection.

Presbycusis: A gradual hearing loss, usually after age 50 years, associated with aging.

Hearing loss may be hereditary (heredity may play a role in up to one third of persons with hearing loss).

▼ ▼ ▼

Procedure

- "Have you had any treatments for your hearing loss— hearing aid or other device? Is it helping?"

- "How has your hearing loss affected your daily life?"

Ask about ear examinations and self-care practices.
- "Have you ever had an audiogram (hearing test)?" If yes, why was this test done; results; testing facility?
- "Do you use a hearing aid?" If yes, does it help; when was last hearing aid examination; how do you care for it?
- "How do you clean your ears?"

Determine if the person has any other ear problems.
- "Do you have earaches or other types of ear pain?" If yes, where do you feel it; describe onset; quality; does the pain increase with talking or chewing?
- "Have you had any ear infections?" If yes, describe age of onset; frequency of infections; treatment.
- "Have you experienced any ear drainage?" If yes, describe color, odor, and relationship to ear pain.

- "Do you ever notice ringing or buzzing in your ears?"

- "Do you ever feel like you or the room is spinning?"

Review the person's medication history for the use of drugs that are potentially ototoxic.

Taste and Smell
Inquire about alterations in taste and smell, which often occur together.
"Have you noticed any changes in your sense of taste or smell?"

Touch
Assess tactile sensation by asking questions about temperature discriminations and unusual skin sensations.
- "Do you have any problems distinguishing temperature changes by touch?"
- "Do you experience any unusual skin sensations, such as tingling, burning, or crawling?"

Clinical Significance

Some people have had poor results with hearing aids and refuse to wear one. The use of a hearing aid may be rejected because of a negative self-image.

Hearing loss may affect a person's ability to work, interact with others, and pursue leisure activities. The person with a hearing loss may become withdrawn, apathetic, and even paranoid.

Recommendations for referral and follow-up can be made according to a person's risk factors. Annual hearing examinations are recommended for people exposed to excessive noise.

Use of sharp instruments in the ears may cause damage; the use of cotton-tipped applicators to cleanse the ears may impact cerumen and result in hearing loss.

Ear pain can be related to disease of the ear or it may be referred pain resulting from a problem with the teeth or oropharynx.

A history of chronic ear infections may be associated with hearing problems.

Otorrhea or ear drainage usually indicates an infection. Purulent, bloody drainage indicates an infection of the external ear (external otitis). Purulent drainage associated with ear pain and a popping sensation indicates eardrum perforation.

Tinnitus is a buzzing, roaring, or ringing sensation in the ear and may indicate an inner ear disorder.

Vertigo is a sensation of rotary movement and may indicate an inner ear disorder.

Common Ototoxic Medications: Antibiotics such as streptomycin, gentamycin, vancomycin; diuretics such as ethacrynic acid and furosemide; aspirin; quinine.

Possible explanations for decreased ability to smell include the common cold, use of tobacco, and a pathologic condition of the frontal lobe of the brain, or in the olfactory bulb tract. Possible explanations for a decreased ability to taste include the common cold and lesions to cranial nerve VII (facial).

People with peripheral neuropathies, such as those associated with diabetes mellitus, may lose the ability to discriminate temperature, which places them at risk for burns, especially from hot water.

Paresthesia: An abnormal skin sensation such as burning, tingling, or "crawling," intense enough to cause considerable discomfort. Associated with nerve damage secondary to diabetes mellitus or demyelinating diseases such as multiple sclerosis.

▼ ▼ ▼

Procedure

- "Do you experience any facial pain or unusual skin sensations over the face? If yes, are painful episodes aggravated by cold or touch?"

3. Teaching and learning evaluation

Determine basic health education learning needs in relation to the following areas:
- Knowledge of condition (if applicable)
- Medications
- Diet
- Activity
- Personal care
- Use of medical equipment

Determine whether there are any barriers to learning, including language barriers, hearing or vision barriers, emotional issues, or problems with motivation or cognitive impairment.

Determine the person's preferred method of learning—written materials, video, demonstration and discussion, or combination of methods.

4. Medical history

Review the person's medical history to identify pathologic conditions that may be associated with cognitive or perceptual dysfunction.

Symptom History

Determine whether the person is experiencing symptoms of neurologic dysfunction.

Interview Questions

- "Do you experience unusual weakness or problems moving body parts?" If yes, describe onset, duration, location, characteristics, and precipitating activities.

- "Have you noticed numbness or tingling in any body part?" If yes, describe location, associated activities, onset, duration, quality—*e.g.*, "pins and needles."

- "Do you have problems with unusually frequent or severe headaches?" If yes, describe onset, how often, where in your head do you feel them, associated activities/events.

- "Do you ever feel dizzy or lightheaded? Have you ever fainted or lost consciousness during an episode of dizziness? Did the dizziness occur with a change in activity or position?"

Clinical Significance

Trigeminal neuralgia: A disease of cranial nerve V (trigeminal) characterized by attacks of severe pain along the trigeminal nerve branches. Pain may be triggered by touch, cold, and chewing.

The identification of specific health education learning needs also may be identified when assessing other functional health patterns. Many health education needs are addressed when assessing the health perception and health management pattern. Learning needs related to diet might be identified during the assessment of the nutritional and metabolic pattern. The categories listed here represent generic health education subject matter. The identification of specific learning needs is only one of several important aspects of teaching and learning evaluation. In addition, the nurse should determine how the person learns and any barriers to an effective learning process.

Learning barriers interfere with the person's ability to receive information.

The person's preferred style of learning will influence the nurse's choice of educational materials.

Indicators of Neurologic Dysfunction: Weakness, numbness, headaches, dizziness, vertigo, loss of consciousness, seizures, lack of coordination or balance, gait problems, falling.

Unilateral (one-sided) weakness or paralysis may be observed with a stroke, compression of the spinal cord, or nerve injury.

Numbness or tingling may accompany pathologic conditions of the brain, spinal cord, or peripheral nerves.

Paresthesia: An abnormal burning or tingling sensation.

Headaches have multiple patterns and causes. Headaches associated with central nervous system pathologic conditions, for example, the earliest stages of a brain tumor, may be noted in the morning and subside after the person has been awake for several hours.

Dizziness accompanied by a loss of consciousness can be due to a lack of cerebral blood flow. If the person has severe atherosclerosis of the carotid arteries, simply turning the head from side to side may obstruct blood flow enough to result in dizziness.

▼ ▼ ▼
G U I D E L I N E S *continued* Cognition and Perception Interview (Health History)

Procedure

- "Do you experience vertigo (sensation of rotary movement)?"

Note: Distinguish true vertigo from dizziness.

- "Have you ever experienced a seizure?" If yes, describe onset, precipitating factors, history of previous seizures, use of anticonvulsant medication, presence of pre-seizure aura.

Medical History

Determine whether the person has a medical history that may affect neurologic function, mental status, or sensory–perceptual functions.

Interview Questions

- "Have you ever had any type of head injury?" If yes, describe when and how it happened, treatment, effects.

- "Have you ever had a stroke, meningitis, or spinal cord injury?"

Other Conditions that May Affect Cognition and Perception

  Altered fluid and electrolyte balance
  Hypoxic states
  Immobility, especially in the presence of sensory overload or sensory deprivation

5. **Medication history**

Determine whether the person is taking any medications or other substances that may affect cognition and perception by taking a medication history. (Note: If the person is unconscious, you can interview others, examine pill containers and medical records, or review toxicology evaluation of blood or urine.)

A medication history may be obtained at some other point in the sequence of the overall health assessment. The medication history should always be analyzed for implications related to cognition and perception.

Medications That May Cause Mental Status Changes at Toxic Levels

Alcohol	Lithium
Antiarrhythmics	Monoamine oxidase
Aspirin	(MAO) inhibitors
Barbiturates	Muscle relaxants
Beta-adrenergic blockers	Narcotics
Calcium channel blockers	Tricyclic antidepressants
Digoxin	

Clinical Significance

Syncope: A sudden, temporary loss of consciousness.

Vertigo is a sensation of rotational spinning associated with neurologic pathologic conditions or inner ear pathologic conditions.

Seizures may occur because of metabolic disorders, high fever, or epilepsy.

Aura: A subjective sensation that precedes a seizure. An aura can be auditory, visual, or a motor sensation.

Head injuries may result in long-term neurologic deficits or changes in mental status.

These conditions may result in long-term neurologic changes and affect cognition and perception functions.

A medication history is especially important when evaluating certain alterations in cognition and perception, such as the following:

- Acute mental status changes. Medication abuse or overdose should always be considered in the initial evaluation of an unconscious person.

- Drug toxicity affecting the special senses (*e.g.*, certain antibiotic toxicities may affect hearing).

▼ ▼ ▼

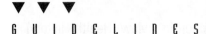

Procedure

Conduct a complete examination of mental status if the person demonstrates mental status changes. If you need to assess the level of consciousness frequently (*e.g.*, more often than every 2 hours), use the Glasgow Coma Scale to help make your assessment more consistent and objective.

1. **Level of consciousness**

   Level of consciousness is evaluated by observing a person's arousability, ability to speak and follow verbal commands, and motor abilities.

   a. Determine the intensity of stimuli necessary to arouse the person.

   If the person is observed to be fully awake, no further testing is necessary.

   If the person appears asleep or unconscious, attempt arousal by applying progressively more intensive stimuli: calling the person by name, touching or gently shaking the person, applying painful stimuli.

   If it becomes necessary to subject the person to painful stimuli, the stimulus should be removed as soon as a response is noted. The following methods may be used:

   Apply pressure to the trapezius muscle by grasping the belly of the muscle between thumb and forefingers and squeezing.

   Apply pressure to the Achilles tendon by grasping the tendon between thumb and forefingers and squeezing.

   Apply pressure to the nail beds by squeezing the nail beds between your thumb and forefinger. Some examiners prefer to place a pen or pencil over the nail plate and squeeze the nail bed between the pen and forefinger.

Clinical Significance

Complete Mental Status Evaluation

- Level of consciousness
- Awareness
- Thought processes
- Communication abilities

Level of consciousness may be quantified in relation to the intensity of the sensory stimuli required to arouse a person.

Avoid unnecessary exposure to painful stimuli by first trying to arouse the person through verbal stimuli.

Certain methods for applying painful stimuli should be avoided, such as vigorously rubbing the knuckles into the sternum ("sternal rub") and pinching the skin. Not only are these methods unnecessarily cruel, they also result in greater tissue damage and bruising.

Normal Findings

Fully Awake: Highest level of consciousness, characterized by the ability to respond to all types of sensory stimuli of minimal intensity. However, a person may be fully awake but still disoriented or forgetful.

Alert: Level of consciousness in which a person is fully awake and oriented as to person, place, time, and environment. Additionally, the person is capable of responding to verbal commands.

Deviations from Normal

Lethargic: Person appears drowsy or asleep most of the time but is capable of making spontaneous movements. It is possible to arouse the person, but gentle shaking of the person is usually required in addition to saying his or her name. Lethargic people tend to fall back to sleep easily and may become disoriented.

Mental Status Evaluation

Procedure

Clinical Significance

Obtunded: The person sleeps most of the time and makes few spontaneous body movements. More vigorous stimulation such as shouting or shaking is needed to arouse the person. The person is still capable of making verbal responses, but is less likely to respond appropriately to verbal commands.

Stuporous (Semicomatose): The person is unconscious most of the time and does not exhibit spontaneous motor activity. Strong, noxious stimuli such as pain are needed to elicit a motor response, which is usually a purposeful attempt to remove the stimuli. Verbal responses are limited or absent. A semicomatose person is rarely oriented or fully awake, even when the examiner is testing responses to sensory stimulation.

Comatose: The person cannot be aroused, even by applying painful stimuli. Some reflex responses to stimuli may be noted, such as the gag reflex. If no reflex responses occur, the person is in a deep coma.

b. Determine motor responses to verbal, or painful stimuli.

A decline in the level of consciousness is associated with a progressive decline in the ability to purposefully respond to a stimulus.

Ask the person to complete a simple task and note response. If the person does not respond to verbal stimuli, apply painful stimuli and observe the motor response.

Normal Findings

Ability to obey verbal commands: The person can move the extremities when asked or perform some other requested task such as squeezing and letting go of your fingers.

Deviations from Normal

Ability to localize or make purposeful movements: The person can withdraw from or attempt to locate and stop a painful stimulus. Any such attempt, whether successful or not, should be classified as purposeful movements.

Semipurposeful response: The person grimaces or briefly flexes the extremities in response to a painful stimulus, but makes no attempt to remove the stimulus.

Flexor or decorticate posturing response: Flexion and adduction of the upper extremities with extension, internal rotation, and plantar flexion in the lower extremities. Decorticate posturing may occur in response to painful stimuli or may be spontaneous.

Decorticate posturing is associated with damage to the internal capsule of the brain or pyramidal tracts above the brainstem.

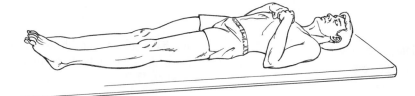

Flexor of decorticate posturing response

▼ ▼ ▼

G U I D E L I N E S *continued*   Mental Status Evaluation

Procedure

Clinical Significance

Extensor or decerebrate posturing: Rigid extension and adduction of one or both arms, and extension of the legs. Decerebrate posturing may occur in response to painful stimuli or may be spontaneous.

Decerebrate posturing is associated with little or no activity above the brainstem level and is a poorer prognostic sign than decorticate posturing.

Flaccid response: No motor response to painful stimuli and a weak or lax appearance of the extremities.

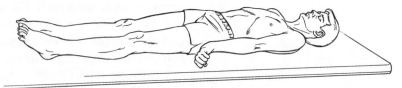

Extensor or decerebrate posturing

Glasgow Coma Scale

Assign a numerical value to level of consciousness by using the Glasgow Coma Scale.

Three behavioral responses are evaluated—eye opening, verbal response, and motor response. The final score is determined by assigning a numerical value to the level of response to individual criteria in each of the three categories and adding these figures to produce a coma score that can have a maximum of 15 points.

The Glasgow Coma Scale is scored in the following manner:

1. Best eye opening response

   Eyes open spontaneously—Score 4

   Eyes open to voice—Score 3

   Eyes open to pain—Score 2

   No eye opening—Score 1

2. Best motor response

   Obeying commands—Score 6

   Localizing to pain—Score 5

   Withdrawing to pain—Score 4

   Flexion to pain—Score 3

   Extension to pain—Score 2

   No response—Score 1

3. Best verbal response

   Oriented to time, person, place—Score 5

   Confused conversation—Score 4

   Inappropriate words—Score 3

   Incomprehensible sounds—Score 2

   None—Score 1

The Glasgow Coma Scale is used to assign a score to level of consciousness. It is used to monitor trends when performing serial assessments of level of consciousness. A decreasing score is associated with neurologic deterioration.

Neurological assessment chart

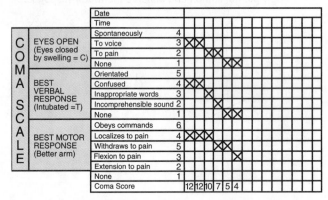

COMA SCALE				
	Date			
	Time			
EYES OPEN (Eyes closed by swelling = C)	Spontaneously	4		
	To voice	3		
	To pain	2		
	None	1		
BEST VERBAL RESPONSE (Intubated =T)	Orientated	5		
	Confused	4		
	Inappropriate words	3		
	Incomprehensible sound	2		
	None	1		
BEST MOTOR RESPONSE (Better arm)	Obeys commands	6		
	Localizes to pain	4		
	Withdraws to pain	5		
	Flexion to pain	3		
	Extension to pain	2		
	None	1		
	Coma Score		12 12 10 7 5 4	

Glasgow Coma Scale documentation

Note: if the person is unable to respond owing to the presence of an endotracheal tube, this is recorded on the record using the letter, "T."

▼ ▼ ▼

G U I D E L I N E S   *continued*   Mental Status Evaluation

___

Procedure

2. Awareness

a. Determine orientation to person, place, and time.

Note responses to the following questions to evaluate *temporal (time) orientation:*

- What is the date (day, month, year)?
- What day of the week is this?
- What time of day is this (morning, afternoon, evening)?
- What was the last meal that you ate (breakfast, lunch, dinner)?
- What season is this?
- What was the last holiday?

Note responses to the following questions to evaluate *locus (place) orientation:*

- Where are you now?
- What is the name of this building?
- What is the name of this city?
- What state is this?

Note responses to the following questions to evaluate *person (personal) orientation:*

- What is your name?
- Who was just here to visit you?
- Who is this? (Indicate visitors or family members who are present)
- What do you do for a living?
- How old are you?
- Where do you live?
- What is your wife's (husband's) name?

b. Evaluate for the occurrence of one-sided neglect.

Observe the person performing daily activities.

Ask the person to read a page-width newspaper headline.

Ask the person to draw a self-portrait or the face of a clock.

Place several small, common objects on a table in front of the person. Ask the person to name the objects.

Observe the person's pattern of ambulation.

Clinical Significance

Deviations from Normal

When awareness is impaired, a person usually loses time orientation first, followed by place orientation, and then person orientation. However, exceptions to this pattern may be noted.

People in unfamiliar environments, without time cues such as clocks, calendars, television, or newspapers, may lose track of time. The last four questions in this list may be a more appropriate means of evaluating such people.

Consider whether the person has been moved several times (*e.g.,* having been transferred through different hospital departments and nursing units). In such cases, the person may have difficulty naming the present or previous location.

Determine personal identity (name) and other personal data, including roles and lifestyle. Asking the person to name various health care providers may be an unreliable technique, especially if the patient has been in contact with many different people in one day, as occurs in acute care settings.

This type of evaluation is indicated for persons who appear to ignore sensory messages from the left side of the body.

Deviations from Normal

Ignoring one side when bathing, combing the hair, shaving, dressing, or eating is a sign of one-sided neglect.

A person with one-sided neglect may omit words from the left side of the page.

The left side of the drawing is incomplete or missing altogether with one-sided neglect.

One-sided neglect is associated with failure to name objects on the left side of the table.

Persons with one-sided neglect often bump into things on the affected side.

▼ ▼ ▼

Procedure	Clinical Significance

3. Thought processes

a. Evaluate abstract thinking or classification.

Test lower-level abilities for abstract thinking by asking the person to classify common objects according to use. For example, spread the following objects on a table: pen, pencil, comb, brush, hairpin, spoon, napkin, and salt shaker. Then ask the person which things go together. Demonstrate by picking up the pen and pencil and explaining that both objects are used for writing.

Another test for lower-level abilities is asking the person to sort a deck of cards according to suit.

Test higher levels of abstract thinking by asking the person to interpret proverbs.

Example: Ask the person what is meant by the expression, "The early bird catches the worm."

Ask the person to describe similarities and differences between objects, such as a tree and a flower.

b. Evaluate the ability to solve problems and concentrate.

Problem solving: Ask the person to perform an arithmetic calculation. For example, ask how many lemons can be purchased for $4 if lemons are priced at 5 for $1.

Concentration: Test concentration by asking the person to count backward from 100 by 7's (the serial 7's test). Alternatively, ask the person to count to 20 by odd numbers only.

c. Evaluate memory.

Test *immediate memory,* Ask the person to remember three numbers, such as 7, 0 and 4. Then, 1 or 2 minutes later, ask the person to recite the numbers.

If the person has difficulty with this task, offer a simpler test of immediate memory or retention. Give the person a set of instructions and observe the response. For example, ask the person to pick up a pencil with the right hand and place it in the left hand.

If the person cannot retain all the parts of this instruction, then simplify again, and ask the person just to pick up the pencil in the right hand.

Clinical Significance (column):

Abstract thinking is the ability to interpret concepts and ideas and enables a person to understand unfamiliar situations. The ability to interpret proverbs, engage in creative conversation, and understand a joke as humorous all require a capacity for abstract thinking.

Choose proverbs that are appropriate to the person's cultural background and educational level.

A response such as "birds eat early in the morning" is considered concrete, whereas the ability to think abstractly is demonstrated by a reply suggesting that people who pursue things in a timely or aggressive manner are more likely to be rewarded for their efforts.

Choose problems that are appropriate for the person's educational level.

Memory is the ability to store thoughts and learned experiences and retrieve previously learned information.

Tests of immediate memory or recall indicate whether a person can register information in the memory cortex. Ability to respond successfully to tests of immediate memory indicates that immediate recall is intact and that the person understands your message. This rules out other problems, such as receptive aphasia and apraxia, which might interfere with the person's ability to make appropriate responses.

Procedure

Test *recent memory.* Ask the person what he or she had for breakfast or if anyone came to visit that day.

Test *distant memory.* Ask the person general questions about the remote past, such as year of birth, types of surgery he or she has had, or where he or she grew up. Verify the person's answers with a family member or the health record.

Ask general questions about the remote past that involve general knowledge. For example, ask the person to name the American president who was assassinated in the early 1960s, or what two countries America fought against in World War II.

Test for *confabulation.*

d. Evaluate judgment.

Observe the person and note whether he or she makes appropriate use of surroundings. For example, check whether the patient knows how to call for assistance with the bedside call light, or whether the person's attire is appropriate for the current weather conditions.

To assess judgment further, ask questions about hypothetical situations. For example, ask the person what he or she would do after noticing that smoke was coming from a trash can.

4. **Communication abilities**

a. Evaluate comprehension.

Ability to hear: Determine whether there is any indication that the person is hearing impaired.

Ability to answer simple questions appropriately: Determine whether the person understands you by asking simple, open-ended questions such as the person's name, age, or address.

Ability to answer yes/no questions appropriately: Continue with closed-ended questions, including some that are not reality-based, such as whether the person has a bird on his or her head.

Clinical Significance

Tests of recent memory indicate whether a person has the ability to recall new information a short time after it is presented.

Deviations from Normal

Recent memory loss is called *anterograde amnesia.* The person may register information (as manifested by repeating phrases) but forgets new information within minutes and does not remember recent events. Ultimately, the person becomes confused. Recent memory must be intact for the person to benefit from teaching efforts.

A person with recent memory loss, however, may have clear recall of temporally distant events.

Deviations from Normal

Retrograde amnesia is characterized by the ability to recall events only from the very distant past, such as childhood. In such cases, the person may live in reference to the distant past as though the recent past has not occurred.

Responses to general questions may be unreliable if the person regards the subject of the questions to be irrelevant to their concerns, or if the person's educational or cultural background is such that they would not have the information needed to answer correctly.

Deviations from Normal

Confabulation is the attempt to compensate for memory loss by using fictional information. In other words, the person may make up answers to questions and may even admit to this practice.

Judgment is the ability to contemplate facts and ideas, and arrive at appropriate decisions or opinions.

Deviations from Normal

Receptive aphasia (Wernicke's aphasia, sensory aphasia) is characterized by impaired comprehension abilities.

Receptive aphasias may occur in varying degrees. In the mildest case, the person may have difficulty naming only certain objects.

▼ ▼ ▼

G U I D E L I N E S *continued*   Mental Status Evaluation

Procedure

Ability to follow simple directions: Ask the person to respond to simple commands such as nodding the head or pointing to the door.

Ability to comprehend but unable to make a verbal reply: Name an object and ask the person to point it.

b. Evaluate verbal expressive abilities.

Ability to speak fluently: Observe the person's speech for use of complete sentences or phrases. Note any slurring of words or facial drooping.

Repetition ability: Observe the ease with which the person repeats words and phrases when instructed to do so. Note whether word substitutions occur with this task.

Naming ability: Point to specific objects, and ask the person to name them.

c. Evaluate written expressive abilities.

Simple writing tasks: Ask the person to write his or her name and address.

Complex writing tasks: Ask the person to write a short paragraph. For example, ask the person to write about what he or she watched on television or what was served for lunch.

d. Evaluate nonverbal communication abilities.

Note the appropriate use of gestures.

Note the range of emotions shown in overall demeanor, facial expression, tone of voice.

Observe for *flat affect* (no signs of emotions).

Observe for *labile affect* (extreme fluctuations of moods or emotions).

Clinical Significance

Deviations from Normal

An inability to follow commands is characteristic of *apraxia* as well as of receptive aphasia. Apraxia is the inability to perform certain motor movements even though paralysis, weakness, or loss of coordination are not evident.

The ability to comprehend in the absence of verbal abilities is evidenced in expressive aphasia.

Deviations from Normal

Expressive aphasia (Broca's motor aphasia, nonfluent aphasia) is characterized by impaired speaking abilities. The speech may be nonfluent or telegraphic, or there may be a paucity of speech. The person may speak in a child-like manner, using only nouns and verbs, for example, "Me hurt," or "Get nurse." The person may struggle to form words, and may hesitate to produce sounds. *Telegraphic speech patterns* are characterized by short, choppy messages. There may be *perseveration*, which is the tendency to repeat words or sounds; for example, "when, when, when."

Deviations from Normal

Repetition ability is poor with expressive aphasias because the person must struggle to form words.

Repetition ability is also poor with receptive aphasias because of *paraphasia errors,* for example, *pink* substituted for *sink,* and use of jargon.

Deviations from Normal

Naming ability may be impaired with both expressive and receptive aphasias.

Deviations from Normal

Writing abilities are poor with expressive aphasias. There is a paucity of written output that parallels speaking ability.

Deviations from Normal

Writing abilities are also poor with receptive aphasias, parallel with speaking ability. The person may be able to write, but the writing will lack meaning.

▼ ▼ ▼

G U I D E L I N E S

Procedure

For persons with acute changes in mental status, a licensed independent practitioner (*e.g.,* physician; nurse practitioner) may request additional diagnostic tests to rule out many processes that should be considered in the differential diagnosis of acute mental status changes.

1. **Laboratory tests**

   Laboratory tests for the initial evaluation of acute mental status changes:
   - Complete blood count (CBC)
   - Serum electrolytes
   - Blood glucose
   - Liver function studies
   - Renal function studies
   - Serum alcohol; blood and urine toxicology screening

2. **Imaging studies**

   A noncontrast CT scan of the brain may be ordered to further evaluate acute mental status changes.

3. **Lumbar puncture**

   A lumbar puncture may be performed if the person has a change in mental status accompanied by fever and meningeal signs (headache, nausea, stiff neck).

Clinical Significance

Acute mental status changes may result from metabolic changes (fluid and electrolyte imbalances; hypoglycemia or hyperglycemia); major organ dysfunctions (liver failure; renal failure); or acute infectious processes. Laboratory results are helpful in the differential diagnosis of mental status changes.

A brain scan can be used to rule out any structural explanations for changes in level of consciousness, including hematomas, brain abscesses, or tumors. A negative result suggests a metabolic abnormality.

A lumbar puncture is ordered to rule out meningitis or subarachnoid hemorrhage as an explanation for altered mental status.

▼ ▼ ▼

G U I D E L I N E S

Procedure

Integrate physical examination findings during the assessment of cognition and perception, with special attention to the following:
- General appearance and environmental surroundings
- The neurologic system
- Sensory organs and systems

(Note: Complete examination guidelines are presented elsewhere in this chapter for mental status, cranial nerves, reflexes, motor system, sensory system, eyes and ears).

Clinical Significance

The primary goals of the physical examination in relation to cognition and perception are to determine the status of the neurologic system and to evaluate sensory organs and related functions. Physical examination findings may help explain cognitive and perceptual dysfunctions. Additionally, the physical examination may reveal secondary problems. For example, you may detect signs of physical injury, such as bruises from bumping into furniture, secondary to visual sensory deficits.

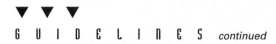

Interpreting Physical Examination Findings Related to Cognition and Perception

Procedure	Clinical Significance
1. General appearance and environmental surroundings Observe the person's general appearance and note whether there are indicators of cognitive or sensory-perceptual problems.	
Note the person's facial expression, especially general affect, level of attentiveness, and symmetry of facial features. When evaluating attentiveness, note whether the person is attentive to various stimuli—do they focus on demonstration activities during patient education; do they startle at loud, unexpected noises; do they listen when you speak?	A flat affect may be associated with apathy or depression that may be a factor influencing cognitive and perceptual functions.
Observe the condition of the skin and grooming practices. Note any skin injuries or burn scars.	Skin injuries may be the result of impaired tactile sensation, poor judgment, or other forms of sensory impairment.
Note whether grooming appears to be neglected on one side of the body.	*One-Sided Neglect:* One-sided neglect is a perceptual dysfunction manifested by the neglect of grooming on one side of the body.
Observe the person's environmental surroundings. Make note of the quality of the sensory stimuli in the person's surroundings, especially if the person is at high risk for sensory perceptual alterations.	Environmental factors may contribute to sensory–perceptual problems, particularly sensory deprivation or sensory overload. *Sensory Deprivation:* Sensory deprivation may occur as a result of decreased sensory input from the surroundings, or inability to extract meaning from sensory input. Risk factors for sensory deprivation include minimal sensory stimulation, especially in the presence of vision or hearing deficits, prolonged bed rest, social isolation, prolonged darkness, and separation from personal objects or familiar surroundings. *Sensory Overload:* Sensory overload occurs when the person is bombarded with meaningless, confusing, or monotonous stimuli, such as frequently happens with patients in intensive care units. Contributing stimuli include noise, continual interruptions to sleep and rest, and constant lighting.
Evaluate the safety of the environment for persons with sensory–perceptual deficits such as impaired vision or impaired hearing.	Surroundings are evaluated to determine whether there are barriers to safe ambulation.

2. The neurologic system
 	
Evaluate the neurologic system by conducting the following examination procedures:
 	
    Mental status examination
    Cranial nerve examination
    Reflex testing
    Motor system assessment
    Sensory system assessment
	Alterations in neurologic systems and functions may have significant effects on cognitive and perceptual functions.

3. Sensory organs and systems Evaluate the sensory organs and systems, with special attention to the eyes and vision and the ears and hearing.	Vision and hearing are major avenues of sensory input. Alterations in vision and hearing can have significant impact on cognition and perception.

Documenting Cognition and Perception Assessment Findings

Data collected in the course of conducting a comprehensive assessment of cognitive and perceptual functions come from many sources, including interviews, mental status evaluations, medication histories, laboratory analyses, and observations. Baseline information about cognition and perception may be recorded on a form such as the one shown in Display 9-2.

Documentation of mental status requires special attention to level of consciousness, awareness, thought processes, and communication. A concise description of a person with no alterations in cognitive functions might be as follows:

> Alert and oriented × 3. Thought processes intact. Comprehension and expressive abilities intact.

(*Note:* "Oriented × 3" means oriented to three things: person, place, and time.)

For persons with altered levels of consciousness, describe your findings in detail in relation to the following assessment parameters: type of stimulus needed to arouse the person, behavior once aroused, verbal and motor responses. Consider the following example:

> Responds only after vigorous shaking and calling by name. Not oriented to person, time, or place when awake. Combative and does not follow verbal commands. Speech garbled—unable to discriminate words. Tries to remove painful stimuli.

Documentation of levels of consciousness, especially when serial evaluations are noted, may be facilitated by using a scoring tool such as the Glasgow Coma Scale.

Nursing Diagnoses Related to Cognitive Assessment

Altered Thought Processes

Altered thought processes refers to a state in which the individual experiences a disruption of cognitive functions such as conscious thought, reality orientation, problem solving, judgment, or comprehension. You should consider a number of factors before concluding that a person has altered thought processes.

First, you should realize that the diagnosis of Altered thought processes is based partly on your observations of the person's ability to make accurate statements about temporal events, his or her physical surroundings, and the people nearby. Use good judgment when interpreting a person's statements about person, place, and time. Some people may respond in a manner that you perceive as inappropriate, when in fact they are thinking clearly. For example, if you ask the person the day of the week, and he or she does not know, do not conclude that the person is disoriented (especially if the person is hospitalized) without further investigation. Concluding that he or she is disoriented might be as erroneous as concluding that a person who asks the date when writing a check is confused.

Second, you should realize that the nursing diagnosis Sensory–perceptual alteration has indicators similar to the diagnosis Altered thought processes. For example, both states may be characterized by disorientation, fear, and altered behavior patterns. Because intervention may differ depending on the diagnosis, you should take care to ensure an accurate diagnosis.

If a person manifests perceptual distortions and such symptoms can be alleviated by helping the person correctly interpret sensory stimuli, the most likely diagnosis is Sensory–perceptual alteration. For example, the person who is exposed to unfamiliar sounds in an intensive care unit may develop auditory misperceptions such as mistaking the sound of aerosol oxygen devices for the sound of falling rain. If you can explain that this sound is not rain but is related to the equipment, and the person develops the insight to interpret the unfamiliar auditory stimuli correctly, the nursing diagnosis would be Sensory–perceptual alteration. Conversely, auditory hallucinations are auditory perceptions with no apparent basis in reality and usually represent altered thought processes. The person is not as likely to have such misperceptions corrected by explanations.

Alterations in thought processes may be characterized by both perceptual distortions and thought disturbances. However, Sensory–perceptual alteration is not characterized by thought disturbances. When choosing between the two diagnoses, you should carefully assess the nature of the person's thought processes and his or her response to your efforts to interpret stimuli.

Unilateral Neglect

A person may be oriented to person, place, and time but still have awareness deficits relative to self and surroundings. Unilateral neglect is an example of altered body and environmental awareness. This condition is associated with damage of the right cerebral hemisphere, particularly when left hemiplegia is present. The person ignores perceptions and sensations relating to or originating from the left side of the body, which has important self-care implications. In extreme cases, the person may eat food from only the right side of his or her dinner plate or may wash only the right side of the body. Homonymous hemianopsia, a visual alteration characterized by blindness of the nasal half of one eye and the temporal half of the other eye, may accompany unilateral neglect.

Impaired Verbal Communication

Impaired verbal communication may be attributable to aphasia, which means a loss of language abilities. Many different types of aphasia have been identified, including Broca's, Wernicke's, conductive, global, transcortical sensory, transcortical motor, transcortical mixed, and anomic. It is helpful to know the type of aphasia a person has so that appropriate interventions can be planned. The diagnosis of a particular aphasia is complicated by the fact that many aphasias have overlapping features or do not fall into discrete diagnostic categories. The specific language symptomatology of the various aphasias is presented in Table 9-1.

PAIN

Definitions of Pain

Pain is a physiologic and sensory process that is influenced by each person's unique experience and responses. Pain may be defined as an unpleasant sensory and emotional experience that is associated with actual or potential tissue damage. In addition, the pain experience is also one that is personal and subjective, not requiring validation by means of objective assessment data. This is consistent with McCaffery's (1979) definition of pain, which stated, "Pain is whatever the person says it is, existing whenever the person says it does." Effective pain assessment is based on defining pain from the person's own perspective. Experts in pain management agree that the single most reliable indicator of the existence and intensity of pain is the individual's own self-report. Other indicators of pain, including physical manifestations such as increased blood pressure or behavioral manifestations such as crying, may serve as indicators of pain, but these manifestations are not required to make the diagnosis of pain.

TABLE 9.1   Differential Diagnosis of Aphasias*

Type of Aphasia	General Speaking Ability	Repetition Ability	Naming Ability	Oral Reading	Auditory Comprehension	Reading Comprehension	Written Expression
Transcortical sensory (isolation aphasia)	Fluent; paraphasia; does not initiate speech on own; ecolalic	Good, despite poor comprehension	Poor	Poor	Poor	Poor	Poor (similar to Wernicke's)
Transcortical motor	Nonfluent; tries to prompt self with hands (like a conductor), does not initiate speech on own	Very good	Poor	Poor	Good	Fair to good	Poor (similar to Broca's)
Transcortical mixed	Nonfluent; ecolalic; does not speak unless spoken to	Relatively preserved in one setting, otherwise limited language skills	Poor	Poor	Poor	Poor	Poor
Anomic	Fluent; vague empty speech; circumlocution	Good	Poor	Good to poor	Fair to good	Good to poor	Good to poor
Broca's (motor, expressive, non-fluent aphasia)	Nonfluent; telegraphic; paucity of spoken output	Poor, struggles to speak	Poor	Poor	Good	Good to poor	Poor (parallels speaking ability) paucity of written output
Wernicke's	Fluent; disorganized; logorrhea (excessive spoken output); incorrect syntax (word order) and paraphasic	Poor due to paraphasia errors (*e.g.*, *pink* for *sink*) and jargon usage	Poor	Poor	Poor	Poor	Poor (parallels speaking ability), excessive, meaningless writing
Conductive (fluent aphasia)	Fluent but with paraphasias, hesitations and repeated trials in approaching certain words	Poor in the context of good comprehension skills	Fair to poor	Poor due to paraphasic errors	Good	Good	Fair
Global (mixed)	Very poor; no output; nonfluent; may repeat one word or syllable	Very poor	Very poor	Very poor	Very poor	Very poor	Very poor

*Clinically, aphasia does not always fall into the discrete categories listed but may have elements of several types.

(Adapted from Pimental, P.A. [1986]. Alterations in communication: Biopsychosocial aspects of aphasia, dysarthria, and right hemisphere syndromes in the stroke patient. *Nursing Clinics of North America, 21* [2], 325)

Pain is classified as *acute, chronic malignant,* and *chronic nonmalignant*. Acute pain follows an injury, surgery, or other medical procedures and has an identifiable source. Acute pain serves as a warning sign (*e.g.,* the chest pain associated with a myocardial infarction). In contrast, no such useful purpose is associated with chronic pain. Chronic malignant pain results from a progressive, possibly fatal disorder such as cancer. The source of chronic malignant pain is organic. Chronic nonmalignant pain is pain of long duration related to conditions that do not directly result in death, such as arthritis. This pain may occur without an organic cause or persist after the initial damage or injury has healed.

Anatomy and Physiology Review

Sensory Component of Pain. Pain is initiated by conditions such as trauma, ischemia, hypoxia, or acidosis, which cause release of endogenous pain substances located in the vesicles or granules of peripheral nerve endings. The endogenous pain substances include substance P, somatostatin, kinins, prostaglandins, histamine, SRS-A, and thromboxanes. The release of these substances stimulates the nociceptors or pain receptors. The lowest-intensity stimulus that initiates the pain impulse transmission along efferent pathways is called the pain (nociceptive) threshold. The pain threshold is the same for all people.

Repeated stimulation of the nociceptors may result in sensitization to pain. Once sensitized, nociceptors continue to respond to painful stimuli, and eventually the pain may be perceived as more intense. Pain relief efforts often involve minimizing continued endogenous pain substance release to prevent sensitization.

Pain sensations are transmitted to the brain primarily by the ascending lateral spinothalamic tracts, where two types of sensory nerve fibers are found. Myelinated *A-delta fibers* transmit sharp, highly localized types of pain that occur immediately with injury. Unmyelinated *C fibers* transmit pain sensations that are more diffuse and aching.

Pain fibers enter the spinal cord through the dorsal roots. The pain impulse then reaches a synapse in the substantia gelatinosa and crosses the cord by way of several short interneurons. Impulse transmission then proceeds along the lateral spinothalamic tract to the brain (Fig. 9-2).

When necessary, pain sensations may bypass the brain and pass through a reflex arc, causing an immediate motor response. For example, the action of quickly removing the hand after touching a hot stove occurs as a result of this mechanism.

Perceptual Component of Pain. Pain perception involves the thalamus and cortical association areas of the brain. Pain may be perceived in the thalamus, or the pain impulse may be projected along diffuse pathways to the cerebral cortex. The threshold for recognizing pain is physiologically the same for all individuals. However, several factors, such as loss of consciousness and inhibition of pain impulse transmission by endogenous opiates (en-

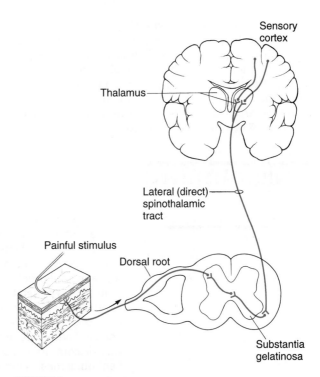

FIGURE 9.2 Sensory pathways and pain.

dorphins) or exogenous opiates (morphine), may alter the perception of pain.

The pain experience, or a person's response to pain, is influenced by memories, personality, culture, and values. Pain tolerance, a learned and socially conditioned human response, is a cortical phenomena and varies among individual people.

Pain Responses. Pain responses, both psychological and physiologic, are initiated at the cortical level. Psychological responses to pain include fear, anxiety, depression, or anger. Neural impulses, conducted along descending pathways, initiate physiologic responses, including cardiovascular responses (increased heart rate and blood pressure), gastrointestinal responses (decreased gut motility and decreased saliva), and musculoskeletal responses (increased muscle tension). Pain responses are probably modulated by signals transmitted from the cerebral cortex.

Pain Theories

The *specificity theory,* first proposed by Max von Frey, holds that pain results from the stimulation of pain-specific fibers, and that when a particular pain fiber is stimulated, a predictable intensity of pain is produced. However, this theory does not account for individual differences in pain perception or the effect of emotions and cognitive processes.

The *pattern theory* proposes that pain results from the stimulation of nonspecific peripheral receptors. A pattern is coded at the peripheral site and then transmitted to the brain, resulting in pain perception. However, this theory does not account for peripheral nerve fiber specialization.

The *gate control theory of pain* (Melzack & Wall, 1965) proposes that the perception of pain is influenced by numerous physiologic and psychological variables. The status of the "gate," located in the dorsal horn in the substantia gelatinosa, affects the pain impulse. In other words, when the gate is open, pain impulses flow freely through the ascending pathways, thereby enhancing pain perception. When the gate is closed, the pain impulse is inhibited, diminishing pain perception. Gates may possibly be closed by factors that stimulate A-delta fibers, such as massage, cold, acupuncture, or transcutaneous electrical nerve stimulation. The gates are opened by C-fiber stimulation, which occurs secondary to tissue damage. Gate activity is also influenced by the cortical perception of pain. For example, distraction and guided imagery may close the gates, consequently altering pain perception.

Pattern Assessment   Pain

PAIN ASSESSMENT ISSUES

Pain is generally poorly assessed and undertreated by health care providers. Some authorities estimate inadequate pain relief in 50% of surgical patients and 80% of cancer patients. Nurses, doctors, and patients can all have mistaken beliefs about pain and pain management that serve as barriers to effective pain management. Health care providers may undertreat pain because of unwarranted fears of establishing opioid addiction or respiratory depression in patients. Patients may be reluctant to report pain because of beliefs that pain is to be expected and tolerated and that treatment will have adverse effects. But undetected and untreated pain can have adverse consequences including unnecessary discomfort and suffering, longer recovery periods, and compromised patient outcomes. A thorough and systematic approach to pain assessment and management is important. With the development of a clinical practice guideline for acute pain management by the Agency for Health Care Policy and Research (AHCPR) in 1992, pain assessment and management became an even more important issue for health policy consideration.

GENERAL APPROACH

Pain assessment is often ill-defined, and clinicians frequently focus on assessing only one or two important dimensions of pain. Researchers who have evaluated the nature of cancer-related pain (Ahles et al., 1983) have characterized pain as an experience with multiple dimensions (Display 9-3). A comprehensive assessment of pain should focus on the multiple dimensions of the pain experience.

A nursing role in pain assessment has been formally delineated by the Oncology Nursing Society (Spross et al., 1991). Although this position paper identifies the nursing role in assessing cancer pain, the concepts can be similarly applied to the nurse's role in assessing acute or other types of chronic pain. By carrying out these pain assessment activities, the nurse will identify dimensions of pain management within the scope of nursing practice. The nursing role in assessing pain includes the following:

1. Describing the pain phenomenon
2. Identifying aggravating and relieving factors
3. Determining the meaning of the pain to the individual
4. Determining the cause of the pain
5. Determining definitions of optimal pain relief
6. Deriving nursing diagnoses
7. Assisting in selecting interventions
8. Evaluating the efficacy of interventions

COMMUNICATION AND INTERACTION

Good communication and a trusting, nonjudgmental relationship between the nurse and the person with pain is essential for the optimal assessment of pain. You should create an environment that allows the person to express their pain. The most important principle to remember is that a person should never be required to "prove" that they are in pain. If you remember that self-reports are the most reliable indicators of pain, you are less likely to impose your own judgments about how much you believe a person is suffering. It is important to sit down with the person, listen actively, and demonstrate that you believe the person and that you can be trusted to help.

(continued)

Pattern Assessment   Pain (continued)

In surgical patients, you should set the stage for effective pain assessment before the operative procedure. The following techniques are helpful in the pre-operative stage:

1. Inform the person and their family that pain reports are valuable, provide information, and may even indicate complications that require immediate attention.
2. Provide accurate information regarding what may be expected in terms of pain.
3. Discuss measures that can be used to manage pain. The person should be informed that a variety of medications as well as nonpharmacologic interventions may be used to manage pain. This type of discussion may help address any concerns the person may have about overmedication or beliefs that opioids should be avoided until the last resort.
4. Determine the person's preferred terminology to describe pain. What words will the person use to describe pain? If the person does not use a term such as *discomfort,* then the nurse should avoid asking, "Do you have discomfort?" when assessing the person for pain.

(continued)

DISPLAY 9.3

Multiple Dimensions of the Pain Experience

1. Physiologic Dimension (the organic cause of pain)
   Assessment Focus: Location, onset, duration, cause, type of pain
2. Sensory Dimension (how the pain feels to the person experiencing it)
   Assessment Focus: Intensity, quality, pattern
3. Affective Dimension (the feelings related to the pain experience)
   Assessment Focus: Mood state, anxiety, depression, well-being
4. Cognitive Dimension (what meaning the pain has and other thought processes)
   Assessment Focus: Meaning of pain, view of self, coping skills and strategies, previous treatments, attitudes and beliefs
5. Behavioral Dimension (the indicators of pain and pain relief)
   Assessment Focus: Communication of pain, pain behaviors, physical activity, interventions, sleep pattern
6. Sociocultural Dimension (other factors that relate to an individual's perception of and response to pain)
   Assessment Focus: Ethnic and cultural background, family and social life, work and home responsibilities, recreation and leisure, attitudes and beliefs, social influences

Pattern Assessment Pain (continued)

5. Choose or review the use of pain assessment tools. A number of tools can be used clinically to help people rate the intensity and quality of pain (see below). Show the tools to the person during the preoperative teaching process. If choices are available, let the person select the tool they prefer.

6. Determine the desired level of pain control. Once a pain assessment tool is chosen, you should discuss with the patient that a score above a predetermined criterion of the patient's choosing (*e.g.,* a score greater than 4 on a 10-point scale) will result in medication or some other type of intervention. The involvement of the person in making such a choice is particularly important if the person fears overmedication or desires to use some alternative interventions before medication is administered.

7. Identify measures that may have been used in the past to successfully manage pain.

PAIN ASSESSMENT TOOLS

A number of tools are available to assist the nurse and patient in the assessment of pain (Fig. 9-3). Most tools used in clinical practice focus on only one to three dimensions of pain, such as location, intensity, and pain relief. Nevertheless, tools can be helpful in communicating pain and pain relief. The use of tools can also prompt utilization of more effective pain-relieving measures. It is especially effective if the nurse and patient can agree what score on a particular pain scale should be considered unacceptable pain in need of some type of intervention.

Visual Analog Scales (VAS) consist of a 10-cm horizontal line with an anchor on each end indicating the absence of pain on one end and the worst possible pain on the other end. The person marks the point along this continuum that represents their pain level. Pain intensity is scored by measuring the distance from the point of no pain to the patient's mark.

(continued)

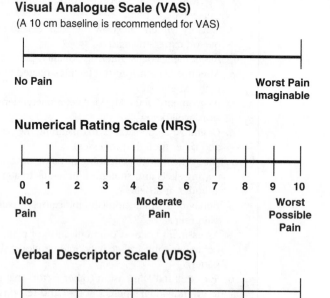

Visual Analogue Scale (VAS)
(A 10 cm baseline is recommended for VAS)

No Pain   Worst Pain
                                 Imaginable

Numerical Rating Scale (NRS)

0   1   2   3   4   5   6   7   8   9   10
No   Moderate   Worst
Pain   Pain   Possible
                                           Pain

Verbal Descriptor Scale (VDS)

No   Mild   Moderate   Severe   Very   Worst
Pain   Pain   Pain   Pain   Severe   Possible
                                      Pain   Pain

FIGURE 9.3 Pain assessment tools.

Pattern Assessment   Pain (continued)

Numerical Rating Scales (NRS) also consist of a horizontal line that is equally divided into increments. The person is asked to rate their pain intensity on a 0 to 5, 0 to 10, or 0 to 100 scale. Zero represents the absence of pain, and the highest number on the scale represents the worst possible pain.

Verbal Descriptor Scales (VDS) consist of a list of adjectives that describe levels of pain intensity by extremes (*e.g.,* "no pain" to "very severe pain"). The person is asked to choose the adjective that best describes their pain.

The *McGill Pain Questionnaire* is an example of a multidimensional pain assessment tool that is widely used as a research tool to measure pain. A shorter format of the tool is also available for clinical use. The short form consists of a front and back body outline used to indicate the exact location of the pain; a pain intensity scale measured from 0 for "no pain" to 5 for "excruciating pain"; and a pain rating index that consists of 78 words that describe the sensory, affective, and evaluative aspects of pain. The patient selects words that describe the type of pain they are experiencing. Numerical scores are then calculated from these selections. This shortened version can still take 15 to 20 minutes to complete.

FREQUENCY OF PAIN ASSESSMENT

Pain should be assessed and findings documented on a regular basis. Pain assessment should always be initiated in the following situations:

1. Preoperatively, to establish a baseline and provide patient education about pain management
2. Postoperatively at routine and regular intervals (*e.g.,* every 2 hours while awake during the first postoperative day)
3. With each new report of pain
4. After each analgesic intervention for pain at an appropriate interval (*e.g.,* 30 minutes after parenteral drug therapy and 1 hour after oral drug therapy).

EXAMINATION AND DOCUMENTATION FOCUS

• Location, including point of origin and radiation
• Intensity
• Quality
• Onset and chronology
• Relieving factors
• Aggravating factors
• Effects of pain on other functions

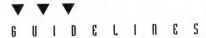

GUIDELINES

Assessment Guidelines   Pain

Procedure

1. Location

a. Ask the person to point to the pain location or to mark the pain location on a figure drawing. Determine whether the pain radiates from its point of origin.

b. If you use a drawing to indicate the location of pain, separate pain sites can be labeled with letters or numbers. For example, headache pain may be #1 and abdominal pain may be #2. These numbers can then be used to categorize descriptive statements made by the person about pain.

c. Ask where the pain is most intense and whether the pain is perceived as internal or external.

Clinical Significance

Pain location often provides clues about the cause of the pain or the type of pain being experienced. The following types of pain may be distinguished on the basis of location:

- *Somatic pain* originates in the trunk, extremities, skin, or bones. Somatic pain that is localized or that originates with cutaneous nerve fibers is called *epicritic pain* (e.g., the pain that occurs after a first-degree burn). Deep somatic pain, which is not as localized, is called *protopathic pain* (e.g., the pain that results from a sprained ankle). The patient may refer to somatic pain as external pain.

- *Visceral pain* originates in the internal organs and is caused by factors such as ischemia, spasm, or acidosis. Visceral pain is often *referred pain* in that the pain radiates away from the pain origin, or the patient feels the pain at a location other than the origin. Unlike somatic pain, visceral pain cannot be sharply localized. The patient may refer to visceral pain as internal pain.

- *Phantom pain* is usually perceived to be in a missing extremity or body part. For example, the patient may feel right-lower-leg pain following an above-the-knee amputation. Nerve fiber alterations at amputation site probably contribute to this particular type of pain.

- *Causalgia* is an intense, burning pain following traumatic injury that involves the peripheral nerves of an extremity. The pain is severe in relation to the initiating trauma. Atrophic skin changes and bone demineralization may occur in advanced stages.

- *Neuralgia* refers to an intense, burning pain along the distribution of a peripheral nerve. The pain may occur after a nerve's "trigger zone" has been stimulated in the area of pain.

▼ ▼ ▼

Procedure

2. Intensity

  a. Ask the person to rate the intensity of the pain being experienced. One of the simplest ways to rate pain is to ask the person to rate the pain on a scale of 1 to 10, with 10 representing the most intense pain ever experienced.

  b. You may ask the person to rate pain and pain relief using visual analog scales. Ask the person to mark an X on each scale representing present pain perception and pain relief. Serial comparisons of visual analog scales help you evaluate the person's pain and pain interventions.

  c. Alternatively, ask the person to describe the intensity of the pain.

3. Quality

Ask the person to describe the quality of the pain.

Approaches such as "Describe what the pain feels like" are preferred over questions such as "Is the pain sharp?"

4. Onset and chronology

  a. Ask about the time of onset and duration of pain.

  b. Ask whether the pain suddenly or gradually became more severe or if the pain is intermittent.

  c. Ask whether the pattern of pain changes within a 24-hour period.

5. Relieving factors

Ask the person what, if anything, relieves the pain. Determine personal preferences in relation to pain relief strategies.

Clinical Significance

If a pain-rating scale is used, the same scale should be used in follow-up assessments to allow for meaningful comparisons.

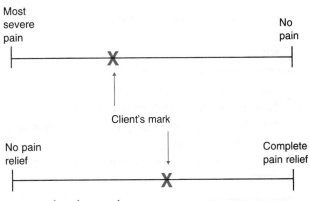

Pain visual analogue scale

Words such as none, mild, moderate, severe, or very severe may indicate intensity.

Words such as pinching, pressing, gnawing, cramping, or crushing may describe pain quality.

The use of open-ended questions will limit cueing or suggesting responses to the person. Limited information may be obtained by asking questions that only require a yes-or-no answer.

Chronic pain may be perceived as having always been present. Acute pain may be associated with a more sudden onset.

Pain that immediately reaches a maximum intensity may indicate tissue rupture. Ischemic pain gradually increases in intensity.

Chronic pain may follow diurnal rhythms. For example, because rheumatoid arthritis pain is aggravated by inactivity, the pain is usually more severe on awakening. *Nocturnal epigastric pain* is associated with peptic ulcer disease.

Colicky pain, which originates in hollow viscera, is a rhythmic, cramping pain.

Pain relief may be obtained through the use of medications or by using alternative pain-management strategies such as guided imagery, massage, music, rest, or position changes.

▼ ▼ ▼

G U I D E L I N E S *continued*   Pain

Procedure

6. Aggravating factors

Ask the person what makes the pain worse.

Note the relationship between activity and pain.

7. Effects

Ask questions such as the following:

"What does this pain mean to you?"

"Tell me how the pain has changed your lifestyle."

"How has the pain influenced your everyday activities—eating, moving, sleeping?"

"How has this pain influenced your relationships with others?"

8. Other observations

a. Note expressions of pain such as crying, withdrawal, moaning.

b. Note physiologic signs of pain:

Autonomic responses: Elevated blood pressure, heart rate, and ventilatory rate; cool, clammy skin; dilated pupils; nausea and vomiting.

Musculoskeletal responses: Clenched fists, restlessness, guarding, muscle rigidity.

c. Note facial expressions of pain: grimacing, "facial mask of pain."

Clinical Significance

Some aggravating factors can be minimized. Consider the effects of sleep deprivation, anxiety, or environmental discomfort such as uncomfortable temperatures or noise.

Ischemic pain (angina, leg claudication) may be precipitated by activity.

Inquiring about the effects of pain helps the nurse identify problems with coping, relationships, and activities of daily living.

Concerns about addiction to narcotics, cost of medications, social interactions, and sexual activities are common in persons experiencing chronic pain.

Pain may be present with or without physical signs.

Facial mask of pain: Flat or fixed facial expression; lusterless eyes; fatigued appearance. Associated with chronic pain.

Documenting Pain Assessment

The initial documentation of pain in the person's record should be thorough because all the qualities of the pain are considered in making a clinical diagnosis. Subsequent references may be more abbreviated, provided the qualities of the pain remain the same. Documentation should include attention to the following: location, intensity, quality, onset and chronology, relieving factors, aggravating factors, and other effects. The pain experienced by a person suffering from angina might be described as follows:

States pain is located in chest beneath sternum and radiates to left shoulder and arm. Pain is described as 8 on a 1-to-10 scale. Feels like pressure or a tight belt around the chest. First noticed pain at 0800 this morning while sitting at desk. Has never experienced this type of pain in the past. Pain was intermittent until 1 hour ago, when it became continuous. Nothing seems to make the pain better or worse. Finds it hard to breathe with the pain and noticed profuse perspiration since the onset of the pain.

Nursing Diagnoses Related to Pain Assessment

Acute Pain

Acute pain is considered self-limiting and purposeful in that it serves to alert a person to possible problems. Numerous factors initiate acute pain by causing tissue damage.

Pain History. The person may or may not verbalize pain perceptions. In the case of acute pain, verbal reports usually indicate that the pain had a sudden onset, and often a precipitating event can be identified (*e.g.,* "I felt the pain in my ankle right after I fell on the stairway."). The person may be able to describe the pain precisely and locate the site.

Observations. Autonomic responses that may be pronounced with acute pain include pallor, diaphoresis, and cardiovascular and respiratory alterations. Guarding is common. Depending on the nature of the pain, the person may decrease or increase the pace of activities or rub the affected part. The person's facial affect usually reflects anxiety or fear. Pain relief strategies are usually effective for acute pain.

Chronic Pain

Chronic pain has a duration of greater than 6 months and may be a result of irreversible tissue damage. In this sense, chronic pain does not serve to warn the person of impending danger.

Pain History. The person may or may not verbalize pain perceptions. However, preoccupation with the pain experience is not uncommon. The pain may be reported as constant or intermittent and may be as intense as any acute pain experience. Rather than describing a specific onset of pain, the person may refer to the pain as being constant. The person may have greater difficulty localizing chronic pain and may describe it as an ache or soreness. Feelings of hopelessness, guilt, and frustration are common. Pain relief efforts may be unsuccessful.

Observations. With chronic pain, there is habituation to the autonomic nervous system responses evoked by pain. Therefore, the person may no longer display acute physiologic signs of stress. The facial expression is frequently characterized by the facial mask of pain. The person may be irritable and angry or depressed.

PART 2
PHYSICAL EXAMINATION TECHNIQUES

THE CRANIAL NERVES
Anatomy and Physiology Review

Nuclei for the 12 paired cranial nerves originate in the brain, differentiating cranial nerves from spinal nerves, whose nuclei originate in the spinal cord. Cranial nerves are distributed mainly to the head and neck. Certain cranial nerves, like all spinal nerves, have both sensory and motor components. However, some cranial nerves have only sensory fibers, and others have only motor axons.

Cranial nerve examination indicates the status of associated sensory or motor functions. Pertinent anatomic, physiologic, and functional features of the 12 cranial nerves are summarized in Table 9-2.

Physical Examination Cranial Nerves

GENERAL PRINCIPLES

Most cranial nerve functions involve the head and neck areas. Therefore, cranial nerve assessment should be performed in the early part of a head-to-toe examination sequence. Generally, cranial nerves should not be assessed alone but in conjunction with other major body areas or systems. For example, cranial nerves II, III, IV, and VI and the ophthalmic branch of cranial nerve V should be tested during eye and vision examination.

EQUIPMENT

- Small vials with familiar odors
- Snellen chart
- Ophthalmoscope
- Tongue blade
- Irrigation syringe (optional)
- Cotton-tipped applicator
- Safety pin

EXAMINATION AND DOCUMENTATION FOCUS

- Responses to external stimuli
- Motor functions
- Visual acuity
- Hearing acuity

TABLE 9.2 Cranial Nerves

Number	Name	Structures Innervated by Efferent Components	Structures Innervated by Afferent Components	Functions
I	Olfactory	None	Olfactory mucous membrane	Nerve of smell
II	Optic	None	Retina of eye	Nerve of vision
III	Oculomotor	Superior, medial, inferior recti; inferior oblique; levator palpebrae superioris; ciliary; sphincter of iris	Superior, medial, inferior, recti; inferior oblique; levator palpebrae superioris; ciliary; sphincter of iris	Motor and muscle sense to various muscles listed; accommodation to different distances; regulates the amount of light reaching retina; most important nerve in eye movements
IV	Trochlear	Superior oblique	Superior oblique	Motor and muscle sense to superior oblique; eye movements
V	Trigeminal	Muscles of mastication	Skin and mucous membranes in head; teeth; muscles of mastication	Nerve of pain, touch, heat, cold to skin and mucous membranes listed; same for teeth; movements of mastication and muscle sense
VI	Abducens	Lateral rectus	Lateral rectus	Motor and muscle sense to lateral rectus; eye movements
VII	Facial	Submaxillary and sublingual glands; muscles of face, scalp, and a few others	Same mucles; taste buds of anterior two thirds of tongue	Taste to anterior two thirds of tongue; secretory and vasodilator to two salivary glands; motor and muscle sense to facial and a few other muscles
VIII	Acoustic (cochlear and vestibular portions)	None	Cochlear organ of Corti; vestibular-semicircular canals, utricle, and saccule	Cochlear division is nerve of hearing; vestibular division is concerned with registering movement of the body through space and with the position of the head
IX	Glossopharyngeal	Superior pharyngeal constrictor; stylopharyngeus muscle; parotid gland	Taste buds of posterior one third of tongue; parts of pharynx; carotid sinus and body; stylopharyngeus muscle	Taste to posterior one third of tongue and adjacent regions; secretory and vasodilator to parotid gland; motor and muscle sense to stylopharyngeus; pain, touch, heat, and cold to pharynx; afferent in circulatory and respiratory reflexes
X	Vagus	Muscles of pharynx, larynx, esophagus, thoracic and abdominal viscera; coronary arteries; walls of bronchi; pancreas; gastric glands	Same muscles; skin of external ear; mucous membranes of larynx, trachea, esophagus; thoracic and abdominal viscera; arch of aorta; atria; great veins	Secretory to gastric glands and pancreas; inhibitory to heart; motor to alimentary tract; motor and muscle sense to muscles of larynx and pharynx; constrictor to coronaries; motor to muscle in walls of bronchi; important in respiratory, cardiac, and circulatory reflexes
XI	Accessory	Sternocleidomastoid and trapezius muscles; muscles of larynx	Sternocleidomastoid and trapezius muscles; muscles of larynx	Motor and muscle sense to muscles listed; shares certain functions of vagus
XII	Hypoglossal	Muscles of tongue	Muscles of tongue	Motor and muscle sense to muscles of tongue; important in speech, mastication, and deglutition

▼ ▼ ▼

GUIDELINES

Assessment Guidelines   Cranial Nerves

Procedure

1. Cranial nerve I (olfactory)

   a. Ask the person to occlude one nostril at a time with the finger and to close the eyes.

   b. Present several familiar odors such as coffee, cloves, peppermint, or soap and ask the person to identify each. Avoid presenting irritating substances such as ammonia or vinegar. Remember that the ability to distinguish between odors is more important than the ability to make exact identifications.

2. Cranial nerve II (optic)

   a. Test cranial nerve II by testing visual acuity (see pp. 435–436).

   b. Examine the optic nerve, which ends in the retina, by using the ophthalmoscope (see pp. 429–434).

3. Cranial nerves III (oculomotor), IV (trochlear), VI (abducens)

4. Cranial nerve V (trigeminal)

   a. Test motor function of the trigeminal nerve. Place a tongue blade between the person's teeth on the right side and ask him or her to bite down. As the person bites, try to pull the tongue blade out. Repeat this procedure on the left side of the mouth.

   b. Alternatively, test motor function by asking the person to clench his or her teeth while you palpate the masseter and temporal muscles for firmness.

Clinical Significance

The olfactory nerve is not tested routinely.

Normal Findings
Identifies common smells with each nostril.

Deviations from Normal
Anosmia: Unilateral loss of smell. Associated with lesions to the olfactory nerve tract on the side being tested.
Bilateral Loss of Smell: Associated with excessive smoking, cocaine use, or a sinus condition.

This nerve should be tested during eye and vision evaluations.

These nerves are tested by evaluating extraocular eye movements. The oculomotor nerve also innervates the intrinsic muscles that control pupillary constriction and accommodation. These functions are tested by evaluating pupillary light reflexes (see p. 429).

Normal Findings
Equal strength of bite bilaterally; no jaw deviation with teeth clenching.

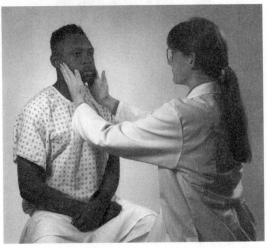

Trigeminal nerve: Testing motor function

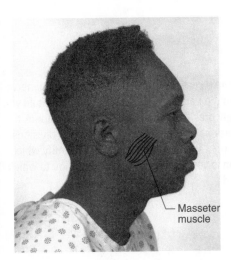

Masseter muscle

▼ ▼ ▼

G U I D E L I N E S *continued*   Cranial Nerves

Procedure

c. Test sensory function.

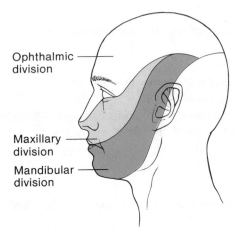

Trigeminal nerve: Three sensory components

Clinical Significance

There are three major sensory components of the trigeminal nerve: ophthalmic, maxillary, and mandibular. All three sensory areas are tested.

---

d. Evaluate the sensory function of the ophthalmic division of the cranial nerve by testing the corneal reflex.

Hold the person's eye open and lightly touch the cornea with the tip of a cotton-tipped applicator that has been pulled into a thin strand. To ensure a reliable test, be careful to touch only the cornea and not the eyelashes or conjunctiva.

This test also indicates the status of the motor division of the facial nerve.

Normal Findings
A strong, forceful blink.

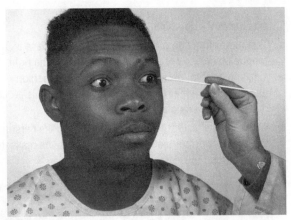

Testing the corneal reflex

---

e. Test all three sensory divisions of the trigeminal nerve by asking the person to keep the eyes closed while you alternately brush cotton across and lightly pinprick the facial areas innervated by the three sensory divisions. As you apply stimuli, ask the person to identify which sensation is being produced and the location to which it is applied.

Normal Findings
Discriminates light touch and pinprick over skin innervated by the three divisions of the cranial nerve.

▼ ▼ ▼
G U I D E L I N E S *continued*   Cranial Nerves

Procedure	Clinical Significance

Procedure

5. Cranial nerve VII (facial)

   a. Test the motor division of the facial nerve by asking the person to perform voluntary facial movements such as frowning, smiling, wrinkling the forehead, puffing cheeks, and whistling.

   b. Test the strength of eyelid closure by asking the person to hold the eyes tightly closed. Then try to open the person's eyes.

   c. Test the sensory division of the facial nerve by evaluating the person's ability to discriminate tastes. Apply salt and sugar to both sides of the anterior tongue.

6. Cranial nerve VIII (acoustic)

   a. Test the cochlear portion of cranial nerve VIII by evaluating hearing acuity (see pp. 444–447).

   b. Test the vestibular portion of cranial nerve VIII by performing the Romberg test (see p. 421).

   c. The vestibular portion of cranial nerve VIII may also be evaluated by performing the caloric test.

     With the person seated or with the head of bed elevated 30 degrees, inspect ear canal with otoscope to ascertain a patent canal and intact tympanic membrane. Irrigate the ear canal with ice-cold water. If client is conscious, use only a few drops.

7. Cranial nerves IX (glossopharyngeal) and X (vagus)

   a. Test cranial nerve IX by touching the palatal arch with a tongue blade to elicit a gag reflex.

   b. Ask the person to open his or her mouth and say "ah."

   c. Cranial nerve X is also tested by evaluating speech quality. Ask the person to say, "kuh, kuh, kuh," "la, la, la," and "mi, mi, mi."

Clinical Significance

Normal Findings
Facial features are symmetric when performing voluntary movements. Symmetry also observed at the nasolabial folds.

Deviations from Normal
Bell's palsy: Lesion to the lower portion of the facial nerve resulting in ipsilateral paralysis.

Upper motor neuron lesions: Upper motor neuron lesions, such as stroke, may produce contralateral facial weakness, drooping, or paralysis.

Taste sensation is not tested routinely.

The caloric test is used to evaluate brain stem function in comatose persons. The test is rarely performed on conscious people, because it may produce nausea.

Normal Findings (conscious person)
Nausea, horizontal nystagmus, vertigo toward unirrigated side, and "past-pointing" on irrigated side (person misjudges distance and points "past" the correct position when instructed to touch your fingertip with his or her fingertip).

These nerves are tested together because both have components that innervate the pharynx. Check them during the oral examination.

Normal Findings
The uvula remains midline, and there is symmetric rising of the soft palate. This indicates normal function of cranial nerves IX and X.

Normal Findings
Speaks with clear voice.

▼ ▼ ▼

GUIDELINES   *continued*   Cranial Nerves

Procedure

8. Cranial nerve XI (spinal, accessory)

   a. Place your hands on the person's shoulders and ask him or her to shrug as you apply resistance.

   b. Inspect and palpate the sternocleiodomastoid muscles, noting tone and symmetry.

   c. Ask the client to turn the head and touch chin to shoulder as you apply resistance. Test both sides.

Clinical Significance

Normal Findings
Raises shoulders against resistance.

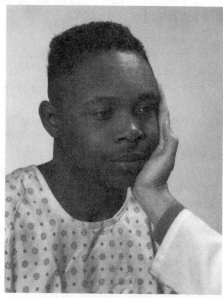

Spinal accessory nerve: Testing motor function

9. Cranial nerve XII (hypoglossal)

   Ask the person to stick out the tongue. Note symmetry, atrophy, and involuntary movements.

This nerve should be checked during the oral examination.

Normal Findings
Extends tongue along midline; no lateral deviation.

NDₓ

Documenting Cranial Nerve Examination Findings

If all 12 cranial nerve functions are normal, you may either specifically describe the normal response of each cranial nerve or make a broad statement indicating normal status of all 12 nerves. A specific description follows:

Cranial nerve VII (facial): Symmetric facial features noted at rest and with performance of facial expressions.

The following is an example of a broad statement:

Cranial nerves I–XII tested. All functions intact and appropriate responses noted.

Any abnormal findings should be described in detail. Record the type of stimuli applied or test performed and the response that was elicited.

NDₓ

Nursing Diagnoses Related to Cranial Nerve Assessment

For persons displaying abnormal responses to cranial nerve testing, the nurse should determine whether the nursing diagnosis Sensory–perceptual alterations is applicable. If a sensory–perceptual alteration is confirmed, you should then attempt to diagnose the response to any deficits. For example, if cranial nerve II (optic) is impaired and the person has a visual deficit, you might diagnose a response such as Potential for injury. Or, if cranial nerve IX (glossopharyngeal) is impaired and the person has lost his or her gag reflex, you might diagnose a response such as Potential for aspiration. Dysfunction of cranial nerve VII (facial) may alter the appearance of the face, and one side may be noted to sag or droop. In this case, you may diagnose the person's response as Body image disturbance.

MOTOR SYSTEM AND REFLEXES

Alterations in motor function may be observed in persons with pathologic conditions of the cerebral cortex or spinal cord. Evaluating the motor system is an important part of a comprehensive neurologic assessment. Neurologic disorders may affect muscle bulk, tone, strength, involuntary reflexes, in addition to a person's ability to perform voluntary movements. Additional guidelines for musculoskeletal assessment are discussed in Chapter 8.

Anatomy and Physiology Review

Voluntary movement is controlled by the motor cortex located in the frontal lobe of the cerebrum and the descending (motor) corticospinal tracts (Fig. 9-4). From the cerebral cortex, the descending tracts pass through the subcortical white matter and the internal capsule, an area between the thalamus and basal ganglia where motor nerve tracts converge before entering the brain stem. Because all motor fibers pass through the internal capsule, a stroke in this area will cause a greater loss of motor function than will occur with a cerebral hemisphere stroke.

Most corticospinal nerve fibers cross to the opposite side (decussate) in the lower medulla and descend the spinal cord as the lateral corticospinal tract. A few fibers continue to descend uncrossed along ventral corticospinal tracts. Motor function is controlled predominantly by the crossed fibers, which accounts for clinical findings such as left-sided paralysis after right cerebral hemisphere damage. Before leaving the brain stem, the corticospinal tract fibers pass through a structure known as the *pyramid,* a compact bundle of nerve fibers in the medulla.

The descending fibers, known as the *upper motor neurons* (UMNs), form synapses with other efferent neurons, the *lower motor neurons* (LMNs), in the anterior horn of the spinal cord. The LMN directly innervates skeletal muscle and transmits the neural impulses essential for movement. Lower motor neurons, called the *final common pathway,* are influenced by one of two neural pathways: descending fibers originating in the brain; or afferent neurons of the reflex arc (neural pathways independent of the brain).

In addition to transmitting neural impulses for voluntary movement through the corticospinal tract, descending cortical fibers transmit neural impulses that control muscle tone. For example, descending rubrospinal tract fibers facilitate flexor muscles and inhibit extensor muscles; pons and medulla descending reticulospinal tracts facilitate and inhibit stretch reflexes, respectively.

Reflexes are involuntary motor movements or glandular secretions that are usually protective and adaptive in nature. The neural pathway involved in reflexes is the *reflex arc.* As noted in Figure 9-5, reflex arcs function independently of the brain. Reflex arcs may be monosynaptic (only two neurons and a synapse) or polysynaptic (more than two neurons). In either case, a sensory receptor in the skin or muscle is stimulated, and a neural impulse travels the afferent neuron to the spinal cord. An efferent

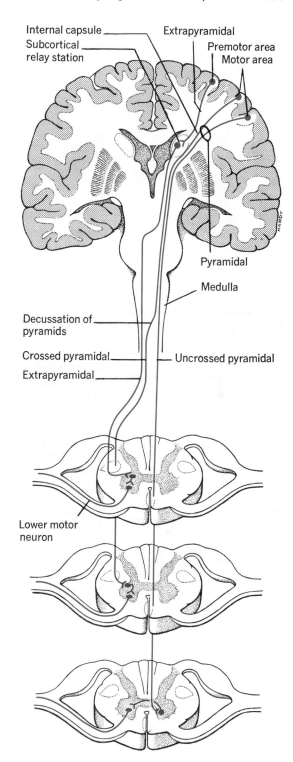

FIGURE 9.4 The motor cortex and motor tracts.

neuron transmits the impulse back to an effector in the muscle or skin, which results in movement or glandular secretion. Were it not for inhibitory descending fibers from the brain, reflex activity would be more pronounced because the sensory receptors involved receive frequent stimulation.

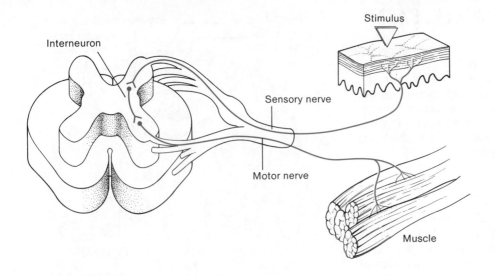

Interneuron

Stimulus

Sensory nerve

Motor nerve

Muscle

FIGURE 9.5   The reflex arc.

Physical Examination   Motor System

GENERAL PRINCIPLES

As a parameter for the assessment of neurologic function, motor system examination should focus on the following areas: degree of movement, strength and equality of movement, muscle tone, deep tendon reflexes, and superficial reflexes. Assessment of general movement or range of motion is described in Chapter 8 in the musculoskeletal assessment guidelines. This chapter section describes evaluation of deep tendon reflexes and superficial reflexes. Included in the deep tendon reflexes are the following: biceps, brachioradialis, triceps, patellar, and achilles. Superficial reflexes do not need to be assessed routinely but should be examined if neurologic or motor deficits are present.

EQUIPMENT

- Reflex hammer
- Tongue blade (optional)

EXAMINATION AND DOCUMENTATION FOCUS

Responses to applied stimuli, including the following:

- Type of movement
- Intensity
- Unexpected movements

▼ ▼ ▼
G U I D E L I N E S

A s s e s s m e n t   G u i d e l i n e s   Deep Tendon Reflexes

Procedure

Note: Reflexes should be compared bilaterally.

Before You Begin

Practice using the reflex hammer. Deep tendon reflexes are tested by striking specific tendons with the reflex hammer. The hammer has a pointed end for small tendons and a blunt end for large tendons. Hold the instrument at the very end of its handle and allow the hammer to swing quickly and freely downward between the first and second fingers. Grasping the hammer too near its head will inhibit free movement.

Remember the principle of reinforcement. The person should be relaxed to elicit a deep tendon reflex successfully. If the reflex is diminished or absent, ask the person to use *reinforcement.* This method involves contracting muscles that are not being tested to relax the effector muscles that are being treated. For example, when testing the patellar reflex, reinforcement is accomplished by asking the person to lock the fingers and attempt to pull the hands apart.

1. **Test the biceps reflex.**
   a. Flex the person's arm slightly at the elbow and rest the forearm in your hand or on the person's leg.
   b. Place your thumb over the biceps tendon in the antecubital fossa.

   c. Strike your thumbnail with the pointed end of the hammer.

Clinical Significance

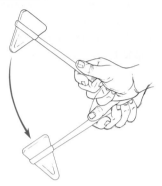

Using the reflex hammer

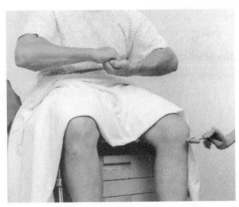

Reinforcement

Stimulates C5–C6 section of the spinal cord.

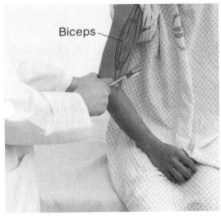

Biceps

Biceps reflex testing

Normal Findings

Person's forearm flexes at the elbow.

▼ ▼ ▼

G U I D E L I N E S *continued*   Deep Tendon Reflexes

Procedure

2. **Test the triceps reflex.**

   a. Flex the person's forearm at the elbow and hold the arm across the person's chest.

   b. Alternatively, allow the person's arm to hang loosely while you support it by placing your hand under the bicep.

Clinical Significance

Stimulates C6–C7 and C7–C8 sections of the spinal cord.

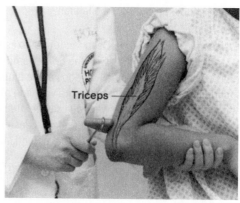

Triceps reflex testing

   c. Strike the triceps tendon, located just above the olecranon process, with the blunt end of the hammer.

3. **Test the brachioradialis reflex.**

   a. The person's forearm should be relaxed, palm facing down, and resting on the leg or supported by your hand.

Normal Findings

Forearm extends slightly at the elbow.

Stimulates C5–C6 section of the spinal cord.

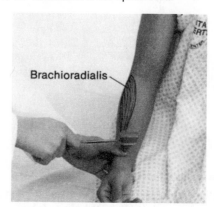

Brachioradialis reflex testing

   b. Strike the brachioradialis tendon, located just above the styloid process of the radius.

4. **Test the patellar reflex.**

   a. The person should be seated with the legs dangling or supine with the knees slightly flexed.

Normal Findings

Slight flexion of forearm at the elbow and forearm pronation.

Stimulates L2–L3 and L3–L4 sections of the spinal cord.

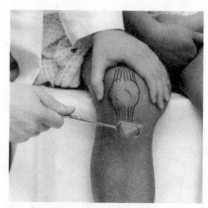

Patellar reflex testing

▼ ▼ ▼
G U I D E L I N E S   *continued*   Deep Tendon Reflexes

Procedure

b. Strike the patellar tendon, located just below the knee-cap. Use the blunt end of the reflex hammer.

5. **Test the Achilles reflex.**

   a. Position the person in the same manner as you would for testing the patellar reflex.

   b. Support the foot in a dorsiflexed position. Tap the Achilles tendon above the heel.

Clinical Significance

Normal Findings

Leg extends at the knee.

Stimulates S1–S2 section of the spinal cord.

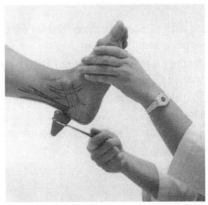

Achilles reflex testing

Normal Finding

Plantar flexion. This may be observed visually or felt by placing your hand against the sole of the foot as the reflex is tested.

▼ ▼ ▼
G U I D E L I N E S

A s s e s s m e n t   G u i d e l i n e s   Superficial Reflexes (Optional)

Procedure

1. **Test the upper/lower abdominal reflex.**

   Lightly scratch or stroke the skin of the upper/lower abdominal quadrant with the handle of the reflex hammer or a tongue blade and note umbilical movement.

2. **Test the cremasteric reflex (males only).**
   Lightly scratch the inner, upper surface of the thigh and note testicular movement.

3. **Test the plantar reflex.**
   a. Firmly stroke the outer border of the sole of the foot with the handle of the reflex hammer.

Clinical Significance

Upper abdominal: Stimulates T7–T8 and T8–T9 sections of the spinal cord.

Lower abdominal: Stimulates T11–T12 section of the spinal cord.

Normal response, upper abdominal: Umbilicus shifts upward toward point of stimulus.

Normal response, lower abdominal: Umbilicus shifts downward toward point of stimulus.

Stimulates T12–L1 and L1–L2 sections of the spinal cord.

Normal response: Testicle on the same side (ipsilateral) of stimulation rises.

Stimulates S1–S2 section of the spinal cord.

▼ ▼ ▼

G U I D E L I N E S   *continued*   Superficial Reflexes (Optional)

Procedure	**Clinical Significance**

Procedure

  b. Note the movement of the toes.

4. **In persons with neurologic deficits, test for the primitive reflexes—grasp, snout, glabellar.**

  a. Test for the *grasp reflex.* Place your fingers in the palm of the person's hand.

  b. Test for the *snout reflex.* Gently tap the side of the person's mouth.

  c. Test for the *glabellar reflex.* Gently tap the person on the forehead.

Clinical Significance

Normal response: Toes should flex (normal *adult* response); record the finding as Babinski negative.

Deviations from normal: If toes fan or extend, record the finding as Babinski positive, indicative in adults of cerebral dysfunction.

The primitive reflexes are indicators of cerebral pathology.

Abnormal reflex finding: The person grasps your fingers but does not release the grasp when instructed.

Abnormal reflex finding: The person puckers the lips.

Abnormal reflex finding: The person blinks repeatedly after being tapped.

ND~X~

Documenting Reflex Examination Findings

The results of reflex testing may be documented by describing the type of movement noted when specific stimuli are applied to elicit a reflex. For example, you may describe a normal plantar reflex as follows:

> Toes flex following stroking sole of foot.

Deep tendon reflexes and plantar reflexes are more often described using a grading scale and diagram, as shown in Display 9-4.

ND~X~

Nursing Diagnoses Related to Reflex Assessment

Persons displaying abnormal reflexes may have neurologic dysfunctions or electrolyte imbalances. Generally,

---

DISPLAY 9.4

Documenting Reflexes

GRADING DEEP TENDON REFLEXES

Deep tendon reflexes are graded on a scale of 0 to 4:

   0 No response
   1+ Diminished (hypoactive)
   2+ Normal
   3+ Increased (may be interpreted as normal)
   4+ Hyperactive (hyperreflexia)

The deep tendon responses and plantar reflexes are commonly recorded on stick figures. The arrow points downward if the plantar response is normal and upward if the response is abnormal.

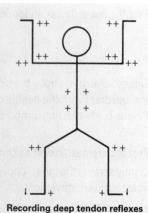

Recording deep tendon reflexes

these problems are not addressed by nursing diagnoses. However, the nurse should consider the types of responses (*e.g.,* anxiety) the person may be experiencing as a result of these problems. The response, rather than the neurologic deficit, becomes the focus when formulating nursing diagnoses related to reflex assessment.

Clinical Problems Related to Reflex Assessment

Reflex testing provides an indication of the status of the central nervous system in the conscious and unconscious person. Reflex responses may be helpful in distinguishing upper motor neuron and lower neuron pathologic conditions.

Damage to upper or lower motor neurons results in altered motor function; the examination findings and type of motor loss associated with each area differ (Table 9-3). Damage to upper motor neurons before decussation in the brain stem usually results in contralateral motor deficits, such as paralysis (hemiplegia) or weakness (hemiparesis). Upper motor neuron damage is also associated with hyperactive reflexes because inhibitory fibers are affected. Cerebral or brain stem dysfunction may result in complete loss of voluntary movements and abnormal reflex development or abnormal motor movements (see Table 9-3). Abnormal reflexes may include a positive Babinski reflex and grasp, snout, and glabellar reflexes. Although the exact mechanism is unclear, abnormal reflexes are believed to be primitive reflexes that are suppressed with nervous system maturation. Pathologic conditions may cause the primitive reflexes to reemerge.

Abnormal motor movements include decortication and decerebration. The clinical significance and assessment of these responses are discussed elsewhere in this chapter with the assessment of mental status using the Glasgow Coma Scale.

SENSORY SYSTEM AND CEREBELLAR FUNCTIONS

Anatomy and Physiology Review

The sensory function tests that are presented in this section provide information about primary or cutaneous sensation and cortical integration of sensory impulses. The structures involved include peripheral spinal nerves, spinal cord sensory pathways, the thalamus, and sensory areas of the cerebral cortex. In addition, cerebellar processing of proprioceptive stimuli is discussed.

The two main types of sensations include exteroceptive, which is caused by stimuli outside the body such as pain, temperature, and touch, and proprioceptive, which is caused by inner body stimuli, such as position, kinesthetic, and vibration sense and touch responses.

TABLE 9.3 *Features of Upper and Lower Motor Neuron Disorders*

Upper Motor Neuron

Spastic paralysis

Hyperactive reflexes

Muscle weakness without atrophy

Decorticate posturing (usually following brain hypoxia)

Possibly frequent urination with reflex bladder emptying (reflex bladder)

Lower Motor Neuron

Flaccid paralysis

Muscle atrophy

Muscle fasciculations

Absence of reflex responses

Possibly urinary retention with overflow incontinence (atonic bladder)

Peripheral Nerves and Dermatomes. Specialized sensory cells in the skin, joints, muscles, and bones detect and then transmit sensory stimuli through peripheral nerve fiber networks. Eventually, fibers join peripheral nerve pathways that enter the posterior portion of the spinal cord as the posterior nerve root. This is the afferent or sensory division of the peripheral nervous system.

Each posterior nerve root is associated with a peripheral sensory network that supplies a strip of skin called a *dermatome* (Fig. 9-6). Although dermatomes appear to have distinct boundaries, some overlap between adjacent dermatomes may exist.

Sensory testing involves applying stimuli to the person's skin surface. Dermatomes should be used to describe specific spinal sensory nerves being tested in comprehensive and specialized examinations. If impaired cutaneous sensation is detected, the examiner should test other areas within the same dermatome. If the entire dermatome is involved but surrounding dermatomes are unaffected, the examiner should suspect a lesion of the posterior nerve root supplying the dermatome, such as posterior nerve root compression secondary to herniated nucleus pulposus. The client may experience pain, tingling, or numbness throughout the dermatome for the affected root.

Dermatomes may be used to explain other sensory phenomena such as referred pain syndromes. For example, clients with ischemic heart pain may feel pain in the jaw, shoulder, and upper extremity as well as the chest. As shown in Figure 9-7, such pain occurs because somatic sensory nerve fibers from the heart have central connections in common with afferent nerve fibers that correspond with arm, shoulder, and jaw dermatomes.

Spinal Cord Sensory Pathways. Sensory impulses enter the spinal cord through the posterior nerve root and travel toward the brain along major spinal cord sensory pathways, most of which cross the midline at some point before reaching the cerebral cortex. Clinically significant as-

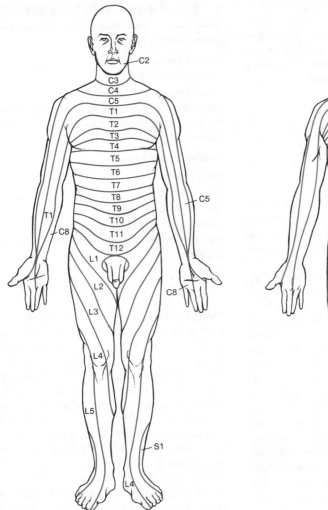
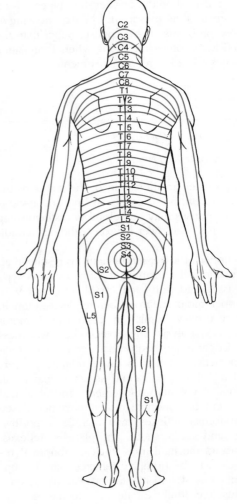

FIGURE 9.6 Dermatomes.

cending sensory pathways include the following (Fig. 9-8):

- *The posterior columns (fasciculus gracilis and fasciculus cuneatus):* Sensory fibers enter the posterior horn of the spinal cord and ascend uncrossed to the medulla. In the medulla, the fibers cross and ascend through the midbrain to the cerebral cortex. Sensations conducted along these pathways include vibratory sense, kinesthesia and proprioception, two-point discrimination, and tactile localization.
- *Lateral spinothalamic tract:* Sensory fibers enter the posterior horn and cross the midline at each segmental level of the cord before ascending toward the brain. Sensations conducted along this pathway include pain and temperature.
- *Anterior spinothalamic tract:* Fibers enter the posterior horn and cross the midline at each segmental level of the cord before ascending toward the brain along a route slightly anterior to the lateral spinothal-

amic tract. Sensations conducted along this pathway include light touch, pain, pressure, and temperature.
- *Posterior and anterior spinocerebellar tracts:* Fibers enter the posterior horn and ascend to the cerebellum, which senses proprioceptive stimuli influencing muscle tone and synergy. Cerebellar sensation impairment affects posture and coordination. Fibers of the ascending dorsal tract do not cross the ventral tract.

Contralateral and ipsilateral sensory deficits can be considered on the basis of sensory tract midline crossings and the location of the causative lesion. A spinothalamic tract lesion located above the crossing point within the spinal cord may cause contralateral sensory losses. For example, a cerebral infarct, causing damage to one side of the sensory cortex, may cause the person to have sensory loss on the opposite side of the body. If the spinothalamic tract is damaged within the spinal cord at the crossing

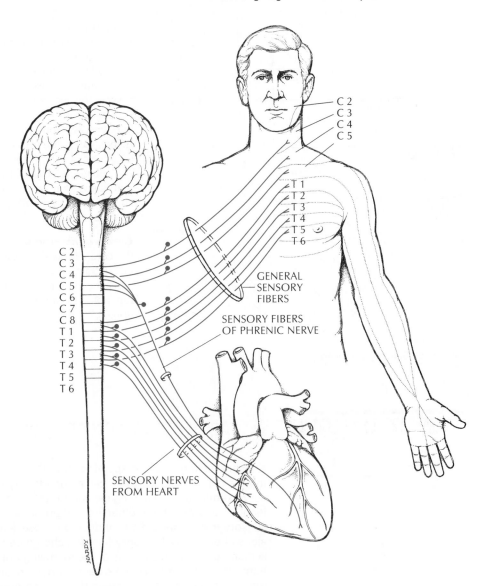

FIGURE 9.7   Referred pain from the heart. (Capell, P.T., & Case, D.B. [1976]. *Ambulatory care manual for nurse practitioners.* Philadelphia: J.B. Lippincott)

point, sensory losses may occur at the dermatome for the affected cord segment. A cord lesion that affects the posterior pathways below the crossing point in the medulla may cause ipsilateral loss of proprioceptive sensations. Because touch is both an exteroceptive and proprioceptive sensation and has alternate pathways to the brain, touch sensation may remain intact after spinothalamic tract lesions.

Thalamus. The thalamus, located in the lower inner portion of the brain, functions as a relay station for sensory and motor impulses traveling to and from the cerebral cortex and plays a role in consciousness and alertness. Incoming sensory stimuli are processed in the thalamus, but conscious interpretation of sensory stimuli, other than pain, does not occur at this level. The thalamus may facilitate cerebral interpretation of sensory stimuli by selectively masking or unmasking cerebral sensory receptive areas and delivering sensory input to the appropriate area

of the cerebral cortex. Olfactory stimuli are the only sensory input that bypass the thalamus.

One type of sensory distortion, known as "thalamic pain," may occur secondary to lesions of the posterior nuclei in the thalamus. The person experiencing such pain may not perceive single sensory stimuli such as light touch (pinpricks). However, repetitive or vigorous stimuli may cause considerable discomfort. Thalamic pain is usually more intensified when the offending stimuli occur in addition to unpleasant emotions.

Sensory Cerebral Cortex. The cerebral cortex, or gray matter at the outer surface of the cerebral hemispheres, is referred to as the sensorimotor cortex because both sensory and motor impulses are processed by cortex neurons.

Brodman divided the cerebral cortex into 47 different areas, correlating functional relations with anatomic locations (Fig. 9-9). Tactile sensations are perceived in the area over the parietal lobe or Brodman's areas 1, 2, and 3.

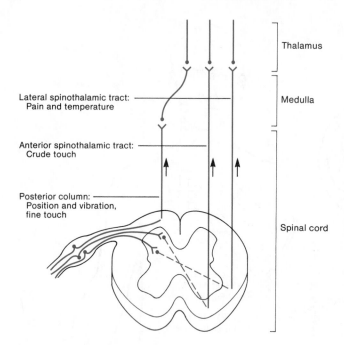

FIGURE 9.8 Sensory pathways.

Besides perceiving sensations, the gray matter makes distinctions between degrees of touch, temperature, vibration, and pain.

Brodman's area 5, a somatic association area, formulates primary sensory stimuli such as tactile sensation into object images and then identifies such images. This process of knowing (or *gnosis*) involves comparing present sensory input with past experience. For example, somatic association areas must be activated when identifying a familiar object on the basis of touch.

Damage to any of these sensory areas may affect primary sensation or the person's abilities to recognize sensory stimuli (agnosia). Sensory examination shows associated deficits.

Cerebellum. Proprioceptive sensory impulses are sent to the cerebellum along the posterior and anterior spinocerebellar tracts. Cerebellar processing of such stimuli maintains coordination, posture, and balance. These cerebellar functions should be tested as part of the sensory examination.

Physical Examination Sensory System and Cerebellar Functions

GENERAL PRINCIPLES

Sensory testing involves applying stimuli to the person's skin surface and noting the person's ability to perceive and identify the stimulus. A complete sensory examination, involving sensation testing over the entire skin surface, is lengthy, and may tire the person and produce unreliable findings. Therefore, sensory testing should be conducted to assess major dermatomes, and conclusions about overall sensory function should be formed accordingly. For gross screening, test skin surfaces at the following areas: foot, lower leg, abdomen, hand, forearm, and face. If no sensory dysfunctions are suspected, fewer areas may be tested. Always compare the left and right sides of the body.

(continued)

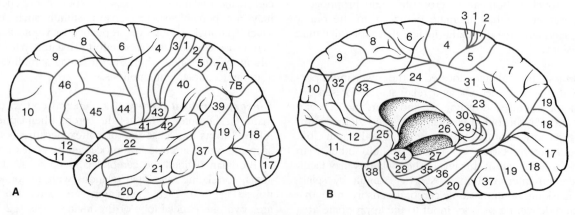

FIGURE 9.9 Brodman's areas. **(A)** Lateral surface. **(B)** Medial surface.

Physical Examination   Sensory System and Cerebellar Functions (continued)

Persons requiring more extensive sensory testing include those who are experiencing rapidly increasing sensory loss, such as occurs with Guillain-Barré syndrome. In such cases, sequential dermatomes should be tested to determine the exact level of sensory deficits. More thorough assessment is also indicated for patients who report numbness, pain, or motor deficits and who have trophic skin changes such as hairless, thin, or shiny skin.

When testing sensation in a particular region, apply the stimulus in a distal-to-proximal manner, such as toes to foot to ankle. Sensation at the most distal site usually indicates that the corresponding spinal nerve tract is intact and precludes further testing within a dermatome. When a sensory deficit exists, you can pinpoint the exact level of dysfunction with distal-to-proximal testing.

EQUIPMENT

Sensory testing may be performed with the following stimuli:

- *Light touch:* Cotton wisps, soft brush, or fingertips
- *Pain:* Safety pin, needles (discard pin/needle after using), deep pressure applied by the examiner
- *Temperature:* Test tubes filled with hot and cold water
- *Vibration:* Tuning fork
- *Stereognosis:* Familiar objects, such as a key, comb, or pencil
- *Two-point discrimination:* Pins, needles, two-pronged caliper

MINIMIZING CUEING

Familiarize the person with each stimulus, such as cotton wisps, pinpricks, or the tuning fork, before the examination and then instruct the person to relax and close his or her eyes for the remainder of the examination. If visual cueing is allowed to occur, responses to tactile stimuli may be rendered invalid. Vary testing patterns and sequence so the person will not simply respond to a predictable pattern. Asking the person to identify a stimulus rather than asking whether the stimulus was felt can help eliminate suggestion. If a tuning fork is used to test vibration sense, eliminate audible vibratory noise by running the tap or turning on a radio.

EXAMINATION AND DOCUMENTATION FOCUS

- Ability to sense and discriminate light touch, pain, temperature, vibration
- Gnosis
- Proprioception and kinesthesia

▼ ▼ ▼
G U I D E L I N E S

A s s e s s m e n t   G u i d e l i n e s   Sensory System and Cerebellar Functions

Procedure

1. **Test light touch sensation.**
   a. Brush the person's skin with cotton, a soft brush, or your fingertips.
   b. Ask the person to identify the sensation and locate the stimuli (Where do you feel this?).

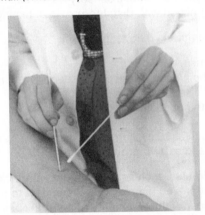

Testing light touch sensation

2. **Test superficial pain sensation and the ability to discriminate sharp and dull pain.**
   a. Alternatively apply a hypodermic needle point (sharp) and hub (dull) against the person's skin and ask the person to identify the stimulus.
   b. Use minimal pressure necessary to elicit a response, being careful not to pierce the skin.
   c. Pause several seconds between applying stimuli to allow the person to perceive each stimulus.

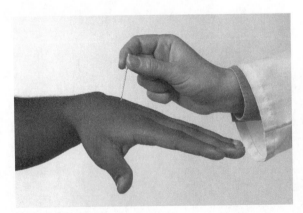
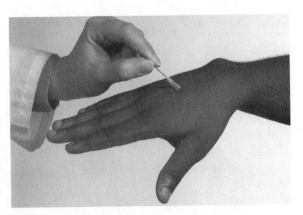

Testing pain sensation

Clinical Significance

Normal Findings
Identifies skin surface touched by the examiner. The ability to discriminate light touch may normally vary at different body areas. Symmetric areas should have comparable responses.

Hypodermic needles are preferred to sharp and dull ends of safety pins, because sterile needles minimize potential for transmitting infection.

Normal Findings
Person can distinguish sharp and dull pain sensations.

▼ ▼ ▼

G U I D E L I N E S *continued*   Sensory System and Cerebellar Functions

Procedure

3. **Test deep pain sensation.**
   a. Grasp a tendon such as the Achilles or biceps between your thumb and forefinger and squeeze hard enough to elicit feelings of pressure or pain.
   b. If the person is comatose, evaluate pain sensation by applying gradual pressure with a pen or reflex hammer handle over the finger or toe nail bed.

4. **Test temperature sensation (optional).**
   a. Test temperature sensation by alternately applying a test tube filled with warm water or cold water against the skin.
   b. Ask the person to identify whether the stimulus is warm or cold.

Clinical Significance

Intact sensory pathways will be indicated by facial grimace or decerebrate/decorticate posturing even when the patient is in a deep coma.

This test is unnecessary if pain sensation is within normal limits.

Normal Findings
Distinguishes warm and cold.

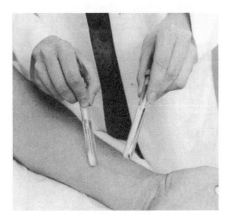

Testing temperature sensation

5. **Test vibration sensation.**
   a. Strike a tuning fork against your hand and apply the base to one of the person's bony prominences, such as the clavicles, sternum, finger joints, wrists, ankles, or toes.

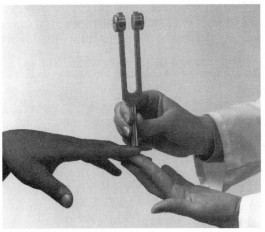

Testing vibration sensation

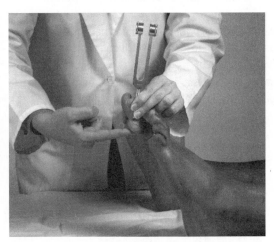

▼ ▼ ▼

Procedure

    b. Place your finger beneath the bony prominence if possible.

    c. Determine whether the person senses the tuning fork vibration while it occurs as well as when the vibration stops. Tell the person to respond "buzzing" when the vibration is sensed and "no" when sensing pressure only.

6. **Test joint position sense.**

    a. Begin testing joint position sense of the most distal joints: the toes and fingers. Grasp a toe or finger on the sides and move it up or down.

    b. If the person does not sense joint position of toes and fingers, test more proximal joints.

Clinical Significance

This enables you to feel the vibration and evaluate the accuracy of the person's response.

Normal Findings

Identifies the vibration starts and stops.

Normal Findings

The person should be able to identify each move, no matter how slight, by the word *up* or *down* relative to the previous stationary position.

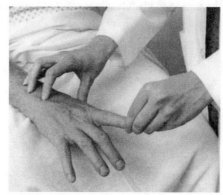

Testing joint position sensation

7. **Evaluate sensory association.**

    a. Evaluate *stereognosis.* Place a familiar object in the person's hand and ask the person to identify it by touch alone.

    b. Evaluate *topognosia.* Touch one of the person's fingers and ask the person to identify which one is being touched.

    c. Evaluate *graphognosia.* Trace a letter or number on the person's palm and ask the person to identify it.

Normal Findings

Gnosis: The ability to comprehend and recognize sensory stimuli.

The ability to identify familiar objects placed in either hand reflects the integrative functions of the parietal and occipital lobes.

Normal response: Client can identify which finger you are touching and whether it is on the left or right side of the body.

The ability to identify numbers indicates a functioning parietal node.

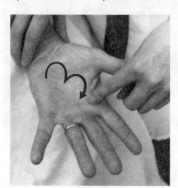

Testing graphognosis

▼ ▼ ▼

Sensory System and Cerebellar Functions

Procedure

Clinical Significance

8. **Check two-point discrimination.**

   Press two needles or two points of a caliper against the person's skin. Ask the person the number of needles being felt.

   Normal Findings

   Person can sense whether one or two areas of skin are being touched.

   Two points are discriminated at the following separations: fingertips, 2.8–5.0 mm; palms, 8–12 mm; dorsal surface of hand, 20–30 mm; chest and forearm, 40 mm; back, 40–70 mm; upper arms and thighs, 75 mm; shins, 30–40 mm.

9. **Evaluate cerebellar function.**

   a. *Finger-to-nose-to-finger test:* Ask the person to touch the index finger to the nose while eyes are closed. Alternatively, ask the person to touch his or her fingertip to your fingertip.

   Normal Findings

   Easily touches nose with finger when eyes are closed, and can touch fingertip.

   b. *Hand movements:* Ask the person to rapidly pronate and supinate the hands.

   Normal Finding

   Diadochokinesia: The ability to perform rapid alternating movements.

   Deviations from Normal

   Adiadochokinesia: Inability to perform rapid alternating movements.

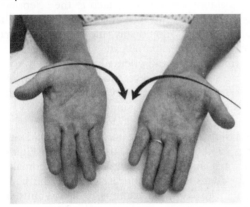

Testing cerebellar function

   c. *Romberg test:* Ask the person to stand with feet close together. First, while the person's eyes are open, note any swaying or difficulty in maintaining balance. Assist person with balance if necessary. Then ask the person to shut the eyes and note if the person moves.

   d. Evaluate gait (see Chap. 8, p. 344).

   Normal Findings

   Slight swaying is normal; if the person maintains balance, the Romberg test is negative.

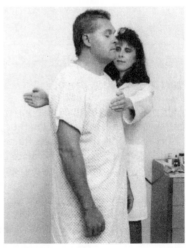

Romberg test

ND_X

Documenting Sensory and Cerebellar Functions

If the examination indicates that sensory and cerebellar functions are normal, document your findings as follows:

> Able to sense and discriminate light touch, pain, temperature, and vibration at major dermatomes. Position sense and two-point discrimination intact. Able to sense joint positions with eyes closed. Can identify objects placed in hand and can identify figure traced on hand. Able to alternate hand movements rapidly. Romberg negative.

Abnormal findings should be described in detail, noting the dermatome(s) affected, the type of stimuli applied to elicit a response, and an exact description of the abnormal response. Descriptive terms used to describe abnormal sensory responses include the following:

- *Anesthesia:* Anesthesia is the absence of sensation and may occur secondary to stroke in varying degrees. A stroke in the thalamic area of the brain may result in complete, contralateral anesthesia. Complete anesthesia is less likely with cerebral hemisphere stroke because alternate sensory pathways remain unharmed. Complete spinal cord transection or pressure from spinal cord tumors may cause incomplete anesthesia. For example, pain and temperature sensation may be lost on one side of the body below the lesion.
- *Paresthesia:* Paresthesia refers to abnormal and unpleasant sensations such as burning, tingling, and crawling, which may occur as a result of contact with sensory stimuli or may occur spontaneously. Paresthesia results from incomplete peripheral nerve damage caused by tumors or diseases such as diabetes mellitus.
- *Hypesthesia (hypoesthesia):* Hypesthesia refers to abnormally decreased sensitivity in the skin and is usually caused by partial damage to peripheral nerves.
- *Hypalgesia:* Hypalgesia refers to a decreased pain sensation.
- *Analgesia:* Analgesia refers to an absence of pain sensation. The person may still feel pressure or touch.

ND_X

Nursing Diagnoses Related to Sensory and Cerebellar Assessment

For persons displaying abnormal responses to sensory testing, the nurse should determine whether the nursing diagnosis Sensory–perceptual alterations (tactile) is applicable. If a tactile sensory–perceptual alteration is confirmed, you should then attempt to diagnose the person's response to any deficits. For example, persons with impaired tactile abilities may be at high risk for injury or tissue damage. Similarly, persons with cerebellar dysfunction also may be at risk for injury secondary to impaired balance or gait.

ND_X

Clinical Problems Related to Sensory and Cerebellar Assessment

Abnormal findings in response to testing sensory and cerebellar functions indicate dysfunction of the central or peripheral nervous system. Additional diagnosis and treatment is directed toward the underlying pathologic condition.

THE EYES AND VISION
Anatomy and Physiology Review

Eye Structures and Functions. The eyes are set in fat-cushioned skull orbits. Openings in the six bones composing each orbit allow the passage of blood vessels and nerves. The major posterior opening, the optic foramen, permits passage of the ophthalmic artery and optic nerve (cranial nerve II), which are visualized during funduscopic eye examination. Visual images are transmitted by the optic nerve to the occipital lobe of the cerebral cortex. Six extrinsic oculomotor muscles attach to the sclera near the anterior portion of the eyeball and facilitate eye movement and rotation. Additionally, the extrinsic eye muscles help maintain a normal conjugate gaze, meaning that both eyes are midposition and oriented in the same direction in the resting state. During eye examination, testing the extraocular eye movements and eye position will enable you to assess the muscles and cranial nerves III, IV, and VI (oculomotor, trochlear, and abducens).

The visible, external eye structures, including ductal openings of the lacrimal sac, are shown in Figure 9-10. The lacrimal apparatus comprises the lacrimal gland, which produces tears to lubricate the eye; the puncta, located lateral to the inner canthus, which drain tears into the lacrimal canaliculus; and the lacrimal sac.

The conjunctiva is membranous tissue covering the inner eyelids (palpebral conjunctiva) and the sclera of the eyeball (bulbar conjunctiva). Except for its most anterior portion, the eyeball is surrounded by a tough, fibrous layer of sclera. The limbus marks the point at which the sclera merges with the cornea, a transparent structure that allows light to enter the eye to stimulate the retinal rods and cones. The sclera becomes discolored or jaundiced from certain systemic diseases such as liver disease.

The pigmented iris surrounds the pupil. The pupil changes size as the iris sphincter and dilator muscles and the ciliary muscle beneath the sclera are stimulated. These muscles, called the intrinsic eye muscles, are innervated by cranial nerve III (oculomotor) and nerve fibers from the ciliary ganglion. Pupil size is determined by the balance between sympathetic and parasympathetic discharge. Alterations in pupillary reflexes and size may indicate oculomotor nerve impairment. Pupillary responses also may be affected by seizure activity and certain drugs.

The anterior chamber, a fluid-filled space, is located between the cornea and pupil. Intraocular pressure (normal, 20–25 mm Hg) is a function of fluid movement and

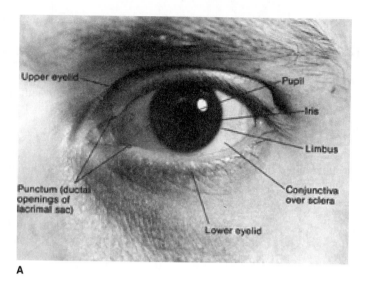

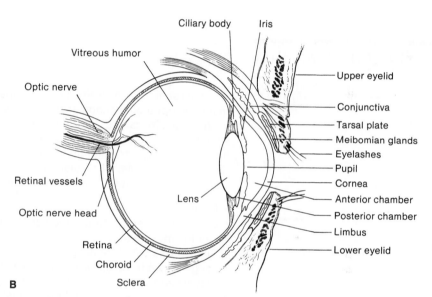

FIGURE 9.10   The eye. (A) Visible landmarks of the external eye. (B) Cross-section of the eye.

B

drainage through the anterior and posterior chambers. If the canal of Schlemm becomes blocked, fluid backup and increased pressure may damage the retina and optic nerve. This condition, glaucoma, may develop slowly and insidiously as a person ages. Intraocular pressure measurements are used to screen for and monitor glaucoma before irreversible damage occurs.

The crystalline lens, which bends incoming light rays to project them to the retina, is not readily visible by inspection. If the lens develops opacities or cataracts, whitened areas may be visible through the pupil. Such changes are seen best through the ophthalmoscope, an instrument for viewing internal eye structures.

The most frequently examined parts of the inner eye include the retina and related structures. The retina, the eye's innermost layer, receives light rays from the lens. Light must pass through the nine retinal layers before reaching the cones (daylight vision receptors), or rods (dim-light vision receptors), which initiate a neural impulse ultimately perceived by the brain as a visual image.

Several retinal structures can be noted when viewing

the optic fundus or the posterior eye wall through an ophthalmoscope. The retina itself is transparent. The orange-red coloration seen through the ophthalmoscope results from the underlying, highly vascularized choroid layer. The optic nerve leaves the retina through a site called the optic disc or the physiologic blind spot, thus named because it has no retinal neurosensory receptors. The optic disc is in the nasal quadrant of the fundus. The central depression in the disc is called the physiologic cup. Optic disc nerve tissues are continuous with brain nerve tissues. Consequently, brain swelling may be associated with visible disc swelling, a condition known as *papilledema.*

Also traveling through the optic disc are four sets of arterioles and veins, which bifurcate and extend toward the peripheral fundus. These retinal vessels are readily identifiable during examination. Systemic vascular changes, especially those resulting from hypertension and diabetes mellitus, may be detected by examining retinal vessels.

The retinal depression, or fovea centralis, is located adjacent to the optic disc in the temporal quadrant of the fundus. The macula surrounds the fovea. The macula, the most darkly pigmented area of the retina, is highly concentrated with cones and represents the area of most highly resolved central and color vision.

Visual Perception. Light rays pass through the refractive eye structures (cornea, aqueous humor, lens, vitreous humor) to the retina. Accommodation occurs when the lens becomes thicker or thinner according to light rays transmitted from near or distant objects. Visual deficits known as refractive errors are common in many individuals. Myopia (nearsightedness) occurs when light rays converge before reaching the retina because the anteroposterior diameter of the eyeball is greater than normal. As a result, visual acuity for distant objects is diminished. Hypermetropia (farsightedness) occurs when the anteroposterior eyeball diameter is shorter than usual, which causes light rays to scatter beyond the retina. Accommodation processes compensate for this refraction error when the person is focusing on distant objects, but close images are blurred as compensation fails. Refractive errors are detected during examination by visual acuity tests.

Retinal neurosensory receptors receive the image refracted through the lens, initiating a photochemical reaction and a neural impulse that travels the visual pathways to the occipital cerebral cortex.

Nerve fibers from the retina enter the optic nerves, which pass through the optic foramen and meet just anterior to the pituitary gland at the optic chiasm. The medial fibers from each eye cross at the chiasm, and fibers from the lateral retina continue toward the brain uncrossed. The manner in which the fibers cross has great clinical and assessment significance. Characteristics of a particular visual deficit may be analyzed to determine what part of the visual pathway has been affected.

Physical Examination   Eyes and Vision

GENERAL PRINCIPLES

The eyes should be examined using inspection and palpation. A special instrument, the ophthalmoscope, is used to inspect the interior ocular structures.

Visual acuity can be determined by special techniques that evaluate far vision, near vision, and peripheral vision. The equipment and procedures for testing visual acuity vary slightly, depending on characteristics of the person being tested. For example, when testing far or near vision in people who cannot read, appropriate substitutions are made for letter charts.

EQUIPMENT

- Penlight
- Cotton wisps and cotton-tipped applicators
- Ophthalmoscope
- Snellen Chart for far-vision testing.
- Jaeger Chart for near-vision testing; newsprint and telephone directory print may be substituted for Jaeger chart
- Occlusive covers for individual eye testing (3 × 5 card, paper cup, or commercially available shields, which must be disinfected between uses)
- Ishihara plates (optional; used to test color vision)

Ophthalmoscope

Although several different brands of ophthalmoscope are available, all have similar features. The handle usually contains batteries for the light source and can be unscrewed from the head and plugged into a wall socket for recharging. All models have a focus wheel to adjust the lens refraction. Initially, the focus is set on 0 diopters, meaning the lens neither converges nor diverges light rays. Depending on both your eyes and the client's, this setting should be adjusted to bring the fundus into sharpest focus. Then the focus wheel should be rotated toward positive numbers to bring near objects into focus. Some ophthalmoscopes have wheels for dialing different lens types. Generally, you will use the lens with the largest beam shining through clear glass. Slit-like beams and red glass are used during special examinations by the ophthalmologist. The ophthalmoscope is discussed further in Chapter 3.

HYGIENE

Wash your hands before palpating the external eye structures. If signs of infection are present in one eye, be careful not to cross-contaminate the other eye. In such a case, wash your hands before examining each eye, and examine the infected eye last.

(continued)

Physical Examination   Eyes and Vision (continued)

PUPIL DILATION

The pupils must be slightly dilated for you to view the interior eye with the ophthalmoscope. Generally, this condition is achieved by darkening the room. Short-acting, mydriatic eyedrops can be used, but it is important for several reasons to first consult a physician. Mydriatics dilate the pupil by inducing temporary cycloplegia (paralysis of the ciliary muscle). Accommodation reflexes also may be lost, and acute glaucoma may be precipitated in a susceptible person. Additionally, iatrogenic pupil dilation may obscure the significant neurologic assessment parameter of pupil size and reactivity.

EXAMINATION AND DOCUMENTATION FOCUS

- *External eye:* Symmetry, shape, eyebrows, eyelids, eyelashes, skin integrity, infestations
- *Lacrimal apparatus:* Lacrimal sac and gland, puncta, tears
- *Conjunctiva:* Palpebral and bulbar
- *Sclera, cornea,* and *iris*
- *Pupil:* Color, size, pupillary reflexes, retinal light reflex
- *Retina:* Color and pigmentation, vessels, macula, optic disc
- *Eye movements:* Conjugate gaze, extraocular eye movements
- *Visual acuity:* Snellen test results, Jaeger test results, peripheral vision, gross vision

▼ ▼ ▼

GUIDELINES

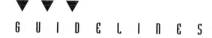

Assessment Guidelines   Eyes

Procedure

1. **Inspect the external eye structures.**

   a. Stand facing the client (who should be sitting on the examining table). Inspect the client's eyebrows, lashes, and eyelids, and note eye shape and symmetry.

   b. Observe blinking, noting whether there is complete closure of the lid. Note the eyeball position and any spontaneous eye movements.

Clinical Significance

Normal Findings

Eye shape and symmetry: Symmetry of the eyes and associated structures. Shape of the eyes varies from round to almond. In Asian persons, the skin fold over the inner canthus (the epicanthus) may cause eye shape to appear narrow. Eyes may appear rounded in some black persons because the eyeball protrudes slightly beyond the supraorbital ridge.

Eyebrows: Appearance may vary according to genetic background. No alopecia.

Eyelashes: Curve outward, away from the eye. No alopecia.

Eyelids: The upper lid does not cover the pupil when open, but may cover the upper portion of iris; eyelids should open and close completely without unilateral drooping or drag; spontaneous blinking should be observed every few seconds.

Deviations from Normal

See Display, "Structural Alterations and Disorders of the Eye."

2. **Inspect and palpate the lacrimal apparatus (optional).**

   a. Look at the punctal openings just lateral to the inner canthus. Gently stretch the bottom eyelids with your thumb to better expose puncta and use a penlight to enhance visualization.

Normal Findings

Puncta visible but without excessive discharge unless the person is crying or the area is momentarily irritated. Lacrimal sac and gland nonpalpable and nontender; eye surface moist.

Deviations from Normal

Excessive tearing

▼ ▼ ▼

G U I D E L I N E S *continued*   Eyes

Procedure   **Clinical Significance**

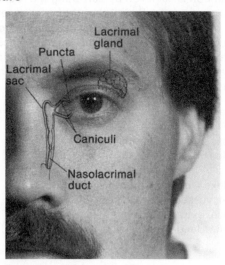
Lacrimal apparatus

b. If you suspect nasolacrimal duct blockage, indicated by excessive tearing, gently press over the duct with your index finger just inside the lower orbital rim. Note any discharge from the puncta. Proceed carefully, because the area will be sensitive if inflamed. Repeat for the other eye.

Deviations from Normal

Dacryoadenitis: Inflammation of the lacrimal gland. The upper, temporal eyelid may be swollen and red.

Dacrocystitis: Inflammation of the lacrimal sac. Associated with profuse tearing (epiphora), redness, swelling, and pain near the inner canthus. Dacrocystitis is associated with an obstructed nasal lacrimal duct, which may be congenital or acquired through trauma or infection.

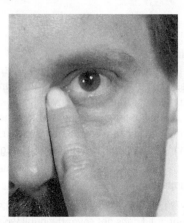
Lacrimal apparatus palpation.

3. **Inspect the lacrimal gland and upper palpebral conjunctiva (optional).**

a. Inspect the lacrimal gland by gently everting the upper lid. Ask the person to look downward with the eyes slightly open. Gently grasp the lid between your thumb and forefinger at the lid/eyelash junction. With your free hand, place a cotton-tipped applicator against the lower portion of the lid while pulling the eyelashes up to evert the lid. Be careful not to press the applicator against the eyeball.

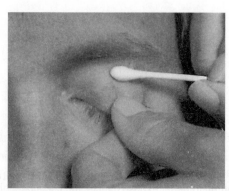
Eyelid eversion: Step a

▼ ▼ ▼
G U I D E L I N E S   *continued*   Eyes

Procedure

b. Move the cotton-tipped applicator away and hold the lid
   against the upper bony orbit to complete inspection.
   Note the small, visible portion of the lacrimal gland and
   at the same time, inspect the upper palpebral conjunctiva. Also note the appearance of exposed sclera.

Clinical Significance

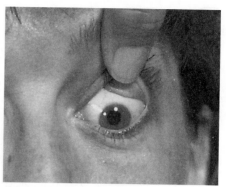
Eyelid eversion: Step b

c. Then, pull the lid lightly forward. The lid will resume
   normal position as you release and the person blinks.

d. Repeat this procedure on the other eye.

4. **Continue inspecting the inner conjunctiva.**

   Gently stretch the lower lid downward to see the lower palpebral conjunctiva. Note the appearance of the exposed
   sclera.

Normal Findings

Palpebral conjunctiva: Pink, moist, and without lesions. Small
vessels may be visible.

Sclera: White, pale yellow cast in some black persons.

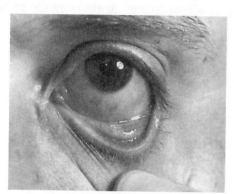
Lower palpebral conjunctiva inspection

5. **Inspect the remaining visible ocular structures.**

   Continue to note the appearance of the sclera. Use a penlight to tangentially illuminate the lens and cornea. Inspect
   from several angles, noting surface features and opacities.
   Note and compare iris shape and color, and pupil shape
   and size.

Normal Findings

Appearance of bulbar conjunctiva: Transparent, allowing white
sclera to show through. Small conjunctival blood vessels may
be visible but normally are not dilated (bloodshot eyes).

Cornea: Smooth, clear, transparent; convex curvature.

Iris: Color varies: blue, brown, gray, green with markings.
Shape is round.

6. **Evaluate extraocular eye movements (EOMs).**

   a. Instruct the person to follow your finger or pen with his
      or her eyes while keeping the head stationary. Move
      your finger or pen through the six cardinal fields of
      gaze, returning to the central starting point before point-
      ing toward the next field. Remember that if you move
      too quickly, the person may have difficulty following.

Tests the function of cranial nerves III, IV, and VI.

Normal Findings

Extraocular movements: Voluntary movement of eyes through
the six cardinal positions without nystagmus (involuntary cyclical movement of the eyeball). However, slight nystagmus
when the eyes are at the far lateral position of gaze is within
normal limits.

▼ ▼ ▼

G U I D E L I N E S   *continued*   Eyes

Procedure

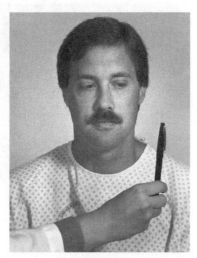

Assessing extraocular eye movements

b. When the person looks toward the most distal point in the lateral and vertical fields, carefully note eyeball movements for normal conjugate movements and nystagmus.

7. **Test for strabismus (cover–uncover test).**
   Ask the person to focus on your pen, which you should hold approximately 1 foot away, while you cover one of the person's eyes. Note any movement in the uncovered eye. As you remove the cover, note any movement in the other eye.

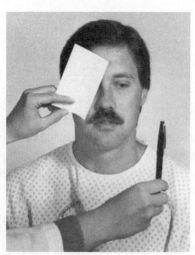

Strabismus testing

Clinical Significance

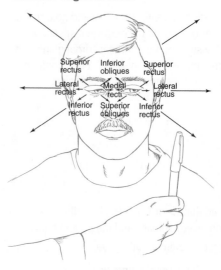

Normal Findings
Conjugate gaze: Eyes midposition when at resting position.

Normal Finding
The gaze remains on the pen during covering and uncovering, indicating good muscle strength.

OPHTHALMOSCOPIC EXAMINATION
Normal Findings
Red Reflex

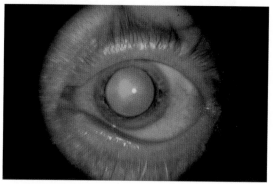

The red reflex is the orange-red coloration of the fundus that occurs when a small circle of light shines through the pupil. (Courtesy of Custom Medical Stock Photo, Inc. [Paula Ihnat])

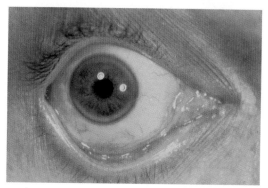

Arcus senilis is a grayish-white ring around the cornea that accompanies normal aging. In younger people it may be the result of hyper-lipoproteinemia. (Courtesy of Custom Medical Stock Photo, Inc. [1993, National Medical Slide Bank])

Common Abnormalities
Cataract

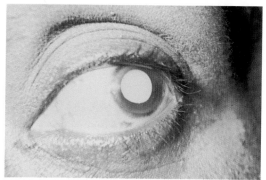

A cataract is a lens opacity that appears as a gray or white opaque coloration behind the pupil. The cataract will result in an absence of the red reflex. (Courtesy of Dr. William C. Byrne, OD, Optometric Eyecare Center, Fairless Hills, PA)

Chalazion

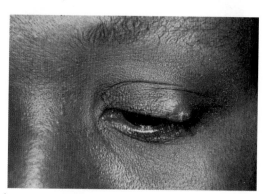

A chalazion is an eyelid mass that results from chronic inflammation of a meibomian gland. (Courtesy of Dr. William C. Byrne, OD, Optometric Eyecare Center, Fairless Hills, PA)

Normal Fundus: Blonde Person

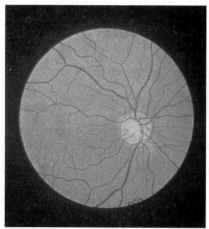

A lighter fundus is normal for a blonde. (Courtesy of American Optometric Association)

Normal Fundus: Brunette Person

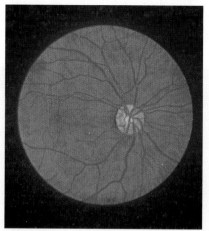

A darker fundus is typical for a brunette. (Courtesy of American Optometric Association)

Normal Fundus: Dark-Skinned Person

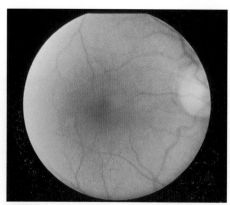

A much darker fundus is normal for a dark-skinned person. (Courtesy of Dr. William C. Byrne, OD, Optometric Eyecare Center, Fairless Hills, PA)

Papilledema

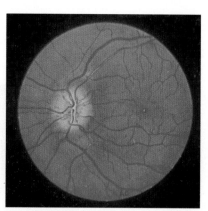

Papilledema is characterized by swelling of the optic disk that obscures the disk margins. The physiologic cup is no longer visible. This abnormality is caused by the venous stasis that occurs with increased intracranial pressure or hypertension. (Courtesy of American Optometric Association)

Hypertensive Retinopathy

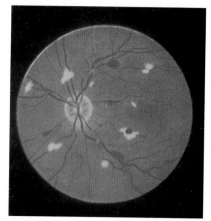

Hypertensive changes result in hemorrhages and bursting blood vessels in the fundus. (Courtesy of American Optometric Association)

Arteriosclerotic Retinopathy

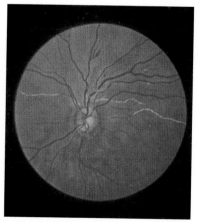

Arteriosclerosis can affect the fundal blood vessels, causing fatty deposits that appear as white streaks along the arteries. (Courtesy of American Optometric Association)

Diabetic Retinopathy

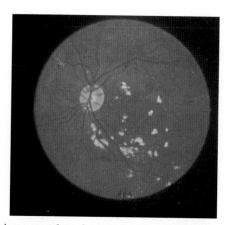

Diabetic changes result in characteristic waxy-looking retinal lesions, microaneurysms of the vessels, and hemorrhages. (Courtesy of American Optometric Association)

Solar Retinopathy

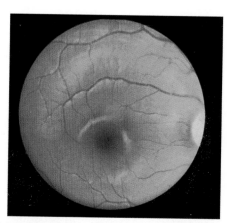

Solar retinopathy results from staring directly at the sun (as could happen when looking at an eclipse with the naked eye). (Courtesy of Dr. William C. Byrne, OD, Optometric Eyecare Center, Fairless Hills, PA)

Glaucoma

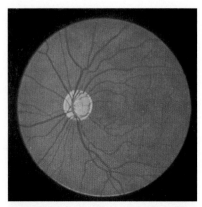

Glaucoma causes cupping of the optic disk when increased intraocular pressure is transmitted to the retina. The physiologic cup enlarges. (Courtesy of American Optometric Association)

Detached Retina

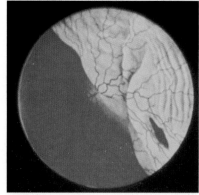

Retinal tears lead to cortical detachment as the vitreous fluid seeps through the hole to the subretinal space, pushing the retina away from the epithelium. (Courtesy of American Optometric Association)

OTOSCOPIC EXAMINATION

Normal Tympanic Membrane

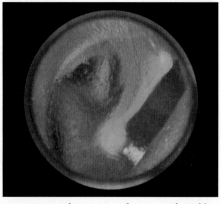

A normal tympanic membrane is pearly gray, with visible structures and light reflex. (Courtesy of Custom Medical Stock Photo, Inc. [1992, Childs])

Red, Bulging Tympanic Membrane

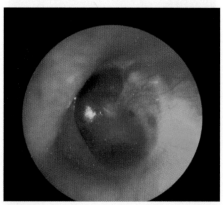

A bulging, red tympanic membrane obscures the typical landmarks, including the light reflex. It typically results from otitis media. (Courtesy of Custom Medical Stock Photo, Inc. [1991, Siu Biomed Comm])

▼ ▼ ▼
GUIDELINES *continued*   Eyes

Procedure	Clinical Significance

Procedure

8. **Evaluate pupillary reflexes.**

   a. *Pupillary light reflex.* Darken the room, or turn the person away from direct light sources. To obtain maximal pupil dilation, have the person focus on a distant object. Ask the person to cover one eye while you shine a light source from the side toward the pupil of the uncovered eye. Repeat testing with the other eye.

   b. *Consensual reaction.* Shine the light source toward one eye from the side and observe both pupils. Both should constrict despite the fact that light is directed toward one eye. The constriction of the eye that is not receiving the direct light is the consensual response.

   c. *Accommodation and convergence.* Hold your index finger approximately 2 feet from the person's eyes. Ask the person to focus on your index finger as you move it toward his or her nose. The person should be able to watch your finger as it moves.

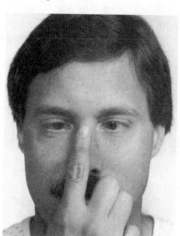

Testing accommodation and convergence

9. **Begin the ophthalmoscopic examination by visualizing the red reflex.**

   a. In a darkened room, instruct the person to look at a distant point and keep his or her eyes focused there throughout the ophthalmoscopic examination.

   b. Grasp the ophthalmoscope with your right hand when you are examining the person's right eye. Check to see that the lens is set at 0, and turn on the light source.

Clinical Significance

Normal Findings

Appearance of pupils: Black, of equal size, round. Five percent of the population have slight inequality in pupil size (anisocoria), which is considered clinically insignificant.

Light reflex: Pupils constrict directly and consensually.

Normal Findings

The pupils should constrict as you move the finger closer (accommodation) and the eyes should converge (cross).

Accommodation is necessary for far-to-near focusing.

Normal Findings

The *red reflex* is the orange-red coloration of the fundus visible through the pupil. (See color photo in this chapter.)

▼ ▼ ▼

G U I D E L I N E S *continued*   Eyes

Procedure

   c. Position yourself at arm's length from the person; to assist your stability, place your left thumb over the person's left eyebrow.

   d. From an angle about 15 degrees lateral to the person's line of vision, shine the ophthalmoscope toward the pupil of the right eye and look through the ophthalmoscope's viewing hole. Note the red reflex.

   e. As you continue to look through the viewing hole and focus on the red reflex, move toward the person until your forehead touches your thumb on the person's forehead.

10. **Inspect the anterior chamber, lens, and vitreous body.**
   Inspect the anterior chamber and lens for transparency. Visualization may be made easier by rotating the lens toward positive numbers (+15 to +20), which are designed to focus objects closest to the ophthalmoscope.

Clinical Significance

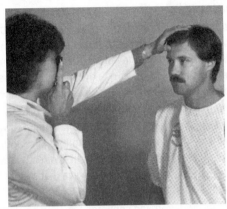

Ophthalmoscopic examination: Visualizing the red reflex

Deviations from Normal

Lens opacities (cataracts) may interfere with red reflex visualization. Cataracts appear as gray or white opacities, or may appear as black spots against the background of the red light reflex. Cataracts vary in size and configuration. (See color photo.)

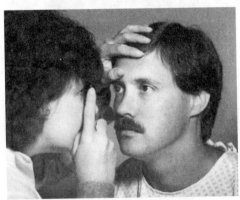

Ophthalmoscopic examination: Inspecting the anterior chamber, lens, and vitreous body

Deviations from Normal

Hyphemia: The appearance of blood in the anterior chamber, which usually results from eye trauma. The red blood cells may settle and cause only the lower half of the anterior chamber to appear bloody.

Hypopyon: The accumulation of white blood cells in the anterior chamber, which causes a cloudy appearance in front of the iris. Secondary to inflammatory response accompanying corneal ulceration or iritis.

▼ ▼ ▼
G U I D E L I N E S   *continued*   Eyes

| Procedure | Clinical Significance |

Procedure

11. Inspect the optic disc.

   a. Rotate the lens back to the 0 setting; then, focusing on a retinal structure such as a vessel or the disc, rotate the lens until you produce the sharpest focus.

   The final setting will vary according to the specific characteristics of your eye structure and the client's eye structure. If the client is myopic, the eyeball will be longer and a negative setting will enable you to focus further back. Use the positive settings to visualize across the shorter eyeball distance that is associated with farsightedness.

   b. If you do not see the optic disc, find a blood vessel and follow it in the direction in which the vessel thickens. This will lead you visually to the disc. Note that vessels have fewer bifurcations toward the disc.

   c. Once the disc is visible, refocus if necessary to obtain the sharpest definition.

12. Inspect the retinal vessels and retina.

   a. Evaluate the retinal vessels that are distributed from the disc to the periphery. Four sets of arterioles and veins pass through the disc.

   b. Systematically inspect the retinal vessels by moving your line of vision through major retinal quadrants, using the person's pupil as an imaginary fulcrum.

Clinical Significance

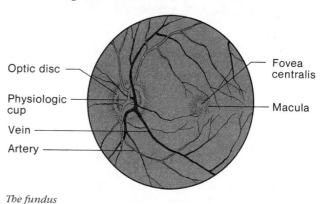

The fundus

Normal Findings

Optic disk: Round to oval with sharply defined borders; whitish or pink; 1.5 mm in diameter when magnified 15 times through ophthalmoscope. Physiologic cup is slightly depressed and lighter in color than the remainder of the disc; cup occupies half of disc diameter.

Deviations from Normal

Papilledema: Swelling of the optic disc that occurs secondary to the venous stasis accompanying hypertension or increased intracranial pressure. Swelling obscures the disc margins, and the physiological cup is no longer visible (see color photo).

Glaucomatous cupping of the optic disk: Occurs when increased intraocular pressure is transmitted to the retina. The physiologic cup enlarges, filling more than half the disc diameter (see color photo).

Normal Findings

Arterioles: Progressively smaller diameter away from optic disk; bright red with narrow light reflex; 25% smaller than veins; no narrowing or nicking.

Veins: Progressively smaller diameter away from optic disc; dark red, no light reflex; occasionally pulsatile.

A-V ratio: Arteriole-to-vein ratio in relation to vessel diameter (A-V ratio) is 2:3 or 4:5.

▼ ▼ ▼

G U I D E L I N E S *continued*   Eyes

Structural Alterations and Disorders of the Eye

Eye examination may reveal alterations or disorders of the external eye. Assessment includes determining if such alterations interfere with visual perception, comfort, or body image.

Exophthalmos

- The eyes appear to bulge with proptosis (downward eye displacement).
- Possible etiologies include cranial tumors and hyperthyroid disease.
- The condition may be detected by direct frontal inspection or by inspecting eye position while looking downward across the surface of the person's forehead.

Exophthalmos

Enophthalmos

- A sunken eye appearance.
- May occur secondary to dehydration or following fracture of the orbital floor.

Ptosis

- Drooping of the upper eyelid.
- The most common causes include oculomotor nerve dysfunction (cranial nerve III) or sympathetic nerve dysfunction.
- May also be congenital.

Ptosis

Epicanthal folds

- Characteristic of certain races, such as Asian persons.
- Also noted in persons with Down's syndrome (trisomy 21).

Ectropion

- Marked eversion of the edge of the eyelid.
- The palpebral conjunctiva is exposed and susceptible to drying.
- If the punctum of the lower lid turns out, the eye no longer drains satisfactorily, and excessive tearing occurs.
- Ectropion may occur after scar formation or secondary to muscle weakness.
- More often occurs in elderly persons.

Ectropion

Entropion

- Inward turning of the eyelid.
- May be associated with *trichiasis,* or eyelash contact with the conjunctiva and cornea.
- Usually painful.
- Causes are the same as for ectropion.

Entropion

Blepharitis

- Infection along the lid margins.
- Usually caused by *Staphylococcus aureus,* seborrhea, or a combination of both.
- The lid margins appear reddened and yellowish.
- Greasy scales may be noted.

Stye

- An infection occurs in the glands around the eyelash hair follicles.
- Associated with localized pain, swelling, and redness.
- A pustule usually forms on the eyelid margin.

Stye

Chalazion (see color photo)

- Infection of the meibomian gland.
- Usually caused by *S. aureus.*
- Swelling and redness occur.
- No pustule formation.
- May be painless.

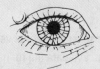
Chalazion

(continued)

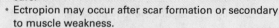

▼ ▼ ▼

G U I D E L I N E S   *continued*   Eyes

Structural Alterations and Disorders of the Eye (continued)

Narrow Angle Glaucoma

- Associated with an anatomically shallow anterior chamber.
- Signs and symptoms include diffuse eye redness, pain, blurred vision, cornea clouding, moderate pupil dilation, and elevated intraocular pressure (40 mm Hg or more).

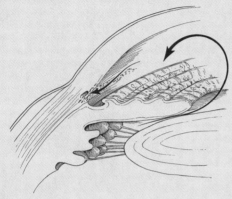

Normal flow

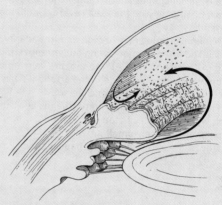

Narrow-angle glaucoma

Open Angle Glaucoma

- The size of the anterior chamber remains normal.
- The diagnosis is based on measuring intraocular pressure, which is usually elevated.

Diabetic Alterations

- Vascular changes associated with diabetes mellitus may contribute to funduscopic changes, including:
- Round and flame-shaped retinal hemorrhages
- Venous dilation
- Microaneurysms
- Retinal detachment
- Neovascularization

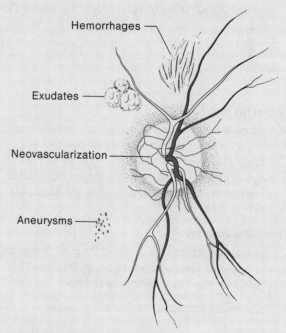

Diabetic alterations of the fundus

(continued)

▼ ▼ ▼

G U I D E L I N E S *continued*   Eyes

Structural Alterations and Disorders of the Eye (continued)

Hypertensive Alterations

The retinal vessels and retinal background may be altered by hypertension. The Keith-Wagner (KW) classification system may be used to describe the severity and prognosis of the hypertension based on retinal changes. KW classifications, beginning with the least severe conditions are as follows:

- *KW1:* Minimal arteriolar narrowing and irregularity.
- *KW2:* Marked arteriolar narrowing and arteriovenous nicking (AV nicking). With AV nicking, the vein appears to stop abruptly on either side of the arteriole. This finding also indicates arteriosclerotic changes.
- *KW3:* Flame-shaped or round hemorrhages and fluffy "cotton wool" exudates noted on the retina. Cotton wool patches represent small infarcts.
- *KW4:* Any of the above signs plus papilledema.

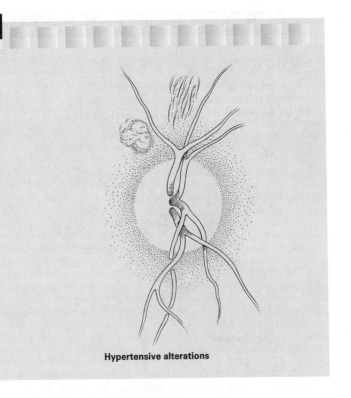

Hypertensive alterations

Procedure

c. Note any underlying retinal lesions as you inspect each quadrant. Also note the crossing points of arterioles and veins.

13. **Inspect the macula.**

Ask the person to look directly into the ophthalmoscope light. Find the macula, which is temporal from the disc. The fovea, the center of the macula, should be approximately two optic disc diameters from the optic disc border. The macula may be difficult to see if the person's pupil is not sufficiently dilated.

14. **Assess the other eye.**

To examine the person's left eye, hold the ophthalmoscope in your left hand. Place your right hand on the person's forehead and repeat the examination sequence.

Clinical Significance

Normal appearance of retina: The retina is transparent, but the diffuse orange-red color of the choroid layer shows through; pigmentation may be darker in black persons. Spotty color alterations such as white patches may be abnormal.

Deviations from Normal
See Display, "Structural Alterations and Disorders of the Eye," and color photo.

Normal appearance: Darker than the surrounding fundus; relatively avascular.

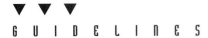

GUIDELINES

Assessment Guidelines   Testing Visual Acuity

Procedure

1. **Test far vision using a Snellen chart or a comparable standardized chart.**

Clinical Significance

The Snellen charts in the center and at right (*below*) may be more appropriate for testing illiterate adults and very young children.

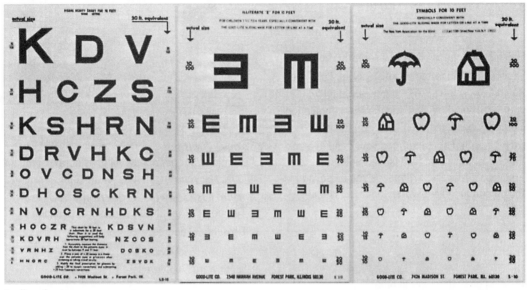

Snellen charts

a. The person should stand 20 feet from the chart in a well-lit area. The person may wear corrective lenses.

Ask the person to cover one eye with a shield while you test the other eye.

b. Ask the person to read the letters as you point to progressively smaller print. Note the last line that the person reads accurately.

c. Report vision acuity as a fraction, such as 20/20. The numerator indicates in feet the distance the person stood from the chart. The denominator indicates the distance at which the normal eye can read the line of letters. (This figure is printed next to each line of letters or figures on the chart.)

If the person wears glasses during testing, note that on the report. Record, for example, "20/30, corrected."

d. Repeat the testing procedure for the other eye.

2. **Test near vision using a Jaeger chart or an appropriate substitute.**

a. Screen near vision acuity by asking the person to read from a Jaeger chart held 12 to 14 inches from the eyes.

b. If a Jaeger chart is not available, ask the person to read from a newspaper or a telephone directory.

Reading glasses should not be worn because they distort far vision.

Covering the eye with the fingers is unreliable because of the possibility of looking through the fingers.

Normal Findings

Normal visual acuity: 20/20 vision (with or without corrective lenses).

Deviations from Normal

Nearsightedness: A larger denominator indicates impaired far vision. For example, if the person's vision is 20/100, this means that he or she needed to be as close as 20 feet to read what the person with normal vision would be able to read at 100 feet.

Normal Finding

Able to read Jaeger chart or newsprint at 12 to 14 inches.

Deviations from Normal

Farsightedness: Inability to focus on near objects due to impaired accommodation of the eye.

▼ ▼ ▼
G U I D E L I N E S *continued*

Testing Visual Acuity

Procedure

Clinical Significance

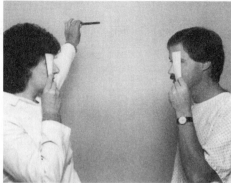

Peripheral vision testing

3. **Test visual fields (peripheral vision) by confrontation.**
   a. Face the person being tested at a distance of 2 or 3 feet.
   b. Ask the person to cover his or her left eye while you cover your right eye. Both you and the client should look at each other's uncovered eye.
   c. Fully extend your left arm and bring your hand in along the main axes of the visual field (superior, inferior, temporal, and nasal). Move your finger as you do so, and instruct the person to indicate when the finger is first seen.

Normal Findings
Assuming your peripheral vision is normal, you and the client should see your finger at the same time.

Normal Visual Fields by Confrontation
- Temporal: extends 90 degrees from midline
- Upward: 50 degrees
- Nasalward: 60 degrees
- Downward: 70 degrees

   d. Repeat testing procedure on the other eye.

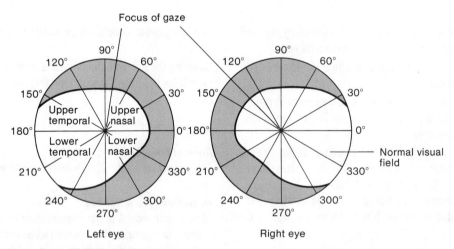

Normal visual fields by confrontation

4. **Test color vision.**
   Ask the person to view Ishihara plates or another color test.

Normal Finding
Able to discriminate and correctly identify different colors.

DISPLAY 9.5

Eye Examination: Common Abbreviations

AV: Arteriovenous crossings in the retina
EOM: Extraocular eye movement
IOP: Intraocular pressure
J₃: Jaeger chart 3 print (print in phone book)
J₅: Jaeger chart 5 print (print in newspaper)
OD: Right eye (oculus dexter)
OS: Left eye (oculus sinister)
OU: Both eyes (oculus uterque)
PERLA: Pupils equal, react to light and accommodation
PERRLA: Pupils equal, round, react to light and accommodation

cc: With correction (wearing glasses or contact lenses)
sc: Without correction (without wearing glasses or contact lenses)
FC: Finger counting (indicates visual acuity—can client discern number of fingers held up by examiner?)
HM: Hand movement (indicates visual acuity—can client discern examiner's hand movements?)
LP: Light perception (indicates visual acuity—can client discern light from dark?)

ND_X

Documenting Eye Examination Findings and Visual Acuity

The results of a normal eye examination (not including visual acuity testing) may be recorded as follows:

External eye structures symmetric, without lesions. Palpebral conjunctiva pink, moist; sclera white without injection. PERLA. Lens clear. EOMs intact and red reflex intact. Lacrimal apparatus nontender to palpation. Funduscopic exam shows A-V ratio 2:3, round disc with sharp borders; no fundal lesions.

Examination findings are often recorded using abbreviations such as those shown in Display 9-5. Results of visual acuity testing may be recorded on appropriate forms

or flowsheets or by using a method such as the one presented in Display 9-6.

ND_X

Nursing Diagnoses Related to Eye and Vision Assessment

Sensory–Perceptual Alteration: Visual

A person's vision may be altered by numerous factors. Some alterations, such as myopia or hyperopia, are relatively benign and do not significantly affect a person's sensory–perceptual abilities if corrective lenses are prescribed and used. Other alterations, such as those that occur with advancing age or secondary to a pathologic

DISPLAY 9.6

Documenting Visual Acuity

DOCUMENTATION	INTERPRETATION
R: 20/200, J₁, s̄c L: 20/100, J₁, s̄c	*Example 1:* Snellen testing indicates 20/200 (right eye) and 20/100 (left eye) when tested without corrective lenses (s̄c). Able to read Jaeger size 1 print (both eyes).
R: 20/20, J₁, c̄c L: 20/20, J₁, c̄c	*Example 2:* Snellen testing indicates 20/20 (right eye) and 20/20 (left eye) when tested with corrective lenses (c̄c). Able to read Jaeger size 1 print with both eyes.
R: FC, HM, LP	*Example 3:* Able to see finger counting (FC), hand movement (HM), and has light perception (LP) with the right eye. No indication in this example of whether corrective lenses were used.

condition such as a stroke, may cause permanent changes in visual perception. Altered visual perception may contribute to loss of functional abilities such as the ability to drive, and may increase a person's risk for physical injury, social isolation, or disorientation.

Environmental or situational factors also may contribute to altered visual perception. For example, a person's position in bed, especially if the person is immobile, may be the sole factor determining his or her visual field. If, for prolonged periods, the person sees only the ceiling, bedrails, or partial views of care providers, sensory input may lose meaning, placing the person at greater risk for sensory deprivation or overload. This situation is especially likely to occur if the person cannot wear his or her corrective lenses. In addition, you should consider the visual overload that may result from excessive glare in a person's surroundings. Elderly people are especially at risk for visual alterations from glare.

Nursing diagnoses are usually formulated to describe the problems the person experiences as a result of visual alterations. For example, rather than the nursing diagnosis Sensory–perceptual alterations: visual, it might be more helpful to diagnose the person's responses such as Potential for injury or Self-care deficit.

Clinical Problems Related to Eye and Vision Assessment

Visual Field Defects Caused by Alterations in Neural Pathways

The visual neural pathways may be pathologically altered by tumors, trauma, infectious diseases, and cerebrovascular accidents. Lesions along the visual neural pathways may result in partial or complete visual losses, depending on the location of the lesion (Fig. 9-11):

- *Unilateral blindness* may be caused by a lesion of one of the optic nerves.
- *Bitemporal hemianopsia* may be caused by lesions at the optic chiasm.
- *Left (or right) homonymous hemianopsia* may be caused by lesions at the right (or left) optic tract.

A person's perception of his or her surroundings will be affected by these changes. With bitemporal hemianopsia, for example, peripheral vision is impaired.

Visual Field Defects Caused by Alterations in Eye Structures

Many alterations in eye structures are associated with increasing age. The cornea may lose translucency, so that more light is required to produce an image on the retina; the sclera may lose opacity, permitting stray light rays to enter the eye and wash out visual images; "floaters," or black spots, may appear in the vitreous humor, distorting visual perception; pupils may dilate more slowly, requiring more time to adapt from light to darker environments. Such alterations may be permanent.

Pathologic alterations in eye structures also may affect visual perception. For example, black spots in the visual field may be an early sign of retinal detachment. As retinal detachment progresses, the person may describe a "black curtain" falling over the visual field. Blind spots or scotomas may occur in the visual field secondary to macular degeneration and glaucoma.

THE EARS AND HEARING
Anatomy and Physiology Review

External Ear. The external ear includes the auricle and external auditory meatus (Fig. 9-12). The auricle, which is curved to receive sound waves, includes the helix, auricular tubercle, antihelix, antitragus, concha, tragus, and lobe. The external auditory meatus (or ear canal) is about 1 inch long and ends at the tympanic membrane, the border between the external and middle ear (Fig. 9-13). The ear canal is curved slightly but may be straightened by gently pulling the auricle up and backward. Cerumen (ear wax) is secreted into the ear canal and may accumulate into a hardened brownish-black plug. The ear canal is supplied by many nerve endings and is extremely sensitive to touch, an important fact to remember during the examination.

The tympanic membrane, or eardrum, is a fibrous, mobile tissue that forms the junction between the external and middle ear. Sound waves entering through the external ear cause the tympanic membrane to vibrate, which in turn transmits sound frequencies to the auditory ossicles of the middle ear.

Middle Ear. The middle ear is a bony cavity within the temporal bone that opens directly to the eustachian tube. The middle ear contains three ossicles or bones (the malleus, incus, and stapes) and mastoid air cells. Except for the imprint of the malleus on the tympanic membrane, the structures of the middle ear are not visible during examination. Vibrations from the tympanic membrane are transmitted and amplified along the ossicles, which join the oval window of the inner ear. The mastoid air cells are air-filled spaces in the temporal bone that communicate with the middle-ear cavity and are lined with mucous membranes. These membranes can become inflamed by organisms transmitted from the upper respiratory tract through the eustachian tube, which connects the middle ear and the nasopharynx. When air enters the eustachian tube, air pressure on both sides of the tympanic membrane is equalized.

Inner Ear. The inner ear consists of the bony labyrinth, the semicircular canals, and the membranous labyrinth. The functions of the inner ear include hearing and equilibrium.

The bony labyrinth is the outer area of the inner ear and contains the vestible, cochlea, and semicircular canals. The membranous labyrinth, the inner area lining the bony labyrinth, contains the canals that transmit sound waves from the oval window. Semicircular canals maintain equilibrium; the utricle and saccule within the inner ear permit an individual to sense changes in gravity and linear

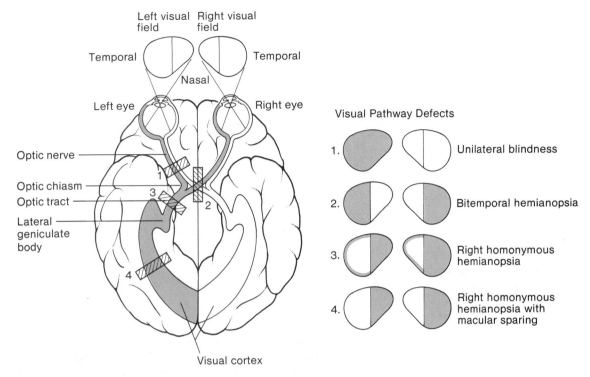

FIGURE 9.11 Visual pathways. Lesions at the numbered points correspond to the visual field defects shown on the right.

acceleration. Auditory sensations are transmitted from the cochlea, which contains sensory cells, to the temporal lobe of the cerebral cortex by the cochlear division of cranial nerve VIII (acoustic). Position sensation is transmitted along the vestibular portion of the same cranial nerve.

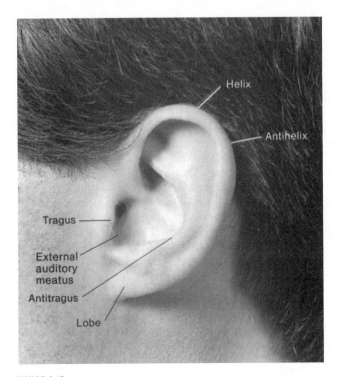

FIGURE 9.12 The external ear.

Hearing Pathway. Sound waves must be conducted to the inner ear before sensory impulses are transmitted to the auditory areas of the cerebral cortex. This can be accomplished by means of air conduction or bone conduction; air conduction is more efficient. In air conduction, sound waves reach the external ear and travel the external canal to the tympanic membrane. The sound waves cause tympanic membrane vibration, which in turn vibrates the ossicles. The oval window vibrates, causing the inner ear fluid to move. This movement affects the basilar membrane of the organ of Corti, which is then activated. When bone conducts sound waves, the organ of Corti is activated, but bone sound waves must be more intense than those required for air conduction.

The neural component of hearing begins at the organ of Corti as the mechanical energy from sound waves is converted to an electrical or neural impulse. Nerve fibers in the cochlear branch of cranial nerve VIII are activated, carrying afferent impulses to the cerebral cortex. Many alternate afferent pathways carry auditory stimuli. Therefore, damage to a single neural pathway will not necessarily cause complete hearing loss.

Equilibrium. The functions of the inner ear are to maintain equilibrium and head position and to direct eye gaze. The three semicircular canals are oriented at right angles in three planes and have specialized cells capable of detecting movement in each plane. These sensations of movement are transmitted to the cerebellum, which rapidly initiates the skeletal muscle movements required to maintain balance and coordination.

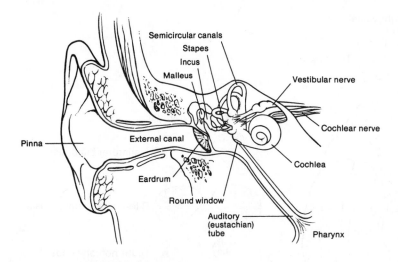

FIGURE 9.13 The middle and inner ear.

Physical Examination   Ears and Hearing

GENERAL PRINCIPLES

The ears should be evaluated by inspection and palpation. The otoscope is used to visualize internal ear structures. Equilibrium, a function of the inner ear, is evaluated as a component of the sensory examination (see pp. 418-421).

A person's hearing acuity may be evaluated during the physical examination by means of gross screening techniques such as observing the ability to hear the ticking of a watch and whispered voice sounds. Additionally, some tests enable you to evaluate the status of the conductive and sensorineural sound pathways. Additional inferences may be made about hearing by observing a person's responses to conversation and instructions. For example, note whether the person must face you to comprehend verbal instructions; this could indicate that he or she is lip reading.

If you identify hearing deficits, refer the person for specialized audiometry testing.

EQUIPMENT

• Otoscope
• Watch (ticking)
• Tuning fork

Otoscope

The otoscope is used to illuminate and inspect the ear canal and tympanic membrane. Although different brands vary, most otoscopes have handles that contain batteries for the light source, a switch for turning on the light, a viewing window, and examining tips that can accommodate differently sized specula (disposable or nondisposable). Choose the largest speculum that can be inserted into the ear without causing pain. Reusable specula need to be thoroughly disinfected. Some otoscopes handles may be unscrewed from the head and plugged into a wall socket to recharge batteries.

A pneumatic otoscope is used to determine the mobility of the tympanic membrane. A rubber bulb is attached to the otoscope, and the examiner squeezes it while visualizing the tympanic membrane. The squeezing action injects air, which normally causes the tympanic membrane to move in and out. Loss of tympanic membrane mobility is associated with middle-ear infection.

Tuning Forks

Tuning forks are used to test for conductive and sensorineural hearing losses. Differently sized tuning forks generate different sound frequencies. Usually, a tuning fork of 512 or 1024 Hz is used in examinations because the human ear can detect frequencies ranging from 300 to 3,000 Hz. The frequency number is usually engraved on the instrument.

(continued)

Physical Examination   Ears and Hearing (continued)

Activate the tuning fork by grasping its stem and striking the ends against your hand or other surface. Hold the instrument by the stem to avoid damping the vibration.

CERUMEN REMOVAL

Normally, cerumen dries and falls out of the ear. However, accumulation and impaction may occur if the ear canal is tortuous or extremely hairy. Attempts to remove cerumen with cotton-tipped applicators may be irritating and may push cerumen further into the ear canal. Cerumen impaction is diagnosed on the basis of symptoms such as feelings of fullness in the ear, tinnitus, and reports of hearing loss (conductive). In such cases, the initial otoscopic inspection will show a large amount of hardened, dark-brown wax. Cerumen impaction interferes with the ability to hear and with visualization of the tympanic membrane, and it may need to be removed by irrigation. However, irrigation is contraindicated if there is a history of eardrum perforation.

Before irrigating the ear, apply protective toweling to the shoulder and neck area. An irrigating syringe is filled with lukewarm water, because cold water may cause dizziness. The tip of the syringe is positioned just inside the ear canal and pointed toward the upper canal wall (Fig. 9-14). This position allows the irrigating fluid to accumulate behind the cerumen and eventually push it from the ear canal. The ear canal can be straightened by gently pulling upward and back on the auricle; irrigating fluid is injected repeatedly until the cerumen mass is dislodged. Discontinue irrigation if any pain or dizziness occurs. An emesis basin may be used to collect the irrigating fluid that will drain from the ear. If the cerumen is not dislodged by irrigation, an earwax-softening solution such as glycerin is applied for several days before the procedure is reattempted.

EXAMINATION AND DOCUMENTATION FOCUS

* *External ear:* Shape, size, position, skin integrity, response to palpation of the mastoid bone and tragus
* *External auditory meatus (ear canal):* Patency, discharge, inflammation, hair growth, cerumen
* *Tympanic membrane:* Color, surface characteristics, landmarks, light reflex, configuration
* *Hearing acuity:* Gross hearing, Weber test results, Rinne test results

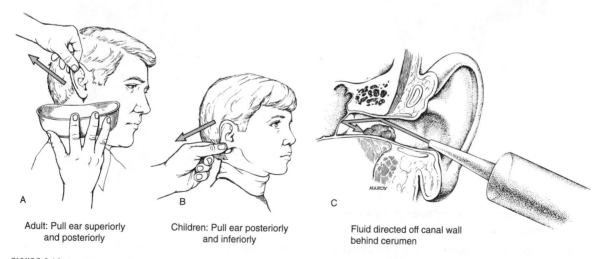

A Adult: Pull ear superiorly and posteriorly

B Children: Pull ear posteriorly and inferiorly

C Fluid directed off canal wall behind cerumen

FIGURE 9.14   Ear irrigation. **(A)** The external auditory canal in the adult can best be exposed by pulling the earlobe upward and backward. **(B)** The same exposure can be achieved in the child by gently pulling the auricle of the ear downward and backward. **(C)** An enlarged diagram showing the direction of irrigating fluid against the side of the canal. *Note:* This is more effective in dislodging cerumen than if the flow of solution were directed straight into the canal. (Brunner, L.S., & Suddarth, D.S. [1991]. *The Lippincott manual of nursing practice* [5th ed.]. Philadelphia: J.B. Lippincott)

▼ ▼ ▼
G U I D E L I N E S

Assessment Guidelines   Ears

Procedure

1. Inspect and palpate the external ear.

   a. Inspect the external ear, noting skin integrity, shape, symmetry, and ear position.

   b. Palpate the auricle between the thumb and forefinger, noting any tenderness or lesions.

   c. Palpate the mastoid process, which should be non-tender. Tenderness is associated with middle ear inflammation.

   d. Press the tragus inward toward the ear canal to detect tenderness, which may indicate inner ear inflammation.

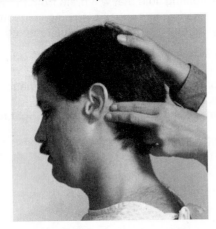

Mastoid palpation

2. Inspect the external auditory canal through the viewing lens of the otoscope.

   Note: If the person has symptoms of an ear infection (ear pain), inspect the unaffected ear first.

   a. Briefly explain the procedure. Ask the person to tip the head slightly toward the opposite shoulder (away from the side being examined).

   b. Choose the largest speculum the ear will comfortably accommodate and turn on the otoscope light.

Clinical Significance

Normal Finding

Left and right ears have equal size and shape. No skin lesions.

Ear position: The top of the ear should just touch or barely cross an imaginary line drawn from the outer canthus of the eye to the occiput.

Deviations from Normal

Lower-set ears may be associated with congenital kidney disorders or other chromosomal abnormalities.

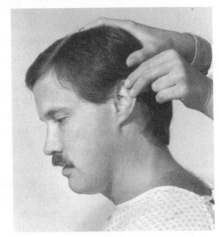

Auricle palpation

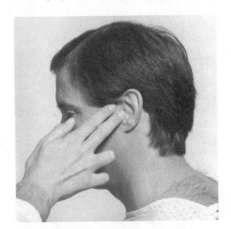

Tragus palpation

Measures should be taken to avoid transferring infective material from one ear to the other on the speculum.

Aligns the ear canal with the examining instrument.

▼ ▼ ▼

Procedure

c. Grasp the otoscope with your dominant hand and hold it in one of two ways:

- For children and restless adults, place the hand that is holding the otoscope handle against the person's head to help stabilize the instrument.
- For cooperative persons, you may hold the handle so the instrument is in an upright position; stabilization efforts are unnecessary.

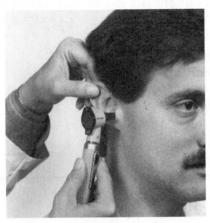

Otoscopic examination: Position for cooperative person

With your free hand, grasp the superior portion of the auricle and gently pull up, out, and back if the patient is an adult. The auricle is pulled downward in young children and infants.

d. Insert the otoscope and gently advance it to inspect the external auditory canal membranes through the lens.

3. **Inspect the tympanic membrane.**

a. Next, move the otoscope to examine the tympanic membrane. If this membrane is not initially visible, pull the auricle up and back again to further straighten the ear canal. Do not force the speculum in too distal a direction.

Cerumen may be present in the canal, partially obstructing the tympanic membrane. Again, gently realign the canal by moving the auricle and try to view around cerumen particles.

Clinical Significance

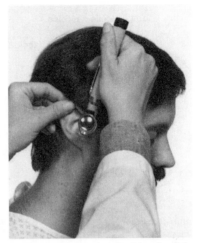

Otoscopic examination: Position for children, restless person

This maneuver should straighten the ear canal so that you can see the tympanic membrane.

Normal Findings

The adult ear canal is about 1 inch long. Skin is intact without redness or discharge. The canal is clear without obstructions. Hair growth is variable; hairs grow near outer third of the canal. Cerumen color and consistency vary depending on length of time since secretion. Fresh cerumen is light yellow, tan, or pink, and is soft. Old cerumen may be light to dark brown and is hard.

Quadrants of the tympanic membrane: Anterosuperior, posterosuperior, anteroinferior, and posteroinferior.

▼ ▼ ▼

G U I D E L I N E S *continued*   Ears

Procedure

b. Inspect the tympanic membrane and note major landmarks and color.

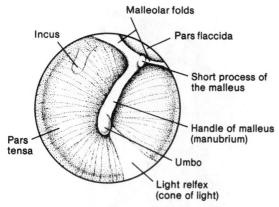

Right tympanic membrane

Labels: Malleolar folds, Incus, Pars flaccida, Short process of the malleus, Handle of malleus (manubrium), Pars tensa, Umbo, Light relfex (cone of light)

c. Observe the movement of the tympanic membrane as the person performs a Valsalva maneuver (or when you inject air with the pneumatic otoscope).

d. Examine the other ear.

Clinical Significance

Normal Findings

Color: Pearly gray; shiny; diffuse white plaques over membrane are scar tissue from previous inflammations (see color figure, this chapter).

Surface: Continuous and intact; slightly transparent.

Landmarks: White light reflex (cone of light) projected over anteroinferior quadrant. Light reflex focused with well-defined borders (not diffuse). following structures are visible: malleus (umbo and short process); pars tensa (taut portion of the tympanic membrane); annulus; pars flaccida (looser, superior fold of tympanic membrane); malleolar folds.

Configuration: Flat or concave (not bulging).

Deviations from Normal (see color figure)

Color: Redness; amber color

Surface: Perforated

Landmarks: No light reflex; inability to see landmarks

Configuration: Bulging or retracted.

Normal Findings

Movement of the tympanic membrane indicates a patient eustachian tube.

▼ ▼ ▼

G U I D E L I N E S

Assessment Guidelines   Hearing

Procedure

1. **Voice/whisper test.**

   a. Stand slightly behind the person, close to the ear that you want to test. Ask the person to cover the other ear with his or her hand.

   b. Whisper a few words, then ask the person to repeat what you said.

Clinical Significance

A test of hearing acuity, especially ability to perceive high-frequency sound.

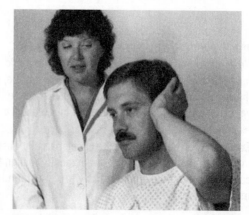

Voice/whisper test

▼ ▼ ▼

G U I D E L I N E S   *continued*   Hearing

Procedure

   c. Repeat the test on the other ear.

2. **Watch-tick test.**

   a. Stand behind the person. Instruct the person to cover the ear that is not being tested.

   b. Hold a ticking watch near the uncovered ear. Ask the person to say "yes" when he or she can hear the ticking and "no" when the ticking becomes inaudible. Move the watch until it is 2 feet from the ear.

   c. Repeat the test on the other ear.

3. **Weber test.**

   a. Strike the tuning fork and place the stem firmly against the middle of the person's forehead or the top of the head at the midline.

   b. Ask the person where the sound is heard.

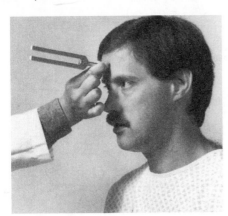

Weber test

Clinical Significance

Normal Finding

Ability to recognize the words of a whispered message from a 2-foot distance.

A test of hearing acuity, especially the ability to perceive high-frequency sound.

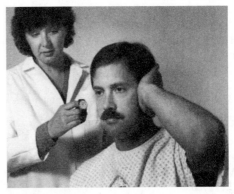

Watch-tick test

Note: Whispers and a watch's ticking are high-frequency sounds. These tests do not indicate a person's ability to perceive low-frequency sounds.

Test perception of sound coming from the body's midline.

Normal Finding

No sound lateralization, meaning the sound of the tuning fork is heard equally in both ears.

Deviations from Normal

In unilateral conduction deafness, the sound is heard best in the affected ear; in sensorineural loss, the sound lateralizes to the unaffected ear. (See Display 9-7, "Types of Hearing Losses").

SENSORINEURAL HEARING LOSS [PERCEPTIVE DEAFNESS]

Associated Conditions

Conditions that disrupt *neural* hearing pathways: the cochlea, cranial nerve VIII, or the auditory portions of the cerebral cortex (bilateral lesions).

Causative Factors

- Congenital defects
- Maternal rubella
- Erythroblastosis fetalis
- Traumatic injury involving the inner ear or cranial nerve VIII
- Vascular disorders involving the inner ear
- Ototoxic drugs
- Bacterial and viral infections (meningitis, encephalitis, mumps, etc.)
- Meniere's disease
- Severe febrile illness
- Posterior fossa tumors
- Multiple sclerosis
- Presbycusis
- Prolonged or repeated exposure to loud sounds

Signs and Symptoms

- Delayed language and speech development (infants)
- Hearing loss that may be more severe in noisy environments
- May be associated with speaking loudly

Hearing Tests

- Whisper test and watch-tick test may indicate hearing loss
- Weber test usually shows sound lateralization to the good ear
- Rinne test should be positive (AC>BC)

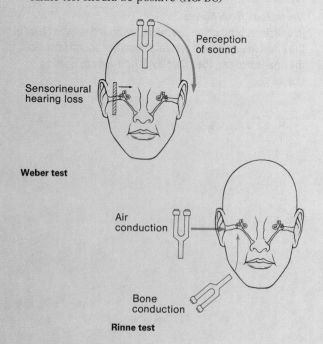

Weber test

Rinne test

CONDUCTIVE HEARING LOSS

Associated Conditions

Associated with external or middle ear problems that prevent normal sound transmission. Otoscopic examination is essential for detecting cerumen impaction, eardrum perforation, and otitis media.

Causative Factors

- Congenital ear malformations
- Traumatic eardrum perforation
- Trauma disrupting the ossicles
- Cerumen impaction
- Middle ear inflammation (otitis media)
- Otosclerosis

Signs and Symptoms

- Hearing loss that may be less noticeable in a noisy environment
- Normal tone of voice usually observed

Hearing Tests

- Whisper test and watch-tick test may indicate hearing loss.
- Weber test usually shows sound lateralization to the affected ear because this ear is less distracted by environmental noise and is therefore more perceptive to vibration.
- Rinne test should be negative (BC>AC) because vibrations passing through bone bypass the obstructive process.

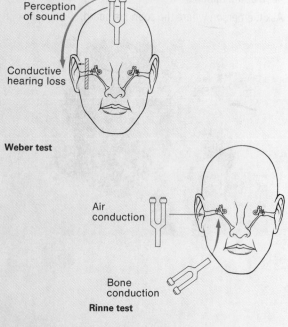

Weber test

Rinne test

Mixed (Combined) Hearing Loss

Hearing losses may be secondary to ineffective conduction and sensory perception. Both air and bone sound conduction are impaired.

▼ ▼ ▼

GUIDELINES   *continued*   Hearing

Procedure

4. Rinne test.

   a. Strike the tuning fork and place the stem firmly against the mastoid process.

Clinical Significance

Tests ability to perceive bone conduction versus air conduction of sound.

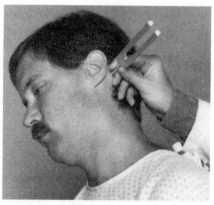

Rinne test: Step a

   b. Ask the person to report when the sound (or "buzzing") stops.

   c. Then move the tuning fork, which will be vibrating weakly, near the external auditory meatus.

Normal Finding

The person should hear the sound of the tuning fork when it is placed in front of the ear. This indicates that air conduction of sound is greater than bone conduction (AC>BC; a normal result, called *Rinne positive*).

Deviations from Normal

Bone conduction of sound is greater than air conduction (BC> AC; an abnormal pattern, called *Rinne negative*). This is associated with a conductive hearing loss. See Display 9-7, "Types of Hearing Losses."

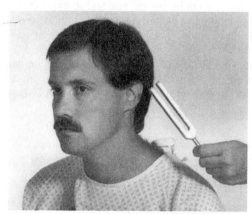

Rinne test: Step c

5. Schwabach's test.

   a. Strike the tuning fork and place it firmly against the person's mastoid process. Note the length of time before the person reports that the sound has stopped.

   b. Then repeat the test, holding the tuning fork against your own mastoid process and note the length of bone conduction.

Compares the person's perception of bone conduction of sound with the examiner's. (The test assumes normal hearing abilities on your part.)

Deviations from Normal

Schwabach diminished: You hear the sound longer than the client, in which case the client may have a sensorineural hearing loss.

Schwabach prolonged: The client hears the sound longer, in which case he or she may have a conductive hearing loss.

Documenting Ear Examination Findings and Hearing

Example 1: Normal Ear

Kay, aged 10 years, had an ear examination as part of summer camp health assessment. The examination was normal and recorded as follows:

External ear skin without lesions; tragus and auricle nontender to palpation. Canals have small amount of soft yellow cerumen; noninflamed. Both TMs pearly gray, shiny; Light reflex intact and landmarks discernible. Able to identify whispered voice, no sound lateralization, AC > BC.

The same examination may be summarized in a problem-oriented format:

S: Mother reports no history of ear infections or hearing problems. Does not use cotton-tipped swabs or similar devices for ear cleaning.

O: External ear skin without lesions; tragus and auricle nontender to palpation. Canals have small amount of soft yellow cerumen; noninflamed. Both TMs pearly gray and shiny. Light reflex intact, and landmarks discernible. Able to identify whispered voice, no sound lateralization, AC > BC.

A: Ear exam and hearing acuity within normal limits.

P: Reinforce current routines and routine screening visits.

Example 2: Cerumen Impaction

Mr. T, aged 79 years, reported to the nurse that his left ear felt full and hearing acuity was diminished. The examination was abnormal and recorded as follows:

Left ear canal impacted with dark-brown, hard cerumen. Unable to visualize TM. BC > AC on left side; AC > BC on right. Sound lateralization to the left side. Does not hear whispered sound on left, but can on right.

The same examination may be summarized in a problem-oriented format:

S: "I don't hear very well on this side [left], and my ear feels plugged."

O: Left ear canal impacted with dark brown, hard cerumen. Unable to visualize TM. BC > AC on left side; AC > BC on right. Sound lateralization to the left side. Does not hear whispered sound on left, but can on right.

A: Tests of hearing acuity indicate conductive hearing loss, probably from cerumen impaction.

P: Consider cerumen removal if no contraindications.

Example 3: Ear Infection

Andrew, aged 8 years, had an upper respiratory infection for the last week and developed left ear pain 12 hours ago. The ear examination was abnormal and recorded as follows:

Right ear canal clear, TM pearly gray with discernible landmarks and light reflex. Left ear canal clear, TM erythematous and slightly convex. Unable to see light reflex or landmarks. Patient reports pain with left tragus palpation.

The same examination may be summarized in a problem-oriented format:

S: Mother reports history of URI for 1 week; began pulling left ear and having ear pain last evening.

O: Temp: 101° F (PO); P: 98; RR: 18. Right ear canal clear, TM pearly gray with discernible landmarks and light reflex. Left ear canal clear, TM erythematous and slightly convex. Unable to see light reflex or landmarks. Reports pain with tragus palpation.

A: Suspect acute otitis media (left side).

P: Consult with physician for treatment. Instruct mother re: antibiotic therapy; worsening of symptoms.

Nursing Diagnoses Related to Ear and Hearing Assessment

Sensory–Perceptual Alteration: Hearing

A person's hearing may be altered by a number of factors, some of which are not amenable to nursing intervention. For example, sensory–perceptual alteration: Hearing related to the effects of aging, may not be a useful diagnostic label in planning nursing care. The nurse would have difficulty identifying realistic outcome criteria for this type of diagnosis. It might not be realistic to say that the person would achieve better hearing acuity as a result of nursing intervention. The nurse should determine the responses the person might have as a result of a hearing loss and specifically label the response, rather than the hearing deficit. For example, people with hearing deficits are at risk for Impaired communication or Social isolation.

Clinical Problems Related to Ear and Hearing Assessment

Otitis Externa (Swimmer's Ear)

Otitis externa is a painful inflammatory condition of the external ear caused by infective organisms, allergic reactions (such as contact dermatitis), or present as a variant of seborrheic dermatitis.

Risk Factors

- Prolonged moisture in the ear, most frequently caused by swimming
- Ear canal trauma, most often caused by cleaning or scratching

Signs and Symptoms

- Ear pain, especially near the external portion of the affected ear; pain may be aggravated by pushing on the tragus, or by chewing and talking
- Itching

- Scaling from the ear canal
- Conductive hearing losses may be noted if ear canal swelling is extensive and causes external canal blockage.
- Low-grade fever possible
- Proximal lymph node enlargement is possible, which may involve preauricular, postauricular, and upper cervical nodes.

Otoscopic Examination

- Inspecting the outer ear and external canal may reveal reddened and swollen skin surfaces.
- Serous exudate may be seen.
- The tympanic membrane should be normal unless otitis media is present.

Acute Otitis Media (Middle Ear Inflammation)

Acute otitis media occurs most commonly in infants and children as a sequela of upper respiratory tract infection.

Pathophysiology

Bacteria, especially beta-hemolytic streptococci, staphylococci, and pneumococci, as well as the *Haemophilus influenzae* virus, are easily transmitted to the middle ear along the eustachian tube.

Signs and Symptoms

- Ear pain (young children or infants may be irritable and pull or hold the affected ear)
- Feelings of fullness, pressure, or roaring in the ear
- Fever and chills are common.

Otoscopic Examination

- During the early stages, the only sign may be hyperemia of the blood vessels across the drum.

- Later, the drum may bulge outward as secretions collect in the middle ear.
- Bulging obscures the tympanic membrane landmarks, including the light reflex.
- The eardrum may be bright red.
- If the eardrum ruptures, purulent drainage may be noted in the canal.
- Eardrum perforation may be directly visible. It places the person at risk for developing chronic otitis media.

Serous Otitis Media

Serous otitis media may occur when sterile fluid accumulates in the middle ear. It may occur secondary to:

- Eustachian tube blockage when pressure changes cause transudation of serous fluid
- Residual exudate accumulation from a bacterial otitis media
- A viral upper respiratory tract infection
- An allergic reaction, causing serous fluid exudation into the middle ear

Signs and Symptoms

- Usually little or no ear pain
- May have feelings of ear fullness or plugging
- Decreased hearing acuity possible, and auditory function tests may indicate a conductive hearing loss
- Unnatural voice reverberation may be noted.

Otoscopic Examination

- The tympanic membrane may be retracted.
- Light reflex may be absent.
- Tympanic membrane color may be amber.
- A fluid demarcation line may be present.
- Air bubbles may be seen behind the tympanic membrane.

CASE STUDY 1

David, aged 25 years, was recovering from a closed head injury received in a motorcycle accident. Recently, he was admitted to a rehabilitation nursing unit. The nurse caring for David noticed that when he was shaving or brushing his teeth, he would attend only to the right side of the body. He frequently appeared disoriented and would bump into things when ambulating.

Case Study Analysis

Observation of David's self-care practices and orientation indicated a need for more thorough assessment and prompted the nurse to ask the following questions:

- What is the nature of the neurologic injury?
- How long has it been since the initial injury?
- How much functional improvement has there been since the injury?
- What is the current level of function in relation to feeding, grooming, and ambulation?

- If current functioning indicates regression, what factors may have influenced the client? Emotional upset? Stress of transfer? Less one-to-one nursing care? Unfamiliarity with caregivers?
- What is the patient's rehabilitation prognosis?

David demonstrated neglect of the left side of his body. The nurse observed that he did not shave the left side of his face or wash the left side of his body. The nature of his neurologic injury, which occurred 3 months ago, helped to explain his behavior. The right parietal lobe had been damaged, which is often associated with perceptual defects. The one-sided neglect had been noted since admission to the rehabilitation unit 1 week before and did not represent a recent change. Previous documentation of such behavior was not available. Disorientation may be associated with one-sided neglect. David had been fully oriented in the last few days, although fatigue and frustration appeared to contribute to transient disorientation.

CASE STUDY *continued*

The rehabilitation team believed that David's chance of recovering normal ability to perform daily living skills was excellent, provided he received continuing therapy.

Possible Nursing Diagnosis

Based on the observed behaviors and history of the neurologic injury, the nursing diagnosis of Unilateral neglect was formulated.

Additional Assessment

The nurse obtained additional data to be used in monitoring David's progress and planning interventions. David was asked to draw pictures of himself and common objects, such as a clock. In both cases, he initially drew only the right half of the image. However, 3 weeks later, he drew similar pictures with some attention to detail on the left side. One morning the nurse asked David to wash the neglected side of his body to see whether he would respond to verbal cueing. Additionally, the nurse had David view himself in the mirror to see if he could identify areas neglected during hygienic care. Eventually, David showed increasing attention to the left side of his body and had fewer episodes of disoriented behavior.

CASE STUDY 2

Mrs. K, aged 75, was brought to the emergency department by her husband because she fell at home and lacerated her scalp. He reported that his wife has been "losing her memory" for the past 2 years and recently had left their home and had been brought back by the police. He reported that she neglected personal hygiene and had occasional fecal incontinence. Her husband stated that he was worried that she would injure herself further.

Case Study Analysis

A more thorough evaluation should be made of Mrs. K's "memory lapses." A thorough health and medication history should be obtained to rule out any potentially reversible contributing factors. Mental status tests may be administered to evaluate judgment, memory, and other cognitive functions. The patient's emotional status and coping responses also should be evaluated. Additional data should be obtained from both the patient and her husband. Finally, the husband's response to the patient's problems should be evaluated.

Possible Nursing Diagnoses

At this point, there are not enough data to make a nursing diagnosis relating to altered cognitive or perceptual functions. The immediate concern is with the patient's safety and emotional response to the emergency department admission. Appropriate diagnoses would include Potential for injury and Possible anxiety.

CHAPTER 9 SUMMARY

Assessment of Cognition and Perception
The assessment of cognition and perception is focused on the following:
- Cognitive functions, including factors related to teaching and learning, level of consciousness, awareness, communication abilities, and thought processes
- Neurologic functions
- The status of the special senses, including vision, hearing, taste, touch, and smell
- Sensory and perceptual experiences such as pain and altered thought processes that may interfere with usual or desired activities

Data Collection Methods
1. Interview and Review of Records
    Mental status
    Status of sensory structures and functions
    Teaching and learning evaluation
    Medical history
    Medication history
2. Pain Assessment (if applicable)
    Perceptions and self-reports of pain
    Physiologic responses
    Behavioral responses
    Cognitive attempts to manage pain

3. Diagnostic Studies Review (to evaluate acute mental status changes)
   Complete blood count
   Electrolytes
   Liver and renal function tests
   Blood alcohol levels
   Toxicology screening
   Radiologic assessment
   Lumbar puncture
4. Physical Examination and Observation
   Neurologic functions
   Mental status evaluation
   Signs and symptoms of neurologic dysfunction detected during the examination of cranial nerves, reflexes, motor and sensory systems
   Physical examination of the eyes and ears

Primary Nursing Diagnoses
   Knowledge deficit (specify)
   Altered thought process

Acute confusion
Chronic confusion
Impaired memory
Impaired environmental interpretation syndrome
Impaired verbal communication
Sensory–perceptual alterations (specify): Visual, auditory, kinesthetic, gustatory, tactile, olfactory
Unilateral neglect
Potential for injury
Risk for autonomic dysreflexia
Pain
Chronic pain

Clinical Problems Related to Cognitive and Perceptual Dysfunctions
   Pathology of the central and peripheral nervous systems
   Structural alterations and disorders of the eye
   Visual and hearing impairments
   Inflammatory processes of the ear

Critical Thinking

The assessment of cognition and perception can be a complex and lengthy process. The assessment is complex because of the broad scope and specialized skill that is required. Also contributing to the complexity is the fact that the people who may be in greatest need of evaluation may be experiencing cognitive or perceptual deficits that interfere with optimal communication. A lengthy assessment is guaranteed if the clinician conducts a complete evaluation of the neurologic system.

Learning Exercises

1. You want to assess cognitive functions of a 32-year-old patient who has suffered a slight concussion. The patient speaks and comprehends only Chinese, and you do not. Select and describe at least three options that might be implemented in this situation. Of these options, which is least likely to be helpful? Why? Which option is most likely to be helpful? Why?

2. Specify how you might use cranial nerve examination findings to plan nursing care.

3. Many nurses do not have time to routinely conduct a comprehensive examination of the neurologic system. Develop some criteria for determining the necessity of conducting an examination of deep tendon reflexes by an emergency room nurse.

4. You are unable to visualize the optic disc during an ophthalmoscopic examination. Identify several reasons why this might happen and recommend whether corrective actions will be helpful.

5. Determine and discuss the primary differences between assessing pain in a patient with a diagnosed condition versus an undiagnosed condition.

BIBLIOGRAPHY

Agency for Health Care Policy and Research. (1992). *Clinical practice guidelines: Acute pain management: Operative or medical procedures and trauma.* (AHCPR Pub. No. 92-0032). Rockville, MD: US Dept. of Health and Human Services.

Ahles, T.A., Blanchard, E.B., & Ruckdeschel, J.C. (1983). The multi-dimensional nature of cancer-related pain. *Pain, 277–288.*

Baillie, L. (1993). A review of pain assessment tools. *Nursing Standard, 7*(23), 25–29.

Bondy, K.N. (1994). Assessing cognitive function: A guide to neuropsychological testing. *Rehabilitation Nursing, 19*(1), 24–30.

Boyd-Monk, H. (1980). Examining the external eye: Part I. *Nursing 80, 10*(5), 58–63.

Boyd-Monk, H. (1980). Examining the external eye: Part 2. *Nursing 80, 10*(6), 58–63.

Camp, L. (1988). A comparison of nurses' recorded assessment of pain with perceptions of pain as described by cancer patients. *Cancer Nursing, 11*(4), 237–243.

Carpenito, L.J. (1985). Altered thoughts or altered perceptions. *American Journal of Nursing, 85*(11), 1283.

Crigger, N., & Forbes, W. (1997). Assessing neurologic function in older patients. *American Journal of Nursing, 97*(3), 37–40.

Crosby, L., et al. (1989). Clinical neurologic assessment tool: Development and testing of an instrument to index neurologic status. *Heart and Lung, 18*(2), 121–129.

Darovic, G. (1997). Assessing pupillary responses. *Nursing 97*(2), 49.

Dick, M.J. (1995). Assessment and measurement of acute pain. *JOGNN, 24*(9), 843–848.

Facione, N. (1990). Otitis media: An overview of acute and chronic disease. *Nurse Practitioner, 15*(10), 11–22.

Folstein, M.F., Folstein, S., & McHugh, P.R. (1975). Mini-mental state: A practical method for grading the cognitive state of patients for the clinician. *Journal of Psychiatric Research, 12,* 189–198.

Forrest, J. (1995). Assessment of acute and chronic pain in older adults. *Journal of Gerontologic Nursing, 21*(10), 15–20.

Hall, G. (1988) Alterations in thought processes. *Journal of Gerontological Nursing, 14*(3), 30–37, 38–40.

Hays, A. (1984). The set test to screen mental status quickly. *Geriatric Nursing, 5,* 96–97.

Hiles, D.A. (1974). Strabismus. *American Journal of Nursing, 74,* 1082–1089.

Jacques, A. (1992). Do you believe I'm in pain? Nurses' assessment of patient's pain. *Professional Nurse, 7*(4), 249–251.

Jess, L. (1988). Investigating impaired mental status: An assessment guide you can use. *Nursing 88, 18*(6), 42–50.

Kaufman, J. (1990). Assessing the 12 cranial nerves. *Nursing 90, 6,* 56–58.

Knight, R.L. (1986). The Glasgow Coma Scale: Ten years after. *Critical Care Nurse, 6*(3), 65–71.

Libow, L.S. (1981). A rapidly administered, easily remembered mental status evaluation: FROMAGE. In L.S. Libow & F.T. Sherman. *The core of geriatric medicine: A guide for students and practitioners* (pp. 85–91). St. Louis: C.V. Mosby.

Lower, J. (1992). Rapid neuroassessment. *American Journal of Nursing, 6*(92), 38–48.

Marr, J. (1992). Acute confusion. *Nursing Times, 88*(21), 31–32.

McCaffery, M. (1979). *Nursing management of the patient in pain.* Philadelphia: J.B. Lippincott.

McGuire, D.B. (1992). Comprehensive and multidimensional assessment and measurement of pain. *Journal of Pain and Symptom Management, 7*(5), 312–319.

Melzack, R. (Ed.) (1983). *Pain measurement and assessment.* New York: Raven Press.

Melzack, R., & Wall, P. (1965). Pain Mechanisms: A new theory. *Science, 150,* 971–979.

Melzack, R., & Wall, P. (1975). Psychophysiology of Pain. In M. Weisenberg (Ed.). *Pain: Clinical and experimental perspectives* (pp. 8–23). St. Louis: C.V. Mosby.

Merskey, H. (1986). International association for the study of pain: Pain terms: A current list with definitions and notes on usage. *Pain, 3,* (s1–s2225).

Russell, J. (1995). Ear Screening. *Community Nurse, 1*(4), 14–16.

Simon, J.M., & McTier, C.L. (1996). Development of a chronic pain assessment tool. *Rehabilitation Nursing, 21*(1), 20–24.

Spross, J.A., McGuire, D.B., & Schmitt, R.M. (1991). *Oncology Nursing Society position paper on cancer pain.* Pittsburgh: Oncology Nursing Press.

Stevens, S.A., & Becker, K.L. (1988). A simple step-by-step approach to neurologic assessment: Part 1. *Nursing 88, 9,* 53–61.

Stevens, S.A., & Becker, K.L. (1988). A simple step-by-step approach to neurologic assessment: Part 2. *Nursing 88, 10,* 51–58.

Sulkowski, J.A., & Judy, K.D. (1997). Acute mental status changes. *AACN Clinical Issues, 8*(3), 319–334.

Walker, J. (1992). Taking pains—pain assessment. *Nursing Times, 88*(29), 38–40.

CHAPTER 10

Assessing Sleep and Rest

ASSESSMENT GUIDELINES

- Sleep and Rest Interview (Health History)
- Sleep Laboratory Evaluation
- Interpreting Physical Examination Findings Related to Sleep and Rest
- Sleep Pattern Observation

CHAPTER ORGANIZATION

Introductory Overview
- Assessment Focus
- Data Collection Methods
- Nursing Diagnoses

Knowledge Base for Assessment
- Stages of Sleep
- Normal Sleep Pattern
- Sleep and Rest Requirements

Sleep is defined in behavioral terms as a state of detachment and unresponsiveness to the environment from which a person can be awakened by sensory or other stimuli. The fact that the person can be stimulated to wakefulness distinguishes sleep from other unconscious states such as coma or anesthesia. *Rest* may be defined in one of two important contexts that have significance to nurses as they evaluate health and functional status. In the context relevant to the assessment of sleep and rest as a functional health pattern, rest refers to a person's general response to a good night's sleep. In this case, rest alludes to feelings of adequate energy for the day's activities, lack of fatigue, invigoration, and cognitive capability. *Rest* also can be described as a state of physical and mental well-being. In this context, being at rest is associated with a state of relaxation, harmony, and freedom from the detrimental effects of stress.

People may experience sleep disruptions at some time or another because of special circumstances such as caring for children, staying up late to complete a task, shift work, sleeping in unfamiliar environments, or travel and "jet lag." Most of these sleep disruptions are insignificant, and a return to a normal sleep pattern can be readily reestablished. But regular disruptions in sleep can be more consequential and have far-reaching detrimental effects on a person's health and functioning. Some people may believe they are obtaining adequate amounts of sleep but they do not feel rested. Regular disruptions of sleep or perceptions of inadequate rest should be carefully assessed to determine an underlying pattern and cause so that appropriate interventions can be recommended. In some cases, the nurse will be able to effectively evaluate sleep and rest disruptions with an individual and assist them in managing the problem. For example, nurses can help identify environmental and stress factors contributing to sleep disturbances and provide appropriate modifications or counseling to promote and improve sleep patterns. In other cases, more specialized evaluation is required to determine the nature of the sleep problem, as in the case of sleep pathologies such as narcolepsy and sleep apnea. The nurse's role in screening for sleep problems and making appropriate referrals for additional evaluation and intervention is important. A basic overview of sleep laboratory evaluation is presented in this chapter to give nurses an understanding of specialized evaluation methods.

As an assessment of sleep and rest is undertaken, the nurse should be especially attentive to the quality and pattern of sleep during major life transitions, the grieving process, and the stresses of acute and chronic illness. Sleep patterns may be significantly disrupted during these life experiences.

ASSESSMENT FOCUS

The assessment of sleep and rest focuses on the evaluation of sleep patterns, habits, and behaviors to determine the overall adequacy of sleep. With a comprehensive assessment of sleep and rest, the nurse will meet the following objectives:

- Identifying individual perceptions about the quantity and quality of sleep and rest
- Evaluating various factors that may influence sleep and rest
- Identifying signs, symptoms, and causes of sleep pattern disturbances
- Evaluating the effect of sleep pattern disturbances on physiological, cognitive, and psychological functions

Data Collection Methods

Data collection is accomplished by the following methods:

1. Interview and/or Review of Records Focus
   Usual sleep patterns
   Altered sleep patterns
   Sleep and bedtime habits
   Medical history
   Caffeine and alcohol intake
   Medication history

2. Sleep Laboratory Evaluation Focus
   Electroencephalogram (EEG)
   Electro-oculogram (EOG)
   Electromyogram (EMG)
   Physiologic event recording and observation
3. Physical Examination and Observation Focus
   Signs and symptoms of sleep deprivation and fatigue
   Direct observation of sleep periods
   Cognitive function and mental status

Nursing Diagnoses

Assessment of sleep and rest may result in the identification of one or more of the following primary nursing diagnoses:

Fatigue
Sleep pattern disturbance
Sleep deprivation

As you explore the factors contributing to sleep and rest problems, you may identify additional problems, especially the following:

Anxiety
Ineffective individual coping
Ineffective family coping
Fear
Pain
Dysfunctional grieving

Stress and other situational factors may have adverse effects on sleep. Sleepless nights or interruptions in sleep may accompany stress. Physical pain, conflict, fear or anxiety, and grief over the death of a loved one all can contribute to sleep pattern disturbances.

KNOWLEDGE BASE FOR ASSESSMENT

Sleep can be defined by behavioral and physiologic criteria. The hallmark behavioral indicator is unresponsiveness to the environment, which can be reversed by stimuli such as noise, physical stimulation, or temperature changes. In addition, the sleeping person is typically observed in a recumbent position with their eyes closed.

Sleep is also defined by a number of physiologic indicators that may be measured by using special data collection procedures and equipment. A sleep laboratory with specially trained personnel is equipped for sleep measurement and monitoring, including the monitoring of effects of abnormal sleep patterns on cardiac rhythms, oxygenation status, and other body systems and processes. A sleep laboratory evaluation includes measuring the electrical activity of the brain by electroencephalography (EEG), the electrical activity of facial muscle groups by electromyography (EMG), and the movement of the eyes by electro-oculography (EOG). Collectively, these measurements are called polysomnographic evaluation (Fig 10-1).

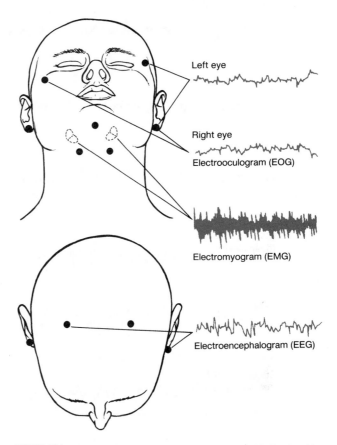

FIGURE 10.1 Sleep laboratory evaluation. Sleep is determined in the laboratory by measuring the electrical activity of the brain and muscles and the movement of the eyes, using techniques of electro-oculography, electromyography, and electroencephalography. Collectively, these measurements are called polysomnographic evaluation.

Stages of Sleep

Sleep has been characterized by polysomnographic evaluation as consisting of two major categories and several well-defined stages. The two major categories of sleep are non–rapid eye movement (non-REM) sleep and rapid eye movement (REM) sleep, during which the eyes appear to move quickly under the eyelids.

Non-REM sleep is further divided into four distinct phases on the basis of EEG waveform criteria (Fig. 10-2). The EEG pattern in non-REM sleep is commonly described as synchronous with characteristic waveforms, including sleep spindles, K complexes, and high-voltage slow waves. The four non-REM stages—stages 1, 2, 3, and 4—roughly parallel a "depth of sleep" continuum, with stage 1 being the lightest sleep stage and stage 4 representing deepest sleep. During non-REM sleep, the body is in a quiet state, but the body's motor tone is such that the person may be observed to change position and move extremities. There is decreased mental activity in the cerebral cortex, meaning the person experiences less vivid dreaming during non-REM sleep, although other brain regulatory functions are active.

REM sleep, in contrast, is defined by more irregular

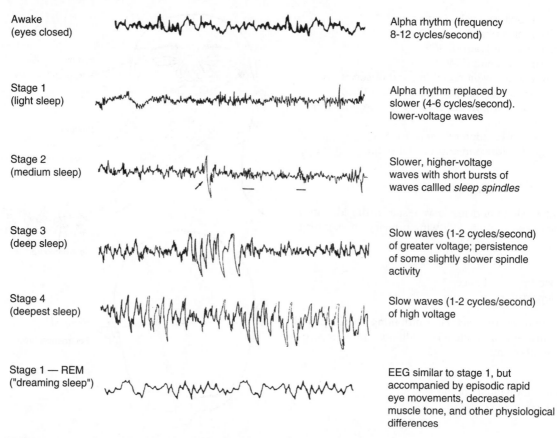

Awake
(eyes closed) — Alpha rhythm (frequency 8-12 cycles/second)

Stage 1
(light sleep) — Alpha rhythm replaced by slower (4-6 cycles/second). lower-voltage waves

Stage 2
(medium sleep) — Slower, higher-voltage waves with short bursts of waves callled *sleep spindles*

Stage 3
(deep sleep) — Slow waves (1-2 cycles/second) of greater voltage; persistence of some slightly slower spindle activity

Stage 4
(deepest sleep) — Slow waves (1-2 cycles/second) of high voltage

Stage 1 — REM
("dreaming sleep") — EEG similar to stage 1, but accompanied by episodic rapid eye movements, decreased muscle tone, and other physiological differences

FIGURE 10.2 Sleep stages and electroencephalographic (EEG) tracings. On the third tracing, the *arrow* indicates a K complex, and the *underlining* shows two sleep spindles.

patterns on the EEG brain wave tracing and episodic bursts of rapid eye movements associated with vivid dreaming. These rapid eye movements are recorded by the electro-oculography electrode in the sleep laboratory, but occasionally, twitching beneath closed eyelids may be directly observed. Dreaming represents active mental activity in the cerebral cortex, and persons wakened from REM sleep usually have accurate recall of their dreams. During REM sleep, the neural impulses from the brain responsible for activating skeletal muscle tone are suppressed, and the extremities and other skeletal muscles appear relaxed. The mind is active, but the body is, in effect, paralyzed. The sympathetic nervous system is activated in REM sleep, which may result in increased blood pressure, increased heart and respiratory rates, and subsequent increased oxygen consumption. In addition, gastric secretion may increase and steroid hormones are released. Penile erections may occur in males of all ages during this stage.

Normal Sleep Pattern

Sleep patterns vary with age and other circumstances. A normal sleep pattern of a young adult is generally used as a frame of reference for describing the typical progression through sleep during a night. The progression through the various sleep stages during an 8-hour sleep period can be graphically depicted by a tool referred to as the sleep his-

togram (Fig. 10-3). The normal adult enters sleep through non-REM sleep with a sequential progression from stage 1 to stage 4 sleep. REM sleep does not occur until about 80 minutes after the initial onset of the sleep period. During an average 8-hour sleep period, a person experiences four or five sleep cycles. An average cycle is 90 to 110 minutes long and is characterized by variable amounts of non-REM and REM sleep.

First Sleep Cycle. The first sleep cycle of the night follows the most orderly and sequential progression through the sleep stages. It begins with stage 1 sleep, which may last only 5 minutes before the onset of stage 2. The eyes will roll slowly from side to side and heart and respiratory rates will usually decrease. Muscle tone is relatively high, and myoclonic jerks or sudden twitching in the face or extremities may be noted. Subjective feelings such as drifting or relaxation may occur. The time it takes to reach stage 1 or "fall asleep" is referred to as sleep latency. A person may be easily awakened from stage 1 by noise or other stimuli, and, if wakened, may deny having been asleep. Brief episodes of stage 1 sleep occur throughout the night, with total time spent in stage 1 constituting approximately 2% to 5% of the total sleep time. After periods of sleep deprivation, there will be an increase in the amount and percentage of stage 1 sleep.

Stage 2 sleep, which lasts from 10 to 25 minutes, is a deeper stage of sleep. Greater effort is required to awaken

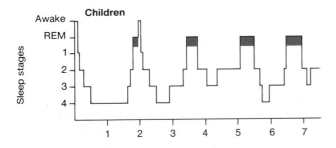

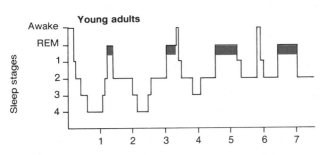

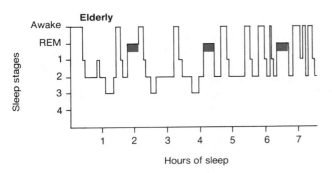

Hours of sleep

FIGURE 10.3 The progression through sleep stages in children, adults, and elders. In children and young adults, stages 3 and 4 are reached early, with progressive lengthening of the first three REM periods and infrequent awakenings. Elderly adults show little or no stage 4 sleep, and awakenings are frequent. (After Kales, A., et al. [1968]. *Annals of Internal Medicine, 68,* 1078)

a person in stage 2 sleep. The EEG pattern is characterized by delta waves, sleep spindles, and K complexes. Little or no eye movement is recorded by the EOG. Metabolic rate and body temperature continue to decrease. Stage 2 sleep generally constitutes approximately 45% to 55% of sleep.

A slowing of the brain wave activity (high-voltage slow wave activity) on the EEG heralds the onset of stage 3 sleep, which usually only lasts a few minutes in the first sleep cycle. This phase of deep sleep is characterized by decreased heart and respiratory rates, decreased blood pressure, and more difficulty in arousing the person. Stage 3 sleep constitutes approximately 3% to 8% of the total sleep period.

Stage 4 sleep, the deepest stage, is entered 15 to 30 minutes after the person falls asleep. The delta waves first observed in stage 2 sleep continue at an even slower rate during stage 4. Stage 3 and stage 4 are sometimes referred to as slow-wave sleep or delta sleep because of the asso-

ciated slow brain wave tracings on the EEG. During stage 4, muscle tone is relaxed, and minimal eye movement is detected. Sleepwalking and bedwetting may occur in this stage. Respiratory and heart rates may be lowered 20% to 50% below waking levels, and the person may be difficult to awaken. Restorative physiologic processes, including increased levels of protein synthesis and increased secretion of growth hormone, occur in this stage. People who

DISPLAY 10.1

Sleep Requirements

FULL-TERM INFANTS
- 14–18 hr/day (newborns)
- 12–18 hr/day (infants)
- Average sleep periods are 3–4 hours
- Nighttime awakenings common
- 50% total sleep time (TST) is REM

1-YEAR-OLDS
- 12 hr/night with AM and PM nap
- 30%–40% TST is REM
- Majority of TST is stages III and IV
- Sleep cycles 45–60 min long

2- TO 5-YEAR-OLDS
- 10–12 hr/night
- Progressive decrease in nap time
- Slight increase in REM sleep time
- Boys require more TST than girls
- Sleep cycles 45–60 minutes long

8- TO 12-YEAR-OLDS
- 8–10 hr/night
- 90-minute adult sleep cycle noted

12- TO 14-YEAR-OLDS
- 8–9 hr/night
- 20% TST is REM (growth spurts increase REM needs)

15-YEAR-OLDS TO YOUNG ADULTS
- 6–9 hr/night
- 20%–25% TST is REM
- 50% TST is stage II

OLDER ADULTS
- 6–9 hr/night
- Progressive decrease in stage IV sleep
- Progressive nighttime awakenings
- Proportion of REM to non-REM sleep remains constant

report they did not sleep well are often found to be deprived of time spent in stage 4 sleep.

REM sleep in the first cycle of the night is relatively short-lived, lasting only 1 to 5 minutes. The duration of REM sleep in subsequent cycles is progressively longer. REM sleep tends to be greater in the last one third of the night or sleep period. REM sleep is a relatively active sleep state that varies in duration and is dominated by sympathetic nervous system activity. EEG waves reflect low-voltage and high-frequency electrical activity, similar to activity associated with wakefulness. At the same time, the muscles may appear relaxed, a sign indicating deep sleep. Because characteristics associated with wakefulness and deep sleep are present, REM sleep is also called paradoxical sleep. Episodic bursts of rapid eye movements, associated with vivid dreaming, are recorded by the EOG. The dreaming that occurs during REM sleep is qualitatively different from the dreaming that occurs during non-REM sleep, in that REM dreams are often bizarre or irrational, whereas non-REM dreams are usually more realistic and logical.

As NREM/REM sleep cycles are repeated during the night, REM sleep predominates. Stages 3 and 4 sleep occupy less time in the second cycle and may disappear altogether in subsequent cycles.

Sleep and Rest Requirements

Although sleep requirements vary and change from infancy to old age, all people need periods of undisturbed sleep and rest during the 24-hour cycle, as outlined in Display 10-1. Sleep needs increase during periods of high metabolic need, such as after surgery or during starvation states. The right amount of sleep is the amount that results in optimal daytime function and minimal drowsiness.

Newborns sleep between 14 and 18 hours in a 24-hour period, and infants sleep 12 to 18 hours a day; for both, 50% of this sleep is REM. By the time a child reaches 1 year of age, REM sleep is reduced to 20% to 30%. Children spend most of their sleeping time in stages III and IV.

Young adults usually sleep 6 to 9 hours at a time and spend 20% to 25% of their sleeping time in REM sleep. Fifty percent of their sleep time is spent in stage II, and the remaining time is spent in stages III and IV.

As people grow older, the amount of deep sleep they obtain decreases, and the total sleep period fragments. However, older adults need amounts of sleep similar to the amount younger adults need, ranging from 6 to 9 hours, depending on the individual. The proportion of REM sleep to the various stages of non-REM sleep remains constant from ages 20 to 60 years. The amount of time spent in stage IV usually declines rapidly, and by the time a person reaches age 50, it is reduced by 50%. Rapid eye movement sleep usually remains constant, but it is patterned more uniformly throughout the sleep cycle.

In elderly people, stage I time increases, but stages II and III remain unchanged. However, elderly women may spend more time in stage III sleep. Interestingly, 25% of 60-year-olds may experience little or no stage IV sleep. With this loss of restorative sleep, then, elderly people may exhibit signs and symptoms associated with sleep deprivation, including fatigue, headache, poor concentration, visual disturbances, forgetfulness, apathy, depression, coordination difficulties, and mood changes.

TABLE 10.1 Sleep Measurement Instruments

Tool	Description	Comments
St. Mary's Hospital Sleep Questionnaire	14-Item multiple-choice and short answer instrument	Designed specifically for hospitalized adults; tests for sleep disturbance, sleep latency, and sleep quality
Baekeland-Hoy Sleep Log	11-Item multiple-choice and short answer instrument	Designed for home use by healthy adults to determine differences between "good" and "bad" sleepers
Verran-Snyder-Halpren Sleep Scale	8-Item visual analog scale	Designed for use by hospitalized and healthy adults; tests for sleep disturbance and sleep effectiveness

Pattern Assessment   Sleep and Rest Assessment Guidelines

GENERAL APPROACH

The foundation for diagnosing sleep disorders is a thorough evaluation of the history of the sleep complaint. The person's medical history, medication use history, and history of contributing stressors also provide essential information for the evaluation of sleep. By interviewing and examining the person you can observe the daytime effects of inadequate sleep. A person's bed partner can provide additional information about nocturnal movements, arousals, and breathing patterns during sleep.

SLEEP LOG

Recording observations about sleep in a sleep log may be a helpful method for characterizing sleep patterns. To keep a sleep log, ask the person to record the number of hours slept each day for a period of a week or more. The following information should be recorded in a sleep log:

- Time the sleep period began (*i.e.,* when the person went to bed)
- Amount of time taken to fall asleep
- Number of awakenings during the sleep period, and their cause, if known
- Time of final awakening
- Number of naps that were taken during the day and how long they lasted

SLEEP LABORATORY EVALUATION

A sleep laboratory evaluation includes an electroencephalogram (EEG), electro-oculogram (EOG), electromyogram (EMG), and evaluation of other physiologic monitors. The procedures that are conducted as part of sleep laboratory evaluation are collectively referred to as polysomnographic evaluation. This type of evaluation is used to refine the diagnosis of sleep disorders such as sleep apnea and narcolepsy. Sleep laboratory evaluation can aid in the differential diagnosis of insomnia by providing an objective assessment of an entire sleep period.

SLEEP MEASUREMENT INSTRUMENTS

Researchers have developed sleep measurement instruments such as questionnaires, self-report methods, and other instruments to refine the measurement of an individual's perceptions of the quality of sleep. The person is asked to respond, usually in writing, to standardized questions about sleep quality and quantity, the number of awakenings, and the time needed to fall sleep. This information is similar to the information that may be obtained by interviewing. Questionnaires may be difficult to complete for someone who is acutely ill, frail, or cognitively impaired. Table 10-1 summarizes some sleep measurement instruments that are used in clinical practice and in the conduct of research studies.

ASSESSMENT AIDS

- Interview Guide to suggest questions and record data (Display 10-2)
- Forms for recording data for a sleep log

Interview Guide: Sleep and Rest Pattern

USUAL SLEEP PATTERNS

Duration of sleep: _____ hours/night
Usual time to retire: _____ Usual time to awaken: _____
Number of awakenings during sleep: _____
Napping: ❑ AM nap ❑ PM nap Other: _____
Usual sleep surroundings: _____ Number of pillows: _____
Usual noise levels: _____

ALTERED SLEEP PATTERNS

Obtain adequate sleep: ❑ yes ❑ no Explain: _____
Difficulty sleeping at night: ❑ no ❑ yes Explain:_____
(If applicable) How long has there been a problem with sleep? _____
Time it takes to fall asleep: _____ Early awakening: ❑ yes ❑ no
Consequences of poor sleep: ❑ fatigue ❑ daytime sleepiness ❑ fall asleep without warning during the day ❑ loss
    of energy ❑ lack of initiative ❑ memory lapses ❑ difficulty concentrating ❑ depression, anxiety, or other
    mood changes
Factors contributing to sleep disturbance: ❑ stress ❑ shift work ❑ jet travel ❑ unfamiliar sleep environment
    ❑ noise ❑ temperature of environment ❑ uncomfortable mattress ❑ other _____
History of sleep problems: ❑ loud snoring ❑ sleep apnea ❑ morning headaches ❑ cataplexy ❑ hallucinations
    with sleep ❑ nightmares ❑ sleep walking

SLEEP AND BEDTIME RITUALS

Usual routine before sleep: _____

MEDICAL HISTORY

Conditions related to problems with sleep and rest: ❑ no ❑ yes
Explain/List: _____

MEDICATION HISTORY

Medications influencing sleep and rest: ❑ no ❑ yes
Explain/List: _____

▼ ▼ ▼

Assessment Guidelines Sleep and Rest Interview (Health History)

Procedure	Clinical Significance

1. Usual sleep patterns

Use the interview to elicit specific information about the person's usual sleep pattern. Determine the following characteristics of the person's sleep pattern:

- Duration of sleep
- Usual time for falling asleep
- Usual time for awakening
- Number of awakenings during the sleep period (and cause, if known)
- Pattern of daytime napping

Determine whether shift work interferes with sleep and rest. Determine what shifts are worked and how frequently shifts change.

Determine whether sleep patterns vary with weekend changes.

Clinical Significance

Sleep patterns vary greatly among people, which may be attributed to differences in culture, family responsibilities, work schedules, and lifestyles.

For a more detailed evaluation of sleep patterns, consider the use of a sleep log (discussed earlier in this section).

People who change work shifts often have difficulty sleeping or do not obtain enough sleep. Frequent changing of shift assignments may interfere more with the sleep pattern than working a straight shift.

2. Altered sleep patterns—insomnia

Interview the person to determine whether there is a perception of inadequate or abnormal sleep.

To screen for insomnia, ask the following:

- "Do you think you obtain adequate sleep?"
- "Do you feel rested on awakening?"
- "Do you have difficulty sleeping at night?"

Ask the person whether there are daytime consequences to poor sleep:

- Fatigue
- Daytime sleepiness
- Loss of energy
- Lack of initiative
- Memory lapses
- Difficulty concentrating
- Depression, anxiety, or other mood changes

Ask the person how long he or she has experienced insomnia to differentiate transient insomnia from persistent insomnia.

Determine whether there are situations or conditions that contribute to sleep disturbance.

Insomnia: The perception of inadequate or abnormal sleep. Insomnia is a *symptom* that includes difficulty falling asleep, a short sleep time, and "nonrestorative sleep."

As a symptom, insomnia should be thoroughly evaluated in a systematic manner to determine its possible cause.

Daytime effects may be attributed to poor sleep. Unless there are daytime consequences to poor sleep, treatment of the insomnia may not be necessary.

Transient Insomnia: Insomnia that lasts for several days (less than 1 week) and affects a person who typically reports normal sleep.

Persistent Insomnia: Insomnia that lasts for weeks or longer.

In a person who typically reports normal sleep, resolution of contributing factors may normalize sleep again.

▼ ▼ ▼

GUIDELINES *continued*   Sleep and Rest Interview (Health History)

Procedure

Contributing factors to transient insomnia:

- Stress
- Shift work
- Jet travel
- Unfamiliar sleep environments
- Noise
- Temperature of environment
- Uncomfortable mattress

Determine the timing of insomnia in relation to the sleep period by asking the following:

- "Do you have difficulty falling asleep?"
- "How long does it take to fall asleep?"

- "Is your sleep interrupted?"
- "Do you wake up frequently during the night?"

- "Are you waking up earlier or later than desired?"
- "Do you wake up early and find that you cannot get back to sleep?"
- "Are you making up for lost sleep during the night by daytime napping or retiring early?"

3. **Sleepiness**

Determine whether the person is experiencing excessive sleepiness that occurs at inappropriate or undesirable times.

- "Do you have difficulty staying awake during the day?"
- "Have you fallen asleep without warning during the day?"

If the person reports excessive daytime sleepiness, determine whether additional associated symptoms are present, including:

- Loud snoring
- Sleep apnea (cessation of breathing during sleep)
- Morning headaches
- Cataplexy (sudden onset of muscle weakness or paralysis)
- Hypnagogic hallucinations (hallucinations that occur at the onset of sleep)

Clinical Significance

Three classifications of insomnia are differentiated on the basis of timing:

Delayed sleep onset (initial insomnia): The person requires more than 30 minutes to fall sleep. Normal sleep onset is within 5 to 15 minutes. Stress and anxiety are common contributing factors.

Latency period: The interval from "lights out" to the beginning of sleep.

Impaired sleep continuity: The sleep period is characterized by several intermittent periods of awakening. The person may not always recall these awakenings but report daytime effects of poor sleep. The most common cause of intermittent awakenings is a stimulus such as noise, the need to void, nightmares, or pain.

Early morning awakening (terminal insomnia): The person awakens in the early morning (or before completion of a typical 8-hour sleep period) and cannot resume sleep. More common in elders, a pattern of early morning awakening is associated with daytime napping or early retiring. Early morning awakening also may be associated with stress or depression.

Excessive daytime sleepiness (EDS) is an indication of a sleep disorder when it occurs at inappropriate or undesirable times such as at work, while driving, or during social activities and when the daytime sleepiness is not relieved by increased amounts of sleep at night.

Sleep laboratory evaluation should be considered for definitive diagnosis.

Identification of these symptoms may aid in the diagnosis of pathological sleep disorders (see "Clinical Problems Related To Sleep and Rest" later in this chapter).

| Procedure | Clinical Significance |

Procedure

4. Sleep and bedtime habits (rituals)

Determine the activities that the person usually engages in before sleep. You can inquire in the following manner:

- "Tell me what you usually do an hour before going to bed."
- "How has your bedtime routine been changed?"

Examples of bedtime rituals:

- Personal hygiene (brushing teeth; washing face; bathing)
- Reading
- Watching television; listening to music
- Bedtime snack

5. Medical history

Screen the person for pathological conditions that may be associated with sleep pattern disturbance.

Conditions Associated With Nocturnal Pain

Arthritis and other rheumatologic disorders

Diabetes with neuropathy (burning foot pain)

Cluster headaches

Angina (chest pain)

Peptic ulcer disease

Hiatal hernia (esophageal reflux)

Tumors and metastatic lesions

Additional cues to sleep disruption secondary to pathologic conditions may come from asking the following:

- "Do you get up at night to take antacids or eat?"
- "Do you elevate the head of the bed or sleep with additional pillows?"

Other Clinical Problems Interfering with Sleep

- Nocturia (nighttime voiding)
- Dyspnea (shortness of breath)

- Paresthesias (numbness, tingling, pain of the extremities)

- Hyperthyroidism; Cushing's syndrome
- Depression, anxiety

6. Caffeine, nicotine and alcohol ingestion; medication history

Any person complaining of insomnia should be evaluated for caffeine or alcohol intake patterns and smoking history. Evaluate caffeine ingestion by inquiring about the type and quantity of caffeinated substances consumed. A food recall (food diary) may be an accurate method for quantifying caffeine ingestion.

Clinical Significance

Regular bedtime behaviors often promote sleep onset. Disruption of bedtime behaviors, such as might occur with travel or hospitalization, can interfere with sleep. Every attempt to maintain bedtime habits or rituals in an unfamiliar environment should be encouraged to set the stage for sleep.

Pain is a common cause of insomnia. Arthritis pain, pain from diabetic neuropathies, and peptic ulcer pain is often worse at night. Peptic ulcer pain is aggravated at night as a result of increased secretion of gastric acid.

Cluster headaches may be precipitated during rapid eye movement (REM) sleep.

Esophageal reflux pain occurs from the movement of peptic acid into the esophagus. Reflux may be aggravated by a recumbent sleep position.

Done to relieve ulcer pain.

Done to alleviate esophageal reflux or dyspnea secondary to heart failure or pulmonary disorders.

Nocturia may be a symptom of obstructive uropathy.

Nighttime dyspnea may occur with congestive heart failure or pulmonary disease, including asthma, bronchitis, and emphysema.

Paresthesias from restless leg syndrome or nerve compressions are usually more troublesome at night.

The endocrine disorders associated with insomnia.

Caffeine Ingestion: Caffeine can decrease total sleep time especially by interfering with the onset of sleep and contributing to nighttime awakenings. Sensitivity to the effects of caffeine can persist for up to 12 hours after ingestion.

Nicotine and Sleep: Nicotine has much the same effects on sleep as caffeine.

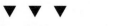

Sleep and Rest Interview (Health History)

Procedure

Average cup of coffee: 100 mg caffeine

Strong cup of coffee: 200 mg caffeine

Tea and cola drinks: 50–100 mg caffeine

Some people will be reluctant to admit to alcohol intake.

Take a medication history to determine whether the person is taking any medications that may affect sleep or that are intended to induce sleep.

Medication

CNS Depressants

  Phenobarbital

  Nembutal

  Seconal

  Demerol

  Valium

  Librium

  Dalmane

  Halcion

  Ativan

  Serax

  Alcohol

CNS Stimulants

  Caffeine

  Amphetamine

  Theophylline

Antipsychotics

  Mellaril

  Haldol

  Thorazine

  Navane

Autonomic Agents

  Nasal sprays

  Cough syrups

  Dextromethorphan

  OTC—Sudafed

Antihypertensives

  Methyldopa

  Reserpine

  Atenolol

  Nifedipine

Clinical Significance

Alcohol and Sleep: Many people believe alcohol promotes sleep because of the initial sedative effect. However, alcohol may contribute to nighttime awakening and REM sleep deprivation. Alcohol withdrawal is associated with severe sleep pattern disturbances, including nightmares and extreme restlessness. Alcohol may contribute to sleep apnea syndrome.

Sleep Aids: Most sleep aids ("sleeping pills") are physiologically effective for 2 to 3 weeks, after which time a placebo effect may occur. People taking sleeping pills may change doctors frequently to acquire access to various sleep-inducing medications.

Effect on Sleep

Decrease the amount of REM sleep.

REM Rebound Sleep: "Catching up" on REM sleep after a period of deprivation or curtailment. When drugs depressing REM and stage IV sleep time are withdrawn, REM rebound sleep and nightmares may occur.

Delay the onset of sleep

Interfere with REM sleep

Contribute to daytime drowsiness

Contribute to daytime drowsiness

Cause drowsiness

▼ ▼ ▼

G U I D E L I N E S *continued*   Sleep and Rest Interview (Health History)

Procedure	Clinical Significance
MAO Inhibitors	Improve sleep in depressed persons
Marplan	Decrease REM time
Nardel	
Parnate	
Diuretics	Nighttime awakenings caused by nocturia

▼ ▼ ▼

G U I D E L I N E S

Assessment Guidelines   Sleep Laboratory Evaluation

Procedure

The sleep laboratory evaluation (polysomnographic evaluation) is a technological process for monitoring and evaluating sleep. This section provides only a summary explanation of polysomnographic procedures. Sleep laboratory evaluation is performed in a dedicated setting with specialized equipment. A specially trained technologist performs the measurement procedures, data are recorded on chart paper that accepts signals from multiple recording channels of the instruments being used, and a specially trained technologist or physician scores and stages the sleep recording.

1. **Electroencephalogram (EEG)**

   The skilled technician applies several EEG leads to the scalp to record brain wave activity during the sleep period. A polygraph recording of the brain wave pattern is obtained on paper.

   The recorded brain waves are analyzed to determine the order and duration of various stages of sleep.

   Sleep EEGs are interpreted and described according to standard methods and nomenclature.

2. **Electro-oculogram (EOG)**

   The EOG records each eyeball position during sleep by measuring the potential difference between the cornea and retina. Small electrodes are placed at the orbital margins, and waveforms representing eye movement are traced on polygraph paper.

3. **Electromyogram (EMG)**

   An EMG is obtained by attaching small electrodes on the chin to record muscle tone.

Clinical Significance

Polysomnography is indicated in the evaluation of sleep-related breathing disorders and periodic limb movement disorders (restless leg syndrome) or when the cause of insomnia is uncertain.

The main sleep functions evaluated by polysomnography are the following:

- Sleep onset latency (time taken to fall asleep)
- Percentage of time spent in each sleep stage
- Sleep disruption over the sleep period

The EEG provides a continuous recording of brain wave activity during sleep. Brain wave characteristics are used to identify and differentiate the various sleep stages.

Criteria for identifying sleep stages by EEG pattern are discussed elsewhere in this chapter (see "Knowledge Base for Assessment—Stages of Sleep and Normal Sleep Pattern.")

Rapid eye movements are associated with REM sleep. Flat waveform lines are usually recorded during non-REM sleep. Frequent eye movements during REM sleep may indicate intense dreaming.

Face and neck muscles are usually hypotonic just before and during REM sleep. However, brief spikes of muscle activity may be noted as a result of electrical discharge from the pons during REM sleep.

▼ ▼ ▼

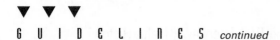

G U I D E L I N E S   *continued*   Sleep Laboratory Evaluation

Procedure

4. Other sleep monitoring

The sleep laboratory evaluation may include additional monitoring during the sleep period, including observation of the following:

- Body movements
- Electrocardiogram
- Respiratory pattern
- Hemoglobin saturation (oximetry)

Clinical Significance

Additional monitoring is indicated to identify sleep-induced cardiac dysrhythmias and the significance of sleep apnea episodes.

▼ ▼ ▼

G U I D E L I N E S

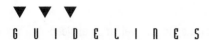

Assessment Guidelines   Interpreting Physical Examination Findings Related to Sleep and Rest

Procedure

Note signs of sleep pattern disturbance and any associated physical effects during the physical examination, with special attention to the following:

- General appearance
- Facial expression
- Speech pattern
- Cognitive functions

1. General appearance

Observe for general behavioral indicators of sleep disruption.

Clinical Significance

Sleep disruption may alter a person's normal physical appearance and behavioral patterns.

Behavioral Indicators of Sleep Disruption

- Restlessness
- Frequent yawning
- Eye rubbing
- Nodding ("nodding off")
- Irritability
- Disorientation
- Lethargy
- Listlessness

2. Face

Observe the facial expression and other facial features.

Indicators of Sleep Disruption

- Flat or expressionless facial affect
- Mild fleeting nystagmus
- Red conjunctivae
- Ptosis of eyelids
- Dark circles under eyes

▼ ▼ ▼
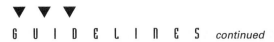

G U I D E L I N E S *continued*   Interpreting Physical Examination Findings
Related to Sleep and Rest

___

Procedure

3. Speech pattern

Listen for signs of sleep disturbance as the person talks, especially thick speech with mispronunciation and incorrect word usage.

4. Cognitive functions

Note any decline in cognitive abilities, especially a decreased level of alertness and awareness. Evaluate the person's attention span and problem-solving abilities.

Clinical Significance

Sleep deprivation is generally associated with progressive disorientation and decline in cognitive functions.

Cognitive Signs of Sleep Deprivation

- Inability to concentrate
- Impaired judgment

___

▼ ▼ ▼

G U I D E L I N E S

Assessment Guidelines   Sleep Pattern Observation

Procedure

In some health care settings, the nurse has the opportunity to actually observe a person's sleep pattern and behaviors as well as the environmental surroundings during sleep.

1. Survey the sleeping person's environment.

Note environmental stimuli that may promote or inhibit sleep.

2. Observe body movements.

Note the person's body movements during rest or sleep periods.

Clinical Significance

A person's reported perceptions about sleep quality provide reliable data about sleep and should be compared with the nurse's perceptions about a person's sleep based on observations.

Sleep Promoters

- Quiet
- Dark or subdued lighting
- Comfortable mattress and pillows
- Room temperature (personal preference varies)
- Presence of usual sleeping partner

Sleep Inhibitors

- Noise (including voices)
- Light
- Irregular or soft mattress
- Uncomfortable pillows
- Extreme room temperatures
- Roommates (especially if requiring treatments or confused)
- Hospital routines (laboratory tests; vital sign measurement; medication administration)

Normal Findings

Expect to see periodic body movements during sleep. Position may be changed 20 to 60 times during an 8-hour sleep period.

▼ ▼ ▼

GUIDELINES *continued*   Sleep Pattern Observation

Procedure	**Clinical Significance**

Procedure

If there is very little body movement observed, ask the person about sleep quality.

3. **Determine the quantity of uninterrupted sleep time.**
   Note the amount of uninterrupted sleep time the person experiences. Uninterrupted sleep time includes periods in which no one enters the patient's room or immediate surroundings.

4. **Observe sleep behaviors.**
   Note general appearance.

   Note specific sleep-related behaviors.

Clinical Significance

Deviations from Normal
Absent or minimal position changes may indicate poor-quality sleep.

People need at least 90 minutes to complete one full sleep cycle including REM sleep. In hospitals, some people are disturbed on an hourly basis and therefore are at high risk for sleep deprivation.

A person who is sleeping will usually lie immobile with eyes closed. Always validate by comparing your observations with the person's reports of sleep.

Normal Findings
Snoring, sleep talking

Deviations from Normal
Snoring associated with sleep apnea syndrome, sleep-walking; night terrors, enuresis; teeth grinding; apnea (see "Clinical Problems Related to Sleep and Rest").

Documenting Sleep Evaluation Findings

Example 1: Normal Sleep Pattern

Ms. G, aged 32 years, was interviewed about sleep and rest patterns as part of a routine health assessment at the community health clinic. Characteristics of her sleep and rest habits were recorded as follows:

> Reports 6 or 7 hours of sleep between 2300 and 0600. Awakens once during night to care for infant but readily falls back to sleep. Awakens feeling refreshed; feels energetic during daytime activities; rarely naps. Presleep routine includes mending or needlepoint while watching television with husband, brushing teeth, checking baby, and letting cat outside.

These findings may be recorded in a problem-oriented record as follows:

S: 6 or 7 hours of sleep per night between 2300 and 0600, with one nighttime awakening to care for infant. Readily falls back to sleep. Rarely naps, feels energetic during day and wakens refreshed. "I feel I get enough sleep."

O: Alert and attentive throughout 20-minute assessment interview. Facial affect animated; eyes bright, clear conjunctivae.

A: Functional sleep–rest pattern; able to maintain desired lifestyle.

P: Follow-up with routine health screening in 1 year.

Reinforce importance of regular daily cycling (regular retirement/wakeup times) in maintaining optimal sleep pattern.

Example 2: Sleep Apnea

Mr. S, aged 49 years, was observed overnight in the coronary care unit (CCU) after hospital admission for chest pain. The nurse observed irregular snoring and periods of apnea. When asked about sleep in the morning, Mr. S. reported long-standing fatigue. This and other data were summarized in the medical record:

> Noted to have apneic periods during sleep lasting 5 to 10 seconds. Irregular, loud snoring. Reports "wife always bothered by snoring": excessive daytime sleepiness, and occasional morning headaches.

These findings may be recorded in a problem-oriented record as follows:

S: "I'm always tired: I must not sleep very well, although my wife says I snore all night long."

O: Obese male: high-risk age-group for sleep apnea; apneic periods during sleep (5–10 sec). Snores irregularly.

A: Sleep dysfunction—possibly sleep apnea.

P: Discuss referral to sleep laboratory for additional evaluation when discharged from hospital. Consider aggravation of cardiovascular problems related to sleep apnea and increase nighttime surveillance while in CCU.

Example 3: Sleep Pattern Disturbance

Ms. P, aged 29, was evaluated at the student health center. Her primary reason for seeking health care was fatigue. She reported: "I'm always tired during the day, but especially on Mondays." Sleep data were recorded as follows:

> Reports 6 hours of sleep on a good night and less than 4 hours of sleep on Friday and Saturday nights. Cites dating and school obligations as interfering with sleep: once asleep, has no difficulty staying asleep "unless I drank too much and then I'm up early, still feeling very tired." Denies use of sleep-inducing medications or caffeine. Reports occasional use of street amphetamines to "give me energy." General appearance: dark circles under eyes; frequent yawning; body slumped; short attention span during interview.

These findings may be recorded in a problem-oriented record as follows:

S: "I'm always tired during the day, especially on Mondays." Usual sleep pattern: "6 hours, uninterrupted, on a good night," and 4 hours on Friday and Saturday nights. Studies and social activities interfere most with sleep time. Occasional alcohol use causes early awakenings. "I take some speed if I get too tired and need some energy."

O: Dark circles under eyes; frequent yawning; body slumped; short attention span during interview.

A: Sleep pattern disturbance—possibly related to ineffective lifestyle management.

P: Discuss usual sleep requirements for age; explore alternative lifestyle patterns that will allow more time for sleep; discuss relationships between amphetamines/alcohol and sleep.

Nursing Diagnoses Related to Sleep and Rest

Sleep Pattern Disturbance

Sleep pattern disturbance can be defined as disrupted sleep that causes discomfort or interferes with a person's desired lifestyle. There are three major types of sleep pattern disturbance, including insomnia, excessive daytime sleepiness, and sleep-related pathophysiology such as sleep apnea or narcolepsy. Some of these disturbances are manifestations of primary sleep disorders or medical illnesses (See also "Clinical Problems Related to Sleep and Rest").

Indicators of sleep pattern disturbance include the following:

- Difficulty falling asleep
- Waking earlier or later than desired
- Experiencing interrupted sleep
- Not feeling well rested
- Demonstrating behavioral or cognitive effects such as irritability, lethargy, restlessness, disorientation

Possible physical indicators include:

- Nystagmus
- Hand tremor

- Eyelid ptosis
- Dark circles under the eyes
- Slurred or otherwise altered speech

Some sleep pattern disturbances are related to unfavorable environmental stimuli that may be obvious if you have the opportunity to observe the person's sleep environment. Stress also may be a contributing factor. The nurse can conduct the interview in such a way as to identify significant stressors. If the person reports periods of insomnia, additional interviewing and, if possible, direct observation of the person's sleep period will be helpful in determining more about the type of insomnia that is occurring. An even more definitive diagnosis may be obtained from a sleep laboratory evaluation. Finally, sleep pattern disturbances may be occurring because of pain or the effects of various medical problems such as cardiac or pulmonary diseases.

Sleep Deprivation

Sleep deprivation is a loss of normally required sleep significant enough to result in a sense of lost sleep, impaired functioning, and physical manifestations. Sleep deprivation results in impaired cognitive function and leads to mental fatigue, impaired memory, inability to concentrate, perception changes, and poor judgment. Personality changes include irritability, withdrawal, increased suspicion, confusion, disorientation, listlessness, and reduced emotional control. Neurologically, sleep deprivation is associated with mild nystagmus, hand tremors, ptosis, flat facial affect, and impaired speech patterns. Finally, sleep deprivation is associated with lowered pain threshold and decreased production of catecholamines and corticosteroids, which are essential for combating stress.

Deprivation of REM period sleep is associated with specific adverse behavioral effects including hyperactivity, mood swings, agitation, and decreased impulse control.

Sleep deprivation can affect subsequent sleep patterns, especially the type and length of the stages of sleep entered. When subjects in controlled studies were prevented from experiencing REM sleep and then were permitted to go back to sleep, they entered REM sleep within 4 to 10 minutes after falling asleep, rather than after the usual 90 minutes (Berger & Oswald, 1962). Furthermore, the amount of REM sleep obtained after REM sleep deprivation may be 50% greater than baseline or normal amounts (REM rebound). Subjects who were deprived of stage 4 sleep tended to gain additional stage 4 sleep in subsequent sleep periods. If after the deprivation of both REM and stage 4 sleep, stage 4 sleep is made up first, the problem of REM sleep deprivation may be aggravated.

Clinical Problems Related to Sleep and Rest

Narcolepsy

Narcolepsy is a sleep disorder characterized by the following:

- *"Sleep attacks"*: Irresistible episodes of daytime sleepiness
- *Cataplexy*: A sudden loss of motor tone that may cause the person to fall
- *Sleep paralysis*: Skeletal muscle paralysis, which occurs during the transition from wakefulness to stage 1
- *Hypnagogic hallucinations*: Nightmares

The cause is unknown but may be related to a central nervous system genetic defect that causes an uncontrollable REM sleep phase.

Involuntary daytime sleep attacks may begin in puberty. Most people with this problem have symptoms for about 15 years before the disorder is accurately diagnosed. The daytime sleep attacks are absolutely irresistible. Cataplexy, especially weak knees, is often precipitated by strong emotion, either positive or negative. Hypnagogic hallucinations or nightmares occur most often as the person falls asleep. Sleep paralysis may affect most skeletal muscles; it is frightening, because the person can neither move nor speak. However, the ability to move the eyes is retained and is usually sufficient to reverse the paralysis, as is someone touching the person or applying other external stimuli. Recovery occurs even if the person is left undisturbed. A small percentage of people who do not have narcolepsy may experience sleep paralysis for unknown reasons. Familial incidence of narcolepsy is 20 times that of the general population.

In addition to the obvious signs of daytime sleep attacks, narcolepsy involves disturbed nighttime sleep, as revealed through sleep laboratory evaluation. The person suffering from narcolepsy tends to enter REM sleep immediately after falling asleep. (Normally, 90 minutes of sleep elapses before the first REM phase.)

Sleep Apnea Syndrome

Temporary cessation of breathing during sleep for short periods of 10 seconds or so is referred to as sleep apnea. In sleep apnea syndrome, as many as 300 episodes of breathing cessation may occur during the sleep period. Most types of sleep apnea are classified as obstructive, or secondary to airway obstruction, which commonly results from enlarged adenoids or tonsils, or obesity. However, the airway is patent during the waking state. Sleep apnea has been linked to sudden infant death syndrome.

History

Men older than 50 years are most frequently affected. Obesity is a risk factor, especially if the person has a short, fat neck. The person usually seeks health care for hypersomnolence or excessive daytime sleepiness, indicating that the disturbance is interfering with his or her lifestyle. Unlike the sleep attacks associated with narcolepsy, the daytime sleepiness that accompanies sleep apnea is resistible. The person may report moving around or slapping himself or herself to stay awake.

Laboratory Evaluation

Sleeping partners of people with sleep apnea syndrome often report that the person stops breathing during sleep for 10 to 20 seconds. Loud snorts follow that increase in intensity until suddenly the person bolts upright in bed and resumes breathing, all without waking. Another possible manifestation is a pattern of irregular snoring. Such behavior is usually confirmed in the sleep laboratory. The person may exhibit typical symptoms of sleep deprivation, including increased irritability, decreased attention span, and impaired memory. The alveolar hypoventilation associated with apneic episodes may contribute to more serious sequelae, including cor pulmonale, pulmonary hypertension, and brain hypoxia.

Kleine-Levin Syndrome

Kleine-Levin syndrome, a rare hypersomnolence disorder unrelated to narcolepsy, is characterized by sleep attacks that last several hours to several days, three or four times a year. Eating patterns vary greatly; the person may gorge with food for several days and gain weight. Often the person suffers from depression or other psychological problems. Sleep laboratory evaluation indicates an otherwise essentially normal sleep pattern.

Nocturnal Myoclonus

Nocturnal myoclonus is a rare form of sleep pattern disturbance whereby the person is awakened by calf muscle spasms, which may occur as frequently as every 30 seconds. Excessive daytime sleepiness or waking feeling unrefreshed may be reported.

Parasomnias

The parasomnias include somnambulism (sleepwalking), pavor nocturnus (night terrors), nocturnal enuresis, talking in one's sleep, and bruxism (teeth grinding). These manifestations originate during non-REM sleep. Parasomnias, which primarily interfere with children's sleep and often appear together in the same child, have a familial tendency.

Somnambulism (Sleepwalking)

Somnambulism, or sleepwalking, occurs most often in children, and boys are affected more frequently than girls. The person usually cannot remember the sleepwalking episode and may not awaken if the episode lasts less than 4 minutes.

Sleepwalking occurs most often in the first third of the sleep period during stage III or IV non-REM sleep. The sleep EEG usually indicates that sleepwalking is preceded by a burst of high-voltage, low-frequency activity similar to that occurring in stage IV. A normal percentage of REM sleep is noted, indicating that the person experiences normal dreaming.

Parvor Nocturnus (Night Terrors)

Night terrors most often affect children younger than age 6. After sleeping a few hours, the child usually bolts up in bed, shakes and screams, and appears terrified, but is difficult to awaken. Children usually do not remember these episodes.

Night terrors occur predominantly in stage IV sleep. They may be treated by administering benzodiazepines, which are known to suppress stage IV sleep.

Nocturnal Enuresis (Bedwetting)

Nocturnal enuresis, or bedwetting, may be either primary or secondary. In primary enuresis, bedwetting has no physiologic basis and persists from birth to age 6 or older. In secondary enuresis, bedwetting occurs because of psychological factors. Nocturnal enuresis is primarily a childhood disorder, occurring especially in boys, although 1% to 2% of some sampled adult groups exhibited the disorder as well.

When assessing enuresis, interview the parent(s) as well as the child. Parents may be frustrated by bedwetting episodes, especially in preschool-age children with daytime control. Ask the parents questions such as, "How do you deal with your child and the bedwetting?" and "Do you feel your child can control the bedwetting?" Sibling jealousy or fear of walking to the bathroom alone in the dark may contribute to the problem. Finally, discuss bedwetting with the child.

Nocturnal enuresis occurs most frequently during the first third of the sleep period, following the transition from stage IV to stage II sleep. Immediately before entering REM sleep, while still in stage II, the child urinates. The child will not usually maintain restful sleep in wet clothing or bed linens.

Usually, talking in one's sleep occurs during non-REM sleep and is associated with body movement. Sleep talking is not considered a disturbance except to someone sleeping in the same room.

Bruxism, or teeth grinding during sleep, occurs in 15% of the population. The teeth may become chipped, and the person may need to wear a nighttime mouth guard to protect the teeth. Bruxism usually occurs during stage II non-REM sleep.

CASE STUDY

Mr. Butcher, a 52-year-old patient who had undergone coronary artery bypass graft surgery complicated by postoperative bleeding, had consented to be a subject in a study to identify sleep pattern characteristics in critical care settings. After Mr. Butcher recovered from general anesthesia, data were collected by continuous EEG recordings and behavioral observations to verify whether he was sleeping. In addition, data were collected about stimuli that could potentially disrupt sleep. Data collection was nearly complete. Mr. Butcher's condition was stable, and he was awaiting transfer to a general surgical ward.

Although comprehensive data analysis for all subjects in the study was to follow, the nurse researcher reviewed the data collected during the previous 48 hours, including the EEG recordings that correlated with the various sleep stages. The data indicated that Mr. Butcher had not entered a sleep state for the previous 32 hours, but rather, had been in a wakeful or aroused state, despite his sleep-like appearance. However, the nurse's charting revealed Mr. Butcher had "slept well throughout the night."

Mr. Butcher displayed a number of behaviors that the nursing staff attributed to the intensive care unit (ICU) environment, such as irritability, inability to concentrate, and mild confusion. For example, he could not state the day or time and had pulled intravenous lines and removed his oxygen cannula frequently during the previous 12 hours. When caregivers approached Mr. Butcher, he asked them to leave him alone so he could get a good night's sleep.

The nurse researcher discussed Mr. Butcher's sleep status with the nursing staff.

Case Study Analysis

It was relatively easy for the nurses to diagnose Sleep pattern disturbance following recovery from heart surgery for Mr. Butcher, because the nurse researcher had documented the problem by EEG recording. Could the nurses have arrived at the same diagnosis without such data? Most experts agree that interviewing and observing provide reliable data about the sleep pattern. However, the diagnostic process involved requires a different cognitive approach than that required to analyze data generated by the EEG.

Assessment Focus

The nurses caring for Mr. Butcher made several observations, even before the nurse researcher shared data collected from the EEG. One nurse described her thinking as follows:

This man had been in the ICU only 2 days, but we had met previously when he visited the unit as part of his preoperative teaching. At that time he was a little anxious but seemed to be coping well. He talked freely, expressing his concerns and asking pertinent questions. After surgery, his behavior changed. He acted paranoid and confused—always picking at lines and equipment. I wanted to focus on problems that might have precipitated his behavior. My initial thoughts focused on several possibilities: Sleep pattern disturbance, Anxiety, Fear, Ineffective coping, and that vague problem area called "ICU psychosis." I realized I needed more information before I could diagnose the problem. It was important to see whether fear was the primary problem causing sleep disruption or whether sleep disruption was the primary problem leading to paranoid behavior. I focused on making the correct differential diagnosis because I knew treatment would be influenced by the final diagnosis.

Sleep deprivation in ICU patients is common, and nurses have begun to place greater emphasis on interventions to promote sleep in such high-risk people. In 1983, critical care nurses were surveyed to determine significant patient problems that could be addressed through nursing research. The survey indicated that critical care nursing research needed to focus on promoting sleep and prevent-

CASE STUDY *continued*

ing sleep deprivation in critically ill clients (Lewandowski & Kotsitsky, 1983).

The expertise and knowledge of nurses in the ICU influenced the types of problems they considered when they noticed behavior changes in Mr. Butcher. The stage of his medical treatment also influenced the direction of nursing assessment. Mr. Butcher was still receiving the type of care associated with multiple stimuli that could interfere with sleep. For example, every hour a nurse measured vital signs, took a pulmonary artery catheter reading, and measured urine output. Once every 4 hours, a nurse, surgeon, intern, or surgical resident performed a head-to-toe examination. Moreover, every 2 hours, Mr. Butcher was turned and positioned and asked to cough, deep breathe, and use the incentive inspirometer. Between 4:00 and 5:00 AM, blood specimens were collected; a chest radiograph was taken; a weight was obtained on the bedscale; and a bath and linen change were provided. Environmental stimuli during daytime and evening hours included bright lights, telephones, cardiac monitors, alarms, intravenous pumps, and ventilators, background talking, and hissing sounds from suction and oxygen equipment.

In addition, Mr. Butcher had experienced some postoperative pain and had required several transfusions of packed red blood cells. Not only could such stimuli interfere with sleep, but they could contribute to additional problems such as anxiety, fear, and ineffective coping.

Preliminary Nursing Diagnoses

The nursing diagnosis of Sleep pattern disturbance was tentatively established for Mr. Butcher based on his difficulty falling asleep, his mood alterations, and his statements concerning sleep loss. Even though there was strong evidence supporting this diagnosis, the nurses remained tentative. Other nursing diagnoses, especially Anxiety, Fear, and Ineffective coping, as characterized by mood alterations, needed to be considered.

Additional Assessment

Additional data were analyzed to select or assign priority to possible nursing diagnoses. To establish a precise diagnosis, the nurses compared the data with defining characteristics and etiologic categories associated with each diagnosis being considered. Occasionally, more data collection was required to make such comparisons. For example:

Anxiety

Assess patient further for the following:

- *Risk factors:* Knowledge deficit, underlying fear, conflict, insecurity, ineffective coping

- *Manifestations:* Verbalized expectation of danger, signs of sympathetic nervous system activation, feelings of apprehensiveness or concern, increased verbalization, sleeping disturbances

Fear

Assess patient further for the following:

- *Risk factors:* Perceived external threat or danger, perceived inability to control events, knowledge deficit
- *Manifestations:* Describes the focus of threat or danger, verbalizes expectation of danger, increased verbalization, restlessness, signs of sympathetic nervous system activation

Ineffective Coping

Assess patient further for the following:

- *Risk factors:* Knowledge deficit, personal vulnerability, situational crisis
- *Manifestations:* Verbalized inability to cope, inability to solve problems, destructive behavior toward self and others, inappropriate use of defense mechanisms

Sleep Pattern Disturbance

Assess patient further for the following:

- *Risk factors:* Environmental stimuli, pain, anxiety, absence of bedtime rituals, previous sleep pattern disturbances, medication effects, periods of interrupted sleep time
- *Manifestations:* Complaints of insomnia, irritability, progressive disorientation, restlessness

Revised Nursing Diagnosis

By comparing information obtained from the patient with information associated with each diagnostic possibility, the nurses decided that Mr. Butcher was most likely suffering from Sleep pattern disturbance. Further assessment was directed toward determining optimal interventions and evaluating interventions. The patient's usual sleep pattern and bedtime rituals were assessed so that as he became more physiologically stable, he could be encouraged to resume previous patterns.

Furthermore, factors that might inhibit sleep, such as excessive environmental stimuli and pain, were identified and modified. Within 48 hours, Mr. Butcher was fully oriented and stated that he was sleeping well. Early nursing intervention and subsequent transfer out of the ICU contributed to resumption of previously functional sleep patterns.

CHAPTER 10 **S U M M A R Y**

Assessment of Sleep and Rest

Sleep and rest assessment should focus on the following:

- The individual's perceptions about the quantity and quality of sleep and rest
- Various factors that may influence sleep and rest
- Signs, symptoms, and causes of sleep pattern disturbance
- The effects of sleep pattern disturbances on physiologic, cognitive, and psychological functions

When assessing sleep and rest, consider the following:

- Sleep deprivation symptoms are general; therefore, the patient may not associate such symptoms with sleep pattern disturbances.
- Self-reports of sleep quantity and quality usually correlate closely with polysomnographic data.
- Sleep requirements vary among people. Sleep adequacy is evaluated relative to age-related norms and the client's perspective.
- Normal progression through sleep stages enhances sleep quality. At least 90 minutes is required for completion of a single sleep cycle.

Data Collection Methods

1. Interview or review of records
   - Usual sleep patterns
   - Altered sleep patterns
   - Sleep and bedtime habits
   - Medical history
   - Caffeine and alcohol intake
   - Medication history
2. Sleep laboratory evaluation
   - EEG
   - EOG
   - EMG
   - Physiologic event recording and observation
3. Physical Examination
   - General appearance
   - Facial expression
   - Speech pattern
   - Cognitive functions
4. Sleep Pattern Observation
   - Environmental stimuli affecting sleep
   - Body movement during sleep
   - Duration of uninterrupted sleep time
   - Sleep-related behaviors

Primary Nursing Diagnoses

- Sleep pattern disturbance
- Fatigue
- Sleep deprivation

Clinical Problems Related to Sleep Pattern Disturbances

- Narcolepsy
- Sleep apnea syndrome
- Kleine-Levin syndrome
- Nocturnal myoclonus
- Parasomnias

 Critical Thinking

Your ICU patient is a 53-year-old man who has a flail chest after an automobile accident. He is intubated and being ventilated mechanically. The nursing staff describes the patient as confused, combative, and agitated. He is kept sedated to control his behavior.

Learning Exercises

1. Plan how you would evaluate your patient's sleep and rest pattern. Given that he is sedated and intubated, determine how this would affect your assessment strategies.

2. One of your colleagues tells you that an assessment of this patient's sleep and rest pattern is irrelevant because there is nothing that you can do about an abnormal pattern. Explain how you would respond. Would you agree or disagree with your colleague? Explain why or why not.

3. Determine what observations you would want to make about this patient's surroundings that would be relevant to sleep and rest.

4. Interventions to improve this patient's sleep and rest cycles are implemented, including the provision of uninterrupted time with the lights dimmed and the room door closed. Propose how you would evaluate the effectiveness of these interventions.

BIBLIOGRAPHY

Assousa, S.N., & Wilson, N.D. (1991). Validation of sleep pattern disturbance. In R.M. Carroll-Johnson (Ed.). *Classification of nursing diagnoses: Proceedings of the ninth conference*. Philadelphia: J.B. Lippincott.

Baekeland, F., & Hoy, P. (1971). Reported vs. recorded sleep characteristics. *Archives of General Psychiatry, 24*(6), 548–551.

Bahr, R.T. (1983). Sleep-wake patterns of the aged. *Journal of Gerontological Nursing, 9*(10), 534–539.

Barndt-Maglio, B. (1986). Sleep pattern disturbance. *Dimensions of Critical Care Nursing, 5*(6), 342–349.

Berger, R.J., & Oswald, I. (1962). Effects of sleep deprivation on behavior, subsequent sleep, and dreaming. *Journal of Mental Sciences, 108*, 457.

Beyerman, K. (1987). Etiologies of sleep pattern disturbance in hospitalized patients. In A.M. McLane (Ed.). *Classification of nursing diagnoses: Proceedings of the seventh national conference* (pp. 193–198). St. Louis: C.V. Mosby.

Buysse, D.J., Reynolds, C.F., Monk, T.H., Berman, S.R., & Kupfer, D.J. (1989). The Pittsburgh Sleep Quality Index: A new instrument for psychiatric practice and research. *Psychiatric Research, 28*, 193–213.

Carskadon, M.A., & Dement, W.C. (1994). Normal human sleep: An overview. In Kryger, M.H., Roth, T., & Dement, W.C. (Eds.). *Principles and practice of sleep medicine* (2nd ed.). Philadelphia: W.B. Saunders.

Closs, S. (1998). Assessment of sleep in hospitalized patients: A review of methods. *Journal of Advanced Nursing, 13*(4), 501–510.

Edell-Gustafsson, U., Aren, C., Hamrin, E., & Hetta, J. (1994). Nurses' notes on sleep patterns in patients undergoing coronary artery bypass surgery: A retrospective evaluation of patient records. *Journal of Advanced Nursing, 20*(2), 331–336.

Ellis, B., Johns, M.W., Lancaster, R., Raptopoulos, P., Angelopoulos, N., & Priest, R. (1981). The St. Mary's Hospital Sleep Questionnaire: A study of reliability. *Sleep, 4*, 93–97.

Foreman, M.D., & Wykle, M. (1995). Nursing standard of practice protocol: Sleep disturbances in elderly patients. *Geriatric Nursing, 16*(5), 238–243.

Frensebner, B. (1983). Sleep deprivation in patients. *AORN Journal, 37*(1), 35–42.

Hartmann, E.L. (1973). *The functions of sleep*. New Haven, CT: Yale University Press.

Hartmann, E.L. (1973). Sleep requirements: Long sleepers, short sleepers, variable sleepers, insomniacs. *Psychosomatics, 14*, 95–103.

Hayter, J. (1983). Sleep behaviors of older persons. *Nursing Research, 32*(4), 242–246.

Helton, M.C., et al. (1980) The correlation between sleep deprivation and the intensive care unit syndrome. *Heart and Lung, 9*(3), 464–468.

Hemenway, J.A. (1980). Sleep and the cardiac patient. *Heart and Lung, 9*(3), 453–463.

Hodgson, L.A. (1991). Why do we need sleep? Relating theory to nursing practice, *Journal of Advanced Nursing, 16*(12), 1503–1510.

Jensen, D.P., & Herr, K.A. (1993). Sleeplessness. *Nursing Clinics of North America, 28*(2), 385–405.

Johns, M.W. (1971). Methods for assessing human sleep. *Archives of Internal Medicine, 127*(3), 484–492.

Kales, A. & Kales, J. (1970). Evaluation, diagnosis, and treatment of clinical conditions related to sleep. *Journal of the American Medical Association, 213*: 2229–2235.

Kales, A., & Kales, J. (1974). Sleep disorders: Recent findings in the diagnosis and treatment of disturbed sleep. *New England Journal of Medicine, 290*(9), 487–498.

Krachman, S.L., D'Alonzo, G.E., & Criner, G.J. (1995). Sleep in the Intensive Care Unit. *Chest, 107*(6), 1713–1720.

Kroenke, K. (1991). Chronic fatigue syndrome: Is it real? *Postgraduate Medicine, 89*(2), 44–46, 49–50, 53.

Lankford, S.R. (1994). Sleep loss in the elderly: Understanding the reasons. *Journal of Gerontological Nursing, 20*(8), 49–52.

Lewandowski, L.A., & Kotsitsky, A.M. (1983). Research priorities for critical care nursing: A study by the American Association of Critical Care Nurses, *Heart and Lung, 12*(1), 35–44.

McNeil, B.J., Padrick, K.P., & Wellman, J. (1986). I didn't sleep a wink. *American Journal of Nursing, 86*(1), 26–27.

Oswald, I. (1976). The function of sleep. *Postgraduate Medicine Journal, 52*, 15–18.

Parrott, C.P., & Hindmarch, I. (1980). The Leeds Sleep Evaluation Questionnaire in psychopharmacological investigations: A review. *Psychopharmacology, 71*, 173–179.

Parsons, L.C., & VerBeek, D. (1982). Sleep awake patterns following cerebral concussion. *Nursing Research, 31*(5), 260–264.

Ream, E., & Richardson, A. (1996). Fatigue: A concept analysis. *International Journal of Nursing Studies, 33*(5), 519–529.

Richards, K. (1987). Techniques for measurement of sleep in critical care. *Focus on Critical Care, 14*(4), 34–40.

Richardson, S.J. (1997). A comparison of tools for assessment of sleep pattern disturbance in critically ill adults. *Dimensions of Critical Care Nursing, 16*(5), 226–242.

Saletu, B. (1975). Is the subjectively experienced quality of sleep related to objective sleep parameters? *Behavioral Biology, 13*, 433–444.

Shaver, J.L.F., & Rodgers, A.E. (1994). Integrating an understanding of sleep knowledge into your practice. Part 2. Screening for sleep-related disorders: Sleep apnea and narcolepsy. *American Nurse, 26*(10), 24–25.

Shaver, J.L.F., & Giblin, E.C. (1989) Sleep. *Annual Review of Nursing Research, 7*, 71–93.

Simpson, T., Lee, E.R., & Cameron, C. (1996). Patients' perceptions of environmental factors that disturb sleep after cardiac surgery. *American Journal of Critical Care, 5*(3), 173–181.

Snyder-Halpern, R., & Verran, J.A. (1987). Instrumentation to describe subjective sleep characteristics in healthy subjects. *Research in Nursing and Health, 10*, 155–163.

Tiesinga, L.J., Dassen, T.W.N., & Halfens, R.J.G. (1996). Fatigue: A summary of the definitions, dimensions, and indicators. *Nursing Diagnosis, 7*(2), 51–62.

Topf, M. (1992). Effects of personal control over hospital noise on sleep. *Research in Nursing and Health, 15*, 19–28.

Topf, M., Bookman, M., & Arand, D. (1996) Effects of critical care unit noise on the subjective quality of sleep. *Journal of Advanced Nursing, 24*(3), 545–551.

Assessing Self-Concept

ASSESSMENT GUIDELINES

Self-Concept Interview
(Health History)

Self-Concept: Physical
Assessment

CHAPTER ORGANIZATION

Introductory Overview
- Assessment Focus
- Data Collection Methods
- Nursing Diagnoses

**Knowledge Base
for Assessment**
- Self-Concept
- Self-Concept Development

- Self-Concept Stability
- Variables Affecting Self-Concept
- A Healthy Personality

INTRODUCTORY OVERVIEW

Self-concept is how a person views or defines his or her own self at a given time and can often be reflected in answers to such questions as "Who am I?" or "What am I?" Self-concept includes the person's view of his or her personality traits, social roles, and physical traits. For example, a person's self-concept may include a personality trait, such as dependable or irresponsible, or a social role, such as community organizer or student. Self-concept is always evolving and is influenced by values, beliefs, interpersonal interactions, culture, and perceptions about how one is perceived by others.

Self-esteem, a part of self-concept, is a personal judgment about self-worth, value, and competence. It is the positive or negative value that one places on oneself. Self-esteem is developed over time, and the value attached to self can be negatively or positively changed through interactions with others. Positive self-esteem can also be enhanced by identifying positive personal traits, decreasing the time with self-devaluation, and focusing on traits respected by others.

When self-concept is threatened or disrupted—such as when a person loses his or her job, does not receive recognition believed deserved, or receives an evaluation perceived to be low—people attempt to maintain their beliefs about self. Defense mechanisms such as rationalization, projection, and displacement are often used to defend self-concept. For example, a person who just lost a job might say "I'm glad I don't work there, it is a very unethical place" (rationalization) or "I should have gotten a better grade on that paper, that teacher just doesn't like me" (displacement). If self-concept is threatened and defenses are not sufficient, stress increases, and the person may experience personality disorganization, a loss of control, and a sense of powerlessness and helplessness.

Assessing a person's self-concept enables the nurse to make judgments about a person's feelings of adequacy in a given situation and the behaviors that might be associated with these feelings. This assessment can provide insight into other problems the person might have. For example, a person in a cardiac rehabilitation program may not participate in recuperation activities because of feelings of inadequacy or feelings that he or she has no control over the outcome (Fig. 11-1).

According to Combs (1971), people "judge the value of their experiences with helpers from the frame of reference of self-concept. What affects the self-concept seems relevant. What appears remote from it seems irrelevant." For example, self-concept influences a person's motivation to learn, so that people who perceive themselves as poor learners, or who have a poor self-concept causing feelings of powerlessness or depression, may not respond to teaching interventions until their poor self-concept is identified and modified.

Assessing a person's self-concept helps reveal how self-perceptions influence behavior and emotional responses. Such an assessment should involve identifying the person's thoughts and feelings about self; factors that have influence on self-concept development; threats to self-concept; and the type of responses demonstrated in the face of threats to the person's self-esteem.

ASSESSMENT FOCUS

Self-concept is evaluated by observing general appearance and body language; listening for statements about personal and social identity as well as statements indicating level of self-esteem; asking pertinent question about self-concept; and interpreting results of questionnaires designed to measure self-perceptions.

Assessing self-concept can be especially difficult if the person uses defense mechanisms to conceal the self. Therefore, special efforts should be made to establish rapport and encourage disclosure.

The goals of assessing the self-concept pattern include:

- Identifying aspects of the person's social identity
- Identifying factors that contribute to the individual's self-concept

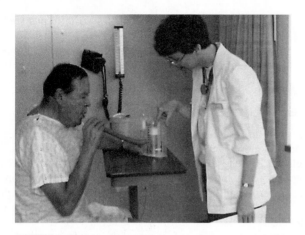

FIGURE 11.1 Patients will feel more in control if they can participate in their own care.

- Identifying the person's perceptions of self-worth
- Identifying actual or potential threats to self-concept

Data Collection Methods

Data collection is accomplished through interview, review of records, and physical assessment.

1. Interview
   Social identity
   Personal identity
   Body image
   Self-esteem
   Threats to self-concept
   Support system
2. Laboratory, x-ray, and diagnostic tools analysis
   There are no specific laboratory test or x-rays for the self-concept pattern.
   Twenty Statements Test
   Locus of Control Scales
   Rosenberg's Self-Esteem Scale
   Piers-Harris Self-Concept Scale
3. Physical assessment
   Observe general appearance
   Observe interactions with others
   Note alterations in body structure or function

Information collected for the self-concept pattern can be analyzed to identify strengths and potential concerns. Conclusions should be based on an understanding of self-concept development across the age span.

Nursing Diagnoses

Primary Nursing Diagnoses

The NANDA-approved nursing diagnoses that address self-concept pattern, as identified by Gordon (1994), include the following:

Body image disturbance
Personal identity disturbance
Self-esteem disturbance
Chronic low self-esteem
Situational low self-esteem
Anxiety
Fear
Hopelessness
Powerlessness

Secondary Nursing Diagnoses

A person with a self-concept disturbance is at high risk for other problems, such as

Ineffective individual coping
Diversional activity deficit
Altered family processes
Altered health maintenance
Self-care deficit
Sexual dysfunction
Impaired social interaction
Spiritual distress
Risk for violence

KNOWLEDGE BASE FOR ASSESSMENT

The assessment of self-concept pattern includes an understanding of the meaning of self-concept, the development of self-concept, and variables that affect self-concept and self-esteem. The self-concept pattern includes the individual's perception of, value of, and feeling toward self.

Self-Concept

According to Rosenberg, self-concept is the "totality of the individual's thoughts and feelings with reference to himself or herself as an object" (Rosenberg & Kaplan, 1982). Self-concept is the individual's synthesis of his or her body, mind, and spirit. Self is "one's own person as distinguished from others . . . It is who one is as a separate and whole person. It consists of physical, cognitive, affective, behavioral, and social dimensions" (McMahon, 1997, p. 144). McMahon (1997) identifies four components of self: public, semipublic, private, and inner self. The public self is what the person presents and is viewed by others. The public self can vary depending on with whom the individual is interacting. For example, a person will project a different self-image when asked about himself or herself on a first date than when on a job interview. The public self can be what the person is willing to divulge in a given situation.

The semipublic self is what others observe and the person may not be aware of. This component of self is the most open to growth through feedback from others. Conversely, the private self is what is known to the individual but generally not shared with others. The private self can include the "ideal-self" or what the individual would like to be—what the person strives toward. The private self may be shared only with others with whom the individual has a close intimate relationship. Different people have different proportions of self that are private. Those individuals with a large private self are at risk for social isolation and misperceptions of self by others.

The inner self is unknown to the individual and to others. It is considered to be unconscious because its content provokes anxiety. Although unknown, it does influence perceptions, thoughts, and behavior. When these influences limit functioning, a counselor or other health professional can assist with gaining insights into the inner self (McMahon).

When assessing self-concept, a challenge is to judge the degree to which the person's self-report of self, and the public display of self, accurately reflect self. Unfortunately, strategies for enhancing such judgments are not well developed, and the nurse may simply have to look for congruence as an indicator of the degree to which the presenting public self correlates with the actual self. For example, a person may report feeling self-confident yet demonstrate behavior that indicates a need for excessive reassurance, thereby revealing a possible discrepancy.

Although theorists differ in the language they use to describe self-concept, nursing models of self-concept generally focus on the following four components: social identity (role and role performance), personal identity (moral/ethical self, intellectual self, and emotional self), physical self (body image), and self-esteem (Kim & Moritz, 1982). Each self-concept component provides a focus for assessment.

Social Identity

Social identity includes sociodemographic characteristics such as age, gender, group membership (*i.e.,* ethnic group, religious affiliation, political group), and cultural identity. Rosenberg and Kaplan (1982) associate social identity with self-concept for two reasons. First, social categories assigned from birth through old age provide structure for life experiences. Social labels may contribute to experiences such as racism, sexism, stereotyping, or discrimination. Second, social labels also define how a person lives and what he or she does. For example, a physician and a migrant farm worker differ not only in what they do but also in the amount of social respect they command; both experiences influence self-concept. Rosenberg (1979) identifies the following six social identity categories:

- *Social status:* Universal classifications such as gender, age, family status, and occupation
- *Membership groups:* Voluntary association groups found within societies such as cultural, religious, sociopolitical, and special interest groups such as Mothers Against Drunk Drivers (MADD)
- *Social labels*: Labels conferred by a socially sanctioned agency or authority, such as alcoholic, criminal, child abuser, or mentally incompetent
- *Derived statuses:* Classification associated with personal history, such as Vietnam veteran, former nun, or reformed alcoholic
- *Types or social types:* Socially defined perceptions, attitudes, or habits that characterize a person, such as a womanizer, hermit, nerd, or ski bum. Various subcultures may use their own terms for social types such as jock, narc, or Deadhead.
- *Personal identity:* In the social sense, a single, unique label, often as simple as the person's first name or nickname

Personal Identity

Bonhan and Cheney (1983) discuss four elements of personal identity: physical self, emotional self, moral/ethical self, and intellectual self. In Rosenberg's schema (1979), personal identity refers to dispositions or inclinations to act in certain ways and becomes part of self-concept as a person becomes aware of such responses or tendencies.

Several categories of disposition are frequently expressed as adjectives such as attitudes (liberal, conservative); traits (stubborn, shy, compulsive); abilities (smart, gifted, expert); values (Islamic; monogamous); habits or acts (reckless, anxious nervous); and preferences.

Body Image

Body image refers to a person's perceptions of personal physical characteristics, including physical attributes, functional abilities, sexuality, wellness–illness state, and appearance. Like other aspects of self-concept, body image develops and evolves over time. For the infant, body image involves sensorimotor experiences in which the body is not perceived as being separate from the surroundings. As a person ages, body image is increasingly influenced by sociocultural beliefs and values. Body image involves not only physical appearance and function but also items associated with the body, such as clothing, jewelry, eyeglasses, and prostheses. For hospitalized individuals, equipment such as cardiac monitors, ventilators, and tubes may be incorporated into body image. In addition to the physical self, body image involves the person's feelings about physical capabilities. This self-concept component is least stable and can readily be altered as a result of illness, surgery, or trauma.

Self-Esteem

Self-esteem refers to how a person feels about the various components of self-concept, including social identity, personal identity, and body image. These perceptions may be reflected in statements of self-approval or disapproval. Negative evaluations may indicate actual or potential low self-esteem. Low self-esteem may be situational or chronic. Situational low self-esteem can occur when one is learning a new task or responding to a loss. Chronic low self-esteem, however, is the result of long-term negative evaluation of self.

Self-Concept Development

Symbolic Interactionism

According to symbolic interactionism, self-concept evolves from infancy through old age. One of the most influential factors is the type of interactions one has with others, such as parents, siblings, peers, authority figures, and with the general sociocultural milieu. In other words, one often becomes what others expect. Cooley (1902) is credited with being the first symbolic interactionist who formulated the idea of a "looking glass self." According to this theory, self-concept is a reflection of one's perceptions about how one appears to others. Self-concept is formed in early childhood when an important person in the child's life exerts such influence that the child adopts that person's judgment of him or her. Therefore, a child who is consistently praised by significant people in his or her life is more likely to develop a positive self-concept than a child who is always criticized.

Mead (1934) expanded on Cooley's theory by stating that self-concept is not merely derived by interaction with significant others but also reflects a "generalized other." In other words, the entire sociocultural milieu influences perceptions of self.

Symbolic interactionist theory suggest that self-concept is a product of what a person believes others think of him or her, regardless of what others may actually think. Any valid assessment of self-concept should be based on the person's perspective of self rather than on social labels or stereotypes.

Developmental Tasks

As a person grows and matures, skills and ability to perform different functions should increase. Different growth periods present specific developmental tasks or tests of strength and ability. The changes inherent in each crucial growth period present the person with developmental crises. Successfully passing through each developmental stage requires that developmental tasks be mastered and subsequent crises resolved to nurture a positive self-image. If developmental crises are not resolved, a negative self-concept may develop, and the ability to master subsequent developmental tasks may be impaired. Erikson's psychosocial stage theory of ego development (1963) provides a theoretical structure for assessing developmental aspects of self-concept. Erikson developed eight different developmental stages: trust versus mistrust (infancy); autonomy versus shame and doubt (toddler); initiative versus guilt (preschool); industry versus inferiority (school age); identity versus role confusion (adolescent); intimacy versus isolation (young adult); generativity versus stagnation (middle adult); and integrity versus despair (older adult). Knowing what stage of development the individual is in, the nurse can enhance assessment of self-concept and choose appropriate interventions to assist with the development or maintenance of a healthy self-concept.

Self-Concept Stability

Despite the influences of interactions with others, the sociocultural milieu, and developmental stages, a person's self-concept is characterized by relative stability, which may be attributed in part to self-consistency. Driever (1976) defines self-consistency as that part of a person that strives to maintain a consistent self-organization and to avoid disequilibrium. Once an inner core of perception, or *phenomenal self*, is formed, the person has a personal frame of reference. The phenomenal self is stable and resistant to change, although the person may not be entirely satisfied with his or her self-image.

The phenomenal self is established at a very young age, when a person may not be aware of the variety of self-perceptions that can be incorporated into overall self-concept. Consequently, self-perceptions consisting of what the person believes others think of him or her become firmly embedded in the overall self-concept. Change may occur as a result of ongoing interactions or events, but resistance to such change is great. Nursing assumes that self-concept changes are possible, for without such an assumption, implementing many nursing interventions would be impossible. However, it is important to remember that changing a person's self-concept is a slow process.

Locus of Control

Personality characteristics or traits that are stable features of a person also may influence self-perceptions and account for a stable self-concept. One such characteristic influencing self-concept is *locus of control*. Locus of control is a social learning theory concept developed by Rotter (1966). According to this theory, locus of control is a relatively stable characteristic developed over time and influenced by social learning experiences. This concept reflects the person's perceptions that the cause of events or behaviors is either within or outside personal control, regardless of the situation. The person is characterized by an internal locus of control if his or her belief is that what happens is largely the result of personal actions and choices. A person who believes that what happens is largely attributable to luck, fate, chance, or powerful beings/people has an external locus of control.

Locus of control characterizes one dimension of a person's self-perceptions. Because internal locus of control is associated with a positive self-concept, this aspect of a person's view of life should be evaluated when assessing self-concept. Knowledge of locus of control also can assist in discovering possible motivators and choosing appropriate interventions.

Variables Affecting Self-Concept

The many factors that influence self-concept can be explained in terms of symbolic interaction theory, developmental theories, and personality theories. The following factors are most influential in the development of self-concept:

- Early bonding experiences
- Physical, cognitive, and interpersonal development and maturation
- Personality characteristics
- Culture
- Environment
- Socioeconomic status

- Historical perspective or person's sense of place in time (cohort effect)
- Physical attributes and capabilities, including present health status
- Interpersonal relationships
- Professional and personal roles

A Healthy Personality

A healthy personality is characterized by a positive self-esteem, meaning that the person perceives self as valuable and worthwhile or has positive regard for self (Stanwyck, 1983). According to Jourard (1968), the term *healthy personality* is not equivalent to the term *normal personality,* which refers to people who play their roles suitably. Rather, a healthy personality is characterized by the ability to play roles satisfactorily and at the same time derive personal satisfaction from one's roles while continuing to grow (Dunn, 1961). The closer a person's self-concept is to the ideal self, the greater the person's self-esteem. The nurse can effectively make judgments about whether a person has a healthy personality by thoroughly evaluating self-perceptions and self-concept. Even the most outwardly successful person may have a poor self-concept.

Physical Examination Evaluating Self-Concept

GENERAL APPROACH

- The establishment of a therapeutic relationship is very important with data collection for self-concept.
- The interview and subsequent interactions may be the primary means of data collection.
- Be careful to avoid stereotyping or labeling—may interfere with ability to be objective.
- In times of crisis, family members may be helpful with providing data.
- Consider whether any drugs (prescribed or not) could influence data collection.
- Consider developmental stage.
- Body language (such as looking down and slouching) and affect can provide cues.
- Be careful not to form a premature opinion.

DIAGNOSTIC AIDS

- Twenty-Statement Test (TST): Unstructured paper and pencil test; person is given blank paper and asked to give 20 answers to the question "Who am I?" within 12 minutes. Score obtained by classifying responses according to a code scheme (Kuhn & McPartland, 1954).

Unstructured format allows spontaneity and allows person to provide relevant self-perceptions (McGuire & Padawer-Singer, 1982).

- Locus-of-control scales. There are several scales available: Rotter's Internal-External (I-E) Scale (1966); the Health Locus of Control Scale (HLC; Wallston, Wallston, & DeVellis, 1978).

These require the person to choose statements that reflect perceptions about the cause of events. The responses are scored in a standardized manner, and judgments are made about locus of control on the basis of the score. For example, the higher the score on Rotter's I-E Scale, the more external the person's locus of control.

- Rosenberg's Self-Esteem Scale (Rosenberg, 1979) consists of 10 statements that people are asked to agree or disagree with.

  See Display 11-1. Responses with asterisks are associated with low self-esteem.

- Piers-Harris Self-Concept Scale measures self-concept in school-aged children. Child responds *yes* or *no* to items such as "I am happy," "I am smart," and "I give up easily."

  The scale is available through Western Psychological Services, 12031 Wilshire Blvd, Los Angeles, CA 90025

(continued)

Physical Examination   Evaluating Self-Concept (continued)

- Depression scales. There are several depression scales available. The easiest to use are self-report instruments; these include Beck Depression Inventory (Beck, et al, 1961), Zung Self Rating Depression Scale (Zung, 1965), and Montgomery-Asberg Depression Rating Scale (Montgomery & Asberg, 1979).

These are standardized assessment scales and should be used in combination with interview and physical assessment.

ASSESSMENT AIDS
- Interview guide to suggest questions and record data (see display 11-2)

DISPLAY II.I

Rosenberg's Self-Esteem Scale

The RSE is a 10-item Guttman scale with a Coefficient of Reproducibility of 92% and a Coefficient of Scalability of 72%. Respondents are asked to strongly agree, agree, disagree, or strongly disagree with the following items (asterisks represent low–self-esteem responses):

1. On the whole, I am satisfied with myself	SA	A	D*	SD*
2. At times I think I am no good at all.	SA*	A*	D	SD
3. I feel that I have a number of good qualities.	SA	A	D*	SD*
4. I am able to do things as well as most other people.	SA	A	D*	SD*
5. I feel I do not have much to be proud of.	SA*	A*	D	SD
6. I certainly feel useless at times.	SA*	A*	D	SD
7. I feel that I'm a person of worth, at least on an equal plane with others.	SA	A	D*	SD*
8. I wish I could have more respect for myself.	SA*	A*	D	SD
9. All in all, I am inclined to feel that I am a failure.	SA*	A*	D	SD
10. I take a positive attitude toward myself.	SA	A	D*	SD*

(After Rosenberg, M. [1979]. *Conceiving the self* [p. 291]. New York: Basic Books.)

DISPLAY II.2

Interview Guide: Self-Concept Pattern

Social Identity

Occupation _____

Please finish the following statements:

My family situation is best described as _____

Groups/clubs/affiliations important to me are _____

People who know me would describe me as _____

(continued)

DISPLAY 11.2

Interview Guide: Self-Concept Pattern (continued)

Personal Identity

How would you describe yourself? _____

What do you like best about yourself? _____

What do you like least about yourself? _____

What achievement are you most proud of? _____

What would you change about yourself if you could? _____

Body Image

My greatest physical health concern is _____

What do you like best about your body? _____

What do you like least about your body? _____

What physical features would you most like to change? _____

Has there been a change in your body or the things you can do? _____

Self-Esteem

Describe how you feel about yourself. _____

Do you feel good or bad about yourself most of the time? _____

Threats to Self-Concept

What types of events or things about your present situation are most distressing? _____

_____

What type of things make you feel angry? _____

Anxious? _____

Fearful? _____

Lose hope? _____

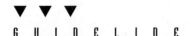

▼ ▼ ▼
GUIDELINES

Assessment Guidelines   Self-Concept Interview (Health History)

1. Social identity

Social identity includes characteristics such as age, gender, roles, and social status. These data are collected by asking questions such as:

"Describe for me the type of work you do"

"My family situation is best described as. . . ."

"Groups/clubs/affiliations important to me are . . ."

"People who know me would describe me as . . ."

The individual's perception of social identity provides a format to view information provided. Roles and relationships are closely connected to social identity (see Chap. 12).

This question also can alert the nurse to health risks that are occupation related (see Chap. 5).

Sometimes one's evaluation of how others perceive oneself is better than self-evaluation, ie, "My friends think I am very successful but I have not accomplished what I wanted." The reverse also can be true.

2. Personal identity

To collect data for this component, ask questions such as:

"How would you describe yourself?"

"What do you like best/least about yourself?"

"What achievements are you most proud of?"

"What about yourself would you change if you could?"

If the person has difficulty responding, you may help by asking questions such as, "Do you see yourself as happy or sad, shy or extroverted, industrious or lazy?"

More structured assessment tools, such as The Twenty Statements Test and the Pier-Harris Self-Concept Scale, may also be used to obtain a more thorough assessment.

▼ ▼ ▼

G U I D E L I N E S *continued*   Self-Concept Interview (Health History)

3. Body image

Body image is the least stable of self-concept components. Ask questions such as:

"Do you have any concerns about your body?"

"What do you like least about your body?"

"What physical features would you like most to change?"

"Has there been a change in your body or the things you can do?"

Determining what body parts have an increased importance to the individual can be helpful; for example, a pianist may value his or her hands, whereas a runner may value leg strength. Adolescents may value overall mobility and physical attractiveness. In clinical settings, body image can be threatened by invasive procedures or devices. How the person reacts in such situations may provide cues to possible body image problems. Machines and other aids that have been assigned names by the individual may be viewed as self-extensions (Fig. 11-2). Because children have difficulty verbalizing perceptions, it may be useful to have them draw a self-portrait and then encourage them to talk about the drawing.

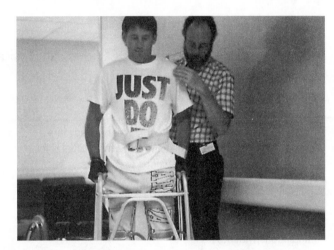

FIGURE 11.2   A walker may be viewed as a self-extension by patients who are regaining their mobility.

4. Self-esteem

Open-ended questions based on a statement the person has already made about self-concept may be useful, for example:

"You identify yourself as a wife and mother; how important is that to you?"

Other questions may include:

"How do you feel about yourself as a person?"

"Do you feel good about yourself most of the time?"

If the responses indicate low self-esteem, the next step is to determine how long the problem has existed. Low self-esteem may be a basic feature of a person's psychological makeup, or it may be related to a specific situation.

The nurse may more thoroughly assess self-esteem by using assessment tools such as the Rosenberg Self-Esteem Scale (see Display 11-1).

Assesssing the person's locus of control also might be helpful; persons who have an external locus of control are at greater risk for negative self-esteem.

Examples of comments indicating low self-esteem are (Miller, 1992):

"I've lost my faith in myself."

"I don't like myself this way."

Blames self excessively

Feels useless

Lacks self-respect

Feels embarrassed about self

▼ ▼ ▼

G U I D E L I N E S   *continued*   Self-Concept Interview (Health History)

5. Threats to self-concept
To identify threats to self-concept, ask the following:

"What types of events or things about your present situation are most distressing?"

"What type of things make you feel angry, anxious, fearful, or hopeless?"

Threats to self-concept can include:
- Significant role change
- Loss of job or significant role
- Deterioration in a meaningful relationship
- Any threat to sexuality (see Chap. 13)
- Loss of a sense of control or independence
- Invasion of one's personal space or privacy

▼ ▼ ▼

G U I D E L I N E S

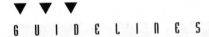

Assessment Guidelines   Self-Concept: Physical Assessment

Procedure

1. Assess self-esteem
To make judgments about self-esteem, observe body language, listen for cues, observe ability to perform usual roles, and note characteristics of interactions with others:
- Does the person make eye contact?
- Appropriate attention span
- Relaxed body posture
- Interactions with others

Clinical Significance

Observations can be done while completing a focused or comprehensive health history interview. Listen carefully for positive and negative self-comments; examples might include feelings of insignificance, difficulty setting goals, and self-doubt in ability to perform tasks (especially important if related to new health care regimen).

Interaction indicators of low self-esteem include the following:
Verbalizations of unworthiness of nurse's time
Hesitance to ask for help
Pessimism
Resentment of others who are well
Lack of self-confidence
Self-consciousness (especially while learning a new skill)
Expression of sense of worthlessness

2. Assess body image
Determine whether the person has experienced a change in body structure of function. Survey for missing body parts or physical alterations. Listen for verbalizations of change in appearance or function.

Note behaviors indicating an altered body image.

Behaviors indicating altered body image include the following:
Not looking at body part
Hiding or overexposing body part
Inability to estimate spatial relationship of body to environment
Focus on past appearance or function
Expressions of fear of rejection
Denial of change
Expressions of helplessness or hopelessness

▼ ▼ ▼

G U I D E L I N E S   *continued*   Self-Concept: Physical Assessment

Procedure

3. Determine whether the person has an internal or external locus of control.
Evaluate locus of control by observing behaviors and listening to statements the person makes about self and others.

4. Threats to self-concept
Identify possible threats to self-esteem, self identity, and body image, for example:

- Scheduled hysterectomy or mastectomy
- Amputations of any limb for any reason
- Recovery from trauma

Clinical Significance

Internal locus of control (ILC) is associated with positive self-concept. The person with an ILC believes that what happens is due to personal actions and choices whereas the person with external locus of control believes other factors/persons are responsible (Table 11-1).

Nurses can anticipate threats to self-concept related to the medical diagnosis of the individual. Even though the individual may be aware of future disfigurement, realizing the extent of the disfigurement may not occur until after a surgical procedure.

TABLE 11.1   Locus of Control: Behavioral Indicators

	Internal Locus of Control	External Locus of Control
Role definition and satisfaction	More clearly defined, more satisfying	Less clearly defined, less satisfying
Relating to authority	Peer-like interactions	Passive interactions
Responsibility for self-care	Active knowledge seeking behavior	Does not actively seek information, accepts what is given
Self-esteem	Higher or more stable	Lower or less stable
Compliance with health care regimen	Manipulates regimen	Compliant
Confidence in abilities	Self-confident	Lacks self confidence
Problem-solving abilities	More successful	Less successful
Goal-setting behavior	Realistic in setting goals	Unrealistic in setting goals
Level of motivation	Motivated	Tends toward helplessness at times
Involvement in decision making	Involved	Little involvement

(Adapted from Miller, J. [1992]. *Coping with chronic illness: Overcoming powerlessness* [2nd ed.]. Philadelphia: F.A. Davis.)

Documentation

Documentation of observations related to self-concept relies on statements made by the individual and corresponding behaviors. It is helpful to quote the person directly.

Example 1: Healthy Self-Concept Pattern

Joseph is a 19-year-old with a left above-the-knee amputation secondary to cancer. He came in for fitting of a new prosthesis. The following data was recorded in SOAP format:

   S: Wants a prosthesis with special foot attachments so he can play basketball and resume running. Wants to see how prosthesis is made and have a decision in the type of prosthesis he will get. Is involved with local organization for individuals with amputations.

   O: Brought in literature regarding different prostheses, sounds excited about resuming athletic activities. Talkative, frequent eye contact. Shows stump and demonstrates how he cares for it.

   A: Good body image, self-concept

   P: Evaluate after arrival of new prosthesis

Example 2: A Self-Esteem Disturbance

Louise, a 37-year-old, recently had a illeostomy related to chronic, uncontrolled ulcerative colitis. She is being taught how to care for her illeostomy at home because she had difficulty with the procedure in the hospital. She infrequently glances at ostomy, refuses to touch the area, and when asked to help states "I just can't do that."

Problem-orientated documentation may be written:

S: "I just can't do that."
O: Glances at illeostomy, does not touch area. Did not assist with ostomy bag change.
A: Possible Body-image disturbance
P: Continue home visits to assess and care for ostomy
  Contact ostomy support group for assistance
  Discuss Louise with psychiatric clinical nurse specialist
  Encourage Louise to discuss illeostomy, plan time to talk at next visit

Nursing Diagnoses Related to Self-Concept Assessment

Self-Esteem Disturbances

Self-esteem disturbance is a result of an individual experiencing a negative self-evaluation about his or her self or abilities. People with self-esteem disturbances do not necessarily respond in typical patterns (Carpenito, 1997). Some people may have self-esteem disturbance because of personal identity problems, whereas others may have an intact personal identity but experience a disruption in social identity.

History

Situational low self-esteem is related to an event in which the individual recently experienced negative feelings toward self, and chronic low self-esteem is a long-standing negative feeling toward self.

Physical Examination Findings

Physical examination findings may include negative verbalizations of self or abilities; there may or may not be a loss of body part, function or disfigurement; rejection of positive feedback; and hesitation to try new skills.

Body Image Disturbance

Individuals with disturbance in body image have negative beliefs about their own body.

History

Negative beliefs may be related to chronic illness, loss of body part or function, trauma with disfigurement, sexual abuse, and body appearance such as obesity, pregnancy, loss of hair related to chemotherapy, unrealistic expectations (anorexia), or deviation from desired body.

Physical Examination

Physical examination will indicate verbal and nonverbal negative responses to the body or body part. The individual may refuse to look at the altered body part. The individual may isolate self so others will not see body change. There may or may not be loss of a body part or function.

Personal Identity Disturbance

This nursing diagnosis is used when the individual is unable to distinguish between self and nonself.

History

The individual may express doubts or confusion regarding self and who he or she is. This is often associated with self-esteem disturbance and early adolescence. The individual may express insecurity, disillusionment, alienation, feelings of fragmentation, isolation, and inconsistent behavior.

Physical Examination

See Self-esteem disturbance.

Anxiety Versus Fear

Fear and anxiety both represent responses to altered self-concept. Making an accurate differential diagnosis between Fear and Anxiety is important because nursing interventions are influenced by the diagnosis. Fear and anxiety as affective responses to danger have some common features, including unpleasant feelings and often accompanying body responses such as those associated with the stress response (see Chap. 14). Physical responses vary among people. On a cognitive level, fear and anxiety can be recognized and verbally expressed. Emotional reactions to fear and anxiety are evident by affective behavior.

Anxiety and fear often coexist. For example, a woman having a breast biopsy may fear having surgery and the associated pain but be anxious about the pathology results of the biopsy. Usually with fear a cognitive component predominates, whereas with anxiety an emotional component predominates. Burke (1982) provides the following additional guideline for differentiating fear and anxiety during assessment:

- Use of the "of" test: this strategy involves asking whether the person has a fear of something. If fear has an identifiable source, the nurse should be able to analyze data and determine the source. For example, the person has a fear of pain, a fear of losing control, or a fear of surgery. Anxiety, although related to some situation, is not always associated with a specific threat. Burke suggests asking whether the person is anxious or does he or she have a fear of . . .

- Evaluate the immediacy and consistency of the threat: Research indicates that fear is expressed immediately and consistently. If behavioral responses to threats, such as crying, physical withdrawal, questioning, or aggression, are noted immediately on exposure to or mention of a particular threat, then the diagnosis is more likely to be fear. When the emotional or behavioral response is less predictable, consider anxiety.

The nurse may wish to consider using the diagnosis Fear/Anxiety Related to . . . as the diagnostic statement.

History

The histories for both anxiety and fear are similar. The person may report a change in status, failure at a task, loss through divorce or death, moving, or threats to self such as death, surgery, assault, disease, trauma.

Physical Examination

On examination, the nurse may note physiologic, emotional, and cognitive findings. Physiologic findings may include fatigue, increased heart rate, restlessness, nausea and vomiting, and body aches and pains. Emotional findings may include crying, lack of self-confidence, helplessness, impatience, and anger. Cognitive findings may include forgetfulness, inability to concentrate, and hypervigilance.

Hopelessness

The nursing diagnosis Hopelessness is used for the response when the individual perceives no alternatives or choices to solve a problem. Additionally, the individual is unable to mobilize any resources on behalf of self to establish goals.

History

The person expresses a profound sense that nothing can be done; there are no options. This may be related to treatments (chemotherapy), diagnosis (cancer, AIDS), failing physical condition, or loss of personal sources of comfort (spouse, enjoyed activity).

Physical Examination

The person may have a flat affect, passive involvement in care, lack of energy, increase in sleeping, and weight loss, and may be withdrawn.

Powerlessness

The nursing diagnosis Powerlessness is similar to Hopelessness. However, with Powerlessness, the individual does discern options but perceives a lack of control over events or the right to choose available options.

History

The patient may express dissatisfaction over his or her ability to control life events. The individual may have a history of a chronic illness (diabetes mellitus, muscular dystrophy) or condition (amputation, cerebrovascular accident) that limits activity,

Physical Examination

There may be no specific physical findings; however, the person may appear depressed, have increased dependence on others, and may be verbally and physically angry.

NDx

Clinical Problems Related to Self-Concept Assessment

Individuals with psychiatric health problems frequently have disturbances of self-concept. For example, bulimia and anorexia nervosa are often related to disturbances

in body-image and self-esteem. Individuals who are clinically depressed might also have disturbances in self-concept. For a more in-depth discussion of clinical problems related to self-concept, refer to a psychiatric nursing text.

Case Study

Malcolm, a 17-year-old high school senior, was admitted to a rehabilitation hospital after a football injury. Malcolm spent several weeks at an acute care hospital until his cervical neck fracture (C2–C3) and health status had stabilized. He is wearing a neck brace, his respirations are assisted with a ventilator, and he is in a wheel chair with all limbs supported. He cannot take care of any activities of daily living (*i.e.,* feeding, toileting, oral care, bathing, dressing). Malcolm's mother is staying with him to learn how to provide care once he is discharged. His father and other siblings are 300 miles away, at home.

He is scheduled for physical therapy but refuses to go. He becomes angry, and his verbal anger increases as his mother attempts to encourage him to go to physical therapy. He has multiple muscle spasms, and the nurse is called in. The decision is made to respect Malcolm's wish not to go to physical therapy this morning.

Case Study Analysis

The nurse recognizes several important cues during the interaction with Malcolm and his mother. Malcolm has commented many times about what he is going to do once he walks again. He has an athletic scholarship for football to a good college (the college has informed Malcolm that they will honor the scholarship, even if he cannot play) and often talks about attending school in the fall and hopefully playing football again. This is the first time Malcolm has expressed anger and refused any therapy. In reviewing the situation, the nurse recognizes that Malcolm's mother has made many decisions for him lately. The nurse describes his thinking as he tries to organize his thoughts about what is going on with Malcolm:

> I realized that if I was 17, couldn't move, and my mother was taking care of me, I would probably be angry, anxious about my future, fearful of what is happening to me, denying that the paralysis is permanent, and powerless to change anything. Also, I could only wonder what or how I felt about my once athletic body that had brought me much recognition—both with my friends and family but also with college athletic teams. What would my future hold? What could I control? I realized that Malcolm might feel that the only thing he could control was whether he went to physical therapy or not at that moment. I also realized that we had allowed Malcolm's mother to make many decisions for Malcolm that he was capable of making. I thought I should schedule Malcolm for a case conference so all the staff could consider what was happening and also thought about inviting Malcolm and his mother to the conference.

Possible Nursing Diagnoses

The nurse identifies the following possible nursing diagnoses for Malcolm in the Self-Concept pattern:

Anxiety related to his future
Fear related to his present treatment and outcomes
Body-image disturbance related to traumatic cervical injury and resultant paralysis

Self-esteem image related to recent trauma and paralysis
Powerlessness related to inability to control events

The nurse does not believe that Malcolm could have a diagnosis of Hopelessness because he still hoped to walk, but knows that when the impact of his injury is realized, hopelessness could become an important diagnosis.

Additional Data Gathering

Before the planned case conference, the nurse makes time to visit with Malcolm when his mother is not present. He talks to Malcolm about his football game and plans for the future, and finally discusses what Malcolm is concerned about. Malcolm starts discussing how he will manage once he gets home. After a few moments, Malcolm stops talking and starts crying as his mother enters the room. The nurse realizes that most of the possible diagnoses probably are appropriate for Malcolm, but he needs to identify which diagnoses take priority. The nurse also recognizes that he should consult with the psychiatric clinical specialist and others to plan appropriate care. He also is aware that the diagnoses will continue to evolve as Malcolm progresses with his rehabilitation and as he realizes the long-term effect of his injury.

CHAPTER 11 S U M M A R Y

Assessment of self-concept focuses on the following:
- Identifying aspects of the person's social identity
- Identifying factors that contribute to the individual's self-concept
- Identifying the person's perceptions of self-worth
- Identifying actual or potential threats to self-concept

When assessing self-concept, the nurse should consider the following factors:
- Self-concept
- Self-concept development
- Self-concept stability
- Variables affecting self-concept
- Healthy personality
- Threats to self-concept

Cues should be analyzed in relationship to meanings relevant to the person. The nurse should collect data pertaining to the Self-Concept pattern by the following methods:
- The interview (health history), which focuses on social identity, personal identity, body image, self-esteem, and threats to self-concept
- Nursing observations, including the person's self-disclosure statements, role performance, interpersonal relationships, general appearance, and affective responses
- Assessment tools such as Twenty Statements Test, Rosenberg's self-esteem scale, the Piers-Harris Self-Concept Scale, and Rotter's I-E Scale

Assessment of self-concept pattern based on these principles and strategies will assist the nurse to identify defining characteristics and risk factors for the following nursing diagnoses:
>   Body image disturbance
>   Personal identity disturbance
>   Self-esteem disturbance
>   Chronic low self-esteem
>   Situational low self-esteem
>   Anxiety
>   Fear
>   Hopelessness
>   Powerlessness

Secondary nursing diagnoses might include:
>   Ineffective individual coping
>   Diversional activity deficit
>   Altered family processes
>   Altered health maintenance
>   Self-care deficit
>   Sexual dysfunction
>   Impaired social interaction
>   Spiritual distress
>   Risk for violence

Critical Thinking Exercise

The assessment of self-concept is considered a crucial element of a holistic nursing assessment. It is through this type of assessment that the nurse begins to truly know the person who is the recipient of nursing care.

1. You are the nurse assigned to a group home for adolescents. Describe to the house parents the normal threats to self-concepts during adolescence.

2. With the house parents, discuss the healthy indicators of a healthy self-concept.

3. Discuss with the house parents why pregnant teens, anorexic teens, and abused teens are at risk for self-esteem disturbances.

4. While discussing your visit and teaching with another nurse, the nurse tells you that assessment of self-concept is a luxury rather than a necessity. Explain how you would respond.

BIBLIOGRAPHY

Beck, A., Ward, C., Mendelson, J., Mock, J., & Erbaugh, J. (1961). An inventory for measuring depression. *Archives of General Psychiatry, 4,* 561–571.

Bonhan, P., & Cheney, P. (1983). Concept of self: A framework for nursing assessment. In P. Chinn (Ed.). *Advances in nursing theory development* (pp. 173–190). Rockville, MD: Aspen.

Bruss, C. (1988). Nursing diagnosis of hopelessness. *Journal of Psychosocial Nursing and Mental Health Services, 26*(3), 28–31, 38–39.

Burke, S. (1982). A developmental perspective on the nursing diagnosis of fear and anxiety. *Nursing Papers, 14*(2), 59–64.

Carpenito, L. (1997). *Handbook of nursing diagnosis* (7th ed.). Philadelphia: Lippincott.

Cooley, C. (1902). *Human nature and the social order.* New York: Scribner's.

Coombs, A. (1971). Self-concept: Product and producer of experience. In D. Avila, A. Coombs, & W. Purkey (Eds.), *Helping relationships.* Boston: Allyn and Bacon.

Driever, M. (1976). Theory of self-concept. In C. Roy (Ed.), *Introduction to nursing:An adaptation model* (pp. 161–191). Englewood Cliffs, NJ: Prentice Hall.

Dunn, H. (1961). *High level wellness.* Arlington, VA: RW Beatty Co.

Dunn, J. (1977). *Distress and comfort.* Cambridge: Harvard University Press.

Erikson, E. (1963). *Childhood and society* (2nd ed.). New York: WW Norton.

Gordon, M. (1994). *Nursing diagnosis: Process and application* (3rd ed). St. Louis: Mosby.

Jones, P., & Jakob, D. (1981). Nursing diagnosis: Differentiating fear and anxiety. *Nursing Papers, 13*(4), 20–29.

Jourard, S. (1968). Health personality and self-disclosure. In C. Gordon & K. Gergen (Eds.), *The self in social interaction. Vol 1: Classic and contemporary perspectives.* New York: John Wiley & Sons.

Kim, M., & Moritz, D. (1982). *Classification of nursing diagnoses: Proceedings of the third and fourth national conferences.* New York: McGraw-Hill.

Kuhn, M., & McPartland, T. (1954). An empirical investigation of self-attitudes. *American Sociology Review, 19,* 68–76.

LeMone, P. (1991). Analysis of a human phenomenon: Self-concept. *Nursing Diagnosis, 2*(3), 126–130.

Long, K. (1988). Use of the Piers-Harris self-concept scale with Indian children: Cultural considerations. *Nursing Research, 37*(1), 42–46.

McGuire, W., & Padawer-Singer, A. (1982). Trait salience in the spontaneous self-concept. In M. Rosenberg & H. Kaplan (Eds.). *Social psychology of the self-concept.* Arlington Heights, IL: Harlan Davidson.

McMahon, A. (1997). The nurse-client relationship. In J. Haper, B. Krainovich-Miller, A. McMahon, & P. Price-Hoskins (Eds.). *Comprehensive psychiatric nursing* (5th ed.). St. Louis: Mosby.

Mead, G.H. (1934). *Mind, self and society.* Chicago: University of Chicago Press.

Miller, J. (1966). *Coping with chronic illness: Overcoming powerlessness* (2nd ed). Philadelphia: F.A. Davis.

Piers, E., & Harris, D. (1969). *Piers-Harris children's self-concept scale (the way I feel about myself).* Nashville, TN: Counselor Recording and Tests.

Rosenberg, M (1979). *Concerning the self.* New York: Basic Books.

Rosenberg, M, & Kaplan, H. (1982). *Social psychology of the self-concept.* Arlington Heights, IL: Harland Davidson.

Rotter, J. (1966). Generalized expectancies for internal versus external control of reinforcement. *Psychological Monographs, 80*(1), 1–25.

Stanwyck, D.J. (1983). Self-esteem throughout the life span. *Family and Community Health, 6*(2), 11–28.

Wallston B., et al. (1976). Development and validation of the health locus of control (HLC) scale. *Journal of Consulting and Clinical Psychology, 44,* 580–585.

Wallston, K., Wallston, B., & DeVellis, R. (1978). Development of the multidimensional health locus of control (MHLC) scale. *Health Education Monographs, 6,* 160–170.

Yocom, C. (1984). The differentiation of fear and anxiety. In M. Kim, G. McFarland, & A. McLane (Eds.). *Classification of nursing diagnoses: Proceedings of the fifth national conference.* St. Louis: Mosby.

Zung, W. (1965). A self rating depression scale. *Archives of General Psychiatry, 12,* 63–70.

ASSESSMENT GUIDELINES

Roles and Relationships:
Interview (Health History)

Roles and Relationships: Physical
Assessment

CHAPTER ORGANIZATION

Introductory Overview
- Assessment Focus
- Data Collection Methods
- Nursing Diagnoses

**Knowledge Base
for Assessment**
- Role Theory

- Social Interaction
- Communication
- Family Process

INTRODUCTORY OVERVIEW

In 1936, Ralph Linton identified roles as collective patterns of behavior socially prescribed within the social structure (Biddle & Thomas, 1979); more recently, Murray and Zentner (1997) defined roles as patterns of behavior expected by others that are learned and performed in social settings. The individual performing the role uses perceived expectations and evaluations of others and self-evaluation to modify behavior. Deutsch and Krauss (1965) proposed that a specific role in any situation is defined three ways: prescribed, perceived, and enacted. Prescribed role is society's expectation—how others intend for the person to behave. Perceived role is what the person in the role perceives as being applicable for the situation. Enacted role is the actual behaviors the individual exhibits (Fig. 12-1). Since the introduction of the role concept, researchers in the behavioral sciences have been concerned with roles and related conflict, strain, behavior, performance, competence, and stress.

Relationships are the feelings of being connected with another through family, friendship, school, work, and society, among others. People establish relationships with others and with pets to meet the need for interaction and contact with others. Roles and relationships provide the structure for family units, friendships, groups, and society (Gordon, 1994). In nursing, roles and relationships are assessed to determine how people manage their particular roles with respect to expectations, social relationships, families, and impact on health status.

ASSESSMENT FOCUS

Assessing role-relationship behavior involves collecting data on the quality and quantity of the roles and relationships of the person. Data collection includes considering the person's role conception, communication patterns, family and social interaction processes, and parenting abilities. Information is collected primarily through interview and observation.

The goals in assessing roles and relationship pattern include the following:

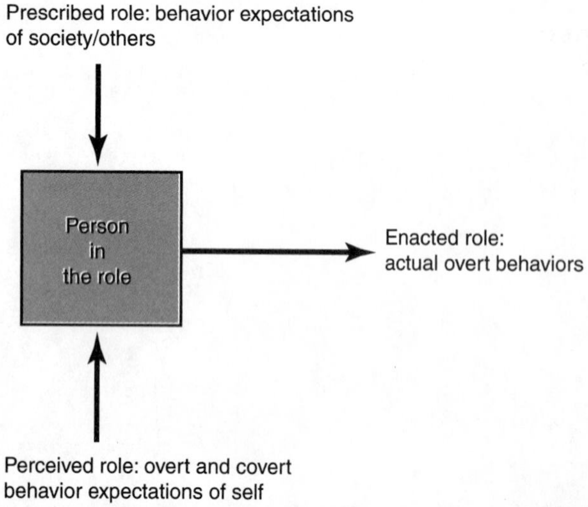

- Identifying perceptions of roles
- Determining the risk for role strain or response to role strain
- Evaluating communication patterns between the person and significant others
- Identifying factors restricting effective communication
- Identifying actual or potential strengths and dysfunction within the family

Data Collection Methods

Data collection is accomplished by:

Interview or Review of Records

1. Interview
   Individual roles
       Perceptions
       Satisfaction
       Role strain
   Family Roles and Relationships
       Family composition and structure
       Family communication patterns
       Family problems or concerns
       Family decision-making process
       Discipline patterns
   Social Relationships
       Individual social relationships
       Family social relationships
       Relationships with helping professionals
   Communication
       Communication skills
       Communication aids

Prescribed role: behavior expectations of society/others

Person in the role

Enacted role: actual overt behaviors

Perceived role: overt and covert behavior expectations of self

FIGURE 12.1 Role: Expectations and behavior.

2. Laboratory/X-ray Analysis
   There are no specific laboratory or X-ray tests for the role-relationship pattern
3. Physical Examination
   General appearance
   Communication skills
   Family interaction
   Parenting skills
   Abuse

Information collected for the roles and relationship pattern can be analyzed to identify strengths or needs in role-relationship behaviors or the need for an in-depth interview to identify possible problems that may arise in these areas. Conclusions must be based on an understanding that role behaviors and expectations vary from individual to individual, family to family, and culture to culture.

Nursing Diagnoses

Primary Nursing Diagnoses

The NANDA-approved nursing diagnoses that address roles and relationship functions include the following:

Altered family processes
Altered parenting, actual
Risk for altered parent–infant attachment
Parental role conflict
Anticipatory grieving
Dysfunctional grieving
Disturbances in role performance
Social isolation
Relocation stress syndrome
Caregiver role strain
High risk for caregiver role strain
Impaired social interaction
Impaired verbal communication
Potential for violence

(Anticipatory and dysfunctional grieving are discussed in the framework of coping and stress; see Chap. 14.)

Secondary Nursing Diagnoses

Other NANDA nursing diagnoses that may be considered with the role-relationship pattern are:

Impaired thought process
Fear
Anxiety
Self-esteem disturbance
Sleep-pattern disturbance
High risk for self-mutilation

KNOWLEDGE BASE FOR ASSESSMENT

The assessment of roles and relationships requires an understanding of role theory, social interactions, communication, and family processes.

Role Theory

Role theory represents a collection of concepts and a variety of hypothetical formulations that predict how actors will perform in a given role, or under what circumstances certain types of behaviors can be expected (Hardy & Conway, 1988).

Social positions are made of two components, status and role. Status refers to a social position that often implies some rank within the social structure. Status is the name of the position, such as daughter, mother, and boss. Role is the performance of the position—the behavior exhibited by or expected from the individual with a particular status. The term *role* has been borrowed from the theater and has been used to describe behaviors that are expected when an individual assumes a particular status. Because role behavior is observable and status is a label, most of the discussion regarding positions focuses on roles. Throughout our lives we perform many roles, both ascribed (assigned) and achieved (acquired). *Ascribed roles*, such as those associated with gender, are usually determined at birth and are often influenced by society. *Achieved roles*, such as professional or occupational status, are obtained through individual effort or competition. Roles such as husband, wife, mother, and father are classified as ascribed, despite the fact that some effort may be necessary to obtain the status.

Each status has a corresponding set of behaviors or role expectations that are socially determined. People often have several roles, ascribed as well as achieved; some of these roles may conflict with one another. Roles are learned in a continuous and cumulative process. Role behaviors of previous developmental stages prepare individuals for future role behaviors. Therefore, role behaviors from one age level to the next remain fairly consistent, and the individual builds a repertoire of behavioral responses to a variety of situational demands (Rosow, 1965). Role learning occurs as the result of assuming new roles or coping with role stress or role strain. In addition, role expectations can change as situations and society change, forcing people to manage several roles while attempting to maintain good health.

Problems experienced in managing role expectation can result in the following situations:

Role conflicts can occur when one or more role expectations compete against one another. For example, a working single parent with a sick child may be conflicted about whether to stay home or go to work. Obviously, one cannot be at both places and may have guilt feelings whatever the decision. Role conflict also occurs when there are different norms for the same role. For example, immigrants may find that acceptable role behavior in their culture of origin is unacceptable in their new social environment. Conflict is to be expected because it is intrinsic to the nature of an ever-changing society.

Role ambiguity may result when role expectations are not clearly identified within society or there is disagreement regarding role expectations. For example, adolescents are often unsure exactly what behavior is expected of them. Role ambiguity is characteristic of professional roles in which expectations are changing and disagreement exists regarding the direction of the change.

Role overload may occur when the individual is unable to handle competing demands of numerous assigned and achieved roles because there is insufficient time or energy to fulfill the obligations of all roles. Simply, the person has more than can be handled. For example, a single parent who works full time may perform all roles adequately until he or she returns to school and assumes the student role. The parent may be unable to find enough time or energy to meet all role expectations adequately. Everyone has numerous roles; for example, a man with three children can be an employee, teacher, father, stepfather, husband, son, brother, son-in-law, brother-in-law, friend, church elder, uncle, grandfather, volunteer, bowler, and so forth. The number of roles a person can successfully fulfill is influenced by situations such as role complexity, disability, and illness.

Role incompetence may occur when the necessary skill or knowledge to fulfill role expectations is lacking. For example, a 14-year-old girl who becomes a mother may not have sufficient maturity or knowledge to care for a newborn.

Role bargaining refers to negotiation with others about acceptable role expectations. A family may abandon society's expectation about traditional responsibilities such as cooking, automobile maintenance, and child care to best meet the individual and family needs. For example, the father may become the primary caretaker of children and the mother may be the primary income-earner. Role reciprocity and role complementarity are components of role bargaining. Role reciprocity refers to a mutual exchange and sharing of decisions regarding responsibilities, whereas role complementarity refers to defining roles and responsibilities in relation to each other. Role bargaining is important in periods of transition and can either enhance growth of all involved or can benefit one at the expense of the other. If roles are rigid, transitions will be difficult and lead to conflict.

Role stress is a sociocultural situation in which role expectations and responsibilities are vague, conflicting, or unrealistic. Role stress is an attribute of the social system and not the individual (Hardy & Conway, 1989). *Role strain* is the individual's response to role stress and other role problems such as overload and conflict; the response can be distress such as anxiety and frustration. Role strain ultimately affects coping abilities.

Role strain can occur when the individual is dissatisfied with a role or roles. Role strain challenges a person's coping capabilities and can cause frustration, insecurity, fatigue, depression, or anxiety (see Chap. 14). Many people experience role strain because of inadequate role preparation, rapid social change, and accelerated technology (Hardy & Conway, 1989). Even when a person is satisfied with his or her status associated with the role, strain can occur. How strain is resolved depends on available resources and options available.

Sick Role

During illness, individuals are often excused from responsibilities of other roles and become dependent on others (family members and health professionals). One of the responsibilities of the sick role is to comply with health advice of others, express a desire to get well, and accept help. During periods of prolonged illnesses, other people may assume a person's role responsibilities. Some people who are sick refuse to assume the sick role, whereas others abuse the sick role, showing little desire to get well. Illness, whether acute or chronic, can alter role capabilities and family functioning and cause role strain for the individual and other family members. The nurse must remember that definitions of legitimate illnesses and role performances vary among societies, and sick role behavior also varies culturally.

The behaviors and attitudes that are associated with various roles are learned at home, in school, at work, and during interaction with others. When a person assumes a role for a length of time, role responsibilities become more refined and may increase. For example, role expectations of a 5-year-old child in school are different than role expectations of a 10-year old. Similarly, a newly graduated nurse will not be expected to perform like a nurse who has been practicing for 6 years. Role strain is reduced when there is clarity of role expectations. Individuals have the choice to conform in role expectations or deliberately not conform to expectations. Sometimes nonconformity is an innovation that brings about social change—for example, the civil rights movement of the 1960s and 1970s.

Social Interaction

Social interaction occurs when two or more people communicate. The characteristics of an interaction are influenced by the relationship between the parties. Relationships are influenced by role status and role hierarchy and can be classified as horizontal (equal), such as husband–wife, friend–friend, or vertical (unequal), such as parent–child, employer–employee, and physician–patient. Relationships are also influenced by culture; for example, some societies encourage a vertical relationship between husband and wife, or expect a parent–child relationship to progress from vertical to horizontal as the child matures.

The degree and depth of a social interaction are dependent on the purpose of the interaction and the degree of trust and familiarity between participants. Relationships between participants can be classified further according to type, such as therapeutic (see Chap. 1), familial, business, or social. Social relationships are formed primarily for pleasure and companionship. No specific knowledge or skill is required, and neither person is responsible for the other. The strength of the relationship is dependent on the amount of energy each party is willing to invest. In any given relationship, the people involved may value the association differently. The number of relationships and interactions people participate in varies greatly from person to person.

An eco-map is a useful tool for assessing social interactions of the individual or family. An eco-map illustrates the individual's or family's contacts with individuals outside of the nuclear family and with agencies such as schools and work places (Fig. 12-2). The eco-map displays important nurturing, neutral, and conflict-laden interactions between the individual or family and society. It

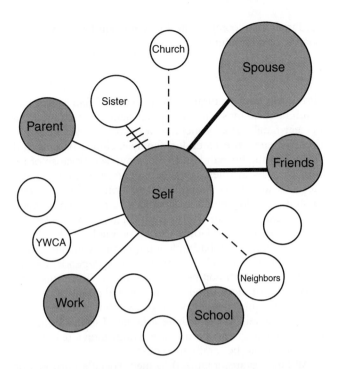

FIGURE 12.2 This ecomap depicting a person's various relationships is completed by labeling additional circles and drawing lines to show the nature of relationships. *Straight lines* indicate strong, positive relationships; *dotted lines* indicate weaker relationships; *slashed lines* represent strained relationships. The wider the line, the stronger the relationship.

also displays the direction of resources into and out of a family or an individual. An eco-map is useful when a family is experiencing stress or a crisis. It can illustrate resources used, those available but not used, and sources of support that are helpful and those that are not helpful.

Relationships With Helping Professionals

The relationship between the health care provider and the individual or family can influence the individual's willingness to interact, plan, seek care, and adhere to mutually

agreed-on health care plans. A positive therapeutic relationship with a health professional is helpful, especially with sensitive problems. The amount of confidence placed in the professional influences a person's willingness to share information. Individuals desire varying degrees of participation in their health care. Some individuals wish to be equal partners on the "health care team," and others desire to play a more passive role. Determining individual expectations and validating findings with the client is helpful in establishing a therapeutic relationship (see Chap. 2).

Communication

Communication, essential to all social interaction, involves sharing information or messages between a sender and receiver through a means of transmission, such as speech, art, writing, or body movements. During a communication exchange, a message is sent, received, and interpreted. Often more than one form of the message is exchanged; for example, with face-to-face exchanges, simultaneous verbal and nonverbal messages are sent and received. Communication can be either circular or linear (Lancaster, 1982) (Fig. 12-3).

Nonverbal communication is as important as verbal communication and includes touch, eye contact, facial expressions, silence, body movement, and posture. Nonverbal communication is more likely to be automatic and less repressed and can provide a more reliable insight into the individual's actual message. Verbal and nonverbal messages are either congruent or incongruent. Many characteristics of nonverbal communication are culturally influenced. In the United States, for example, eye contact is important with face-to-face exchanges; however, some Native American cultures avoid eye contact. In certain Eastern cultures, a smile conceals emotions and unpleasant news and does not necessarily represent agreement with the message.

Besides verbal and nonverbal communication, Wright and Leahey (1994) have identified emotional and circular types of communication. Both emotional and circular communication have elements of verbal and nonverbal communication. Emotional communication refers to the expression or demonstration of emotions and feelings that

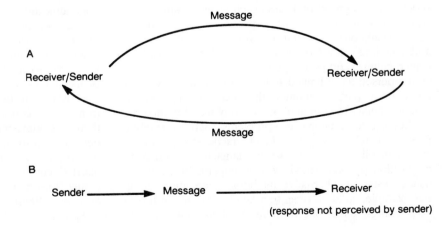

FIGURE 12.3 Communication patterns. In circular communication *(A)*, receivers and senders transmit messages and return messages in response to messages received. In linear communication *(B)*, one person sends a message to another, who receives it but does not respond.

range from sadness and anger to happiness. Circular communication is the reciprocal communication between people. It can be functional/adaptive or dysfunctional/nonsupportive. Functional circular communication occurs when one person makes a conclusion and acts positively to relay support for the other. The other person perceives that the first person cares and reacts positively. The positive response by the second person encourages the first person and so forth. With dysfunctional circular communication, the first person again makes a conclusion but acts negatively with the showing of nonsupport or anger. The second person perceives that the person is angry and either responds in anger or avoids the situation, which causes increased anger in the first person and so forth.

For effective communication to occur, the receiver and sender must be effective. Common problems with the receiver that lead to ineffective communication include (Friedman, 1994):

- Failure to listen
- Disagreeing with the message (yes-but)
- Reacting defensively to the message
- Change of issue—"counterattack"
- Premature advice—offering advice without exploring sufficiently
- Cutoff or curtailment of communication

Some common problems with the sender that lead to ineffective communication include (Friedman, 1994):

- Assuming what the receiver is thinking or feeling without validating
- Speaking for another
- Sending incomplete messages
- Assuming others feel or believe the same
- Sarcasm
- Expressing hurt as anger
- Inability to express needs
- Silent when angry
- Verbal–nonverbal incongruence

Assessing communication involves noting the message as well as related behaviors and influencing factors. The communication process is not static but changes in relation to family, social systems, role expectations, and age/maturity of the people involved. Furthermore, as the number of persons involved in the interaction increases or decreases, the process changes. The communication process is influenced by factors such as environment; the type of relationship that exists between the sender and receiver; status of sender and receiver (emotional, physical, and cognitive); level of development of sender and receiver; culture; and past experiences.

If a person has a limited ability to speak, write, read, or move body parts, communication may be impaired. A person's ability to communicate verbally may be impaired by hearing loss, neurologic problems such as cerebral palsy or cerebrovascular accident, tracheostomy, stuttering, or inability to speak a second language. When communication is complicated by such impairments, families usually establish alternative methods of communicating. For example, children often translate for parents in health care settings. When one or more members cannot speak,

the family may compensate by using sign language, word boards, or computers.

Family Process

Historically and culturally, the concept of family has had different meanings. In the United States, for example, a nuclear family usually includes a husband, wife, and children, whereas the extended family includes parents and siblings of the husband and wife. However, because of recent changes in roles, laws, economic opportunities, and lifestyles, alternative family configurations have come into existence. Multigenerational families in one home, which were common in the 19th century, have recently seen a resurgence. Today a family can be defined as a living social system, usually sharing living quarters, with significant emotional bonds such as affection, interdependence, responsibility, or commitment (Levitt, 1982). Given this definition, two or more unrelated, unmarried adults of the opposite or same gender with or without children who reside together may constitute a family. Essentially, members of a family can be anyone whom individuals mutually consider to be family members.

All families are organized to meet specific purposes or common goals. Some purposes or family functions are determined by society, such as education and socialization of children and nurturing and support of family members as well as provision of clothing, shelter, and nourishment. The family is the foundation for the child's development and is responsible for the growth and development of children. Murray and Zentner (1997) have identified six tasks of healthy families:

- A feeling of togetherness that promotes the ability to change
- Balance between mutual and independent activities for family members
- Nurturing and resources for growth
- Stability of family structure
- Adaptation
- Encouragement of mastery of developmental tasks of members and family

Families can be defined in terms of structure and function. Family structure is the way a family organizes to meet the needs of family members and social expectations. Structure includes form, power structure, values, communication process, and role structure. Family structure is influenced by socioeconomic status, cultural background, age of members, and situational events such as illness and death. Poverty negatively affects the family's ability to provide the basic economic and emotional needs of its members. Because of increased stress, families in poverty tend to be more rigid and less open than families from other economic levels. Family form is varied; today there are numerous forms, such as homeless, single parent, gay or lesbian, multigenerational, grandparents as surrogate parents, communes, families without children, unmarried couples, and of course the traditional nuclear family (Friedman, 1994; Edelman & Mandle, 1998; Wright & Leahey, 1994).

Spradley (1990) classified divergent family structures

into three main types: single parent, merged, and elderly families. The single-parent family that has an adolescent mother as head of house often has numerous problems related to the mother's own developmental level and needs, her immaturity, and her lack of parenting skills. The merged family has been a growing phenomenon in the United States as individuals (divorced or widowed) with children marry others with or without children. Frequent problems in these families are adjustment and relearning of roles, relationships, and communication patterns for all family members. The third group, elderly families, consists of elderly couples or elderly individuals (most often women) living alone. These families have the task of leading healthy lives while dealing with multiple losses. Losses can be retirement; the death of spouse, friends, or other relatives; and loss of one's own functional abilities and health.

To clearly identify a client's family structure, consider diagramming the family unit (Fig. 12-4). The family structure diagram can be accomplished at the same time as the genogram (see Fig. 12-4 and Chap. 5). A written narrative also may be helpful if the structure is complex. Family function is how the family meets the needs of its members, with emphasis on socialization of children, reproduction (continuing the family over generations), economic resources, and provision of physical and physiologic needs. Within a family system, family functions are not identical but are influenced by mutual expectations of members, repetitive and reciprocal patterns of behavior, roles, communication, power structure, boundaries, and individual capabilities. Assigned family roles are dependent on the number of family members. The fewer the members, the more roles one must assume. Roles determine task, influence communication and relationships, and define power within the family (Phipps, 1980). Family roles may be either ascribed or achieved. Role expectations may be rigid or flexible, clear or vague, and complementary or conflicting. In healthy families roles are flexible, allowing members to shift roles efficiently.

Family roles reflect family structure and values and determine behaviors, which in turn influence interactions and relationships. Unstable families tend to have covert, excessive, or ambivalent rules. Moreover, rules usually influence the roles family members are expected to perform. If a member fails to perform as expected, family stability is threatened. Punishment is an attempt to encourage conformity and ensure stability. The family unit usually depends on communication for function as well as stability. Family functioning also can be threatened by illnesses, abuse, divorce, or members leaving the family.

Additionally, family roles can be overt or covert. Overt roles (also known as formal roles) are critical to the family's functioning, have explicit behaviors, and are present in most families. According to Nye and Gegas (1976), there are eight basic formal family roles: *provider, housekeeper, child-care, child-socialization, recreational, kinship* (maintaining extended family relationships), *therapeutic* (meeting affective needs), and *sexual*. Covert roles (also known as informal roles) are often not evident to people outside the family but do meet the emotional needs of individuals and families (Friedman, 1994). Some covert roles are adaptive, and others have a negative impact on the family's well-being. Examples of covert roles are martyr, scapegoat, black-sheep, placater (trying to please), peacemaker, troublemaker, blamer, dominator, compromiser, harmonizer, encourager, and caretaker. Friedman identified eight informal roles assigned to children: the responsible one, the popular one, the ambitious one, the studious one, the family isolate, the irresponsible one, the sickly one, and the spoiled one. These roles generally have inverse pairs; for example, the irresponsible one and the responsible one, and the studious one and the goof-off. Children learn behaviors associated with informal role as a result of being labeled by the parents or other significant individuals such as teachers and grandparents. Negative labels are particularly detrimental because the child internalizes the negative perceptions of others, has lowered self-esteem, and is at risk for physical and mental illnesses.

Identifying achieved roles within the family is also helpful when assessing composition and structure. For example, how many members are labeled as income earners or identified as being the troublemakers? Such information may be added to the family diagram. Determining the composition of the family and the ages of its members also establishes a basis for assessing individual and family developmental status. Duvall (1977) has identified eight stages of family development: marital, childbearing, preschool, school age, teenage, launching, middle age, and aging. Murray and Zentner (1997) have defined four developmental stages: establishment, expectant, parenthood, and parental disengagement. Awareness of stages of development alerts the nurse to developmental role transitions that can lead to role strain. However, not all families experience these developmental stages,

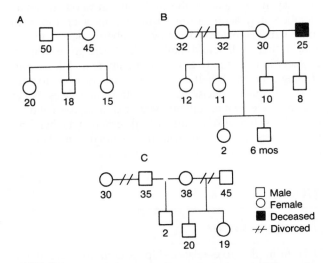

FIGURE 12.4 Possible family configurations include *(A)* a traditional nuclear family including a married couple and their three children; *(B)* a marriage between two people whose previous marriages ended by divorce or death, and who have children both from this marriage and the previous marriages; and *(C)* a family that includes an unmarried heterosexual couple, their child, and the woman's two children from a previous marriage. The numbers indicate peoples' ages.

which are based on procreation and children's ages (*e.g.*, childless families).

Friedman (1994) has identified characteristics within families that are related to functional or dysfunctional communication patterns. Functional communication patterns are characterized by a wide range of emotional communication, including expressions of caring and spontaneous responses; mutual respect for others' feelings and beliefs; ability to discuss personal and social issues; few areas of closed communication (subjects that cannot be talked about); and distribution of power according to the developmental level and needs of family members. Dysfunctional communication is characterized by low self-esteem of family members, self-centeredness (focusing on one's needs while excluding needs of others), need for total agreement by continually pleasing another (agreeing to prevent arguments and burying negative feelings), and lack of empathy (inability to understand other family members' needs). Dysfunctional communication is frequently confusing, vague, indirect, and defensive.

Parenting, a basic function of the *traditional* family, involves the responsibility of physically and emotionally caring for dependent children. Parents are charged with the socialization of their children by transmitting cultural knowledge, values, and rituals. Parenting and family functioning are influenced by the ages of the dependent children, culture, and outside demands such as employment. Society may remove children from their parents' care if such roles are unmet. Conversely, society allows parents to relinquish their roles, rights, and responsibilities to others through adoption and guardianship.

Socialization of children refers to teaching children behaviors, values, and roles they must learn to survive and be effective within their society. In addition to families, day care centers, schools, and even the mass media play an important role in the socialization of children. Children are socialized through role modeling, teaching/learning, and discipline (positive and negative). For a family to function optimally, its members need to follow predetermined guidelines and rules. Generally, discipline involves parents teaching their children acceptable behavior, values, and attitudes, thereby giving them appropriate limitations. Rewards or positive discipline reinforce desired behavior. Punishment (negative discipline), a method of controlling undesirable behavior, relies on making a child feel guilty about a misdeed. Punishment may be verbal, physical, or restrictive. Extreme punishment is considered abuse. Abuse is a pattern of abnormal interactions that often result in physical, emotional, or sexual attacks. Next to children, women and elders are most at risk for abuse in the home. However, men also can be victims of abuse, as can people with developmental disabilities. Occasionally, adolescents abuse adults in their family.

Family Problems or Concerns

Socially, families have the responsibility to provide for the physical, emotional, and social well-being of every member. Because financial resources are necessary to satisfy many of these needs, housing and income should be evaluated in relation to the family's needs. Outside resources such as food stamps and federally funded low-income housing are sometimes not used because family members are unaware of their availability, do not know how to apply for such assistance, or are too proud to ask for help.

Families have numerous concerns that can become stressors and interfere with family health. Concerns may include relationships with in-laws, education of children, inadequate income to meet needs, disability/illness, unemployment or underemployment, disagreement on child rearing, substance abuse, interfamily relationships, environmental hazards, and religious/spiritual disagreements. The health of all family members has a direct effect on the family and family members. The altered health status (whether it be short-term or long-term) of one family member affects all family members and alters the family process. If children of working parents become ill, for instance, then one parent may need to stay home, which could affect income and employment. The death of a family member or moderate to severe disability may cause role responsibilities to change, and other family members may need to assume new roles rapidly.

Yura and Walsh (1978) developed a topology of family problems that classifies problems as (1) no apparent problems; (2) potential problems; (3) problems adequately handled by family; (4) problems that require intervention; (5) problems that require health professional intervention; (6) problems that require further data collection; and (7) temporary problems that involve short-term dependency that might occur during acute illness or death. In general, most family problems are brief in duration and can be adequately handled within the family.

Family Decision-Making Process

How families make decisions varies. In one family, a parent may have most of the authority; in another, family members may act as a unit in making most decisions. In some families, extended family members, such as uncles and brothers-in-law and family elders, participate in making decisions that may range from naming a child to purchasing a house. Whether families react passively to situations or make decisions to control their lives is an important element to identify when assessing roles and relationships. It is also important to determine whether family members are satisfied with their particular methods of making both minor and major decisions.

Documentation

Data from the role–relationship pattern may be documented as follows:

Example 1: Healthy Role–Relationship Pattern

Irma, aged 36, a single mother with two children ages 12 years and 6 weeks, was interviewed as part of a comprehensive postpartum visit. Documentation of the role–relationship pattern was as follows:

Physical Examination   Evaluating Roles and Relationships

GENERAL PRINCIPLES

The foundation for the role–relationship pattern is the interview.

Evaluation of stress, social support, and transition to new roles (such as parenting) is important in assessment of roles–relationships.

The interview and physical examination can provide information about role strain.

Other family members or significant others may provide additional information regarding role strain.

If the client does not report any problems with roles, family, or relationships, a screening assessment is indicated (Display 12-1).

Any interpretation of roles and relationships is subject to change as the person's situation changes.

A comprehensive interview is indicated whenever a person reports role–relationship problems or is at high risk for problems, as reflected in a family history of abuse, adolescent parenting, insufficient resources, or changes in family structure or roles.

LABORATORY / X-RAY EVALUATION

There are no specific diagnostic studies for roles and relationships. However, some diagnostic tests, such as for vision and hearing, may be useful with communication problems.

ASSESSMENT AIDS

Eco-map (see Fig. 12-2)
Genogram (see Fig. 12-4)
Interview guide to suggest questions and record data (see Display 12-1)

Denies any difficulty with identified roles of mother and waitress. Both she and older child (Rosa) are adjusting to new infant. Irma's mother stayed with family for 4 weeks just before and after infant's birth. States "getting up at night again and diapers takes some getting used to, but he is such a good baby." Has adequate child care for infant, but some concerns about Rosa, as she no longer wishes to attend "after-school program." Has numerous friends, two whom she can confide in and discuss problems. Currently satisfied with life, thinking of returning to school to get a high school diploma and possibly a college degree. Her mother would like for her to return "home" so mother could help with child care and expenses. No longer sees infant's father. Talkative, expresses self freely and adequately with appropriate affect.

These findings may be recorded in a problems-oriented record as follows:

S: Roles identified—daughter, mother, waitress; denies difficulty with these. Numerous friends, two that she can confide in. Good relationship with children, using child care. Some concern about continuing after-school program for daughter. Considering moving home to be near her mother and returning to school and possibly college. No contact with children's fathers.

O: Communicates easily, easy to understand, smiles when talking of children

A: Functional role–relationship pattern

P: Reassess in 1 year during routine screening. Provide information about adult education programs in area. Explore alternatives to after-school program for Rosa with social worker.

Example 2: Altered Role–Relationship Pattern

Nancy and Tim have a 5-year-old son, David, and an 8-month-old daughter, Nicole. The son, never completely toilet-trained at night, started bed-wetting every night after the birth of Nicole. David has been evaluated by a urologist. The parents have tried everything without success to reduce enuresis. During the process of the assessment, an ecomap was completed. Parents use babysitters at night four to five times per week. This family has a large social support system; however, every member except Nicole is involved in one to two major activities daily, more on the weekends, and they infrequently have meals together.

These findings may be recorded in a problem-oriented record as follows:

S: Nancy express concern about David's persistent enuresis, which has increased since Nicole's birth. Family infrequently eats meals together, and they are involved in numerous activities during the week and more during the weekend. David involved in karate, soccer, T-ball, church club, after-school program, and basketball. Large circle of friends. Use babysitters four or five times per week at night and also on weekends.

O: Nancy nonverbally expresses frustration with enuresis and appears tired.

A: Possible family process, altered

P: Talk with Tim and David to obtain their input. Encourage Nancy to reduce David's activities to two or

(continues on p. 506)

DISPLAY 12.1

Interview Guide: Roles and Relationships

ROLES

Describe your roles with family/friends/coworkers: _____

How satisfied are you with all of your responsibilities? _____

Do you ever feel overwhelmed, incompetent, or under a lot of stress? If yes, describe: _____
_____

How has your health status altered your roles or relationships with others (if ill)? _____
_____

How are you preparing for your new role? (*e.g.*, new parent, new job) _____
_____

FAMILY/RELATIONSHIPS

Describe your family structure (genogram, Fig. 12-4): _____

Whom do you live with? _____

Whom do you turn to for help? _____

Describe your relationships with others (ecomap, Fig. 12-2): _____

How do you make individual/family decisions? _____
_____

For Parents

Tell me what you do when (name) does something you consider to be a minor wrong. Give an example of a minor
wrong: _____

Tell me what you do when (name) does something you consider to be a major wrong? Give an example of a major
wrong: _____

Do you have any problems with communication? (explain) _____

Do you use any communication aids such as corrective lenses or hearing aids (identify)? _____

Do you have any concerns about: parenting _____ relationships _____

physical or emotional abuse _____ finances _____ marital issues _____

discipline_____

Explore any positive findings:

▼ ▼ ▼

GUIDELINES

Assessment Guidelines Roles and Relationships: Interview (Health History)

Procedure	Clinical Significance
1. Individual roles Interview to elicit specific information about the person's roles:	
• Number of roles To assess roles, ask the person to identify and discuss all pertinent roles and responsibilities.	Individuals are able to perform numerous roles; however, too many roles/responsibilities can result in role overload. Examples of statements regarding role overload may include expressions of insufficient time, reduced quality of work, or being overwhelmed.
• Role perception Does the person think the number of roles and responsibilities are appropriate?	
• Role satisfaction/dissatisfaction Ask questions such as: "Is there any thing about any of your roles you would like to change?" "How satisfied are you with all of your responsibilities?"	Role conflict occurs when role responsibilities compete for time or resources. Expression of role conflict may include one set of responsibilities interfering with another set of responsibilities, for example, "I don't get to spend enough time with my kids because of work."

▼ ▼ ▼

Roles and Relationships: Interview (Health History)

Procedure

- Role strain
  Ask the following:
  "Do you ever feel overwhelmed, incompetent, or under a lot of stress?"

2. Family roles and relationships

Interview the person to determine quality of family relationships. It is often helpful to interview more than one family member if the focus of the assessment is the family.

- *Family composition and structure:* draw a genogram (see Fig. 12–4)
- *Covert family roles*
  Ask questions such as:
  "Does anyone in the family have any roles such as peacemaker, martyr, the smart one, or caretaker?"
- *Family communication patterns*
  Ask questions related to usual patterns, such as:
  "Would you say that more anger or happiness is expressed in your family?"
  "Who does most of the talking in the family?"
  "What is the quality of the communication within the family?"
  "How well do others listen?"

- *Family problems or concerns:*
  "Are there any current family problems or concerns?"
  "How well are family problems discussed?"

- *Family decision-making process*
  "How are family decisions made?"
  "Is there one person who makes most of the decisions?"
  "Is there one person who makes the final decision?"

Clinical Significance

Role incompetence occurs when the individual does not have sufficient knowledge or skill to adequately meet responsibilities. Expressions of role incompetence may include doubts about performance, feelings of failure, or inability to do a good job.

Expressions that may indicate role strain include being overwhelmed, doubts about ability, feelings of inferiority in performing role, feelings of failing, not accomplishing anything, letting others down, lack of self-confidence, not enough time, and insufficient knowledge or skill. Physical signs of role strain might include fatigue, frequent headaches, depression, gastric and duodenal ulcers, anxiety, neglect of self, and physical illnesses.

The genogram diagrams the composition of the family and provides an overview of the family structure.

Identification of roles that may be detrimental to the individual's or family's well-being can alert the nurse to the need for specific interventions.

The focus of the assessment is the interaction among all family members and not just individuals. Different members may have different perceptions. By viewing the interaction of family members and not focusing on the individual, the nurse can evaluate relationships and behavior within the context of the family and not in isolation (Wright & Leahey, 1994). From these and follow-up questions the nurse gains insight into the degree of functional and dysfunctional communication patterns within the family.

Family concerns may be financial, social, or health related. Some may be beyond the scope of nursing and require referral to other professionals such as a social worker. This may be difficult to discover, because some families do not discuss specific problems such as sexual orientation, adoption, and abuse.

How decisions are made provides cues to family structure (power) and function.

▼ ▼ ▼

G U I D E L I N E S   *continued*   Roles and Relationships: Interview (Health History)

Procedure

- *Discipline patterns*

  Inquire into discipline patterns if minor children are in the family.

  "Tell me what you do when (name) does something you consider to be a minor wrong. Give me an example of a minor wrong."

  "Tell me what you do when (name) does something you consider to be a major wrong. Give me an example of a major wrong."

3. Social relationships

- *Individual social relationships*

  Social relationships can be assessed by exploring the person's perceptions about the adequacy of his or her relationships.

  How satisfied is the person with the quality and quantity of relationships? The variety of relationships? The use of an ecomap (Fig. 12–2) is helpful in illustrating this information.

- *Family social relationships*

  The family's social relationships are evaluated similarly to the individual's; however, there are more people to consider, and the ecomap can become quite large.

- *Relationships with helping professionals*

  Ask questions such as:

  "Do you feel comfortable discussing health problems with health care providers such as nurses and doctors?"

  "Who do you think should decide and plan your health care?"

4. Communication

- *Communication skills*

  Determine the individual's perception of his or her ability to express self and understand written communication.

  Is there a history of an eye or hearing injury, stroke (cerebrovascular accident [CVA]), presence of a tracheostomy, or loss/injury to the vocal cords?

  Does the individual relate problems with reading or understanding what is read? This can be discovered by asking questions such as:

  "What do you like to read?"

  "Do you have trouble understanding health information pamphlets?"

  If the person's primary language is not English, you should ask about their ability to read English.

Clinical Significance

Methods of punishment indicate much about family relationships and beliefs about acceptable methods of discipline. Consider if family rules are clear to everyone. Behavior limits, expectations, and punishment patterns should be consistent and appropriate for the child's age and developmental level.

Types of punishment the family uses—physical, such as spanking; behavior modification such as time-out; or emotional, such as belittling—can provide cues to appropriate discipline patterns when there is a risk for abuse.

People vary in their need for social interaction and social support. If a person has few sources of support and if they all come from the same source (such as work), during times of stress or crises the amount of social support may not be sufficient. An ecomap illustrates the quality, quantity, and diversity of an individual's social interactions and available social support.

This information provides cues to the nurse regarding the amount of involvement the person desires in his or her health care and the level of comfort in discussing health problems.

A CVA can interfere with an individual's ability to speak (aphasia) and ability to read because of visual field loss (see Chap. 9). Visual losses can interfere with the person's ability to read and also limit or prevent lip reading, which many people find helpful while listening to others. Hearing loss can limit a person's ability to understand spoken communication. A tracheostomy and injury or removal of the vocal cords can profoundly affect one's speech.

Knowing what a person likes to read can provide a clue to his or her reading level. Many health education and discharge instructions are given in written form. If a person has a low reading level or does not read English, the nurse needs to find alternative sources of education, for example, videos and pamphlets in languages other than English. Keep in mind that many people who can speak English cannot read English.

▼ ▼ ▼

Procedure

- *Communication aids*
  Does the individual use any of the following as a primary means of communication:
    Corrective lenses (glasses)
    Hearing aids
    Artificial voice device
    Computer
    Word board
    Sign language

5. Roles and relationships
Diagnostic aids
There are no specific laboratory or x-ray tests that aid with the evaluation of the roles and relationship pattern. Indirectly, diagnostic aids from other patterns can provide clues to the evaluation of this pattern.
Examples of diagnostic tests from other patterns include:
- Vision screening
- Hearing screening
- X-rays of the skeleton

- Diagnostic tests for stress-related problems such as headaches and possibly gastric ulcers (see Chaps. 7 and 14)

Clinical Significance

Knowledge of an individual's use of aids can assist the nurse in using aids to provide care and in assessing the effectiveness of the aid in communication.
There are many types of sign languages, such as American Sign Language; however, as with spoken language, there are regional differences. Some individuals and families develop their own sign language.

Vision and hearing are important in written and spoken communication (see Chap. 9).

X-rays can show broken bones; bones in various stages of healing are a sign of physical abuse (see Chap. 10).

Stress-related problems may indicate role strain.

▼ ▼ ▼

Assessment Guidelines Roles and Relationships: Physical Assessment

Procedure

A nurse makes observations for the role–relationship function during the entire contact with the person and family. Cues from other functions, such as problems with coping and stress, sleep, self-concept, and values and beliefs, can alert the nurse to potential problems within the role–relationship pattern.

1. General appearance
Observe for indicators of role strain.

Clinical Significance

Indicators of Role Strain
- Fatigue
- Feelings of being overwhelmed
- Expressions of anxiety
- Headaches
- Gastric upset
- Anger
- Reports of stress
- Depression
- Self-neglect
- Signs of sleep disruption (see Chap. 10)

▼ ▼ ▼

G U I D E L I N E S *continued*

Roles and Relationships: Physical Assessment

Procedure	Clinical Significance

Procedure

2. Communication skills

Observe and listen for communication abilities.

Observe skill with communication aids.

3. Family interaction

Observe family interaction, noting:
- Who answers questions
- Pattern of communication
- Who is silent
- Who makes decisions
- Signs of affection

Clinical Significance

Normal Findings
- Speech understandable
- Vocabulary appropriate for age
- Appropriate responses
- Congruence between verbal and nonverbal communication

Findings That May Cause Problems With Communication
- Inability to speak dominant language
- Use of sign language
- No access to communication aid such as hearing aid, corrective lenses, and computer

Deviations from Normal
- Stuttering
- Weak or absent voice
- Slurring
- Unable to remember
- Inappropriate responses
- Inability to read

Normal Findings
Individual can demonstrate use of aid, *i.e.,* how to insert hearing aid and change battery, how to use computer, how artificial voice equipment works.

Indicators of poor family relationships include:
- Expression of frequent verbal hostility
- Physical violence
- Inability to talk with other members
- Lack of nurturing environment (needs are not met)
- Rigidity in family members and family rules
- One individual answering all questions, even those directed to others
- Ignoring of family member(s) by others
- Lack of touching
- Belittling comments
- Evidence of physical violence
- Little verbal interaction among members

Care must be taken not to make quick judgments. For example, some families use little physical contact such as touching and hugging; this does not always indicate a problem.

▼ ▼ ▼

Procedure

When possible, observe interactions of individual/family with others.

Clinical Significance

Expressions indicating difficulty with relationships include:
- Feelings of aloneness or loneliness; not being worthy of friends
- Lack of self-confidence in groups or in one-to-one relationships
- Feelings of inferiority
- Fear of groups of people or of meeting new people
- Insufficient support group

Observations of difficulty with relationships with others might include:
- Avoiding interactions; limited verbal communication
- Lack of eye contact
- Allowing others to speak for self

4. Parenting skills

Observe for parental role adequacy:
- Signs of affection
- Reaction of child to parent
- Verbal and nonverbal communication between parent and child
- Note how child is disciplined during visit

Parents who are not having difficulty with the parenting role will express overall satisfaction with their role and pleasure with their children. Although they may have questions, generally they actively seek guidance from professionals, books, or friends.

Individuals having difficulty parenting may express the following:
- Inadequacies in the role
- Frustration with parenting
- Anger with children
- Inappropriate discipline for child's age
- Dissatisfaction with child
- Use of negative labels—"the stupid one"
- Conflict with other roles
- Feelings of being overwhelmed, with little or no time for self

Behaviors that may be observed include:
- Hitting children
- Inappropriate anger expressed
- Lack of touching
- Little or infrequent emotional support
- Lack of nurturing

Children who are inappropriately parented may demonstrate the following:
- Signs of physical violence
- Abusive behavior to others or to animals
- Inappropriate dress
- Unkempt appearance
- Poor hygiene
- Delay of physical and psychosocial development
- Clinging to or avoiding others
- Malnourishment

▼ ▼ ▼

Procedure

5. Abuse

Observe for signs of physical abuse:
- Bruising
- Multiple injuries, including fractures and burns

Clinical Significance

Signs of physical abuse include bruising, especially between the elbows and knees; multiple injuries in various stages of healing; burn scars, especially those that are round and cigarette-shaped; history of broken bones; reports of clumsiness; frequent falls; report of how injury occurred inconsistent with injury; history of using numerous different hospitals and physicians for injury treatment; and expressions indicating the victim is "bad" or deserving of injury. Individuals who perform acts of violence may demonstrate or express the following: low frustration tolerance, physical expressions of anger, chemical substance use, or history as an abuse victim.

---

three per week. Encourage Nancy and Tim to spend quality time with David. Discuss case at next case conference for suggestions.

Example 3: Altered Role–Relationship Pattern

Otto, age 80, had a stroke 2 days ago that affected his speech and resulted in left-sided paralysis. The discharge planning nurse documented the following about the role–relationship pattern:

> Unable to speak, words garbled, speech therapy daily—to continue as outpatient two times per week after discharge. Becomes frustrated rapidly when trying to express self. Wife, Geneva, concerned about how they will manage, as husband pays all the bills and does the yard work and most of the driving. Geneva has arthritis, uses a walker, and depends on Otto for assistance with household tasks. Will refer to home health agency to evaluate home environment and needs before discharge.

These findings may be recorded in a problem-oriented format as follows:

S: Tries to communicate, garbled speech. Wife concerned about how family will manage. Otto's roles include: pay bills, yard worker, driver, helper with household tasks. Wife's activity limited—arthritis, needs help with instrumental activities of daily living.

O: Otto's speech not understandable, speech therapy daily, to continue two times per week on discharge, left-sided paralysis, becomes frustrated after a few moments of trying to move or speak. (Wife) Geneva's hands gnarled, uses walker.

A: Probable diagnosis: Otto—verbal communication impaired, related to recent neurologic insult. Otto and Geneva: Family process, altered, related to recent debilitating illness of Otto.

P: Gather additional data to support diagnosis. Refer to home health agency to evaluate home environment and needs before discharge, consider support group for both Otto and Geneva. Visit in 2 days to note progress and additional concerns.

ND$_x$

Nursing Diagnoses Related to Roles and Relationships

Altered Family Process

Altered family process occurs when the family system that has been functioning effectively becomes unable to meet the physical and emotional needs of family members adequately, perform family responsibilities, or maintain communication for mutual growth and development. Ineffective family coping is the correct diagnosis for the family that has a history of inappropriate functioning (Carpenito, 1997).

History.   The person reports an inability to communicate with other family members, disharmony between family members, and disagreement in family about family rules, and is having difficulty adapting positively to a crisis that may be maturational, situational, or related to illness. Altered family process may occur any time a family member is hospitalized; leaves the family by death or divorce or by attending college; a new member enters the family by birth, adoption, or marriage; or there is a change in economic status such as unemployment, retirement, or obtaining employment.

Physical Examination Findings.   The nurse may observe behaviors such as limited or no verbal exchanges between family members, self-blaming or blaming others, sudden outbursts of emotions, and verbal abuse. Family members may show physical evidence of Altered family process, such as weight loss or gain, alcohol and drug use, and stress-related conditions such as headaches, lack of sleep, and physical abuse.

Altered Parenting

Altered parenting is an actual inability by parents or caregivers to provide an environment that supports optimal physical and emotional growth and development of a dependent child. Risk for altered parenting occurs with normal maturational processes of adjustment to parenting. Risk factors may become evident during the prenatal period or during normal transitions of the dependent child such as from infant to toddler and from school age to adolescent.

History. An individual experiencing altered parenting may verbalize disappointment, resentment, or shame about a child; feelings of being an inadequate parent; or frustration with being a parent. There may be a documented history of numerous injuries that may be poorly explained. There is a lack of parental attachment behavior.

Physical Examination Findings. The nurse may observe inappropriate parenting behaviors such as hitting, verbal abuse, and ignoring the child. Other observations may include lack of touching or holding, no eye contact, and hostility of child to the parent. The physical examination may show wounds in various stages of healing and poor correlation of how injury occurred between parent and child. With a hospitalized child, the parents may not visit or visit infrequently.

Risk for Altered Parent–Infant Attachment

This nursing diagnosis is used when significant risk factors are present that may interfere with the normal maturational process: nurturing, protecting, and interacting between a parent/caregiver and infant.

History. Individuals at high risk for alterations in parent–infant attachment may be identified by interruption of the normal bonding process because of parent or infant illness, unrealistic expectations of the infant or self, unwanted pregnancy, disappointment with the infant because of gender or congenital anomalies, economic problems, lack of knowledge of parental role, and physical disability of the parent.

Physical Examination Findings. The presence of physical or mental illness may interfere with the individual's ability to parent. The presence of physical illness of the child also may interfere with the adult's ability to parent. Observations of problems in family process, such as communication and support received within the family, can increase the risk for alterations in parenting. The parent may be unable to hold, talk to, or make eye contact with the infant. The parent also may refuse to participate in the infant's care and verbalize negative feelings about the infant.

Parental Role Conflict

The nursing diagnosis Parental role conflict is used when the parent is experiencing role confusion and conflict in response to crises experienced by one or both parents. The conflict can be between values/beliefs and societal expectations or between two or more role obligations. This diagnosis is used to describe a situation in which previously effectively functioning parents are having difficulty because of external factors such as illness. If not resolved, alteration in parenting may occur (Carpenito, 1997).

History. During the interview, parents with role conflict may express their concerns about changes in their roles. Verbalizations regarding frustration in not being able to meet their perceived responsibilities may be ex-

pressed. Parents also may report the occurrence of acute, chronic, or life-threatening illnesses/conditions of a family member that interfere with the ability to perform the parenting role as the parent desires.

Physical Examination Findings. The parent may verbalize feelings of guilt or inadequacy in meeting role obligations. If the parent needs to learn a new skill to provide care to a child, he or she may demonstrate poor technique or verbalize an inability to perform the skill. You may be able to observe feelings of fear, anger, anxiety, or frustration regarding the effect of illness, death, or separation on family process and the ability to parent all children.

Disturbances in Role Performance

The nursing diagnosis Disturbances in role performance is used when there is a change, conflict, or denial of role responsibilities or when the individual is unable to fulfill role obligations.

History. The history includes any verbalization of difficulty or frustration with role responsibilities, such as an increase in the number of duties, forgetting to complete required tasks, or reports of conflicts between two or more roles, such as needing to attend two different meetings at the same time. The individual also may report a role but is unable to describe the responsibilities associated with it. With denial, the individual would not report a particular role.

Physical Examination Findings. Physical findings would be limited. Physical signs of stress may be evident (*e.g.,* fatigue, headaches, and poor attention span). Denial of role may be evident in others; for example, the child of a parent who denies a parenting role may have evidence of physical and psychosocial neglect.

Social Isolation/At Risk for Loneliness

Social isolation is used when the individual or family perceives a need but is unable to obtain greater social involvement. Carpenito (1997) poses that the nursing diagnosis Social isolation is a condition of the response to loneliness and that the diagnosis Loneliness or At risk for loneliness is a more appropriate diagnosis. To experience social isolation, one must express feelings of aloneness and a desire for more social contact. The nursing diagnosis At risk for loneliness is used when an individual desires more contact with others.

History. The history includes any fear of rejection for physical reasons such as obesity, cancer, developmental disability, or incontinence. Other factors that may place an individual at risk are the loss of a significant other or relationships because of death, divorce, loss or transportation, or relocation. An ecomap illustrates few interactions.

Physical Examination Findings. Because feelings of loneliness are subjective, there may be no physical findings. However, some physical findings may be sadness, depressed affect, withdrawal, poor eye contact, inability to concentrate, and evidence of drug or alcohol abuse.

Relocation Stress Syndrome

Relocation stress is experienced by individuals who move from one environment to another, whether it be across the hall or across the country. The diagnosis is appropriate when a person or family experiences psychological or physiologic disruptions because of the move.

History. Besides mentioning a recent move, the individual expresses loneliness, depression, anxiety, or changes in normal habits such as eating and sleeping.

Physical Examination. Physical findings may include weight loss, fatigue, sad affect, depression, restlessness, and confusion (in elders).

Caregiver Role Strain/High Risk for Caregiver Role Strain

With Caregiver role strain, the individual can experience physical, emotional, social and financial burdens because of care provided to another person. An individual is at risk for caregiver role strain when the possibility exists for him or her to experience a burden in caregiving.

History. The individual is providing care to another and expresses difficulty in performing activities required, interference of caregiving with other important roles, concern about the future, and feelings of guilt, anger, and being overwhelmed. The individual at risk may report a history of a poor relationship with the care receiver, ineffective coping, chronic health problems, and insufficient finances or support.

Physical Examination. The physical assessment may identify depression, anxiety, fatigue, and previously undetected chronic illnesses.

Impaired Social Interaction

The nursing diagnosis Impaired social interactions is used when the individual experiences, perceives, or is at high risk for experiencing negative, insufficient, or unsatisfactory interactions with others. Interactions may be unsatisfactory because the individual is overwhelmed by numerous interactions that are considered superficial, and time is not sufficient to have meaningful interactions.

History. The client may verbalize being uncomfortable in social interactions, avoiding people either individually or in groups, lacking the ability to have satisfying encounters with others, lacking friends or close confidants, and identifying few persons who can provide social support.

Physical Examination Findings. Individuals who have a mental illness such as schizophrenia and depression may have difficulty in sustaining social relationships and interactions. Findings may include physical evidence of panic or anxiety attacks during interactions with others, inappropriate communication pattern and content, or lack of communication with others. Additionally, language barriers, visual and hearing deficits, impaired mobility, and speech impediments are physical findings that may contribute to impaired social interactions.

Impaired Verbal Communication

Impaired verbal communication occurs when the individual has a reduced, changed, or absent ability to use verbal communication. This nursing diagnosis may be situational. For example, an individual goes to a clinic where the providers do not speak his or her native language; this may not be a problem at another clinic, where providers do speak that language.

History. In individuals with severe impaired communication, the history may need to be obtained in writing or by a family member. A history of conditions such as cerebral palsy, cerebrovascular accident, or surgery for laryngeal cancer may be present. In children, there may not be a change in communication ability but a delay in or lack of verbal development. In individuals with a history of Alzheimer's disease, there may be nothing wrong with the ability to speak; however, the content of the words is inappropriate. Individuals may verbalize frustration or inability to say certain sounds, speak the dominant language, or speak loudly enough for others to hear.

Physical Examination Findings. Findings may include the presence of a tracheotomy, scars from laryngectomy, shortness of breath, cleft lip or palate, infected or inflamed throat, or polyps on the vocal cords. Diagnostic screening may identify difficulty with hearing or vision. Listening closely to the individual, you may document confusion, stuttering, slurring, inappropriate word use, incoherent speech, and the use of another language. You also may find that although the individual has a hearing aid, it is not used or it is malfunctioning.

Potential for Violence

Potential for violence exists when the individual is at high risk for self- and other-directed physical aggression. Self-directed violence is closely related to the nursing diagnosis Risk for self-harm (abuse, mutilation, and suicide).

History. The history consists of reports or verbalizations of physical harm or attempts to harm self, others, or property. The individual also may report increased stress and difficulty handling stress.

Physical Examination Findings. The physical examination of the individual or others, such as children or spouse, may reveal wounds and bruises in various stages of healing, and x-rays may show old and new fractures. Other findings may include observations of low frustration level, verbal threats, and expressions of helplessness, hostility, and fear of loss of control. There may be evidence of drug and alcohol abuse. Body language may indicate intent to harm, such as rigid posture, tense facial expression, and clenched hands. Laboratory results may indicate a toxic response to drugs (prescription and others), altered electrolytes, presence of blood alcohol, and altered blood gases in individuals with potentially violent behavior.

ND$_x$

Clinical Problems Related to Roles and Relationships

Assessment of roles and relationships provides indicators for nursing diagnoses; however, clinical problems with roles and relationship are often associated with clinical problems in other assessment areas. For example, gastric ulcers are clinical problems in the elimination pattern, and fatigue is a clinical problem in the sleep–rest pattern. Ineffective coping is often a symptom of role strain. During the assessment, the nurse should consider any clinical problems from other patterns that may have an effect on roles and relationships. Some clinical problems the nurse may encounter primarily in roles and relationships include physical abuse (musculoskeletal system), aphasia (cognitive/perceptual pattern), tracheotomy (respiratory system), agoraphobia (stress and stress response pattern), social isolation of elders (mobility/cognitive impairment and other factors), and adolescent parenting.

Physical Abuse

Physical abuse of an individual by another can occur at any age and with any gender; however, children, women, and elders are at higher risk than other groups. Signs of physical abuse include frequent trauma injuries from fists; objects such as electric cords, belts, and household items; and cigarettes (burns). Injuries between the elbows and knees are especially suspicious. The use of numerous physicians and different emergency rooms is also significant. Generally, the injury presented and the explanation for the injury do not correspond. An atypical form of child abuse is *Munchausen syndrome by proxy,* in which the parent invents signs and symptoms of illnesses in the child and may induce some symptoms such as vomiting. The child is then subjected to numerous medical tests, hospitalization, and, in some situations, exploratory surgery. During the process, the parent receives desired attention. Recently, several cases of pseudo–sudden infant death syndrome (SIDS) have been uncovered, in which the parent kills the infant in a way that appears to be SIDS, thereby receiving the attention allocated to a grieving parent.

Aphasia

Aphasia is a defect or loss of the ability to express oneself by speech or in writing or to comprehend the spoken language. Aphasia is the result of disease or injury in the speech center in the brain. *Broca's aphasia,* also known as expressive aphasia, often occurs as a result of a stroke. With this aphasia, the person can understand and knows what he or she wants to say but cannot find the correct words (see Chap. 9).

Tracheostomy

Tracheostomies interfere with the individual's ability to speak words. Air is diverted from the larynx, preventing the vocal cords from vibrating and making sounds. If not connected to a respirator, tracheostomies can be plugged by a finger or cork to allow the individual to speak. When temporarily closing the tracheostomy opening, you must be observant for signs of respiratory distress (see Chap. 8).

Cancer of the Larynx

Generally, when cancer of the larynx occurs, the larynx is surgically removed. The individual may use an electronic device to simulate speaking. The nurse needs to listen very carefully, as speech can be difficult to understand (see Chap. 6).

Agoraphobia

With agoraphobia, the most severe phobia, the individual fears open spaces, eventually becomes house bound, and all social interactions outside the home stop. In the most severe forms, the individual cannot leave the house without experiencing a severe panic attack. If health care is needed outside the home, the health professionals must also assist the individual in dealing with panic attacks (see Chap. 14).

Social Isolation Associated With Age

As an individual becomes very old and frail, social isolation often occurs as the result of loss of transportation, loss of mobility, and loss of friends to death. Some elders may seek medical care and hospitalization to avoid feelings of aloneness (see Chap. 17).

Adolescent Parenting

Adolescents, especially young adolescents, experience stress and role strain while attempting to parent an infant or child. The child may suffer from neglect or abuse because of the parent's lack of maturation and skill. Neglect can be purposeful or benign. Benign neglect occurs when individuals do not desire to neglect the child but are unaware that they are causing harm.

CASE STUDY 1

John, age 34, lives with his mother, stepfather, and 17-year-old sister to save money. He recently lost his job to downsizing and has a new job that pays significantly less. Six months ago he learned he has human immunodeficiency virus (HIV)—the AIDS virus. He chose not to tell his family, but did advise his sexual partner in another city. He is now hospitalized with pneumonia and has been told that he has AIDS. When his family was informed of his diagnosis, they stopped visiting. John's lover makes a trip as often as possible to visit, but he is now concerned about his own health. He recently tested negative for the virus but knows this can change.

To assess John's role–relationship status, the nurse reviews the available data and concludes that, in addition to other health problems, John is probably experiencing a problem with roles and relationships. The nurse bases this judgment on the following: John did not tell his family of his HIV status; when his family discovered his status they stopped visiting; he lives with his family to save money; he has an alternative lifestyle; he has recently learned that he has a life-threatening disease; and he maintains a relationship with a significant other who lives in another city and is concerned about his own health. After considering the initial data, the nurse identifies the following possible

CASE STUDY 1 *continued*

diagnoses: Loneliness, Altered family process, and Disturbances in role performance.

After identifying these possibilities, the nurse collects
additional data to either support or reject the diagnoses.
The nurse also considers alternative diagnoses. Once all
the data are collected and analyzed, a final diagnosis can
be made. In this situation the nurse makes the final nursing diagnoses of Anticipatory grieving related to ap-
proaching death; Altered role performance related to increased dependency; Loneliness related to others' fears
and beliefs about AIDS; and Ineffective family coping, dis-

abling, related to nonacceptance of John's illness and
lifestyle.

John does not do well on medication, and his life expectancy is limited. After a family conference involving
John, his lover, and his sister (his mother and stepfather
refuse to come), it is decided to discharge John to his
lover's residence and to make a referral to Hospice's home
health program. The nurse is concerned about John's
lover's risk for caregiver strain and encourages him to attend a support group. John dies 11 months later with his
lover and sister at his bedside.

CASE STUDY 2

Letty is a 30-year-old legal immigrant and the mother of
four children ages 6, 4, 3, and 1. Her husband died 18
months ago. All the children were born in the United
States. She speaks little English. She is currently receiving
Aid to Families with Dependent Children (AFDC). She has
been advised that because of welfare reform, she must
start looking for employment. Through an interpreter Letty
states, "Some days it is just too much with no money, all
the pressure, the kids crying and fighting. I just don't
know what to do! How will I find a job, who will take care
of my children, who wants to hire someone who can't
speak English? What will become of me and my children?"
Both of her parents are dead, and she is unaware of her
dead husband's family. She does receive social support
from her cultural community.

In preparing for this visit, the public health nurse reviews the child health conference records of the four children, including their height, weight, and developmental
status. Within the role–relationship pattern, the nurse decides to identify the diagnosis of Possible alteration in parenting based on the mother's stated distress and the children's growth lag; Altered role performance related to
increased responsibilities as a single parent; and Altered
family process related to the husband/father's death. Addi-

tionally, the nurse speaks with the social worker and explores community services available to the family. Because
of the mother's stress, the nurse also is concerned about the
potential of violence toward the children.

The nurse continues to make home visits, enrolls the
two younger children in the nutrition program Women,
Infants, and Children (WIC), and provides Letty with information about an English as a second language program that will provide day care while she attends classes
during the day. Three months after the first home visit,
Letty is attending English classes and the three younger
children are in day care. Learning English makes Letty
feel better about herself, and she appears to be less stressed.
The nurse no longer considers the diagnosis Potential for
violence. Letty's plans are to finish the English program
and then study for a GED so that she will be employable.
The nursing diagnoses Alteration in parenting and Altered family process remain relevant, although they are revised as new data emerge. When Letty does go to school
and eventually seek employment, this will affect the family
process and her parenting behavior. Continuous data collection and analysis are indicated so that appropriate interventions can be added to modify or resolve problems.

CASE STUDY 3

Glenn and Suzi were both looking forward to spending
time together after they retired. However, 3 months after
their retirement Suzi's father died, and shortly thereafter
her mother, Martha, became ill. Suzi had helped Martha
care for her father and found it to be rewarding. As
Martha deteriorated, Suzi became aware that she could no
longer remain at home alone. After much discussion, Suzi

and Glenn had Martha move in with them. Suzi continued to care for Martha for the next 2 years without help.

Suzi comes into the hospital emergency room late one
night with complaints of chest pain and a terrible
headache. During the course of the interview the nurse
discovers that Suzi has not been anywhere except to the
grocery store for the last 12 months, feels incompetent and

CASE STUDY 3 *continued*

overwhelmed by Martha's care, and has no time for house-cleaning or for herself. Martha no longer speaks or recognizes anyone and has become incontinent of bowel and urine in the last month.

The nurse makes the diagnosis of Caregiver role strain and refers Suzi and Glenn to the social worker. After seeing the emergency department physician, a medical diagnosis of anxiety attack is made. The nurse and social worker talk to Suzi and Glenn about getting assistance in the form of home health nursing and respite care to give

them some free time. They are also referred to a caregiver support group. After 2 months the home health nurse makes an evaluation visit and determines that continued in-home care is necessary. Suzi is getting out regularly and has attended some support group meetings. The home health nurse revises the nursing diagnosis to Risk for caregiver role strain and talks to Suzi about temporary nursing home respite admissions for Martha, so that Suzi and Glenn can have some time alone.

CHAPTER 12 SUMMARY

Assessment of roles and relationships focuses on the following:

- Identifying role, role perception and role performance
- Determining the risk for role strain or response to role strain
- Evaluating communication patterns between person and significant others
- Identifying factors restricting effective communication
- Identifying actual or potential dysfunction and strengths within the family

When assessing roles and relationships, the nurse considers:

- People assume many roles during the course of their lifetimes.
- Roles are either ascribed or achieved.
- Role strain can occur because of conflict, ambiguity, overload, and incompetence.
- Social interaction is influenced by the number of people interacting and the relationships between those people.
- Communication is verbal and nonverbal, effective and ineffective, and influenced by social interaction.
- The term *family* may be defined as a human group with significant emotional bonds, interdependence, and (usually) shared housing.
- Family structure, function, and role responsibilities are culturally influenced.
- Parenting involves the responsibility of providing physical and emotional care to minor children.

The following methods are used for data collection:

Interview or Review of Records

1. Interview
   - Individual Roles
     - Perceptions
     - Satisfaction
     - Role strain

Family Roles and Relationships
- Family composition and structure
- Family communication patterns
- Family problems or concerns
- Family decision-making process
- Discipline patterns

Social Relationships
- Individual social relationships
- Family social relationships
- Relationships with helping professionals

Communication
- Communication skills
- Communication aids

2. Laboratory/X-ray Analysis
   There are no specific laboratory or x-ray tests for the role relationship pattern.

3. Physical Examination
   - General appearance
   - Communication skills
   - Family interaction
   - Parenting skills
   - Abuse

Role and relationship assessment based on these principles and methods helps the nurse to identify characteristics and risk factors for the following nursing diagnoses:

- Altered family processes
- Altered parenting, actual
- Risk for altered parent–infant attachment
- Parental role conflict
- Anticipatory grieving
- Dysfunctional grieving
- Disturbances in role performance
- Social isolation
- Relocation stress syndrome
- Caregiver role strain
- High risk for caregiver role strain
- Impaired social interaction
- Impaired verbal communication
- Potential for violence

Additionally, you should develop skill at detecting and monitoring the following clinical problems:
- Physical abuse
- Communication problems associated with
  - Aphasia
  - Tracheostomy
  - Cancer of the larynx
- Agoraphobia
- Social isolation associated with age
- Caregiver strain
- Adolescent parenting
- Role strain

 Critical Thinking

You are an elementary school nurse. One of the teachers expresses concern for one of her students, Olivia. Last year Olivia's brother Markus was also in this teacher's class. The teacher states that both children were frequently late to class, often appeared tired, at times were poorly dressed, and often had bruises on their arms; Olivia has had some on her legs as well. The teacher does not know whether she is seeing signs of abuse and asks the nurse to make a home visit.

1. Explain to the mother why you are making a home visit.

2. What observations would you make during the home visit?

3. The mother denies abuse, but you note bruises of various levels of healing on her arms and legs also. The infant and toddler at home do not have any obvious injuries, but all three are not dressed warmly enough for the climate, and the house is cold. What would you do next?

4. Discuss how you would include the entire family in the assessment of potential abuse. Are there any others outside of the family you would talk with to gather additional information?

5. If you strongly suspect abuse, what are your legal obligations?

BIBLIOGRAPHY

Biddle, B., & Thomas, E. (1979). *Role theory: Concepts and research.* New York: John Wiley & Sons.

Butcher, L., & Gafney, M. (1995). Building health families: A program for single mothers. *Clinical Nurse Specialist, 9,* 221–226.

Carpenito, L. (1997). *Handbook of nursing diagnosis* (7th ed.). Philadelphia: Lippincott.

Deutsch, M., & Krauss, R. (1965). *Theories in social psychology.* New York: Basic Books.

Duvall, E. (1977). *Marriage and family development* (5th ed.). Philadelphia: Lippincott.

Edelman, C., & Mandle, C. (1998). *Health promotion throughout the lifespan* (4th ed.). St. Louis: Mosby.

Friedman, M. (1994). *Family nursing: Theory and practice* (3rd ed.). Norwalk, CT: Appleton & Lange.

Gilliss, C., Highley, B., Roberts, B., & Martinson, I. (1989). *Toward a science of family nursing.* Menlo Park, CA: Addison Wesley.

Gordon, M. (1994). *Nursing diagnosis: Process and application* (3rd ed.). St. Louis: Mosby.

Hardy, M., & Conway, M. (1988). *Role theory: Perspectives for health professionals* (2nd ed.). Norwalk, CT: Appleton-Century-Crofts.

Lancaster, J. (1982). Communication as a tool for change. In J. Lancaster & W. Lancaster (Eds.). *Concepts for advanced nursing practice: The nurse as a change agent* (pp. 109–131). St. Louis: Mosby.

Levitt, M. (1982). *Families at risk: Primary prevention in nursing practice.* Boston: Little, Brown.

Murray, R., & Zentner, J. (1997). *Health assessment and promotion strategies through the life span* (6th ed.). Stamford, CT: Appleton & Lange.

North American Nursing Diagnosis Association. (1996). *Nursing diagnoses: Definitions and classification (1997–1998).* Philadelphia: NANDA.

Nye, F., & Gegas, V. (1976). The role concept: Review and delineation. In F. Nye (Ed.). *Role structure and analysis of the family* (Vol. 24). Beverly Hills, CA: Sage.

Pender, N. (1996). *Health promotion in nursing practice* (3rd ed.). Stamford, CT: Appleton & Lange.

Phipps, L. (1980). Theoretical frameworks applicable to family care. In J. Miller & E. Janoski (Eds.). *Family-focused care.* New York: McGraw-Hill.

Rosow, I. (1965). Forms and functions of adult socialization. *Social Forces, 44*(1), 35–40.

Spradley, B. (1990). *Community health nursing: Concepts and practice* (3rd ed.). Glennview, IL: Scott Foresman/Little, Brown.

Stanhope, M., & Lancaster, J. (1996). *Community health nursing: Process and practice for promoting health* (4th ed.). St. Louis: Mosby.

Wright, L., & Leahey, M. (1994). *Nurses and families: A guide to family assessment and intervention* (2nd ed.). Philadelphia: F.A. Davis.

Yura, H., & Walsh, M. (1978). *The nursing process* (3rd ed.). New York: Appleton-Century-Crofts.

Assessing Sexuality and Reproductive Patterns

ASSESSMENT GUIDELINES

- Sexuality and Reproduction: Interview (Health History)

- Sexuality and Reproduction: Physical Assessment

- Female Genitalia: Physical Assessment

- Breasts: Physical Assessment

- Physical Examination of Fundal Height, Fetal Heart, and Fetal Lie

- Male Genitalia: Physical Assessment

CHAPTER ORGANIZATION

Introductory Overview
- Assessment Focus
- Data Collection Methods
- Nursing Diagnoses

Knowledge Base for Assessment
- Sexuality
- Sexual Health
- Gender Identity
- Sexual Response Patterns
- Health Status Effect on Sexuality
- Discussing Sexuality

The Female
- Female Genitals and Pelvic Structure

Breasts and Axillae
- Anatomy and Physiology Overview

Physical Changes During Pregnancy
- Anatomy and Physiology Overview
- Physical Changes During Pregnancy

The Male
- Genitalia and Inguinal Area
- Assessment and Documentation Focus

Human sexuality, a complex phenomenon that involves physical, psychological, cultural, and social aspects, is the behavioral presentation of sexual identity. It is influenced by lifelong attitudes and reflects individual perceptions of that identity. Although reproductive development and function are determined at conception, reproductive patterns are influenced by the individual's perception of maleness and femaleness and by social and cultural norms.

Until recently, an individual's sexual and reproductive functions were not routinely assessed or considered essential components of a complete health history. Sexual assessment continues to be the function most frequently omitted from the health history. Such an omission is alarming because many illnesses, surgical procedures, physiologic aging processes, and medications affect sexual function and satisfaction.

Unfortunately, certain taboos against discussing sexuality have pervaded the Western healthcare fields. In the 1960s, Masters and Johnson's studies, which promoted an understanding of normal sexual responses in men and women, were initially rejected by publishers of obstetric and gynecology journals. Eventually, these studies were published in the *Western Journal of Surgery*.

The work of Masters and Johnson encouraged health professionals to assess their clients' sexuality and, when indicated, to initiate sexual counseling. Additional factors that opened the subject to discussion include social forces such as the women's movement, the availability of reproductive control and abortion, and the prominence of sexually transmitted diseases (STD), including human immunodeficiency virus (HIV) disease (acquired immune deficiency syndrome [AIDS]).

Sexual and reproductive functions are evaluated during health assessment to assist individuals to express sexual or reproductive concerns, identify teaching needs, identify problems that need to be treated, and monitor normal development of reproductive structures and functions from birth to senescence.

ASSESSMENT FOCUS

Although human sexuality is now considered a legitimate focus of nursing practice, many nurses have not received the education required for effective sexual counseling. Logically, health assessment should be guided by actual or potential problems identified. However, because registered nurses without graduate education or other specialized training are not qualified to offer sexual counseling, the appropriateness of nurses assessing sexual behaviors is often questioned. Nevertheless, nurses are qualified to perform screening assessments and refer when the problem identified is beyond the nurse's scope of practice.

One approach to assessing sexual and reproductive functions is offered by the PLISSIT sexual health model, which was developed by psychologist Jack Annon (1976). The PLISSIT model establishes guidelines for assessment and interventions that nurses with different levels of educational preparation are qualified to perform. The model establishes a scale of complexity for sexual problems, indicates the treatment suitable for each level of complexity, and indicates who is qualified to offer treatment. PLISSIT is an acronym for four levels of therapeutic approach in dealing with sexual concerns of problems: permission,

limited information, specific suggestions, and intensive therapy (Table 13-1). All professional nurses should have the educational foundation to assess sexual function to intervene at the first level of approach, giving permission to discuss sexual concerns and offering limited information. Therapeutic interventions involve providing specific factual information to deal with sexual problems. For example, the individual may express uncertainty or may reveal misconception arising from myths about sexual matters or ask about a new medication available for impotence. The individual may express fears and uncertainties about suitable sexual behavior after illness or surgery, such as a myocardial infarction or a hysterectomy. A preadolescent girl may need information about menstruation and physical development, and an adolescent boy may need information about wet dreams. People with such concerns can benefit extensively from health teaching. More intensive assessment and therapy should be performed by advanced practitioners (see Table 13-1). However, all nurses should be able to identify individuals who need this level of intervention and make appropriate referrals.

Concerns and problems related to reproductive structure and function also should be assessed to detect signs or symptoms of specific clinical problems such as genital

TABLE 13.1   PLISSIT Sexual Health Model*

	Professional Preparation Required[†]	Levels of Assessment	Levels of Therapeutic Intervention
Level 1	Professional nurse	Takes health history: screens for sexual functions and dysfunctions	Provides limited sex education, including information about sexual feelings, behaviors, and myths Refers client to level 2 or 3 professional if necessary
Level 2	Professional nurse with postgraduate training in sex education and counseling	Takes sexual history	Provides sex education and counseling, including specific informaiton about sex and sexuality; concise suggestions about sexual fears and adaptations to illness; and anticipatory guidance Refers client to level 3 professional if necessary
Level 3	Professional nurse, physician, pyschologist, or social worker who has received training as a sex therapist	Takes sexual problem history	Provides sex therapy: individual, group, or couple Refers client to level 4 professional if necessary
Level 4	Masters prepared psychiatric nurse clinician, physician, or social worker who specializes in sex therapy	Takes psychiatric and pyschosexual history	Eclectic approach: may provide intensive individual psychotherapy, sex therapy, or marital therapy

*Developed by Jack Annon, 1976.
[†]The more serious the client's sexual problem, the more advanced is the level of professional preparation required to treat the problem.
(Watts, R.J. [1979]. Dimensions of sexual health. *American Journal of Nursing*, 79(9), 1570)

infections, menstrual problems, physiologically related aging problems, or malignant processes involving reproductive organs. In these cases, appropriate referral for treatment should be made.

The assessment of sexual and reproductive function should focus on the following objectives:

- Identifying any immediate sexual concerns
- Evaluating the person's understanding of sexual and reproductive function
- Determining the stage of sexual development with associated and expected physical changes
- Identifying any sexual or reproductive problems

Data Collection Methods

Data collection is accomplished by the following methods:

1. Interview and Record Review
   Gender identification and role
   Lifestyle and protective practices
   Sexual satisfaction
   Sexual abuse
   Sexually transmitted diseases
   Family risk factors for cancer of breast and ovaries
   Reproductive history: Men and Women
2. Laboratory and X-ray Analysis
   Sexually transmitted diseases
   Cervical/uterine cancer
   Breast anomalies
   Pregnancy-related tests
   Infertility tests

   Pelvic ultrasound
   Prostate-specific antigen
3. Physical Examination
   Examination of genitalia: Male and female
   Examination of breasts
   Examination of inguinal area
   Physical signs and symptoms of normal and abnormal alterations of pregnancy
   Signs and symptoms of fetal distress

Nursing Diagnoses

Primary NANDA nursing diagnoses for the sexual and reproductive pattern are:

Sexual dysfunction
Altered sexual patterns
Breast-feeding: effective
Breast-feeding: ineffective
Breast-feeding: interrupted
Rape–trauma syndrome

Dysfunctions in sexual and reproductive function may be related to other health problems. Secondary nursing diagnoses related to sexual and reproductive function include the following:

Altered family process
Altered role performance
Body image disturbance
Incontinence
Ineffective family coping

Ineffective individual coping
High risk for infection
Spiritual distress
Altered nutrition: less than body requirements

KNOWLEDGE BASE FOR ASSESSMENT

Sexuality

Sexuality refers to a person's perceptions, thoughts, feelings, and behaviors related to sexual identity and sexual interaction with others. Expressions of sexuality are not limited to sexual intercourse or coitus but include the manner in which people project themselves as sexual beings, and the way they respond to others as sexual beings.

Expressions as a sexual being begin at birth or when parents discover the gender of a fetus. Moral, religious, social, cultural, and political forces influence how the individual behaves and how others behave toward the individual. Individuals develop their sexual identity throughout their life span as they adapt to physiologic changes of aging and social changes.

Adult sexuality has been broadly classified as procreative or nonprocreative. Procreative expressions of sexuality are associated with childbearing. In women, these expressions cease with menopause. Nonprocreative sexuality refers to behaviors involving sexual satisfaction that are noted in persons of all ages, regardless of whether they are involved in sexual relationships with others.

Sexual Health

The World Health Organization defines sexual health as follows:

> The integration of the somatic, emotional, intellectual and social aspects of sexual being in ways that enhance personality, communication, and love. Every person has a right to receive information and to consider accepting sexual relationships for pleasure as well as for procreation.

Sexual health is promoted when the individual has the ability to control sexual behavior and reproduction in harmony with personal and social values. There should be freedom from psychological factors such as fear, shame, and guilt that may inhibit sexual responses and sexual relationships. In addition, physiologic factors such as organic disease, deficiencies, and disorders should not interfere with sexual and reproductive functions.

Gender Identity

Gender and gender identity are two different concepts. Gender is traditionally assigned at birth and is based on external genitalia ("It's a boy"). Gender identity is a sense of being male or female; it usually develops in children between the ages of 2 and 3 years ("I'm a girl"). Although gender and gender identity are generally in harmony, it is not unheard of for some men and women to feel "trapped" in the wrong gender body. It is possible with surgical and hormonal intervention to change the external gender of an individual from male to female or female to male. However, it is not currently possible to change the genetic structure of an individual from one gender to the other.

Sex Role (Gender Role)

Roles involve a set of expectations about a person's position in life (see Chap. 12 for a more thorough discussion of roles). Sex roles, based on gender, are assigned at birth. Assigning maleness or femaleness establishes expectations for appropriate role behaviors. In the United States, for example, female babies are often dressed in pink and males are dressed in blue. Infant clothing for girls may be trimmed with flowers or laces, whereas clothing for boys is frequently adorned with athletic symbols such as footballs or with boats. Parents often choose names for newborns that are considered either boy or girl names. Because of these early attempts to establish a child's sex role on the basis of anatomy, sex roles are learned through socialization. Consequently, cultural norms, role models, personal values, sexual experiences, and other factors ultimately influence individual performance of the sex role.

During the 1960s, attention began to focus on the impact of negative influences associated with male and female roles in the United States. Stereotypical male behavior (masculine) expectations can be identified as aggressiveness, strength, dominance, endurance, toughness, and orientation to achievement. Conversely, stereotypical female behavior (feminine) can be identified as submissiveness, delicacy, passivity, sensitivity, and emotionalism (teary). Such stereotypes promoted myths about appropriate masculine and feminine behaviors, which may have a negative impact on both sexual and physical well-being.

Forrester (1986) has suggested that sex role stereotypes are a contributing factor to higher mortality rates and lower life expectancies in men than in women. For example, cardiovascular disease may be linked to type "A" behavior, which is described as aggressive and competitive. Also, because men have been told during most of their developing years not to cry and to "act like a man," they may be more likely to ignore signs and symptoms of health problems and delay preventive or palliative health care. Traditionally, men receive less health care than women during their adult years, even when differences in life expectancy are considered. Similarly, sex role stereotypes have had a negative impact on women. For example, the "super-mom" who attempts to do it all (i.e., have a career and family) is placed under undue stress when attempting to perform *all* of her wife–mother sex role along with her career role. Also, women who have experienced menopause are often viewed (even by women themselves) as having lost their feminine appeal; as a result, middle-aged women are at higher risk for depressive disorders and low self-esteem.

In the last 30 years, sex role expectations have been changing and have been open to negotiation. Men are beginning to be more active in traditional female roles such as nurturing and caregiving of small children. Women are also beginning to be more represented in traditional male roles such as corporate executive and politician. This blending of sex role behavior (androgynous role—expression of both masculine and feminine characteristics) is becoming more common and is becoming synonymous with health. Sex roles, even if changing, vary among people and may have a profound impact on sexuality and overall health.

Sexual Response Patterns

An understanding of normal sexual responses assists with identifying misconceptions and the need for information about sexual matters. For example, elderly men often believe that impotence accompanies the aging process. This myth is based on the misconception that certain physiologic changes associated with aging prevent sexual activities. The changes that occur may alter sexual response but do not lead to impotence. Many adolescents incorrectly believe that women do not ovulate for the first few years after menarche. This belief could result in an undesired pregnancy. Because sexual myths may cause unnecessary anxiety or unsafe sexual practices, identification and discussion of such myths should occur when assessing a person's sexual functions and beliefs.

The Sexual Response Cycle

The sexual response cycle reflects an interaction between sexual function, sexual identity, and sexual relationships. Masters and Johnson's (1970) ground-breaking studies during the 1960s showed that response to sexual arousal was related to genital changes, extragenital changes, and subjective or feeling states. Four phases of sexual response were identified: excitement, plateau, orgasm, and resolution. Normal variations were noted between men and women as well as among persons of the same gender. For example, some women experience multiple orgasms after sexual arousal, and others do not reach orgasm at all.

Excitement. Sexual response is characterized by two main physiologic changes that begin during the excitement phase: vasocongestion and myotonia. Vasocongestion, the primary response to sexual stimulation, results from localized pooling of venous blood, occurs in response to erotic stimuli, and is influenced by steroid sex hormones. In men, penile erection and increased scrotal size are attributed to vasocongestion. Vasocongestion in women includes enlargement of the clitoris, elongation of the clitoral shaft, and vaginal lubrication. Vaginal lubrication is the result of fluid transudating across vaginal mucous membranes. Bartholin's glands secrete no lubrication during the excitement phase.

Myotonia involves an increase in muscular tension resulting in involuntary muscle contractions that occur throughout the body. In men, the testes elevate in response to contraction of the cremaster muscle and retraction of the spermatic cord. In women, irregular contractions of the vaginal vault occur, increasing the vaginal vault in width and length. The uterus may rise in response to muscle contractions in the surrounding tissues. Extragenital myotonic responses of both genders include nipple erection, tension of the long muscles of the arms and legs, and involuntary contraction of the abdominal and intercostal muscles.

The excitement phase may last from minutes to hours. Erotic stimuli may be psychic or sensory. For example, reading erotic literature, rubbing lotion on the body, smelling a particular fragrance, fantasizing, dreams, or giving verbal messages are stimuli capable of causing excitement. Interpretation of erotic stimuli varies greatly among people. For instance, some people may be socially conditioned to find certain stimuli offensive rather than erotic.

The excitement phase may be interrupted by distracting stimuli such as a baby crying or the telephone ringing. Psychic stimuli, such as guilt feelings, anxiety, or stress, also may interrupt this phase. For men, distracting stimuli may cause loss of erection. The person may become anxious about sexual performance during the excitement phase, especially if he or she does not understand the effects of distracting stimuli on normal sexual function.

Plateau. The plateau phase follows excitement and is characterized by an increase in sexual tension as vasocongestion and myotonia intensify. A woman will experience increasing vasocongestion in the labia and lower vagina and retraction of the clitoris. The vagina continues to expand in length and width. Bartholin's glands may excrete lubricant to augment vaginal lubrication. The plateau phase does not always lead to orgasmic resolution. Many factors, including the amount of sexual stimulation and psychological factors such as stress, can affect the nature of the plateau response.

During the plateau phase, the penis increases in circumference at the coronal ridge. The testes also continue to enlarge and are fully elevated just before ejaculation. A small amount of mucoid lubricating fluid containing active spermatozoa may be secreted from Cowper's glands. Typically, the plateau phase lasts from 30 seconds to 3 minutes.

Extragenital responses occur in both sexes. Breast engorgement and marked nipple erection may occur. The skin may become flushed, a phenomenon sometimes referred to as "sex rash." Hyperventilation usually occurs toward the end of the plateau phase. Heart rates increase from 100 to 175 beats/min. The average heart rate increases up to 120 beats/min or more for relatively short periods of approximately 15 seconds. Systolic blood pressure may elevate 20 to 80 mm Hg, and diastolic pressure may increase by 10 to 40 mm Hg. Generally, men have higher blood pressure elevations during the plateau phase than women.

Orgasm. Orgasm involves the involuntary resolution of vasocongestion and muscle tension through a series of 5 to 12 muscle contractions. The contractions decrease in intensity and frequency during orgasm, which last from 3 to 15 seconds. Female orgasmic response is most intense in the area called the orgasmic platform, which includes the outer third of the vagina and labia minora. Male orgasmic contractions are felt most intensely along the penile urethra and help propel ejaculate. In men, the internal bladder sphincter is closed during ejaculation, preventing retrograde ejaculation into the bladder. Extragenital responses parallel those occurring during plateau. Heart and respiratory rates increase, blood pressure elevates, there is involuntary muscle contraction and skin flushing, and diaphoresis may occur.

Resolution. During the resolution phase, vasocongestion and myotonia dissipate entirely. If orgasm has not been achieved, the resolution phase will be longer. In women, genital organs gradually return to their normal positions, swelling subsides, and skin color returns to preexcitement tones. In men, genital organs return to their preexcitement size. Heart and respiration rates and blood pressure return to baseline levels. The length of the refractory period varies, usually between 10 and 30 minutes.

Influencing Factors

Sexual response is an integrated biologic function involving the entire body, sexual identity, and sexual relationship. Anything affecting any one component can influence the sexual response cycle. Fear and pain are strong antagonists of sexual desire. Other factors, such as illness, medications, environmental changes, and emotional stimuli, can influence the sexual response cycle. If sexual desire is not perceived as appropriate or other behaviors are seen as more important, it is possible to diminish sexual response urges.

Health Status Effect on Sexuality

Intercourse is a physical activity. Individuals with health alterations such as cardiovascular, respiratory, and musculoskeletal impairments may have difficulty engaging in intercourse. People with recent myocardial infarctions or their spouses may fear that sexual activity could be deadly. Individuals who easily fatigue or who have shortness of breath or problems such as rheumatoid arthritis may have difficulty with sexual satisfaction. Education regarding risks and alternative coital positions could be helpful to these individuals and their sexual partners.

Emotional concerns also impact people's sexuality concerns. For example, individuals with new abdominal ostomies may fear leakage during sexual contact and avoid coitus. Paraplegics and quadriplegics may fear loss of sexual ability and sexuality self-identity changes. Additionally, an individual with disfiguring injuries or surgeries may experience a change in sexual identity and fear being sexually repulsive to his or her mate. Education and counseling can assist these individuals and their partners to have active sexual lives.

Discussing Sexuality

Certain attitudes or assumptions on the part of the nurse can act as barriers to obtaining adequate data and establishing a therapeutic relationship. These barriers should be overcome to ensure accurate collection of relevant data. It is important not to allow personal prejudices or aversions to develop toward the individual or to inject the nurse's values, morals, or beliefs into the discussion. Also, the nurse should not assume that sexuality or sexual matters are not important to the individual or that certain sexual behaviors are practiced or preferred. For instance, do not assume on the basis of appearance or stereotypes that a person is monogamous, homosexual, or asexual. Waterhouse and Metcalfe (1991) found that the overwhelming majority of individuals (regardless of gender, age, educational level, and marital status) reported that nurses should discuss sexual concerns with clients.

Being sure of your own knowledge of sexual matters and making every effort to understand the views, perceptions, and language of the person will help open communication and will convey a professional attitude about the importance of sexual function in health promotion. Questions about sexuality should be incorporated into the initial interview. Frequently, this aspect of assessment is postponed until a sense of rapport exists between the individual and the interviewer. Many people need time to develop a trusting relationship with a nurse before they are comfortable discussing personal matters. However, including questions about sexuality in the initial interview conveys the message that sexuality is a natural part of life and has health implications in the same way that nutrition, elimination, and activity do. Introducing the subject early in the assessment process also gives the person permission to discuss any sexual concern or problems.

Introductory questions may encourage further discussion; however, the person may have no perceived sexual concerns to discuss or may be reluctant to continue the discussion because of embarrassment or discomfort. Whatever the response, it is wise to accept it and to invite further questions at a time when the individual feels more comfortable about discussing such matters.

Privacy and Confidentiality

One reason people are reluctant to discuss sexual matters is the fear that their conversation will be overheard or divulged to others. To ensure privacy in the hospital setting, the interview should be conducted where other people, including roommates, will not overhear the conversation. Waiting until others have left the room or using a private conference room can avoid the possibility of embarrassment. The discussion should be initiated without family or sexual partners present. With the person's permission, the family or partners may be included during subsequent discussions or teaching sessions.

The interview on this subject should be conducted by one care provider rather than several. Asking a person to discuss intimate subjects repeatedly may cause anxiety, embarrassment, or guilt and is unnecessary. Ideally, one person should interview the individual and share pertinent information with other care providers. Based on the person's response to initial sexuality screening questions, a decision should be made about who should initiate an in-depth interview if indicated. For example, if the person states that impotence is a problem with his spouse but not with other partners, a referral may be made to a sex therapist.

If notes are recorded during the interview, the person may become concerned about confidentiality. Such concerns can be alleviated by stating at the beginning that parts of the interview are to be entered on the record and the reason for doing so. Requesting permission is also appropriate and may be phrased as follows: "It would be helpful to record some of your concerns in your health record. Is that okay with you?" If a referral seems in order, the nurse might state, "A specialist in this clinic may be most helpful in answering some of your specific concerns about sexual relations. May I put some of our conversation in your record so that he or she can follow through?" Be careful to document only data necessary for ensuring continuity of care, ensuring the person's privacy.

Structure

Extensive guidelines and interview questions have been developed for obtaining and recording a sexual history. Usually, specialized professionals such as sex therapists will use a more structured, lengthy approach. For the initial assessment and screening interview, questions about sexual matters should be kept to a minimum. The purpose of the screening interview is to identify any specific sexual concerns or problems and to determine whether the individual needs further information or referrals.

The need for more extensive questioning may be indicated by the presence of specific sexually related problems. For example, if the nurse is interviewing someone seeking treatment for a sexually transmitted disease (STD), it is essential to ask specific questions about his or her sexual partners and knowledge of disease transmission and prevention.

Facilitating Communication

When asking about sexuality, phrase questions in a nonthreatening manner so as not to stir guilty feelings or resentment. The nurse should preface certain questions in a specific way to indicate that the behavior is normal. Consider the following examples:

"Many people find masturbation a way to . . ."
"Many people feel uncomfortable discussing sexual problems . . ."

"It is not unusual to feel unsure about resuming sexual relations . . ."
"In Kinsey's study over half of the men had at least one homosexual experience . . ."

Generally, questions that require a yes or no answer should be avoided. For example, "Are there any concerns about your sex life?" may elicit less information than a more open-ended question such as "Can you tell me how the accident has affected your sexual relations?"

Choosing Appropriate Terminology

Derogatory or judgmental terms should be avoided during the interview. Using terms such as *promiscuous, unfaithful,* or *inadequate* may convey a judgmental attitude and block further discussion. Using words such as *wife, husband,* or *girlfriend* also may reflect incorrect assumptions. Using more general terms such as *sexual partner* or *mate* will help the nurse maintain a more neutral approach.

Technical terms such as *erection* or *orgasm* may sound intimidating or may not be understood. Conversely, slang terminology may be offensive or embarrassing. Finding a common ground for understanding or describing sexual activity will allow for a more natural flow of information. It is essential that the terms be clarified and understood. For example. a woman may state that her "bottom" feels itchy after sexual intercourse. Does *bottom* refer to rectum, vagina, or labia? A person may use slang to describe sexual practice. If the meaning is not clear to you, take a matter-of-fact approach, such as asking the person to explain the terms.

Even legitimate-sounding terms may need to be defined. For example, if a man reports that he is "impotent," it is important to determine whether this means that he is unable to obtain an erection or that he has a problem only with certain partners or in certain circumstances. Perhaps he is referring to something totally different, such as infertility.

Children require a different approach because they use a special vocabulary to refer to sexual matters or genitalia. If a 5-year-old boy refers to his penis as "pee-pee," then the nurse should use this term with him to ensure understanding. If necessary, the child's parents can help clarify and identify such terms.

Physical Examination   Sexuality and Reproductive Pattern

GENERAL PRINCIPLES   The nurse should avoid injecting his or her own values, morals, or aversions into discussions about sexual behaviors and beliefs.

Open communication will convey a professional attitude about the importance of sexual function in health promotion.

People may fear divulging information because of concerns about confidentiality.

Asking a person to discuss intimate issues can cause anxiety.

Phrase questions in a nonthreatening manner.

(continued)

Physical Examination   Sexuality and Reproductive Pattern (continued)

The individual may be embarrassed about exposing himself or herself or about the discovery of an infection. The nurse should explain in detail what will be done throughout the assessment and the reason for each segment of the assessment.

Genital structures and breasts are examined by inspection and palpation.

With any unexpected finding, such as a rash or lump, identify when it was first noted, whether it changes (especially with the menstrual cycle), whether it has gotten worse or better, and what has been done to treat the problem.

Individuals may feel more comfortable if a nurse of the same gender performs the examination.

If a male client has an erection during the assessment, reassure him that this is a normal response to genital palpation.

Nurses need to work through their own feelings and not convey anxiety or embarrassment to the client.

COMPREHENSIVE REPRODUCTIVE ASSESSMENT

A comprehensive assessment includes the following components:
Interview
Assessment for STDs
Laboratory analysis
Physical assessment

EQUIPMENT

No equipment is needed to assess sexuality; however, equipment is needed for male and female genitalia assessment and is noted in those sections later in the chapter.

ASSESSMENT AIDS

Interview guide to suggest questions and record data (Display 13-1)

DISPLAY 13.1

Interview Guide: Sexuality and Reproductive Patterns

A structured interview guide may be used to facilitate data collection. The headings correlate with major interview areas discussed in the text. Items may be deleted if deemed inappropriate for age or situation. Items also should be adapted to correlate with developmental age and sexual activity of the individual. Items also may be added to get a full explanation of problems. If a problem is identified, ask when it started, whether anything makes it better or worse, pattern of occurrence (this is important for some hormone cyclical–influenced problems), and what the person is currently doing for the problem.

SEX ROLES AND GENDER IDENTIFICATION

Gender _____
Sexual lifestyle (preference and activity)_____
Has any health problem interfered with your ability in your role as wife/husband, mother/father? _____
_____

What does this surgery/illness/condition mean to you as a woman/man?_____
_____

What questions do you have regarding your sex role or activity? _____
_____

KNOWLEDGE ABOUT SEXUALITY AND REPRODUCTION

Do you have any questions about reproduction or sexuality? _____
What would you like to know more about regarding reproduction and sexuality? _____

(continued)

Interview Guide: Sexuality and Reproductive Patterns *(continued)*

People sometimes experience changes in sexual function with (name of illness/disability/injury); have you received any information about this? _____ What concerns do you have about this? _____
People sometimes have questions about how their illness/condition/injury will affect sexual aspects of their lives; what type of concerns do you have? _____

SEXUAL PERFORMANCE AND SATISFACTION

Are your sexual relationships satisfying to you? _____
Has anything changed that interferes with your ability to achieve satisfying relationships? _____
What concerns do you have about your sexual performance? _____

SEXUAL ABUSE

Have you ever been abused as an adult or child? _____

SEXUALLY TRANSMITTED DISEASES

What do you use for protection against sexually transmitted diseases and HIV? _____
Have you ever had a sexually transmitted disease (for those at risk)? _____

FAMILY HISTORY OF REPRODUCTIVE CANCER

Before menopause, has your mother or any close relative had breast, ovarian, or uterine cancer? _____
Is there any history of ovarian or prostate cancer in your family? _____
Do you know if your mother took DES to prevent miscarriage? _____

REPRODUCTIVE HISTORY

Males and Females

How many children do you have? _____ How many would you like? _____
Are you or your sexual partner currently using any form of birth control (type)? _____
Do you experience any pain or discomfort during intercourse? _____

Males Only

Have you ever had any surgery to your penis or scrotum, or hernia repair? _____
Do you have problems urinating (prostate problems)? _____
How often do you perform testicular self-examination? _____

Females Only

Age at menarche _____
Menstrual pattern: interval between menses _____; duration of menses _____; amount of flow _____; last menses _____
Associated discomforts: cramps _____; tension _____; pain _____; bloating/swelling _____
Premenstrual symptoms _____ Identify _____
Pregnancy: number _____; number of live births _____; number of stillborns _____; number of abortions/miscarriages _____; number of living children _____
Any pregnancy or delivery complications? _____
Any surgeries to cervix, ovaries, uterus? _____
Last Pap smear _____; results _____
Last mammogram _____; results _____
Do you perform a breast self-examination? _____ How frequently? _____
Do you have any questions about your ability to find lumps? _____
Detection of lumps: Location _____; size _____ Does size change with menstrual cycle? _____
When found _____; any breast surgery? _____
Menopause onset _____ Any symptoms such as dry vagina? _____
Hot flashes? _____ Mood swings? _____
Describe—pattern, trigger, degree of lifestyle disruption _____

▼ ▼ ▼
GUIDELINES

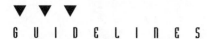 Sexuality and Reproduction: Interview (Health History)

Procedure

1. Gender identification and role

Inquire into feelings and beliefs about sexuality and gender-related roles.

- Tell me your beliefs about yourself and sexuality.
- Has any health problem interfered with your ability in your role as wife/husband or mother/father?

When appropriate, the following approaches may be helpful when interviewing the person about usual sex roles and role transitions caused by events such as hospitalization, illness, or normal growth and development:

- What does this surgery (illness, disability) mean to you as a woman (or man)?
- How do you think this pregnancy will change your life or your feelings about yourself or family?
- How do you think this illness (surgery) will alter your sexual functioning after you leave the hospital?
- How do you expect your ability to function as a wife (husband, lover, mother, father) will change?

2. Knowledge about sexuality and reproduction

Current knowledge and understanding, language used, and myths can alert the nurse to learning needs of the individual. The following questions can elicit this information:

- Do you have any questions about sexuality or reproduction?
- What would you like to know more about regarding sexuality?
- What concerns do you have about your knowledge of sex?
- People sometimes experience changes in sexual function as a result of conditions like yours. Have you received information about this? What concerns do you have?
- People sometimes have questions about whether their illness will affect the sexual aspects of their lives; what type of concerns do you have?

3. Sexual performance and satisfaction

Determining sexual behavior and satisfaction with activity alerts the nurse to possible risk factors and health care needs of the individual. Information can be obtained by asking questions such as:

Clinical Significance

Understanding the manner in which a person perceives his or her sex role contributes to a broader understanding of the person. For example, a married woman may perceive her sex role in terms of being a wife and mother. She may see herself as providing guidance and help to their children and giving and receiving emotional support and sexual companionship from her husband.

Both sexes may feel threatened by relationship transitions, such as pregnancy, marriage, or the loss of a lover through divorce, separation, or death. Because of stereotyped sex roles that emphasize invulnerability and strength, many men feel less masculine after life-threatening illnesses such as a myocardial infarction. Any illness or surgery involving reproductive organs, such as a vasectomy, hysterectomy, or prostate surgery, may threaten sex roles. Finally, changes in body image after hair loss, mastectomy, ostomy surgery, amputation, or other disfigurements or disabilities may cause concern or conflict about sex roles and function, not only for the individual but also for his or her partner.

Inadequate knowledge may contribute to sexual dysfunction; genital disease, including STDs; HIV disease; unwanted pregnancy; or anxiety about sexual functioning.

Certain illnesses and physiologic alterations, such as cancer, ostomies, cardiovascular disease, diabetes mellitus, spinal cord injury, and multiple sclerosis, have sexual ramifications that necessitate patient teaching. The types of sexual problems and teaching needs associated with these disorders are presented in Table 13–2. Each person has unique needs and should be encouraged to express such needs. If additional information is needed, consultation with a specialist may be indicated.

Multiple sexual partners can place the individual at risk for STDs and HIV; women are at increased risk for cervical cancer.

TABLE 13.2 Physiologic Alterations, Sexual Function, and Teaching Needs

Sexual Activity Problems	Teaching Needs
Cancer and associated treatment (surgery, radiation, chemotherapy)	
Decreased physical energy	Fatigue and debilitation commonly alter libido and forms of sexual expression
Fears about touching and causing harm	Alternative coital positions to avoid physical contact with painful surgical or radiation sites.
Fear of inducing bleeding if thrombocytopenic	Alternative forms of sexual expression.
Fear of infection if immunosuppressed	Good oral and perineal hygiene; "safe sex" practices.
	Avoid anal intercourse, which is associated with greater risk of abscess formation.
Body image disturbance	Depression is a common reaction to changes in body image and may alter libido.
	Full impact of mutilating surgery on body image may not be felt for 2 or 3 months.
Oral mucosa ulceration after chemotherapy or radiation	Avoid oral contact.
Anger	Anger secondary to cancer diagnosis may be directed toward healthy sexual partner.
Ostomy	
Concerns about stoma leakage, odors, and possible stoma damage during sexual activity	Empty stoma before sexual activity.
	Dietary means to control stoma discharge and odors.
	Sexual activity will not harm stoma.
Body image disturbance related to stoma	Open communication with sexual partner is important.
	Stoma can be covered during sexual activity.
Decreased physical energy and libido after ostomy surgery	May affect potency; may take several months after surgery to regain strength and functional abilities; alternate sexual positions may conserve energy.
Cardiovascular disorders	
Fear of additional cardiac damage	Resumption of sexual activity usually safe 5 to 8 weeks after MI (patient should consult physician).
	Symptoms indicating adverse cardiac response to intercourse: rapid heart and respiratory rates persisting 10 minutes after orgasm, or extreme fatigue the following day are indications to consult physician.
	Avoid intercourse immediately after large meals, excessive alcohol intake, in hot or humid weather, when extremely anxious or tired, or with unfamiliar partners.
Partner's fear of causing the other harm	A common response; open discussion of fears important.
Depression	Depression is a common postMI response that may persist for several months; may adversely affect libido.
Spinal cord injury/multiple sclerosis	
Paralysis and weakness, making sexual activity difficult and certain coital positions impossible	Alternate forms of sexual expression and alternate coital positions.
Inability to achieve or maintain an erection	Patients with upper motor neuron involvement have high percentage of reflexogenic erections (physically stimulated erections); psychogenic erections (stimulated by thought or emotion) are rare.
	Patients with lower motor neuron involvement have higher incidence of psychogenic erections and lower incidence of reflexogenic erections.
	Erectile ability after spinal cord injury is highly variable.
Loss of pelvic sensation (men and women)	Sexual enjoyment is often decreased; loss of sensation and pelvic vasocongestion may cause lack of orgasm.

(continued)

TABLE 13.2 Physiologic Alterations, Sexual Function, and Teaching Needs [continued]

Sexual Activity Problems	Teaching Needs
Spinal cord injury/multiple sclerosis (continued)	
Concerns about involuntary bowel or bladder emptying during sexual activity	Empty bowel or bladder before sexual activity; indwelling catheters may be removed before sexual activity or left in place (men can fold and tape catheter back along penis and wear a condom; women can tape catheter to one side.) Good hygiene is important to reduce transmission of chronic urinary tract infections.
Diabetes mellitus	
Males: erectile dysfunction	Affects 50% males, 33% females
Females: orgasmic dysfunction	Sexual desire usually remains constant. Increased foreplay may be helpful.
Frequent vaginitis interferes with sexual activity	Avoid pantyhose, wear cotton underwear, monitor vaginal pH; a water-soluble lubricant useful if dyspareunia present
Concerns about having children: fear of pregnancy for diabetic women related to higher still birth and risk of neonate health problems; for diabetic father, concerns about fertility—reduced sperm count and volume; and concerns of either parent for genetic transmission.	Adequate diabetic control and physician supervision should decrease risk of stillbirth and health problems. Genetic counseling may be helpful. Having intercourse on day of ovulation and abstaining before ovulation may increase chance of fertilization.

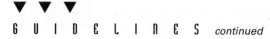

GUIDELINES *continued*

Sexuality and Reproduction: Interview (Health History)

Procedure

- Describe your current sexual activity.
- How satisfied are you with your sexual relations?
- Do you have any concerns about your sexual performance?
- Has anything changed that interferes with your sexual performance?

Questions about medications should be posed in a manner that will not suggest a problem where one does not exist. For example, it is not wise to say, "Most men become impotent from this drug. Has this happened to you yet?" Rather, the question can be rephrased to allow for a more extensive response: "Some people, taking similar medications, experience changes in sexual function. What concerns do you have about this?"

Clinical Significance

Sexual dysfunction often can be attributed to problems or dissatisfaction with sexual performance, which in turn may affect or be affected by other problems. For example, fatigue, anxiety, and depression can interfere with sexual performance or even sexual desire and should be discussed. The perception of poor sexual function may also reinforce a low self-concept ("I can't do anything right").

Medications and normal, healthy aging can also contribute to alterations in sexual performance (Display 13–2).

DISPLAY 13.2

Medication and Sexual Function

ALCOHOL

May release inhibitions and promote relaxation. May interfere with sexual function because it may act as central nervous system depressant, suppress motor activity, and induce diuresis.

AMYL NITRATE

Questionable effect on sexual function. May potentiate intensity of orgasm by genitourinary tract vasodilation and smooth muscle relaxation.

ANTIDEPRESSANTS

(amitriptyline, desipramine, imipramine, nortriptyline, pargyline, phenelzine sulfate, protriptyline)
May interfere with sexual performance and libido because of central nervous system depression and peripheral blockade of nerve innervation of sex glands/organs.

ANTIHISTAMINES

(chlorpheniramine, diphenhydramine, promethazine)
May have negative effect on sexual function due to blockade of parasympathetic innervation of sexual glands or organs.

ANTIHYPERTENSIVES

(clonidine, methyldopa, beta-blockers, reserpine, trimethaphan)
May impair sexual performance by peripheral blockade of nerves involved in sexual function.

ANTISPASMODICS

(glycopyrrolate methobromide, hexocyclium, methantheline, poldine)
May impair sexual performance by ganglionic blockade of nerves involved in sexual function.

BARBITURATES

May impair sexual function secondary to central nervous system depression, suppression of motor activity, and hypnosis.

CAFFEINE

Questionable effect on sexual function; acts as central nervous system stimulant.

CANTHARIS [SPANISH FLY]

Considered an aphrodisiac by some although there is no basis for this claim; generally irritating and inflammatory to genitourinary tract mucosa; may result in systemic poisoning.

CIMETIDINE

Associated with reduced sperm counts (though still within the normal range), gynecomastia, and loss of libido or impotence (rare).

DIURETICS

May interfere with sexual activity secondary to diuresis.

LITHIUM CARBONATE

Specific effects questionable; may interfere with sexual function secondary to broad endocrine alterations and diuresis.

NARCOTICS AND PSYCHOACTIVE DRUGS

(amphetamines, cocaine, heroin, LSD, marijuana, methadone, morphine)
May transiently enhance sexual function by releasing inhibitions, increasing suggestability, and promoting relaxation. May interfere with sexual function secondary to central nervous system depression, loss of libido, and impotence.

SEDATIVES AND TRANQUILIZERS

(chlordiazepoxide, chlorpromazine, diazepam, methaqualone, prochlorperazine, thioridazine)
May promote sexual function by relaxation. May interfere with sexual function secondary to central nervous system depression, blockade of autonomic innervation of sex glands or organs, suppression of hypothalamic and pituitary function.

VITAMIN E

Questionable effects—promotes fertility in laboratory animals.

▼ ▼ ▼

GUIDELINES *continued*   Sexuality and Reproduction:
Interview (Health History)

Procedure	Clinical Significance
4. Sexual abuse Sexual abuse is a very sensitive topic and may not be discussed or reported by the individual. The nurse may ask questions such as: • Have you been abused as a child or adult?	If abuse is suspected, an in-depth interview and possible examination (if recent) needs to be performed by an experienced professional. Signs of sexual abuse include • Depression/withdrawal • Poor self-image • Vague physical complaints • Substance abuse • Suicidal tendencies • Post-traumatic stress syndrome • Sexual promiscuity • Flashbacks For a more in-depth discussion of sexual abuse, see Display 13–3.
5. Sexually transmitted diseases With individuals who have more than one sexual partner, determine how the individual protects him- or herself from STDs by asking: • What do you use for protection against sexually transmitted diseases and HIV? With individuals at risk, inquire into history of STDs.	Protection during intercourse and foreplay can provide some protection from these diseases if used appropriately. Contraceptive methods other than condoms and spermicides do not provide protection from STDs. Some STDs such as chlamydia and gonorrhea are responsible for infertility and pelvic inflammatory disease.

6. Family history of reproductive cancer
Inquire into the family history of the following conditions:
• Before menopause, has your mother or grandmothers had
  • Breast cancer
  • Ovarian cancer
• Did your mother take DES while pregnant with you to prevent miscarriage?
	Cancer of the breast and ovaries in first-degree relatives (mother, grandmother) increases the risk of breast and ovarian cancer two to three times (U.S. Preventive Services Task Force, 1996).
	
	The use of DES in women to prevent miscarriage has been associated with vaginal cancer in female and reduced fertility in male offspring.

7. Reproductive history Males: • Inquire into the number of children the individual has and method of family planning/birth control. • Inquire into the presence of endocrine disorders such as diabetes mellitus. • History of genital surgery • Frequency of testicular self-examination (TSE) • How frequently do you perform testicular self-examination? • Do you have any questions regarding what you detect?	There are a few methods of male birth control available; these include: • Condom • Coitus interruptus (withdrawal)—has high failure rate • Vasectomy Diabetes mellitus is a frequent factor in impotence. Types of genital surgery include vasectomy, correction of undescended testicles, testicular torsion, and testicular tumors. TSE should be performed monthly. Any lump should be referred to a specialist for evaluation of the possibility of testicular cancer.

DISPLAY 13.3

Interviewing Sexual Abuse or Assault Victims

Male and female victims of sexual abuse or assault often experience extensive psychological and emotional trauma. The expression of the psychological trauma may be delayed for years if sexual abuse occurred during early childhood. The interview should be directed at eliciting specific details for medical and legal purposes. In addition, specialized crisis intervention techniques should be used to support the victim's feelings and associated behaviors. Generally, nurses who interview sex crime victims have received special education and are frequently available through emergency departments on a 24-hour, emergency basis. Understanding the basic interviewing principles will help the nurse who has initial contact with such victims. In general, the following principles are applicable:

- The most qualified available staff member should conduct the interview.
- The number of people who interview the victim should be kept to a minimum.
- The interview should be conducted before the physical examination.
- A quiet, private setting free from interruptions should be selected for the interview.
- Time should be taken to establish rapport with the victim and explain the purpose of the interview.
- According to institutional policy, the nurse may have to ask about the following: characteristics and identity if known, of the assailant: type of assaultive activity that took place, including orifices that were penetrated; time and place of the assault: threats made by the assailant: significant others the victim wants contacted; immediate emotional needs of the victim; and extent of any injuries.

Because of lack of maturity and vulnerability, any sexual activity, with or without consent, between a minor child and an adult (or another child significantly older than the minor child) is considered sexual abuse. Minor children cannot legally provide consent because they cannot fully understand the consequences of their consent. Mentally retarded adults, depending on cognitive ability, may or may not be able to give consent and are vulnerable to sexual abuse and assault. Violence is rarely needed to force children into sexual acts because they can be easily coaxed, bribed, enticed, or intimidated. Usually a child is told that such acts are part of a special game that must be kept secret. A secrecy pact is often made through threats or coercion. The abuser may say, for example, "If you tell anyone, I won't love you any more," or "If you tell anyone, I'll kill your mother."

In such cases, effective interviewing skills are needed to obtain information from the victim, who has already been told not to talk and who may feel shame and guilt. Additionally, children do not have the adult vocabulary to describe the abuser's actions. However, one should be suspicious when a child is sexually precocious in speech, mannerism, and dress. Children may also be reluctant to discuss sexual abuse because the threat of being removed from the parents' care is greater than the threat of continued abuse. Special techniques such as drawing or playing with anatomically correct dolls may facilitate communication. Children and mentally retarded adults may find such approaches helpful and less threatening when describing abusive acts. Important principles to keep in mind when interviewing sexually abused children and lower-functioning mentally retarded adults include the following:

- Parents, other family members, or friends should not be present until it is certain that such persons are not the abuser. The parent's presence may heighten the child's feelings of guilt and shame.
- The parents and family members should be interviewed separately at the same time the child is interviewed. Parents need an opportunity to ventilate feelings and receive emotional support.
- Use sexual language comprehensible to the child's language development, preferably their own terms.
- Asking a child to draw pictures may be less threatening than asking him or her to describe incidents of sexual abuse. Encourage the child to draw himself or herself, the offender, and what happened, and to describe their drawings.
- Anatomically correct dolls may be used to encourage the child to describe the assault or assaults.

Victims of sexual assault, both males and females, may experience delayed reactions to the incident. Female adult incest survivors often seek professional help as adults because of relationship problems, depression, and substance abuse. Sexual assault victims may have problems with somatic symptoms and psychological and sexual functioning. Victims often report an absence or reduction of sexual feelings and desires after an attack. Other common emotional reactions include anger, fear, guilt, helplessness, feeling "dirty," numbness, and not wanting to be alone. Some individuals may react through hostile behavior to others. In some cases, either peer or professional counseling is indicated.

The primary responsibility of the nurse is to identify manifestations of Rape trauma syndrome and to make appropriate referrals. It is also important to be aware that trauma from sexual assault can be a long-standing phenomenon that persists for months or years after the assault. The victim also may have a short-term fear of pregnancy (pregnancy testing can be performed in less than 2 months after the assault) and the long-term fear of contracting HIV (AIDS) disease (an incubation period of several years). Equally important is the prompt, precise documentation of data; all of the victim's records as well as the professional staff are likely to be subpoenaed if there is a court case.

▼ ▼ ▼

Procedure

Females:
Inquire into menstrual history:
- Age of menarche
- Menstrual cycle, interval between cycles, duration of flow, amount and pattern of flow
- Last menstrual period
- Any associated discomfort
- Cramps
- Tension
- Pain
- Bloating/swelling
- Premenstrual syndrome (PMS)
- For women in their late 40s, inquire into signs and symptoms of menopause:
- Irregular menses
- Hot flashes
- Cessation of menses
- Mood swings
- Vaginal dryness

Inquire as to irregular bleeding such as vaginal bleeding between periods.

Inquire into pregnancy history:
- Number of live births
- Number of stillborn births
- Number of miscarriages/abortions
- Any pregnancy or delivery
- Complications
- Type of contraceptive

Inquire into history of any gynecologic surgeries.

Inquire into preventive health care:
- Date of last Pap smear and results
- Date of last mammogram and results
- Frequency of breast self-examination (BSE) and confidence in ability to detect abnormalities
- If lump present, collect the following data: location, size, when found, any changes with menstrual cycle

Clinical Significance

Menarche usually occurs between 11 and 16 years, with the average age of 12.5 years; a normal cycle is normally 22–34 days. Menstrual flow is usually 3–7 days.

Some cramping, headaches, and bloating are common complaints before and during menstruation. However, when symptoms interfere with daily function, this is typically diagnosed as PMS. Have the individual describe any symptom for frequency, when it begins, how long it lasts, what she does for relief, and how effective relief efforts are.

Menopause typically occurs between the ages of 35 and 58, with an average of 50 years.

Irregular bleeding may indicate several health problems, such as ovarian cysts, uterine fibroids, and uterine cancer.
This provides important baseline data and can alert the nurse to possible pregnancy if contraceptives are not being used and if medications are to be prescribed for other health problems.

Examples of gynecologic surgeries include:
- Tubal ligation
- Hysterectomy
- Laparosocopy
- Rectoecele and cystocele repairs

This provides baseline data and also indicates the need for health prevention teaching.

This information is important if the nurse is going to verify findings and make appropriate care decisions.

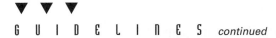

Sexuality and Reproduction:
Interview (Health History)

Procedure	Clinical Significance

Laboratory/X-Ray Evaluation

A complete sexuality and reproductive assessment includes consideration of laboratory values and x-rays. Not all tests are performed on all individuals—only those individuals at risk for diseases or specific conditions such as genetic disorders.

1. **Sexually transmitted diseases**
   - VDLR (Venereal Disease Research Laboratories)
   - Cultures

   - Wet mounts or slides

   - EIA (enzyme immunoassay) and Western blot

   - Syphilis (*Treponema pallidum*)
   - Gonorrhea (*Neisseria gonorrhoea*), chlamydia (*Chlamydia trachomatis*), vulvovaginitis (*Gardernerella vaginalis*)
   - Trichomoniasis (*Trichomonas vaginalis*), candidiasis (Moniliasis)
   - HIV (human immunodeficiency virus)

2. **Cervical/uterine cancer screening**
   - Papanicolaou smear

   - A cytology test for cervical cancer. There are five levels of findings that range from cells that are not abnormal to those that are conclusive for malignancy (Table 13–3). Viral, fungal, and parasitic conditions also can be identified with Pap smears.

   - Cervical biopsy

   - Cervical tissue is removed and examined microscopically for cancerous cells.

   - Colposcopy

   - A speculum with a magnifying glass is used to identify atypical areas of the vagina and cervix.

   - Endometrial biopsy

   - A sample of endometrium is removed for pathology report—used for endometrial cancer and some infertility assessments.

3. **Breast anomalies**
   - Mammogram

   - X-rays of the breasts to detect the presence of tumors and cysts. Benign cysts are generally well defined and tend to be bilateral, whereas malignant tumors are irregular, poorly defined, and tend to be unilateral. Abnormalities can be detected with mammograms before they are palpable.

   - Ultrasonography

   - Ultrasounds beamed into the tissue and reflected by body tissue are also used to detect breast abnormalities.

   - Fine-needle aspiration and excisional biopsy

   - Fine needle usually removes small portion of a lump, whereas biopsy removes the entire lump for pathology evaluation.

TABLE 13.3   Pap Smear Classification

Class I	Absence of atypical cells
Class II	Atypical cells but no signs of malignancy
Class III	Suggestive but not conclusive of malignancy
Class IV	Strongly suggestive of malignancy
Class V	Conclusive for malignancy

▼ ▼ ▼

G U I D E L I N E S *continued*

Sexuality and Reproduction:
Interview (Health History)

Procedure	Clinical Significance
4. Pregnancy-related tests	
• Pregnancy test (urine)	• Tests for elevated levels of hCG secreted by the chorionic villi. Levels begin to increase 6–8 days after conception and peak in 8–12 weeks.
• Maternal alpha-fetoprotein	• Used to screen (not detect) neural tube defects such as spina bifida. Fetus excretes alpha-protein into amniotic fluid that can be detected in maternal blood. Optimal time for testing is 16–18 weeks' gestation. May also be useful to screen for Down syndrome. If test is positive, amniocentesis is necessary for diagnosis.
• Amniocentesis	• Amniotic fluid (15–20 mL) is aspirated to develop fetal genetic profiles between 16 and 20 weeks' gestation. Detects genetic diseases/conditions such as neural tube defects, Down syndrome, and sex-linked disease.
• Chorionic villus sampling	• Chorionic villi are obtained at 9–12 weeks' gestation to develop genetic profiles. Use is similar to amniocentesis but can be done earlier.
• Ultrasound	• Ultrasound uses high-frequency sound waves to create an image. Used to determine normal development, can detect gender, gestational age, multiple fetuses, and some anomalies such as anencephaly and pyloric atresia.
5. Infertility tests	
• Hysterosalpingoraphy	• X-ray of the uterus and fallopian tubes, 2–6 days after menses (to avoid possible pregnancy). Outlines uterine shape and patency of fallopian tubes.
• Pelvic ultrasonogram	• Use of ultra-high-frequency sound waves to create an image of pelvic structures. Can be used to monitor follicular development.
• Sperm antibody agglutination	• Semen of partner mixed with woman's serum; if agglutination occurs, demonstrates antibodies against partner's sperm.
• Semen analysis	• Evaluates number, motility, volume, and pH of sperm.
• Sperm penetration assay	• Evaluates the ability of the sperm to penetrate the ovum.
6. Pelvic ultrasound	Ultra-high-frequency sound waves used to create an image of pelvic structures. Uterine fibroids, ovarian disorders, and other problems can be identified.
7. Prostate-specific antigen (PSA)	Blood test for prostate-specific antigen. Levels increase with benign prostatic hypertrophy and with age. However, levels are substantially higher with prostate cancer and increase proportionally to the size of the tumor. The use of PSA, however, remains controversial.

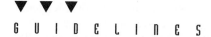

▼ ▼ ▼
G U I D E L I N E S

Assessment Guidelines   Sexuality and Reproduction: Physical Assessment

Procedure

General appearance:
Are there any obvious factors that can affect a person's sexuality, for example:
- Shortness of breath
- Paraplegia
- Neurologic disorders such as Parkinson's disease, multiple sclerosis
- Extreme obesity
- Fatigue
- Ostomies

When discussing sexuality, are verbal communication and nonverbal communication congruent?

Physical assessment of reproductive structures:
Female:
    Genitalia and pelvic assessment
    Breast assessment
    The pregnant abdomen
Male
    Genitalia assessment

Clinical Significance

Generally, most of the data collected regarding sexuality are obtained from the interview and how the individual presents him- or herself. However, some conditions can interfere with physical functioning and self-image related to sexuality.
If the individual is uncomfortable talking about sexuality, he or she may demonstrate being uncomfortable nonverbally or provide only brief answers.

These guidelines follow a brief overview of anatomy and physiology.

Nursing Diagnoses Related to the Female

Currently, five nursing diagnoses in the sexuality pattern are related to assessment of the female: Rape–trauma syndromes, Altered sexuality pattern, Sexual dysfunction, Effective breast-feeding, and Ineffective breast-feeding.

Rape–Trauma Syndromes

The nursing diagnosis of Rape–trauma syndrome is appropriately used when an individual experiences a forced sexual assault against one's will and without consent. Sexual assault can be vaginal, anal, oral, or a combination. The reaction to rape has short- and long-term implications. The nursing diagnosis Rape–trauma syndrome: compound reaction is noted when an individual, after a rape event, experiences the reactivation of previous physical or psychosocial problems or a reliance on drugs and alcohol. The nursing diagnosis Rape–trauma syndrome: silent reaction is used when the individual exhibits signs and symptoms of rape trauma but does not tell anyone about the event. If the assault is recent, the nurse may wish to refer this individual to another nurse or health professional with advanced education.

History.   The individual may or may not report a sexual assault. During the acute phase of the rape–trauma syndrome, the individual may report gastrointestinal up-

set, genitourinary discomfort, and skeletal muscle discomfort. Verbalization of other responses may include insomnia, fear, anger, guilt, panic attacks, change in sexual behavior, and a distrust of others of the same gender as the rapist. Long-term effects of the rape may continue if resolution does not occur. In these situations, the individual may report phobias, nightmares, anxiety, and depression.

Physical Examination Findings.   Recent rape victims should be examined by an individual with expertise in rape victim examinations for legal purposes (see discussion on interviewing sexual abuse or assault victims in this chapter). Observe injuries such as ecchymoses, lacerations, and abrasions in recent victims. Observe emotional status and responses as well. After the initial examination, victims may avoid, refuse, or experience increased discomfort during future genital and pelvic examinations.

Altered Sexuality Pattern

The nursing diagnosis Altered sexuality is used when the individual experiences or is at risk of experiencing a change in sexual health or is concerned with her own sexuality.

History.   During the health history or the examination, the individual may verbalize concerns about possible or actual difficulties, limitations, or changes in sexual behavior. Verbalizations about these concerns may be about fear of pregnancy or health problems or conditions (such as pregnancy, cancer, new ostomy, paraplegia, and multiple sclerosis), change in sexual response or reaction of partner, or sexual orientation or identity.

Physical Examination Findings. The individual's perception of the existence or probability of a problem may have more significance than physical findings. You may discover the presence or absence of pregnancy or sexually transmitted diseases, which may either distress or reassure the woman. Observing the individual during a discussion of sexuality may provide information about the presence of depression, withdrawn behavior, and low self-esteem.

Sexual Dysfunction

The nursing diagnosis Sexual dysfunction is used for the individual who is experiencing or is at high risk for experiencing a change in sexual function that is perceived as undesirable. The individual experiences a dissatisfaction with sexuality.

History. During the health history or the physical examination, the individual may verbalize problems with sexuality, difficulty in fulfilling the sex (gender) role, inability to achieve sexual satisfaction, alteration in relationship with significant partner(s), or value/belief conflicts with others regarding sexual expression and practice.

Physical Examination Findings. There may be no direct genital or pelvic structure findings for this diagnosis; however, the woman who is unable to get into a lithotomy position because of discomfort or hip mobility restriction may experience difficulty in traditional sexual intercourse positions. Other physical findings that may indicate the necessity of different positions include pregnancy, abdominal obesity, and spinal cord injuries. The presence of Foley catheters may interfere with satisfaction. While examining the vagina, note excessive dryness or inflammation that can be a cause of pain during coitus.

Effective Breast-Feeding

The nursing diagnosis Effective breast-feeding is used when both the woman and infant exhibit proficiency and satisfaction with the breast-feeding process.

History. Verbalizations by the breast-feeding woman that indicate effective breast-feeding include satisfaction with breast-feeding, infant contentment after feeding, and regular breast-feeding times.

Physical Examination Findings. Observations indicating effective breast-feeding include effective maternal–infant communication patterns and signs of oxytocin release (let-down reflex when infant cries). Physical findings may include appropriate weight for age of infant and strong sucking reflex.

Ineffective Breast-Feeding

This nursing diagnosis is used when the woman or infant or child experiences dissatisfaction or difficulty with the breast-feeding process.

History. For ineffective breast-feeding, the woman may report difficulty or lack of satisfaction with breast-feeding, sore nipples, or insufficient milk for the infant.

She may report that the infant is fussy shortly after feeding, has poor sucking, and does not like to nurse.

Physical Examination Findings. Nipples may be sore, cracked, or inverted. There may be no signs of oxytocin release (letdown reflex), and the breast may not be engorged just before regular feeding. The woman may show signs of insufficient nutrition and fluid intake (see Chap. 6). The infant may not be gaining weight for age. When possible, observe the breast-feeding event and note the following: Does the woman appear uncomfortable or tense? How is the infant sucking? Is sucking sustained? Is each breast emptied at feeding? Does the infant resist sucking?

ND_X

Nursing Diagnoses Related to Males

Currently, three nursing diagnoses in the sexuality pattern are related to assessment of the male: Rape–trauma syndromes, Altered sexuality pattern, and Sexual dysfunction. Characteristics unique to men for these diagnoses are considered here.

Rape–Trauma Syndromes

Although rape occurs more frequently to women, men also experience rape. Men at high risk are adolescents and younger men in abusive situations and adult men in prison or jails. Men are generally subjected to anal penetration and sometimes oral penetration. The male response to rape is similar to the female response; male rape also has a low report rate.

Sexual Dysfunction and Altered Sexual Pattern

In addition to the problems experienced by women, men may report difficulty attaining or sustaining an erection (impotence) and ejaculation problems, including premature, retarded, and retrograde ejaculation. The nature of these problems may be psychogenic, or disease- or medication-related. In male diabetics, erection problems are common. Men with erection and ejaculation problems should be assessed by a specialist.

THE FEMALE

Female Genitals and Pelvic Structure

The female reproductive structures involve the external genitals and internal structures.

External Genitals

Visible external genitalia include the mons pubis, labia majora, labia minora, clitoral prepuce, clitoral glans, urinary meatus, vaginal orifice, hymen, and perineum (Fig. 13-1). The labia can be separated to bring the clitoral glans, urinary meatus, and vaginal orifice into view. The

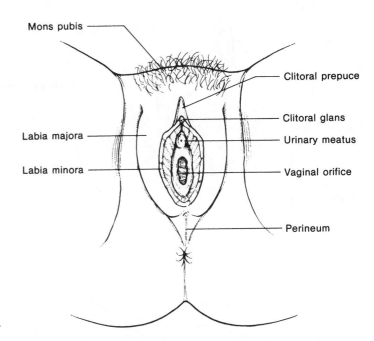

Mons pubis

Clitoral prepuce

Clitoral glans

Urinary meatus

Labia majora

Labia minora

Vaginal orifice

Perineum

FIGURE 13.1 External female genitals.

appearance of female genitalia varies depending on the stage of growth and development and individual differences. Therefore, graphic drawings or photos of female genitalia should be used as general guides. The mons pubis is a fatty pad over the symphysis pubis and is usually covered with hair after puberty. However, hair may be sparsely distributed in women who shave this area and in older women.

Vulva is a term used to refer collectively to the following structures: labia major and minora, clitoral prepuce and glans, and vaginal orifice. The labia majora are large folds of adipose tissue extending from the mons pubis to the perineum. The outer surfaces are covered with hair after puberty, and the inner surfaces are smooth and moist. The labia minora are thinner skin folds that surround the vaginal and urethral openings. The boat-shaped area between the two labia minora is also known as the vestibule.

Just below the mons pubis is the clitoral prepuce, a small fold (or folds) of tissue covering the clitoris. The clitoris has erectile properties and is homologous to the male penis. The urinary meatus is located approximately midway between the clitoris and vaginal orifice. Although the sphincter-like structure is often represented as a small, circular, doughnut-shaped orifice on drawings and models, it is not easily visualized because it may blend with surrounding skin folds (see Fig. 13-1). In some cases, however, trauma from catheters, assault, or other factors may exaggerate the opening. The meatus may be more visible if the skin is stretched with the fingers or if the woman bears down as though having a bowel movement. The ducts of Skene's glands, on either side of the urinary meatus, may be visible if the margins of the meatus are gently spread apart.

The vaginal orifice may be partially occluded by a mucous membrane, the hymen. The hymen usually tears in response to trauma such as that associated with tampon use, sexual intercourse, or other vaginal penetrations. Occasionally, the hymen may be elastic enough to remain intact after penetration. The ruptured hymen shrinks in size and may appear as a fringe of skin around the vaginal opening. The ductal openings of Bartholin's glands, located on each side of the lower vaginal opening, secrete small amounts of mucoid lubrication during the plateau phase of sexual arousal and are rarely noted on examination. The perineum refers to the area between the lower border of the vaginal opening and the rectum.

Internal Structures

The internal structures include the vagina, cervix, uterus, and adnexa. The vagina is tubular, rugated, 11 to 15 cm long, and extends from the vaginal orifice to the uterus (Fig. 13-2). This structure is lined with mucous membrane composed of squamous epithelial cells, is surrounded by layers of longitudinal and circular muscles, and has a rich arterial and venous blood supply. When not aroused, the vagina is collapsed. The angle of the vagina is directed backward and then upward over the pelvic floor or slanted toward the small of the back. At the terminal end, the projection of the cervix produces the posterior, anterior, and two lateral fornices. Uterine structures may be palpated through the thin fornix walls.

The cervix is the lower neck of the uterus and projects into the terminal portion of the vagina. The cervical opening to the vagina, the cervical os, is visible when the vagina is examined with a speculum. A nonparous cervical os, which has not been dilated by childbirth, appears as a small, round depression. A parous cervical os, dilated by childbirth, will appear larger and irregularly shaped, usually as a slit. The uterus is an inverted, pear-shaped, muscular organ oriented at a right angle to the vagina, or

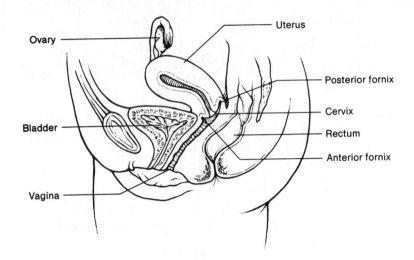

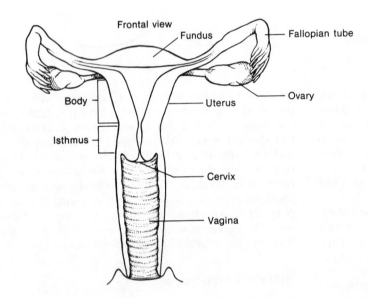

FIGURE 13.2 Internal female genital structures.

anteverted in most women, and located between the bladder and rectum. In some women the uterus may be retroverted and the body of the uterus may be felt immediately above the posterior fornix. The top of the uterus is known as the fundus. The fallopian tubes, each approximately 10 cm long, extend between the fundus and the ovaries and allow ova to pass into the uterus. The two ovaries are almond-shaped and vary in size among women, with the average size being 4 cm in length, 2 cm in width, and 2.5 cm thick. They are usually located near the lateral pelvic wall, in line with the anterosuperior iliac spines. The term *adnexa* refers collectively to the ovaries, fallopian tubes, and supporting muscles and ligaments.

Musculature

The three major groups of pelvic muscles include the superficial muscles, the urogenital diaphragm, and levator ani muscles (Fig. 13-3). Contractions of the pelvic muscles enhance orgasm and affect the ability to control urinary flow. The levator ani muscles are composed of several

muscles that form a hammock-like support to the pelvic floor. Poor muscle tone in this area has been associated with urinary stress incontinence. People can be taught to exercise the levator ani muscles by voluntarily contracting these muscles as though stopping the flow of urine or by tightening the anal sphincter (Kegel exercises). Not only do such exercises help control stress incontinence, but several weeks of toning also may result in stronger orgasms.

Examination and Documentation Focus

- External genitals: Color and pigmentation, contour and symmetry, discharge, lesions, masses, infestations
- Vaginal structures: Skin integrity, cervical contour and position, color, lesions or discharges of the cervix and vagina, vaginal muscle tone
- Uterus: Position, contour, and consistency; mobility; masses; pain or discomfort on palpation
- Adnexa: Size, contour, and consistency of the ovaries; masses; discomfort on palpation

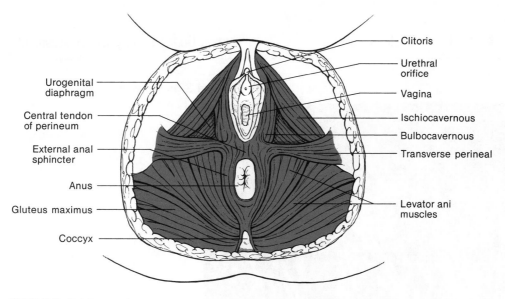

FIGURE 13.3   Pelvic muscles.

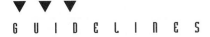

GUIDELINES

Assessment Guidelines   Female Genitalia: Physical Assessment

Procedure

1. **Equipment needed:**
   - Gloves: nonsterile, examination type
   - Water-soluble lubricant (KY jelly, Lubrifax)
   - Vaginal speculum
   - Hand-held mirror
   - Goose-neck lamp
   - Glass slides, sterile cotton-tipped applicators, wooden spatulae, fixative (for specimens), culture media (if screening for STDs)
   - Feminine napkin

Clinical Significance

The vaginal speculum is used to inspect the vagina and cervix and may be metal or disposable plastic. The plastic specula, although they are clear, are usually more uncomfortable. Specula vary in size and shape (Fig. 13–4). Graves specula are somewhat larger than Pedersen specula, which are used if the vaginal orifice is very small. The speculum has two blades that are spread to open the vaginal orifice and a level or screw device for opening and closing the blades. Proficiency in using the speculum can be gained by practicing opening and closing the blades. Before the speculum is inserted, it is warmed by running the blades under warm water. The person's natural vaginal secretions are usually sufficient lubrication to allow the speculum to be inserted. If additional lubrication is necessary, warm water poured over the blades is usually sufficient. Lubricating cream, jellies, and lotions are not advisable because they interfere with specimen collection for analysis. Furthermore, such substances may irritate vaginal tissues.

Procedure   **Clinical Significance**

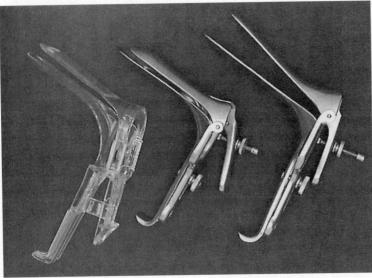

FIGURE 13.4   Vaginal specula.

2. **Preparation for genitalia assessment**
   - Begin explaining the examination procedure before the examination rather than after the woman is in the lithotomy position, so she has an opportunity to anticipate what will happen and thereby maintain a sense of personal control. The purpose of the assessment, the basic steps of the procedure, and any associated discomfort should be described before the assessment. This is especially important if it is the woman's first experience.
   - In the United States, male examiners often have a female associate present. Any conversation between the examiner and the associate should include the woman. Joking during the assessment may cause the woman to feel degraded or embarrassed.
   - One way to help the woman understand the assessment is to give her a hand-held mirror so she can view her genitals as the nurse explains anatomy and physiology during the procedure (Fig. 13–5). Some women prefer not to view the assessment with a mirror; their decision should be respected.

Women often have negative feelings about pelvic assessments and may even avoid recommended health screening practices because they dread the assessment. Some women are anxious because they believe their genitals are unclean or shameful, or they fear the genitals emit embarrassing odors or secretions. Some women have adverse feelings because they feel a loss of control during the procedure (Domar, 1986). Because of cultural or personal beliefs, some women feel more comfortable with a woman performing the assessment than a man. The lithotomy position may be viewed as having a sexual implication or associated with feelings of helplessness and vulnerability. The woman is usually draped during the examination, preventing her from seeing what is being done. Lack of eye contact between the examiner and the woman may inhibit communication, causing feelings of depersonalization. Feelings of discomfort can be compounded by a lack of understanding about the procedure.

Basic instructions for relaxing pelvic muscles during the assessment will help give the woman time to implement relaxation techniques. In addition, if she wishes to have someone present during the assessment, every effort should be made to accommodate this request.

▼ ▼ ▼
Female Genitalia: Physical Assessment

Procedure

Clinical Significance

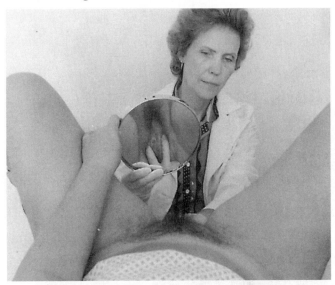

FIGURE 13.5 Use of a mirror during the pelvic examination.

3. **Positioning:**
   - Before the pelvic assessment, instruct the individual to empty her bladder.
   - Have woman undress, place a gown on; may wear socks.

   - Assist her into dorsal lithotomy position—lying supine on the examining table. Place her feet in the stirrups to help support the legs. When stirrups are used, the buttocks should be at the edge of the examining table, with the knees dropped to the sides and the heels in the stirrups. The nurse should be seated, facing the genitals, while inspecting and assessing with the speculum (Fig. 13–6). The nurse may stand to perform bimanual palpation.
   - Place a small pillow under her head or raise the examination table and instruct her to place arms at side or folded across chest. She should not lie with arms over her head.

To reduce bladder discomfort

Stockings help keep her warm, which prevents additional muscle tensing that could increase discomfort.
Although uncomfortable, it is the most effective position for the pelvic assessment.

These actions decrease tensing of the abdominal muscles.

▼ ▼ ▼

GUIDELINES *continued*   Female Genitalia: Physical Assessment

Procedure

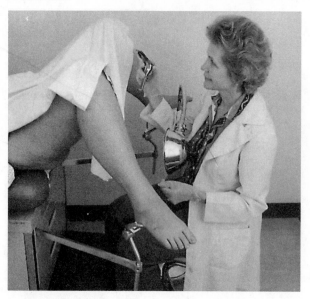

FIGURE 13.6   Pelvic examination: position of patient and examiner.

- Drape a small sheet over her legs and push down the center of the drape

- Place a goose-neck lamp at the end of the table.

4. **Inspect the external genitals.**
   a. Glove both hands.

   b. Touch the back of her thigh with the back of your hand before touching the genitals.
   c. Use the fingers of the nondominant hand to gently spread the labia so the clitoris, urinary meatus, and vaginal opening are clearly visible. Note any skin lesions or discharge and pubic hair distribution.

Clinical Significance

If the woman prefers to watch or does not want a drape, the drape is eliminated. Pushing the drape down allows eye contact between the nurse and the woman, and the nurse can observe for facial expressions of pain or anxiety.
Good lighting is essential, especially while inspecting the vagina and cervix.

Gloves are used to protect both the examiner and the individual.
Reduces pelvic muscle tensing

Normal Findings
a. Pubic hair distribution should be in the shape of an inverted triangle, although in some cultures pubic hair is shaved.
b. The color of the labia minora varies from pale pink to red. Bluish or brown pigmentation may be noted. It should be slightly darker than the rest of the skin color, sometimes resembling lip color. The skin surrounding the labia should have pink or brown undertones. The labia majora usually appears symmetric, and the labia minora ranges in shape from triangular to semicircular. Edges of the labia minora appear smooth or irregular and may protrude through the labia majora.

▼ ▼ ▼

Procedure

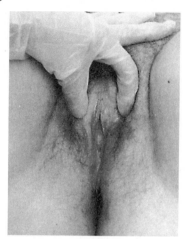

External genital inspection

5. Palpate Skene's and Bartholin's glands.

   a. While spreading the labia with nondominant hand, insert the index finger of your other hand into the vagina. Palpate Skene's glands by gently exerting pressure against the anterior vaginal wall, moving your finger from inside to outside the vagina. This maneuver is also known as "milking the urethra."

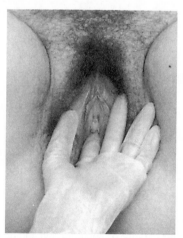

Skene's gland palpation

   b. Palpate Bartholin's glands on each side of the posterior vaginal opening by placing your index finger inside the vagina at the lower lateral aspect and your thumb opposite the labia majora. Gently squeeze the skin between the thumb and index finger.

Clinical Significance

   c. Odorless, nonirritating vaginal discharge is normal with appearance varying according to the menstrual cycle. After menstruation, a slight, white discharge may be noted. Toward ovulation, a thin clear discharge usually occurs. After ovulation, the discharge may again be thickened and appear white. Some women note changes in discharge or cervical mucus color and consistency, to estimate ovulation for either pregnancy or contraception purposes.

Deviations from Normal
Bright red skin color is abnormal and commonly associated with vaginal yeast infections. Abnormal vaginal discharge is strong smelling, discolored, or purulent and may be associated with vaginal itching. Asymmetric labia may indicate abscess. Genital lesions, masses, and lice infestations (nits at base of hair) are abnormal.

Normal Findings
Should be nontender, with no discharge

Deviations from Normal
Discharge is abnormal, and any discharge should be cultured. Discharge could be from a gonorrhea or chlamydia infection.

Normal Findings
The gland should be soft, not tender, and not palpable.

Deviations from Normal
Discharge or discomfort may indicate inflammation of the gland. Swelling is abnormal and may indicate a plugged duct.

▼ ▼ ▼

G U I D E L I N E S   *continued*   Female Genitalia: Physical Assessment

Procedure   **Clinical Significance**

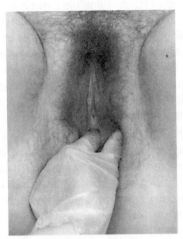

Bartholin's gland palpation

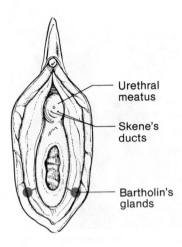

Urethral
meatus

Skene's
ducts

Bartholin's
glands

6. Evaluate vaginal musculature.
  a. Insert index finger 2–4 cm into vagina; ask individual to
     squeeze the finger.

Normal Findings
The nurse should be able to feel the finger being squeezed.
Muscle tone is usually firmer in nulliparous women.

Deviations from Normal
Absent or weak squeeze indicates poor muscle tone.

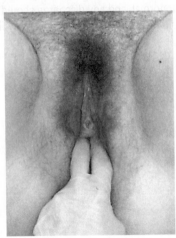

Evaluating vaginal musculature

  b. Insert middle and index finger in the lower border of the
     vagina and spread the labia by displacing the fingers
     laterally. Ask the individual to bear down "like having a
     bowel movement."

Normal Findings
No bulges, either anterior or posterior, felt and no discharge of
urine.

Deviations from Normal
  a. An anterior bulge may be a cystocele. A cystocele is caused
     by herniation of the posterior bladder wall into the vagina
     and is more common in multiparous women (see Chap. 7).
     Pelvic examination usually reveals a soft, reducible mass
     that bulges into the vagina and is accentuated by straining.
  b. A posterior bulge may be a rectocele. A retocele is a recto-
     vaginal hernia caused by rupture of the fibrous structures
     between the vagina and rectum, which usually occurs during
     childbirth. Bulging of the lower, posterior portion of the
     vagina may be noted, often without using a speculum (see
     Chap. 7).

▼ ▼ ▼

G U I D E L I N E S *continued*   Female Genitalia: Physical Assessment

Procedure

7. Insert the speculum.

 a. Select an appropriate-sized speculum.

 b. To insert the vaginal speculum, open the vaginal orifice by placing your index and middle fingers just inside the lower vagina and gently press down.

 c. Direct the closed, prewarmed (with warm, not hot, water) speculum blades over your fingers into the vagina at a 45-degree angle, following the natural contour of the posterior vaginal wall. Insert the blades obliquely to minimize discomfort. Be careful not to scrape or pinch genital tissue or pull pubic hairs. Insertion may be difficult if the woman tenses the pelvic muscles. If this occurs, stop advancing the speculum momentarily and remind the woman to relax. Instruct her to take slow, deep breaths and exhale through slightly pursed lips to relax. Then continue advancing the speculum.

 d. When the speculum is inserted, remove your fingers holding the lower vagina open, and gently rotate the speculum so the blades are oriented horizontally: Partially open the blades by pressing the speculum lever with your thumb.

 e. Look through the open blades at the cervix. The cervix will be in full view if the blades are correctly located in the anterior and posterior fornices. If the cervix is not fully visible, slowly close the blades, withdraw the speculum slightly, and reinsert at a slightly different angle.

 f. Once the cervix is clearly visible, lock the blades in the open position by turning the thumbscrew (metal speculum) or completely depressing the lever (plastic speculum).

Clinical Significance

Virgins and some postmenopausal women may need small speculums if there is a narrow vaginal orifice.

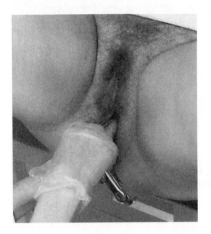

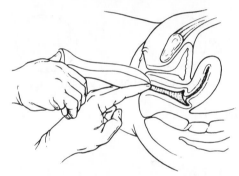

Vaginal speculum insertion

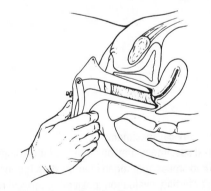

Vaginal speculum in place

▼ ▼ ▼

G U I D E L I N E S   *continued*   Female Genitalia: Physical Assessment

Procedure

8. Inspect the cervix.

a. Look through the open blades to inspect the cervix. Adjust external light source if necessary

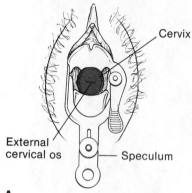

Cervix

External cervical os — Speculum

A

Nonparous external os   Parous external os

B

The cervix

9. Obtain cervical specimens.

Cervical specimens may be obtained for cytology evaluation (Pap smear), pathogen identification (gonorrhea culture), or fertility evaluation (postcoital, cervical mucus evaluation). Three techniques may be used to obtain specimen:

a. The cervical scraping technique involves inserting a specially designed wooden spatula (Ayre spatula) through the open speculum blades. Place the spatula against the cervix and scrape by rotating the instrument 360 degrees against the cervical surface. Withdraw the instrument and smear both sides of the spatula end gently across a glass slide. Spray the specimen with a fixative solution.

Clinical Significance

Normal Findings

Shape and position: The *cervix* is a rounded structure, 3 to 4 cm in diameter, protruding about 2.5 cm into the vagina. The position of the cervix is determined by the configuration of the uterus. For example, in most women the cervix is directed posteriorly. However, when the uterus is retroverted, the cervix is directed anteriorly. Normally, the cervix appears midline rather than laterally displaced. The cervical os, or opening, appears as a small round depression in the nulliparous woman and as a flat slit in the parous woman.

Color: The cervix is usually pink and generally appears paler after menopause. In the pregnant woman, bluish pigmentation usually occurs by the sixth week. Oral contraceptives may cause dark pink to reddish cervical pigmentation.

Discharge: Should be odorless and may be white to clear and thin to thick.

Deviations from Normal

Cervix size: A cervix larger than 4 cm in diameter or a lateral diversion is abnormal and should be evaluated. This may indicate a tumor or prolapse of the uterus.

Color: The following colors may indicate the corresponding problems: pale—anemia; red—inflammation/infection; blue—cyanosis or pregnancy. Any white spots, strawberry patches, or asymmetric red areas need evaluation.

Lesions: Because the cervix may tear during childbirth, the parous woman may have cervical scarring from healed lacerations. Cervical lesions may indicate serious pathology or infections and should always be thoroughly evaluated. A relatively benign lesion, nabothian cyst, appears secondary to cervical gland duct obstruction. Such cysts may occur in groups as small, yellowish papules less than 1 cm in diameter. A string protruding from the cervical os usually indicates an intrauterine device (IUD) used for contraception.

Discharge: Colored or purulent discharge is abnormal and should be cultured. Bloody discharge except during menses is abnormal.

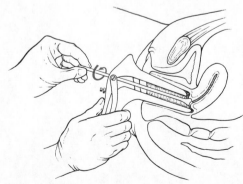

Cervical scraping with wooden spatula

▼ ▼ ▼

G U I D E L I N E S *continued*   Female Genitalia: Physical Assessment

Procedure

b. The endocervical swab technique involves inserting a sterile, cotton-tipped applicator through the cervical os about 0.5 cm. Rotate the applicator 360 degrees with your fingers and leave the applicator tip in place several seconds to allow saturation. Withdraw the applicator and gently brush the speculum across a glass slide and spray with a fixative.

c. The vaginal pool technique is performed with the wooden spatula. Insert the spatula through the speculum blades to the posterior fornix. Scrape this area and remove the spatula; transfer the material to a glass slide and spray with a fixative.

d. Following laboratory procedures, collect additional specimens for cultures or slides from any suspicious discharges.

10. Inspect the vagina.

Inspect the walls of the vagina as the speculum is removed. Release the locking device that holds the speculum open, being careful to manually hold the speculum open as you begin to withdraw. Removing a partially open speculum may cause pain or pinch tissue if the blades are suddenly snapped shut at the vaginal opening. Once the cervix is no longer visible, allow the speculum to close slowly so that the blades are completely closed when the speculum is withdrawn through the vaginal opening.

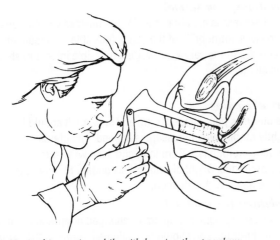

Vaginal inspection while withdrawing the speculum

Clinical Significance

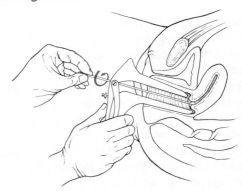

Endocervical swab technique

Normal Findings

Vaginal appearance: The walls of the vagina appear pinkish with rugae, ridge-like structures caused by folding of the mucous membranes. Normal vaginal secretions may give the vagina a shiny or wet appearance. The walls may be pale pink with fewer rugae in postmenopausal women.

Deviations from Normal

Discharge. Any discharge other than clear or white-creamy and thin should be described according to color, consistency, amount, odor, and appearance. May indicate infection. Vagina: A pale vagina may indicate anemia. A red vagina is indicative of an inflammation process and should be evaluated.

▼ ▼ ▼

Procedure

11. Palpate the vagina and cervix.
   a. Lubricate glove with water-soluble lubricant.
   b. While standing, use index finger and middle fingers to palpate the vagina.
   c. Insert fingers, following the natural vaginal contour, by exerting slight posterior pressure. Hold thumb abducted and flex the other fingers. If the vaginal opening is very small, you can use one finger.
   d. Palpate the vaginal wall and note nodules, masses, or tenderness. Palpate the cervix and note position, mobility, consistency, and tenderness.

12. Bimanually palpate the pelvic structures.
   a. Remain standing with the index and middle fingers in the vagina.
   b. Place your other hand—which now may be ungloved—on the woman's abdomen between the umbilicus and symphysis pubis.
   c. Use two hands to "trap" deeper pelvis structures such as ovaries, making palpation possible.

Clinical Significance

Water-soluble lubricant should be placed on the gloved fingers to facilitate vaginal penetration during the bimanual assessment. Ideally, the lubricant is dispensed from small, disposable tubes intended for single use that lower the risk of contamination of the lubricant. Lubricant obtained from a large tube that is used repeatedly should be squeezed in a manner that allows lubricant to drop to the gloved fingers. The gloved fingers should not be placed against the opening of the tube, which could contaminate the contents.

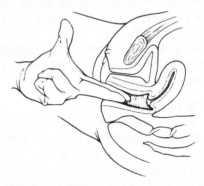

Vaginal palpation

Normal Findings
The cervix is firm, like the tip of the nose, nontender, and mobile.

Deviations from Normal
Palpable masses are abnormal. Do not mistake vaginal rugae for masses. Immobility of the cervix (possible malignancy) or tenderness of the cervix and vagina (possible infection) should be evaluated.

Normal Findings
The uterus is pear-shaped, firm, and smooth. It should be slightly mobile when pressure is applied. The uterus of a nonpregnant woman is 7–8 cm long and 5 cm wide across the body of fundus. Slight discomfort secondary to muscle tensing may be noted with palpation.

Deviations from Normal
Masses, sharp pain, cramping, or enlarged nonpregnant uterus are all abnormal and should be evaluated. *Retroverted uterus:* A retroverted uterus is usually not palpable with this approach. A fixed or tender uterus may indicate masses, fibroids, or infection.

▼ ▼ ▼

Female Genitalia: Physical Assessment

Procedure

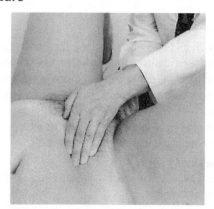

Bimanual palpation: Pelvic structures

d. Palpate the uterus by pressing the abdominal hand downward toward the vaginal hand, which is held firmly in the vagina, by exerting slight pressure against the perineum with your flexed, outside fingers. The uterus should be palpable just above the symphysis pubis. Palpate the anterior wall and fundus of the uterus and note any masses or tenderness.

e. Move the vaginal fingers toward the left, lateral fornix and rotate this hand so that your palm is facing upward. Move the abdominal hand to the left lower quadrant. The ovary and adnexa, which are not always palpable, are now trapped between your two hands for evaluation. Use the vaginal hand for palpation. Press the abdominal hand toward the vaginal hand. Note any masses or tenderness as well as ovary size if palpable. Repeat on the right side.

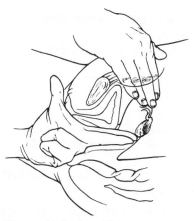

Bimanual palpation: Adnexa

Clinical Significance

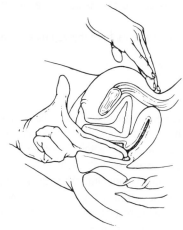

Bimanual palpation: Uterus

Normal Findings

The fallopian tubes are usually not palpable. The ovaries may or may not be palpable and should feel small, firm, almond-shaped, mobile, and smooth, without masses. Slight discomfort on palpation is common.

Deviations from Normal

Palpation of ovaries larger than 6 cm, irregular or round shape, and pain on palpation should be evaluated. May indicate ovarian cyst or other mass.

▼ ▼ ▼

Procedure

13. Palpate the uterus and adnexa using the rectovaginal approach.

a. Remove your fingers from the vagina and change the glove.

b. Lubricate the index and middle fingers of your newly gloved hand. Explain the procedure and ask the individual to use relaxation breathing. Tell her she may feel sensations associated with having a bowel movement.

c. Insert your index finger into the vagina and your middle finger into the rectum. Keep your index finger against the cervix so the rectal finger does not mistake the cervix for a rectal wall mass.

d. Repeat the maneuvers used during bimanual palpation to evaluate the uterus and adnexa. With this technique, use the rectal finger to palpate the uterus and adnexa.

14. Complete the examination.

Remove fingers and wipe perineum, using a front-to-back stroke. Help the woman out of the stirrups and provide additional tissues for cleansing.

Clinical Significance

- The vagina should never be examined after the rectum unless hands are rewashed and gloves changed. Gloves should be changed between the vaginal and rectal assessments to prevent inadvertent spread of infection from the vagina to the rectum.
- Lubrication aids the finger insertion into the rectum.
- Deep breathing helps to relax the anal sphincter.

Normal Findings:
The posterior wall of the uterus is palpated and should be smooth, firm, and mobile.

Deviations from Normal:
Tenderness, immobility, and masses are abnormal.

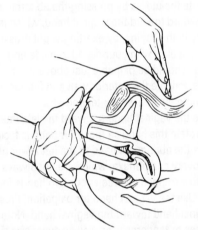

Rectovaginal examination

- Front-to-back strokes prevent contamination of the vaginal area from the rectum.
- The woman may desire to cleanse herself.

Documenting Female Genital and Pelvic Examination Findings

Example 1: Normal Findings

Ms. K, aged 33, had a pelvic assessment and Pap smear as part of the routine health assessment. The assessment findings were normal and were recorded as follows:

External genitals and vagina moist, pink, without lesions or discharge. Cervical specimen for Pap obtained by endocervical swab.

No visible cystocele or rectocele. Bimanual exam reveals no palpable masses, no tenderness: uterus midline, mobile, and anteverted.

The same findings may be summarized in the following problem-oriented format:

S: Denies vaginal itching, pain, or discharge. Non-parous; uses barrier contraception; satisfied with method; regular menstrual periods with LMP 15 days ago. Here for annual exam and Pap smear. All previous smears normal; no family history of pelvic cancer.

O: External genitals and vagina moist, pink, without lesions or discharge. Nonparous cervical os, pink, midline with trace of clear discharge. Cervical specimen for Pap obtained. No visible cystocele or rectocele. Bimanual exam reveals no palpable masses or tenderness. Uterus midline, mobile, and anteverted.

A: Normal genital pelvic assessment.

P: Follow-up with routine exams. Notify about Pap results.

Example 2: Vulvovaginitis

Mrs. L., aged 23. had a genital–pelvic assessment after noticing vaginal itching and discharge. The findings were abnormal and were recorded as follows:

Vulva and vagina erythematous, covered with patchy, white, thick exudate. Parous cervical os, midline without discharge. Bimanual palpation reveals no masses; marked tenderness over right adnexa.

The same findings may be summarized in a problem-oriented format as follows:

S: Reports intense vaginal pruritus accompanied by thick white discharge for 1 week. Denies history of similar problem, recent use of antibiotics, and diabetes mellitus. Taking oral contraceptives for 2 years. Treatment: vinegar douche with only short-term relief.

O: Vulva and vagina erythematous and covered with patchy, thick, white exudate. Parous cervical os midline without discharge. Bimanual palpation reveals no masses; marked tenderness over right adnexa.

A: Vulvovaginitis—suspect monilial vaginitis.

P: Refer to nurse practitioner in clinic for confirmation and treatment. Instruct about administration of vaginal suppositories. Discuss risk factors for monilial vaginitis. Instruct to return if treatment ineffective.

Clinical Problems Related to Female Genital and Pelvic Assessment

Sexually Transmitted Diseases (STD)

Many organisms are transmitted by sexual contact. A person who contracts an STD may or may not have multiple sexual partners. For example, *Trichomonas* infections may develop in the vagina when the normal vaginal flora is altered. A male sex partner of a woman with *Trichomonas* infections may become infected but have no symptoms and therefore may not receive treatment. The woman may then be reinfected by the partner, meaning that the disease is sexually transmissible even in sexually monogamous relationships. Table 13-4 summarizes clinical features of major STDs. Often, clinical findings differ between genders because of anatomic differences in reproductive organs.

Gonorrhea. Gonorrhea, also called clap, is caused by the *Neisseria gonorrhoea* bacterium. The organism invades and inflames the columnar and transitional epithelium of the urethra, cervix, fallopian tubes, and Skene's and

Bartholin's glands. Because the disease rarely affects the vulva, vagina, or uterus, many women are asymptomatic during the acute phase. In some women, the condition is first diagnosed when their male partner is treated for the disease.

In symptomatic women, gonorrhea has variable courses. Usually cervicitis develops. Symptoms range from slightly increased vaginal discharge to purulent discharge, urethritis, inflammation of Skene's and Bartholin's glands, and acute salpingitis, or pelvic inflammatory disease (PID). The diagnosis may be confirmed by isolating the gonococcus. A culture specimen should be obtained and applied to a Thayer-Martin culture medium.

Additional findings include discharge or tenderness during palpation of Skene's or Bartholin's glands. Salpingitis is indicated during bimanual pelvic palpation if cervical movement or adnexa palpation causes marked pain. Rectal infection may be characterized by rectal pain, itching, and purulent discharge.

Systemic manifestations include fever, prostration, and abdominal tenderness and guarding accompanying acute salpingitis; leukocytosis with left shift, nausea, and vomiting; gouty arthritis; and skin lesions. Fallopian tube damage may cause infertility.

Syphilis. Less common than gonorrhea, syphilis is caused by sexual transmission of the bacterium *Treponema pallidum*. If untreated, the disease is disseminated through the bloodstream, ultimately affecting all body systems. The disease has five stages: incubation, primary, latency, secondary, and tertiary. Incubation and primary syphilis are noted by a primary lesion (called a chancre), a painless, ulcerated papule up to 2 cm in diameter. In women, the chancre most commonly occurs on the cervix or vagina and heals spontaneously within weeks. Regional lymph node involvement may cause enlargement and swelling of inguinal lymph nodes at this stage. Primary and secondary stages are separated by an asymptomatic latency period.

Secondary syphilis is characterized by systemic manifestations, especially the development of lesions on the skin and mucous membranes. These lesions are usually rash-like, bilateral, and symmetric. The hallmark of tertiary syphilis is the gumma lesion, a granulomatous lesion affecting the skin, bones, and viscera. Syphilis bacteria do not grow on routine culture media; therefore, the disease is diagnosed based on chancre appearance and serologic testing (VDRL).

Herpes. The *herpes simplex virus type 2 (HSV-2)* is most often implicated in genital infections, although HSV-1 also may be the infective agent. In both cases, similar genital lesions may be noted. The lesions are a grouping of small vesicles that eventually rupture and may ulcerate. Intense pain and itching are usually reported. Lesions usually heal in 4 to 6 weeks. In women, genital lesions are commonly distributed on the cervix, labia, vagina, and clitoris. Sexually transmitted herpes lesions also may occur in the mouth and anus.

Venereal Warts. Warts occurring on the genitalia and perineal area are known as *condyloma acuminata,* a human papillomavirus (HPV). Rarely, venereal warts occur before puberty or after menopause. The dry, wart-

TABLE 13.4 Sexually Transmitted Diseases

For treatment of sexually transmitted diseases, refer to an appropriate text, because treatments change as new medications and knowledge become available.

Incidence	Clinical Presentation	Diagnosis	Complications
Syphilis: Treponema pallidum (spirochete)			
7,787 new cases reported in 1997 (fewer than reported in 1996—a reportable disease). Syphilis is increasing among women of child-bearing age.	Incubation 10–90 days. *Primary syphilis:* Classic chancre is painless, eroded lesion with a raised, indurated border. Atypical lesions common; multiple lesions may occur. Extragenital chancres may appear. Unilateral or bilateral lymphadenopathy may accompany. *Secondary syphilis:* Highly variable cutaneous and mucous membrane lesions, alopecia, generalized lymphadenopathy, mild cold symptoms	Demonstration of *T palidum* from exudate of primary or secondary lesions by dark-field microscopy is definitive. Typical lesions and a reactive (positive) reagent test result for syphilis (VDLR or RPR) FAT/ABS or MHA-TP can confirm questionable reagent test results. If the initial reagent test is nonreactive, repeat test 1 week, 1 month, and 3 months later. Individuals with HIV have unreliable test results.	Complications at all stages are secondary to gumma lesions. Gummas, resulting from treponemal tissue invasion, are granulomatous lesions with necrotic centers. Gummas occur in visceral, cardiovascular, and nervous tissue. Associated clinical manifestations during late syphilis include the following: *Visceral gummas:* alteration in liver, esophagus, stomach, intestines. *Cardiovascular gummas:* aortic valve incompetence, aneurysms, coronary artery disease. *Neurologic gummas:* general paresis; dementia, euphoria, mania depression, schizoid reactions. Argyle Robertson pupils, optic nerve atrophy. *Tabes dorsalis:* loss of sensation, locomotor ataxia, incontinence, constipation, swelling joints, pathologic fractures. *Congenital syphilis:* fetus affected—crippling blindness, facial abnormalities, deafness, fetal demise.
Gonorrhea: Neisseria gonorrhoeae			
In 1997, there were 284,427 new cases reported (reportable disease). This is slightly less than in 1996. Highest rates in late adolescents and young adults.	Incubation: Male, 3–30 days; female, 3–indefinite. Men have dysuria, frequency, and urethral discharge. This is usually purulent and often more severe in the morning. Women experience vaginal discharge and cystitis. 10–40% of men and 10–80% of women have no symptoms.	Presumptive identification: Microscopic identification of typical gram-negative, intracellular diplococci on direct smear of urethral exudate from men. Because sensitivity is low in females, smears cannot be substituted for culture or positive oxidase reaction of typical colonies from specimen obtained from anterior urethra, endocervix, and anal canal, or oral pharynx and inoculated on selective media.	*In both genders:* Primary infections may affect the pharynx, conjunctivae, and anus. May cause blindness in infants infected at birth. Disseminated infections may result in meningitis, septicemia, arthritis, and endocarditis. *In men:* epididymitis, urethral stricture, prostatitis. *In women:* inflammation of Skene's and Bartholin's glands, pelvic inflammatory disease, tubo-ovarian abscesses.

(continued)

TABLE 13.4   Sexually Transmitted Diseases [continued]

Incidence	Clinical Presentation	Diagnosis	Complications
Genital Herpes (Herpes Genitalis): Herpes Simplex Virus (HSV), Types I and II			
300,000–500,000 cases estimated (nonreportable disease). Caused by HSV I and II. HSV II is more commonly associated with recurrent outbreaks. Highest occurrence in young adults.	*Incubation:* Virus can be dormant for 3 days to years. Migrates along sensory nerves to dorsal root ganglia, remaining inactive, nonreplicating until reactivated. Multiple shallow vesicles, lesions, or crusts can occur on genital area, including buttocks and inner thighs. Inguinal adenopathy, dysuria, local pain, edema, fever are more severe with primary infections. Initial infections lasts 7–10 days, recurrent 3–10 days.	Clinical appearance of herpetic lesions. Pap smears from lesions stained to show multinucleated giant cells with intranuclear inclusion bodies (40% sensitivity). Tissue culture most definitive test.	Neonatal herpes infection. Associated with cervical cancer. Neuralgia, meningitis, ascending myelitis, urethral stricture, lymphatic suppuration. Can be infectious even without lesions. Can be fatal to infants exposed during birth.
Chlamydia: Chlamydia trachomatis			
Estimated 2–4 million cases per year (nonreportable disease). Caused by *Chlamydia trachomatis* bacteria. Most common STD in the Untied States.	Frequently asymptomatic. Men may have urethritis; women may experience yellowish endocervical discharge, dysuria, and acute salpingitis.	Isolation of bacteria on culture or antigen detection; difficult to diagnosis.	*Women:* Pelvic inflammatory disease (PID), which increases risk for sterility and ectopic pregnancy; can develop into chronic PID. If pregnant, risk of spontaneous abortion, stillbirth, and postpartum fever. *Men:* see NGU below.
Nongonococcal Urethritis (Nonspecific Urethritis, NSU, NGU)			
Primarily caused by *C trachomatis* (23–55%) and by *N gonorrhoeae*. Also can be caused by Trichomonas. Nonreportable disease. Age distribution similar to other STDs.	Incubation period appears to exceed 10 days in half of cases. Urethral discharge varies from profusely purulent to slightly mucoid. Dysuria may or may not be present. Some men are asymptomatic. Women frequently have cervitis, and urethritis in women often appears after gonorheal infections.	Clinical picture of dysuria, or urethral discharge with ≥5 polymorphonuclear leukocytes on smear. If this is not confirmed, then individual should be tested for *N gonorrhoeae* and *C trachomatis*.	Epididymitis, sterility, prostatitis, proctitis, urethral strictures, neonatal ophthalmia, or pneumonia.
Vulvovaginitis: Gardenerella vaginalis			
The incidence is unknown. Caused by the bacteria *G. vaginalis.*	Nondescript thick or thin, occasionally frothy vaginal discharge, usually gray–white.	The pH of the vagina is >4.5, may have a fishy odor; Gram stain or KOH wet mount may show tiny gram-negative coccobacilli (clue cells) adhering to vaginal epithelial cells.	Pregnant women are at risk for preterm deliveries. The bacteria has been associated with PID (see above).
Candidiasis (Moniliasis): Candida albicans			
A yeast infection; it is estimated that 75% of all women will have at least one infection, with about 50% having 2 or more incidences. Individuals with diabetes mellitus have a higher risk for this infection than other women.	Vulva erythematous and edematous. Vaginal discharge may be thick, white, and resembling cottage cheese. Occasionally discharge is thin and watery. Many women have no symptoms. Men may develop balanitis or cutaneous lesions on the penis.	Microscopic examination of gram-stained smears of introital or vaginal wall scrapings. Also examination of KOH wet mount of vaginal discharge. Culture on Sabouraud's modified agar.	Risk for neonatal thrush.

(continued)

TABLE 13.4   Sexually Transmitted Diseases [continued]

Incidence	Clinical Presentation	Diagnosis	Complications
Trichomoniasis: Trichomonas vaginalis			
Incidence ranges from as low as 5% of private gynecologic patients to as high as 75% in prostitutes. Colonization rates are higher in women than men. Caused by a protozoa.	Mostly women have symptoms of this infection. Women have diffuse malodorous yellow-green discharge with vulvar irritation. Men may have NSU. Incubation period is unknown. Vagina and cervix have strawberry appearance. Postcoital bleeding may occur.	Microscopic examination of wet mount of vaginal discharge. Pap smears may show the parasite. Culture methods are not available.	Epididymitis and prostatitis in men. Pregnant women may experience preterm delivery.
Human Immunodeficiency Virus (HIV, the AIDS virus)			
In 1887 53,031 new cases of AIDS, the end stage of HIV infection, were reported to CDC. 87% of all infected with HIV convert to AIDS within 17 years. There are currently two types of HIV virus, I and II. I is the predominate type in the United States and type II is unusual (occurring primarily in West Africa). The virus does pass the placental barrier, infecting the fetus.	*Early:* may be asymptomatic with serologic conversion from HIV negative to positive. *Mid:* Reduced resistance to diseases, malaise, fatigue, and enlarged lymh nodes, especially of groin and axilla. *Late:* compromised immune system, opportunistic diseases such as *Pneumocystis carinii* pneumonia (PCP), tuberculosis, and candidiasis.	Serologic testing: Enzyme immunoassay (EIA); if positive then Western blot test. Can be diagnosed without serologic testing if diagnosis of conditions such as Kaposi sarcoma, PCP, candidiasis of esophagus.	Death is the most severe complication. Other complications include blindness, dementia, muscle wasting, PCP, Kaposi sarcoma, and high risk for opportunistic diseases such as tuberculosis, influenza, pneumonia.
Genital Warts: Human Papillomavirus			
Incidence unknown; not a reportable disease. There are more than 20 viruses that cause genital warts.	Warts in the vagina, on the cervix, penis, urethra, anus (anal sex); can appear on, in, or near any orifice used in sexual activity.	Biopsy, usually not needed—observation is sufficient, may resolve on their own.	Cervical dysplasia.
Hepatitis: Types A and B			
Hepatitis A (HAV) and hepatitis B (HBV) can be transmitted during sexual activity and can be prevented through immunizations available at health care facilities. 33% of the US population has had HAV. 30–60% of HBV is transmitted sexually. 36,621 people in the United States had either HAV or HBV in 1997.	Fatigue, jaundice, fever; however, the individual can be asymptomatic. Male homosexuals, individuals with multiple sex partners, and IV drug abusers are at high risk for these infections.	Blood test for liver enzymes, and presence of virus or antibodies for the virus.	HAV—usually self-limiting. Without long-term complications. HBV—chronic infection and liver failure. Chronic HBV occurs in 90% of infants infected in utero.

Adapted from Centers for Disease Control and Prevention (1998). 1998 guidelines for treatment of sexually transmitted diseases. *MMWR 47* (Nu. RR-1); Centers for Disease Control and Prevention (1998). Provisional cases of selected notifiable diseases, United States weeks ending December 27, 1997 and December 26, 1996 (52nd week). *MMWR, 46* (52 & 53), 1260–1261; Centers for Disease Control and Prevention (1998). Provisional cases of selected notifiable diseases, preventable by vaccination, United States weeks ending December 27, 1997 and December 26, 1996 (52nd week). *MMWR, 46* (52 & 53), 1262–1263.

like growths may appear on the vulva, vagina, cervix, or rectum. They may occur singularly or in clusters large enough to occlude the vagina. They are highly infectious and can be transferred to a fetus during a vaginal delivery.

Vaginitis. Vaginitis is a general term referring to infections characterized by vaginal discharge. Organisms causing vaginitis may originate from several sources, including normal vaginal flora, the large intestine (as a result of cross-contamination), and exogenous sources, including sexual transmission. The most common cause of altered vaginal flora is douching, which causes the normally acidic pH to become more alkaline. Antibiotic therapy and diabetes mellitus also can alter the normal vaginal flora and predispose women to infection.

General assessment findings related to vaginitis include odorous vaginal discharge, genital pruritus, dyspareunia (painful intercourse), and dysuria. Multiple infections may be noted.

Trichomonas caused by the *Trichomonas vaginalis* organism is easily transmitted between sexual partners but is endogenous and may cause infections in persons who do not contract it through sexual activity. The vaginal discharge is watery, yellow, or yellow-green. The organisms are easily identified under the microscope by placing a few drops of vaginal discharge on a glass slide and applying normal saline. Genital examination may indicate erythematous mucous membranes, and reddened papules may be noted on the cervix and vaginal walls.

Candida albicans is a yeast organism that is part of the natural vaginal flora. However, certain conditions such as taking oral contraceptives, receiving antibiotic or corticosteroid therapy, pregnancy, and poorly controlled diabetes mellitus predispose women to this type of infection. *Candida* infections are characterized by intense genital pruritus and a thick, white, curd-like vaginal discharge. The genitals appear bright red and are covered with whitish exudate.

Atrophic vaginitis, an inflammation of the vaginal walls associated with estrogen deficiency, occurs most frequently in postmenopausal women. The vaginal walls become thin, and accompanying pH changes may predispose women to bacterial infections. Vaginal discharge, if present, may be mucoid and occasionally flecked with blood. Vaginal inspection shows a smooth, thin, and glistening vaginal mucosa unless infection is present, in which case the vaginal walls appear red.

BREASTS AND AXILLAE

The examination of the breast and axillae is the same for men and women. Because the woman has more breast tissue, this discussion is female-oriented.

Anatomy and Physiology Overview

The breasts are paired, modified sebaceous glands located between the second and sixth ribs and between the sternal border and the midaxillary line on the anterior chest wall. A nipple, surrounded by the areola, is centrally located on each breast.

The breast is composed of glandular tissue, fibrous tissue, and retromammary and subcutaneous fat. Variation in breast size is a result of the amount of fat present. The amount of glandular tissue is about the same in all women and is organized into some 12 to 25 lobes in a circular pattern around the nipple. These lobes are composed of lobules containing acini, the milk-producing glands. The lobes have a duct that terminate on the nipple (Fig. 13-7). Most of the glandular tissue occurs in the upper lateral quadrant of the breast. A portion of the glandular tissue, known as the tail of Spence, extends toward the axilla. The breasts also contain fibrous tissue or Cooper's ligaments, which connect the skin and fascia to the pectoralis muscle. Although breasts are usually symmetric, slight variation in shape between the breasts is normal. Breast size in a woman may vary with age, menstrual cycle, and pregnancy. Breasts should be fairly mobile, and the skin should be the same as that of the abdomen.

The areolae are pigmented areas surrounding each nipple. Color may vary from pink to brown and may change during pregnancy. The size of the areolae vary greatly; it may enlarge during pregnancy and remain enlarged. Montgomery's tubercles, sebaceous glands, are found within the areolae. Nipples are projectile tissue that contain the ducts from the glandular milk-producing tissue. Nipples are the same color as or a little darker than the areolae, and generally "point" up and laterally.

The breast contains several lymph node groups (Fig. 13-8). Most but not all of the lymph drains toward the axilla. The lymphatic system within and proximal to the breasts frequently serves as a vehicle for the spread of cancer.

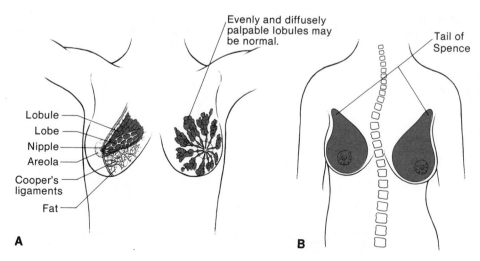

FIGURE 13.7 Female breast anatomy. *(A)* Internal tissues and support structures. *(B)* Tail of Spence extends to support axilla. Note normal asymmetry of breasts due to scoliosis.

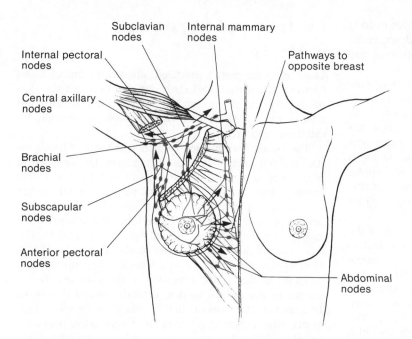

FIGURE 13.8 Lymphatic drainage of the breast. *Arrows* indicate direction of lymph flow.

The breast examination has two components—inspection and palpation—that are performed with the person in sitting and supine positions. The chest and breast must be completely exposed for inspection. The nurse should provide appropriate explanations during the breast examination. Cold hands can interfere with the individual's comfort and with the interpretation of examination findings. During inspection the breast can be described using two mapping methods: the clock and the quadrant. In the clock method, the breast is compared with the face of a clock, with the nipple at the center. Lesions or other findings should be located by their position on the clock face such as 11 o'clock or 2 o'clock. The quadrant method divides the breast into four areas: upper inner, upper outer (including the tail of Spence), lower outer, and lower inner. Horizontal and vertical lines cross at the nipple (Fig. 13-9).

Examination and Documentation Focus

- Size, shape, and symmetry
- Skin color, texture, lesions, and vascular patterns
- Tissue quality

- Breast lymphatics
- Nipple discharge

ND_x

Documenting Breast and Axilla Examination Findings

Record breast examination findings carefully so that comparison with subsequent findings will be meaningful and reliable. Any changes noted by the person should also be recorded. If a breast lump is discovered, document the following characteristics:

- Location, using clock orientation or quadrants, and distance from nipple in centimeters
- Size (length and width), in centimeters
- Shape
  - Consistency (soft, hard, rubbery)
  - Discreteness (are borders easy to distinguish from surrounding tissue?)

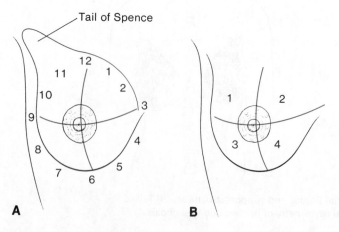

A **B**

FIGURE 13.9 Breast examination landmarks. *(A)* Breast clock landmarks, including tail of Spence; *(B)* breast quadrants.

▼ ▼ ▼
G U I D E L I N E S

A s s e s s m e n t G u i d e l i n e s   Breasts: Physical Assessment

Perform breast inspection with the person in five different positions: seated with arms at side, with arms over head, leaning over, with hands pressed onto hips, and supine. Inspecting the breast in these five positions enables the nurse to assess the quality of fibrous tissue stretching limits, to determine whether any part of the breast is fixed, and to detect asymmetry or decrease in breast mobility as positions are changed.

Procedure

1. **Inspect breasts with the person in the following positions:**
   a. Seated with arms at side. Ask the person to sit comfortably with both arms at the side. Observe breasts for symmetry, size, shape, skin color, texture, vascular patterns, presence of moles, nevi, lesions, and visible lymph nodes. Note direction and symmetry of nipples and any discharge.

      If you detect abnormalities, ask the person when the finding was first noted and whether there have been any past evaluations or treatment. Inspect the breast from different angles and positions.

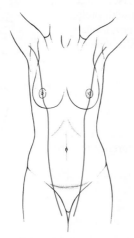

Milk lines

   b. *Arms over head.* Ask the person to raise both arms over the head, and continue to inspect the breasts.

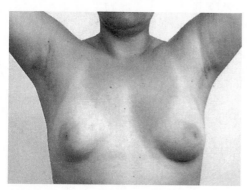

Breast examination: Arms over head

Clinical Significance

Normal Findings

Breast size and shape may vary according to age and body type, but breasts should be symmetric. Slight asymmetry may be normal if not a recent development. The nipples should look the same on each breast and point slightly up and laterally. Inverted nipples may be congenital and are insignificant if the condition existed before puberty. Inverted nipples may make breast-feeding difficult. Note the exact location of any supernumerary nipples (extra congenital nipples found along milk lines from the axilla to the groin). During movement, breast size and shape should remain symmetric.

Normal skin color: Skin color should be the same on each breast and similar to that of the abdomen. Areolae should be pink to brown. Nipples and Montgomery tubercles may be slightly darker than areolae. There may be a few hair follicles around the areolae.

Normal vascular patterns on the skin: Vascular patterns should be symmetric. Vascular patterns may be difficult to note on dark-skinned persons. Increased vascularity, indicated by bluish or reddish hues, may occur during pregnancy. Such vascular changes should be symmetric and diffuse.

Deviations from Normal

Skin: The breast should be without lesions; however, moles and nevi are common. The breasts are susceptible to the same lesions as the rest of the skin. Prominent or asymmetric venous pattern or peau d'orange (edema of the skin) may indicate malignancy.

Change in breast size/shape: A unilateral change in size, shape, or symmetry of the breast is abnormal. When the arms are raised or lowered or when the person is lying down or leaning over, any change in symmetry may be the result of a mass or lesion restricting the stretching ability of the ligaments. Note whether one breast seems to be fixed to the chest wall or shortens, dimples, or bulges with movement.

Nipples: Recent nipple inversion is abnormal and is a sign of retraction. Bright red nipples and areola may be an indication of Paget's disease (see Display 13–4, "Deviations from Normal Breast Findings").

DISPLAY 13.4

Deviations from Normal Breast Findings

RETRACTION SIGNS

- Signs include skin dimpling, creasing, or changes in the contour of the breast or nipple
- Secondary to fibrosis or scar tissue formation in the breast
- Retractions signs may appear only with position changes or with breast palpation.

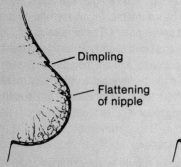

Dimpling

Flattening of nipple

Retraction signs   *Retraction with compression*

BREAST CANCER MASS [MALIGNANT TUMOR]

(See Chapter 5 for risk factors)
- Usually occurs as a single mass (lump) in one breast
- Usually nontender
- Irregular shape
- Firm, hard, embedded in surrounding tissue
- Referral and biopsy indicated for definitive diagnosis

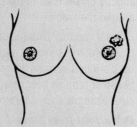

Breast cancer mass

BREAST CYST [BENIGN MASS OF FIBROCYSTIC DISEASE]

- Occur as single or multiple lumps in one or both breasts
- Usually tender (omitting caffeine reduces tenderness); tenderness increases during premenstrual period
- Round shape
- Soft or firm, mobile
- Referral and biopsy indicated for definitive diagnosis, especially for first mass; later masses may be evaluated over time by a specialist

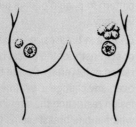

Breast cysts

FIBROADENOMA [BENIGN BREAST LUMP]

- Usually occurs as a single mass in women aged 15–35 years
- Usually nontender
- May be round or lobular
- Firm, mobile, and not fixed to breast tissue or chest wall
- No premenstrual changes
- Referral and biopsy indicated for definitive diagnosis

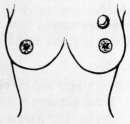

Fibroadenoma

INCREASED VENOUS PROMINENCE

- Associated with breast cancer if unilateral
- Unilateral localized increase in venous pattern associated with malignant tumors
- Normal with breast enlargement associated with pregnancy and lactation if bilateral and bilateral symmetry

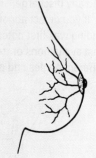

Increased venous prominence

PEAU D'ORANGE [EDEMA]

- Associated with breast cancer
- Caused by interference with lymphatic drainage
- Breast skin has "orange peel" appearance
- Skin pores enlarge
- May be noted on the areola
- Skin becomes thick, hard, immobile
- Skin discoloration may occur

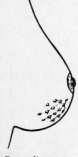

Peau d'orange

NIPPLE INVERSION

- Considered normal if long-standing
- Associated with fibrosis and malignancy if recent development

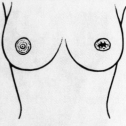

Nipple inversion

Deviations from Normal Breast Findings *(continued)*

ACUTE MASTITIS [INFLAMMATION OF THE BREASTS]

- Associated with lactation but may occur at any age
- Nipple cracks or abrasions noted
- Breast skin reddened and warm to touch
- Tenderness
- Systemic signs include fever and increased pulse

PAGET'S DISEASE [MALIGNANCY OF MAMMARY DUCTS]

- Early signs: Erythema of nipple and areola
- Late signs: Thickening, scaling, and erosion of the nipple and areola

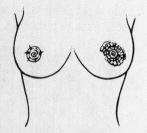

Paget's disease

▼ ▼ ▼

G U I D E L I N E S *continued*

Breasts: Physical Assessment

Procedure

c. *Leaning over.* Ask the person to lean over. You may need to support the person's arms to help with balance. If preferred, the person may stand and lean over. Continue to inspect the breasts.

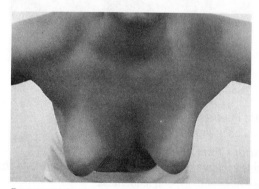

Breast examination: Leaning over

Clinical Significance

▼ ▼ ▼

GUIDELINES *continued*   Breasts: Physical Assessment

Procedure

d. *Pressing hands onto hips.* Ask the person to place hands on hips and press in. An alternate method is for the person to put palms together and press to cause the pectoral muscles to contract. Inspect as before.

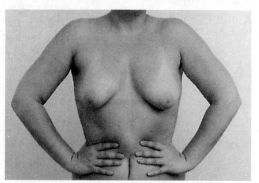

Breast examination: Pressing hands onto hips

2. **Palpate the breasts and axillae with the person in a sitting position.**
   (Option: see procedure for palpation in the supine position). The sitting position is optional unless the person reports an abnormal finding, has a history of breast abnormalities, has a high risk for breast cancer (family history), or has pendulous breasts.

a. Bimanually palpate pendulous breast. Use one hand to support the inferior side of the breast while palpating the breast with the dominant hand, moving from the chest wall toward and including the nipple.

Clinical Significance

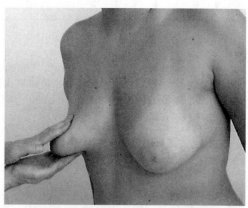

Bimanual breast palpation

Normal Findings
Lymph nodes should not be palpable.

Deviations from Normal
Palpable axillary nodes are abnormal. If palpated, note size, consistency, mobility, and tenderness.

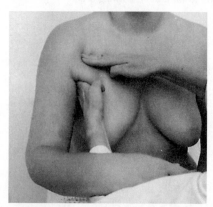

Axillae palpation: Seated position

▼ ▼ ▼

Procedure

b. Palpate the axillae while the muscles are relaxed. To relax the muscles, adduct and support the person's arm on top of your arm. Place the hand of the arm that is supporting the individual's arm in the axillae with the dominant hand on the anterior surface of the chest. Most of the lymphatic drainage of the breast is toward the axillae. Locate the nodes of the axillae according to their anatomic position. Evaluate the nodes by rolling the soft tissue against the chest wall and between your hands. Examine the anterior, posterior, medial, and lateral aspects of the axillae. Bimanually palpate the anterior aspect of the axillae to obtain access to the nodes near the pectoralis muscle. Also palpate the subclavian and supraclavicular nodes.

Clinical Significance

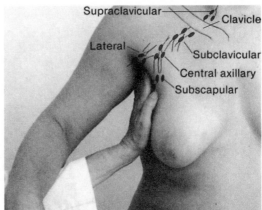

Axillae nodes: Palpatory areas

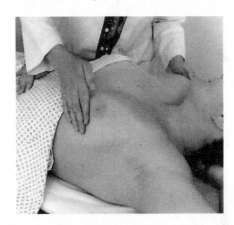

Breast palpation: Supine position

3. **Inspect and palpate the breasts with the person in the supine position.**

   a. Position the person on the examination table in the supine position. Place the arm on the same side as the breast being examined comfortably over and behind the person's head. For women with moderate to large breasts, place a folded towel or small pillow under the shoulder and upper back. Inspect each breast.

   b. Palpate to evaluate tissue texture and detect masses. Light palpation is followed by deep palpation. With deep palpation the breast tissue is pressed against the chest wall. Palpate all four quadrants and the tail of Spence. When palpating use the distal finger pads, the fingers held together, and move the fingers in a circular motion without lifting until the assessment is complete. Use a systematic approach. If person reports abnormal findings in one breast or inspection indicates possible problem, begin palpation in the nonsuspected breast. Give special attention to the upper outer quadrant and the tail of Spence, because most breast changes develop in the upper outer quadrant and the tail of Spence.

• Placing the arm over the head or a small pillow aids in displacing tissue evenly over the chest wall and enhances the examination.

• Keeping fingers continuously on the breast helps ensure that all breast tissue will be examined. A systematic approach helps ensure a consistent and complete evaluation. Begin palpation at the same location on both breasts. Use same clockwise, spoke, or vertical lines approach so findings from one breast can be compared with the other.

• Palpating the nonsuspicious breast first allows the nurse to establish a baseline for comparison.

▼ ▼ ▼

G U I D E L I N E S   *continued*   Breasts: Physical Assessment

Procedure

Clinical Significance

Normal Findings

Breast tissue should be smooth, elastic, soft, and easily moved. During palpation, the normal breast feels glandular and lumpy. The lumpiness is the result of glandular tissues, lobes, fat, and connecting fibers. The closer to the menstrual period, the more lumpy the breast may feel. Generally, the breast is not uniform in quality, but the two breasts are symmetrically uniform. A firm ridge, which is normal, may be noted along each breast between the 4- and 8-o'clock positions. Nipples should be smooth and may become erect during palpation.

Deviations from Normal

Palpation of any unusual *masses* or notation of differences in quality and quantity of breast tissue between breasts. All lumps should be referred for further evaluation. Tenderness may be due to a fibrocystic condition (see Display 13–4) or to malignancy. Increased temperature may indicate inflammation.

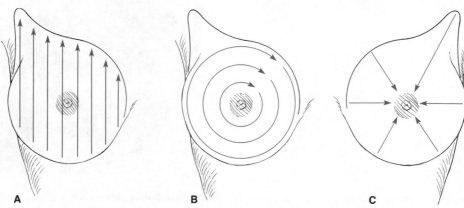

(A) Vertical lines approach; (B) clockwise approach; (C) spoke approach

c. Palpate the areola for underlying masses, and compress the skin around the nipple to assess for masses and discharge. If you note discharge, compress the breast along the suspected ducts to identify the lobe producing the discharge. Note color, consistency, and odor of discharge.

You may wish to use a glove on the hand that compresses the nipple.

Normal Findings

There should be no discharge from the nipple of a nonstimulated breast. A milky discharge (galactorrhea) may be normal during pregnancy and lactation; near or during the menstrual period; during sexual breast stimulation; as a side effect of some psychotropic drugs; and as a symptom of either hyper- or hypothyroidism.

Deviations from Normal

Any bloody nipple discharge should be considered the result of cancer until proved differently. Any discharge other than noted in normal findings should be evaluated and cultured.

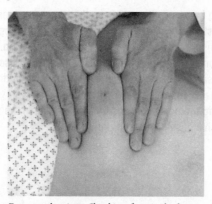

Breast palpation: Checking for nipple discharge

▼ ▼ ▼

G U I D E L I N E S   *continued*   Breasts: Physical Assessment

Procedure

4. The male breast

The male breast examination is essentially the same as the female breast examination. The breast should feel flat and smooth, and glandular breast tissue should not be present. The size and shape of the male breast vary according to body structure and fat distribution. The axillae are evaluated in men as in women.

Clinical Significance

Deviations from Normal

Gynecomastia, enlargement of the male breast, has multiple causes, such as drugs, illnesses, and pubertal changes. In adults this condition should receive prompt attention if the enlargement is a recent development.

- Mobility
  - Skin color over the lump
  - Tenderness to palpation
- Any retraction signs

If a lymph node in the axillary area or any other area is palpated, document the following:

- Location
- Size
  - Contour
  - Consistency
  - Discreteness
- Mobility
- Tenderness

Example 1: Normal Breast Assessment

Ms. M., aged 29, had a breast assessment when she came to the clinic for contraception and a cervical Pap smear. The examination results were normal and recorded as follows:

States she performs monthly breast self-examination (BSE) and has noted no changes, lumps, or tenderness except for a few days before menses. No palpable masses; no nipple discharge. No palpable axilla or supraclavicular nodes.

The same findings may be summarized in a problem-oriented format as follows:

S: Performs monthly BSE; no lumps or changes noted; slight breast tenderness a few days before menses every month.
O: Breasts symmetric with intact skin; no dimpling or edema. No symmetry changes in breast shape with movement. No palpable masses; no nipple discharge; no palpable axillary or supraclavicular nodes.
A: Practices and understands appropriate health screening activities; breast assessment within normal limits.
P: Reinforce appropriateness of BSE; advise next professional breast exam should be in 3 years unless

changes noted with BSE; consider baseline mammogram in 5 years.

Example 2: Breast Masses

Mrs. C, aged 40, reported to the clinic for a breast assessment after she found a single lump in her left breast. The assessment findings were recorded as follows:

Breasts symmetric with no visible masses, slight dimpling noted in upper outer quadrant when hands pressed on hips. No complaints of tenderness. No masses noted on palpation of right breast. In upper outer quadrant at 11 o'clock and 6 cm from nipple, firm mass, nonmobile, difficult to distinguish borders; approximately 0.5 by 0.25 cm, slight retraction with compression.

The same findings may be summarized in a problem-oriented format as follows:

S: Performs BSE every 3 to 4 months, found mass in left breast, upper outer quadrant, 3 days ago. Denies tenderness. LMP 10 days ago. No family history of breast cancer. No baseline mammogram.
O: Right breast—no visible or palpable masses, no changes in symmetry with movement, no dimpling. Vascularity symmetric bilateral. Left breast—slight dimpling upper outer quadrant only when hands pressing on hips; on palpation, noted firm mass in upper outer quadrant at 11 o'clock and 6 cm from nipple, nonmobile, difficult-to-distinguish borders approximately 0.5 by 0.25 cm, slight retraction with compression.
A: Abnormal breast assessment, need to rule out malignancy.
P: Refer to physician for diagnostic testing and treatment. Follow-up with phone call in 2 days.

ND$_X$

Clinical Problems Related to Breasts and Axillae

Clinical problems related to breasts and axillae generally are related to the integumentary system, the lymphatic system, and glandular tissue. Problems include breast cancer, fibrocystic and fibroadenoma disease, nipple inversion, and mastitis. These clinical problems are illustrated in Display 13-4.

PHYSICAL CHANGES DURING PREGNANCY

Anatomy and Physiology Overview

Observable physical changes occur throughout pregnancy, especially in the skin, breasts, abdomen, and pelvis. Less noticeable changes occur in other body systems, including the cardiovascular, gastrointestinal, genitourinary, respiratory, and musculoskeletal systems. Physical assessment of the pregnant woman is similar to that of other people and requires only occasional modification of technique.

Prenatal assessment involves periodic evaluation throughout pregnancy. Although the frequency of professional assessments depends on the person, the following schedule for clinic visits is generally recommended:

- First 28 weeks: every 3–4 weeks
- Last 12 weeks: every 1–2 weeks

At each prenatal visit, the following aspects of maternal and fetal health are evaluated:

- Weight
- Blood pressure
- Glucose and protein in the urine
- Fluid retention (edema)
- The height of the fundus
- The position of the fetus (Leopold's maneuvers)
- Fetal heart sounds

Other evaluations are conducted as needed and include the following:

- A complete head-to-toe physical assessment at the first prenatal visit
- Pelvic assessments at the first prenatal visit and during the last trimester
- Evaluation and measurement of the bony pelvis at the first prenatal visit and again at 32 to 36 weeks
- Specific examinations indicated by the condition of the mother or the fetus, such as abdominal ultrasound, amniocentesis, or antibody titers (some serologic testing may be required by state law)

See Display 13-5 for preventive services recommended for pregnant women by the US Task Force on Preventive Services.

DISPLAY 13.5

US Preventive Task Force Screening Recommendations for Pregnant Women

FIRST VISIT

Blood pressure
Hemoglobin/hematocrit

Hepatitis B surface antigen (HbsAG) to detect acute or chronic hepatitis
Rubella serology or vaccination history

STD screening
  Chlamydia <25 years
  Gonorrhea (high risk)
  VDRL/RPR (syphilis)
Pap smear
D(Rh) typing, antibody screen
HIV testing if high risk
Assess for problem drinking
If 35 and over and <13 weeks; gestation, offer chorionic villus sampling (CVS); if 15–18 weeks' gestation, offer amniocentesis for chromosomal defects.
Offer hemoglobinopathy screening (sickle cell) if high-risk group

FOLLOW-UP VISITS

Blood pressure
Urine culture (12–16 weeks)—untreated bacteriuria increases risk for preterm delivery
Offer amniocentesis if >35 years and 15–18 weeks' gestation.

Offer serum alpha-fetoprotein at 16–18 weeks (neuro tube defect)
Counseling
Tobacco cessation—effects of passive smoke
Alcohol and drug use
Nutrition
Breast feeding
Car seat restraint for self and infant
STD prevention
Chemoprophylaxis
Multivitamin with folic acid (neuro tube defect).

Adapted from US Preventive Task Force. (1996). *Guide to clinical preventive services* (2nd ed.). Baltimore: Williams & Wilkins.

Pregnancy is confirmed on the basis of characteristic subjective symptoms, physical signs, and laboratory values. Signs and symptoms are grouped into categories called presumptive signs, probable signs, and positive signs.

Presumptive signs of pregnancy include symptoms reported by the woman, such as the following:

- Amenorrhea 10 days or more past the date the menstrual period was expected to begin
- Morning sickness (nausea or vomiting persisting 3 weeks or more past the missed period)
- Tingling, soreness, or heaviness of the breasts

Probable signs of pregnancy include many physical assessment findings, including the following:

- Uterine enlargement
- Hegar's sign (softening of the uterine isthmus)
- Piskacek's sign (asymmetric enlargement of one uterine cornua)
- Chadwick's sign (bluish pigmentation of the vagina and cervix)
- Godell's sign (cervical softening)
- Internal ballottement of the uterus
- Urine or serum that is positive for human chorionic gonadotropin (hCG). The urine test for hCG can be done at home with an over-the-counter pregnancy test kit.

Positive signs of pregnancy confirm the presence of a fetus and include the following:

- Auscultation of a fetal heartbeat
- Palpation of fetal movement
- Identification of fetal parts by x-ray or ultrasound

Physical Changes During Pregnancy

Documenting Measurement of Fundal Height

Example 1: Normal Findings

J.A., 6 months pregnant, returns to the clinic for a regular visit. Findings are recorded as follows:

S: Now wearing maternity outfits—most of clothing no longer fits.
O: Has gained 3 pounds since last visit, fundal height 24 cm.
A: Fundal height growth and weight gain appropriate.
P: Return in 4 weeks for follow-up and repeat measurements.

Example 2: Abnormal Findings

S.S., 4 months pregnant, returns to the clinic for a regular visit. Abnormal Findings are recorded as follows:

S: Now wearing maternity outfits—most of clothes do not fit; with last pregnancy, did not change over until 6 to 7 months.
O: Has gained 4 pounds since last visit, fundal height at umbilicus, believe possibility of two different fetal heart sounds.
A: Possibility of more than one fetus.
P: To be seen by certified nurse midwife in 1 week, will follow up at that time.

Documenting Abdominal Palpation During Pregnancy

Example 1

S: Feels "butt" under ribs.
O: Nonengaged head presenting to pelvic outlet, spine along left side of uterus, feet palpated on right side.
A: Left, occipital, transverse position.
P: Assess in 3 weeks for engagement.

Example 2

S: Last baby was breech.
O: 30 weeks' gestation, fetal spine parallel to maternal spine, head palpated at fundus, nonengaged fetus.
A: Breech presentation.
P: Recheck position at next appointment in 3 weeks. Advise nurse midwife of findings today.

Documenting Fetal Heart Auscultation

Example 1: Normal Findings

Suzanne, 6 months pregnant, comes to the clinic for a regular visit. Findings are recorded as follows:

S: No data.
O: Fetal heart sounds 144 beats/min, and strong; uterine bruit 74/min heard in right upper outer quadrant of uterus.
A: Appropriate fetal heart rate.
P: Return in 1 month and repeat.

Example 2: Abnormal Findings

Diane, 7 months pregnant, comes to the clinic for her regular appointment. Abnormal findings are recorded as follows:

S: Last felt fetus move 1 week ago; before that, movement infrequent.
O: Unable to hear fetal heart sounds or uterine bruit where last heard: fundal height 2 cm less than 4 weeks ago.
A: Suspect possibility of fetal demise.
P: Refer to physician for immediate follow-up and diagnosis.

Physical Changes During Pregnancy

Changes

Clinical Significance

1. **Integumentary changes**
   a. Color and pigmentation
      (1) Month 2 through term, generalized hyperpigmentation develops, especially over the bony prominences and breast nipples and areola.
      (2) Week 16 through term: *linea nigra,* a brownish-black line extending from the umbilicus to the pubic bone, may appear.
      (3) Chloasma, mottled hyperpigmentation over the cheeks and forehead, may develop (called the mask of pregnancy).

   - Skin changes during pregnancy are common. The degree to which these changes occur varies from woman to woman and from pregnancy to pregnancy. Changes in the color and pigmentation of the skin during pregnancy are associated with an increased blood level of melanocyte-stimulating hormone. The resulting hyperpigmentation is benign, although body image may be altered.

   b. Moisture
      Increased perspiration (especially during the first trimester)

   - Secondary to increased output of the exocrine glands

   c. Thickness
      Gums hypertrophy

   - Secondary to proliferation of blood vessels in oral mucosa

   d. Turgor and mobility
      (1) Localized edema or ankle edema

   - Usually not considered pathologic; secondary to an increase in venous pressure in the lower extremities

      (2) Generalized edema

   - Caused by sodium and water retention secondary to elevated levels of steroid hormones

   e. Vascular alterations
      Palmar erythema; spider nevi over the face, chest, or abdomen

   - Secondary to the effects of estrogen and usually insignificant except for possible effects on body image

   f. Skin lesions
      Striae gravidarum (stretch marks), especially over breasts, abdomen, and thighs

   - Caused by stretching of the skin as weight is gained and fetus grows; pink or red during pregnancy and turning silvery white after delivery

2. **Breast changes**
   Breast changes are normal during pregnancy and include changes in size, shape, color, vascularity, and tissue quality.

   - Breast self-examinations should be practiced during pregnancy (see Chap. 5 for detailed breast self-examination techniques)

   a. Size and shape
      Month 2 through term and lactation: breast and nipple enlargement

   - Accompanies the increase in glandular and ductal tissue occurring because of hormonal influences and later because of milk production

   b. Skin color
      Hyperpigmentation of the nipple and areolae; the areolae may increase in size; secondary areolae may develop

   - Secondary to increased levels of melanocyte-stimulating hormone

   c. Vascularity
      Venous engorgement of the breasts; venous patterns should remain bilaterally symmetric

   - Causes the breast to appear larger, caused by the venous pressure increases during pregnancy. Venous engorged breasts may feel slightly warmer than surrounding skin and may be tender.

   d. Tissue quality
      Increased nodularity

   - The breasts may feel generally lumpy as glandular and ductal tissue become more prominent during pregnancy. Other breast lumps should be considered and ruled out.

   e. Lesions
      Striae gravidarium

   - Secondary to skin stretching as breasts change and enlarge

   f. Discharge
      Week 16 through term: colostrum may be secreted from the nipples. Amount secreted increases in the third trimester.

   - Colostrum, a yellowish premilk fluid, is secreted from the mammary glands. Milk is secreted 49–96 hours after delivery

(continued)

Physical Changes During Pregnancy (continued)

Changes

   g. Breast-feeding
      Preparation for breast feeding
      Feelings and nipples

Clinical Significance

- Understanding and feelings about breast-feeding should be explored during the third trimester. The nipples would also be assessed to determine whether they are everted or inverted. If the nipples are inverted, the woman should be shown how to roll the nipple to promote eversion. Ascertain whether she is toughening the nipples (preparing the nipples to withstand infant suckling) by methods such as rubbing them vigorously with a rough, dry washcloth.

3. Genital and Pelvic Changes

Changes in the genitals and pelvis are noted throughout pregnancy and include alterations in the appearance of the genitals, vagina, and cervix and changes in the consistency of the cervix and uterus.

- Generally, the pelvic assessment is conducted in the same manner for pregnant and nonpregnant women. Special variations in the technique of bimanual palpation may be required to elicit pregnancy signs, for example, Hegar's sign (see below). Advanced nurse practitioners and nurse midwives learn additional assessment techniques to determine pelvic configuration and size. Such techniques are discussed in most maternity textbooks.

   a. Genital pigmentation
      May note hyperpigmentation of labia or vulva

- Secondary to increased levels of melanocyte-stimulating hormone during pregnancy

   b. Vaginal discharge
      Moderate to profuse, thick, clear, odorless mucus is present from 6 weeks through term.

- Discharge is associated with increased vascularity of the vagina.
- Leukorrhea may be noted and represents discharge secondary to hypertrophied cervical glands.
- Any bloody or excessive water discharge may represent impending termination of pregnancy.

   c. Vaginal walls
      (1) Rugae become more pronounced.
      (2) Vaginal tissue becomes more edematous.
      (3) Vaginal skin develops a bluish pigmentation (Chadwick's sign).

- Caused by increased vaginal vascularity

   d. Cervix
      (1) By 6–8 weeks, the cervix has a bluish pigmentation (Chadwick's sign).
      (2) By 5–8 weeks, the cervix softens (Goodell's sign).

- Secondary to increased vascularity and venous congestion
- Secondary to increased vascularity

   e. Uterus
      (1) after 6 weeks, asymmetric uterine enlargement (Piskacek's sign)
      (2) By 6–8 weeks, softening of the uterine isthmus (Hegar's sign) (see Fig. 13–10). Modification to bimanual pelvic palpation: Place index and middle fingers into anterior vaginal fornix in front of the cervix. Use abdominal palpating hand to compress the uterus slightly above the symphysis pubis so that the isthmus is trapped between both hands.

- Related to rapid uterine enlargement at site of ovum implantation
- Secondary to increased vascularity

      (3) After 6 weeks, the cervix and uterus may be flexed at the junction during bimanual palpation (McDonald's sign).

- Secondary to increased vascularity

      (4) After 16 weeks, uterine ballottement is possible; elicited by tapping 2 fingers against the cervix.

- The rebounding of the fetus against the uterus

4. Miscellaneous physical changes

Miscellaneous changes occur throughout the body during pregnancy.

   a. Posture
     • Increased lumbar lordosis

- The expanding uterus contributes to lumbar lordosis.

(continued)

Physical Changes During Pregnancy (continued)

Changes

Clinical Significance

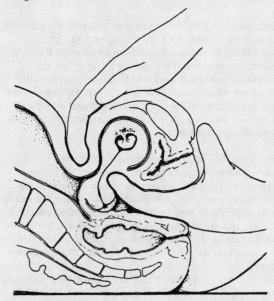

FIGURE 13.10   Bimanual palpation: Hegar's sign.

- Increased dorsal kyphosis and cervical lordosis

b. Gait
   Waddling gait
c. Weight
   Progressive weight gain; optimal weight gain is 15–40 pounds, depending on age, height, and body mass index before pregnancy. Pattern of weight gain is more important than total weight gain—usually 2–4 pounds first trimester and 1 pound per week thereafter.
d. Vital signs
   (1) Heart rate may increase slightly—10–15 beats per minute more.
   (2) Systolic blood pressure usually unchanged; diastolic may decrease slightly. In last trimester, there may be a slight fall.
   (3) Respiratory rate may increase; after 7 months thoracic breathing replaces abdominal breathing.

e. Heart sounds
   A physiologic systolic murmur (grade II/IV) may be heard during the third trimester. Apical pulse may be displaced laterally 1 cm.
f. Hair
   Loss or straightening of scalp hair, increased facial or abdominal hair
g. Elimination
   (1) Reduced peristalsis

   (2) Urinary frequency—more evident during first and third trimesters
5. **Abdominal Changes**
   The abdomen is evaluated at regular intervals during pregnancy to determine fetal growth and development, gestational age, fetal position and lie, and fetal heart rate.

- These changes represent compensation for lumbar lordosis and are necessary to maintain a safe center of gravity.
- Secondary to postural alterations and slight instability of the pelvis
- Secondary to fetal growth, placenta, amniotic fluid, maternal fat storage, breast enlargement, increased blood volume, extracellular fluid

- Secondary to increased blood volume and increased oxygen consumption
- A decreased peripheral vascular resistance alters the diastolic blood pressure.

- Secondary to increased oxygen consumption and breathing pattern changes due to displacement of the diaphragm by the growing fetus

- Results from increased blood flow secondary to an increased blood volume. Displacement is a result of fetal growth

- Secondary to increased amounts of androgens and corticotrophic hormones

- Secondary to relaxation of the muscles of the large intestines
- The uterus compresses the bladder against the pelvis, thereby reducing capacity.

The following Assessment Guidelines provide information on how these are assessed.

▼ ▼ ▼
G U I D E L I N E S

Assessment Guidelines   Physical Examination of Fundal Height, Fetal Heart, and Fetal Lie

Procedure

1. Equipment needed
Measuring tape in centimeters
Fetoscope or Doppler ultrasound stethoscope

2. Measuring fundal height

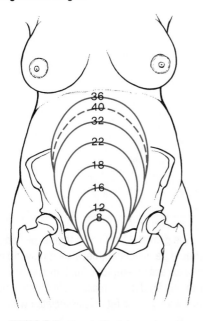

FIGURE 13.11   Fundal height and gestational age.

a. Before 13 weeks' gestational age, the height of the fundus is evaluated by bimanual pelvic examination

b. After 13 weeks
   1) The fundus is palpable with one hand over the abdomen. With the woman supine, place your fingers over the abdomen as shown in the figure. Start to palpate from above the point where you expect the fundus to be palpable; then progressively palpate downward

Clinical Significance

• The term *fundus* refers to the body of the pregnant uterus. During pregnancy, the height of the fundus is measured at each prenatal visit to evaluate fetal growth. The height of the fundus correlates with gestational age (Fig. 13–11).

• This procedure is usually performed by a professional nurse with additional advanced education, such as a certified nurse midwife and nurse practitioner.

Normal Findings
When you note a change in tissue consistency from soft to firm, you have palpated the fundus. Slight measurement variations may occur with different examiners. Nevertheless, expect progressive increases of approximately 1 cm per week in fundal height until week 37–40, then a decrease. Increasing size is associated with fetal growth. A decrease in fundal height at 37–40 weeks is associated with pelvic engagement of presenting part.

▼ ▼ ▼

Physical Examination of Fundal Height, Fetal Heart, and Fetal Lie

Procedure

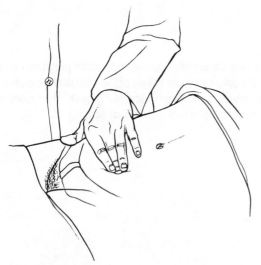

Fundal height palpation

2. When the fundus expands above the umbilicus, the height of the fundus may be measured with a tape measure. Place the end of the tape measure at the top of the symphysis pubis and measure the distance in centimeters to the height of the fundus.

Clinical Significance

Deviations from Normal

Excessive uterine growth (4 cm more than expected for gestational age) should be evaluated, because it may indicate more than one fetus, excessive amniotic fluid, or a very large fetus. Excessive amniotic fluid is often associated with congenital anomalies, and a very large fetus is associated with maternal diabetes mellitus.

A stoppage of growth may indicate fetal death, whereas slow uterine growth may indicate incorrect calculation of gestation or retarded growth.

An ultrasound of the uterus is indicated with unusual uterine growth.

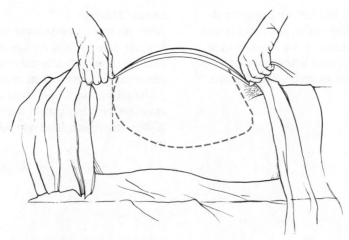

Fundal height measurement

▼ ▼ ▼

G U I D E L I N E S   *continued*

Physical Examination of Fundal Height, Fetal Heart, and Fetal Lie

Procedure

3. Fetal position and lie

Leopold's maneuvers consist of four abdominal palpation techniques for determining fetal position and lie.

a. Assist the woman into a supine position on the examining table. Tensing of the abdominal muscles may be minimized by slightly flexing the knees and supporting them with a pillow.

b. Begin with fundal palpation to determine what fetal part occupies the fundus. Stand beside the woman, *facing* her head. Place both hands on top of the fundus and palpate to determine which fetal part is presenting.

Clinical Significance

The fetal lie can be longitudinal (fetal spine fairly parallel to mother), transverse (fetal spine somewhat perpendicular to mother's spine), and oblique (fetal lie is between longitudinal and transverse). Leopold's maneuvers are performed routinely after 26 weeks' gestation, when the fetal parts are more discernible.

• The buttocks of the fetus, the most frequently presented part, will feel soft and slightly irregular with limited side to side mobility. The head will feel firm, hard, and round and may be more freely movable.

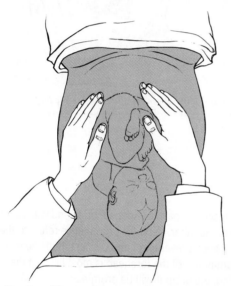

First Leopold's maneuver: Fundal palpation

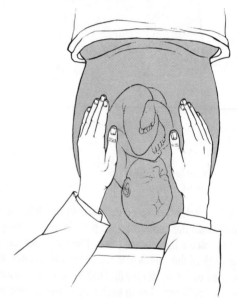

Second Leopold's maneuver: Lateral palpation

c. Next determine the position of the spine by *lateral palpation.* Move your hands from the fundus to the sides of the abdomen. Support one side of the fetus with one hand while using your other hand to palpate the opposite side of the uterus. Then palpate the other side of the abdomen in a similar fashion.

d. The third maneuver, called *Pawlik palpation,* determines what fetal part lies over the pelvic inlet. Place your right hand just above the symphysis pubis, then grasp the skin firmly between your thumb and third finger.

• The fetal spine will feel bony and continuous, whereas the limbs will feel irregular or nodular.

• A nonengaged head is palpable as a movable, round hard, smooth mass. If the head is engaged, you may feel a shoulder as a bony, nonmovable nodule.

▼ ▼ ▼
G U I D E L I N E S   *continued*

Physical Examination of Fundal Height, Fetal Heart, and Fetal Lie

Procedure

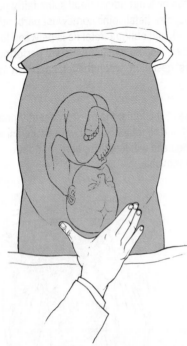

Third Leopold's maneuver: Pawlik palpation

e. Finally, perform *deep pelvic palpation* to determine the position of the head (cephalic prominence). Change position to face the woman's feet. Place both hands over the neck of the uterus just above the pelvic inlet. Ask the woman to inhale deeply and exhale slowly. During exhalation, apply pressure to each side of the uterine neck.

f. During palpation you may note occasional abdominal movement or contractions.

Clinical Significance

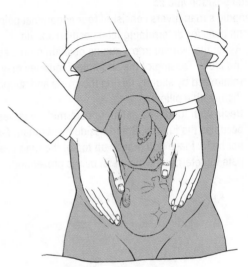

Fourth Leopold's maneuver: Deep pelvic palpation

- If the presenting part is engaged, one hand will descend further than the other. Cephalic prominence refers to that part of the fetal head preventing hand descent. If the head is flexed, the prominence of the forehead is most likely. If the head is extended, the occiput will be prominent.
- While performing these procedures, you may feel the head or buttocks during the second maneuver. The head may be felt with the first maneuver and the buttocks with the third or fourth maneuver. All of these positions indicate that the fetus may have a breech or transverse lie. Such findings need further evaluation by a specialist because of risk to the mother and fetus.
- Abdominal movement is fetal movement and is felt especially after 6 months' gestation. The nurse also may feel contractions while performing Leopold's maneuvers. Intensity of contraction may be mild to strong. Note frequency, length, and strength. Stop performance of maneuvers until contraction is complete.

Physical Examination of Fundal Height, Fetal Heart, and Fetal Lie

---

Procedure

4. Fetal heart assessment

Fetal heart tones are an indicator of the health of the fetus throughout pregnancy beginning at about 10–12 weeks, when heart sounds are first detected by Doppler flow devices. After 16 weeks, heart tones may be detected by the fetoscope.

Clinical Significance

- The intensity of fetal heart sounds varies depending on the position of the fetus.

Normal Findings

Fetal heart rates are between 120 and 160 beats/minute. A uterine bruit (also called uterine souffle), representing increased uterine blood flow, is a normal variation and will occur at the same pulse rate as the woman's pulse rate.

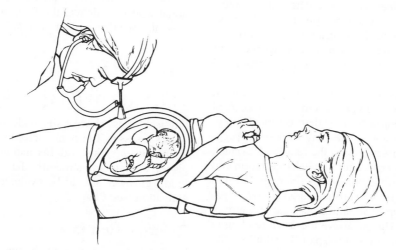

Fetal heart auscultation

Generally, heart sounds are auscultated by placing the fetoscope over the area between the symphysis pubis and umbilicus. Occasionally, heart tones are heard slightly above the umbilicus.

Deviations from Normal

A heart rate lower than 120 or greater than 160 may indicate fetal distress. A soft or absent uterine bruit may indicate poor uterine blood flow and placental function.

Nursing Diagnoses Related to Special Examinations for Pregnancy

Pregnancy is a time of great adjustment (physical as well as psychosocial) for the woman and her partner. Nursing diagnoses from other functional areas would include Altered nutrition (see Chap. 6), Health-seeking behavior (see Chap. 5), Fatigue (see Chap. 8), Sleep pattern disturbance (see Chap. 10), Altered family process and Potential for altered parenting (see Chap. 12), Spiritual distress (see Chap. 15), and Ineffective individual and family coping (see Chap. 14). Pregnancy also can alter or challenge perceptions regarding sexuality. Nursing diagnoses in the sexuality pattern that apply to pregnant women include Rape–trauma syndromes, Sexual dysfunction, and Altered sexual patterns. A discussion of these diagnoses is included in the section on female genitals and pelvic structures in this chapter. Characteristics unique to pregnancy for these diagnoses are addressed here.

Rape–Trauma Syndromes

Pregnancy may be an outcome of the rape event. This can place an additional burden on the woman: Should the pregnancy be aborted, or should the infant be placed for adoption or kept in the family? The stresses that normally occur after rape are compounded by the necessity of this decision.

Sexual Dysfunction and Altered Sexuality Patterns

During pregnancy, many factors can affect sexual functioning. There may be a fear of damage to the fetus or breast leakage with coitus, fatigue, cultural beliefs regarding coitus and pregnancy, changes in sexual drive and satisfaction, and discomfort (dyspareunia) during coitus with traditional positions. Sexual identity confusion is common during pregnancy and in the postpartum period (Carpenito, 1997). Sexual partners also may affect the woman's perception of her own sexuality. The partner also may fear hurting the fetus or the pregnant woman. If the pregnancy was unplanned, both partners may experience feelings of guilt.

ND_X

Clinical Problems Related to Pregnancy

During pregnancy, women can experience any clinical problem they could have when not pregnant. The risks and occurrences of sexually transmitted diseases are the same for the pregnant woman as the nonpregnant woman. (Refer to the discussion of sexually transmitted diseases and women in this chapter.)

Clinical problems related solely to pregnant women include pregnancy-induced hypertension (toxemia), fetal demise, and fetal presentation other than occipital. Pregnancy-induced hypertension is the only disease of pregnancy and can be life-threatening to the fetus and woman. This problem generally occurs after 24 weeks' gestation and is characterized by a systolic blood pressure over 140 mm Hg or a 30 mm Hg rise above the usual reading in two measurements at least 6 hours apart, and a diastolic pressure of 90 mm Hg or a 15 mm Hg rise above the usual reading in two measurements at least 6 hours apart. In addition, the woman will have protein in her urine, excessive weight gain, and edema of her face or hands. In the later stages of toxemia, convulsions and death can occur. This condition is considered a medical emergency, and the woman should be seen by a specialist immediately.

Fetal demise can occur for numerous reasons and often results in a natural abortion (miscarriage). Sometimes a natural abortion does not occur, and a therapeutic abortion must be performed. Mummification of the fetus can occur if the fetus is not aborted. Cardinal signs of fetal demise include no fetal heart sounds, no fetal movement, and no growth or decreasing fundal size. With natural abortions, signs and symptoms include increased vaginal secretions, vaginal spotting or bleeding, and uterine contractions before fetal survivability.

Fetal presentations other than occipital are not of great concern until engagement occurs. The fetus can and does change position. Fetal positions that can cause trauma for the woman and fetus include breech (buttock), shoulder presentation, and transverse lie. With breech presentation, the buttock is engaged; if the fetus delivered vaginally, the legs and feet are generally delivered with the body and the head is last. Shoulder presentation can cause the most difficulty, and generally the fetus is delivered by cesarean section. With shoulder presentation, the shoulder is in the pelvic outlet and the body lies horizontally (transverse lie) in the uterus. With complete transverse lie, the fetus can only be delivered by cesarean section. The health professional who is to deliver the fetus should be advised of all presentations that are not occipital.

THE MALE

Genitalia and Inguinal Area

Physical assessment of the male reproductive system involves assessing the penis, scrotum, and the groin area for lymphatic integrity and herniating masses. The prostate gland, an internal structure that contributes to seminal fluid formation, should be evaluated during the rectal examination (see Chap. 7).

External Genitals

The visible external reproductive structures include the penis, urinary meatus, and scrotum. The *penis* is a hairless, cylindrical organ that is normally flaccid, except during sexual arousal. The *glans penis* is the bulbous end of the penis. In an uncircumcised man, the glans may be partially or completely covered by a loose fold of skin called the *foreskin* or prepuce (Fig. 13-12). The *coronal ridge* or *corona* forms the border between the glans penis and the penile shaft. The *frenulum,* a fold of tissue between the glans and shaft that joins the foreskin to the glans, is extremely sensitive to erotic stimuli. The urethral opening, located near the ventral tip of the penis, appears as a small, horizontal slit. Tyson's

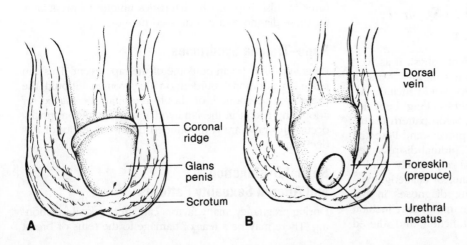

A

- Coronal ridge
- Glans penis
- Scrotum

B

- Dorsal vein
- Foreskin (prepuce)
- Urethral meatus

FIGURE 13.12 External male genitals. *(A)* Circumcised; *(B)* uncircumcised.

glands are modified sebaceous glands located around the corona and on either side of the frenulum. Secretions from the glans are one of the components of smegma, an odorous, cheese-like material that is a good bacterial growth medium if not removed.

The penis has three columns of erectile properties secondary to vascular engorgement: the corpus *spongiosum,* which surrounds the urethra, and the left and *right corpus cavernosum,* which are located along the dorsal half of the penis and terminating at the glans.

The *scrotum* is the pendulous sac of tissue behind the penis that holds the testicles. The scrotal skin, which has a darker pigment than surrounding skin, is hair-covered, with a medium ridge or *raphe* extending from the base of the penis to the anus. The raphe divides the scrotal sac into two sections. The left side of the scrotum usually hangs slightly lower than the right because the spermatic cord is longer in the left testicle. The cremasteric or dartos muscle surrounds the testicles and spermatic cord. These muscles contract in response to cold, causing the scrotum to appear smaller than usual.

Internal Structures

The internal male genitalia are designed for sperm production and propulsion as well as urinary excretion. Sperm forms in the *testes,* enters the coiled tubules of the *epididymis,* and is propelled by muscle contraction through the *vas deferens* and *ejaculation duct,* and through the *prostate gland.* During ejaculation, sperm leaves the prostate and passes through the urethra and urinary meatus (Fig. 13-13). *Cowper's glands,* located near the prostate, are homologous to female Bartholin glands and secrete mucus into the sperm during sexual arousal. Additional secretions are produced by the *seminal vesicles.*

The Inguinal Area

The term *inguinal* refers to the groin region. Several inguinal structures are routinely assessed as part of the male

genital examination. The *inguinal ligament* is an important assessment landmark that extends from the anterior iliac spine to the pubic tubercle. Above and parallel to the inguinal ligament is the *inguinal canal,* which carries the spermatic cord (Fig. 13-14). The distal opening of the inguinal canal is called the *external inguinal ring,* a structure accessible to palpation. Occasionally, because of weakness in the abdominal wall, the visceral contents protrude through the inguinal canal and, in some cases, extend through the external inguinal ring into the scrotum. This is called an *inguinal hernia.* The femoral canal, although not generally palpable, represents another potential route for herniation. The femoral canal lies below the inguinal ligament, medial to the femoral artery. Lymphatic chains are located below the inguinal ligament and medial to the femoral vein.

Assessment and Documentation Focus

Penis: skin color and pigmentation, skin lesions, masses, or discharge; discharge from urinary meatus
Scrotum: skin integrity, consistency of testicles, epididymis, and vas deferens
Inguinal area: bulges, masses

ND

Documenting Male Genital and Inguinal Examination Findings

Example 1: Normal Findings

Mr. L, age 26, had a complete physical assessment, including genital and hernia assessment. The findings were normal and recorded as follows:

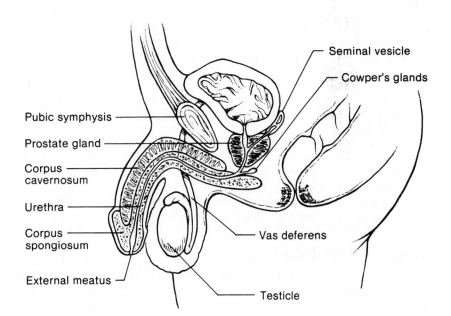

FIGURE 13.13   Internal male genitals.

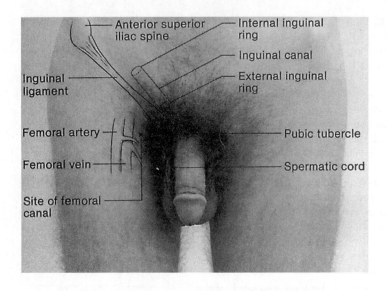

FIGURE 13.14   Male inguinal structures.

External genital skin smooth without lesions or discharge. Testes descended and equal size, scrotal contents smooth, nontender. No palpable masses in inguinal or femoral canals.

These same findings may be recorded in a problem-oriented format as follows:

S: Denies genital lesions, dysuria, or urethral discharge.
O: External genital skin smooth; no lesions or discharge. Testes descended and equal size, scrotal contents smooth, nontender. No palpable masses in inguinal or femoral canals.
A: Normal male genitals, no inguinal or femoral hernias.
P: Evaluate teaching needs regarding TSE, STDs, reproductive management. Routine annual follow-up.

Example 2: Suspected Inguinal Hernia

Mr. B., age 45, had an inguinal assessment in an occupational health clinic. He had recently been treated for low back pain. The findings were abnormal and recorded as follows:

No visible inguinal masses. Small, firm mass palpated in right inguinal canal with Valsalva maneuver. Nonpalpable when relaxed.

These findings may be recorded in a problem-oriented format as follows:

S: Job responsibilities include heavy lifting. Denies genitourinary problems such as dysuria, lesions, or urethral discharge.
0: No visible inguinal masses. Small, firm mass palpated in right inguinal canal with Valsalva maneuver. Not palpable when relaxed.
A: Suspect indirect inguinal hernia.
P: Evaluate teaching needs regarding hernia complications and preventive treatment—proper body mechanics while lifting. Refer to physician.

Example 3: Genital Skin Lesions

Mr. M., age 18, came to the student health clinic for evaluation and treatment of genital skin lesions. The physical assessment findings were recorded as follows:

Nit-like particles on shaft of pubic hair concentrated at base of penis and scattered on pubic hair of scrotum. No lice or other parasites noted. Small cluster of multiple vesicles noted at base of penis. Skin otherwise intact. Reports burning at lesion sites and generalized genital area itching.

ND_X

Clinical Problems Related to Male Genital and Inguinal Examination

Sexually Transmitted Diseases

Gonorrhea.   Although the clinical course and presentation of the disease vary, men with gonorrhea, unlike women, are seldom asymptomatic. Usual symptoms are related to urinary elimination and appear early as the organism invades the urethra. The man may report urgency, frequency, burning, and a serous or purulent urethral discharge. Within a week of exposure, the discharge may become profuse, yellow, and blood-tinged. The discharge should be cultured on a Thayer-Martin medium to identify the organism. Rectal infection may be noted in homosexual men and is associated with rectal pain and burning as well as purulent discharge. Infection of the oropharynx should not be overlooked. Untreated gonorrhea affects the epididymis, prostate, and periurethral glands, causing acute inflammation, and can result in infertility.

Syphilis.   As with women, untreated syphilis in men advances through five stages (see discussion earlier in this chapter). During early stages, a syphilitic chancre appears, usually on the glans penis or shaft. The chancre is a round, ulcerated papule that may be palpated with a gloved hand as a firm, hard mass, usually not painful. For those who engage in oral or anal intercourse, the chancre may be found near the mouth or anus.

Herpes.   Genital herpes presents as a cluster of small painful vesicles on the penis, which eventually rupture and heal. Recurrence is common. Viral shedding, even when vesicles are not present, can infect others during intercourse.

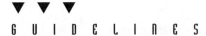

Assessment Guidelines   Male Genitalia: Physical Assessment

Procedure

1. Equipment
- Gloves: nonsterile
- Examination-type flashlight

2. Preparation and positioning
- Before starting, explain the procedure and answer any questions.
- The individual should stand for the assessment. The nurse should be seated, facing the individual's genitals.

3. Inspect and palpate the penis.
- a. Ask individual to expose genitals by lifting gown.
- b. Inspect hair distribution; look for any infestations.

- c. Inspect penis and note skin integrity of glans, foreskin, and shaft. If the individual is uncircumcised, ask him to retract the foreskin so that you can inspect the underlying area. Inspect the base of the penis and pubic hair; note any signs of infestation.

- d. Inspect the urinary meatus by grasping the glans between your thumb and forefinger and gently squeezing to expose the meatus.

Clinical Significance

Both hands should be gloved during the assessment. Gloves offer protection from inadvertent exposure if an infection is present. Gloves should be changed before the rectal assessment to avoid cross-contamination in the case of genital infections.

The inguinal area can be palpated easily in this position. The person may wear an examining gown that is easily lifted during the assessment.

Normal Findings
Normal hair distribution—covers the entire groin area, extending to thighs and toward the umbilicus. Free of infestations and erythema.

Deviations from Normal
Chemotherapy may cause loss of hair. Nits are often found at the base of the penis and pubic hairs.

Normal Findings
The size and shape of the penis normally vary considerably among adult men but are often a source of concern. Although penis size may vary considerably in the flaccid state, considerably less size variation exists in the erect penis. The glans penis varies in size and shape and may appear rounded, broad, or even pointed. Assist the individual to understand normal variations if he expresses concern. Smegma may be present (explain the need to clean this material from the penis).

Deviations from Normal
The presence of any rash, lesions, or lumps may indicate malignancy or an infection. A ventral curvature (chordee) of the penis shaft is abnormal and is the result of a fibrous band of tissue constricting the penis.

Normal Findings
Normally, the urinary meatus is free of drainage and discharge.

▼ ▼ ▼

GUIDELINES   *continued*   Male Genitalia: Physical Assessment

Procedure

If the person reports a history of discharge from the urethra but none is revealed by the above maneuver, ask him to milk the shaft of the penis from the base to the tip with his fingers.

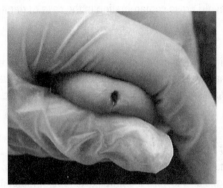

Inspecting the urinary meatus

e. Palpate the shaft of the penis between your thumb and forefinger, noting any masses or tenderness (optional in the young asymptomatic boy or man).

4. Inspect and palpate the scrotum.
  a. Displace the penis to one side or ask the person to do so, to inspect the scrotum.
  b. Lift the scrotal sac and inspect the posterior side. Note skin integrity. If the scrotum is enlarged, place a flashlight next to the scrotum and observe for transillumination of the scrotum.

  c. Palpate one scrotal compartment at a time by grasping the scrotum between your thumb and forefinger. Gently squeeze to detect the testicle, remembering that this maneuver may be slightly painful.

Clinical Significance

Deviations from Normal

Any discharge noted with this maneuver is abnormal and should be cultured. A yellow discharge may be gonorrhea. Any time the meatus is not found centered on the glans, it should be noted. The meatus may be found on the shaft of the penis; this is known as hypospadias.

Normal Findings

Masses should not be palpable along the shaft of the penis. The penis is not normally tender to palpation and should not be tender when the glans is squeezed gently to assess the urinary meatus.

Normal Findings

Scrotal size and shape vary considerably, and this may cause anxiety in men who believe the sexual myth that a large scrotum is associated with virility. Some scrotal sacs hang below the penis, whereas others are above. The left side of the scrotum is usually lower than the right. The scrotum is held high and appears smaller when scrotal muscles contract in response to fear or cold. Scrotal skin has scattered hairs. The skin should be thin and rugated, causing a wrinkled appearance.

Deviations from Normal

Lesions should be noted as abnormal. The absence of rugated skin, red color, warmth to touch, and an enlarged scrotum indicate inflammation and possibly infection. An enlarged scrotum that is not red may indicate excessive fluid or a mass in the scrotum. A scrotum that is enlarged with fluid (except for blood) will transilluminate. A scrotum enlarged by a mass such as intestines or tumor will not transilluminate.

Normal Findings

Two testicles that feel about 3.5–5 by 2.5 cm by 2.5 cm in size, ovoid in shape, smooth, and homogeneous in consistency should be palpable through the thin scrotal skin. The testicles should be freely movable, rubbery in consistency, equal in size, and slightly sensitive to compression.

▼ ▼ ▼

G U I D E L I N E S   *continued*   Male Genitalia: Physical Assessment

---

Procedure

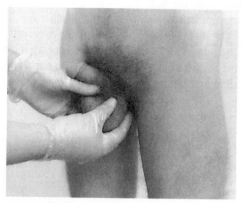

Scrotal palpation

d. Palpate the epididymis by grasping the posterior portion of the scrotum between your thumb and forefinger and feeling for a firm, comma-like structure. If not found in the posterior portion, it may be found in the anterolateral or anterior areas of the testes.

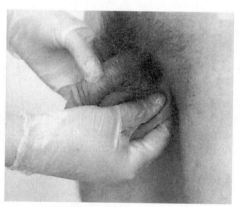

Palpating the epididymis

e. Finally, palpate the vas deferens by moving your thumb and forefinger from the epididymis to the vas in an anterior direction. Palpate the inguinal ring.

5. **Inspect for inguinal and femoral hernias.**
   a. Inspect the inguinal area and note any bulges. Ask the person to bear down "like having a bowel movement" so you can detect any bulges.

Clinical Significance

Deviations from Normal
Any inconsistency of homogeneity between the two testes should be evaluated. Malignant nodules are usually nontender. *Any mass should be referred immediately because testicular cancer metastasizes rapidly.* Absence of testes may indicate cryptorchidism.

Normal Findings
The epididymis should be firm. In 7% of men, the epididymis is located in the anterolateral or anterior portions of the testes.

Deviations from Normal
A nonfirm or very tender epididymis may indicate inflammation.

Normal Findings
The vas should feel cord-like and move freely. The epididymis should be discrete, smooth, nontender, and without masses. The vas deferens should feel like smooth cords and are movable and nontender.

Deviations from Normal
Palpable veins may indicate the presence of a varicocele. A thickened or tender cord may indicate an inflammation/infection.

Normal Findings
Bulges should not be noted on the skin overlying the inguinal and femoral canal or during coughing or straining.

▼ ▼ ▼

G U I D E L I N E S *continued*   Male Genitalia: Physical Assessment

Procedure

b. Palpate the area overlying the femoral canal with and without the person bearing down.

c. Palpate the skin overlying the superficial inguinal lymph nodes, noting enlargement and mobility of palpable nodes.

Clinical Significance

Deviations from Normal

A bulge may indicate a hernia. Enlarged nodes may indicate an infection distal to the area (legs and feet). If a mass is felt, have the person lie down and see whether it disappears. If it remains, auscultate for bowel sounds and try to push it upward into the abdomen. Do not do this if the area is extremely painful.

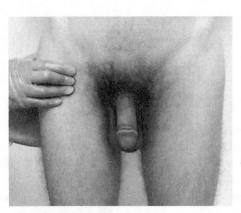

Femoral canal palpation

6. Palpate the inguinal canal.

a. To palpate the right inguinal canal, approach the person from the right side. Palpate the inguinal canal by invaginating the loose scrotal skin with your right index finger at the bottom of the scrotal sac. Follow the spermatic cord with your finger to the external inguinal ring, a triangular, slit-like opening. If the inguinal ring is large enough, continue advancing your finger along the inguinal canal. Ask the person to cough or bear down. Repeat the procedure on the left side.

Normal Findings

You should not feel a bulge in the inguinal canal or a mass moving down the canal when the person coughs or bears down.

Deviations from Normal

Palpable masses in the inguinal canal may represent hernias. See note above regarding evaluation of masses. See Display 13–6 for types of hernias in the inguinal–femoral area.

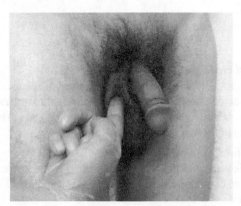

Inguinal canal palpation

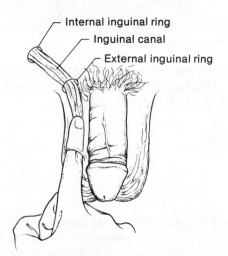

┌ Internal inguinal ring
┌ Inguinal canal
┌ External inguinal ring

Inguinal canal palpation

DISPLAY 13.6

Inguinal and Femoral Hernias

INDIRECT INGUINAL HERNIAS

An indirect inguinal hernia is a herniation through the inguinal canal. The hernia may be felt with the fingertip as a bulge in the canal or may extend beyond the canal into the scrotum. Indirect inguinal hernias may be detected by inserting your index finger into the inguinal canal.

DIRECT INGUINAL HERNIA

A direct inguinal hernia does not travel through the inguinal canal; rather, the hernia sac protrudes anteriorly through the abdominal wall. During inguinal canal palpation, the hernia displaces the examining finger forward.

Alternatively, a direct hernia may be felt as a bulge between the thumb and forefinger when palpating the skin around the external canal as the person bears down. Direct inguinal hernias rarely descend into the scrotum.

FEMORAL HERNIA

A femoral hernia may be detected below the inguinal ligament and medial to the femoral pulse as a visible or palpable bulge. Femoral hernias are more common in women.

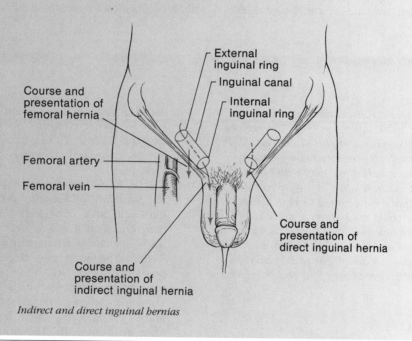

Indirect and direct inguinal hernias

Genital Warts. In men, warts appear on the penis as a single lesion or multiple elongated lesions. Occasionally, the warts proliferate to the extent that they appear as large cauliflower-like lesions. They may heal spontaneously or may undergo malignant transformation.

Nonspecific Urethritis. Affecting only men, nonspecific urethritis refers to urethritis from which specific organisms such as Gonococcus cannot be isolated. In many cases, *Chlamydia* may be the responsible organism. Men with nonspecific urethritis are usually sexually active with multiple partners. With physical assessment, a urethral discharge may be noted, ranging from a slight watery discharge to a copious, purulent discharge. The infection may spontaneously resolve within 8 weeks, although recurrences are common.

Other Conditions

Phimosis. In phimosis, the foreskin of an uncircumcised man cannot be retracted because of stenosis. Circumcision is indicated.

Carcinoma of the Penis. Malignant lesions are noted more often in uncircumcised men. The lesion, often covered by the foreskin, appears as a hard, nontender nodule.

Impotence. Impotence is the inability either to have an erection or to sustain an erection. Causes of impotence include diabetes mellitus, prostatectomy, arteriosclerosis, some medications for hypertension and depression, and any injury to the penis. On inspection and palpation, no abnormalities may be noted. Erectile devices are available; however, new medications such as alprostadil are available, and several new drugs are being tested that can produce an erection.

Scrotum Abnormalities

Hydrocele.   A hydrocele is a collection of fluid in the tunica vaginalis of the testicle. This abnormality is associated with many clinical conditions that involve inadequate fluid reabsorption, including local inflammation and injury, cirrhosis, congestive heart failure, and testicular tumor. On physical assessment, the scrotum is enlarged, and if transilluminated with a penlight, transmits light. Hydroceles are usually painless until large enough to create excessive pressure or scrotal pulling.

Varicocele.   A varicocele is a mass of varicose veins in the scrotum, usually around the spermatic cord. The mass is palpable, feels like a "bag of worms," and may dissipate after the person has been supine. It usually appears at puberty.

Scrotal Edema.   The scrotal skin can become edematous; palpation causes pitting. With any generalized edema associated with such conditions as congestive heart failure, scrotal edema is common.

Testicular Cancer.   Any palpable mass or nodules on the testicles should be suspected of malignancy. The testicular self-examination should be taught to adolescent men as a means of early detection (see Chap. 5). Tumor masses are often painless.

Epididymitis.   Epididymitis may result from the spread of an STD or from an infected prostate or urethra. The scrotum is usually diffusely tender, edematous, and erythematous. Localized scrotal pain may be noted, especially during palpation.

Torsion of the Spermatic Cord.   Torsion is an axial rotation or twisting of testicle on the spermatic cord. A mass is felt anterior to the testicle. Extremely painful, the scrotum may become edematous and erythematous. This condition is considered a surgical emergency because of obstructed circulation and eventual infarction of the testicle. It occurs most frequently in adolescents.

CASE STUDY 1

Manuel, aged 47, was recently discharged from the hospital after an acute myocardial infarction (MI). Although he has suffered no serious complications, his illness has frightened him and his wife. Before his discharge, many health care providers discussed his recovery with him and assessed his teaching needs in relation to diet, exercise, medications, and gradual resumption of work activities. His wife Tanya, age 40, could not be present for most of the teaching because she had to work. No one addressed sexual concerns. Manuel and Tanya both fear that sexual intercourse could be fatal to Manuel. Tanya is concerned about how she would take care of their four children without Manuel.

Profile Analysis

Manuel and Tanya both have the potential for sexual dysfunction because of the following risk factor: They are uninformed about sexual function after an MI. Moreover, the health care providers failed to elicit an important cue, so his potential problem has not been diagnosed and preventive measures have not been initiated.

Several factors may have contributed to failure to diagnose the problem. Factors that may have influenced assessment and, ultimately, diagnosis include the following.

1. *Failure to perceive sexual functions as part of the nursing domain.* The profile indicates that many other functions were evaluated before Manuel's discharge, but sexual functions were not. Possibly, sexuality assessment was not a usual part of the data collected by nurses at this institution. Such an omission may prevent the nurse from asking both Manuel and Tanya a simple screening question such as "What concerns do you have about sex after this illness?" Failure to ask the question could indicate that sexual matters were not a nursing concern.

2. *Failure to use pre-encounter patient data to notice the possibility of sexuality problems.* According to Carnevali and coworkers (1993), pre-encounter patient data such as age, gender, and medical diagnosis may be used to narrow or direct data collection. The nurse may decide on probable diagnoses and focus data collection by looking for cues to confirm diagnoses. It is well documented in nursing and medical literature that middle-aged men and their spouses often have sexual concerns after an acute MI. Therefore, the nurse should assess the sexual concerns of such individuals even though they may not initiate the discussion. Failure to use pre-encounter data may indicate a deficit in the nurse's knowledge base about acute MIs.

3. *Failure to extract meaning from the available cues.* Often the most meaningful cues are those that indicate well-known signs or symptoms of specific problems. Other cues may be more elusive or may be perceived by the nurse as unreliable, particularly if they do not correlate with textbook representations of a problem. For example, the most obvious cues indicating actual or potential sexual dysfunction include the defining characteristics for this nursing diagnosis specified by NANDA. Apparently, Manuel or Tanya did not reveal any such signs or symptoms to health care providers. However, other cues were significant. Manuel had risk factors for

CASE STUDY 1 *continued*

sexual dysfunction, including a major health problem, acute MI. Manuel and Tanya's failure to discuss
sexual concerns may serve as an indication of potential sexual dysfunction. The nurses also may have
believed that Manuel would be attending a cardiac
rehab program where he would receive information
regarding sexual activity. However, cardiac rehab is
not covered by his limited health insurance, and he
cannot afford to pay for it himself.

CASE STUDY 2

*Paul, age 62, is recovering from prostate surgery. He is
concerned because his long-term relationship had recently
ended, and he has had little emotional support while recovering and dealing with the fact that he has cancer.
When the nurse attempts to discuss sexual aspects with
him, Paul denies having any problems because he thinks
the nurse might not understand that his sexual partners
are usually men.*

Profile Analysis

Paul is unlikely to discuss sexual aspects of his health care
with providers he perceives might be judgmental about
his sexual lifestyle. The nurse should initiate the topic of
sexuality again and provide him with some written material even though no concerns have been expressed. If a
trusting relationship has developed between the nurse
and client, information is more likely to be shared. At all
times, avoid judgmental language such as "How do you
think your surgery will affect your relationships with
women?"

CASE STUDY 3

*Rebecca, age 19, is a freshman at a large university, living
away from home for the first time in campus housing. She
is taking 16 credits and has one night class. She is sexually active, having a total of three different partners. She
has not consistently used contraception but has avoided
pregnancy. She has come to the student health clinic for
oral contraceptives.*

Profile Analysis

1. *Identifying the problem.* The nurse considers the diagnosis Altered sexual pattern because of inconsistent use of contraception that places Rebecca at risk
   for unintended pregnancy.
2. *Pre-encounter knowledge.* The nurse recognizes that
   college students are sexually active and that many
students away from home for the first time experiment with a number of different sexually risky behaviors. The college nurse also has additional concerns for Rebecca and other college students. These
include unintentional pregnancy, STDs, and the
increase of heterosexually transmitted HIV (AIDS).
Additionally, there are always a few rapes on
campus.
3. *Cues in the profile.* The following cues indicate that
   Rebecca is at risk for Altered sexual pattern: living
   on campus—has night class, living away from home
   for the first time, has unprotected sexual intercourse. The nurse discusses with Rebecca her risks
   and examines alternatives with her to reduce those
   risks.

CASE STUDY 4

Ana, aged 72, is recovering from a mastectomy; because of the size of the tumor, a lumpectomy was not possible. She is an attractive woman who enjoys dressing fashionably, trying different hairstyles, and using cosmetics. A widow for 5 years, Ana is devoted to her children and grandchildren and is expecting her first great-grandchild. After surgery, Ana becomes depressed and withdrawn and finally tells the nurse that even though she has no desire to remarry, she feels she has lost her sexual identity. "Even an old woman like me needs to feel like a woman," she cries.

Profile Analysis

1. *Identifying the problem.* The nurses caring for Ana recognize cues indicating a potential problem with sexual health. Additionally, the diagnostic process is influenced by pre-encounter knowledge.
2. *Pre-encounter knowledge.* Ana is receiving care from the professional staff of a surgical oncology unit. The nurses realize that most cancer surgery, especially if disfiguring, threatens body image and influences sexuality, regardless of a person's age. Sexual health is especially threatened when cancer surgery affects organs such as breasts.

   Although younger people often express concerns related to sexual performance and procreative functions, the older person is also concerned with feeling like and being perceived by others as a sexual being. Both body image and sexuality contribute to a person's overall self-concept (see Chap. 11). On the basis of this knowledge, the nurses realize that because Ana has had a mastectomy, she is at greater risk of developing an altered body image, an altered sexuality, and an altered self-concept. Therefore, they collect data relevant to such diagnostic possibilities. The nurse considers the following questions: What does this surgery mean to Ana? How does she perceive self and body? What body parts have the greatest importance for the self-concept?
3. *Cues in the profile.* The following cue indicates that Ana is at risk for self-concept alterations: Loss of a body part (breast) by surgery. A subjective indicator of this problem is Ana's statement: "Even an old woman like me needs to feel like a woman." Other cues suggesting strengths that might promote recovery include strong family ties and Ana's previously

healthy body image, as manifested by her pride in her appearance. Additionally, the nurses note that Ana is widowed and states that she has no desire to remarry. This cue suggests that Ana is not concerned with the immediate reaction of a sexual partner to her changed appearance. However, they would need to validate this inference with Ana.

Possible Nursing Diagnoses

One of Ana's nurses describes her thoughts leading to a definitive nursing diagnosis.

Ana kept making references to her sexual identity or feelings about being a woman, so I first considered a diagnosis related to sexual dysfunction. Knowing that radical surgery can be a causative factor also influenced my diagnosis. I wanted confirmation of her sexual desirability, which is a defining characteristic for sexual dysfunction. My first diagnosis was sexual dysfunction related to mastectomy.

Then I began to ask why Ana's sexual health was threatened. It seemed to make more sense to focus nursing interventions on the underlying factors threatening sexuality, in which case a more specific diagnosis was needed. I began to consider the diagnosis Body image disturbance, and reevaluated the data with this diagnosis in mind. She indicated that she now views herself differently, a cue consistent with this diagnosis; she had lost a body part, which can be a causative factor. She showed signs of grieving (depression, withdrawal, and weeping) as well as negative feelings about her body, which are defining characteristics. It seemed to me that we should focus on the body image disturbance, keeping in mind that failure to resolve the problem could alter sexual health.

Final Nursing Diagnosis

The definitive nursing diagnosis, Body Image Disturbance related to loss of body part, is recorded on the nursing care plan, and interventions and outcomes are formulated.

Prognosis

Planning interventions require further assessment. Assessment focuses on factors known to influence adaptation to body image alteration, including the reactions of significant other and Ana's interpretation of such reactions; the meaning of the body change to Ana; and Ana's coping style and ability. The nurse also refers Ana to Reach for Recovery (a support group for breast cancer survivors).

S U M M A R Y

Sexuality and reproductive function assessment focuses on the following:
- The person's concerns related to sexual and reproductive functions
- The person's sexual and reproductive teaching needs
- Identification of sexual or reproductive problems requiring nursing intervention or referral
- Evaluation of reproductive growth and development

When assessing sexuality and reproductive functions, the nurse should consider the following:
- A trusting, nonjudgmental nurse–client relationship facilitates the assessment process.
- Data collection is initiated by giving the person permission to discuss sexual concerns.
- Sexuality assessment is important regardless of the person's age, marital status, sexual activities, or physical status.
- The nurse's values or personal beliefs may influence assessment, especially when they conflict with the client's.
- Some sexual problems should be treated by health professionals with advanced education. The nurse should facilitate appropriate referrals.

Data collection is accomplished by the following methods:

Interview and Record Review
- Gender identification and role
- Lifestyle and protective practice
- Sexual satisfaction
- Sexual abuse
- Sexually transmitted diseases
- Family risk factors for cancer of breast and ovaries
- Reproductive history: men and women

Laboratory and X-Ray Analysis
- Sexually transmitted diseases

- Cervical/uterine cancer
- Breast anomalies
- Pregnancy-related tests
- Infertility tests
- Pelvic ultrasound
- Prostate-specific antigen

Physical Examination
- Examination of genitalia: male and female
- Examination of breasts
- Examination of inguinal area
- Physical signs and symptoms of normal and abnormal alterations of pregnancy
- Signs and symptoms of fetal distress

Nursing Diagnoses
The following nursing diagnoses are associated with sexual and reproductive function:
Sexual dysfunction
Altered sexual patterns
Breast-feeding: effective
Breast-feeding: ineffective
Breast-feeding: interrupted
Rape–trauma syndrome

Dysfunctions in sexual and reproductive function may be related to other health problems. Nursing diagnoses related to sexual and reproductive function include the following:
Altered family process
Altered role performance
Body image disturbance
Incontinence
Ineffective family coping
Ineffective individual coping
High risk for infection
Spiritual distress
Altered nutrition: less than body requirements

Critical Thinking

Historically, nurses did not venture into the assessment of sexuality and sexual function with patients, but since the publication of Masters and Johnson's work on human sexuality in the 1960s, the assessment of sexuality has become increasingly sanctioned. Currently there is a public emphasis on issues relating to sexuality and reproductive function, including the AIDS epidemic, abortion, homosexuality, and implications of welfare reform. Health professionals have an increasing need to obtain accurate data about sexual and reproductive functioning.

1. At the hospital you work at, you note that most physicians defer all pelvic examinations on older women and most nurses do not collect data regarding sexuality on people older than 50. Explain to your coworkers why sexuality is a lifelong issue and concern.

2. Explain how health problems, chronic and acute, can affect sexuality.

3. You have an adolescent in the clinic for the first time for reproductive assessment. How would you put this adolescent at ease for the first-time assessment?

4. Identify and describe circumstances under which you would not feel comfortable discussing sexual functions. How would you assist the client in obtaining necessary care? Evaluate and discuss your reasons for feeling uncomfortable.

BIBLIOGRAPHY

Aiken, M. (1990). Documenting sexual abuse in prepubertal girls. *MSN, 15* (5), 176–177.

Andrews, J. (1992). How we do it: Sexual assault aftercare instructions. *Journal of Emergency Nursing, 18* (2), 152–157.

Annon, J. (1976). The PLISSIT Model: A proposed conceptual scheme for the treatment of sexual problems. *Journal of Sex Education and Therapy, 2,* 1–15.

Brink, P. (1987). Cultural aspects of sexuality. *Holistic Nursing Practice, 1* (4), 12–20.

Bullard, D., & Knight. (1981). *Sexuality and physical disability: Personal perspectives.* St Louis: Mosby.

Carlson, K., Eisenstat, S., & Ziporyn, T. (1996). *The Harvard guide to women's health.* Cambridge, MA: Harvard University Press.

Carnevali, D., et al. (1993). *Diagnostic reasoning in nursing* (3rd ed.). Philadelphia: J.B. Lippincott.

Carpenito, L. (1997). *Handbook of nursing diagnosis* (7th ed). Philadelphia: Lippincott.

Castiglia, P. (1991). Sexual abuse of children. *Journal of Pediatric Health Care, 4* (2), 91–93.

Centers for Disease Control and Prevention. (1998). 1998 Guidelines for treatment of sexually transmitted diseases. *MMWR, 47* (Nu. RR-1).

Domar, A. (1986). Psychologic aspects of the pelvic exam: Individual needs and physician involvement. *Women and Health, 10* (4), 75–90.

Forrester, D. (1986). Myths of masculinity: Impact on men's health. *Nursing Clinics of North America, 21* (1), 15–23.

Friend, R. (1987). Sexual identity and human diversity: Implications for nursing practice. *Holistic Nursing Practice, 1* (4), 21–41.

Hogan, R. (1985). *Human sexuality: A nursing perspective* (2nd ed.). Norwalk, CT: Appleton-Century-Crofts.

Kinsey, A., et. al. (1965). *Sexual behavior in the human female.* New York: Pocket Books.

Kinsey, A., Pomery, W., & Martin, C. (1948). *Sexual behavior in the human male.* Philadelphia: Saunders.

Koshti-Richman, A. (1996). The role of nurses in promoting testicular self examination. *Nursing Times, 92* (33), 40–41.

Lasater, S. (1988). Testicular cancer: A nursing perspective of diagnosis and treatment. *Journal of Urological Nursing, 7* (11), 329–349.

Masters, W., & Johnson, V. (1970). *Human sexual inadequacy.* Boston: Little, Brown.

Nichols, F., & Zwelling, E. (1997). *Maternal-newborn nursing: Theory and practice.* Philadelphia: W.B. Saunders.

Paul E., & O'Neill, J. (1983). A sexual health model for nursing intervention. *Issues in Health Care for Women, 4* (2.3), 115–125.

Waterhouse, J., & Metcalfe, M. (1991). Attitudes toward nurses discussing sexual concerns with patients. *Journal of Advanced Nursing, 16,* 1048–1054.

Wilson, P. (1991). Testicular, prostate, and penile cancers in primary care settings: The importance of early detection. *Nurse Practitioner, 16* (11), 18–26.

Woods, N. (1987). Toward a holistic perspective of human sexuality: Alterations in sexual health and nursing diagnoses. *Holistic Nursing Practice, 1* (4), 1–11.

Assessing Stress and Coping

ASSESSMENT GUIDELINES

- Stress and Coping Interview (Health History)
- Suicide Potential
- Interpreting Physical Examination Findings and Stress Responses

CHAPTER ORGANIZATION

Introductory Overview
- Assessment Focus
- Data Collection Methods
- Nursing Diagnoses

Knowledge Base for Assessment
- Stressors
- Stress Response
- Coping

- Coping Styles
- Effective Coping
- Crisis
- Diagnostic Studies (Measurement) of Coping and Stress

INTRODUCTORY OVERVIEW

Stress, as defined by Lazarus (1966), is the disruption of meaning, emotional stability, physical balance, or smooth functioning in a person's life, resulting in threat, loss, or challenge. Stressors include stimuli with potentially adverse or threatening effects, such as physical, mental, or emotional trauma. Stressors induce emotional arousal, leading to activation of the central nervous system, increased production of hormones along the hypothalamic–pituitary axis, and coping reactions on the psychological and behavioral level.

People respond to stress in a variety of ways. Depending on the type, intensity, or duration of a particular stressor, as well as the personal and psychosocial resources of the individual, stressful situations may have adverse effects on health.

Some people may respond to stress with feelings of tension or anguish, others may interpret stress as normal and something to be endured, and still others might learn a new skill that helps them adapt to the new situation. Selye (1976) emphasized that stress is inevitable and that stress can affect a person's health either positively or negatively. Positive stress, which Selye calls *eustress*, is associated with adaptation and is necessary for growth and development. An example of positive stress might be the initial pressures and anxiousness felt by an individual when promoted into a new job with added responsibilities. Another example is the normal anxiousness of adolescents as they strive to be accepted by their peers and the opposite sex.

In contrast, negative stress, called *distress*, is potentially harmful and may exhaust one's ability to adapt. In the example above, the positive stress might turn into negative stress if the newly promoted individual realizes that the new boss requires that he works 60 hours a week and meanwhile, at home, his wife is expecting a third child, is having a difficult pregnancy, and he faces time and energy demands at home to help out with the other young children in the evenings and weekends.

Stress may interfere with a person's abilities to meet basic needs, function on the job, or solve daily problems. Negative stress can become excessive and cumulative. It can build up over time, spanning several different events or problems, and become overwhelming to the individual and reach a crisis stage. Such unresolved negative stress can adversely affect individuals both physically and emotionally. It can contribute to serious illness such as hypertension, coronary artery disease, and peptic ulcer, in addition to unpleasant feelings of powerlessness, helplessness, or fear. In worst cases, unresolved negative stress can lead to despondency, depression, or even suicide.

Coping includes psychological and behavioral responses to stress. In general, coping styles can be classified as problem-focused or emotion-focused in nature. Problem-focused coping involves taking direct actions to solve a particular problem. Emotion-focused coping is characterized by a greater tendency toward avoidance of the stressor or taking action to reduce the tension associated with the stressor.

Stress, stress responses, and the effectiveness of coping processes can have a significant impact on health and quality of life. Therefore, the nurse's evaluation of an individual's health status should always address stress and coping.

ASSESSMENT FOCUS

The assessment of stress and coping focuses on determining an individual's exposure to stress, the person's appraisal of stressful events, and the overall effectiveness of their coping styles. A comprehensive assessment of stress and coping will focus on the following:

- Identifying situations or events causing stress
- Understanding the meaning of stressful situations or events to the individual
- Identifying the person's coping style and other responses to stress
- Evaluating the overall effectiveness of coping processes
- Recognizing signs of crisis or threats to safety brought on by stress

Data Collection Methods

Data collection is accomplished by the following methods:

1. Interview or Review of Records Focus
   Stressor identification
   Stress perception
   Coping styles
   Resolution of stress
2. Diagnostic Studies (Measurement) of Stress and Coping Focus
   Stress audit instruments
   Coping style/coping effectiveness measurement instruments
3. Physical Examination and Observation of Stress Responses Focus
   General survey and observation of behavior
   Physiologic manifestations of stress noted during the examination of various body systems
4. Suicide Risk Evaluation

Nursing Diagnoses

Assessment of stress and coping patterns may result in the identification of one or more of the following primary nursing diagnoses:

Ineffective individual coping
Impaired adjustment
Defensive coping
Ineffective denial
Decisional conflict (specify)
Dysfunctional grieving
Anticipatory grieving

Diagnoses pertaining to family coping (Ineffective family coping) are discussed more thoroughly in the chapter on roles and relationships (see Chap. 12).

Grieving is a normal process that a person uses to adapt to a significant loss, whether the loss pertains to a person, an animal, a role, or a valuable function. In addition to grieving for the loss of a loved one, a person also may grieve the loss of a home, job, or health. Grieving is a complex emotional response, incorporating numerous and varied coping strategies. Because grieving represents a specific stressful experience, nursing diagnoses pertaining to grieving are listed here.

Nursing diagnoses related to grieving also may be evaluated in relation to roles and relationships, in which case the emphasis is on evaluating the meaning of terminating significant relationships and roles.

Other, secondary nursing diagnoses related to the assessment of stress and coping responses may be identified, including the following:

Risk for violence: Self-directed or directed at others
Risk for self-mutilation
Post-trauma response
Risk for post-trauma syndrome
Rape–trauma syndrome
Rape–trauma syndrome: Compound reaction
Rape–trauma syndrome: Silent reaction
Anxiety
Fear
Hopelessness
Powerlessness
Altered self-concept
Spiritual distress

KNOWLEDGE BASE FOR ASSESSMENT

To assess stress and coping, it is helpful to first understand the concept of stressors, the stress response, and what is meant by coping.

Stressors

Selye's (1976) classic work on stress refers to stressors as noxious stimuli, such as cold or injury, that arouse the body from a resting state into a state of readiness to combat or deal with the stressor. This initial response is the alarm phase of the stress response. Physiologically, stressors activate the hypothalamic-pituitary-adrenal axis, thereby stimulating hormones and other substances that enable a person to initiate a psychophysiologic stress response.

There are a number of ways to classify stressors. In general, stressors may be divided into the following broad categories: threat, loss, or challenge. Use of the category "challenge" implies that stress can have a positive nature and that not all stress should be thought of as "noxious stimuli," nor is all stress deleterious. Challenges that activate the stress response may includes life events generally thought of as positive, such as marriage, the birth of a child, or the start of a new job. These types of stressors provide opportunities for growth, enjoyment, and further development. They also involve change, added responsibility, and adjustment.

Another consideration in the classification of stressors is to determine whether the stress is acute and time-limited in nature or chronic and repeated. When stressors are chronic and repeated, the person may develop some level of emotional habituation to the stressor, and the overall impact of the stressor may be diminished.

Stressors are classified by Guzzetta and Forsyth (1979) as physiologic, psychological, environmental, and sociocultural (Display 14-1). This classification is particularly useful for nursing practice because of its emphasis on factors having relevance to health, illness, and the healthcare environment. Nursing and other clinically oriented disciplines have also found it helpful to identify the particular types of stressors affecting different patient groups. For example, in the classification work of Guzzetta and Forsyth (1979), myocardial infarction patients were studied to determine the specific types of stressors they experienced (Display 14-2). For the patients in this study, the nature of the stressors listed in Display 14-2 were found to change over the course of their illness and convalescence. In the critical care environment, patients experienced stressors that were predominantly physiologic and environmental in nature, such as loss of sleep, the development of cardiac complications, lack of privacy, and exposure to frightening machines and noises. Before hospital discharge, however, common stressors experienced by this group of patients were mainly psychological or social in nature, such as alterations in body image, feelings of hopelessness, worry about work, and financial concerns.

Another nursing study identified and rank-ordered the specific types of stressors experienced by hemodialysis patients (Baldree, Murphy, & Powers, 1982). As can be seen in Display 14-3, this study found that fluid limitation, muscle cramps, fatigue, and uncertainty about the future were the predominant, treatment-related stressors.

Stressors experienced by elders in long-term care facilities were identified by Wolanin and Phillips (1981). These stressors reflected changes related to aging and social milieu (Display 14-4).

More recently, clinical research to identify specific stressors has been conducted on persons with human immunodeficiency virus (HIV) infection (Grassi, Righu, Sighinolfi, Makoui, & Ghinelli, 1998; Linn, 1997; Moneyham, Seals, Sowell, Hennessy, Demi, & Brake, 1997; and Thompson, Nanni, & Levine, 1996), victims of emotional trauma, (Stuber et al., 1997), and persons having caregiver roles for dependents, especially aging or demented family members (Haley et al., 1996; Vitaliano, Russo, Young, Becker, & Maiuro, 1991). This type of clinical research aimed at identifying stressors common in various situations provides important knowledge for the health assess-

---

DISPLAY 14.1

Classification of Stressors*

PHYSIOLOGIC

Trauma
Surgery
Radiation
Body chemistry alterations (drugs, hormones, abnormal secretions, dietary, poisons)
Infectious processes (bacterial, viral, fungal)
Pain
Sleep deprivation or fatigue

ENVIRONMENTAL

Pollutants
Urbanization
Changes in physical environment (relocation, hospitalization, poverty, incarceration)
Sensory deprivation
Sensory overload
Loss of privacy
Frightening or unpleasant noises, odors
Untidy surroundings

PSYCHOLOGICAL

Distressing emotions (fear, anxiety)
Psychological distress (helplessness, powerlessness, loneliness, poor self-esteem, lack of motivation)

SOCIOCULTURAL

Change
Financial status
Vocational pressures
Family dysfunction
Difficulty with developmental tasks
Child rearing
Aging
Retirement
Religious beliefs

*Physiologic stressors disturb primarily tissue systems; the other categories of stressors are evaluated cognitively before stressor recognition occurs.

(After Guzzetta, C.E., & Forsyth, G.L. [1979]. Nursing diagnostic pilot study: Psychophysiologic stress. *Advances in Nursing Science,* 2[10], 27–44)

DISPLAY 14.2

Stressors Identified by Patients After Acute Myocardial Infarction

This list represents stressors identified by the researchers before the study. At least 1 of the 50 stressors listed was identified by each subject in the study.

PHYSIOLOGIC

Acute myocardial insult
Severity of illness
Related heart complications
Severity of symptoms
Previous history of heart disease
Other coexisting illness
Other complications
Rapid eye movement sleep deprivation
Other

PSYCHOLOGICAL

Fear of death
Fear of hospital procedures
Weakness
Altered body image
Loneliness
Powerlessness
Helplessness
Hopelessness
Loss of virility
Transfer from coronary care unit
Other

ENVIRONMENTAL

Observation of cardiac arrest
Observation of other procedures
Lack of structure; boredom
Lack of privacy

Sensory deprivation/overload
Inability to sleep
Untidy surroundings
Unpleasant odors
Frightening noises
Multiple sounds
Lack of windows/clocks
Frightening machines
Restricted visitation
Altered daily routine
Other

SOCIOCULTURAL

Age
Social class
Financial status
Ethnic origin
Religious beliefs
Education
Fear of family reaction
Family conflicts
Concern for self
Concern for family
Interpretation of symptoms
Loss of peer respect
Inability to work
Other beliefs/attitudes
Other

(Guzzetta, C.E., & Forsyth, G.L. [1979]. Nursing diagnostic pilot study. Psychophysiologic stress. *Advances in Nursing Science, 2*[10], 27–44)

ment process. Nurses usually identify the nature of stressors confronting a person before planning and implementing interventions to support coping. Knowing about the typical kinds of stressors facing persons with particular health issues or problems can facilitate this aspect of the assessment process.

Stress Response

The stress response is initiated when a stressor is present in the body or perceived by the mind. Physiologically, the stress response involves the nervous system (sympathetic branch of the autonomic nervous system), the endocrine system (pituitary and adrenal glands), and the immune system. Cognitively, a person's appraisal (perception) of the stressor will influence the overall physiologic aspects of the stress response as well as the person's ability to effectively cope with stress.

The stress response is initiated by stimulation of the sympathetic nervous system (Fig. 14-1). This stimulation affects the endocrine system by causing the adrenal gland to secrete catecholamines (epinephrine, norepinephrine, and dopamine) into the bloodstream. At the same time, the pituitary gland is stimulated, causing release of additional hormones, including adrenocorticotropic hormone, which, in turn, stimulates the adrenal cortex to secrete cortisol.

In general, the catecholamines prepare the body to act

DISPLAY 14.3

Hemodialysis Stressors: Rank Ordering of 29 Stressors According to Frequency of Occurrence by 35 Hemodialysis Patients

STRESSOR	CLASS	RANK
Limitation of fluid	PS	1.0
Muscle cramps	P	2.5
Fatigue	P	2.5
Uncertainty concerning the future	PS	4.5
Limitation of food	PS	4.5
Interference in job	PS	6.0
Itching	P	9.0
Limitation of physical activities	PS	9.0
Changes in bodily appearance	PS	9.0
Arterial and venous stick	P	12.0
Nausea and vomiting	P	12.0
Length of treatment	PS	12.0
Limit on time and place for vacation	PS	12.0
Dependency on staff members	PS	12.0
Decrease in social life	PS	16.0
Changes in family responsibilities	PS	16.0
Cost factors	PS	16.0
Loss of bodily function	PS	18.0
Decrease in sexual drive	PS	19.5
Stiffening of joints	P	19.5
Limited to styles of clothing	PS	21.5
Dependency on physicians	PS	21.5
Transportation to and from the unit	PS	23.5
Frequent hospital admissions	PS	23.5
Sleep disturbances	PS	25.0
Reversal in family role with spouse	PS	26.5
Fear of being alone	PS	26.5
Reversal in family role with the children	PS	28.5
Decreased ability to procreate	PS	28.5

PS, psychosocial stressor; P, physiological stressor.

(Baldree, K.S., Murphy, S.P., & Powers, M.J. [1982]. Stress identification and coping patterns in patients on hemodialysis. *Nursing Research, 31*[2], 107–112)

in response to the stressor. Catecholamines support the so-called "fight or flight" mechanisms of the stress response. Cortisol causes the mobilization of energy (glucose) and other substances needed for energy during the stress response.

The catecholamines secreted in response to stress primarily affect the cardiovascular and pulmonary systems. As a result, cardiac output and blood flow to the heart, brain, and skeletal muscles is increased. At the same time, blood flow is shifted away from the skin and visceral organs. The pulmonary airways dilate, and oxygen delivery to the bloodstream is enhanced.

These aspects of the stress response can be appreciated during the physical examination of major body systems (cardiovascular, pulmonary, and integumentary). Changes in these systems may relate to variations observed in the vital signs and appearance of the skin.

The cortisol secreted during the stress response mobilizes glucose that is needed to fuel the body's "fight or flight" mechanisms. Cortisol also suppresses the body's inflammatory response and promotes secretion of acid in the gastrointestinal tract. Excessive gastric secretion may result in ulceration of the gastric mucosa. This condition has commonly been called a "stress ulcer."

The manner of interaction between the neuroendocrine and immune systems during stress is not completely understood. However, it is believed that the interaction of these systems plays a role in the pathogenesis of many so-called stress-related diseases (*e.g.,* coronary artery disease, hypertension, tension headaches, ulcers, irritable bowel syndrome, and others).

The physiologic response to stress is mediated by the individual's appraisal (perception) of the stressor. Lazarus (1966) has labeled this perceptual element the cognitive appraisal of the stressor. Cognitive appraisal includes a primary as well as a secondary appraisal of the stressor. During the primary appraisal, the focus is on the evaluation of the significance of the stressful event or situation to the individual. As a result of primary appraisal, the person will conclude that the event is (1) a threat, (2) a loss, (3) a challenge, or (4) benign and irrelevant. Secondary appraisal of a stressor occurs when the person determines the degree of control they believe they have over the situation. Strong feelings of personal control are exemplified by characterizations such as having a "fighting spirit." Conversely, low feelings of control are associated with feelings of helplessness or powerlessness. In general, the stronger the feelings of personal control, the more likely it is that the person will positively respond and adapt to the stress.

Coping

Coping is defined by Weisman (1979) as follows: "what one does about a problem in order to bring about relief, reward, quiescence, and equilibrium . . . what one does or does not do about that problem, constitutes how one copes." Coping, as a distress-relieving process, may lead to one of two outcomes: problem resolution or tension reduction. Both problem resolution and tension reduction are adaptive in the sense that both approaches involve enabling the person to adjust to the environment. Each method represents a different level of adaptation, with problem resolution generally viewed as more adaptive.

Tension reduction involves coping strategies that provide some type of distraction to relieve the preoccupation with the stressor. Common negative examples include overeating, ingesting alcohol, and using drugs. A positive example is engaging in exercise or a fitness program to

DISPLAY 14.4

Stressors Experienced by Elders in Long-Term Care

- *Threats to life and health:* Client's apprehension about fate, whether in the form of the fear of death following acute trauma or surgery, the fear of permanent disability, or the fear of the dying process.
- *Discomforts:* The physical complaints of the client in regard to pain, cold, fatigue, poor food, lack of care, etc.; Client's apprehension regarding ability to regulate discomforts and being assured staff will attend to discomforts.
- *Loss of a means of subsistence:* Client's concern about economic conditions in general, economic conditions of significant others, own economic conditions, and economic concerns about illness.
- *Deprivation of intimacy:* Loss of physical closeness, sexual satisfaction, close affiliations, and friendships.
- *Enforced idleness:* Client's concern about inability to perform usual tasks, engage in necessary tasks for survival, such as cooking and shopping, and engage in recreational activities.
- *Restriction of movement:* Physical immobility, monotony of daily encounters, and the absence of personal privacy.

- *Isolation:* Separation of client from usual environment, and acquaintances or friends, and perception that caregivers are uncaring.
- *Threats to family structure:* Fear of loss of family status or family role, and realization of failing health and loss of resources of close family members.
- *Capricious behavior of those in charge:* Client's perception that caregivers are unpredictable.
- *Propaganda:* Client's lack of accurate information about status, feeling that information is being withheld, and pressure to do something not wanted or believed.
- *Awareness of personal degeneration:* Client's awareness of own physical and mental failings.
- *Rejection:* Feelings of being forgotten, or significant others not caring, and perception of the ridicule and dislike of others.
- *Unknown duration:* Feelings that the confinement will never end and that time drags.

(Adapted from Wolanin, M.O., & Phillips, L.R. [1981]. *Confusion: Prevention and care* [p. 273]. St. Louis: C.V. Mosby)

redirect one's attention. Tension reduction may be an intermediate process eventually leading to problem resolution, or it may be the only coping process used to respond to the stressor. The resulting behaviors may be viewed as maladaptive. As an intermediate process, tension reduction is employed to reduce stress to a more manageable level. Subsequently, the stress is alleviated, and effective coping processes are initiated leading to a higher level of adaptation.

Lazarus (1966) defined coping as cognitive and behavioral processes used to deal with threats. This definition offers no distinction between coping and defending. In contrast, Weisman (1979) views coping and defending as two different processes that may occur, to some extent, simultaneously. According to Weisman, coping is a response to a recognized problem, whereas defending is a response to some unknown or unspecified concerns. Defending may occur as a reflex or autonomic response, as would happen when the sympathetic nervous system prepares a person for fight or flight, or it may involve psychic processes of defense, such as denial, regression, and repression. Once the instigating problem is understood, defending mechanisms become coping responses. Health care providers occasionally have the tendency to label coping strategies of which they do not approve as defense mechanisms, implying that such responses are an inferior way of dealing with stressors.

Coping Styles

An individual's coping style refers to the overall approach the person uses to deal with stress. Coping styles are influenced by personality, resources available to the person, and the person's past experiences with stress. The appraisal of the stressor, especially the process of secondary appraisal whereby the individual determines their degree of personal control over a situation, also influence an individual's coping style.

Coping styles are generally categorized as (1) problem-focused, (2) emotion-focused, or (3) dualistic, having features of both problem-focused and emotion-focused styles. Problem-focused coping involves dealing directly with the stressful situation or stressor in an active (as opposed to passive) manner. It involves both planning and taking action. Actions may include changing the effects of a stressor by finding a way to eliminate it or reevaluating its effect and significance. Another course of action might be to confront the stressor or find positive features in the situation. The overall effect of a problem-focused coping style is problem resolution.

Emotion-focused coping is characterized by a tendency to avoid or ignore the stressor. It often involves tension-reducing thoughts or behaviors such as denial or redirecting one's effort to activities that can take the mind off the stressor such as overeating or using drugs or alcohol. Dis-

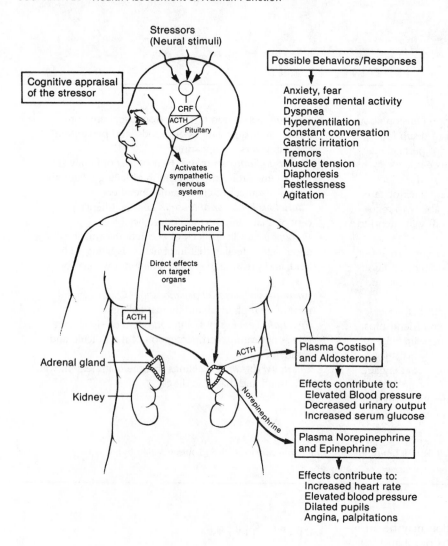

Stressors
(Neural stimuli)

Cognitive appraisal
of the stressor

CRF
ACTH
Pituitary

Activates
sympathetic
nervous
system

Norepinephrine

Direct effects
on target
organs

ACTH

ACTH

Adrenal gland

Kidney

Norepinephrine

Possible Behaviors/Responses

Anxiety, fear
Increased mental activity
Dyspnea
Hyperventilation
Constant conversation
Gastric irritation
Tremors
Muscle tension
Diaphoresis
Restlessness
Agitation

Plasma Costisol
and Aldosterone

Effects contribute to:
Elevated Blood pressure
Decreased urinary output
Increased serum glucose

Plasma Norepinephrine
and Epinephrine

Effects contribute to:
Increased heart rate
Elevated blood pressure
Dilated pupils
Angina, palpitations

FIGURE 14.1 The stress response.

tancing oneself from the stressor also may be observed in emotion-focused coping styles. The overall effect of an emotion-focused coping style is tension reduction.

A personality trait that is especially predictive of an individual's coping style is locus of control. Locus of control refers to an individual's self-concept of personal control over situations and events. People with a self-concept of high personal control have an internal locus of control (internals). Conversely, a self-concept whereby the person believes they have little or no personal control over events characterizes people with an external locus of control (externals).

Different coping styles are associated with each personality type. The more self-reliant, internal locus of control individual tends to adopt a problem-focused coping style. People with an external locus of control, who feel controlled by forces outside themselves, are more likely to adopt an emotion-focused coping style. Characteristics associated with each of these personality types are listed in Display 14-5. Determining a person's locus of control may indicate which coping style the person will adopt.

Overall, effective coping patterns are more strongly associated with problem-focused approaches. The emotion-focused style may be helpful if it provides temporary relief

from tension so that the person can eventually activate problem-solving skills. In the long run, sustaining an emotion-focused style tends to produce greater anxiety and depression and may contribute to abusive or self-destructive behavior patterns.

Problem-solving and tension reduction are embodied in four coping strategies identified by Lazarus and Launier (1978): direct action, information seeking, intrapsychic mode, and action inhibition.

Direct Action. Direct action includes the common coping strategy of fight or flight. The role of the sympathetic nervous system is paramount in preparing the body systems for this type of action. The body provides additional oxygen to the skeletal muscles, which facilitates the actions of the appropriate muscles for either fleeing or fighting; the bronchioles of the lungs dilate, allowing more oxygen to enter the body; the heart beats more forcefully to deliver the oxygen to the skeletal muscles; and glucose levels rise in response to the need for fuel for the activities of fight or flight.

Direct action may also involve goal-directed, problem-solving approaches to a situation, such as beginning a diet or joining an exercise class to resolve the stressor of poor

DISPLAY 14.5

Coping Behaviors Associated with Internal and External Locus of Control

"Internals" showed more problem-solving, active coping behaviors associated with effective coping, whereas "externals" tended to show passive or defensive behaviors associated with ineffective coping.

INTERNAL

- Is active on self-care.
  Examples: Helps others recognize self-care strides. Boasts of ability. Plan for care needs. Makes suggestions to health workers.
- Interacts socially.
  Example: Shows active interest in others and helps them solve problems.
- Sets goals.
  Examples: Modifies environment. Plans for safety needs. Uses problem-solving skills.
- Seeks information.
  Examples: Asks specific, relevant questions. Reads about condition.
- Shares perception of self as being important.
  Example: Describes positive role as strong person in family.
- Deliberately uses prayer to provide strength.
- Uses purposeful distraction.

EXTERNAL

- Is passive and dependent.
  Example: Sleeping more than usual.
- Has little or no interest in acquiring self-care skills.
- Demonstrates social withdrawal (isolation).
- Focuses on unrealistic cures.
- Refuses therapies that increase mobility (*e.g.,* physical therapy).
- Expresses verbally that nothing more can be done.

(After Miller, J.F. [1992]. *Coping with chronic illness* (2nd ed.). Philadelphia: F.A. Davis)

---

self-esteem related to obesity. Using these approaches, the person confronts and acts on the stressor.

Information Seeking. Generally, information seeking is a cognitive coping strategy applied to dealing with potential stressors as well as existing stressors. It involves considering the potential stressor and associated unpleasant sensations and then developing advance strategies to deal with these sensations. Information seeking may help eliminate frightening misconceptions about the stressor and may be useful when information about the potential stressor's sensations are provided in advance. For example, the sensations associated with abdominal surgery include feeling incisional pain after surgery, fatigue with minimal activity, and cramping from abdominal gas. Providing this information preoperatively may help the patient in coping with the stress of surgery.

The process of providing information, also referred to as providing preparatory sensory information, represents a nursing intervention to promote coping based on the need for information seeking. Whether this method of coping is more effective than any other method has not yet been decided.

Intrapsychic Mode. The intrapsychic processes involve directing one's attention to other considerations. This coping strategy, which includes defense mechanisms, helps reduce the tension and anxiety associated with a stressor and involves distractions, such as daydreaming or fantasizing. Many "psychological" coping mechanisms are intrapsychic in nature, including the defense mechanisms of displacement, projection, suppression, repression, rationalization, regression, and denial.

Intrapsychic processes may be viewed as either effective or ineffective coping strategies. Intrapsychic defensive processes may provide a reprieve from the overstimulating and exhausting aspects of stress, allowing the person's energy to be directed toward developing other, more effective and long-term coping mechanisms.

Prolonged use of intrapsychic processes may encourage continual avoidance of stressors or denial, with no attempt at resolving the threats or problems. For example, many people use denial after various diagnoses such as cancer or myocardial infarction. Denial is also recognized as an aspect of the coping process observed with bereavement. Often, using denial temporarily eliminates intense negative effects of the stressor until the person is able to develop effective coping strategies.

Action Inhibition. When using this coping strategy, a person will refrain from activities that are impulsive, dangerous, or embarrassing. For example, some people may cope by acting out behaviors such as driving recklessly or initiating an argument. Action inhibition may be used to prevent such impractical behavior.

Effective Coping

Regardless of the coping strategy employed, effective coping is manifested by high levels of adaptation to stress or the development of stress tolerance. Effective coping has the following results:

- Distress is maintained within manageable limits.
- Hope and encouragement are generated.
- A sense of personal worth is maintained.
- Relationships with significant others are maintained or restored.
- Prospects for physical recovery are enhanced.
- Prospects for favorable situations (interpersonal, social, and economic) are enhanced.

Coping effectiveness varies greatly among people and may be influenced by the following factors (Cohen, 1981; Kobasa, 1979; Selye, 1976):

- *Number of stressors confronting a person:* In the presence of multiple stressors, stress may be perceived as an insurmountable obstacle, and crisis may result.
- *Access to social or financial support resources:* People with such resources usually perceive themselves as more able to cope.
- *Stressor duration:* Chronic exposure to stressors predisposes a person to chronic stress or tension.
- *Stressor intensity:* An intense stressor may be perceived as insurmountable and may precipitate crisis.
- *Past experience with stressors:* If the person has coped successfully in the past, the stressor may be perceived as less threatening.
- *Personality:* Certain people are more stress resistant—especially those who view change as a challenge and believe they can influence events.

Crisis

Crisis occurs when the person feels overwhelmed by stressors and unable to resolve the problem. It is an acute, self-limiting state that is usually resolved within a period of 4 to 6 weeks. Although crisis may be associated with major disorganization of the personality, it is also viewed as a potential growth process. People in crisis may be more willing to accept help toward developing effective coping skills. Crisis intervention processes have been developed, based on crisis theory, to help people move through crisis and achieve the same levels of stress adaptation as existed before the crisis (Infante, 1982).

Fink (1967) identified four observable crisis stages that may be recognized during health assessment:

- *Shock (stress):* Stressors are perceived as overwhelming. The person may experience powerlessness, anxiety, and altered thought processes.
- *Defensive retreat:* Attempts are made to maintain usual structures, often by employing coping strategies to reduce tension and to reorganize one's thoughts. Being challenged at this stage may result in anger because it interferes with coping attempts.
- *Acknowledgment:* The person can no longer be distracted from the overwhelming stress. Feelings of hopelessness and powerlessness may be strong, and suicide may be considered. Thought processes are altered as perceptions must become more reality oriented.
- *Adaptation and change:* New or precrisis structures are established, and the person gains a feeling of control and increasing self-worth. Thought processes return to normal.

Pattern Assessment Stress and Coping Assessment Guidelines

GENERAL APPROACH

An assessment of what is stressful and a person's responses to stress begins by asking the person to describe stressful events or situations encountered presently or in the past. How specific stressors are perceived by the individual also should be explored. These aspects of the health history are usually established by interviewing the person. You also should review the person's medical diagnosis and prognosis, the quality of significant relationships, and social or work history to gain insights about stress and coping.

Some people find it difficult to discuss stress and coping. Whether the person responds to direct questioning during the interview may depend on what coping mechanism is being used to handle stress, as well as the stage of the stress reaction. For example, a person who is using denial as a coping mechanism may offer little relevant information about his or her problems. Not every person will be ready to discuss stressors and coping at the moment the subject is raised in the interview. Even in the absence of denial, people may be reluctant to express their anxiety about the problems that confront them, or they may have difficulty openly discussing their coping methods. Drug and alcohol use are examples of coping mechanisms that people may be reluctant to discuss.

(continued)

Pattern Assessment   Stress and Coping Assessment Guidelines (continued)

Injecting one's personal bias into the situation may interfere with objective evaluation of the person's statements and should be avoided. Keeping an open mind will provide an opportunity to evaluate fairly and rationally all coping mechanisms employed by the person.

REVIEW THE MEDICAL HISTORY AND ASSOCIATED PROBLEMS

High-risk conditions include childbirth, pain (chronic), chronic renal failure, HIV or any other chronic or life-threatening illness, and heart disease. Determine whether the person experienced cancer as a child. This type of past experience could contribute to posttrauma stress.

Researchers have found that different groups of patients experience different types of stressors. The groups studied by nurses include people who have had a myocardial infarction, those who are undergoing hemodialysis for chronic renal failure, and those recently admitted to long-term and short-term nursing care facilities. Knowing the nature of potential stressors in these types of situations, as well as others, is one means of anticipating possible problems and psychological reactions.

STRESS AND COPING MEASUREMENT INSTRUMENTS

In addition to interviewing, formal assessment tools, such as the Social Readjustment Rating Scale (SRRS) developed by Holmes and Rahe (1967), and the Everyday Hassles Scale (EHS) developed by Lazarus (1981), may be used to help identify and rank everyday stressful events (see "Diagnostic Studies").

ASSESSMENT AID

Interview guide to suggest questions and record data (Display 14-6).

DISPLAY 14.6

Interview Guide: Stress and Coping Pattern

CURRENT STRESSORS

Major concerns/problems—Specify: _____

Lift Changes: ❏ None ❏ Change in relationship
❏ Change in job ❏ Financial
❏ Death of family member
❏ Birth of a child ❏ Move
❏ Other _____

History of abuse (physical, emotional, sexual). If you suspect abuse, ask the following: Have you ever been the victim of violence or abuse? ❏ yes ❏ no

STRESS PERCEPTION

Do you feel like you can cope with the present stress you face? _____
Any problems sleeping? ❏ yes ❏ no
Loss of weight or appetite? ❏ yes ❏ no
Currently under the influence of drugs or alcohol? ❏ yes ❏ no
Coping strategies: ❏ Talking to others ❏ Drugs/ alcohol/tobacco (circle) ❏ Physical activity ❏ Avoidance
❏ Other _____

Diagnostic Studies (Measurement) of Coping and Stress

Diagnostic tools may be used to measure stress and coping. The diagnostic evaluation of stress may include the administration of questionnaires or surveys to determine the magnitude and type of stress experienced by the respondent. There are many types of assessment tools available. Several examples are presented.

The Social Readjustment Rating Scale. The Social Readjustment Rating Scale (SRRS) developed by Holmes and Rahe (1967) is a diagnostic tool designed to identify stressors and quantify the degree of stress a person is experiencing. The SRRS presents a list of major stressful life events and assigns a numerical stress quotient to each event (Display 14-7). The stress quotients are added to provide a score indicating mild, medium, or high levels of stress. The score may be used to predict the person's susceptibility to illness.

Although the SRRS has received wide recognition since it was first introduced, some researchers challenge its reliability. Thorson and Thorson (1986) question the general application of the scale to all age-groups, because older people may perceive and deal with stress differently from how younger people do. Also, the tool does not take into account sociocultural background and personality, even though these factors may greatly influence the way a person perceives stress. Similarly, Baker and colleagues (1985) believe that some events listed on the SRRS are irrelevant to certain groups, such as the chronically mental

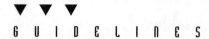

▼ ▼ ▼
G U I D E L I N E S

Assessment Guidelines Stress and Coping Interview (Health History)

Procedure	**Clinical Significance**

Procedure

1. Stressor identification

Begin the interview process by identifying the presence of major life stressors, minor life stressors (daily hassles), and traumatic events experienced in the past.

Identify events or situations precipitating stress, by asking the person questions such as the following:

- "What do you see as the major causes of stress or problems for you right now?"
- "What is changing in your life right now?"
- "What types of stress are you experiencing as a result of this illness (or hospitalization, life change, family change, etc.)?"
- "What types of everyday events are causing you stress or problems?"
- "Tell me about any losses you have experienced lately."

A person's surroundings, especially if they are unfamiliar, also can elicit a stress response. Determine whether environmental stressors are present by asking the following questions:

- "What frightens or annoys you in this setting?"
- "In what ways does this setting affect your usual lifestyle and routines?"

Identify stressful events related to family relations, career, and financial concerns by asking the following questions:

- "How would you describe your relationship with your spouse (or children, parents, girlfriend, boyfriend, etc.)?"
- "How has this situation (*e.g.,* illness) affected your family?"
- "How do present circumstances in your life interfere with work or school?"
- "How has this situation affected your financial status?"
- "Do you have a caregiver role?"

Determine whether there is a history of traumatic events in the person's past, such as a history of abuse and victimization, rape, assault, disasters, war, or catastrophic illness or accident.

People may repress their memories of traumatic events. Therefore, a history of trauma cannot always be reliably obtained through a typical interview process. Post-traumatic stress symptoms include intrusive memories, avoidance of talking about the vent or the environment where the event took place, and hypervigilence.

Clinical Significance

Identifying stressors and problems is usually necessary before the person can learn to develop effective coping strategies. Understanding the nature of stressors enables the nurse and patient to plan appropriate interventions. For example, a person who is scheduled for open heart surgery may be faced with fear of the unknown. Preoperative teaching (preparatory sensory information) would be an appropriate nursing intervention aimed at providing information and encouraging coping. If the stressor is tension from conflict with a coworker, problem-solving strategies or assertiveness training techniques may promote effective coping.

Stressors: Events or situations in a person's life that may result in stress.

Daily Hassles: Stressors that are recurrent and relatively minor in nature. People may view daily hassles as very stressful or they may view them as minor irritants.

Environmental Stressors (Examples): Unfamiliar sights, smells or sounds; changes in daily routine; lack of privacy, heat, or cold; sensory deprivation or overload.

Significant Stressors Related to Family and Relationships: Sexual and physical abuse history; death of a significant other; turmoil in the childhood family.

Caregiver Roles and Stress: More people are assuming caregiver roles for aging parents and others in our society. This may contribute to high levels of stress within the entire family.

The adverse psychological effects of traumatic events can persist for many years after the actual experience of the event.

Post-traumatic Stress Syndrome (PTSS): The delayed effects of severe psychological trauma. Persons experiencing PTSS may initially repress their recall of the traumatic event as a coping mechanism. Later, they may be affected by intrusive and disturbing memories of the event.

▼ ▼ ▼
Stress and Coping Interview (Health History)

Procedure

If you determine that the person is dealing with many stressful events, it may be helpful at this time to rate the stressors, from the most distressing to the least distressing. This will help in prioritizing any problem-solving efforts in a manner that is consistent with the individual's most pressing concerns.

2. Stress perception

Determine the manner in which the individual perceives or appraises the stressor.

Determine the person's primary appraisal of the stressor by asking questions to evaluate the significance of the stressful event to the individual such as the following:
- "What does this situation mean to you?"
- "Do you see this event as positive or negative?"
- "What is the most upsetting problem you face as a result of this situation? Least upsetting?"

Determine the person's secondary appraisal of the stressor by asking questions to explore feelings of control or helplessness.
- "Do you feel like you can cope with this situation?"
- "Do you feel like you can control some of these stressful events and any distressing feelings that have occurred?"
- "How do you feel when things seem to be out of your control?"

3. Coping style

Determine how the person typically responds to stress, including what methods are used to reduce tension. Ask the person:
- "How do you relieve tension or deal with stress?"
- "Tell me which of the following approaches best describes your coping style:
  - Talking to others
  - Trying to solve the problem
  - Blaming someone else for the problem
  - Seeking help
  - Engaging in physical activity
  - Praying
  - Trying to forget
  - Trying to relieve tension with drugs, alcohol
  - Going to sleep
  - Doing nothing
  - Accepting the situation
  - Other (Describe)"

Clinical Significance

Determining the number of stressors confronting a person at once is important because more effort to adapt is needed when multiple stressors are present.

Reactions and adaptations to stress are influenced by how the stressor is perceived by the individual. A person's perception of stress is influenced by several factors such as other concurrent events, the person's feelings about his or her ability to cope, and the degree of distress experienced.

Primary Appraisal of a Stressor: An individual's evaluation to determine whether a particular stressor is negative or positive.

Secondary Appraisal of a Stressor: An individual's evaluation of his or her sense of control over events and ability to cope effectively. People with an internal locus of control, who see themselves as active participants in determining their fate, tend to cope positively with stress.

Classification of Coping Styles (Weisman & Worden, 1979)
- *Rational-intellectual:* Seek more information about the situation.
- *Shared concern:* Talk with others to relieve stress.
- *Reversal of effect:* Laugh it off, make light of the situation.
- *Suppression:* Try to forget; put it out of mind.
- *Displacement:* Do other activities for distractions.
- *Confrontation:* Take firm action based on present understanding.
- *Redefinition:* Accept, but find something favorable in the situation.
- *Fatalism:* Submit to and accept the inevitable.
- *Acting out:* Do something—anything—no matter how reckless or impractical.
- *Problem solving:* Negotiate feasible alternatives.

▼ ▼ ▼

G U I D E L I N E S *continued*   Stress and Coping Interview (Health History)

Procedure	Clinical Significance
	• *Tension reduction:* Reduce tension by drinking, overeating, or drugs.
	• *Stimulus reduction:* Withdraw socially into isolation.
	• *Disowning responsibility:* Blame someone or something.
	• *Compliance:* Seek direction from an authority and comply.
	• *Self-Pity:* Blame self, sacrifice, or atone.
Identify the person's support system (family, friends, clergy) and determine their role in helping the person deal with stress.	Support given by significant others may contribute to a stable emotional state. It helps to determine whether a person has turned to other professionals in the past, such as clergy, a nurse, psychologist, or marriage counselor. A person who had done so may be willing to accept this type of support again.
4. Resolution of stress	
During the interview, you can ask the person whether they feel they have effectively adapted to stress:	Compare the individual's observations with your own. People who are effectively coping will meet the usual expectations of their roles and responsibilities, meet basic needs for themselves and others, demonstrate problem solving skills, and demonstrate constructive personal behavior.
• "Do you feel like you usually solve your problems?"	
• "Are your coping methods effective against current stressors?"	
• "Do the methods you have just described for relieving tension seem to help?"	

ill, who tend to perceive a different set of life events as stressful.

The Everyday Hassles Scale. Lazarus' Everyday Hassles Scale (EHS) lists, in rank order, items associated with stress and behaviors and feelings that promote well-being (Display 14-8). The EHS emphasizes common, everyday irritants that contribute significantly to stress levels, especially if positive stimuli or events do not occur to buffer the stressor effects. Similar concerns have been raised for the Everyday Hassles Scale as were noted for the Social Readjustment Scale. However, such tools are still useful for assessment if their limitations are recognized and considered.

The Stress Audit. The Stress Audit, developed by Miller, Smith, and Mehler (1991), is a self-administered questionnaire designed to assess experienced and anticipated stressful events. Unlike most tools, the Stress Audit focuses on stressful events anticipated in the future as well as situations from the past. The tool also identifies stress symptoms and responses to stress. The person's overall vulnerability to stress is also identified.

Coping Measurement. The Jaloweic (1981) Coping Scale is a survey instrument designed to measure the use and efficiency of various coping strategies. The Coping Inventory for Stressful Situations was developed by Kurokawa and Weed (1998). The tool measures three basic coping styles: task-oriented; emotion-oriented; and avoidance-oriented.

Nursing Observations   Suicide Potential

Suicide or suicide attempts may be a person's response to stress or crisis states. The greatest suicide risks occur in the following groups: alcoholics, adolescents, elderly persons, accident-prone persons, those with a history of suicide attempts, minority groups, police, and physicians (McClean, 1983).

When evaluating suicide potential, consider the following risk factors:

(continued)

DISPLAY 14.7

Holmes and Rahe's Social Readjustment Scale

The person selects from the scale life events that have occurred during the past year. Add the stress unit values associated with each event to determine the final score.

LIFE EVENT	STRESS UNIT VALUE	LIFE EVENT	STRESS UNIT VALUE
Death of spouse	100	Children leaving home	29
Divorce	73	Trouble with in-laws	29
Marital separation	65	Outstanding personal achievement	28
Jail term	63	Spouse begins or stops work	26
Death of close family member	63	Begin or end school	26
Personal injury or illness	53	Change in living conditions	25
Marriage	50	Revision of personal habits	24
Fired at work	47	Trouble with boss	23
Marital reconciliation	45	Change in work hours or conditions	20
Retirement	45	Move or change in residence	20
Change in health of family member	44	Change in schools	20
Pregnancy	40	Change in recreation	19
Sexual difficulties	39	Change in church activities	19
Gain of new family member	39	Change in social activities	18
Business readjustment	39	Mortgage or loan less than $10,000	17
Change in financial status	38	Change in sleeping habits	16
Death of close friend	37	Change in number of family gatherings	15
Change to different line of work	36	Change in eating habits	15
Arguments with spouse	35	Vacation	13
Mortgage or loan more than $10,000	31	Christmas	12
Foreclosure of mortgage or loan	30	Minor law violations	11
Change in responsibilities at work	29		

Score interpretation:

150–199	Mild stress
200–299	Medium stress
300+	High stress: Associated with high rates of illness

(Adapted from Holmes, T.H., & Rahe, R.H. [1967]. The social readjustment rating scale. *Journal of Psychosomatic Research, 11*[2], 213–218)

Nursing Observations   Suicide Potential (continued)

- *Age:* Suicide is the third leading cause of death in the age-group of 15 to 24 years. Elderly persons (especially those in the eighth decade of life) also are at higher risk for suicide. The suicide rate for elderly men is four times the national suicide rate.
- *Sex:* Men commit suicide more often than women by a ratio of 3:1. Most male suicides occur after age 45 years. Women attempt suicide more often than men by a ratio of 3:1. Most female suicides occur after age 55 years.
- *Recent loss:* Loss of loved ones, social status, health, independence, income, employment (especially if elderly person)—all may precipitate a suicidal crisis.
- *Drug and alcohol abuse:* Drug and alcohol abuse may precipitate suicide or be considered a type of passive suicide.

(continued)

DISPLAY 14.8

Lazarus's Everyday Hassles Scale

The following scale rank-orders "hassles," which contribute to stress, and "uplifts," which contribute positively to stress management, as evaluated in several middle-aged groups. The nurse may determine the person's hassles and uplifts for purposes of providing anticipatory guidance. Individual person may perceive hassles and uplifts differently from the groups studied by Lazarus.

HASSLES [RANK ORDERED]

1. Feeling concern about weight
2. Worrying about health of a family member
3. Worrying about rising cost of living
4. Dealing with home maintenance
5. Having too many things to do
6. Misplacing or losing things
7. Doing yard work or outside home maintenance
8. Worrying about property, investment, or taxes
9. Worrying about crime
10. Feeling concern about physical appearance

UPLIFTS [RANK ORDERED]

1. Relating well to spouse or lover
2. Relating well with friends
3. Completing a task
4. Feeling healthy
5. Getting enough sleep
6. Eating out
7. Meeting responsibilities
8. Visiting, telephoning, or writing someone
9. Spending time with family
10. Home pleasing to you

(Adapted from Lazarus, RS. [1981]. Little hazards can be hazardous to your health. *Psychology Today, 15*[7], 58–62)

Nursing Observations   Suicide Potential (continued)

- *Social isolation:* Those who live alone or who have never married are at greater risk.
- *Depression:* You should be especially concerned if the person exhibits the triad of hopelessness, helplessness, and worthlessness.
- *Previous suicide attempts:* Evaluate seriousness of attempts in terms of lethality and intent.

Assess suicide risk by interviewing the person, listening to statements for suicide ideation, and observing behaviors and appearance.

GENERAL PRINCIPLES

The quickest and most direct assessment method is to interview the person. Although a person may not volunteer an intent to commit suicide, he or she may discuss it when asked. Questioning should be conducted in a direct but caring manner. For example, it is better to ask the person, "Are you thinking of taking your own life?" than to say, "You would not harm yourself, would you?"

Establish rapport. Be empathetic by carefully listening to the person and being supportive. Avoid using language that is accusatory.

EXAMINATION AND DOCUMENTATION FOCUS

- Intent and suicide ideation
- Plan
- Means
- Previous attempts
- Additional risk factors

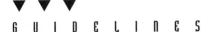

▼ ▼ ▼
GUIDELINES

Assessment Guidelines   Suicide Potential

Procedure	Clinical Significance
1. Determine intent.	
Ask the person whether he or she has, or has had, suicidal thoughts.	Expression of suicide thoughts is referred to clinically as "suicide ideation."
Direct questioning is usually most effective.
Ask the person whether he or she is currently contemplating suicide.	
Listen for statements such as the following:	Statements may indicate that the person has made a decision to attempt suicide.
"They'll be sorry when I'm gone."	
"I'm such a burden."	
"I don't deserve to live anymore."	
Verbal statements may be less direct, such as:	
"Everything's okay now."	
"I've finally found the solutions to my problems."	
Look for behaviors that are out of character for the person. For example, someone who has been depressed may suddenly appear cheerful and animated and talk about the future. The person may give away prized possessions, suddenly decide to write a will, or contact friends and relatives as though saying goodbye. Behaviors associated with depression, such as sleep disturbances, use of drugs or alcohol, and feelings of hopelessness, are also significant.	Behaviors are more difficult to analyze in terms of suicide intent but may be the only clue.
Not all of these behaviors indicate a suicide threat, but further assessment is always warranted.
2. Determine whether the person has a plan for how to commit suicide.	If the person has a plan, suicide risk increases.
Ask the person questions such as the following:	
"How would you take your own life?"	
"When would you do it?"	
3. Evaluate means.	
Determine whether the person has the means to carry out the plan.	A person with a plan and the means to carry out the plan is considered high risk for suicide.
Ask questions such as the following:	If the means is highly lethal, the person should be considered high risk for suicide.
"Do you have a gun? How would you get a gun?"	
"Do you have the sleeping pills?"	
4. Note previous attempts.	
Determine whether the person has a history of suicide attempts. If so, identify method.	
5. Note additional risk factors.	
Observe whether the person is under the effects of drugs or alcohol.	Drugs and alcohol may alter judgment and increase the risk of suicidal behavior.
Ask the person whether he or she has been or is being abused (physically, emotionally, or sexually).	Abuse may be an indicator of a poor social support system.
Having an unsatisfactory support system increases suicide risk.

▼ ▼ ▼
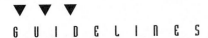
G U I D E L I N E S

Assessment Guidelines   Interpreting Physical Examination Findings and Stress Responses

Procedure

1. Integrate findings

Integrate the physical examination findings and observations of behavior into the overall assessment of stress and coping with special attention to the following:

- General appearance and behavior
- Cardiovascular system
- Respiratory system
- Gastrointestinal system
- Musculoskeletal system
- Integumentary system

2. General appearance and behavior

Conduct a general survey and note general indicators of stress.

Identify general physical symptoms associated with stress, including the following:

- Nausea, anorexia, gastrointestinal pain, overeating
- Fatigue, insomnia, sleeping more than usual
- Headache, chest pain, back pain, neck pain

Observe the person's facial expression.

Note cognitive responses to stress.

Note affective responses to stress.

Look for patterns of defensive coping, including denial, displacement, projection, rationalization, regression (dependence), repression, suppression (see Display 14-9).

Avoid abrupt confrontation when first recognizing signs of defensive coping.

Clinical Significance

Stressors activate the sympathetic nervous system and hypothalamic-pituitary-adrenal axis, resulting in behavioral and physiologic alterations that may be observed during the physical examination.

(Note: Complete physical examination methods for the cardiovascular, respiratory, and musculoskeletal systems are found in Chapter 8; the GI system and skin assessment are discussed in Chapter 6).

General appearance may or may not be affected by stress.
Acute Stress Indicators: Sense of panic, hypervigilance, feelings of being "nervous" or "jittery," hyperactivity, preoccupation with frightening images, ineffective problem solving or decision making, stereotyped thinking.

Facial Indicators of Stress: Anxious or alarmed facial expressions.
Cognitive Indicators of Stress: Decreased perceptual ability, narrowing of focus, thought disorganization, decreased problem-solving abilities, impaired decision making.
Cognitive Indicators of Stress Reduction: Increased participation in decision making and problem solving.
Affective Indicators of Stress: Feeling overwhelmed, helplessness, loss of control, anxiety, guilt, anger, low self-esteem.
Affective Indicators of Decreasing Stress: Ability to express doubts, fears, and concerns; increased self-esteem.
Defending is a means of protecting against an unspecified problem. The defensive response, however, results in avoidance of the problem, rather than problem solving.
Defensive mechanisms are protective and may actually promote eventual development of adaptive coping behaviors. Abruptly removing a defense mechanism can predispose the person to a severe stress reaction when the defense is penetrated and no other coping strategies have been developed. However, some defensive behaviors are potentially harmful, and the defense may need to be penetrated. For example, a person who denies having had a myocardial infarction and persists in being fully ambulatory even though such activity is potentially dangerous may need to be confronted about the severity of his or her illness.

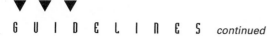

GUIDELINES *continued*

Interpreting Physical Examination Findings
and Stress Responses

Procedure	Clinical Significance
3. Cardiovascular system Observe the heart rate and rhythm, and blood pressure. Determine whether there are ECG changes indicating myocardial ischemia or chest pain.	***Cardiovascular Indicators of Stress*** • Increased heart rate (more than 10 beats/min greater than baseline) • Increased systolic blood pressure • Cardiac dysrhythmias such as premature ventricular contractions and premature atrial contractions • ECG changes consistent with cardiac ischemia • Chest pain sensations or palpitations *(Note: a person with underlying cardiovascular system disease is more likely to exhibit these signs and symptoms during periods of stress.)*
4. Respiratory system Observe the ventilatory pattern and rate. Determine whether there is a history of a greater incidence of upper respiratory infections that may be associated with the effects of stress on the immune system.	***Respiratory Indicators of Stress*** • Hyperventilation • Reports of "air hunger," shortness of breath
5. Gastrointestinal system Listen to bowel sounds for signs of increased motility of the gastrointestinal tract. Determine whether there is a history of ulcers or other gastrointestinal symptoms.	***Gastrointestinal Indicators of Stress*** • Hyperactive bowel sounds • Excessive bowel movements • Nausea • Abdominal pain
6. Musculoskeletal system Observe the overall muscle tone and body movements.	***Musculoskeletal Indicators of Stress*** Skeletal muscle tension, restlessness, constant movement of a body part.
7. Integumentary system Observe the appearance of the skin. Determine whether there are skin conditions that are associated with stress.	***Integumentary Indicators of Stress*** Variations in normal skin temperature and moisture. Skin lesions, including herpes, eczema, and dermatitis, may recur during periods of stress.

DISPLAY 14.9

Defensive Behaviors

- *Denial.* Consciously or unconsciously ignoring symptoms and avoiding discussion about a stressor to allay anxiety and reduce stress. (*Example:* The patient states, "It's only gas," when in fact he or she has had a myocardial infarction. Failure to follow activity restrictions after an illness or injury may represent denial.)
- *Displacement.* Unconsciously transferring emotional feelings from the actual stressor to a substitute. (*Example:* "None of you knows anything about taking care of sick people.")
- *Projection.* Attributing personal ideas or characteristics to others. (*Example:* "My wife thinks I am going to die.")

- *Rationalization.* Justifying behaviors or decisions to maintain self-respect and eliminate guilt. (*Example:* "I am glad I didn't get promoted because I would have had to work extra hours.")
- *Regression or Dependence.* Adopting behaviors used at an earlier level of emotional development. (*Example:* "I cannot give myself a bath. Will you do that for me?")
- *Repression.* Involuntarily blocking painful thoughts or memories from consciousness. (*Example:* "I do not remember yelling at you.")
- *Suppression.* Consciously and deliberately dismissing thoughts or feelings. (*Example:* "I do not want to talk about my illness; it would only upset me.")

NDx

Documenting Stress Response and Suicide Potential

Document your observations with special attention to (1) observations you make regarding degree of vigilance, problem solving, judgment, and decision-making abilities, and (2) statements and behaviors indicating poor self-esteem, feelings of helplessness, defensive coping behaviors, or suicide ideation. It may be helpful to quote the person directly. A description of a person displaying defensive coping might be as follows:

> Does not verbalize reason for hospitalization. Physician discussed with him earlier. Continues to state, "I'm here for a couple of routine tests and I wouldn't be here at all if my kids weren't such worriers."

A description of a person displaying low self-esteem might be as follows:

> Does not initiate conversation. Keeps head lowered when talking to others. Participates minimally in activities and only after persuasion from staff. Told roommate, "I'm no use to anybody anymore."

A description of a person showing a decreased stress reaction might be as follows:

> Discussing discharge and return to family and work. States she wants to continue with outpatient physical therapy. Talks about accident. Appearance well-groomed. Less dependent on staff for assistance with activities of daily living.

A description of a person with suicide ideation might be as follows:

> States "Life just isn't worth it anymore." Denies having plan for suicide but states he has stockpiled approximately 40 "downers."

NDx

Nursing Diagnoses Related to Stress and Stress Responses

Nursing diagnoses addressing coping include the following: Ineffective individual coping, Defensive coping, and Ineffective denial. Benner and Wrubel (1989) question the use of terms such as *effective* or *ineffective coping* or *defensive coping,* which bring to mind a dichotomy of "good" coping versus "bad" coping. According to Benner and Wrubel, the use of this terminology suggests that someone outside the stressful situation, such as the nurse, has a clearer view and can pass judgment on whether the person is coping effectively. They go on to say that this approach might cause the nurse to fail to consider the individual's interpretation of the stressful situation. They suggest that the nurse focus on understanding personal meanings and why a particular way of coping may have been right for the person at the time. Although Benner and Wrubel discourage the use of terms such as *effective* or *ineffective coping,* such diagnoses are considered clinically useful by others. Ineffective coping is officially recognized as a nursing diagnosis.

Ineffective Individual Coping

Ineffective individual coping is a state of inadequate response to stressors because of lack of physical, psychological, and behavioral resources necessary to promote effective coping strategies. Dysfunctional coping behavior is not the same as a single instance of overreacting to a stressor but rather represents a prolonged and debilitating pattern of ineffective coping.

Dysfunctional coping is identified if the person fails to adapt to a stressor within a 3- to 6-month period. Failure to adapt is manifested as follows:

- Persistence of distressing symptoms such as depression or anxiety
- Impaired social functioning such as drunken or reckless driving, abusive behavior toward others, failure to obey the law, truancy
- Inadequate performance on the job or at school or excessive procrastination

Other dysfunctional behaviors include self-destructive behavior, overuse of defense mechanisms, and verbalizing an inability to cope.

Dysfunctional or Anticipatory Grieving

Grieving, a normal process of coping, is the response to an actual or perceived loss of a person, object, function, status, or relationship. Grieving also may be anticipatory, in response to the realization of a future loss. If grieving is *dysfunctional,* more active intervention may be indicated.

Normal grieving consists of four stages: shock and disbelief, awareness, restitution, and resolution. Assessment is focused on evaluating the person's progress through the grief stages:

- *Shock and disbelief:* The person may feel numb to all unpleasant emotions or deny that the loss has occurred. Denial represents a defense mechanism used to alleviate the intense feelings precipitated by the loss.
- *Awareness:* The person may become increasingly and painfully aware of the reality of the loss and may express anger toward others. This coping mechanism is a form of displacement, or the unconscious transfer of feelings to others.
- *Restitution:* In this stage, the person begins to mourn the loss.
- *Resolution:* Finally, the person resolves the loss by using intrapsychic methods and, perhaps, becoming

less preoccupied with the loss. The stage may last for many months.

Post-trauma Response

Trauma is the occurrence of extraordinary life events such as war, rape or other assault, natural disasters, accidents, or catastrophic illness. The trauma victim has usually been exposed to multiple stressors directly associated with the traumatic event, not to mention threats to life and safety, and increased feelings of vulnerability. Assessing a person who has experienced trauma includes evaluating coping mechanisms as well as the need for crisis intervention or other forms of emotional support. In the period immediately after the trauma, the person may use various defense mechanisms such as denial, regression, and suppression as a defense against overwhelming and possibly unknown threats. The use of such defense mechanisms in this phase is a normal stage of the post-trauma response.

Clinical Problems Related to Stress and Stress Responses

Stress is believed to be a causative factor in a number of illnesses and conditions. In the cardiovascular system, stress has been linked to coronary artery disease, hypertension, and cardiac dysrhythmias. In the pulmonary system, stress is associated with asthmatic reactions. Stress affects the gastrointestinal system by contributing to ulcers, irritable bowel syndrome, diarrhea, nausea and vomiting, and ulcerative colitis. Stress may affect sexual functions, resulting in impotence or frigidity. Stress-related skin disorders include eczema and acne. Additionally, stress has been linked to headache, backache, and immunosuppression.

CASE STUDY

Tim Jensen, aged 38 years, believed that he was too young to be in the hospital for a bleeding ulcer. He thought this disease occurred only in people who were excessive drinkers or who had been overworked for years. It seemed like the older men he was acquainted with inevitably had either heart attacks or ulcers. Although he did not drink alcohol, he had a stressful job selling real estate and worked long hours. He had been experiencing heartburn for the last 6 years, used antacid tablets frequently, and was slightly overweight. His diet included soda and processed foods, because he was rarely home at his family's usual mealtime, and his relaxation activities included smoking marijuana. Tim believed the recurring heartburn, or what the physician had called an ulcer, was due to being overweight. After receiving a blood transfusion and ulcer medication, Tim signed himself out of the hospital. After all, he could not close any real estate deals

and keep up with his competitors while lying in a hospital bed.

Mr. Jensen's medical diagnosis was hemorrhagic peptic ulcer, a stress-related illness. Peptic ulcers have been described as a 20th-century disease, especially in men younger than 50 years. The pathogenesis of peptic ulcer is related to hypersecretion of hydrochloric acid and high concentrations of corticosteroids, which are associated with long-term stress and anxiety. Recognizing and modifying stress are important nursing concerns.

Case Study Analysis

Many people seeking health care are confronted by significant stressors and demonstrate various responses. The nurse evaluates stress and responses to stress to identify nursing intervention needs.

CASE STUDY *continued*

Mr. Jensen showed signs of significant stress. Although the nurses caring for him after his hospital admission for hemorrhagic peptic ulcer identified stress, Mr. Jensen's decision to refuse health care prevented immediate nursing care.

Identifying the Assessment Focus

Once Mr. Jensen's physiologic status was stabilized, the nurses caring for him began evaluating stressors and stress perceptions. The decision to evaluate this area was based on knowledge of the role of stress in the disease etiology. Furthermore, Mr. Jensen's nutritional patterns were targeted for priority assessment because dysfunctional eating behaviors, often a response to stress, can further potentiate ulcer formation by adversely affecting digestion.

Assessment of Mr. Jensen's stress response focused on identifying what he perceived to be the stressful conditions in his life and his usual methods of coping with them.

Possible Nursing Diagnoses

Nursing diagnoses of Ineffective individual coping, Defensive coping, and Ineffective denial were tentatively established for Mr. Jensen, based on the following cues the nurses had detected since his hospital admission:

- Self-destructive behavior. He repeatedly stated he would leave the hospital against medical advice, saying, "Dying might be better than not making a living."
- Denial of obvious health problems. He continued to attribute gastrointestinal symptoms to "just a little gas" rather than ulcer disease.
- Inability to ask for help

Additional Data Gathering and Analysis

The nursing diagnoses prompted further investigation. Specifically, the nurses needed to identify causative or contributing factors. Important factors to consider and evaluate further included career and financial concerns as well as Mr. Jensen's usual coping strategies. A more thorough assessment was planned to identify or rule out other stressors such as strained family relationships, poor self-esteem, sleep loss, and health concerns.

Additionally, Mr. Jensen's use of denial and other attempts at coping warranted further investigation and analysis. The ulcer pain represents a stressor that Mr. Jensen may not have accepted; therefore, he chose to deny the significance of the pain. Rather than interpreting his pain as a signal of illness, he chose to reduce emotional distress by attributing the pain to being overweight. Although using denial is not always harmful, continually using such a mechanism represents an ineffective coping strategy. Furthermore, Mr. Jensen coped with tension by using drugs. Inasmuch as denial evades dealing with the cause of the symptoms, drugs only temporarily induced relaxation. Mr. Jensen's coping strategies may not be effective for dealing with stress.

CHAPTER 14 SUMMARY

Assessment of Stress and Coping

The assessment of stress and coping is directed toward the following:

- Identifying stressors and situations that precipitate stress
- Understanding the meaning of the stressful situation to the individual
- Identifying the person's strengths and coping skills
- Identifying responses to stress
- Recognizing signs of crisis or threats to safety brought on by stress

Key Assessment Principles: Stress and Coping

- Assessment of stress and stress responses is optimal when nurse and client have an open and trusting relationship.
- Stressors vary among people because stressors are interpreted from each person's perspective.
- Individual responses to stress are varied and are influenced by personal values, culture, perception, socioeconomic resources, and experience with the stressor.
- Physiologic signs of stress are varied and are usually not as reliable as information obtained by client interview and observation.
- Coping should be judged in terms of distress reduction and adaptation. Nurses should take care not to judge coping strategies with respect to their own personal values.
- Many different coping strategies may facilitate effective coping, including the temporary use of defense mechanisms.
- Crisis or suicide ideation detected during assessment represents an emergency situation in need of immediate intervention.

Data Collection Methods

1. Interview and Review of Records
   Stressor identification

Stress perception
Coping styles
Resolution of stress
2. Diagnostic Studies (Measurement) of Stress and Coping
Social Readjustment Rating Scale
Everyday Hassles Scale
Stress Audit
3. Physical Examination
General appearance
Body system indicators of stress
4. Suicide Risk Evaluation

Primary Nursing Diagnoses
- Ineffective individual coping
- Impaired adjustment
- Defensive coping
- Ineffective denial
- Decisional conflict (specify)
- Dysfunctional grieving
- Anticipatory grieving

 Critical Thinking

A 45-year-old woman is returning to the orthopedic outpatient clinic for evaluation of continued low back pain and discussion of therapeutic options. She also complains of being "stressed-out" and tired.

Learning Exercises

1. Describe how you would identify the sources of stress for this person. What is the significance of evaluating stressful life events?

2. Describe several barriers to communication that could occur during the assessment of this person. How would you overcome each barrier?

3. Explain how you would identify a defensive coping pattern. What are typical characteristics?

4. Describe the self-concept that is associated with ineffective coping patterns; Identify some indicators of self-concept you could observe during the assessment process.

BIBLIOGRAPHY

Baker, F. et al. (1985). The impact of life events on chronic mental patients. *Hospital and Community Psychiatry, 36*(3), 299–301.

Baldree, K.S., Murphy, S.P. & Powers, M.J. (1982). Stress identification and coping patterns in patients on hemodialysis. *Nursing Research, 31*(2), 107–112.

Benner, P. & Wrubel, J. (1989). *The primacy of caring: Stress and coping in health and illness.* Menlo Park, CA: Addison-Wesley.

Bjorck, J.P., & Klewicki, L.L. (1997). The effects of stressor type on projected coping. *Journal of Traumatic Stress, 10*(3), 481–497.

Bromberger, J.T., & Matthews, K.A. (1996). A longitudinal study of the effects of pessimism, trait anxiety, and life stress on depressive symptoms in middle-aged women. *Psychology of Aging, 11*(2), 207–213.

Burns, K.R., & Egan, E.C. (1994). Description of a stressful encounter: Appraisal, threat, and challenge. *Journal of Nursing Education, 33*(1), 21–28.

Cohen, F. (1981). Stress and bodily illness. *Psychiatric Clinics of North America, 4,* 269–286.

Cronqvist, A., Klang, B. & Bjorvell, H. (1997). The use and efficacy of coping strategies and coping styles in a Swedish sample. *Quality of Life Research, 6*(1), 87–96.

Crow, C.S., Olivet, L.W., Burry-Stock, J., & VanderMeer, J.L. (1996).

Assessment of pain coping styles: Development of an inventory. *Journal of Advanced Nursing, 24*(5), 890–898.

Ehlert, U., & Straub, R. (1998). Physiological and emotional response to psychological stressors in psychiatric and psychosomatic disorders. *Annals of the New York Academy of Science, 851,* 477–486.

Fink, S.L. (1967). Crisis and motivation: A theoretical model. *Archives of Physical Medicine Rehabilitation, 48,* 592–597.

Friedman, M.J. (1997). Posttraumatic stress disorder. *Journal of Clinical Psychiatry, 58,* Supplement 9, 33–36.

Gignac, M.A., & Gottlieb, B.H. (1996). Caregiver's appraisals of efficacy in coping with dementia. *Psychology of Aging, 11*(2), 214–225.

Grassi, L., Righu, R., Sighinolfi, L., Makoui, S., & Ghinelli, F. (1998). Coping styles and psychosocial-related variables in HIV-infected patients. *Psychosomatics, 39* (4), 350–359.

Guzzetta, C.E. & Forsyth, G.L. (1979). Nursing diagnostic pilot study: Psychophysiologic stress. *Advances in Nursing Science, 2*(10), 27–44.

Haley, W.E., et al. (1996). Appraisal, coping, and social support as mediators of well-being in black and white family caregivers of patients with Alzheimer's disease. *Journal of Counseling and Clinical Psychology, 64*(1), 121–129.

Holmes, T.H. & Rahe, R.H. (1967). The Social Readjustment Rating Scale. *Journal of Psychosomatic Research, 11*(2), 213–218.

Infante, M.S. (Ed). (1982). *Crisis theory: A framework for nursing practice.* Reston, VA: Reston Publishing.

Jaloweic, A., & Powers, M.J. (1981). Stress and coping in hypertensive and emergency room patients. *Nursing Research, 30*(1), 10–15.

King, K.B., Rowe, M.A., Kimble, L.P., & Zerwic, J.J. (1998). Optimism, coping and long-term recovery from coronary artery surgery in women. *Research in Nursing and Health, 21*(1), 15–26.

Kobasa, S.C. (1979). Stressful life events, personality and health: An inquiry into hardiness. *Journal of Perspectives on Social Psychology, 37*(1), 1–11.

Kurokawa, N.K.S., & Weed, N.C. (1998). Interrater agreement on the coping inventory for stressful situations. *Assessment, 5*(11), 93–100.

Lazarus, R.S. (1966). *Psychological stress and the coping process.* New York: McGraw-Hill.

Lazarus, R.S. & Laurier, R. (1978). Stress-related transactions between person and environment. In Pervin, L.A. & Lewis, M. (Eds.), *Perspectives in interactional psychology* (pp. 287–327). New York: Plenum Press.

Lewis, K.S. (1998). Emotional adjustment to a chronic illness. *Lippincott's Primary Care Practitioner, 2*(1), 38–51.

Lindqvist, R., & Sjoden, P.O. (1998). Coping strategies and quality of life among patients on continuous ambulatory peritoneal dialysis (CAPD). *Journal of Advanced Nursing, 27*(2), 312–319.

Linn, J.G. (1997). Stress, appraisal and coping in HIV-infected African-American men and women. *Cellular and Molecular Biology, 43*(7), 1123–1130.

Low, J. (1996). The concept of hardiness: A brief but critical commentary. *Journal of Advanced Nursing, 24*(3), 588–590.

Marmar, C.R., Weiss, D.S., Metzler, T.J., & Delucchi, K. (1996). Characteristics of emergency services personnel related to peritrau-matic dissociation during critical incident exposure. *American Journal of Psychiatry, 153*(7) (Suppl.), 94–102.

McClean, L. (1983). Guilt and fear of self-destruction. In Haber, J. et al. (Eds.), *Comprehensive psychiatric nursing* (2nd ed.) (pp. 577–597). New York: McGraw-Hill.

Miller, L.H., Smith, A.D., & Mehler, B.L. (1991). *The stress audit.* Brookline, MA: Biobehavioral Associates.

Moneyham, L., Seals, B., Sowell, R., Hennessy, M., Demi, A., & Brake, S. (1997). The impact of HIV on emotional distress of infected women: Cognitive appraisal and coping as mediators. *Scholarly Inquiry in Nursing Practice, 11*(2), 125–145.

Selye, H. (1976). *The stress of life* (2nd ed.). New York: McGraw-Hill.

Simoni, P.S., Paterson, J.J. (1997). Hardiness, coping, and burnout in the nursing workplace. *Journal of Professional Nursing, 13*(3), 178–185.

Stewart, M.J., Hirth, A.M., Klassen, G., Makrides, L., & Wolf, H. (1997). Stress, coping, and social support as psychosocial factors in readmissions for ischaemic heart disease. *International Journal of Nursing Studies 34*(2), 151–63.

Thompson, S.C., Nanni, C., & Levine, A. (1996). The stressors and stress of being HIV-positive. *AIDS Care, 8*(1), 5–14.

Thorson, J.A. & Thorson, J.R. (1986). How accurate are stress scales? *Journal of Gerontological Nursing, 12*(1), 21–24.

Vitaliano, P.P., Russo, J., Young, H.M., Becker, J., & Maiuro, R.D. (1991). The screen for caregiver burden. *Gerontologist, 31*(1), 76–83.

Weisman, A.D. (1979). *Coping with cancer.* New York: McGraw-Hill.

Wijma, K., Soderquist, J., & Wijma, B. (1997). Posttraumatic stress disorder after childbirth: A cross-sectional study. *Journal of Anxiety Disorders, 11*(6), 587–597.

Wolanin, M.O. & Phillip, L.R. (1981). *Confusion: Prevention and care.* St. Louis: C.V. Mosby.

Assessing Values
and Beliefs

**A S S E S S M E N T
G U I D E L I N E S**

Values and Beliefs: Interview
(Health History)

Values and Belief Pattern

C H A P T E R   O R G A N I Z A T I O N

Introductory Overview
- Assessment Focus
- Data Collection Methods
- Nursing Diagnoses

**Knowledge Base
for Assessment**
- Culture
- Cultural Sensitivity

- Culture and Health
- Spirituality
- Nurse's Self-Assessment of Values
  and Beliefs

INTRODUCTORY OVERVIEW

In a society with more than 270 subcultures and 200 religious groups, nurses need to be aware of cultural and religious beliefs and values to provide culturally competent care. People of all ages and backgrounds may face situations or crises that cause them to question the meaning and value of life. How these experiences are viewed may be influenced by the cultural and spiritual beliefs and values of the individual and the nurse.

Values and beliefs greatly influence a person's attitudes and moral outlook, which help guide behavior and establish life goals. A value is defined as "an effective disposition toward a person, object, or idea" (Steele & Harmon, 1979). Values are used in decision making and generally persist over a long time. Beliefs are "a special class of attitudes in which the cognitive component is based more on faith than fact. They represent a personal confidence in the validity of some idea, person, or object" (Steel & Harmon, 1979).

The values and beliefs of an individual are influenced and shaped by one's culture. Cultural values "are unique expressions of a particular culture that have been accepted as appropriate over time" (Giger & Davidhizar, 1995). The values of a culture and the beliefs and values of an individual guide and influence individuals in forming goals, opinions, and decisions every day. Values and beliefs influence health-related decisions, health practices and priorities, and behavior in life-threatening situations. Behaviors that initially seem inappropriate or illogical to an observer may be logically explained once the values and beliefs of the individual are examined.

A value and belief system is the basis of a person's philosophy of life, whether conscious or unconscious, religious or secular. Such a philosophy is intimately connected with spirituality. Spirituality is a complex abstract concept. After a literature review and concept analysis, Julia Embers (1992) defined spirituality as a personal life principle that animates the transcendent quality of a relationship with God or god being. Each person's spirituality is highly variable, individualistic, and ever-changing.

The pattern of a person's values and beliefs is closely related to self-concept, coping abilities, stress tolerance, and role–relationship behaviors. Values and beliefs must be considered in the assessment process to provide holistic care that takes into account not only the physical needs of a person but the emotional, psychological, and spiritual needs as well. Understanding a client's values and beliefs also helps the health professional to understand the client's health-related decisions and to plan coping strategies and interventions that support those values and beliefs.

When providing care to people from different cultures, subcultures, and religious groups, it is important to avoid generalizing. Although particular values and beliefs may be associated with a certain group of people, they are not necessarily the values and beliefs of each member of that group. When assessing clients from different cultural or religious groups, the nurse should try to learn as much as possible about the individual's values and beliefs, and what impact they may have on his or her health.

ASSESSMENT FOCUS

Value and belief assessment is the process of collecting and analyzing data for the purpose of identifying satisfying levels of spirituality, risks to spirituality, and the desire to enhance spirituality. A comprehensive value and belief assessment includes the following objectives:

The purposes for assessing values and beliefs are as follows:

- Identifying the person's cultural and ethnic background and the degree to which traditional ethnic values are maintained
- Identifying the person's values and beliefs about life, death, health, illness, and spirituality
- Determining whether the person's values and beliefs are in conflict with those of the health care system providing care
- Identifying culturally based health practices
- Recognizing any evidence of spiritual distress

Data Collection Methods

Data collection is achieved by the following methods:

1. Interview or Review of Records
     Cultural and ethnic background
     Identification of risk factors associated with ethnic background
     Use of folk remedies
     Verbalization regrading spiritual beliefs
     Participation in religious activities
2. Physical Examination Focus
     General appearance
     Note use of cultural/spiritual adornments

Nursing Diagnoses

Assessment of the value and belief pattern may result in one of the following NANDA-approved nursing diagnoses that has been identified for the value and belief pattern:

Spiritual distress (distress of the human spirit)
Potential for enhanced spiritual well-being

Secondary NANDA-approved nursing diagnoses for a person with spiritual distress also may include the following:

Anxiety
Decisional conflict
Dysfunctional grieving
Hopelessness
Impaired social interaction
Ineffective individual coping
Personal identity disturbance
Self-esteem disturbance
Sleep pattern disturbance

KNOWLEDGE BASE FOR ASSESSMENT

Culture, spirituality, values, and beliefs are closely interrelated and must be considered together during the assessment process. These factors can greatly influence the outcome of treatment and the success of nursing interventions. Often these factors are not assessed by the nurse unless a problem occurs, for example, the person does not comply with the established regimen or is unable to make a decision. It is important for the nurse to know how variables such as culture, values, and spirituality affect health and health behaviors.

Culture

Culture is "a patterned behavioral response that develops over time as a result of imprinting the mind through social and religious structures and intellectual and artistic manifestations" (Girer & Davidhizar, 1995). Every person's definitions of health, optimal health, illness, and communication patterns are influenced to some extent by cultural background. Culture is socially inherited and represents a complex system of values, beliefs, customs, rituals, taboos (laws), and norms shared by a group of people. Although cultures are always evolving, changes are often slow; nonetheless, culture is passed down from generation to generation. Even though a person may not be totally influenced by all aspects of his or her culture, the influence of culture on a person's behaviors and a person's interpretation of others' behaviors is inevitable and usually discernible.

According to Spector (1996), culture has the following characteristics: culture is the medium of all relationships; conscious and unconscious; an extension of biological capabilities; interlinked web of symbols; creates and limits choices; can be internal (in the mind) and external (in the environment). Culture is complex; each part is linked to every other part. Language and behavior are the symbols of culture. Additionally, culture determines the types of experiences encountered by an individual and influences the response to those experiences. For example, until recently, in the United States, women's hockey, professional women's basketball, and men staying home to care for children were not socially sanctioned.

Cultural Sensitivity

Being aware of a person's cultural background is important in assessing values and beliefs and in determining a plan of care. More important is determining the degree to which people identify with their ethnic heritage. Nurses should be careful not to stereotype individuals into a particular ethnic group because of their last name or physical appearance, because these factors are often not accurate indicators. Asian-Americans or Hispanic-Americans may identify more with the culture of the United States than they do with their foreign ethnic heritage (Fig. 15-1). Also,

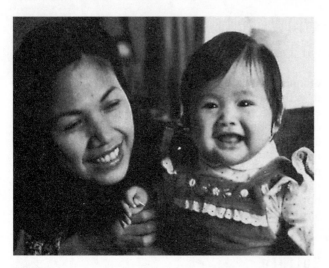

FIGURE 15.1 The entrance of Mexican-Americans into politics, new perspectives on their culture, and new opportunities have helped Mexican-American families come out of isolation into the "American" society.

individuals adopted as infants in another country may know nothing of their birth culture.

Immigrants to a different culture face not only external changes but also changes within the family. With each succeeding generation from the original immigrants, individuals tend to be less affiliated with the original culture and more affiliated with their surrounding culture. At times, this difference between generations causes family strain. Families whose members have more than one set of cultural values, beliefs, and customs generally experience more distress than families with one cultural orientation.

Because the United States and Canada are nations inhabited by native and immigrant peoples from numerous places, nurses frequently encounter clients from different ethnic groups. It is not unusual for nurses to encounter health beliefs and practices that differ or conflict with their own beliefs and practices. Therefore, it is essential that the nurse be sensitive to persons from different cultures and adapt intervention strategies to deliver effective, efficient care and avoid misunderstanding. Practicing competent cultural sensitivity includes (1) using nursing interventions based on the individual's culture rather than on stereotypes; (2) understanding implications of culturally specific health beliefs and attitudes; (3) incorporating folk health practices when possible; and (4) acting as an advocate for a person of another culture who has been denied quality care (Clark, 1996; AAN Expert Panel, 1992). Avoiding cultural blindness, ethnocentrism, cultural imposition, and stereotyping is crucial in providing effective care (see Display 15-1 for definitions).

Cultures share similar components in the shaping of values and beliefs. Five dimensions of orientation basic to all cultures have been identified as the nature of human beings, relationship between human beings and nature, time focus, purpose of life, and relationship with others (Kluckhorn, 1961).

Nature of Human Beings. Some cultures view people as basically good, others as basically evil but having a potential for good, or as a combination of good and evil. In the United States, the dominant view is that human beings are both good and evil and are able to practice self-control in the interest of promoting good. Subcultures may reflect more polarized viewpoints; for example, the Society of Friends, which represents Quaker beliefs, views human beings as good (Spector, 1996).

Relationship Between Humans and Nature. Cultural groups vary in their views as to how much control people have over their surroundings. Some groups believe that people have no control over the environment, whereas others believe they can eventually master the environment. In the middle are groups that believe in living harmoniously with nature.

Time Focus. All cultures have ideas about the past, present, and future. In the United States, however, the dominant culture is oriented to the future, whereas many Native American and Hispanic subcultures believe in concentrating on the present. The traditional Chinese subculture emphasizes the past.

Purpose of Life. Views about the purpose of life are closely identified with values. Cultural expectations of the dominant culture in the United States include continual achievement. Subcultures such as the Hispanic and Appalachian peoples place a higher value on personal development.

Relationship to Others. Interpersonal relations are influenced by cultural values. Views about relationships may be linear, collateral, or individualistic. Linear relationships emphasize the family and extended family; group goals take precedence over individual goals, and the continuum through generations is important. An example of a linear relationship is a closely knit Korean family that may include several generations. Individuals work toward family goals and often have joint ownership in a family business in which everyone is employed. The needs of the family business often take precedence over individual goals. Collateral relationships also emphasize family and group goals, but the valued family unit is nuclear, and in some groups the people are the same age. Collateral relationships exist in kibbutzim in Israel and in some communes in which the individual is responsible to the group and the group is responsible to the individual. Within individualistic relationships, individual goals take precedence, and autonomy and self-responsibility are highly valued. In the United States, individualistic relationships are the most frequent.

Interpersonal relations and role expectations within the family are also influenced and defined by cultural values. Family structure and decision-making power are often prescribed. In the United States, family structure, prescribed roles, and relationships have seen a dramatic change in the last 25 years, and there appears to be no dominant pattern. Male dominance remains common in Hispanic and fundamentally religious families, however. The importance of extended families is common among Native American and

DISPLAY 15.1

Definitions Related to Culture

Acculturation: The process of minimizing cultural differences when a member or members of one culture are a minority within another. Generally, members of the minority culture adapt to survive. The majority culture may adopt some aspects of the minority culture. For example, foods of other cultures (ethnic foods) are easily assimilated into American culture.

Assimilation: The end product of acculturation is assimilation. The individual has become a member of the dominant group in all aspects: culture, behavior, values, beliefs, rituals.

Cultural blindness: Ignoring cultural differences and interacting as if no difference exist.

Cultural relativity: The belief that all cultures are equal; no culture is better than another.

Culture conflict: Conflict occurs when people from different cultures are aware of the cultural differences and feel threatened by the differences.

Culture imposition: The belief that everyone in a society must conform to the dominant culture.

Culture shock: Immobilization and disorientation of a person that results from the awareness that the behavior, values, and beliefs of others in the community are different. For example, a particular gesture may have different meanings in different cultures, which may inhibit interaction and intensify culture shock and isolation.

Enculturation: The process of passing culture from one generation to another. Enculturation is accomplished through socialization.

Ethnicity: Belonging to an identified cultural or ethnic group.

Ethnocentrism: The belief that a particular way of life, beliefs, and culture are superior to all others.

Heritage consistence: The degree to which a person's values, beliefs, and behaviors reflect his or her culture.

Race: A biological term referring to physical features and inherited traits. Race is not necessarily related to culture.

Stereotype: Assumption that all people in an ethnic group or race are the same, and ignoring differences and uniqueness among individuals.

Subculture: A group that has a set of behaviors, values, and beliefs different from the dominant group. Also called an ethnic or minority group.

Transcultural nursing: The study of different cultures in relationship to health, illness, beliefs, values, lifestyle, and behaviors. Analysis of data enables the nurse to provide culture-specific nursing care and to become culturally competent. Introduced by Madeleine Leininger in 1960s.

Xenophobia: The fear of strangers or people who are different.

Amish families. For some ethnic groups, such as Vietnamese and Koreans, the family may be the only social network for its members. For a more detailed discussion of roles and relationships, see Chapter 12.

Culture and Health

Cultural values influence an individual's behavior, beliefs, and attitudes about health and illness. In the United States, people place a high value on youth, health, and personal responsibility. When illness occurs, people tend to look to themselves, the environment, or other people for a cause. Six cultural phenomena that vary among cultural groups and influence health include communication, space, social organization, time orientation, environmental control, and biological variations (Giger & Davidhizar, 1995).

Communication. Communication is an essential component of all stages of nursing care; however, communication, both verbal and nonverbal, often presents barriers when the nurse and client are from different cultures. In some cultures it is not appropriate to discuss personal information with individuals of the opposite gender. For ex-

ample, Arabic women do not feel comfortable discussing sexual issues with men. When effective communication is not possible because of language differences, a cultural barrier exists, and both nurse and client become frustrated. Clients who cannot communicate often become isolated, withdrawn, hostile, or uncooperative. The use of competent interpreters can lessen the effect of communication barriers (Giger & Davidhizar, 1995; Murry & Zentner, 1997; Spector, 1996).

Space. Personal space is the area around the individual and is an extension of the body. Territoriality is the behavior and attitude people have about their personal space. Territoriality and space serve four functions: security, privacy, autonomy, and self-identity. Individuals have control over their personal space and feel threatened when control is endangered. Personal space varies among ethnic groups. Americans, Canadians, and British individuals require more personal space when compared with members of other cultures such as Latin Americans, Japanese, and Arabic persons (Giger & Davidhizar, 1995; Watson, 1980).

Social Organization. Social organization is the environment in which children learn their culture and all people behave. It is composed of the family unit and social organizations such as religious groups and schools. Definitions of the family unit vary among different cultures. For example, among Native Americans and families of Mexican heritage, the family often is composed of extended family members that may include several households. In the United States and Canada, there are numerous family types (see Chap. 12) (Giger & Davidhizar, 1995; Spector, 1996).

Time. Time can be viewed in the past, present, and future. Different cultures place different emphases on the concept of time. Individuals in future-oriented cultures such as the United States and Canda tend to make long-term goals and plan ahead. Other cultures, such as many Native-American and Mexican groups, tend to be present oriented. The Chinese culture, however, tends to be past oriented. Whereas for people in the United States time often flies, for Mexicans time walks and the bus misses the person, the person does not miss the bus. Time orientation can influence health teaching that promotes health and prevents diseases. People with present-time orientation have difficulty finding time to prevent something that can occur in the future (Giger & Davidhizar, 1995; Spector, 1996).

Environment. Environment refers to the ability of an individual or society to plan activities that control nature. Included in environment are the health and illness beliefs and health care activities people use. Cultures that possess a high level of internal locus of control (see Chap. 11) believe that diseases can be prevented and health promoted by efforts of the society. The cultures of United States, Canada, and most of Europe possess an internal locus of control. The Mexican, Appalachian, and Puerto Rican cultures possess an external locus of control. Some cultures that believe in harmony with nature fall outside of the locus of control concept, for example, Japanese, Chinese, and Native Americans (Giger & Davidhizar, 1995; Spector, 1996).

Biological Variations. Physically and genetically, people from one culture vary from other peoples. There is a direct relationship between race, body structure, skin color, enzymatic and genetic variations, susceptibility to diseases, and nutritional variations (Giger & Davidhizar, 1995)

- ***Body structure.*** Body structure, including height, bone density (higher in African and Polynesian and lower in Asian heritage people), eyelid variations (epicanthic fold in Asian heritage people), nose shape, and muscle size and mass, all vary among ethnic groups.
- ***Skin color.*** Skin variations include color, texture, and hair. The palms of hands and soles of feet have the least amount of pigment. It may be difficult to assess slight skin color changes in dark-skinned individuals. Usually the darker the skin, the darker the oral mucosa (mucosa is always lighter). Cyanosis may be difficult to determine in some individuals of African heritage because of a normal blue tone to their lips, whereas eye sclera may naturally be yellowish. Mon-

golian spots (a bluish discoloration; see Chap. 16) may be present in infants of the following heritages: African, Native American, Mexican, and Asian. Individuals of African heritage are also more likely to have keloids (excessive scar tissue) than other ethnic groups (Giger & Davidhizar, 1995).
- ***Enzymatic and genetic variation.*** Variations include genetic differences as well as responses to medications and drugs (including alcohol). Twins are more common in individuals of African heritage and less in individuals of Asian heritage. Drugs for hypertension, tuberculosis, and psychosis are metabolized differently by racial groups (Giger & Davidhizar, 1995).
- ***Susceptibility to disease.*** Some ethnic groups have higher morbidity and mortality for specific diseases than other groups. Tuberculosis is higher in African Americans, Asians, Native Americans, and Hispanics than in non-Hispanic white Americans (environmental factors and poverty also may influence these higher rates). Diabetes mellitus is higher in Native Americans (except Alaskan Eskimos), Mexican Americans, other Hispanics, and African Americans. Hypertension is highest among African Americans and is also a problem for Mexican-Americans. Sickle cell anemia is the most common genetic disorder in the United States and occurs primarily in African Americans (Giger & Davidhizar, 1995).
- ***Nutritional variations.*** Most nutritional variation is dependent on what is available within the environment. Some food intolerances such as lactose (milk sugar) intolerance are common in Mexican-Americans, African Americans, Native Americans, and Asians. There are also some nutritional variations related to religious groups, such as kosher diet among Jewish and Islamic people and a vegetarian diet among Seventh Day Adventists (Giger & Davidhizar, 1995).

How Various Cultures Define Health and Illness

Definitions of health vary from culture to culture. Rachel Spector (1996) has documented definitions from numerous cultural groups. Some examples follow:

Chinese: Health is a state of spiritual and physical harmony with nature; the human body is a gift from ancestors and must be adequately maintained.

Hispanic: Health is a reward for good behavior, a gift from God.

Native Americans: Health is living in harmony with nature.

African Americans: The mind, body, and spirit are inseparable. Health is maintained by living in harmony with nature, a gift from God.

Cultural groups may view illness as resulting from a pathologic process within the body or from external sources such as the "evil eye." Illness definitions from various cultures include the following:

Chinese: Illness represents an upset in the balance of yin and yang. Yang is the male or positive energy, producing light, warmth, and fullness. Yin is female or negative energy, producing darkness, cold, and emptiness. To heal disharmony, yin and yang must be brought into harmony. Yin treatments are for yang illnesses, and vice versa. Yin treatments include acupuncture, herbal teas, and vegetables. Yang treatments include spicy foods and burning incense.

Hispanic: Illness represents either physiologic imbalance or punishment for wrongdoing. Imbalances may be viewed as "hot" or "cold." Hot illnesses are treated with cold substances, and vice versa. It is believed that imbalances may occur because of dislocation of body parts, resulting, for example, in abdominal cramping (*empacho*) or depression of the anterior fontanel in infants (*caida de la mollera*). Supernatural forces such as witchcraft and bad eye (*mal ojo*) also may cause imbalances, as may fright (*susto*). Finally, causing others to envy oneself (*envidia*) can produce an imbalance and cause bad luck.

Native Americans: There are over 400 different Native American groups. When working with a specific group, identify meanings for the group. The sources of illness are defined in various ways, such as the result of evil spirits, disharmony between positive and negative forces, cause-and-effect relationships, displeasure of holy people, and misuse of sacred ceremonies. Illness affects the person's spiritual as well as physical nature; both must be treated.

African Americans: Illness may be viewed as a disharmony of the mind, body, and spirit with nature, or the will of God. Prayer, laying of hands, and home remedies (folk medicine) may be used for treatment.

For members of many religious groups, such as Church of the Nazarene, Church of Christ, Christian Scientist, and Assemblies of God, divine intervention through prayer is sought during illnesses.

Although these definitions should only serve as a guide and are broad generalizations, they represent an overview of the different perspectives about health and illness. The perception and experience of health and coping with illness are based on cultural values and beliefs and provide an expectation of health care (Meleis, Lipson, and Paul, 1992). Therefore, the individual's viewpoint and expectations are important and need to be considered when health care is provided. Incorporating culturally and religiously appropriate beliefs into the treatment plan encourages the client to accept the plan and participate in its implementation.

Cultural Health Customs and Rituals. In addition to shaping views about health and illness, cultural beliefs serve as the basis of customs and rituals. Customs include sexual identity practices, such as circumcising males (and females in some African/Middle East cultures) or wearing certain clothing or ornaments; dietary regulations, such as avoiding meat or certain combination of foods; and folk remedies, such as wearing garlic necklaces or copper bracelets to guard against certain illnesses or conditions. Folk medicine represents a system of self-care, even if not formally recognized, that relieves the health care system.

For example, people will eat chicken soup, take aspirin, and increase fluid intake for a cold rather than seek professional care. If people sought professional care for every illness or adverse condition, there would be no space in the waiting rooms of health care facilities. Folk medicines are used for promoting health and dealing with short-term conditions, chronic and incurable conditions, and psychosomatic conditions (Bushy, 1992). Recent studies on folk medicines used by Mexicans and Mexican-Americans show that there is scientific evidence to support the use of some of these medications.

Dietary practices and beliefs about folk medicines are especially important considerations when collecting assessment data and designing plans of care. Here, too, recognizing a person's preferences and beliefs can assist in planning interventions and facilitating a client's acceptance with a prescribed treatment. Dietary customs and usual mealtimes should be considered if a client is taking medications with meals.

Some families use folk or home remedies to prevent and cure health problems. Folk remedies may be made by the family or require the help of special folk practitioners such as lay midwives, herbalists, *curandera* and *curandero* (medicine men and women), and faith healers. Folk practitioners have various educational backgrounds and usually learn their skills and obtain their knowledge through apprenticeships. Chicken soup exemplifies a popular American folk remedy for the common cold and flu. Other remedies include drinking herbal teas, cleansing the system with enemas or laxatives in the spring, taking extra vitamin C in the winter, eating raw onions and garlic, rubbing goose fat on the chest, drinking hot lemonade with whiskey and honey, wearing charms or medals, praying, and sitting in sweat baths or saunas.

Folk remedies are used for a variety of problems. For example, people of Mexican heritage along the border use garlic and tincture of marijuana for arthritis; garlic and papaya for hypertension; and *nopales* (prickly pear cactus) and aloe vera for diabetes (Long, 1996). Folk remedies are passed down from generation to generation. Usually wives or mothers are the providers of health care in the family and are responsible for providing folk remedies. In some cultures, older women assume responsibility for dispensing health care advice to the extended family. Families also may rely on cultural health providers. Knowledge of who assumes responsibility for the health of the individual and the providers used for specific problems can assist in a greater understanding of the individual's health practices.

Cultural rituals are usually associated with major life events such as birth, puberty, marriage, and death and should be discussed whenever possible. Some rituals impact health practices, such as circumcision of males in Jewish families.

Because individuals from many ethnic minorities have a foreshortened life span and increased prevalence of chronic illnesses, careful assessment of cultural beliefs and practices becomes important to establish effective and efficient nursing services. Identification of individuals of specific ethnic groups also alerts the nurse to possible health risks (Table 15-1). Statistics also show that Native Ameri-

TABLE 15.1 Health Risks for Selected Ethnic Groups

Ethnicity	Health Risks
African Americans	Cerebrovascular accident (stroke), hypertension, end-stage renal disease, sickle cell disease, HIV, homicide, cancer
Native Americans	Infant mortality, alcoholism, homicide, suicide, diabetes, liver diseases, arthritis, tuberculosis, and heart disease
Southeast Asians	Lung cancer, liver cancer, tuberculosis, hepatitis B, adult lactase deficiency
Japanese Americans	Cancer of stomach, esophagus, and liver
European Americans	Cardiovascular disease, osteoporosis, cancers, emphysema, breast cancer, diabetes mellitus, phenylketonuria, cystic fibrosis
Mexican-Americans	Diabetes mellitus, tuberculosis, communicable diseases, adolescent pregnancy, obesity
Filipino Americans	Hypertension, diabetes mellitus, thyroid cancer
Poor European Americans	Tuberculosis and other communicable diseases, heart diseases, diabetes mellitus, infant mortality, nutritional deficiencies, dental caries, adolescent pregnancy, obesity

Adapted from Giger, J., & Davidhizar, R. (1995). *Transcultural nursing: Assessment and interventions* (2nd ed.). St. Louis: Mosby; and Spector, R. (1996). *Cultural Diversity in health and illness* (4th ed.). Stamford, CT: Appleton & Lange.

cans are more likely to die of diabetes, cirrhosis, and pneumonia/influenza; Hispanics are more likely to die of diabetes, HIV (AIDS), and prenatal conditions; and African Americans are more likely to die of heart disease, cancer, and stroke.

In addition to ethnic risk factors, poverty is an added risk factor for many minorities. Poverty often denies people access to health care. Even among those who do manage to gain access to health care services, many are reluctant to seek health care because of fear and distrust of the health care system and providers who may seem unfamiliar, impersonal, or strange to them. There may be a language barrier or lack of understanding when interventions are described. When interventions are first presented to people, many will seem polite and agreeable, but often they fail to follow through with prescribed interventions or regimens, particularly if interventions are complicated, expensive, or long-term. The nurse should know that just because a person agrees to a plan of care at the outset does not always mean that he or she fully understands or is willing to follow through with prescribed care.

Spirituality

The dimensions of spirituality include a continuous interrelationship between the inner being of a person, the supreme values that guide the person, and the relationship with self, others, and the environment (Carson, 1989). Spirituality interacts with all aspects of the person and is "expressed through interpersonal relationships between persons and through a transcendent relationship with another realm; [it] involves relationships and produces behaviors and feelings which demonstrate the existence of love, faith, hope, and trust, therein providing meaning to life and a reason for being" (Labun, 1988). Carson (1989) defines spirituality as going beyond religion and tapping deeper beliefs about the meaning of life, love, hope, forgiveness, and life after death. Supreme values are most commonly placed with God but may be placed in science, nature, or whatever the individual believes. Most people have spiritual beliefs in some form, whether these beliefs are part of a formal religious creed or a more amorphous component of a general philosophy of life.

Embers (1992) defined religion as a system of organized beliefs and worship that the person practices. Organized religions provide a set of values, beliefs, norms, a frame of reference, and a perspective that can be used to organize information and govern daily activities. When numerous cultures exist within one society, religious values, beliefs, and norms will vary. In many societies, one set of religious beliefs dominates, such as Judaism in Israel and Islam in Saudi Arabia.

Spiritual beliefs and values may or may not be linked with an organized religion. Atheists and agnostics have spiritual beliefs and values to the same extent as devout Baptists and Moslems. Individual values and beliefs vary greatly. Spiritual values and beliefs go beyond belief in a being or "force" and include beliefs about death, sin, illness, health, the existence of a soul, life after death, and responsibilities to others.

Religious beliefs can have a strong influence on views about health and illness (Table 15-2). In some instances,

TABLE 15.2 Selected Health Care Issues and Religious Beliefs

Abortion prohibited	Roman Catholic, Jehovah's Witnesses, Baptist, Pentecostal
Blood and blood products prohibited	Jeohovah's Witnesses
Medications restricted	Christian Science
Organ donation restricted	Jehovah's Witnesses, Judaism (questionable), Christian Science
Active euthanasia, assisted suicide prohibited	Judaism, Islam, Roman Catholic, Jehovah's Witnesses
Withdrawal of live support supported if condition medically hopeless	Judaism, Islam, Roman Catholic, Protestant, Jehovah's Witnesses
Birth control restricted	Roman Catholic, Buddhism, Church of Jesus Christ of Latter Day Saints

illness may be interpreted as punishment for certain deeds. Conversely, some religious codes, such as the Latter Day Saints of Jesus Christ (Mormons), promote healthy lifestyles by advocating that certain potentially harmful substances such as tobacco and alcohol be avoided. Most religions have beliefs and practices that influence health and illness, such as dietary habits, birth control, birth, and death (beliefs regarding autopsies and cessation of life support). For example, gelatin capsules cannot be ingested by Jews and Seventh Day Adventists, who practice Old Testament dietary laws. Pork insulin is prohibited for Jews and Islamics. Diabetic diets that require eating three meals a day may interfere with religious fasts. Taking daily medication for a chronic condition may conflict with a devout Christian Scientist's belief in "Divine Mind" and spiritual truth. Religion also may provide a sense of identity and equilibrium, promoting the development of a person's strengths and a positive lifestyle.

Individuals throughout their life span experience spiritual and religious development. Spiritual development is a dynamic process of gaining awareness of the meaning, purpose, and values in life. Religious development is the process of accepting a specific system of beliefs, values, norms, and rituals. Spiritual and religious development may or may not parallel each other. At the heart of religious or spiritual beliefs is the faith that one's beliefs are true and valid. The concept of faith can be viewed in a broader context of intellectual, philosophical, and developmental growth. Several stages of faith development have been advanced. Fowler (1983) has identified seven developmental stages of faith (Display 15-2). It is Fowler's belief that most people do not move into the higher stages of development.

Knowing a person's current developmental stage of faith can provide insight into his or her spiritual needs and can serve as a guide in planning appropriate interventions of care. Once spiritual and religious beliefs are developed, they usually do not change significantly. A crisis such as serious illness or the death of a loved one, however, may cause spiritual distress. At the same time, such a crisis can provide an opportunity for growth by forcing the person to rethink beliefs and values. Understanding a person's spirituality and religious beliefs can assist the nurse in providing support during such a crisis.

Nurse's Self-Assessment of Values and Beliefs

Awareness of possible conflicts in value–belief systems between the nurse and a client is possible only if the nurse understands his or her values, beliefs, and spirituality. Nurses who evaluate their own life philosophies, values, and beliefs may be less vulnerable to stressors. If a nurse understands his or her spirituality, he or she will be more comfortable discussing the meaning of life and death with clients. It is difficult to provide holistic care and promote spiritual well-being if the nurse is unaware of his or her own value and belief system and lacks spiritual well-being.

Nurses should assess and question their own spirituality to gain and maintain the necessary reserves to assist clients

DISPLAY 15.2

Fowler's Stages of Faith Development

- *Primal faith* (Stage 0—infancy). Prelanguage; characterized by the formation of trust relationships with significant others.
- *Intuitive–projective faith* (Stage 1—early childhood). Beliefs based on imagination, perceptions, and feelings; beliefs involve positive and negative powers affecting the child.
- *Mythic–liberal faith* (Stage 2—childhood and beyond). Characterized by development of logical thinking, which assists with understanding world order and meaning of life. The perspectives of others, especially family and religious figures, are usually accepted.
- *Synthetic–conventional faith* (Stage 3—adolescence and beyond). Personal, mostly unreflective synthesis of values and beliefs; evolves as the person attempts to reduce internal conflict by relying on conventional belief systems.
- *Individualistic–reflective faith* (Stage 4—young adulthood and beyond). Characterized by critical reflection on values, beliefs, and understanding of self and the social system. Choices made about ideology and lifestyle.
- *Conjunctive faith* (Stage 5—middle life and beyond). The recognition of multiple interpretations of reality; reinterpretation of life and appreciation of symbols, metaphor, and myth for understanding truth.
- *Universalizing faith* (Stage 6—middle life and beyond). Grounded in oneness with the powers of being. Visions free the individual to devote self to overcoming division, oppression, and brutality.

in facing spiritual crises and to maintain their own well-being. The purpose of questioning beliefs is not to determine whether they are good or bad, but rather to determine how beliefs influence one's behavior and relationships with others. Spiritual assessment is one of the most omitted assessments in health care. Nurses need to know how to assess and support clients' spiritual needs. Supporting clients' spiritual needs can be done by the nurse or by others such as ministers and rabbis when the nurse is unsure of the need or the need is beyond his or her abilities or resources.

ND$_X$

Documenting Assessment Findings

Assessment data and clinical judgments are documented from the client interview and nurse observations. Assess-

Physical Examination   Value and Belief Assessment

GENERAL PRINCIPLES

There is no universally accepted evaluation tool for cultural heritage, spirituality, and values and beliefs.

A person's values, beliefs, cultural heritage, and spirituality are revealed throughout the health assessment interview and become more apparent through language, behavior, and appearance.

Accurate cultural assessment leads to appropriate interventions and culturally competent nursing care.

Although each individual is culturally unique, general baseline data regarding a specific group form a starting point for providing care (Giger & Diaidhizar, 1995).

Use interpreters during the assessment if the nurse does not speak the language of the client (Display 15-3).

Show respect for the individual and his or her culture.

Do not rush the interview; be patient, speak slowly and clearly.

COMPREHENSIVE VALUE AND BELIEF ASSESSMENT

Culture
  Ethnic background
  Beliefs about health and illness
  Use of folk remedies
  Orientation to time
  Biological variations
Spirituality
  Philosophy of life
  Spiritual beliefs and values
  Spiritual support

EQUIPMENT

No specific equipment is needed for the assessment of the Values and Beliefs Pattern; if language is a problem, an interpreter may be helpful.

ASSESSMENT AIDS

Interview guide (Display 15-4)
Language dictionary

DISPLAY 15.3

Enhancing Communication with Individuals of Other Cultures

- Determine the level of English fluency—if the individual does not speak English and the nurse does not speak the language of the individual, an interpreter is essential.
- When using an interpreter, speak to the individual, not the interpreter. Also, watch the individual while he or she is responding for nonverbal communication.
- Allow the individual to choose seating for comfort, with private space and eye contact.
- Choose a speech rate and sentence structure that promotes understanding and demonstrates respect.
- Avoid use of slang, jargon, medical terms, and metaphors.
- Use open-ended questions; may need to rephrase in several ways to obtain desired information; when in doubt ask for clarification.

- Validate information, do not assume meaning is understood without distortion.
- Provide reading material and other media (videotapes) in appropriate language.
- If an interpreter is used, try to use the same interpreter with every encounter.
- Do not use children to interpret culturally sensitive issues/concerns such as sexuality.
- Avoid offensive body and verbal language.
- Use caring tones and body expressions.
- Use an appropriate language dictionary.
- Try to learn the language of the individual or at least a few phrases, such as "hello."
- Develop a trusting relationship; give your full attention to the individual during the visit.

Adapted from Spector, R. (1991). *Cultural diversity in health and illness* (3rd ed.). Norwalk, CT: Appleton & Lange; and Giger, J., & Davidhizar, R. (1995). *Transcultural nursing: Assessment and interventions* (2nd ed.). St. Louis: Mosby.

DISPLAY 15.4

Interview Guide: Values and Beliefs

CULTURE:

Ethnicity

How long have you been in this area? _____

Where were you born? _____ Your parents? _____

Do you identify with any specific group (*i.e.,* Cubans, Sioux, Korean)?_____

Health Beliefs

How would you define health?_____

How would you define illness?_____

When you become ill, whom do you consult? _____

In your culture, are there some health practices that are important to you? _____

Folk Remedies

Many people use home remedies when they don't feel well. Could you describe what you do when you aren't feeling well?_____

When you were growing up, what types of home remedies did your mother or grandmother use? _____

When you are not feeling well, whom do you consult with first? Usually, how effective is their advice? _____

Could you describe remedies you use to help you stay healthy? _____

ORIENTATION TO TIME

How important is time to you? _____

Do you like to make plans for the future? _____

Would you desire life support? What are your views on organ donation? _____

Do you have an advanced directive or living will? _____

SPIRITUAL BELIEFS

Are there any foods you eat or avoid because of your religious beliefs? _____

Is there anything that is forbidden by your beliefs I should be aware of? _____

Would you describe how important your religious beliefs are to you?_____

Has anything recently changed your belief in your religion or God? _____

SPIRITUAL SUPPORT

Who else in your family shares your religious beliefs? _____

What religious books or religious articles are helpful to you? _____

When you need spiritual help, who assists you? _____

Do you find prayer or meditation helpful? (describe) _____

ment pertaining to values and beliefs may be documented as a part of a comprehensive assessment, entered in progress notes, or incorporated into problem-oriented records. Examples of narrative and problem-oriented types of documentation follow.

Example 1: Normal Value and Belief System

Mrs. S., an 84-year-old, was admitted to the rehab unit after a minor stroke. She had slight right-sided weakness and needed to learn to use a walker. She always appeared cheerful, frequently said "praise Jesus," "we all have a friend upstairs who looks over us," and "things could be worse." Her well-used Bible was always at her bedside.

S: Praise Jesus, We all have a friend up stairs who looks over us, things could be worse.

O: Cheerful, minister a frequent visitor, Bible at bed-side—well worn, active participant in rehab program.

A: Spiritual well-being.

P: Evaluate only if a change occurs. Support Mrs. S.'s spiritual beliefs.

Example 2: Spiritual Distress

Mr. K., a 22-year-old college student from Malaysia, was in the hospital with a severe fracture of his leg and pelvis after an auto accident 300 miles from the college he was attending. The day after he started on solid foods, he

▼ ▼ ▼
GUIDELINES

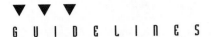

Assessment Guidelines   Values and Beliefs: Interview (Health History)

Procedure

Clinical Significance

1. Culture

a. Ethnic background

Data related to ethnic background can be collected through a combination of open and closed questions. If the person does not speak a language adequately known by the nurse, an interpreter may be needed. If an interpreter is not available, the interview should be rescheduled for a time when one is available.

- How long have you lived here?
- Where have you lived?
- Where were you born?
- Where were your parents born?
- Do you identify with any specific group?

If you are interviewing families, the nurse may wish to explore place of grandparents' birth.

The nurse may wish to further explore ethnicity by asking questions such as:

- I don't know much about the way of life in (insert country/area). Could you tell me a little about that?
- What was it like growing up in _____?
- Are there any special foods from _____ that you like to fix?
- Are there any special traditions or activities that you participate in?
- How closely do you identify with the culture of your parents or grandparents?
- How close are you to your aunts, uncles, cousins, and grandparents?

b. Health beliefs

Open-ended questions will reveal more information regarding health practices. Ask the following type of questions:

- How would you define health?
- How would you define illness?
- When you become ill, whom do you consult?
- In your culture, are there some health practices that are important to you?

c. Folk remedies

- Many people use home remedies when they don't feel well. Could you describe what you do when you aren't feeling well?
- When you were growing up, what type of home remedies did your mother or grandmother use?
- When you are not feeling well, whom do you consult with first? Usually, how effective is their advice?
- Could you describe remedies you use to help you stay healthy?
- Are there any special things you do when a baby is born? (if woman is pregnant)

The place of the individual's and parents' birth will give the nurse cues about the possibility of a different cultural orientation. If a person or his or her parents were born in a different culture, the nurse may wish to do a more extensive cultural interview. Assuming that a person from an ethnic group will automatically share that group's views can lead to incorrect conclusions. Knowing where the person has lived can provide cues to health risks endemic to specific regions. Remember that not all cultural groups are defined by ethnicity; for example, gangs and some groups such as the Hell's Angels also have unique cultures.

It is believed that it takes at least three generations for a family to completely assimilate into the dominant culture.

This information will assist the nurse in planning culturally competent interventions. With these open-ended questions, the nurse can discover important dates such as holy days and foods preferred by the individual. Additionally, family availability for social support also may be discovered. Some of this information already may have been collected for other patterns such as roles and relationships, health perceptions and health management, and self-concept. If this information is already available, the nurse may wish to omit these questions or verify the information.

All cultures define health and illness differently. Some groups (many Asians, Hispanics, and Arabs) believe that illness is caused by imbalances. Knowing what it means to be ill or well will assist in understanding why individuals prefer certain treatments and refuse others.

Individuals use remedies to prevent illnesses and to treat illnesses. It is useful to discover what the individual does for common health problems (such as cold, fevers, and headaches) and for chronic illnesses (such as hypertension and diabetes). Individuals often use remedies similar to what their mothers and grandmothers used and may be more willing to discuss their remedies. Some remedies have scientific evidence to support effectiveness. When a new remedy is identified, the nurse should attempt to discover its benefit or harm without dismissing the remedy's value.

▼ ▼ ▼
G U I D E L I N E S   *continued*   Values and Beliefs: Interview (Health History)

Procedure

- Is there anything special you do in your culture when someone is dying?

d. Orientation to time
To elicit this information, the nurse may wish to ask:
- How important is time to you?
- Do you like to make plans for the future?

e. Biological variations
The nurse will get information about biological variations from knowing the individual's ethnic/racial background. There are no interview questions for this component of the health history.

2. Spirituality

a. Philosophy of life
How a person views life can affect physical and emotional well-being. Assessing this dimension includes determining whether the client is satisfied with life, has plans for the future, and sees a purpose for own life.
- Ask a question such as "Would you describe for me what you believe is the meaning and purpose of life?" Use follow-up questions to clarify and verify your understanding.
- Also inquire into the individual's desire for life support and views of organ donation.
- Does the individual have an advanced directive or living will?

b. Spiritual beliefs
Most health history forms contain a question about religious preference.
Interview questions that elicit data about spirituality beliefs include the following:
- Are there any foods you eat or avoid because of your religious beliefs?
- Is there anything that is forbidden by your beliefs that I should be aware of?
- Would you describe how important your religious beliefs are to you?
- Has anything recently changed your belief in your religion or God?

Clinical Significance

The incorporation of safe cultural practices into the delivery of care is necessary if care is to be culturally competent and enhances compliance (Bushy, 1992). The nurse should use judgment when asking about cultural rituals and ask these questions when appropriate.

Knowing a person's time orientation is important—it provides information regarding making schedules and setting goals. Individuals with future orientation like schedules and long-term goals, and those with present orientation prefer short-term goals and may be late to appointments.

Knowing the ethnic background of the individual and the biological variations associated with the ethnicity is important while performing the physical assessment for other patterns. For example, while examining the external genitalia of a woman from Somalia, the nurse may find the external genitalia has been surgically removed (female circumcision). The nurse may wish to do screening or education for specific conditions related to the individual's ethnicity (see Table 15–1).

Life philosophies are culturally and spiritually influenced and are related to time orientation, beliefs about the relationship of human beings to nature, interpersonal relationships, and life purposes.

Organ donation, life support, and advanced directives are all associated with spiritual beliefs. These are decisions that should be explored before a need arises so an individual's wishes can be honored, and the individual has time to contemplate what their wishes are.

Additional questions to ask during the interview concern actual religious activities and the degree to which the client subscribes to religious beliefs or values.
Do not assume, because people indicate that they identify with a particular religion, that they follow religious codes. For example, some Roman Catholics use oral contraceptives, and some Jewish people eat pork. The nurse needs to discover what is important to the individual to provide holistic care.

▼ ▼ ▼

GUIDELINES *continued*   Values and Beliefs: Interview (Health History)

Procedure

c. Spiritual support

The following open-ended questions are useful to collect data regarding spiritual support:

- Who else in your family shares your religious beliefs?
- What religious books or religious articles are helpful to you?
- When you need spiritual help, who assists you?
- Do you find prayer or meditation helpful? (describe)

d. Diagnostic studies

There are no specific diagnostic studies for spiritual distress. Spiritual distress and culture shock may be manifested as symptoms in other patterns such as nutrition (weight gain or loss) and stress (difficulty coping).

Clinical Significance

People who lack sufficient spiritual support or a sense of spirituality are at greater risk for spiritual distress during a crisis. Many individuals receive spiritual support from prayer, reading a religious book such as the Bible, wearing or having special symbols such as rosary beads nearby, and wearing special garments.

The nurse may wish to consult with the individual's spiritual provider (minister, rabbi, or priest) to find additional ways to spiritually support the individual.

Several assessment tools are available that are similar to the interview guide display, for example, "Guidelines for Spiritual Assessment" (Stoll, 1979); "Spiritual Well-Being" (Ellis, 1983); and "Spiritual Assessment Guide" (O'Brian, 1982). Cultural assessment tools include Spector's (1996) Heritage Assessment Tool, and Bloch's (1983) Ethnic/Cultural Assessment Guide, which may be used if more information is desired; however, there are similar components in the interview guide.

---

stopped eating. The nurse discovered from his records that he was Islamic. After talking with him, she discovered the reason he did not eat was because bacon had been on the plate, and he now considered all eating utensils unclean.

 S: Islamic; because bacon had been on plate believes all utensils unclean.
 O: Stopped eating day after started on solid foods; bacon served with breakfast.
 A: Possible spiritual distress related to observation of religious dietary laws.
 P: Talk to Mr. K. regarding his dietary habits and what is possible and what is not.

Talk to the dietitian to get appropriate foods and utensils.

Consult with Imam (religious leader) at local mosque for ways to reduce spiritual distress and other possible cultural disturbances.

ND_x

Nursing Diagnoses Related to Values and Beliefs

There are only two nursing diagnoses for values and beliefs: Spiritual distress and Spiritual well-being.

Spiritual Distress

Spiritual distress occurs when there is a disruption in the life principle that pervades a person's entire being and integrates and transcends one's biologic and psychosocial nature (NANDA, 1996).

History. The individual express a disturbance in his or her belief system. This may be expressed by questioning credibility or fairness of beliefs, inability to perform previous religious activities, sense of emotional vacuum, anger at life events, and request for spiritual assistance.

Physical Examination Findings. Physical findings may be totally absent. Sign and symptoms of anxiety or stress such as palpations, sleeplessness, and gastric upset may be present. The nurse might observe a sudden increase or decrease in the amount of spiritual activity or interest.

Potential for Enhanced Spiritual Well-Being

The individual experiences confirmation of life through an interconnectedness with higher power and inner strength (NANDA, 1996).

History. The individual is content and in harmony with self and higher power; the individual has a sense of self-awareness.

Physical Examination Findings. There may be no physical findings. The individual should not have signs of stress or anxiety.

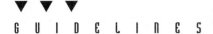

Assessment Guidelines   Values and Belief Pattern

1. General appearance

The nurse can gather much information from general appearance; however, one must be careful not to jump to conclusions before validating observations.

- *Dress.* The way an individual dresses may indicate cultural or religious background.

For example, orthodox Jewish men wear a yarmulke (skullcap), adult Mormons wear sacred undergarments, Mennonite women wear long-sleeved dresses and a cap, Indian women may wear native dress, and Islamic Arab women cover their hair.

- *Facial expressions.* Facial expressions can provide information during the interview and physical examination.

For example, a questioning expression, frown, or grimace may lead the nurse to wonder whether the individual really understands what is being asked. Lack of eye contact may represent normal behavior in some Native American people.

- *Touch.* A person's avoidance of a handshake or other touching may indicate cultural customs.

For example, the only women Orthodox Jewish men touch are their wives, children, and mothers, and Islamic Arabs do not touch anyone considered unclean (Carson, 1989).

- *Speech.* An individual's speech can provide much information, such as the presence of an accent, fluency in verbal English, or whether the individual speaks another language to others.

Accents or use of another language should alert the nurse to explore cultural beliefs and the individual's ability to understand and read English. If written material is provided, when possible provide it in the language the person prefers to read.

2. Observe for folk remedy use.

Physical signs of folk remedies used include copper bracelets, a coin on the navel wrapped with a belly binder in a Mexican-heritage infant, strong garlic breath smell, a small pouch tied to a cord around the neck or attached to a belt, and a bracelet made of hair.

3. Evaluate spiritual beliefs.

- Actively listen for remarks regarding spiritual belief.
- Observe for spiritual symbols.

Types of statements indicating spiritual distress include (Carson, 1989):

- Expression of anger, hurt; disappointment in God, religious representatives, church/temple/synagogue
- Verbalization of inability to sleep, stay asleep, nightmares
- Questions about belief system or meaning/purpose of life
- Verbalizing inability to exercise usual religious practices
- Asking for spiritual guidance or assistance
- Expressions of unworthiness

People may wear religious symbols or charms; observe for crucifix, crystals, angels on the shoulder, presence of religious statues or paintings, speaking in tongues, taviz (black string with word of the Koran attached), and wearing sacred undergarments (Mormons).

- Observe for participation in religious activities such as praying, reading Bible/Koran

- Observe for abrupt change in religious practices.

For example, a person who usually reads the Bible or watches religious programs suddenly stops, or a person who claims to have no religious beliefs suddenly begins to read holy books or watch religious programs.

ND_X

Clinical Problems Related to Values and Beliefs

Assessment of values and beliefs is useful for making nursing diagnoses and to determine appropriate interventions for clinical problems. Clinical problems such as miscarriage, death, and diagnosis of a potentially fatal disease can be factors in the nursing diagnosis of Spiritual distress.

Understanding values and beliefs will allow the nurse to determine areas of potential conflict between the client's values and beliefs and the health care options. Selecting and modifying appropriate options that reinforce, or at least do not conflict with, the client's values and beliefs enhances adherence to a health regimen. Charting out the client's beliefs and the possible health options may be useful in determining the most appropriate intervention (Display 15-5). In the example, option 3 has less of a chance of adherence even if scientifically it is the best option. The nurse may desire to use the same chart to insert his or her own values and beliefs or those of the health agency to determine where conflicts may occur between the client and nurse, the client and agency, and the nurse and agency.

DISPLAY 15.5

Comparing Values and Beliefs with Health Options

VALUES AND BELIEFS	OPTION #1	OPTION #2	OPTION #3
Value #1	+++	+	--
Value #2	+	+	+
Value #3	+++	+	0
Belief A	-	+	---
Belief B	+++	+++	+
Belief C	+	+	-
Belief D	+	+	+

Key: agreement with client, +; disagreement, –; neutral, 0. Adapted from Tripp-Reimer, T., Brink, P., & Saunders, J. (1984). Cultural assessment: Content and process. *Nursing Outlook, 32* (2), 78–82.

CASE STUDY

Mr. and Mrs Ramirez have recently discovered that the child Mrs. Ramirez is carrying has anencephaly (lacking most of the brain). This condition is not compatible with life. The physician wants Mrs. Ramirez to have a therapeutic abortion. The nurse and the Ramirez's talk about their options to have an abortion or not. Mrs. Ramirez states that she is Catholic and it is a mortal sin to have an abortion; however, Mr. Ramirez is not Catholic, and he believes that abortion is an option. Mrs. Ramirez agrees to return the next day to talk to the clinical nurse specialist about her options. The next day, Mrs. Ramirez tells the nurse that her mother and husband had a terrible argument about the possible abortion. She does not know what to do. She has been trying for 3 years to get pregnant. She asks many questions about the causes of anencephaly. She begins crying and wonders why this has to happen to her.

As Mrs. Ramirez's nurse, I realized she had the potential for numerous problems, including spiritual distress that was increased because of differences in belief between herself and her husband. I answered Mrs. Ramirez's questions as best I could and got some material she could take home to read. I also realized I needed more information about Mrs. Ramirez's beliefs and how active she was in her religion.

Additional data include that Mrs. Ramirez attends Mass weekly and on holy days. Her religious beliefs are very important to her, and she tries to be a good Catholic. She attended parochial school for 12 years. She has not yet talked to her priest about the baby. Mrs. Ramirez is now 20 weeks' gestation.

I prepared for my next meeting with Mr. and Mrs. Ramirez by discussing with the physician the procedure to be used for the abortion, and other options such as carrying to term and donating organs. I also talked with a priest regarding the religious implications of abortion and organ donation. During the visit I explained the procedure, options available, and what their health insurance would cover, because Mr. Ramirez seemed concerned with cost. Mr. and Mrs. Ramirez agreed to discuss this problem with her parish priest.

Mrs. Ramirez decides to carry the infant to term and donate organs. When she goes into labor, her priest is called to support Mr. and Mrs. Ramirez with the birth, baptism, and death of their infant girl, named Maria Louise. Maria's organs are donated to other infants. Organ donation helps Mrs. Ramirez believe that God had a purpose for Maria's short life.

CHAPTER 15   S U M M A R Y

A comprehensive value and belief assessment includes the following objectives:

- Identifying the person's cultural and ethnic background and the degree to which traditional ethnic values are maintained
- Identifying the person's values and beliefs about life, death, health, illness, and spirituality
- Determining whether the person's values and beliefs are in conflict with those of the health care system providing care
- Identifying culturally based health practices
- Recognizing any evidence of spiritual distress

Data collection is achieved by the following methods:

Interview and/or Review of Records
- Cultural and ethnic background
- Identification of risk factors associated with ethnic background
- Use of folk remedies
- Verbalization regrading spiritual beliefs
- Participation in religious activities

Physical Examination Focus
- General appearance
- Note use of cultural/spiritual adornments

Nursing Diagnoses
Assessment of the value and belief pattern may result in one of the following NANDA-approved nursing diagnoses that has been identified for the value and belief pattern:
- Spiritual distress (distress of the human spirit)
- Potential for enhanced spiritual well-being

Secondary NANDA-approved nursing diagnoses for a person with spiritual distress also may include the following:
- Anxiety
- Decisional conflict
- Dysfunctional grieving
- Hopelessness
- Impaired social interaction
- Ineffective individual coping
- Personal identity disturbance
- Self-esteem disturbance
- Sleep pattern disturbance

Critical Thinking

Amy, a 24-year-old, delivered a 32-week gestation female (Marguerite) 18 hours ago. Surgery is indicated for the infant. After explaining the procedure to Amy, the physician gets consent and then advises her that Marguerite may need blood. Amy and her family are Jehovah's Witnesses, and it is against their religious beliefs to receive blood or blood products. You enter the room as the physician leaves.

1. Amy asks you what could happen if Marguerite does not get blood. What would you tell Amy?

2. Amy also asks you to help her with this problem. What would you do?

3. Whom could you consult with regarding Amy and her baby?

4. What could/should a nurse do if he or she did not believe that the cultural/religious belief the client desired was morally correct?

BIBLIOGRAPHY

American Academy of Nursing Expert Panel on Culturally Competent Nursing Care (1992). AAN expert panel report: Culturally competent health care. *Nursing Outlook, 40* (6), 277–283.

Andrews, M., & Boyle, J. (1995). *Transcultural concepts in nursing care* (2nd ed.). Philadelphia: Lippincott.

Bloch, B. (1983). Bloch's assessment guide for ethnic/cultural variations. In M. Orque, B. Bloch, L. Monrroy (Eds.). *Ethnic nursing care: A multicultural approach.* St. Louis: Mosby.

Bushy, A. (1992). Cultural considerations for primary health care:

Where do self-care and fold medicine fit? *Holistic Nursing Practice, 6* (3), 10–18.

Carpenito, L. (1997). *Handbook of nursing diagnosis* (7th ed.). Philadelphia: Lippincott.

Carson, V. (1989). *Spiritual dimension in nursing process.* Philadelphia: Saunders.

Clark, A. (1996). *Community nursing.* Philadelphia: Saunders.

Dawes, T. (1986). Multicultural nursing. *International Nursing Review, 33* (5), 148–150.

Eddy, M. (1994). *Science and health with key to the scriptures.* Boston: The First Church of Christ, Scientist.

Ellwood, R. (1995). *Many peoples, many faiths* (5th ed). Englewood Cliffs, NJ: Prentice Hall.

Embers, J. (1992). Religion and spirituality defined according to current use in nursing literature. *Journal of Professional Nursing, 8*(1), 41–47.

Fowler, J. (1983). Stages of faith. *Psychology Today, 17*(11), 56–62.

Giger, J., & Davidhizar, R., (1995). *Transcultural nursing: Assessment and interventions* (2nd ed.). St. Louis: Mosby.

Kluckhorn, F. (1976). Dominant and variant value orientations. In P. Brink (Ed.). *Transcultural nursing* (pp. 63–91). Englewood Cliffs, NJ: Prentice-Hall.

Labun, E. (1988). Spiritual care: An element in nursing care planning. *Journal of Advanced Nursing, 13*(3), 314–320.

Leininger, M. (1978). *Transcultural nursing: Concepts, theories and practice.* New York: John Wiley & Sons.

Long, L. (1996). *Remedios Casero used for treatment of arthritis, hypertension, and diabetes.* (Masters' thesis, University of Texas at El Paso). El Paso, Texas.

Meleis, A., Lipson, J., & Paul, S. (1992). Ethnicity and health among five Middle Eastern immigrant groups. *Nursing Research, 41* (2), 98–103.

Murray, R., & Zentner, J. (Eds.) (1997). *Nursing concepts for health promotion* (6th ed.). Englewood Cliffs, NJ: Prentice-Hall.

North American Nursing Diagnosis Association. (1996). *Nursing diagnoses: Definitions and classification.* Philadelphia: NANDA.

O'Brian, M. (1982). The need for spiritual integrity. In H. Yura & M. Walsh (Eds.). *Human needs and the nursing process* (pp. 85–116). Norwalk, CT: Appleton-Century-Crofts.

Pender, N. (1996). *Health promotion in nursing practice* (3rd ed.). Stamford, CT: Appleton & Lange.

Ripley, G. (1986). Mexican-American folk remedies: Their place in health care. *Texas Medicine, 82* (11), 41–44.

Spector, R. (1996). *Cultural diversity in health and illness* (4th ed.). Stamford, CT: Appleton & Lange.

Steele, S., & Harmon, V. (1979). *Value clarification in nursing.* New York: Appleton-Century-Crofts.

Stoll, R. (1979). Guideline for spiritual assessment. *American Journal of Nursing, 79*(11), 1574–1577.

Watson, O. (1980). *Proxemic behavior: A cross-cultural study.* The Hague, Netherlands: Mouton.

UNIT THREE

Health Assessment Across the Life Span

16. Assessing Infants, Children, and Adolescents

17. Health Assessment of Elderly Persons

18. Assessing in Special Situations

CHAPTER 16

Assessing Infants, Children, and Adolescents

ASSESSMENT GUIDELINES

- Pediatric Interview (Health History)
- Physical Examination of Newborns
- Physical Examination of Infants
- Physical Examination of Young Children
- Physical Examination of Older Children and Adolescents

CHAPTER ORGANIZATION

Introductory Overview
- Assessment Focus
- Data Collection Methods
- Nursing Diagnoses

Knowledge Base for Assessment
- Age Classifications
- Health Perception and Health Management
- Nutrition and Metabolism

- Elimination
- Activity and Exercise
- Cognition and Perception
- Sleep and Rest
- Sexuality and Reproduction
- Coping and Stress Tolerance
- Roles and Relationships
- Self-Concept
- Values and Beliefs

Health assessment of infants, children, and, to a lesser extent, adolescents differs from assessment of adults in approach, techniques, and interpretation of findings. Infants and children grow physically and develop cognitively and emotionally at a rapid pace. The nurse is challenged to evaluate growth and development in the pediatric population in relation to developmental norms that may be quite different for children only a few months apart in chronologic age.

Healthy children should be assessed at frequent intervals that change as the child ages. For example, during the first year of life the child, who is rapidly growing and changing, is usually assessed five to six times, whereas the school-aged child is assessed yearly. Developmental and anthropometric changes are evaluated in relationship to previous assessments of the child, in comparison to standards of growth and development, and are conducted to detect deviations from normal ranges as soon as possible. In extreme cases, screening can mean the difference between mental retardation and normalcy. For instance, a child with a hepatic enzyme deficiency (phenylalanine hydroxylase) has abnormal amino acid blood and tissue levels, which can lead to brain damage and mental retardation. If the child is placed on a special diet during brain development, mental retardation can be avoided.

Health assessment of the child also involves evaluating other family members and their ability to provide care for and nurture the child. Because most children are accompanied by one or more family members, the nurse has the opportunity to assess many aspects of family functions that affect the children, including family relationships, values and beliefs, childrearing and punishment practices, and health management practices. Parents or other caretakers may need nursing interventions regarding their concerns for, and their ability to meet, the needs of the child. The needs of caretakers will change as the child grows and develops.

ASSESSMENT FOCUS

This chapter focuses on well-child assessment, not deviations related to congenital, acquired, or genetic anomalies, or the preterm newborn. In such cases, a comprehensive assessment should be performed by a pediatrician specialist, and the child then may be followed by a pediatric nurse practitioner.

The nurse's ability to interpret observations of children is facilitated by an understanding of normal growth and development processes. For example, findings such as lordosis, Snellen screening of 20/40, and umbilical hernia are considered normal at one age but abnormal at another age. Being aware of normal ranges for various ages will assist the nurse to determine whether intervention or referral is necessary.

The wide variation among individual children in growth and development makes interpretation of assessment findings especially difficult. For example, although most children learn to walk between ages 11 and 15 months, some children walk as early as 9 months and others not until 22 months. The range of 9 to 22 months is considered normal for learning to walk. Furthermore, children vary greatly in height, weight, and rates of developing motor, language, and social skills. Also, individual variations and ranges of normal become greater as people age.

With a comprehensive assessment of newborns, infants, children, and adolescents, the nurse will meet the following objectives:

- Evaluating the individual's growth
- Evaluating the individual's developmental status to identify strengths, variations, and delays
- Identifying parental/caretaker knowledge about childcare and development
- Identifying risk factors that threaten health

Data Collection Methods

Data collection is accomplished by the following methods:

1. Interview Child or Parent or Review of Records
    History, including gestational age and pregnancy and delivery problems if infant or child with developmental delays
    Developmental milestones
    Parental or caretaker concerns
2. Diagnostic Studies and Screening Tests
    Developmental screening
    Screenings recommended by US Task Force for Preventive Services
    Age-specific diagnostic tests

3. Physical Examination
    Head-to-toe or focused physical assessment with age-appropriate modifications

Nursing Diagnoses

Although all nursing diagnoses are appropriate for children, not all nursing diagnoses are used for each age group. For example, Self-care deficit and Incontinence would be the maturational norm for infants and toddlers. In place of the nurse emphasizing what the child cannot naturally accomplish, the nurse would be assessing parenting skills. Some nursing diagnoses applicable to children that are often overlooked include Rape–trauma syndrome, Potential for violence, Alteration in parenting (especially the adolescent mother), and Grieving.

Some nursing diagnoses focus on the family, thereby implying an effect on children. These diagnoses include Altered parenting, Alteration in family process, and Ineffective family coping. Additionally, children at specific ages are at higher risk for some nursing diagnoses than at other ages. For example, infants and toddlers are at higher risk for poisoning and suffocation than school-aged children or adults. Adolescents are at higher risk for Disturbance in personal identity, self-esteem, and body image than the preschool and school-aged child.

The nursing diagnosis Altered growth and development is used almost exclusively with children younger than 22 years. If an adult has not accomplished a developmental task, the focus is then on what has been altered because of this delay (Carpenito, 1997). For example, the individual with altered motor development may have the diagnosis of Impaired physical mobility or Self-care deficits.

For the diagnosis Altered growth and development, the child must exhibit an inability to perform or difficulty performing a task or behavior typical of his or her age group, or the child's weight must be two standard deviations below what it should be for height, or the child must have experienced an undesired drop in weight/height ratio. Reasons for altered growth and development can be related to health problems of the child or environmental conditions. Health problems might include congenital heart defects, neurologic impairments (cerebral palsy, mental retardation), muscular dystrophy, nutritional deficits (inadequate intake or disease processes such as cystic fibrosis), and prolonged casting of an extremity. Environmental factors may include lack of stimulating environment; parental lack of nurturing knowledge; abuse or neglect; loss or separation of family member, friend, or pet; hospitalization; and stress.

KNOWLEDGE BASE FOR ASSESSMENT

Age Classifications

From a growth and development perspective, children are evaluated with respect to norms for a particular age range. The following categories are widely used:

- Newborn: birth to 1 month
- Infant: 1 month through 11 months
- Toddler: 12 months through 35 months
- Preschool: 3 years through 5 years
- School age: 6 years through 12 years
- Adolescence: 13 years through 17 to 20 years

Judgments are made about the health status of newborns, infants, children, and adolescents on the basis of observations made during the interview and physical assessment. In babies and young children, functional abilities are rapidly evolving. Health assessment is focused on determining the acquisition and mastery of necessary skills such as motor and social skills, including language, speech, and intellectual development. Developmental screening tests such as the Denver Developmental Screening Test 2 (DDST2) and the Denver Articulation Screening Examination (DASE) may provide a reliable means of determining the development of motor, cognitive, social, and speech abilities (see Appendix D) and those children in need of diagnostic evaluation.

Health Perception and Health Management

For *babies* and *young children,* the responsibility for health promotion and health maintenance activities lies with parents or other caregivers. Health promotion activities for infants begin with the mother's health habits and exposure to harmful substances before and during the prenatal period. *Adolescents* usually have developed a perception of their own health status and generally assume more responsibility for their health maintenance.

The assessment of health perceptions and health-promoting activities requires an evaluation of the following:

- Common health concern or problems
- Immunization status
- Screening for diseases and disease risk factors
- Safety practices

Common Health Concerns or Problems

Healthy infants may experience few problems except for common colds and ear infections. First-time parents may have more questions and concerns about their children because of lack of previous experience and not knowing what is normal and what is not. As children interact with other children in environments such as day care, school, and playgrounds, the incidence of communicable diseases increases. More frequent colds, ear and throat infections, skin infections, and parasite infestation (pediculosis or lice) may occur. School-aged girls may develop urinary tract infections related to improper hygiene after bowel elimination. In addition, young children often develop vision and hearing problems. The most common adolescent health problems are accidents, nutritional disorders (including obesity, anorexia nervosa, and bulimia), acne, substance abuse, pregnancy, sexually transmitted diseases, and stress-coping problems.

Immunizations. Childhood immunizations are commonly initiated shortly after birth for protection against communicable diseases such as hepatitis, diphtheria, pertussis, tetanus, poliomyelitis, measles, mumps, and rubella. Table 16-1presents a recommended immunization schedule for infants and children. The recommended immunization schedule has had several revisions in the last several years. Health professionals are encouraged to use this as a guide only, because other revisions may follow. Parents should be encouraged to keep written immunization histories or charts to remind them of the schedule and for proof of immunization status for entry into day care, school, and college.

Screening for Disease or Disease Risk Factors. Children from families with positive histories for genetic-re-

TABLE 16.1 Childhood Immunization Schedule

Recommended Childhood Immunization Schedule United States, January–December 1997

Vaccines[1] are listed under the routinely recommended ages. Bars indicate range of acceptable ages for vaccination. Shaded bars indicate *catch-up vaccination:* at 11–12 years of age, hepatitis B vaccine should be administered to children not previously vaccinated, and Varicella vaccine should be administered to children not previously vaccinated who lack a reliable history of chickenpox.

Age ▶ Vaccine ▼	Birth	1 mo	2 mos	4 mos	6 mos	12 mos	15 mos	18 mos	4–6 yrs	11–12 yrs	14–16 yrs
Hepatitis B[2,3]	Hep B-1		Hep B-2		Hep B-3					Hep B[3]	
Diphtheria, tetanus pertussis[4]			DTaP or DTP	DTaP or DTP	DTaP or DTP		DTaP or DTP[4]		DTaP or DTP	Td	
H influenzae type b[5]			Hib	Hib	Hib[5]	Hib[5]					
Polio[6]			Polio[6]	Polio		Polio[6]			Polio		
Measles, mumps, rubella[7]						MMR			MMR[7] or MMR[7]		
Varicella[8]						Var				Var[8]	

Approved by the Advisory Committee on Immunization Practices (ACIP), the American Academy of Pediatrics (AAP), and the American Academy of Family Physicians (AAFP).

[1]This schedule indicates the recommended age for routine administration of currently licensed childhood vaccines. Some combination vaccines are available and may be used whenever administration of all components of the vaccine is indicated. Providers should consult the manufacturers' package inserts for detailed recommendations.

[2]**Infants born to HBsAg-negative mothers** should receive 2.5 µg of Merck vaccine (Recombivax HB) or 10 µg of SmithKline Beecham (SB) vaccine (Engerix-B). The 2nd dose should be administered ≥ 1 mo after the 1st dose.

Infants born to HBsAg-positive mothers should receive 0.5 mL hepatitis B immune globulin (HBIG) within 12 hrs of birth, and either 5 µg of Merck vaccine (Recombivax HB) or 10 µg of SB vaccine (Engerix-B) at a separate site. The 2nd dose is recommended at 1–2 mos of age and the 3rd dose at 6 mos of age.

Infants born to mothers whose HBsAg status is unknown should receive either 5 µg of Merck vaccine (Recombivax HB) or 10 µg of SB vaccine (Engerix-B) within 12 hrs of birth. The 2nd dose of vaccine is recommended at 1 mo of age and the 3rd dose at 6 mos of age. Blood should be drawn at the time of delivery to determine the mother's HBsAg status; if it is positive, the infant should receive HBIG as soon as possible (no later than 1 wk of age). The dosage and timing of subsequent vaccine doses should be based on the mother's HBsAg status.

[3]Children and adolescents who have not been vaccinated against hepatitis B in infancy may begin the series during any childhood visit. Those who have not previously received 3 doses of hepatitis B vaccine should initiate or complete the series during the 11–12-year-old visit. The 2nd dose should be administered at least 1 mo after the 1st dose, and the 3rd dose should be administered at least 4 mos after the 1st dose and at least 2 mos after the 2nd dose.

[4]DTaP (diphtheria and tetanus toxoids and acellular pertussis vaccine) is the preferred vaccine for all doses in the vaccination series, including completion of the series in children who have received ≥ 1 dose of whole-cell DTP vaccine. Whole-cell DTP is an acceptable alternative to DTaP. The 4th dose (DTaP or DTP) may be administered as early as 12 mos of age, provided 6 mos have elapsed since the 3rd dose, and if the child is considered unlikely to return at 15–18 mos of age. Td (tetanus and diphtheria toxoids, absorbed, for adult use) is recommended at 11–12 years of age if at least 5 years have elapsed since the last dose of DTP, DTap, or DT. Subsequent routine Td boosters are recommended every 10 years.

[5]Three *H influenzae* type b (Hib) conjugate vaccines are licensed for infant use. If PRPOMP (PedvaxHIB [Merck]) is administered at 2 and 4 mos of age, a dose at 6 mos is not required. After completing the primary series, any Hib conjugate vaccine may be used as a booster.

[6]Two poliovirus vaccines are currently licensed in the US: inactivated poliovirus vaccine (IPV) and oral poliovirus vaccine (OPV). The following schedules are all acceptable by the ACIP, the AAP, and the AAFP, and parents and providers may choose among them:
  1. IPV at 2 and 4 mos; OPV at 12–18 mos and 4–6 yr
  2. IPV at 2, 4, 12–18 mos, and 4–6 yr
  3. OPV at 2, 4, 6–18 mos, and 4–6 yr

The ACIP routinely recommends schedule 1. IPV is the only poliovirus vaccine recommended for immunocompromised persons and their household contacts.

[7]The 2nd dose of MMR is routinely recommended at 4–6 yrs of age or at 11–12 yrs of age, but may be administered during any visit, provided at least 1 mo has elapsed since receipt of the 1st dose and that both doses are administered or at after 12 months of age.

[8]Susceptible children may receive Varicella vaccine (Var) at any visit after the first birthday, and those who lack a reliable history of chickenpox should be immunized during the 11–12-year-old visit. Children ≥ 13 years of age should receive 2 doses, at least 1 mo apart.

After American Academy of Pediatrics (1997). *Redbook: Report of the Committee on Infectious diseases* (24th ed.). Elk Grove Village, IL: AAP.

lated diseases such as cardiovascular disease and diabetes mellitus should receive appropriate screenings such as blood pressure and education regarding the effects of lifestyle. Cholesterol screening of young children is considered controversial in part because the normal range of cholesterol is not known for children. Adolescents should begin to practice self-examination techniques such as breast self-examination or testicular self-examination. Sexually active female adolescents should have a pelvic examination and Papanicolaou's (Pap) smear.

Safety Practices. Accidents are the leading cause of morbidity and mortality in babies, children, and adolescents. Home safety should be carefully evaluated for infants and young children. Measures should be taken to prevent falls, burns, and ingestion of poisons. Learn whether the preschool-aged child knows how to avoid traffic. Check whether the child can recite his or her name, address, and telephone number. How does the child perceive police and firefighters; are they feared or seen as helpful adult figures? The nurse may directly interview older children about safety measures. Ask the child questions such as, "What would you do if a fire started in the kitchen? What would you do if a stranger wanted you to go with him or her?"

Automobile safety is a concern for all age groups. Is the child restrained in an automobile and is the restraining device appropriate for the child's age and size? Infants and toddlers should be restrained in infant seats with a five-point harness. The infant seat should face the back of the car seat until the infant is several months old or above a particular weight. Children more than 4 years of age or weighing more than 40 pounds may use a standard lap belt. The shoulder harness should not be used until the child is taller than 55 inches because the strap may cause neck injuries. Small children should not sit in the front seat of a car with air bags.

For children and adolescents who participate in sports activities, are appropriate measures taken to prevent sports-related injuries? Do adolescents drive under the influence of drugs or alcohol? Driving while intoxicated is a common risk factor for trauma or death.

Nutrition and Metabolism

Evaluation of nutritional status in the infant, child, or adolescent can be accomplished by the following methods:

- Interview parents or older child to obtain diet history and insight into any nutritional problems.
- Use anthropometric evaluation, including height, weight, and head and chest circumferences, in infants. Midarm muscle circumference and skinfold thickness may be measured in older children.
- Perform physical assessment to detect problems interfering with nutritional process and to detect signs of malnutrition.

Development of Eating Functions

At birth, babies can only suck and swallow liquids that are introduced into the back of the throat, as occurs with nip-

ple feeding. By age 2 months, the infant is usually able to swallow semisolid foods because the tongue can be brought against the palate. Between age 4 and 6 months, the gag reflex decreases, which facilitates swallowing solid foods. Teeth eruption usually occurs before the infant can ingest solid foods. The first teeth to erupt, between ages 5 and 6 months, are the lower central incisors. By 1 year, the infant usually has 6 to 8 teeth. Problems related to the development of eating functions include problems with weak sucking, bottle/breast weaning, appetite control, and food allergies.

Eating Behaviors. According to Erikson's developmental theory, the conflict facing children from ages 1 to 3 years involves autonomy versus shame and doubt. The young child usually resolves this conflict by asserting independence from parental control. Eating behaviors exemplify this need for autonomy beginning with weaning, when the child no longer takes breast or bottle feedings and begins to use a cup and eat at the table. These changes usually occur by the end of the first year. Early self-feeding is frequently associated with messiness, with almost as much food on the child as in the child. By the end of the second year, the rate of physical growth decreases, and children can tolerate longer periods between meals. The young child also may demonstrate autonomy by refusing certain foods or insisting on self-feeding.

Older children may find mealtime distracting because they are preoccupied with other activities. As children become older, their eating habits and food preferences are increasingly influenced by advertising and social/peer pressure. Children on special diets, such as diabetic diets, may experience difficulty in adhering to the diet while attempting to eat foods their friends eat, especially at certain events such as birthday parties.

Adolescents are particularly likely to engage in fad diets or unusual eating habits. Self-esteem is often tied to self-image; female adolescents often seek the ideal model-thin appearance, and male adolescents often aspire to a muscular, athletic appearance. These perceptions and other pressures place adolescents at risk for eating disorders of anorexia (not eating), bulimia (gorging followed by forced vomiting), and steroid abuse to build muscles with increased weight.

Caloric Needs. Caloric needs and nutrient requirements change throughout the life span. Caloric and nutrient needs for different age groups are in Appendix A. Caloric needs are further evaluated in relation to the child's rate of physical growth, stage of sexual maturity, and usual levels of physical activities.

Anthropometric Measurements. Anthropometric measurements of infants include measurement of height, weight, and head and chest circumference. In older children, height and weight are evaluated, and skinfold thicknesses may be evaluated. Measurements should be graphed. On a graph, children establish a normal curve for growth that should be consistent. Regardless of height and weight measurements, height should be proportional to weight. Because of age-related variations in the amount and distribution of subcutaneous fat, anthropometric norms vary across age groups and gender. Tables are available with norms for different age groups (see Appendix F).

Elimination

Patterns of bowel and bladder elimination should be evaluated in relation to age-related norms and expectations. The nurse should determine the following:

- The child's pattern of bowel and bladder elimination
- Characteristics of feces and urine
- Development of control of bowel and bladder elimination and related behaviors
- Problems with bowel and bladder elimination

Elimination Patterns. The character of feces is evaluated in infants to determine whether the gastrointestinal tract is functioning normally and whether bowel elimination problems such as diarrhea or constipation are present. Meconium, a tarry, odorless stool, is usually the first bowel movement after birth. Passage of meconium before birth is usually indicative of fetal distress and places the baby at risk for pneumonia. During the first week of life, the baby usually has transitional stools, which may be loose, green or yellow, and infiltrated with mucus. Two to four bowel movements a day are considered normal.

Differences in the infant's stool may he attributed to diet. Babies receiving formula will usually have feces that are more yellow and harder than the feces of breast-fed babies. Formula-fed infants average one to two bowel movements a day, whereas breast-fed babies may have as many as four per day. As other foods are added, the infant's feces becomes more adultlike. Initial voiding usually occurs within the first hour after birth; frequency depends on the total fluid intake and hydration status.

Control of Elimination. Children usually indicate a readiness for bowel and bladder training between ages 2 and 3 years. Bowel training usually occurs before bladder training, and daytime bladder control is usually achieved before nighttime dryness. Periodic loss of daytime bowel and bladder control is considered normal in young children and may occur during stressful periods or intense play. Complete control of elimination is usually achieved by age 4 to 5 years, although bed-wetting may occur through the preschool and school-age years.

Once bowel and bladder control are developed, children generally have few problems related to elimination. Young girls may develop occasional urinary tract infections because of poor hygienic practices.

Activity and Exercise

The developmental aspects of activity and exercise functions one should consider when evaluating children include the following:

- Nature of play, exercise, and leisure activities
- Developmental and maturation of self-care abilities in relation to eating, dressing, and attending to personal hygiene

- Actual or potential problems that may be associated with activity

Motor Development. Motor functions develop rapidly and eventually mature during adolescence and young adulthood. Motor functions are easily evaluated during the physical assessment of the child and by the administration of screening tools such as the DDST2 (see Appendix D). With the development of motor abilities, increasing independence occurs in the performance of self-care activities such as feeding, dressing, and attending to personal hygiene. School-age children and adolescents are usually completely independent in their performance of self-care activities.

Play. Play is the major activity of early childhood, providing opportunities for social interaction, learning, and developing gross and fine motor function. Playing house, for example, encourages role playing with socialization, and computer games and playing musical instruments increase hand–eye coordination. Toy safety and age-appropriate toys and leisure activities should be discussed with parents. Inappropriate toys can be harmful or fatal, especially for young children. An object that can fit through a cardboard toilet roll poses choking risks for children younger than 3 years.

By the end of the second year, children begin to exhibit parallel play, which involves playing near other children but not always interacting with them. Preschoolers (ages 3–5 years) move to cooperative play patterns and begin to participate in group activities that require mutual cooperation with other children. Team games such as softball/baseball and soccer are enjoyable to school-age children and adolescents.

Cognition and Perception

Evaluation of cognitive and perceptual functions can be accomplished by the following:

- Administration of appropriate screening tools such as the DDST2 and DASE
- Interaction with the child
- Interview of parents about any cognitive and perceptual problems
- Physical assessment of sensory and hearing systems and special senses

Cognitive Functions. Piaget's theory of cognitive development (1969) describes four sequential stages of cognitive development in infants, children, and adolescents. Application of this theory assists in understanding how children of different ages think and learn, which has implications for anticipatory guidance as well as nursing interventions of a teaching–learning nature.

According to Piaget, infants are in the sensorimotor stage of cognitive development. Learning occurs by repeated exposure to stimuli that are perceived through the senses of sight, hearing, smell, and touch. As the infant grows, other factors influence the learning process, especially the child's innate intellectual capacity, exposure to language, social interactions, and physical health.

The development of the infant's cognitive functions is evaluated by determining the age when certain learned responses first occurred. For example, by age 3 months the infant should recognize and respond to the primary caregiver; at age 4 months the bottle-fed infant can associate the appearance of a bottle with feeding; at age 6 months, the infant can recognize people as familiar or strange. Also at 6 months the infant begins to imitate behaviors demonstrated by others. Some of these behaviors, such as waving bye-bye, are not well developed until the infant has developed greater coordination. The infant learns object permanence by 7 months and will demonstrate this understanding by looking briefly for a hidden object. The search for hidden objects will continue for a longer period at 9 months and makes "peek-a-boo" a fun game.

Children aged 2 to 7 years are viewed by Piaget as being in the preoperational stage of cognitive development. The child is inquisitive and learns by imitating others. Thought processes are concrete, and the child's attention span is short. Children in this age group should be screened for problems with vision and hearing that may interfere with cognitive development. Physical problems, mental deficits, and shorter-than-usual attention span also may influence the rate of cognitive development.

Older children and adolescents enter the stages of concrete and formal operations, respectively. Cognitive development usually proceeds without major problems as long as appropriate adaptations have been made to any sensory deficits, the child is motivated to learn, and the child is exposed to stimulating learning environments. Consideration should be given to school performance as well as the effects that watching television and playing with computer video games may have on learning.

Language Development. The ability to comprehend and speak the dominant language develops with cognitive abilities. Language comprehension precedes the ability to speak or write the language.

Several screening tools, the Early Language Milestone Scale (ELM Scale) and Denver Articulation Screening Exam (DASE), are available to assess speech abilities. The ELM Scale is used for children from birth to 36 months, and the DASE is used for children from 2.5 to 6 years. The DDST2 also has a language development component. Generally, the DDST2 is sufficient unless a more extensive screening is desired (*e.g.,* correct articulation of specific word sounds). The DASE is presented in Appendix D. It is helpful to evaluate the age that the child acquired various verbal skills. For example, almost all children should coo by 2 to 3 months and babble beginning at 4 months. Infants begin verbalizing "ma" or "da" sounds around 7 months. After 12 months, children begin to verbalize rather than cry some of their needs, although this communication may be in the form of jargon that may only be understood by family members. Twins and other multiple-birth children may develop their own unique jargon.

Understandable speech begins between 15 and 24 months in the form of two- to three-word phrases and plurals. By age 2 years, the receptive vocabulary consists of about 900 to 1,200 words and expressive vocabulary consist of approximately 250 words. The child knows some 2,000 words by 6 years (this doubles by sixth grade); some of these words may include profanities learned by imitating others. Verbal communication skills and the ability to write continue to develop during the school-age years and adolescence.

The development of language skills is influenced by factors other than innate cognitive abilities. It is especially important to determine the possible influences of other factors when speech development appears delayed. Factors that optimize language development include a consistent and satisfying relationship with a parent or other caregiver, a sense of security, verbal stimulation (*e.g.,* storytelling, descriptive conversation), and positive response to attempts to verbalize. Speech delays may be secondary to hearing problems and lack of verbal communication within the family.

Sleep and Rest

Evaluation of sleep and rest in babies, children, and adolescents should focus on the following:

- Amount of time the child sleeps each day, including naps and nighttime sleep
- Child's or parent's perceptions of sleep pattern disturbances
- Identification of factors that contribute to sleep and rest problems

Sleep Patterns. Sleep patterns vary greatly from the newborn period through adolescence (for a description of the normal sleep cycle, see Chap. 10). Newborns generally spend more time asleep than awake, requiring as much as 18 hours of sleep per day. Such long sleep periods are believed to support the infant's rapid growth rate. Infants gradually develop individual nocturnal sleep patterns. Some infants may sleep through the night as early as 6 weeks of age, and most sleep all night by age 3 months. Premature infants may develop nocturnal sleep patterns more slowly than full-term infants. Morning and afternoon naps are common through the first year. The infant may sleep 12 to 14 hours during the night and 1 to 4 hours during the day.

Toddlers and preschool-aged children generally sleep 12 to 14 hours a day, including one or two daytime naps. By age 5, children may need only one daytime nap or rest period. Nighttime awakenings are normal. Presleep routines or rituals such as bath, snack, or bedtime story may help ease the transition from activities to sleep and rest. Sleep pattern disturbances related to nightmares, bedtime fears, sleepwalking, and bed-wetting may develop in preschool-aged children and may persist through early school-age years.

School-aged children may require only 9 hours of sleep per day, although great variability exists among children. School-aged children commonly resist bedtime at a specific hour because they want to continue favorite activities such as watching television and playing games.

The adolescent's sleep–rest needs usually increase because the rate of physical growth accelerates. Daytime naps and late awakening on weekends are not unusual because this age group is subject to fatigue.

Sexuality and Reproduction

Sexuality and reproduction are evaluated in children and adolescents primarily to determine the following:

- Parental and child teaching needs in relation to sexual development and sexual myths
- Development and maturation of secondary sex characteristics
- Sexuality self-esteem

Sexual Development. The development of a person's sexuality begins during infancy and continues throughout the life span. Infants derive bodily pleasure from sucking and being touched. The manner in which the infant is fed, washed, stroked, kissed, and hugged provides messages related to sexuality. Infants explore their own bodies, including genitalia.

Toddlers explore their own bodies and begin to differentiate between males and females at about age 2. They develop an interest in viewing the genitals of adults and other children of either gender. Normally, gender identity is firmly established by age 3 as the child explores bodily functions, especially elimination. Between the ages of 3 and 4, children may begin to masturbate; this may represent one way the young child deals with stress.

Preschool children develop a curiosity about reproduction and the differences between men and women, boys and men, and girls and women. Children continue to ask questions through early school-age years about such topics as where babies come from, breast-feeding, and why women have breasts and men have penises. During this developmental phase, children require simple and factual explanations.

School age is generally a quiet time for sexual development. Children usually have same-sex friends. They continue to learn more about the anatomy of their bodies and experiment with different sexual roles.

Puberty. Anticipatory guidance for school-age children may focus on preparing the child for the physical changes associated with puberty. The nurse may ask parents questions about how they plan to prepare their children for changes such as menstruation. Generally, girls begin puberty between ages 10 and 12, and boys between ages 12 and 14. For girls, sign of puberty include changes related to breast development, pubic and axillary hair growth, menarche and menstruation, and height increases (Table 16-2). For boys, puberty changes include genital development; ejaculation from masturbation or nocturnal emissions (wet dreams); pubic, axillary, chest, and facial hair growth; voice changes; and height increases (Table 16-3).

Adolescent Sexuality. The development of sexuality involves more than experiencing and responding to the physical changes of puberty. During adolescence, the further developments of one's personal identity and sexuality are closely associated. Adolescents are concerned with attitudes, behaviors, and feelings toward themselves and the opposite sex; relationships, affection, and caring between

---

TABLE 16.2   Physical Changes with Puberty and Adolescence in Girls

Age	Physical Changes
8–13 yr (average, 11 yr)	Breast development *Sequence:* Stage 1: Preadolescent—no glandular tissue Stage 2: Breast bud stage Stage 3: Further breast tissue growth with nipple protrusion Stage 4: Nipple and areola form a mound distinct from breast tissue Stage 5: Mature breast (average age, 14–16 yr)
8–13 yr (average, 1 yr after breast bud stage)	Pubic hair growth *Sequence:* Stage 1: Preadolescent—no pubic hair Stage 2: Sparse, long, silky, pigmented hair, mainly along the labia Stage 3: Coarser, darker, curlier hair spreading sparsely over pubic symphysis Stage 4: More hair growth and distribution than stage 3, but hair does not yet extend to medial surface of thighs Stage 5: Adult pattern with hair growth to medial aspect of thighs
9–14 yr (average, 1 yr after stage 2 pubic hair)	Axillary hair growth
10–15 yr (average, during stage 3 or 4 breast development)	Menarche: initial cycles may be anovulatory; ovulatory cycles begin within 2 yr of menarche
	Height increase: average American adolescent grows 24 cm (9 in), with peak growth spurt at age 12 yr
Puberty through adolescence	Increased apocrine gland secretion, sometimes resulting in acne

TABLE 16.3   Physical Changes with Puberty and Adolescence in Boys

Age	Physical Changes
10–13 yr (average, 11 yr)	Genital development
	Sequence:
	Stage 1: Preadolescent—no enlargement of testes or penis
	Stage 2: Enlargement of testes; scrotal skin becomes more pigmented; no significant enlargement of penis
	Stage 3: Penis enlarges in length; continued enlargement of testes
	Stage 4: Penis grows in length and width with glans development; enlargement of testes
	Stage 5: Mature genitals (average age, 15–16 yr)
10–13 yr (average onset with stage 2 genital development)	Pubic hair growth
14–15 yr	Facial hair growth
	Voice changes
	Height increase: Average American adolescent grows 34 cm (13.5 in), with peak growth spurt at age 14 yr
Approximately 3 yr after onset of stage 2 genital development	Ejaculation (masturbation or nocturnal emissions); mature sperm produced between ages 14–16 yr
Puberty through adolescence	Increased apocrine gland secretion, sometimes resulting in acne

people; and recognition and acceptance of themselves and others as sexual beings. They also must deal with incorporating the physical changes of sexual development into their self-image and sexual identity. Adolescents may question their sexual identities and sexual orientations.

Adolescents usually have educational needs in relation to sexuality and reproduction. Parents may or may not be able to meet these needs. The nurse should determine whether parents and children discuss sexual matters, including sexual values, sexual roles, and related behaviors. Additional evaluation may include determining the adolescent's knowledge about risks of sexual intercourse, including pregnancy and sexually transmitted diseases.

Coping and Stress Tolerance

During assessment of children in relation to stress and coping, the nurse focuses on the following:

- Common stressors associated with childhood stages of growth and development
- The child's perception of stressors
- Behavioral manifestations of coping or responding to stress
- Support systems during times of stress or crisis

Stress Response. The infant's response to stress is commonly manifested by crying. By age 2, children can respond to simple stresses by expressing impatience and imitating some adult displays of emotions. When overwhelmed, the response to stress can be excessive and manifested in a "temper tantrum." Preschool children begin to use adaptive mechanisms such as denial, reaction formation, regression, projection, suppression, and sublimation, which help the child develop stress tolerance as well as a sense of independence. Striking out by hitting, biting, and hair pulling is a frequent response to stress in

the toddler and preschool child. Because physical activity is a method of handling stress, children with high levels of stress may be hyperactive.

Young children usually learn to imitate the feelings, emotions, and responses to stress from family members. This process, called *identification,* helps children learn how persons of like gender experience and cope with stress. Imagination, as well as play and participation in sports activities, may be used to alleviate stress.

School-age children can identify stressors, and they begin to reason with others regarding how to cope, using past experiences and advice from others. They also may engage in ritualistic behavior to reduce anxiety. Fantasy can compensate for feelings of inadequacy or inferiority. Projection, rationalization, regression, sublimation, and malingering may help protect the ego when children are unable to perform at expected levels. Using such defense mechanisms in moderation can help children handle anxiety and grow emotionally.

Adolescence is a transition period from childhood to adulthood and is generally considered a stressful period for both adolescents and their families. Coping styles are fairly established by mid-adolescence, although adolescents can learn new ways to cope from peers and adult role models. Alcohol and other chemicals may be used by adolescents in attempts to cope with stressors.

Roles and Relationships

During the health assessment of infants, children, and adolescents, determine the following pertaining to roles and relationships:

- Nature of the child's important relationships and who fulfills the child's needs for nurturing, protecting, and helping

- Dynamics among family members
- Roles enacted by the child

Important Relationships. The infant's most important relationships are usually with the parents or primary caregiver. A major developmental task for a new family involves attachment. *Bonding,* the most significant relationship between the mother and infant, refers to the attachment that is usually initiated after the infant's birth. *Engrossment* refers to the father's initial parental response to the baby. Instruments are available to assess the quality of mother–infant bonding (*The Neonatal Behavioral Assessment Scale* and *Neonatal Perception Inventory*; see Bishop, 1976; Clark, 1976; Brazelton, 1973).

Behavioral indicators of a positive relationship between the infant and primary caregiver include the following:

- Response to caregiver's voice by making sounds (by age 2 months)
- Visual recognition of caregivers (by age 3 months)
- Preference for being with others during waking hours, and initiation of social interaction by smiling (by age 4 months)
- Separation anxiety, or fear of being with strangers (by age 6 months) or fear of being separated from primary caregiver (between 7 and 10 months)

The most important relationship for the toddler usually continues to be with parents. During this developmental phase, separation anxiety resurfaces and is most stressful, especially between 18 and 24 months. A major developmental task for the toddler is learning that parental separation does not mean abandonment and can be tolerated for short periods. By age 3, most toddlers can tolerate short separations but may still cry when first left in the care of another. Toddlers begin to establish play relationships with other children, although some parallel play continues.

Preschool children begin to participate more fully as family members but may prefer to spend play time with same-age children. Cooperative play is the primary interaction with other children. Preschool children frequently play games such as house that imitate future roles. By ages 4 or 5, children usually identify strongly with the parent of the same gender and the focus of love may be with the parent of the opposite gender. Other significant adults include relatives, parental friends, and adult caregivers or babysitters.

School-age children begin to demonstrate decreased dependence on family and increased interaction with peers, especially neighborhood children and other adults such as teachers. Even so, family relationships are important and continue to influence emotional and social development. Interactions and frustrations with peers and adults outside the home help the child in this growth phase to learn more complex social responses.

The preadolescent usually spends more time in the community. At this age, children begin to develop pride in family, school, and community. Older children may earn a small income for services such as yard care or newspaper delivery. They learn to appreciate that parents are individuals with different ideas as well as specific attributes. Gender or sex roles usually develop or are identifiable by

school age. The best friend becomes very important, and friends are usually of the same gender.

Adolescent relationship patterns include interacting with peer groups and forming relationships with members of the opposite gender. Dating behaviors vary considerably across cultures and among families. The adolescent becomes very concerned about appearance and looking like others in the peer group. Achieving independence from parents and other adults while maintaining affection is an important concern. Adolescents may have many conflicts with parents, especially between ages 13 and 15. Such conflicts may develop because of crisis or the child's need to express his or her own identity. Conflicts may decrease later as adolescents begin to view parents as acceptable role models.

Adolescents may form strong relationships with other adults such as teachers, clergy, sports coaches, and parental friends. Adolescents may further identify with adult roles through part-time work or career plans.

Self-Concept

Self-concept can be evaluated by doing the following:

- Observing the child's overall appearance and body language
- Interpreting self-disclosing statements about self and self-esteem
- Observing quality of social interactions
- Identifying potential threats to self-esteem and the child's response patterns

The development of a child's self-concept (beliefs and feelings about self) is influenced by cognitive and intellectual abilities, the actions and reactions of others (especially the family), moral development, and emotions.

According to Erikson (1963), a positive self-concept in the child is achieved through successful resolution of developmental crises experienced as the child passes through each stage. Evaluation of self-concept is difficult when the child is too young to verbalize feelings about self. Young infants do not differentiate self from others. Infants establish the basis of a positive self-concept by learning to trust others through the communication of love and acceptance by caregivers. Infants who demonstrate weight loss, excessive colic, and difficulty sleeping may be apprehensive and have difficulty establishing trusting bonds with others.

Toddlers know themselves as separate beings, although the boundaries of self may be vague. Toddlers who are frustrated in their attempts to establish autonomy may have feelings of self-doubt and anger toward themselves and others. Between 18 and 36 months, children conceptualize themselves as being either "good" or "bad." The self-concept of the preschool-age child may be threatened by feelings of guilt that occur when the child senses doing something wrong. Guilt feelings may be indicated by the child's behaviors, including lack of coordination, verbalization of fears, stammering speech, eating and elimination problems, fear of strangers, or a disinterest in playing with other children. The preschool child may start comparing his or her own accomplishments with those of older siblings or feel threatened by new siblings.

The greatest threats to self-esteem of school-age children include a sense of inferiority, inadequacy, difficulty learning or performing tasks, an inability to concentrate, or being different. If the child is not doing well in school, he or she may perceive self as stupid. When evaluating self-concept in school-age children, it may be helpful to ask children to draw a picture of themselves. The nurse and the child can then discuss the child's interpretation of the drawing.

Adolescents encounter many potential threats to self-esteem as they go through the process of forming a unique identity and adjusting to a new body image. Failure to become independent and responsible and to have friends during adolescence may threaten self-confidence and self-esteem.

Values and Beliefs

Evaluation of values and beliefs can be accomplished by doing the following:

- Identifying signs of interpersonal conflict and confusion
- Identifying level of faith and moral development
- Identifying anticipatory learning needs of parents

Theories that suggest developmental norms in relation to children's values and belief systems include Fowler's (1974) theory of stages of faith development and Kohlberg's (1981) theory of level of moral development.

Stages of Faith. Fowler classifies the infant as being in the primal stage of faith. The infant does not have values or beliefs but does understand bodily comfort and the relief of tension. "Good" and "bad" are defined in terms of physical consequences to the self. Preschoolers and young children go through the intuitive stage of faith. The child develops an awareness of parental values, beliefs, and any associated religious practices, conforming to such patterns to gain acceptance and love. Preschoolers may misinterpret parental value and belief patterns because of limited experience or concrete thinking patterns.

School-age children enter the mythical–literal stage. The child's value and belief system can be influenced by storytelling. Symbolic meanings are still difficult to interpret for this age-group. Adolescents enter the synthetic–conventional stage and may never advance further in faith development.

Moral Development. The conscience begins forming about age 4 years and is analytical as well as judgmental in relation to moral development. Kohlberg classifies sequential levels of moral development. The first level (preconventional stage) is characterized by a punishment and obedience orientation. This orientation is characteristic of young children who engage in right or wrong behavior depending on the consequences of the behavior. Children at this stage generally view rules as unchanging and imposed by adults. Children begin to value fairness, agreement, and equal exchange, although self-interests are still the most important.

The second level (conventional stage) is characterized by conforming to the expectations and behaviors of others. The child's conduct is influenced more by social expectations than by the threat of punishment. School-age children display these types of behaviors. As the child enters adolescence, a law-and-order orientation to right and wrong may develop. Rules may be accepted without question, because the person believes that the particular rule is best for all concerned.

Physical Examination   Pediatric Assessment

GENERAL PRINCIPLES

The Interview

Interviewing is an important means of obtaining health assessment data.

Use the child's name or preferred nickname; identify the people accompanying the child. If they are not the parents, determine whether there is a consent to treat for legal purposes.

Encourage the child to participate in the interview process. School-age children and adolescents should be very involved.

Establish Rapport

Be alert to the interaction between the child and others.

Regardless of the child's age, address the child directly, as well as adults.

Many children feel threatened by white uniforms or lab coats, strange equipment, and a hurried, abrupt, or uncaring attitude.

Save more intrusive procedures (*e.g.,* ear examination) until last. Try to do cardiovascular and respiratory evaluation while the child is quiet.

Praise the child during the health assessment (*e.g.,* "You're helping by holding so still" or "Thank you for opening your mouth so wide"). This makes the child feel more comfortable.

In general, the younger the child, the more concrete is his or her thinking.

Both comprehension and the ability to communicate verbally are related to age and emotional status.

(continued)

Physical Examination   Pediatric Assessment (continued)

DIAGNOSTIC TESTS

Displays 16-1 and 16-2 provide screening recommendations for children. Most tests that can be performed on adults also can be used with children; values may differ.

Display 16-3 summarizes recommendations for preventive pediatric health care.

ASSESSMENT AIDS

Most aids used for adults can also be used for children. Additional equipment includes:

Head circumference tape measure (infants)
Stethoscope with infant diaphragm and bell
Infant scale
Measurement board to measure length (infants)
Development assessment kit

Documenting Newborn Examination Findings

Example 1: Normal Findings

S: Mother reports no difficulty with pregnancy (gravida i, para i), labor (12 hours), or delivery. Family history negative for genetic disorders. Intends to breast-feed.

O: 3 hours old, Apgar 8 at 1 minute and 10 at 5 minutes. Heart rate 121, no murmurs, respirations 40, weight 3500 g, length 50 cm, head circumference 34 cm, chest circumference 31 cm, anterior and posterior fontanel soft, good sucking reflex, mouth without defects, ears at same angle as eyes, spine intact, no hair tufts, extremities symmetric, urinary meatus at center of glans, testes descended, meconium stool present, urinated.

A: Normal newborn.

DISPLAY 16.1

US Preventive Services Task Force Recommendations: Newborn to 10 Years

SCREENING

Height and weight
Blood pressure
Vision (3 years and up)
Hemoglobinopathy screen (birth)
T4 and or TSH (birth)
Blood lead level (high risk)

COUNSELING

Car safety seats (under 5 years)
Lap–shoulder car restraint (5 years +)
Bicycle helmet use
Smoke detector, flame-retardant sleep wear
Hot water temperature (less than 120–130°F)
Window/stair guards
Safe storage of drugs, toxic substances, matches, lighters, firearms
Syrup of ipecac, poison control number
CPR training for caretakers
Breast feeding/iron-enriched formula and foods (infants & toddlers)

Limit fat and cholesterol, maintain caloric balance, emphasize grains, fruits, and vegetables (over 2 years)
Regular physical exercise/activity
Effects of passive tobacco smoke (parents)
Effects of tobacco use (children)
Regular dental care
Baby bottle tooth decay

IMMUNIZATIONS [SEE IMMUNIZATION SCHEDULE]

Diphtheria-tetanus-pertussis (DPT) polio
Measles-mumps-rubella
H influenzae type b (Hib) conjugate
Hepatitis B
Varicella

CHEMOPROPHYLASIS

Ocular prophylaxis (birth)

US Preventive Services Task Force. (1996). *Guide to clinical preventive services* (2nd ed.). Baltimore, MD: Williams & Wilkins.

DISPLAY 16.2

US Preventive Services Task Force Recommendations: 11–24 Years

SCREENING

Height and weight
Blood pressure
Pap test (18 or sexually active)
Chlamydia screen (females <20)
Vision
Problem drinking

COUNSELING

Lap–shoulder car restraint
Bicycle/motorcycle helmet use
Smoke detector
Safe storage of firearms
Tobacco avoidance
Avoidance of alcohol and illicit drug use
Avoid alcohol while driving, swimming, etc.
STD prevention: abstinence and condoms

Pregnancy prevention: contraception
Limit fat and cholesterol, maintain caloric balance,
   emphasize grains, fruits and vegetables
Adequate calcium intake (females)
Regular physical exercise/activity
Regular dental care
Baby bottle tooth decay

IMMUNIZATIONS [SEE IMMUNIZATION SCHEDULE]

Diphtheria–tetanus (Td booster every 10 years)
Measles-mumps-rubella (11–12 yrs)
Hepatitis B
Varicella (11–12 yrs)

CHEMOPROPHYLASIS

Multivitamin with folic acid (females)

US Preventive Services Task Force. (1996). *Guide to clinical preventive services* (2nd ed.). Baltimore, MD: Williams & Wilkins.

P: Provide discharge teaching to mother:
   a. Care of circumcision (to be performed later)
   b. Breast-feeding
   c. Newborn care
   d. To be reassessed by regular health care provider in 4 weeks

Example 2: Deviation From Normal

For a complete newborn assessment a check sheet is beneficial. Normals are checked, and abnormalities are described. Below is an example of this type of documentation.

S: Mother denies any difficulty with pregnancy, labor (8 hours), or delivery. Two living children with no congenital defects. No history of genetic disorders.
O: See Newborn Assessment Form for normals. Heart rate 152 while sleeping; S3 heart sound loudest at third left intercostal space; lips, hands, and feet blue. Respirations 50 at rest.
A: Needs follow-up by physician for possible heart problems.
P: Advise pediatrician of findings.

ND$_x$

Clinical Problems Related to Newborn Examination

Common clinical problems related to newborns include normal physiologic jaundice (see discussion under Diag-

nostic Tests), heart murmurs, respiratory distress syndrome, prematurity (see discussion under Gestational Screening), and diseases transmitted from the mother. Newborns experience numerous congenital disorders; refer to any nursing pediatric textbook for a complete description of these problems.

Heart Murmurs

Heart murmurs are usually transitory (see Chap. 8 for a discussion of murmurs). They are frequently heard in newborns until age 48 hours. The murmurs resolve with the transition from fetal to systemic pulmonary circulation. S3 sounds are normal and occur in 30% of all newborns; however, S4 sounds are never normal in newborns. Murmurs lasting more than 48 hours or associated with cyanosis can represent congenital heart malformations.

Respiratory Distress Syndrome

Respiratory distress syndrome occurs in newborns when the lungs are not mature. Signs of respiratory distress syndrome include difficulty with inspiration, see-saw pattern of breathing (thorax, then abdominal), flaring of the nostrils, and noisy respirations. Respiratory distress syndrome can be life-threatening.

Diseases Transmitted From Mother

In utero or during delivery, neonates can be exposed to numerous diseases. Of the sexually transmitted diseases, gonorrhea can cause blindness, herpes simplex can be life-threatening, and syphilis infection can occur. The HIV virus can be transmitted (most cases of AIDS in children are a result of in utero transmission).

DISPLAY 16.3

Recommendations for Preventive Pediatric Health Care

Age[4]	INFANCY[3]											EARLY CHILDHOOD[3]		MIDDLE CHILDHOOD[3]				ADOLESCENCE[3]										
	New born[1]	2–4 d[2]	By 1mo	2 mo	4 mo	6 mo	9 mo	12 mo	15 mo	18 mo	24 mo	3y	4y	5y	6y	8y	10y	11y	12y	13y	14y	15y	16y	17y	18y	19y	20y	21y
History Initial/Interval	•	•	•	•	•	•	•	•	•	•	•	•	•	•	•	•	•	•	•	•	•	•	•	•	•	•	•	•
Measurements Height/Weight	•	•	•	•	•	•	•	•	•	•	•	•	•	•	•	•	•	•	•	•	•	•	•	•	•	•	•	•
Head Circumference	•	•	•	•	•	•	•	•	•	•	•																	
Blood Pressure												•	•	•	•	•	•	•	•	•	•	•	•	•	•	•	•	•
Sensory Screening Vision	S	S	S	S	S	S	S	S	S	S	S	O⁵	O	O	S	O	O	S	O	S	O	S	O	S	O	S	S	S
Hearing[6]	S/O	S	S	S	S	S	S	S	S	S	S	O	O	O	O	S	O	S	O	S	O	S	O	S	O	S	S	S
Developmentl./ Behavioral Assessment[7]	•	•	•	•	•	•	•	•	•	•	•	•	•	•	•	•	•	•	•	•	•	•	•	•	•	•	•	•
Physical Examination[8]	•	•	•	•	•	•	•	•	•	•	•	•	•	•	•	•	•	•	•	•	•	•	•	•	•	•	•	•
Procedures— General[9]																												
Heriditary/ Metabolic Screening[10]	←	—•	•																									
Immunization[11]	←		—→	•	•	•		•	←		—→	←	—→					←					—→					
Lead Screen[12]						←	—→				•																	
Hematocrit or Hemoglobin				←				—•										←¹³										—→
Urinalysis				←								•						←¹⁴										—→
Procedures— Patients at Risk																												
Tuberculin Test[15]									*	*	*	*	*	*	*	*	*	*	*	*	*	*	*	*	*	*	*	*
Cholesterol Screening[16]											*	*	*	*	*	*	*	*	*	*	*	*	*	*	*	*	*	*
STD Screening[17]																		*	*	*	*	*	*	*	*	*	*	*
Pelvic Exam[18]																		*	*	*	*	*	*	←*	*	—*¹⁸	*	*
Anticipatory Guidance[19]	•	•	•	•	•	•	•	•	•	•	•	•	•	•	•	•	•	•	•	•	•	•	•	•	•	•	•	•
Injury Prevention[20]	•	•d[2]	•	•	•	•	•	•	•	•	•	•	•	•	•	•	•	•	•	•	•	•	•	•	•	•	•	•
Initial Dental Referral[21]								←			—•																	

Key • = to be performed   S = subjective, by history   ←→ = the range during which a service may be,
     * = to be performed for   O = objective, by a standard   provided with the dot indicating the preferred
         patients at risk   testing method   age.

NOTE. Special chemical, immunologic, and endocrine testing is usually carried out on speciic indications. Testing other than newborn (e.g., inborn errors of metabolism, sickle disease, etc.) is discretionary with the physician.

The recommendations in this publication do not indicate an exclusive course of treatment or serve as a standard of medical care. Variations, taking into account individual circumstances, may be appropriate.

(continued)

Assessment Standard for General Professional Nursing Practice (continued)

1. Breastfeeding encouraged and instruction and support offered.

2. For newborns discharged in less than 48 hours after delivery.

3. Developmental, psychosocial, and chronic disease issues for children and adolescents may require frequent counseling and treatment visits separate from preventive care visits.

4. If a child comes under care for the first time at any point on the schedule, or if any items are not accomplished at the suggested age, the schedule should be brought up to date at the earliest possible time.

5. If the patient is uncooperative, rescreen within 6 months.

6. Some experts recommend objective appraisal of hearing in the newborn period. The Joint Committee on Infant Hearing has identified patients at significant risk for hearing loss. All children meeting these criteria should be objectively screened. See the Joint Committee on Infant Hearing 1994 Position Statement.

7. By history and appropriate physical examination: if suspicious, by specific objective developmental testing.

8. At each visit, a complete physical examination is essential, with infant totally unclothed, older child undressed and suitably draped.

9. These may be modified, depending on entry point into schedule and individual need.

10. Metabolic screening (e.g., thyroid, hemoglobinopathies, PKU, galactosemia) should be done according to state law.

11. Schedule(s) per the Committee on Infectious Diseases, published periodically in Pediatrics. Every visit should be an opportunity to update and complete a child's immunizations.

12. Blood lead screen per AAP statement "Lead Poisoning: From Screening to Primary Prevention" (1993).

13. All menstruating adolescents should be screened.

14. Conduct dipstick urinalysis for leukocytes for male and female adolescents.

15. TB testing per AAP statement "Screening for Tuberculosis in Infants and Children" (1994). Testing should be done on recognition of high-risk factors. If results are negative but high-risk situation continues, testing should be repeated on an annual basis.

16. Cholesterol screening for high-risk patients per AAP "Statement on Cholesterol" (1992). If family history cannot be ascertained and other risk factors are present, screening should be at the discretion of the physician.

17. All sexually active patients should be screened for sexually transmitted diseases (STDs).

18. All sexually active females should have a pelvic examination. A pelvic examination and routine Pap smear should be offered as part of preventive health maintenance between the ages of 18 and 21 years.

19. Appropriate discussion and counseling should be an integral part of each visit for care.

20. From birth to age 12, refer to AAP's injury prevention program (TIPP) as described in "A Guide to Safety Counseling in Office Practice" (1994).

21. Earlier initial dental evaluations may be appropriate for some children. Subsequent examinations as prescribed by dentist.

From Hay, W. et al. (Eds.). (1997). *Current pediatric diagnosis and treatment* (13th ed.). Stamford, CT: Appleton & Lange.

Documenting Infant Examination Findings

Example 1: 9-Month-Old Male

S: Mother states Wesley is a happy baby, standing unsupported, eats three meals/day, breast-feeds four times a day for 20 minutes, plans to wean to cup in next 2 to 3 months. No specific problems.

O: Normal DDST2; see form. Weight for height at 50th percentile, weight and height in 75th percentile—see chart and graphs. Urine negative for glucose, protein, and red blood cells and white blood cell counts. No abnormal physical finding—see exam check sheet. Immunization status: OK.

A: Normal growth and development.

P: Return in 3 months for follow-up. Anticipatory teaching: safety precautions for 9 to 12 months and weaning to cup.

Example 2: Deviations From Normal

S: Has been fussy all night, unusual, pulling at right ear, has had a cold for 2 days. Here for regular 6-month checkup and immunizations. Attends day care 5 days per week for 9 hour per day. Other children at center have colds.

O: Temperature 100. Right ear: tympanic membrane bulging and red, fluid present. Left ear: tympanic membrane red around edges, no fluid or bulging, landmarks and light reflex present. Green nasal discharge, nasal membranes bright red. Normal lung sounds—no crackles or wheezes.

A: Suspect otitis media.

P: Refer to nurse practitioner in clinic this AM. Defer

▼ ▼ ▼

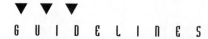

Procedure

For interview guidelines the following five age groups are used: newborn, infant, young children, older children, and adolescents.

Clinical Significance

For interviewing and performing physical examinations, there is little difference in approach for the toddler and preschool child. The preschool child has a longer attention span and may be more cooperative than the toddler; however, the approach to the interview and examination is similar. The same is true for the school-age and adolescent child. However, the adolescent does become more independent from parents and relies less on parents in answering health questions.

1. Newborns

The health history of the newborn primarily addresses the following:

- Prenatal care
  - General health
  - Number of pregnancies (gravida and para)
  - Prenatal diseases or conditions (such as hypertension, eclampsia, vaginal bleeding, and infectious diseases)
  - Use of medication
  - Attitude toward pregnancy and children
  - Perceptions of fetal movement
- Labor and delivery
  - Duration of pregnancy and labor
  - Place of delivery
  - Nature of labor (analgesia or anesthesia use and any spontaneous or induced complications)
  - Nature of delivery (presentation, unassisted or assisted, and any complications)
  - Any concerns of the parents
- Apgar scores at birth, 1 and 5 minutes

- Anthropometric measurements
  - Height and weight
  - Head circumference

Prenatal care and health problems can alert the nurse to potential problems and risk to the newborn. For example, mothers with diabetes often have newborns who weigh more than 9 pounds and are at risk for hypoglycemia and congenital anomalies. This information also provides baseline data.

Knowledge of labor and delivery problems can alert the nurse to possible developmental delays as the child grows if distress occurred.

The Apgar score assesses neonate vigor. A low score indicates problems (Table 16–4).
Anthropometric measurements and other data provide baseline data for future assessments as well as evaluating nutritional status.

TABLE 16.4   Apgar Score

Heart Rate	Respirations	Muscle Tone	Reflex Irritability	Color
0 = None detected	0 = Absent	0 = Flaccid	0 = No response	0 = Cyanosis
1 = Less than 100	1 = Shallow, irregular	1 = Some tone, weak response	1 = Weak cry	1 = Acrocyanosis (blue hands and feet)
2 = Above 100	2 = Strong cry, regular	2 = Full flexion	2 = Vigorous cry	2 = Totally pink

A score from 0 to 2 is assigned to each category for a score range of 0–10.

▼ ▼ ▼

G U I D E L I N E S   *continued*   Pediatric Interview (Health History)

Procedure   **Clinical Significance**

- Other data
  - Complications or anomalies noted
  - Feeding characteristics and type (breast or formula—specify type).
  - Duration of hospitalization
  - Use of medications
  - Usual daily schedule
  - Any illnesses or problems such as jaundice or convulsions

2. **Infants and toddlers**

   If the interview is initiated to assess the health status of an infant, obtain the same data as for the newborn, as well as developmental milestones.

   Ask parents open-ended questions such as:

   "Tell me what your child is doing now." After determining the child's present developmental status as perceived by the parent, obtain data regarding appropriate milestones such as when the child smiled, rolled over, sat unsupported, stood unsupported, used words, and cut deciduous teeth. Ask parents about safety practices: storage of chemicals, medications, presence of stairs, use of car seat restraint.

   This information provides a baseline to evaluate the infant's growth and development.

   Such an approach will elicit information without alarming parents if the child is not able to perform a particular skill. Age of performing developmental tasks provides cues to developmental status.

   During the interview, try to become familiar with the child and assess parent–child interactions.

   Accidents are a leading cause of death in small children.

   Toddlers have a short attention span and may find it difficult to be held during the interview; they prefer to explore. Ensure that the environment during the interview is safe for the child.

3. **Preschool children**

   Ask questions of the child that are appropriate for his or her age. In addition to the usual data, record data on the age when the child first walked, language development, and toilet training.

   If the child has no history of congenital problems or developmental delays, you may decide to collect little or no information about pregnancy, labor and delivery, and Apgar scores.

   The preschool child probably will be able to participate in the interview, although very young or shy children may have limited interaction.

   If abnormal findings are noted during the assessment, the judgment can be made to solicit and record such information.

4. **School-aged children**

   Usually, a great deal of interaction occurs between the nurse and the school-aged child during the interview. When interviewing a child, ask questions simply and directly.

   If the child is not experiencing congenital problems or developmental delays, the birth data and early developmental milestones are optimal. At the end of the interview, ask both child and parent to contribute any further information that may be helpful.

   Spend some time alone with an older child to determine whether he or she has any concerns that require privacy.

   Although this child is capable of relaying a current history, the parent should validate data and provide remote history.

   Stories and dolls may be helpful if the child is experiencing difficulty with providing information (this technique is especially useful if sexual, emotional, or physical abuse is suspected and the parent is not present).

   This is particularly important if any type of abuse is suspected.

5. **Adolescents**

   Usually the adolescent can participate fully in the interview process without parental assistance. Ask the adolescent whether the discussion may include parents. If parents are present, direct interview questions to the adolescent and not the parent.

   Often adolescents have questions or concerns they would like to discuss with the nurse privately about sexual activities or concerns, alcohol, tobacco, or drugs. In such cases, advise the adolescent what information must be shared with other health professionals or parents.

▼ ▼ ▼

Procedure

At some point in the interview, parents should be included and afforded the opportunity to discuss concerns either with or without the adolescent present.

Clinical Significance

The joint interview period may be the only time the nurse will be able to assess the parent–child relationship. In some instances, an adolescent may seek health care without a parent's presence or knowledge.

Diagnostic and Screening Tests: Pediatrics

1. Newborns

Some diagnostic studies are mandated by state law. Generally, these are phenylketonuria (PKU) and thyroxine (T_4) levels.

Other studies, such as bilirubin, blood type, sickle cell, HIV testing, hearing, Apgar score, and gestational age, are often performed.

Phenylketonuria: This is a blood test that measures the amount of phenylalanine amino acids in the blood. Condition occurs once in every 15,000 live births.

This test is performed 1 to 4 days after the newborn has ingested breast milk or formula. Excessive phenylalanine in the body causes tissue and brain damage resulting in mental retardation.

Thyroxine. This test is performed at the same time as the PKU. Newborns with low values (hypothyroidism) risk permanent brain defects. Congenital hypothyroidism occurs once in every 4,500 live births.

Thyroxine is a thyroid hormone necessary for normal growth, development, and metabolism.

Bilirubin. Bilirubin is a result of red blood cell breakdown. The liver cannot metabolize all of the bilirubin produced; therefore, plasma bilirubin increases.

The high plasma bilirubin results in jaundice (a yellowing of the skin). Most infants experience normal physiologic hyperbilirubinemia beginning about the third day. If bilirubin level rises above 12 mg/dL, it is considered excessive, and central nervous system damage may occur.

Blood Type. A newborn's blood type may be tested, especially if the mother is Rh-negative and the father is Rh-positive. Blood type also may be tested if ABO incompatibility is suspected.

Blood typing also occurs to determine possible paternity. Rh and ABO incompatibility causes red blood cell destruction and jaundice (see above).

Sickle Cell (hemoglobinopathy screen). Sickle cell testing detects the presence of hemoglobin S. If hemoglobin S is present, hemoglobin electrophoresis should be performed to determine whether the newborn has the trait or the disease. Occurs once in every 400 African-American infants.

Sickle cell disease, a hemolytic anemia, is a genetic blood disease that primarily affects individuals of African, Mediterranean, Middle Eastern, or Indian ancestry.

HIV Testing. Newborns of mothers with HIV or at risk for HIV are usually tested for presence of HIV. HIV antibodies are present in all infants born to infected mothers.

Test for HIV virus in the blood or nucleic acid detection test differentiates between infants who do not have HIV and those who do. Maternal HIV may remain in the newborn's blood for up to 18+ months (not all of these will develop the disease).

Hearing. Special audiometric testing of newborns is available.

Some hospitals routinely test hearing of all newborns.

Apgar Score. This screening is done at 1, 5, and sometimes 10 minutes after birth. The neonate receives a score from 0 to 2 for each of the five assessment areas.

A score below 6 is considered abnormal. See Table 16–4.

Gestational Age. Normal gestation is between 38 and 42 weeks. A newborn of less than 38 weeks' gestation is considered to be premature. Several gestational screening tools are available, such as the New Ballard Score for assessment of fetal maturation of newly born infants (Ballard, 1991).

Some newborns are large for gestational age (common when mother has diabetes), and some are small for gestational age. Determining gestational age is an important consideration.

▼ ▼ ▼

2. Diagnostic studies for infants

Routine diagnostic and screening studies performed on infants include developmental screening, urine screening, and hemoglobin.

Developmental Testing. Because infants grow and develop, regular developmental testing should occur. Denver Development Screening Tool 2 consists of four components: Personal–Social, Fine Motor, Language, and Gross Motor.

Urine Screening. A complete urine analysis can be performed to determine the presence of any anomalies such as glucose, protein, and red or white blood cells.

Hemoglobin or Hematocrit. Hemoglobin tests measure the amount of hemoglobin in the blood. Hemoglobin is a protein found in red blood cells that carries oxygen. Hematocrit measures the percentage of red blood cells in a blood sample.

See screening recommendations by the US Task Force for Preventive Services for infants and children to age 10 (see Display 16–1).

If delays are noted, the child should be referred for diagnostic testing by a specialist. The Bayley Scales of Infant Development—Second edition (BSID-II) are used for diagnosing developmental delays and planning and evaluating intervention strategies. They consist of three scales that evaluate mental and motor status and behavior.

Generally, a urine dipstick screening test is sufficient. If any of the above is positive, a routine urinalysis should be performed. This is usually performed when the infant is aged 6 months.

A hemoglobin level below 10 WdL is considered low, and the infant would be anemic. Low hematocrit levels are frequently associated with anemia. For infants, a reading below 29% is considered low.

3. Diagnostic studies for young children

Diagnostic and screening studies routinely performed during young childhood are similar to those done in infants.

Developmental Testing. DDST2; also DASE (Denver Articulation Screening Examination)

Vision and Hearing. At age 4, vision and hearing screening is done (see discussion of these tests in Chap. 9).

A dental examination performed by a dentist

Tuberculin Skin Test. A diagnostic screening to determine the presence of tuberculosis antibodies.

See Recommendations of US Preventive Services Task Force, Display 16–1; generally occurs at each well child visit.

Because young children have difficulty following directions and communicating appropriately, screening before this age is very difficult. Vision screening charts include Snellen E and HOTV. Normal visual acuity is 3 years, 20/40; 4 years, 20/30, and 5 years, 20/20.

Usually recommended to begin between ages 2 and 3 years and then every 6 months.

This is usually recommended at 24 months and whenever the child is exposed to tuberculosis. A false-positive result is possible if the skin test is given up to 3 months after a measles, mumps, or rubella immunization. The two can be given simultaneously.

4. Diagnostic studies for older children and adolescents

The only routine diagnostic or screening studies performed on older children are tuberculin skin testing, hemoglobin, and urine screening (these have been discussed previously in this chapter).

Other diagnostic tests may be appropriate because of risk factors such as sexual activity. Most diagnostic tests appropriate for adults are also appropriate for adolescents if indicted. See US Preventive Services Task Force Recommendations for children 11–24 years (Display 16–2).

▼ ▼ ▼
GUIDELINES

Assessment Guidelines   Physical Examination of Newborns

Procedure

Newborns

Birth to the first 29 to 30 days of life is considered the newborn or neonate period. The functional pattern associated with examination procedure is identified in parentheses.

Keep the newborn warm, exposing only those parts being assessed (Fig. 16–1). When possible, perform assessment with mother or father present (Fig. 16–2).

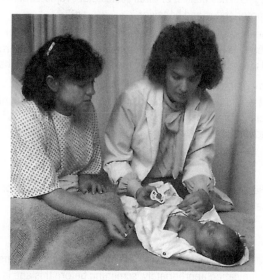

FIGURE 16.1   The newborn baby is kept warm during the examination by exposing body parts only as necessary.

Clinical Significance

Birth requires rapid adjustment to a new environment, making this assessment critical to the detection of possible problems.

Because of large surface area, newborns lose body heat easily. Take advantage of teaching opportunities.

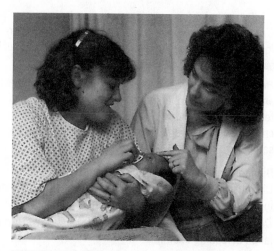

FIGURE 16.2   The parent may discuss concerns with the nurse during the newborn examination.

1. **Anthropometric measurements**
   (Nutrition Pattern)
   a. With newborn on examining table or in mother's arms, measure head and chest circumference by applying a tape measure around the widest part of the head (just above the eyebrows) or chest (at nipple line) as shown in the photo. Maintain records of serial measurements on standardized graph tables and compare to normal ranges. Tables for head and chest are shown in Appendix E.

The full-term newborn's head circumference should be about 33 to 35 cm; the chest circumference, 30 to 33 cm.

Deviations from Normal

Head circumference should not be more than 3 cm larger or smaller than the chest circumference. If larger, may be hydrocephalus; if smaller, may be microcephaly.

▼ ▼ ▼
G U I D E L I N E S   *continued*   Physical Examination of Newborns

---

Procedure   **Clinical Significance**

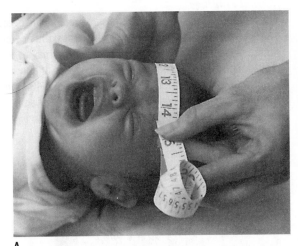
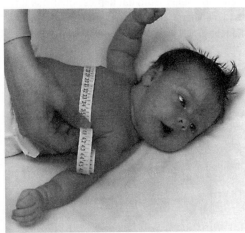

A   B

Measuring head circumference (a) and chest circumference (B)

b. Measure length of newborn from head to heels, extending as much as possible without forcing.

c. Weigh newborns without any clothing, including diaper. Record weight on growth chart. Record height to weight on growth chart (See Appendix E for examples).

Normal Findings
Length usually between 45 and 55 cm (18–22 inches)

Normal Findings
Weight is generally between 2,500 and 4,000 g (5 lbs 8 oz and 8 lbs 13 oz). Weight should be proportional to height.

Deviations from Normal
Less than 2,500 g may represent prematurity; more than 4,000 g is frequent when mother is diabetic and newborn may be large for gestational age.

2. Assess head.

a. Assess hair (nutrition pattern)

Normal Findings
Hair may vary in amount and color; more copious amounts of hair are seen on preterm infants. Lanugo (fine hair) may appear on the body, especially the upper arms, shoulders, back, and pinna of the ears.

b. Face and skull (cognition and perception pattern)
(1) Observe for symmetry and position of head.
(2) Try to transilluminate skull if newborn has high-pitched cry. This is evaluated by holding a flashlight with a protective foam collar against the baby's head from several different angles.

Normal Findings
Asymmetry of the face or skull may be associated with molding caused by accommodation of the skull to the birth canal. This problem usually resolves within 1 week. The newborn is unable to hold the head erect. The head will lag when the baby is pulled to a sitting position. The skull should not transilluminate.

Deviations from Normal
Caput succedaneum, swelling of soft scalp tissue from birth trauma, may be noted. *Cephalhematoma,* unilateral edema over parietal bones, may occur after birth and resolves in 6 weeks. *Complete transillumination* of the skull is abnormal. Localized bright spots or glowing of the entire skull may indicate severe pathology.

▼ ▼ ▼

Procedure

(3) Palpate fontanelles (soft, flat depressions); use fingers to palpate skull, noting anterior and posterior fontanelles.

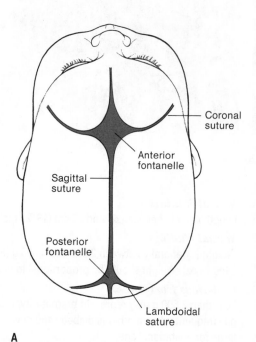

A

Palpating the fontanelles

Coronal
suture

Anterior
fontanelle

Sagittal
suture

Posterior
fontanelle

Lambdoidal
sature

c. Examine the oral cavity (nutrition pattern). Examination of the newborn's oral cavity is important to determine whether congenital anomalies exist.

(1) Inspect and palpate the palate with finger; inspect, when possible, using a tongue blade and light. Assess sucking strength while finger is in newborn's mouth.

Clinical Significance

Normal Findings

The fontanelles may pulsate at the same rate as the heart. The anterior fontanelle is 2.5 to 4.0 cm across; the posterior fontanelle is not greater than 2 cm across and may even be closed. The posterior fontanelle usually closes at about 2 months, and the anterior closes between 12 and 18 months. Suture ridges may be felt until about 6 months of age.

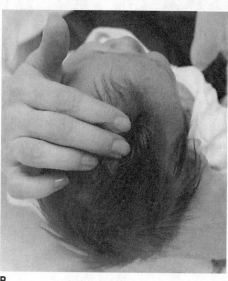

B

Deviations from Normal

A depressed fontanelle may indicate dehydration, and bulging may indicate hydrocephalus or increased pressure within the brain. A closed anterior fontanelle is not normal.

Inspecting the newborn's oropharynx may be difficult because of the strong reflex protrusion of the tongue when depressed with a tongue blade. Although the uvula may be retracted upward and backward during crying, observations of the oral cavity may still be possible.

Normal Findings

The palate is slightly higher and narrower than in the adult. The palate and oral cavity is moist; generally, no salivation is present.

▼ ▼ ▼

G U I D E L I N E S   *continued*   Physical Examination of Newborns

Procedure

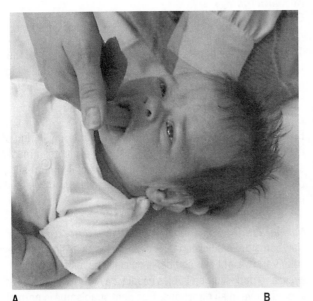
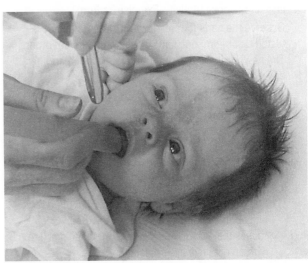

A   B

Examining the oral cavity. (A) Paplating the palate with the finger. (B) Inspecting the palate using a tongue blade and light.

(2) Inspect the tongue.

(3) Inspect and palpate the gums.

Clinical Significance

Deviations from Normal
A high palate or narrow arch or holes in the palate are considered abnormal, and referral is indicated. *Epstein's pearls* (Bohn nodules) may be observed along both sides of the hard palate midline. These small, whitish nodules cause no problems and usually disappear by age 2 or 3 months. A cleft in the palate—involving the soft and/or hard palate and the gums and lips—is not normal. Newborns with this defect have difficulty with eating.

Normal Findings
The tongue should fit in the mouth and be pink and not coated. Sucking reflex should be strong and coordinated.

Deviations from Normal
A large protruding tongue may be a sign of congenital defects and should be referred. Newborns with Down syndrome or with hypothyroidism typically have enlarged tongues. A white, cottage cheese–like coating on the tongue and cheeks may be thrush caused by *Candida albicans.*

Normal Findings
The gums of dark-skinned babies may have accumulations of patchy brown pigment; this is usually insignificant.

Deviations from Normal
Epstein's pearls may be noted on the gums. Occasionally a newborn will be born with a tooth (natal tooth) or one erupts shortly after birth; these teeth are usually removed because the infant could aspirate the tooth when it falls out.

▼ ▼ ▼

Procedure

(4) Inspect the tonsils.

d. Inspect the nose (Activity–Exercise Pattern).
Observe the naris for patency and flaring. Patency is tested by holding one naris closed and then the other. The newborn's sinuses are poorly developed and generally are not assessed.

e. Inspect the eyes (Cognition and Perception Pattern).
(1) The external eye may be assessed by holding the infant supine with the head gently lowered, which causes the eyes to open. Bright light will interfere with an effective eye assessment.

(2) Inspect eyelids. Upper and lower lid eversion is usually not performed during newborn assessment.

(3) Inspect the lacrimal apparatus.

(4) Inspect the bulbar conjunctiva and sclera.

(5) Elicit light reflexes. The corneal light reflex, red reflex, and pupil: constriction to light should be observed. An ophthalmoscopic examination is not usually performed on newborns unless some type of anomaly is present; in such cases, an ophthalmologist should conduct the examination.

Clinical Significance

Normal Findings
Generally the tonsils are not observed.

Normal Findings
The nose may be flattened. There should be no flaring of the nares. The newborn is an obligatory nose breather. Sneezing may be frequent and is a normal attempt to clear nasal passages.

Deviations from Normal
Bruising of the nose may occur during delivery. Any flaring of the nares may indicate respiratory distress; evaluate immediately. Nasal obstruction may indicate congenital abnormality, presence of a foreign body, or congestion. Newborn will be irritable.

Normal Findings
Newborns generally keep their eyes closed. As with adults, eye color varies. Light-skinned babies usually have gray to blue eyes, and dark-skinned babies usually have brown eyes. Eyes should move in all directions. Transient strabismus is normal, related to lack of binocular vision.

Normal Findings
Eyelids may be edematous for the first 2 days; frequent bilateral blinking is normal. Epicanthal folds are normal in Asian infants.

Deviations from Normal
If epicanthal folds are large in Asian babies or are noted on children of other ethnic backgrounds, Down syndrome may be suspected.

Normal Findings
No tearing is evident for the first month. Purulent discharge is abnormal and indicates infection.

Normal Findings
Bulbar conjunctiva and sclera may be blue tinged; small vessels may be visible in the sclera.

Deviations from Normal
Yellow discoloration occurs with jaundice. Subconjunctival hemorrhage may be present, caused by rupture of vessels during birth. Dark blue sclera may indicate congenital anomalies such as ontogenesis imperfecta.

Normal Findings
Pupils should constrict; the baby should blink at bright light. Pupils should be round and equal in size. Red reflex and bilateral symmetric corneal light reflex can be noted.

Deviations from Normal
The absence of a **red** reflex may indicate congenital cataracts (white pupil) or retinal hemorrhage. Dilated or fixed pupil may indicate anoxia or brain damage.

▼ ▼ ▼
G U I D E L I N E S   *continued*   Physical Examination of Newborns

Procedure

(6) Check for visual acuity.

Clinical Significance

Normal Findings

Nystagmus may be present. The older neonate may be able to follow an object to midline; however, acuity is difficult to assess. Visual acuity is about 20/100 to 20/500. Response to visual stimuli should include not immediately reopening eyes in response to bright light; after 2 weeks, neonate is capable of fixation on an object.

Deviations from Normal

Lack of blinking or sensitivity to bright light may indicate blindness. Absence of normal findings may indicate visual or neurologic problem.

f. Inspect the ears and assess hearing (Cognition and Perception Pattern).

(1) Determine the position of the external ears. An imaginary line is drawn from the inner and outer canthus of the eye to the vertex. The pinna of the ears should be at the level of this line.

Normal Findings

The pinna of the ears should be at the level of the eye-to-ear line.

Deviations from Normal

Low-set ears are associated with congenital kidney defects and other problems.

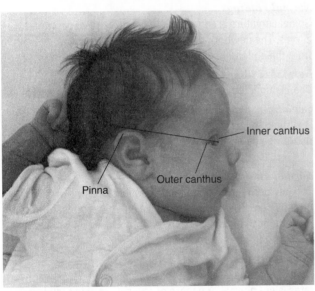

Checking ear position

(2) To assess the newborn with the otoscope, the baby should be held immobile, with special effort taken to maintain head immobility during the assessment. The following positions may be helpful: (1) prone with arms restrained at side and head secured by another or (2) supine with arms over head and head secured. The otosocope should be held with the handle directed toward the top of the head. Children younger than age 3 years have an upward curvature of the canal. Therefore, to visualize the structures, you should pull the lower auricle or pinna down and back.

Normal Findings

Tympanic membrane visualization is usually not performed on newborns because the canal is usually filled with vernix caseosa and amniotic fluid. When the canal is clear, the tympanic membrane and other structures should be visualized. There is no cone of light; the light reflex is usually diffuse.

▼ ▼ ▼

G U I D E L I N E S *continued*   Physical Examination of Newborns

Procedure

(3) Hearing screening. Check hearing by ringing a bell or making a similar noise near the newborn.

3. **Examine the chest and back (Activity and Exercise Pattern).**
   a. Inspect and palpate the shoulders and neck, including the clavicular area.

   b. Inspect the back.

   c. Examine the sacral area for dimpling, bulging, masses, or tufts of hair.

4. **Assess the lungs (Activity and Exercise Pattern).**
   a. Observe rate with chest exposed and auscultate for lung sounds, using appropriate-sized diaphragm and bell attachments.

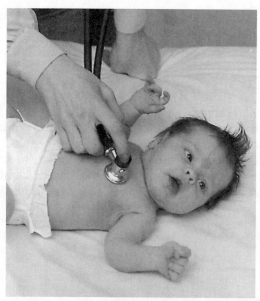

Auscultation of the anterior chest. Note the small bell and diaphragm attachments on the stethoscope.

Clinical Significance

Normal Findings
The newborn should display the startle reflex in response to a bell or other loud noise. This is an indirect measure of hearing and not accurate.

Deviations from Normal
If no startle reflex occurs, refer the baby for further hearing evaluation.

Normal Findings
The neck is short, and it is difficult to determine landmarks or the thyroid gland; the neck should be able to turn 80 degrees to the left and right.

Deviations from Normal
A broken clavicle is a common complication of birth; signs include local swelling, visible dislocation, crepitus, and tenderness.

Normal Findings
Spinal curvature is convex; there are no cervical or lumbar curves. The newborn has a C-shaped appearance when held from the abdomen.

Normal Findings
There should be no blemishes.

Deviations from Normal
Any dimpling, bulging, masses, or **tufts** of hair may indicate a neurotube defect.

Normal Findings
The newborn has abdominal respirations at a rate of 30–60 breaths/min. Brief periods of apnea (10–15 seconds) may be present for the first 4 weeks. Clear bronchovesicular breath sounds are normal throughout the lungs.

Deviations from Normal
Apnea for longer than 20 seconds accompanied by lower heart rates is not normal. A pattern of seesaw breathing (abdominal–thorax breathing with sternal and supraclavicular retractions), flaring of the nostrils, and noisy respirations (grunting) indicates respiratory distress. Stridor (high-pitched sound on inspiration) is indicative of upper airway obstruction.

Procedure

b. Palpate the back with two fingers while the newborn is crying.

c. Percuss the chest lightly with one finger.

5. **Assess heart (Activity and Exercise Pattern).**
   a. Observe apical impulse.

   b. Auscultate the heart while the baby is quiet and before proceeding to more intrusive measures. Use an appropriate-sized diaphragm and bell to auscultate the newborn. Auscultate the five precordial landmarks: (1) aortic second right intercostal space by the sternum; (2) pulmonary, second left intercostal space near the sternum; (3) third left intercostal space right and left of the sternum; (4) tricuspid area, fifth interspace, right of the sternum and (5) apex, lateral to midclavicular line at fourth/fifth interspace.

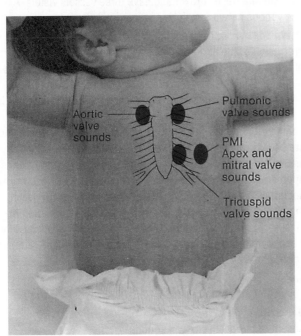

Precordial landmarks

c. Assess blood pressure and peripheral pulses—carotid, brachial, femoral, and pedal—using only one finger to avoid obliterating the pulse. Vasoconstriction from chilling will make pulses less intense. Blood pressure should be taken with Doppler or 1-inch blood pressure cuff.

Clinical Significance

Normal Findings
Fremitus findings **are** similar to those in the adult.

Normal Findings
Hyperresonant sounds are normal.

Normal Findings
Should be seen at fourth intercostal space to the immediate left of the midclavicular line.

Normal Findings
A normal heart rate is 120 to 170 beats per minute. The rhythm may be slightly irregular, with an increased heart rate on inspiration and a decreased heart rate on expiration. Heart sounds of newborns are louder than adults because of the thinner chest wall and the larger-size heart in proportion to the chest. Heart sounds are shorter in duration and higher in pitch. An S3 may be heard as a normal finding and occurs in 30% of all newborns.

Deviations from Normal
An S4 is never considered a normal finding. Murmurs are frequently heard in newborns until age 48 hours. Most murmurs resolve with the transition from fetal to systemic pulmonary circulation. Murmurs also can represent congenital heart malformations, especially if persisting more than 2 days and accompanied by other signs such as cyanosis. Marked cyanosis that occurs after birth may indicate congenital problems such as transposition of great vessels, severe septal defects, or pulmonic stenosis. All murmurs persisting more than 2 days require further evaluation.

Normal Findings
Pulses should be of same intensity in corresponding limb; amplitude should be same in limbs. Capillary refill is very rapid. Slowed refill may indicate dehydration.

Deviations from Normal
A difference in the amplitude of pulses between the lower and upper extremities is considered abnormal and may represent coarctation of the aorta.

▼ ▼ ▼

Procedure

6. Assess the abdomen (Nutrition Pattern).
Assessment will be easier if the newborn's abdomen is relaxed. Allowing the crying or restless baby to suck a pacifier and flex the knees relaxes the abdomen.
   a. Inspect the abdomen.

   b. Auscultate the abdomen using appropriate-size stethoscope attachments.

   c. Percuss the abdomen.

Clinical Significance

Normal Findings
A newborn's blood pressure ranges between 40 and 50 mm Hg systolic but will vary depending on cuff size and whether a Doppler is used. By age 4 weeks, the baby's blood pressure averages 80 systolic and 40 diastolic.

Deviations from Normal
If the systolic blood pressure is 96 or greater for the first 7 days or 104 or greater between 8 and 30 days, referral is warranted for significant hypertension. Before referral, get three elevated readings while the infant is quiet and not crying.

Normal Findings
The contour of the abdomen is rounded and dome-shaped. The umbilical cord should be dry in 5 days and drop off by 2 weeks. The end of a fresh cord should have three vessels visible. A fine venous network may be observed.

Deviations from Normal
Protrusion of the abdomen above the chest may be the result of feces, masses, or organ enlargement. Further evaluation is required. Visible peristalsis may indicate pyloric stenosis. Prominent venous networks along with taut skin appearance is abnormal, and in such cases the abdomen should be transilluminated. Small (1–2 cm) umbilical hernias may be noted and are usually considered normal in children before age 2 years and in African-ancestry children until age 7 years. If the skin is open around the hernia, immediate attention is required from a pediatrician. Herniation through the diastasis rectus muscle may result in a midline bulging between the xiphoid and umbilicus, especially when the baby is crying. This hernia usually disappears during the early school years. Inguinal and femoral hernias are not normal.

Normal Findings
Bowel sounds are heard every 10 to 30 seconds.

Deviations from Normal
Absent or hypoactive bowel sounds

Normal Findings
Tympany is heard and may be increased secondary to air swallowing. The upper edge of the liver should be located by percussion within 1 mm of the fifth intercostal space. The spleen may be located by percussion 1 or 2 cm below the costal margin.

Deviations from Normal
Hepatomegaly is associated with congestive heart failure secondary to congenital heart defect.

▼ ▼ ▼

GUIDELINES *continued*   Physical Examination of Newborns

Procedure

d. Palpate the abdomen. Perform light and deep palpation, gently, with fingertips. It may be difficult to differentiate pain and tenderness, especially if the baby is already crying. If fluid is suspected in the abdomen, use a flashlight to transilluminate the abdomen.

7. **Examine the hips and lower extremities (Activity–Exercise Pattern).**

a. Inspect the foot.

b. Inspect legs with the newborn supine on the examining surface; place the knees together and note how far apart the legs are at the ankles.

c. Test range of motion. Perform range-of-motion testing of the lower extremities while palpating over involved joints.

d. Examine hips. There are two tests for the hips: Ortolani's test and Barlow's test. Both are used to detect congenital hip dislocation; because it is often missed, repeat these tests through infancy.

Ortolani's test: With the baby supine on the examining surface and the knees and hips flexed, place your first two fingers over the greater trochanter and your thumb over the lesser trochanter. With both hands placed in this manner, abduct both hips by pulling the knees toward the examining surface.

Clinical Significance

Normal Findings

The abdomen should feel soft during inspiration. There should be no transillumination.

Deviations from Normal

The light will glow through the skin if fluid or air is present but will not glow if solid masses or blood is present.

Normal Findings

The foot appears flat, and the soles have creases. Shortly after birth, the feet may remain in the same position they were in utero, appearing deformed. Full range of motion and manipulation can bring the foot back to normal position if a true deformity is not present.

Deviations from Normal

Lateral deviation of the forefoot (metatarsus varus) and inversion of the foot with the forefoot adducted (talipes varus), polydactyly, syndactyly (extra or webbed toes/fingers), talipes equinovarus (club foot—fixed deformity of the ankle) are all deviations from normal.

Normal Findings

Some bowing of the legs is considered normal. The legs should be equal in length. Creases of legs and gluteal folds should be symmetric and even.

Deviations from Normal

Severe bowing is not normal; uneven creases may indicate congenital hip dislocation.

Normal Findings

The hip abducts to 170 degrees and can be put through full range of motion. The knees and ankles should perform full range of motion.

Deviations from Normal

Clicking sounds or crepitus *are* considered abnormal, as is the inability to abduct the hip past 160 degrees.

Normal Findings

The movement over the the greater trochanter should be smooth, without a click or slip of the femoral head.

▼ ▼ ▼

G U I D E L I N E S   *continued*

Physical Examination of Newborns

Procedure

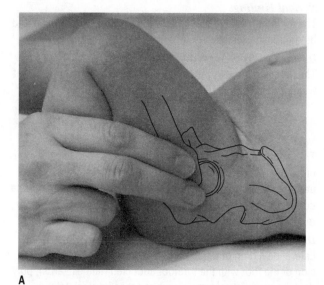

A

Clinical Significance

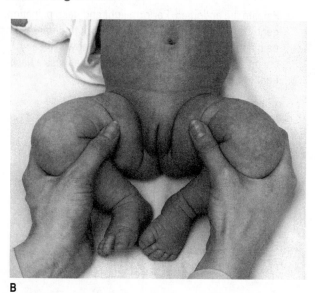

B

Ortolani's test for congenital hip dislocation. (A) Placement of examiner's hands. (B) Abduction of infant's hips.

Barlow's test: Place the baby supine on the examining surface. Use one hand to steady the pubis by placing the fingers over the greater trochanter of the hip being tested and gently pressing your hand over the symphysis pubis. Grasp the outer thigh with your other hand, placing your thumb over the lesser trochanter. Test by applying backward and outward pressure in a motion that moves the femur away from the joint socket.

Deviations from Normal
Movement should be smooth. If slipping movements are felt, the hip may be unstable or dislocated.

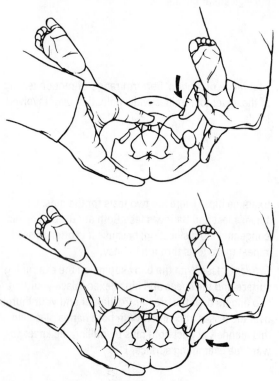

Barlow's test for congenital hip dislocation

▼ ▼ ▼

GUIDELINES   *continued*   Physical Examination of Newborns

Procedure

8. Examine the genitalia (Sexuality Pattern).

  a. Male:

    (1) Inspect the penis and gently retract the foreskin (prepuce). Do not force; may cause a tear in the prepuce.

    (2) Inspect and palpate the scrotum. If testes are not felt, place a finger over the inguinal ring and push gently toward the scrotum. The testes may descend into the scrotal sac with this maneuver.

  b. Female:

    (1) Inspect the external genitalia. Assess the genitals by placing the baby supine with the hips abducted (frog position). Gently, with thumbs on either side of labia majora, push out and down.

Clinical Significance

Normal Findings

The shaft of the penis should be straight. Erections are common, with the usual nonerect length of the penis being 2 to 4 cm and about 1 cm wide. The urethral opening should appear as a midline slit. The prepuce is loose and may cover the urethral opening in the uncircumcised baby. The prepuce becomes more mobile as the child ages. Urine stream should be strong.

Deviations from Normal

A dorsal or ventral urethral opening on the shaft of the penis is abnormal.

Normal Findings

The scrotum appears large in comparison with the penis. Each scrotal sac should be 1 or 2 cm across and contain a testicle. If testes descend into scrotum, consider this a normal finding. The spermatic cord is smooth on palpation.

Deviations from Normal

If the testes are palpable in the inguinal canal but will not descend, consider them undescended and refer. Scrotal rugae may be absent in preterm infants. Edema and bruising of the scrotum are commonly observed with breech delivery. A deep cleft in the scrotum may be related to genitourinary anomalies or ambiguous genitals. Transillumination of the scrotum may be conducted to differentiate fluid from mass lesions. Lumps or roughness in the scrotum may indicate a hernia. Hydrocele is most common in children younger than 2 years and usually resolves as the child ages.

Normal Findings

The labia majora and minora may be edematous but should separate. The size of the labia is influenced by maternal hormones, and decreases in size may be noted within 2 or 3 weeks. If the baby was born breech, more edema and possibly bruising of the labia may be observed. The color of the labia will be light pink in light-skinned newborns and darker than the skin of the abdomen in dark-skinned newborns. The clitoris appears large (0.3–0.5 cm) in proportion to the rest of the genitalia. A vaginal opening is present in newborns and may drain a mucoid, white discharge for 4 weeks. Vaginal secretions may be blood-tinged the first week after birth. Skene and Bartholin glands are not visible or palpable in newborns and should not have discharge. The urethral meatus is usually midline, anterior to the vagina, and emits an uninterrupted stream when the baby is voiding.

Deviations from Normal

If the clitoris is larger than 0.5 cm, the appearance ambiguous, or the vaginal orifice unusual, the baby should be evaluated further. The absence of a vagina is abnormal.

▼ ▼ ▼

G U I D E L I N E S   *continued*   Physical Examination of Newborns

Procedure

(2) Assess pelvic structures.

9. **Examine the anus and rectum (Elimination Pattern).**
   For newborns, this part of the assessment is restricted to inspection. The rectum is not usually digitally assessed.

10. **Examine the upper extremities (Activity–Exercise Pattern).**
    a. Inspect arms and hands.

11. **Examine the skin.**
    a. Inspect the skin as each body part is assessed. During the assessment of specific body parts, all creases and skin folds should be carefully examined.

Clinical Significance

Pelvic structures are not usually evaluated in newborns and young children.

Normal Findings

The passage of meconium stool is associated with patency of the gastrointestinal tract. Feces from breast-fed babies are mustard colored and watery to soft in consistency, whereas formula-fed babies have yellowish-green feces that are more formed. If the anus is stroked, it should quickly contract.

Deviations from Normal

A child who has not passed a meconium stool or seems to pass meconium through the urinary meatus or vagina, or who does not have an anal opening (imperforate anus), should be referred immediately.

Normal Findings

The nails are soft and pliable, usually longer than wide. Nails may be long enough to scratch the skin. Vernix caseosa may be observed under the nails.

Deviations from Normal

These include polydactyly (extra fingers) and syndactyly (fused or webbed fingers). transverse palmar creases (simian lines) with a curving and shortened fifth finger are associated with Down syndrome.

Normal Findings

The skin color may change rapidly in response to activity and temperature changes. Normal variations in skin color and pigmentation include the following:

- An *erythematous flush* may be noted, especially during the first 8 to 24 hours.
- Children of *dark-skinned parents* may appear lighter in the newborn period because melanin concentrations have not developed except on nail beds and the scrotum.
- *Cyanosis* or *acrocyanosis* (cyanosis of hands and feet) may appear, especially if the baby is chilled.
- *Physiologic jaundice* occurs in about half of all newborns and is noted as slight yellowing of the skin occurring 3 or 4 days after birth. It usually disappears within 1 week. Physiologic jaundice is more common in breast-fed newborns.
- *Transient mottling (cutis marmorata)* is noticed on the trunk and extremities in response to cold.
- *Mongolian* spots are areas of dark blue or black pigmentation that are observed more frequently in dark-skinned infants, especially in the sacral and gluteal regions.
- *Vernix caseosa* is a white, cheese-like substance that covers the skin of the fetus. It is present in varying degrees and is almost always seen in skin folds and creases.
- *Lanugo* is a fine, silky covering of hair present in varying degrees after birth, more commonly in preterm newborns.

▼▼ ▼▼ ▼

Procedure

Clinical Significance

- *Telangiectatic nevi* (commonly called "stork bites" or "angel kisses") are macular red or deep pink lesions at the back of the neck, eyelids, or forehead. These lesions may blanch to touch and usually fade with age but may be noted when excessive skin flushing occurs, even in adults.

Deviations from Normal

A beefy red color lasting more than 24 hours may be related to hypoglycemia. Persistent cyanosis may represent a congenital heart problem. If jaundice occurs earlier than 3 days or is a darker yellow, it may represent hemolytic disorders. Transient mottling may be pronounced in preterm bodies or Down syndrome infants. Common benign lesions that may be noted on the newborn's skin include the following:

- *Milia* appear as small white papules on the face, especially on the nose, cheeks, and chin. Milia represent sebaceous cysts and usually disappear within 2 months.
- *Cavernous hemangiomas* are cystic lesions with a reddish-blue hue. The lesion may grow at variable rates and may require medical treatment.
- *Strawberry hemangiomas* are red or purple, raised areas on the skin caused by dilated capillaries. Although the lesion may increase in size, it is usually no greater than 2 or 3 cm wide. The lesion may appear at birth or shortly thereafter and disappear by age 5 years.
- *Port wine stains* are purplish, sharply demarcated macular lesions that can occur on any skin surface or mucous membrane. The lesion is related to excessive proliferation of the capillary bed of the skin; it may invade the nervous system, and additional evaluation may be necessary.
- *Café-au-lait* are small, light-brown (coffee with cream color) macules. If fewer than six are noted over the entire body, the lesion has little clinical significance. If six or more are present, a high correlation exists with neurofibromas; further evaluation is warranted.
- *Erythema toxicum* (fleabite rash) is a diffuse rash characterized by small, red papules, 2 to 4 mm in size, with small, white, pinpoint centers. Commonly appears within 24 hours after birth on the trunk and diaper area and disappears spontaneously in 7 to 10 days.

b. Assess moisture and turgor. Skin turgor of the newborn should be evaluated using the skin of the lower abdomen. Skin turgor is a good indicator of the degree of hydration.

Normal Findings

The skin of the newborn should appear soft and smooth. Dry, flaky skin may indicate prolonged gestation. It is not uncommon to observe a transient puffiness or edema of the hands, feet, legs, eyelids, pubis, or scrotum. This condition usually disappears within 2 or 3 days.

▼ ▼ ▼

G U I D E L I N E S *continued*   Physical Examination of Newborns

Procedure

12. Perform a neurologic examination (Activity–Exercise, Nutrition, and Cognition–Perception Patterns).

   a. Assess muscle strength and function. Hold the newborn upright at the axilla with feet on a flat surface.

   b. Assess sensory functions.

   c. Assess reflex movements. It is not always necessary to test all the newborn reflexes. The most important to elicit include the Moro, stepping, palmar grasp, plantar grasp, Babinski, and rooting reflexes. The methods of testing these reflexes and the expected responses are shown in Display 16–4.

   d. Assess cranial nerves. The cranial nerves are difficult to evaluate in newborns and infants because cooperation is usually required. Observation of certain behaviors may help with judgments about cranial nerve function.

Clinical Significance

Deviations from Normal

Any alteration in neurologic findings, such as weakness, absence of normal reflexes, or asymmetry, may reflect neurologic problems.

Normal Findings

If the baby can maintain this position, muscle strength is considered adequate.

Deviations from Normal

Muscle weakness is apparent if the baby slips through the nurse's hands. Some muscle paralysis may occur as a result of pressure during vaginal delivery. Paralysis may disappear spontaneously or within 3 months with therapy, or may be limited to no recovery. Paralysis of any area needs to be assessed by a physician.

Normal Findings

The sensory assessment of newborns is nonspecific; vision and hearing screening were discussed earlier. The response to painful stimuli may be the only sensory function tested during the newborn assessment. Limbs should withdraw in response to painful stimuli.

Normal Findings

Several reflex movements are noted in newborns that are not present in other age groups. These primitive reflexes normally disappear by a specific age range. Failure to elicit one of these reflexes or persistence of the reflex beyond the usual time may be related to neurologic problems.

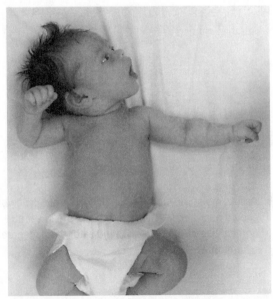

The fencing response, or tonic neck reflex, elicited by turning the infant's head to the side when the infant is supine. Note the skin mottling secondary to cold exposure.

▼ ▼ ▼
G U I D E L I N E S   *continued*   Physical Examination of Newborns

Procedure

(1) Assess cranial nerves III, IV, and VI by observing a blink reflex and eliciting a doll's eye response (rotation test). To check this response, hold the baby up under the axillae at arms' length facing you. Turn the baby in one direction and then the other; the head is restrained by your thumbs.

(2) Assess cranial nerve by observing the newborn's rooting and sucking reflexes.

(3) Assess cranial nerve VII.

(4) Assess cranial nerves IX, X, and XII.

Clinical Significance
Normal Findings
The eyes should turn in the same direction as the body.

Movements of the facial muscles should appear smooth, symmetric, and without tremors or spasticity.

Normal function of cranial nerve VII is indicated by wrinkling of the forehead when the baby is crying and by symmetric mouth movements.

The ability to swallow and a gag reflex indicate normal functioning of cranial nerves IX and X. Function of cranial nerve XII is required for the coordination of sucking and swallowing.

---

developmental testing and immunizations until well. Mother will reschedule appointment in 2 weeks.

Clinical Problems Related to Infant Examination

The most common clinical problems of infants are otitis media, upper respiratory infections, diaper rash, allergies, and colic.

Otitis Media

Otitis media is discussed in Chapter 9. Infants are at high risk for otitis media because their eustachian tubes have a horizontal connection between the inner ear and the pharynx. As the child ages, this tube becomes more vertical.

Upper Respiratory Infections

Upper respiratory infections with accompanying otitis media occur frequently in infants. Most upper respiratory infections are viral and are either nasopharyngitis (involve nose and pharynx) or pharyngitis (throat and tonsils). Elevated temperature, cough, and runny nose (rhinitis) are common. Parents should avoid the use of aspirin because of the risk of Reye's syndrome (acute encephalopathy with degeneration and a high mortality rate). Types of lower respiratory infections include *bronchitis* (an inflammation of the bronchi almost always occurs with upper respiratory problems) and *pneumonia* (an inflammation of the lungs can be viral or bacterial).

Diaper Rash

Diaper rash or diaper dermatitis results from urine and feces excoriating the skin. If urine and feces are allowed to remain on the skin, denudement and bacterial infection may occur. Plastic pants and plastic covers on disposable diapers increase warmth and decreases air circulation, enhancing conditions that promote dermatitis. Prompt changing of the diaper and adequate cleansing will inhibit diaper dermatitis.

Allergies

The most common allergies of infants are to foods, primarily eggs, wheat, vegetables, and fruit. When infants start eating more foods, they are exposed to numerous new antigens, and the immature intestinal tract absorbs many of these antigens, producing allergic reactions. As the intestinal tract matures, the infant may outgrow some food allergies. Symptoms of food allergies include rash, irritability, diarrhea, abdominal bloating, flatus, and respiratory coughing or wheezing. Food allergies can be controlled by avoiding foods that cause allergic reactions.

Colic

Colic is a paroxysmal abdominal pain or cramping. Infants with colic have loud crying, are irritable, and draw legs up to the abdomen; they are not easily comforted. Colic is more common in infants younger than 3 months. The exact cause of colic is unknown. Parents become very frustrated with the daily routine of colic, have guilt feelings about not being able to relieve infant, and become irritable from lack of sleep and prolonged crying of infant.

Newborn and Infant Reflex Evaulation*

RELFEX	METHOD OF TESTING	EXPECTED RESPONSE	APPEARANCE	DISAPPEARANCE
Moro	Hold the infant, supporting the head and neck with one hand and the buttocks and lower legs with the other; lower head by several cm, suddenly, being careful not to hyper-extend	1. Sudden, symmetrical abduction of arms and shoulders 2. Elbows extend 3. Hands open with semiflexion of index finger and thumb to form a C 4. Arms return over body with clasping motion	Birth	Diminishment in 3 or 4 mo, disappearance by 6 mo
Startle	Expose to loud noise, sudden position change (see Moro testing); jar crib	Similar to Moro but hands are clenched	Birth	4 mo
Tonic neck	Hold the infant supine and turn the head to one side so the jaw is over the shoulder	1. Extension of arm and leg on the side to which head is turned 2. Flexion of opposite arm and leg	Birth	3–4 mo
Stepping (dancing or walking)	Hold infant under axillae, allowing feet to contact firm surface	Legs move up and down as though infant were walking	Birth	4 mo
Placing	Hold infant under axillae and move one foot to touch the edge of a table	Flexion of knee and hip, and placement of stimulated foot on table surface	Best after 4 days	Variable
Palmar grasping	Place finger or small object in infant's palm	Fingers curl tightly around finger or object	Birth	4 mo
Plantar grasping	Place thumb firmly against ball of infant's foot	Plantar flexion (curling) of all toes	Birth	12 mo
Babinski	Stroke lateral aspect of foot from heel toward little toe with tongue blade or other edged object	Big toe rises (dorsiflexion and other toes fan out (positive Babinski sign)	Birth	24 mo
Rooting	Touch edge of infant's mouth or lightly stroke cheek	Mouth opens, and head turns toward stimulus	Birth	Usually 4 m but variable
Sucking	Touch infant's lips	Sucking movements	Birth	3–4 mo
Blinking	Expose to sudden, bright light	Eyelids close	Birth	12 mo
Acoustic blinking	Expose to sudden, loud noise	Bilateral eyelid closing	Birth	Variable
Parachuting	Thrust body downward, suddenly in head-first position	Arms and fingers extend in a protective motion	4–6	Indefinite
Neck righting	Turn head to one side and observe body movement	Body will turn toward same direction as neck	3 mo	
Body righting	Turn hips or shoulders to one side and observe body movement	Other body parts turn in same direction as hip or shoulder	6 mo	24–36 mo
Landau	Hold infant suspended prone, in horizontal position; raise head	Extension of legs and spine	6–8 mo	12–24 mo

*Failure to elicit a reflex may be abnormal. Try again to elicit the reflex before deciding it is absent. Persistence of reflexes beyond usual time of disappearance may indicate neurologic dysfunction. Refer infants if abnormal findings exist.

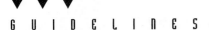

G U I D E L I N E S

Assessment Guidelines   Physical Examination of Infants

Procedure

Approach: Before age 6 months, the infant may be assessed similar to the newborn. As the infant develops better body control, he or she may become uncooperative. Therefore, the assessment may be less threatening if the infant is held on the parent's lap.

There are many similarities between newborn and infant assessment. Some findings are the same; others change as a result of growth and development.

1. Anthropometric measurements (Nutrition Pattern)

   a. Measure the head and chest circumference, using the same procedure as for newborns. Older infants may be afraid of the tape measure; have the parent assist in restraining infant's arms if necessary, and perform as quickly and as accurately as possible.

   2. Measure height and weight to evaluate physical growth. Chart all measurements on an appropriate growth chart; this will allow evaluation of growth according to standardized ranges and determine the child's own growth curve.

2. Examine the head.

   a. Inspect the cranial scalp, hair, face, and ear pinnae. Note the symmetry of facial structures as the baby cries or smiles.

   b. Palpate the fontanelles.

   c. Assess the eyes (Cognitive–Perceptual Pattern).

   (1) Evaluate visual acuity. Much of visual acuity can be tested while performing the DDST2. The ophthalmoscopic assessment may be difficult or impossible to perform if the infant is uncooperative. To focus on the retina, the initial lens settings on the ophthalmoscope should be between 0 and 5 diopters. If unable to perform a funduscopic assessment, test for the red reflex, corneal light reflex, pupillary constriction, and blinking.

Clinical Significance

Babies at this age are not generally afraid of strangers and will quickly forget the more intrusive parts of the assessment. After age 6 months, the infant is more fearful of strangers and may be anxious about separation from the parent. Try to create a game-like atmosphere to encourage cooperation. Performing the DDST2 before the physical examination often provides the infant a chance to get used to surroundings, and many examination findings can be observed.

Normal Findings
The head circumference normally increases by 1.5 cm each month for the first 6 months and by 0.5 cm per month between 6 and 12 months. Chest circumference is almost equal to head circumference by age 12 months.

Normal Findings
Birth weight should double by 6 months and triple by 12 months. Height should increase by 50% by 12 months. Height-to-weight proportions should be stable.

Normal Findings
The face, skull, and hair distribution should be fairly symmetric. The amount of scalp hair varies.

Normal Findings
The posterior fontanelles should be closed by age 2 months. The anterior fontanelle is usually closed by age 18 months.

Deviations from Normal
A sunken fontanelle may indicate dehydration, whereas a bulging fontanelle may indicate increased intracranial pressure. Premature closing of the anterior fontanelle is not normal.

Normal Findings
The infant's eyes should be able to rotate 180 degrees to follow an object in the field of vision by age 3 months. By age 5 months, the infant will focus on objects that are 3 feet away or further. Normally, infants have full binocular vision, depth perception, and visual acuity of 20/100.

Deviations from Normal
Inability to follow or fix the eyes on objects may be abnormal. Strabismus may be noted at age 3 months but should resolve by age 6 months; persistence of strabismus after 6 months is abnormal and should be evaluated. Internal eye structures appear smaller than in the adult, and the macula is poorly developed and not discernible until age 1 year. Blinking is frequent and bilateral.

Deviations from Normal
Unilateral blinking is considered abnormal; other abnormal findings are the same as in the newborn.

▼ ▼ ▼

Procedure

(2) Assess lacrimal apparatus.

(3) Assess eye color.

d. Inspect the ears. Assess the inner ear with the otoscope (perform this procedure near the end of the assessment because of its intrusive nature). Place the infant supine on the examining table. The parent may help restrain the baby by holding the arms over the head and holding the head between the hands. Children younger than 3 years have an upward curvature of the ear canal; therefore, pull the auricle down and back to visualize the tympanic membrane.

Using a small speculum, closely assess the tympanic membrane for abnormalities. Pneumotoscopy is performed by gently forcing air into the ear canal by squeezing a bulb that is attached to the otoscope via a small rubber tube.

Clinical Significance

Normal Findings
The lacrimal apparatus continues to develop, and true tearing begins between 1 and 2 months.

Deviations from Normal
If no tearing occurs after 2 months, the lacrimal apparatus may be plugged, and additional intervention is necessary to unplug them.

Normal Findings
The infant's permanent eye color is developed by age 12 months. Bulbar conjunctiva and sclera that were blue-tinged in the newborn period gradually lose this coloration. A slight yellow cast may be noted over the sclera and conjunctiva of dark-skinned infants.

Deviations from Normal
Continuation of blue coloration may indicate ontogenesis imperfecta.

Normal Findings
By age 6 months, findings should be the same as with adults. With pneumotoscopy, the normal tympanic membrane will move in and out as positive and negative pressure is applied.

Deviations from Normal
Tympanic membrane redness, bulging, and loss of the light reflex or other landmarks are abnormal. When inflammation or fluid is behind the tympanic membrane, it will move little or not at all with pneumotoscopy.

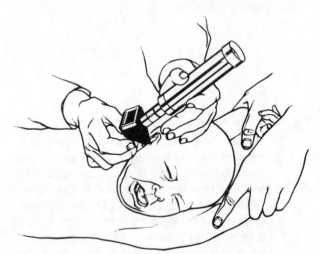

Restraining the infant during the physical examination

Procedure

e. Assess oral cavity and throat (Nutritional Pattern). With the infant supine on an examining table or parent's lap, have the parent restrain the baby by holding arms overhead. If the infant will not open the mouth, hold the nose closed, which causes the mouth to open. Gently insert a tongue blade between the upper and lower teeth/gum line, moving toward the midline of the tongue. The gag reflex will be stimulated when the blade is back far enough. The infant should quickly open the mouth, and oral structures may be inspected. Use of a penlight facilitates inspection. Observe the palate, teeth, tonsils, and oral mucosa, and note any lesions.

Clinical Significance

Normal Findings

Tooth eruption begins with the lower central by age 6 months. The pattern of tooth eruption is summarized in Display 16–5. Tonsils may seem large but should be the same color as surrounding tissue.

Deviations from Normal

Tooth eruption delayed beyond 12 months should be evaluated. Deviations for infants are the same as for newborns and adults.

DISPLAY 16.5

Pattern of Tooth Eruption in Infants and Children

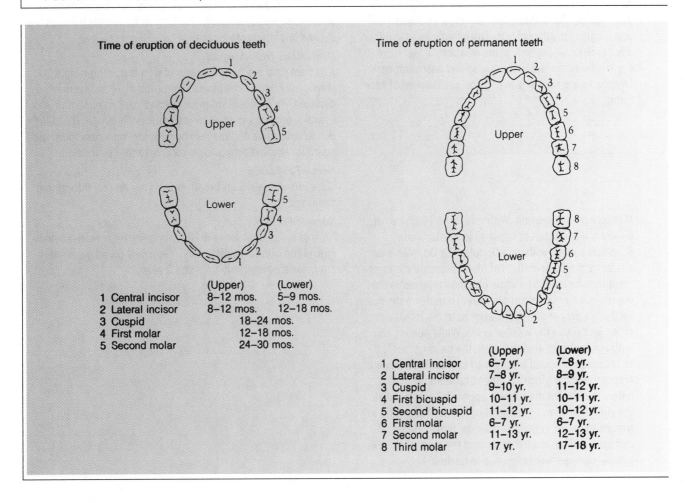

Time of eruption of deciduous teeth

		(Upper)	(Lower)
1	Central incisor	8–12 mos.	5–9 mos.
2	Lateral incisor	8–12 mos.	12–18 mos.
3	Cuspid		18–24 mos.
4	First molar		12–18 mos.
5	Second molar		24–30 mos.

Time of eruption of permanent teeth

		(Upper)	(Lower)
1	Central incisor	6–7 yr.	7–8 yr.
2	Lateral incisor	7–8 yr.	8–9 yr.
3	Cuspid	9–10 yr.	11–12 yr.
4	First bicuspid	10–11 yr.	10–11 yr.
5	Second bicuspid	11–12 yr.	10–12 yr.
6	First molar	6–7 yr.	6–7 yr.
7	Second molar	11–13 yr.	12–13 yr.
8	Third molar	17 yr.	17–18 yr.

▼ ▼ ▼

G U I D E L I N E S *continued*   Physical Examination of Infants

Procedure	Clinical Significance

Procedure

3. **Examine the chest and back (Activity–Exercise Pattern).**
   Assessment of the chest and back is similar to that in the newborn.

4. **Examine the heart and lungs (Activity–Exercise Pattern).**
   a. Observe the ventilatory rate and pattern.

   b. Auscultate the heart and lungs while the baby is quiet, before proceeding to more intrusive procedures. The infant may remain on the parent's lap or be held in the parent's arms in a chest-to-chest position for posterior auscultation. Auscultate heart sounds with a small bell and diaphragm attachments. The infant's heart is generally in the same position as the newborn's; therefore, the locations of the apical impulse and auscultatory landmarks are similar (see physical assessment of newborn).

   c. Measure blood pressure. With infants and some small children, it is difficult or impossible to auscultate Korotkoff sounds without a Doppler. If a Doppler is not available, the flush method of blood pressure measurement may be used. The value obtained represents the approximate mean blood pressure. To perform the flush method, a proper-size cuff is applied to the infant's arm or leg just above the wrist or ankle. While holding the limb above the level of the heart, the hand or foot is squeezed or wrapped snugly with an elastic bandage to empty the underlying capillaries and veins. The skin below the level of the cuff will appear blanched. Inflate the cuff, then unwrap the hand or foot and allow the extremity to return to the infant's side. Slowly deflate the cuff and read the manometer when the color of the extremity changes from blanched to flushed.

Clinical Significance

Normal Findings
The cervical curve of the spine develops at age 34 months; lumbar curve develops and lordosis becomes evident as the baby begins to walk (12–18 months).

Deviations from Normal
Same as with newborn.

Normal Findings
The infant has abdominal respirations at a rate of 25–50 breaths/min. Apnea is less common in infants than in newborns. Infants remain obligatory nose breathers and are irritable with nasal congestion.

Deviations from Normal
Nasal flaring, stridor, and sternal retractions are all signs of respiratory distress in the infant.

Normal Findings
The infant's heart rate ranges from 80–160 beats/min. The heart rhythm is frequently irregular (sinus dysrhythmia), especially during sleep. *Heart sounds:* A physiologic or normal third sound may be auscultated. This is most frequently heard at the second left intercostal space.

Deviations from Normal
An infant who is a poor sucker and who is gaining weight slowly may have a cardiovascular problem. Murmurs may be detected. An innocent murmur, a soft blowing sound that is not heard in other areas, may be insignificant; however, it is difficult to determine seriousness by auscultation alone. Murmurs heard for the first time should receive further evaluation.

Normal Findings
Clear bronchovesicular breath sounds are normal throughout the lungs.

Normal Findings
Normal systolic pressure is 70–80 mm Hg. Be sure that a pediatric blood pressure cuff is used. Generally blood pressure is not measured regularly until age 3 years.

▼ ▼ ▼

Procedure	Clinical Significance

Procedure

5. Examine the abdomen (Nutritional Pattern).

   a. Inspect the abdominal contour and look for hernias in the supine position and as the infant is held in a standing position. Also inspect for abdominal hernias when the baby is crying. Avoid vigorous deep palpation if the baby has just finished feeding.

   b. Auscultate the abdomen, using appropriate bell and diaphragm.

   c. Percuss the abdomen to identify abdominal organs.

6. Examine external genitalia (Sexuality Pattern).

   Place the infant supine and hold the hips adducted (frog position). Carefully inspect the genitals and perineum for skin lesions and rashes. Many findings are similar to those in the newborn (see Examination Guidelines for newborns).

   a. Females:

   (1) Inspect labia.

   (2) Inspect vaginal and urethral orifices. Part the labia with the thumb and forefinger.

   (3) Internal structures are not assessed unless molestation is suspected, and then a qualified physician should perform the assessment.

   b. Males:

   (1) Inspect the penis.

Clinical Significance

Normal Findings

The infant's abdomen is dome-shaped and moves with respiration. The diastasis recti muscle remains split as in the newborn period. A fine venous network may be observed over the abdomen. The umbilicus should appear dry and inverted.

Deviations from Normal

Visible peristaltic waves moving across the upper abdomen are abnormal and may be secondary to pyloric stenosis. Prominent venous networks along with a taut skin appearance are abnormal. In such cases, the abdomen should be transilluminated (see newborn). Umbilical eversions over 2 cm wide represent hernias and may require further evaluation. Smaller umbilical hernias, however, are common in this age group.

Normal Findings

Bowel sounds are normally heard every 10 to 30 seconds. Percussion may reveal increased tympany, which is secondary to air swallowing during feeding.

Normal Findings

After age 6 months, the liver span is 2.4–2.8 cm at the midclavicular line; by age 12 months, the span is 2.8–3.1 cm at the midclavicular line.

Deviations from Normal

Liver more than 3 cm below rib margin, palpable spleen, or enlarged kidney

Normal Findings

The labia minora are more prominent than the labia majora.

Deviations from Normal

Redness and swelling of the labia may indicate sexual molestation or infection.

Normal Findings

No redness or discharge should be noted.

Normal Findings

Erections are common during infancy. The foreskin may not be fully retractable until age 1 year in the uncircumcised male.

Deviations from Normal

Severe inflammations of the skin of the penis may occur with diaper rash.

▼ ▼ ▼

G U I D E L I N E S *continued*   Physical Examination of Infants

Procedure

(2) Inspect and palpate scrotum. If testes are not descended, try to descend them by placing fingers over the inguinal ring and gently pushing the testes toward the scrotum.

7. **Examine the anus and rectum (Elimination Pattern).**
Generally these are not assessed except externally. Inspection is the same as for adults.

8. **Examine the skin.**
Inspect the skin as each body part is being assessed. Examine skin creases and folds carefully.

Clinical Significance

Normal Findings

Testes may move back and forth between the inguinal canal and scrotum until age 4 years. If the undescended testes easily descend into the scrotum, this finding may be normal.

Deviations from Normal

Hernias and hydroceles are common problems in this age group. The scrotum may appear enlarged or asymmetric. The scrotum may transilluminate. Transillumination occurs across a hydrocele (fluid) but not across hernias (mass). Failure to palpate or descend the testes is abnormal and should be evaluated.

Normal Findings

Infant should be having bowel movements without difficulty; there should be no anal fissures or tears.

Normal Findings

The skin should be moist, have good turgor, and be without blemishes.

Deviations from Normal

If the infant becomes cold, mottling of the skin may occur. Any scars, bruises, or abrasions in various stages of healing, particularly above the knees and below the elbows and in the diaper area, may indicate child abuse. Skin pallor and cyanosis are abnormal in the infant. Pallor may be a sign of anemia. Cyanosis is often associated with congenital malformations of the heart or great vessels. The most common skin deviations in infants include the following:

Diaper dermatitis (diaper rash) is noted early as erythema in the diaper area. If severe, papules and skin excoriation may be noted. The skin folds in the inguinal and gluteal areas are especially sensitive to the irritating effects of urine. Secondary infections with *Candida* (yeast) may occur. *Candida* lesions appear as bright red, circumscribed, scaling patches. Satellite lesions may be present.

Atopic dermatitis (eczema) is noted in infants with skin hypersensitivity and allergic tendencies. Exposure to various allergens, irritants, moisture, temperature changes, excessive dryness, and even fear and stress can cause the skin to itch intensely. Itching causes scratching, and eventually the skin develops eczematous lesions and lichenification. Eczematous lesions appear as erythematous papules and vesicles that may have a discharge and become crusted. In infants, eczema usually appears on the face and in skin folds.

Seborrheic dermatitis (cradle cap) appears on the scalp or diaper area as flat, adherent, greasy scales. This condition is fairly common, and exact causes are unknown; however, a relationship to infrequent shampooing of the hair may exist. Secondary bacterial infection may occur, especially if pruritus causes scratching of the lesions.

▼ ▼ ▼

G U I D E L I N E S   *continued*   Physical Examination of Infants

___

Procedure

9. Assess musculoskeletal structures and functions (Activity–Exercise Pattern).

The muscutoskeletal system is best evaluated with the infant supine and unclothed except for a diaper.

a. Assess the upper extremities and the manner in which the infant uses the hands and fingers. Many of the hand and finger functions can be evaluated during the administration of the DDST2 (see Appendix D).

b. Examine the lower extremities. The infant's hips should be assessed for dislocation and deformities at every health assessment until age 1 year. The diaper should be removed for this assessment. Perform Ortolani's and Barlow's tests (see Examination Guidelines, for newborns).

c. Move the infant through several position changes to evaluate other musculoskeletal functions.
  (1) First, gently pull the infant from the supine to the sitting position. If necessary; prop the infant into a sitting position.

  (2) Test appropriate reflexes for the infant's age (see Display 16–4).

Clinical Significance

Normal Findings
The hands will be held in tight fists until after age 1 month, when they are held loosely fisted. The infant's grasp should be strong and equal. After age 3 months the infant can hold objects placed in the hands, and by age 4 months objects in the hands will be taken directly toward the mouth. At age 5 months the infant will voluntarily grasp objects and clasp the hands together. Objects will be transferred from one hand to the other by 7 months. The ability to pick up objects between the thumb and forefinger (pincer grasp) begins to develop at age 8 months. The ability to hold a crayon is developed by age 11 months.

Deviations from Normal
Shoulder or elbow dislocations may be the result of pulling, lifting, or twirling the infant by the arms.

Normal Findings
Joints should be smooth and without any clicks. See findings for newborns.

Deviations from Normal
Other indicators of hip problems include asymmetry of hip abduction, unequal leg lengths, and unequal skin creases and folds of the legs. The legs have a bow-legged appearance throughout infancy.

Normal Findings
By age 4 months the infant can maintain balance when propped. Observe the infant's ability to maintain the position, hold the head upright, and control back position. Most infants can sit unsupported by 6–7 months. Crawling movements begin by age 6 months. By age 7 months, greater mobility is possible by crawling. By 9 months, most infants begin to pull themselves to a standing position and stand easily by holding onto something. Walking by holding onto furniture may be observed at age 11 months. Momentary standing without support occurs by age 1 year, and most infants walk unsupported by 14 months.

Normal Findings
Infants will lose various reflexes during this period, such as tonic neck and Moro. However, they will gain new reflexes, such as neck righting, Landau, and parachuting. Persistence of reflexes beyond normal time of disappearance or failure to elicit new reflexes at the appropriate age may indicate neurologic defects.

▼ ▼ ▼

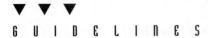
GUIDELINES

Assessment Guidelines   Physical Examination of Young Children

This section includes the toddler (12 months to 3 years) and the preschool child (3–6 years). This is the age of upright locomotion, self-expression, autonomy, and gaining independence in self-care. Children between the ages of 1 and 5 years may be the most challenging to assess because of their fear of strangers, fear of bodily injury, and the need to be in control of the situation. Engaging the child in a story or game may be helpful. Older children in this age group may be anxious because they anticipate an injection. If the child asks about this possibility, honest discussion should be encouraged. Younger children may feel more comfortable sitting on a parent's lap during most of the assessment.

The ability to speak and comprehend language increases dramatically. Children learn to count, distinguish and name colors, and define simple concepts such as what is a ball or lake. Some of the child's anxiety may be alleviated by talking to the child and parents throughout the assessment. Also, starting with the DDST2 gives the child a chance to become familiar with the nurse and environment. It may be helpful to demonstrate the use of equipment on the parent, a doll, or the nurse to ease the child's fears. For example, place the blood-pressure cuff on the parent before using it on the child. Allow the child to handle equipment as much as possible. Using the equipment in a playful manner is also helpful.

Procedure

1. Anthropometric measurements (Nutrition Pattern)
   a. Measure height and weight. If the child is walking, standing height measurement is preferred over lying length.

   b. Head and chest circumference may continue to be evaluated until the child is 3 years old.

2. Examine the head (Cognitive–Perception Pattern).
   a. Examine the eye.
      (1) Inspect the external eye. Perform the cornea light reflex test by shining a light approximately 13 inches level with the eye brows; observe where the light falls. Also perform the cover/uncover test for amblyopia.

      (2) Ophthalmoscopic assessment is difficult to perform on children in this age group. Determine whether the red reflex is present. If the child cooperates, the macula and retinal vessels may be visualized.
      (3) Assess visual acuity. Refractive visual errors do occur in young children, so evaluation of visual acuity is an important part of the assessment. The traditional Snellen chart needs to be modified for this age group, although the procedure for Snellen testing is similar to that used with adults. The child may not be able to cooperate until age 3–4 years. The 3-year-old child should be screened for visual problems with an "HOTV" chart. At age 4, some children can use the illiterate "E" version.

Clinical Significance

When the child's height as opposed to length is measured, a new graphic form for height and weight should be used. Physical growth is slower than in the infant—about 4–6 pounds/year (about 3 in/y).

Normal Findings
Weight should be proportional for height.

Normal Findings
Chest circumference exceeds head circumference at 24 months.

Most assessments of head shape and hair distribution are the same as for adults.

Normal Findings
The external eye should have a similar appearance in adults and children.

Deviations from Normal
Strabismus may be noted in this age group. In a child without strabismus, the light should be observed in the center of each pupil. It is important to test for strabismus to prevent blindness in one eye secondary to amblyopia. If one eye wanders with the cover/uncover test, refer for possible amblyopia.

Normal Findings
The retina and macula should appear similar to the fundus of the adult. A red reflex should occur.

Normal Findings
Visual acuity at age 3–4 years is 20/40; by age 5 it is 20/30 to 20/20.

▼ ▼ ▼

G U I D E L I N E S   *continued*   Physical Examination of Young Children

Procedure

b. Examine the ears. The child may need to be restrained while assessing the ears. Children younger than 3 years have an upward curvature of the ear canal; therefore, pull the lower auricle down and back to visualize ear structures. For older children, use the same techniques as for the adult to visualize the ear structures. The speculum is inserted only ¼ to ½ inch in young children because their ear canals are short. Use the largest speculum the ear will accommodate. If it becomes necessary to restrain a young child, use one of the following positions: (1) lying prone with arms restrained at side and head secured by another, (2) lying supine with arms over head and head secured, or (3) sitting on the parent's lap with the arm restrained, head held against the parent's chest, and the legs restrained by the parent's legs. To avoid trauma to the ear canal, immobilize the child's head during otoscopic assessment if the child is unable to cooperate.

c. Assess the oral cavity and nose. Children in this age group may perceive this part of the assessment as threatening and refuse to cooperate. In some cases, it may be necessary to restrain the child. If the child will not open the mouth, hold the nares shut. When the mouth opens, insert the tongue blade to elicit a gag reflex. Quickly visualize the mouth and throat.

Clinical Significance

Normal Findings

The appearance of the ear and related structures is similar in all age groups.

Deviations from Normal

If fluid in the inner ear is suspected or if the child is not hearing well by history or standardized testing, determine whether the tympanic membrane is mobile (see pneumotoscopy in the Examination Guidelines for infants for technique).

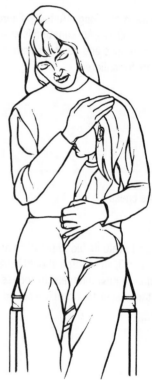

Restraining the young child during the physical examination

Normal Findings

Assessment findings are similar in infants and young children (see Examination Guidelines for infants).

Deviations from Normal

Teeth that are worn may be the result of teeth grinding. Dental caries are common in this age group. Children in this age group frequently have upper respiratory infections associated with otitis media and enlarged tonsils.

▼ ▼ ▼

Procedure	Clinical Significance

Procedure

d. Examine the throat and neck.

(1) Palpate the cervical lymphatic structures.

(2) Inspect the tonsils.

3. **Examine the heart and lungs (Activity–Exercise Pattern).**

a. Auscultate the chest. Auscultation is easiest when the child is cooperative and quiet. Use smaller stethoscope attachments for children.

b. Percuss the chest.

c. Measure and evaluate blood pressure and peripheral pulses. At age 3, all children should have blood pressure measured at regular intervals. In some small children, it is difficult to auscultate Korotkoff sounds.

4. **Assess the abdomen.**

a. Inspect the abdomen. The general appearance of the abdomen should be observed while the child is standing, sitting, or playing in the room. Assessment of the 4- or 5-year-old may be easier with the child on the examination table rather than on the parent's lap.

b. Percuss and palpate the liver. Most organs are fairly mature by this age. The liver and intestines are functioning.

Clinical Significance

Deviations from Normal
Tender lymph nodes may be an indication of infection.

Normal Findings
Tonsils may seem enlarged but should be the same color as surrounding tissue. Tonsils reach peak size by age 6 years.

Deviations from Normal
The tonsils may become so enlarged that they obstruct the airway.

Normal Findings
The average heart rate in a 2-year-old is 80 to 130 beats/min; from 3–5 years, it is 80 to 120 beats/min. An irregular heart rhythm characterized by a higher rate during inspiration than expiration (sinus dysrhythmia) is normal in young children. At the second left intercostal space, a splitting of the second heart sound is common in young children. *Breathing pattern:* Young children continue to have an abdominal breathing rate of 20–40 breaths/min. By age 6, other respiratory sounds can be identified, as with adults (bronchial and vesicular).

Normal Findings
The lung percussion note is slightly more resonant than that noted in the adult.

Normal Findings
The blood pressure reading should be less than 116/76 for children up to 5 years. Peripheral pulses should be palpable with a 3+ quality when graded on a 4-point scale. Pulses should be equal bilaterally.

Deviations from Normal
If a child has two consecutive readings above 116/76 after a 5-minute rest period, additional evaluation is necessary. In children, hypertension is most commonly related to kidney disorders.

Normal Findings
Young children have a rounded abdomen (potbelly appearance) in standing and supine positions that appears exaggerated secondary to lordosis. Any splitting of the diastasis rectus muscle begins to resolve at this age.

Deviations from Normal
Umbilical hernias that were present during infancy begin to resolve in light-skinned children by age 2 years and in black children by age 6 or 7 years.

Normal Findings
The liver span at the midaxillary line is 3.5–3.6 cm at age 2 years and 4.3–4.4 cm at 4 years. The liver may normally be palpable 1 or 2 cm below the costal margin in this age group. Use only one hand to palpate the liver.

▼ ▼ ▼
G U I D E L I N E S   *continued*   Physical Examination of Young Children

---

Procedure

5. Examine the genitals (Sexuality Pattern).

a. Inspect the external genitals. A pelvic assessment is rarely performed on young girls and requires special instruments as well as expertise. The child younger than 3 years old may assume the frog-leg position. Older children may be seated on the examination table. The head is raised 30 degrees so the child may comfortably lean against the table while assuming a frog-leg position. The child may be modest and feel more comfortable with a drape. Boys older than 3 years may sit on a chair or table in the tailor position, with the knees bent and feet flat or knees bent and ankles crossed.

6. Examine musculoskeletal functions (Activity–Exercise Pattern).

a. Musculoskeletal functions can be evaluated during the DDST2 and by watching the child playing or moving around the room. Asking the child to demonstrate activities such as hopping on one foot, throwing a ball, and getting onto a chair will help evaluate muscle development and skeletal functions.

b. Note muscle strength,hands, and nails as you would for an adult.

Clinical Significance

Normal Findings

The appearance of the external genitals is similar to that noted during infancy (see Assessment Guidelines for infants). Although most organs are fairly mature, reproductive organs remain immature.

Deviations from Normal

By 4 years, any boy whose testicles are not continuously descended into the scrotum should be evaluated by a physician for possible treatment. The risk for testicular cancer increases if testes do not descend.

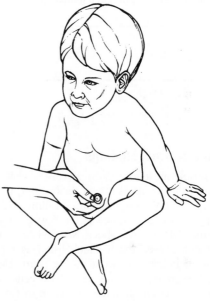

Tailor position

Normal Findings

The young child has spinal lordosis, but this becomes less noticeable as the child grows. The child should be able to get up from a supine to a standing position without having to place the hands on the thighs for extra leverage.

Deviations from Normal

The inability to get into a standing from a supine position could indicate certain types of muscular dystrophy.

Normal Findings

Similar to adults, muscle strength increases with age to adult levels.

Deviations from Normal

Children with cardiovascular problems may have clubbing of the fingers.

▼ ▼ ▼

G U I D E L I N E S *continued*   Physical Examination of Young Children

Procedure

c. Examine the hips and lower extremities. Evaluation of the hips for deformities or dislocation continue as routine screening until age 4.

7. Perform neurologic assessment.
The young child will not be able to cooperate with neurologic testing; however, the 3- to 4-year-old will cooperate with testing if done as part of a game.

Clinical Significance

Normal Findings
The bow-legged appearance of infancy disappears by age 2 to 3 years. A knock-kneed appearance is normal between the ages of 2 and 4. Feet pronation is common until age 30 months. The arch of the foot develops by age 3 years. When checking the feet, also observe the child's shoes for patterns of wear and proper fit.

Normal Findings
Neurologic findings should be similar to those for adults.

ND_X

Documenting Young Child Examination Findings

Example 1: Normal Findings

S: No problems; in for regular 3-year-old visit, eats three meals per day but is now a picky eater, plays house with other children. Just started riding a trike. Enjoys helping mother with new sister (6 weeks old).

O: Normal DDST2; see sheet. No deviations from normal noted—see exam check list. Has remained at 60% for height and weight—see chart. Urine negative for protein glucose, red blood cells, and white blood cell count. Immunizations up to date.

A: Normal growth and development.

P: Return in 1 year for health assessment. Return to clinic as needed for illness or problems. Anticipatory teaching—safety ages 3 to 4, discussed bike helmet use.

Example 2: Deviations From Normal

S: Child 4 years old. Was 3 weeks premature, Apgar 6 and 8. Discharged from hospital at 10 days. Mother doesn't remember anything "really" being wrong with Mike. Quiet child, rarely talks, and often ignores mother.

O: Only deviations reported—see exam checklist and DDST2 for normals. Unable to test vision or hearing. 1 caution and 1 delay in language. DASE only correctly pronounced 14 sounds, for a score in the 5th percentile.

A: Altered growth and development, language; etiology unknown.

P: Refer to speech-hearing clinic for hearing and speech assessment. Mother to call after speech and hearing evaluation and nurse to follow up at that time.

ND_X

Clinical Problems Related to Examination of Young Children

In addition to the clinical problems that occur in infancy except for colic, young children have health problems that include poisoning (usually the 2- to 3-year-old) and infectious diseases such as chicken pox and strep throat. Immunizations can prevent the infectious diseases of measles, rubella, mumps, chicken pox, poliomyelitis, pertussis (whooping cough), tetanus, diphtheria, *Haemophilus influenza* B, and hepatitis B and A.

Poisoning occurs in the young child when toxic substances such as medication, plants, household cleaning agents, and insecticides are within reach. The sense of taste is not well developed in the toddler, and one means to explore the world is to taste it. Poisoning is preventable, and parents should receive anticipatory guidance regarding how to childproof their homes.

Strep throat is caused by the group A beta-hemolytic *Streptococcus*. If untreated, it can progress to scarlet fever and cause complications, or to rheumatic fever with corresponding heart and glomerulus damage. Incubation is approximately 10 days. It begins with a sore throat usually covered with white patches. A throat culture should be performed with all suspicious sore throats. Treatment is usually a full course of an antibiotic such as penicillin and erythromycin.

ND_X

Documenting Examination Findings

Example 1: 10-Year-Old Male

S: No problems, enjoys school, favorite subjects math and art. Occasionally has difficulty seeing black-

▼ ▼ ▼
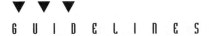

The school years generally refer to the period between 6 and 12 years, and adolescence between the ages of 13 and 18 to 19 years. Cognitive and emotional development are the hallmarks for this group. Older children and adolescents usually cooperate during the physical assessment; therefore, the assessment may be performed in a manner similar to adults. Procedures and findings for these age groups are similar to adults; only those procedures and findings that vary from adults are discussed in this section.

The school-aged child may be cooperative during the assessment if he or she knows what to expect. The child should be dressed in underclothes and a gown for modesty, if desired. The school-aged child usually wants parents present. The adolescent may or may not wish to have parents present during the physical assessment. Such a decision may be influenced by the gender of the nurse and the parent.

Procedure

1. **Anthropometric measurements (Nutrition Pattern)**
   a. Measure weight and height.
   b. Muscle circumference and skinfold thickness may be evaluated.

2. **Examine the head (Cognitive–Perception Pattern).**
   The assessment of the head is the same as in adults.
   a. Assess the eyes and evaluate visual acuity. This assessment is essential to ensure optimal visual acuity during cognitive development and learning. The assessment is conducted in a manner similar to that for adults. Older children will usually cooperate, follow instructions during evaluation of eye movements and visual acuity, and focus their eyes as instructed by the nurse. Children who wear corrective lenses should be tested with lenses on. Inquire as to when the last refractive change occurred. Be sure to ask about contact lenses before performing eye assessment.
   b. Assess the ears in the same manner as you would for the adult. The ear pinnacle is pulled upward and outward during the otoscopic assessment. Hearing acuity is also tested, by either standard testing or the whisper test.
   c. Examine the oral cavity. Children in this age group usually will cooperate with assessment of the oral cavity. Inquire about teeth brushing, flossing, and regular dental assessments.
   d. Examine the neck. Carefully palpate the cervical lymph nodes.

Clinical Significance

Normal Findings
School-age children grow about 3–6 pounds/year and 1–2 inches/year. Adolescence is marked by rapid growth spurts. Young men can grow 4–12 inches and gain 15–65 pounds. Young women usually grow 2–8 inches and add 15–55 pounds.

Deviations from Normal
Be alert for rapid weight changes. Excessive weight loss or inadequate weight gain may be signs of anorexia nervosa or bulimia.

Normal Findings
Ophthalmoscopic findings are the same as for adults.

Normal Findings
Should be similar to those in the adult

Normal Findings
Assessment findings are similar to those noted in adults.

Normal Findings
Nodes should not be enlarged.

▼ ▼ ▼

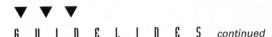

G U I D E L I N E S   *continued*   Physical Examination of Older Children
                                                       and Adolescents

---

Procedure

3. Examine the heart and lungs (Activity–Exercise Pattern).
   a. Perform auscultation, percussion, and inspection as for
      the adult.

   b. Measure blood pressure.

4. Examine breasts.
   Examine breasts as in the adult.

5. Examine the skin (Nutrition Pattern).
   a. Inspect the skin during the general survey and while as-
      sessing each body part.

6. Examine the abdomen.
   Conduct the assessment of the abdomen in a manner similar to that used with adults. Ticklishness may interfere with
   the assessment. Placing the child's hand under the nurse's
   during palpation may help reduce ticklishness. Depending
   on size and abdominal musculature, use one or both hands
   for palpation.
   a. Percuss and palpate the liver.

7. Examine the genitals.
   Children in this age group should be assessed on an examining table and may feel more comfortable if draped. Older
   children and adolescents may or may not desire the parent's presence and should be given a choice after an explanation of the assessment. A frog-leg position is used for
   school-age children. Girls should not be placed in a lithotomy position, which may be frightening and uncomfortable. This position may be used for girls older than age 15
   years.

Clinical Significance

Normal Findings
The heart rate at 6 years is 75–115 beats/min, with the average
being 95. From age 7 years to adolescence, the heart rate is 70
to 110 beats/min, with the average being 85. Older adolescents
have heart rates similar to those of adults at 60 to 100 beats/
min, with the average being 82. The respiratory range for this
age-group should be 16 to 20 breaths/min. Abdominal breathing is observed until age 6 or 7 years. After this age, girls begin
to develop a thoracic pattern, whereas boys continue to have
an abdominal pattern.

Normal Findings
For children ages 6 to 9 years, blood pressure should be less
than 122/78; ages 10 to 13, less than 130/80; girls age 14, less
than 133/82; girls age 15, less than 137/85; girls 16 to 20,
less than 140/85; boys 14 to 19, less than 128/84.

Normal Findings
The female breast develops to maturity during adolescence.
See Table 16–2 for breast development.

Deviations from Normal
Infectious skin disorders are noted in this age group, including
impetigo, rashes, and fungal infections. Seborrhea and acne
are common skin problems of adolescents.

Normal Findings
The potbelly contour may be observed in younger children in
this group when the child is standing. The abdomen may have
a scaphoid contour when the child is supine. All umbilical hernias should be resolved by age 7.

Normal Findings
The liver span at the midaxillary line at age 6 is 4.8–5.1 cm; at
age 8, 5.1–5.5 cm; and at age 12, 9 cm. The liver may be palpated 0–2 cm below the costal margin in school-age children.
The findings for adolescents are the same as for adults.

▼ ▼ ▼

G U I D E L I N E S   *continued*   Physical Examination of Older Children
and Adolescents

Procedure	**Clinical Significance**

Boys may be seated and placed in the tailor position (see Examination Guidelines for younger children). *Girls* usually experience their first pelvic assessment during adolescence. Explain the procedure, including any uncomfortable sensation that may be experienced (see Chap. 14). *Boys* should be assessed for hernias in the same manner as an adult. Prostate assessment is rarely performed on children and adolescents. Refer to Tables 16–2 and 16–3 regarding physical changes with puberty.

a. Females:

　(1) Inspect pubic hair.

Normal Findings

Soft, downy hair may be first noted along the labia majora at age 9–12 years. Darker hair appears on the mons pubis at age 10–12. Abundant, coarse hair appears by age 12–13.

　(2) Inspect the external genitalia.

Normal Findings

The labia minora recede to their adult configuration before puberty. The clitoris is about 1 cm wide in school-age children and 2 cm wide in adolescents. The hymen membrane may develop a 1-cm opening by age 10–12 years. Bulging behind the hymen may indicate the presence of blood. A watery vaginal discharge may be noted 2 or 3 years before the onset of puberty. Skene's and Bartholin's glands should not be visible and should not have any associated discharge.

Deviations from Normal

With the presence of sexually transmitted diseases in older children and young adolescents or enlarged vaginal orifices, sexual abuse should be considered.

b. Males:

　(1) Inspect pubic hair.

Normal Findings

Fine, downy pubic hair first appears at the base of the penis between ages 10 and 12. By age 13, darker, coarser hair is noted at the base of the penis. The distribution of pubic hair is similar to that noted in adult males between the ages of 14 and 16, with a spread to the inner thigh by age 16.

　(2) Inspect the penis.

Normal Findings

Penile growth begins at approximately 11 years. The penis reaches adult size and shape by age 17.

　(3) Inspect and palpate the scrotum and inguinal canal.

Normal Findings

The scrotum enlarges starting at age 10, with the left side usually appearing longer. The scrotum reaches adult size by approximately age 17. The adolescent should be taught how to do a testicular self-examination. Inguinal findings are the same as in the adult.

▼ ▼ ▼

G U I D E L I N E S *continued*

Physical Examination of Older Children and Adolescents

Procedure

8. Assess musculoskeletal function.

a. Inspect and palpate the spine. It is important to evaluate the spinal configuration carefully in this age group, with an emphasis on scoliosis screening. Inspect the exposed spine with the child in standing and bending forward positions. Stand behind the child and note structural symmetry when standing. Then ask the child to bend at the waist, allowing the arms to hang forward.

b. Assessment of the musculoskeletal function is similar to that in the adult, and findings are similar.

Clinical Significance

Normal Findings
The shoulder heights should be equal, and bony prominences such as the scapulae should be at the same horizontal level.

Deviations from Normal
Scoliosis is a lateral curvature of the spine. Scoliosis is most commonly noted during and after growth spurts in the adolescent.

---

board. Grades are OK (mostly Cs and Bs). Plays soccer after school on a community team. Has one best friend of same age and gender and several other friends at school. Rarely reads but watches TV 3 to 4 hours per night. Mother states no problems, pleasant child, no colds or ear infections this year, had chicken pox last year, believes immunizations up to date.

O: Physical examination findings: no deviations except for vision—see exam check sheet. Vision on Snellen screening 20/40 right eye and 20/60 left eye. Able to follow directions, cooperative. Weight-to-height proportion has increased from 50th percentile to 60th.

A: Visual impairment possible. Weight gain greater than desired over last year.

P: Refer to eye specialist for further evaluation. To return in 2 years for follow-up. Teaching: Need to decrease empty calorie foods and increase activity, encourage reduction in high cholesterol foods and increase in fruits and vegetables. Encourage reading.

Example 2: 17-Year-Old Female

S: Wants to play volleyball, here for sports physical, LMP 2 weeks ago, regular cycle of 28 days, flows 5 days. Not sexually intimate with anyone. No health problems. Denies recent weight loss. Came by self.

O: Genital and pelvic examination deferred. Physical findings normal—see exam check sheet. Weight-to-height proportion 40th percentile.

A: Healthy; however, possible nutritional deficiency as evidenced by low weight to height.

P: Return as needed. At next visit assess weight and height proportion and dietary intake.

Clinical Problems Related to Examination of Older Children and Adolescents

School-age children can develop the same infectious diseases as younger children. Colds, upper respiratory infections, and otitis media are less common than at younger ages. Common eye problems such as near- and far-sightedness occur (see Chap. 9). Adolescents can experience numerous health problems. Sexually active adolescents are at risk for all sexually transmitted diseases, and young women are at risk for pregnancy (see Chap. 13). Other problems may include anorexia and bulimia and drug abuse. *Anorexia nervosa* is characterized by severe weight loss in the absence of a physical cause. Anorexia is more common in women, occurring most frequently around 12 to 13 years and again at 19 to 20 years. With severe weight loss, amenorrhea, bradycardia, decreased blood pressure, and cold intolerance may occur. Bulimia is a similar disorder, although severe weight loss may or may not occur. The individual may gorge herself or himself on food and then force vomiting. This disorder is more common in women; however, it has recently been recognized in men who participate in wrestling.

Drug abuse is a major concern with adolescents. Types of drugs abused include alcohol, prescription drugs, and street drugs such as crack. The use of intravenous drugs also places adolescents at risk for HIV disease, as does prostitution to purchase drugs. Signs of drug abuse may include depression, withdrawal behavior, skipping or cutting school, change in usual behavior, friends who use drugs, and increased moodiness.

DISPLAY 16.6

Guidelines for Recording the Pediatric Database
Using Functional Health Patterns

This form was developed for use in acute care settings but could be adapted to other health care settings.

FUNCTIONAL HEALTH STATUS

Nursing History/Examination—Children

Date: _____ Time: _____ Name: _____ Source of Infomation: _____
Admitting Diagnosis: _____ Age: _____
Reason for Admission: _____

I. Health Perception and Health Management = Subjective Data	Objective Data
A. What is the problem? Why did you seek help today? Describe the problem. How has the problem been managed at home?	General appearance Child/parents
B. Current health	

A. What is the problem? Why did you seek help today? Describe the problem.
   How has the problem been managed at home?
B. Current health
   Preventive and safety practices
   Health today as related to past months, years
   Family/parent health
C. Past health
   1. Birth history
      Prenatal: Planned pregnancy
         Emotional response   Wt. gain
         Complications   Alcohol use; medication
      Natal: Length of labor   Spontaneous/induced
         Vaginal/cesarean   Anesthesia
         Complications
         Bonding   Support person
      Neonatal: Wt.: _____ Length: _____ Head circ.: _____
         Apgar
         Nursery course:
   2. Immunizations: DPT   Polio   Measles   Mumps   Hep B
                     Rubella   TB test   Flu   Hib   Other _____
   3. Growth and development:
      Motor: Rolling over _____
                           Sitting _____
                           Crawling _____
                           Standing _____
                           Walking _____
                           Sports _____
      Social–cognitive: Smiling _____
                           First word _____
                           Sentences _____
                           Playing _____
                           School _____
      Early behavior patterns as viewed by parents
   4. Frequency of health assessments and checkups—date of last visit
   5. Hospitalizations: Date, reason, length, diagnosis
   6. Accidents or injuries: Time, place, reactions, physical response
   7. Allergies/reactions: Drugs, foods, contactants, inhalants
D. Family history: Familial, inherited, genetic disorders (use back of sheet to illustrate)
      Parents   Heart
      Siblings   Hypertension

(continued)

DISPLAY 16.6

Guidelines for Recording the Pediatric Database
Using Functional Health Patterns (continued)

	Objective Data
D. Family history (*continued*)	
Aunts, uncles (maternal, paternal) Arteriosclerosis	
Cousins Coronary artery disease	
Maternal grandparents Blood disorders	
Paternal grandparents Renal disease	
Cancer	
Diabetes	
Obesity	
Arthritis	
Gout	
Mental illness	
Epilepsy	
Allergies	
Migraines	
Race–culture	
Environmental history:	
Type of housing	
Seasonal changes	
Pollution effects	
Economic	
Employment of parents	
Adequate means for family needs	
Community resources used: Associations, organizations, foundations, HHC, CHNC, PHN	
II. Nutrition	
Recall of intake past 24 hours: Food, fluids, vitamins	Wt.: _____
	Ht.: _____
Meal patterns	Head: _____
	(attach growth chart)
	Temp: _____ AX-R-O
	B.P.: _____
Eating behavior	Skin
First tooth How many now?	Teeth
Likes Dislikes	Rash, odors
Food allergies/behavioral changes toward certain food	Nodes
III. Elimination Patterns	
Bowel and bladder pattern; Daytime; nighttime control	Bowel sounds
Usual time of BM	Appearance of feces, urine
Words used for BM; Urination	
Recent changes in elimination	Hernia
Excess perspirations? Odor?	
IV. Activity–Exercise Patterns	
Describe usual day	Reflexes, ROM, gait, strength
Level of self-care/routine	
Feeding	Pulses
Dressing	Capillary refill
Toileting	Breath sounds
	(continued)

Guidelines for Recording the Pediatric Database
Using Functional Health Patterns (continued)

	Objective Data
Bathing	Respiratory sounds
	Heart sounds
	Coordination
Mobility	Motor skills
Use of free time	

V. Sleep–Rest Patterns

Usual pattern Naps	Appear rested?
	Child/parent
Sleeping arrangements	Attentive
Bedtime items Blanket/stuffed toy	
Easy to awaken?	

VI. Cognitive–Perceptual Patterns

Variations in vision, hearing, taste, smell, touch, pain	PERRLA
Response to noise, touch, talking, music	Cover test
Educational experience (includes infant stimulation)	Acuity Glasses
Speech pattern	Hearing Ears
Ability to cooperate, communicate	Speech DASE
	Pain
Behavior as viewed by parents	Sensory functions
	Oriented

VII. Self-Perception–Self-Concept Patterns

Outstanding personality trait	Body posture/movement
Overall behavior	Eye contact
Interests	Behavior changes
What causes fears, strong emotions How handled?	Self-confidence
Sense of humor	

VIII. Role Relationship

Usual caregiver/parent–child interaction	Observed interaction with
Siblings:	significant others
Sibling–child relationship	
Grandparents	
Peer interactions	
Favorite person	
Security objects	
Additional members of household	
Response to separation	
Dependency	
School adjustment	

IX. Sexuality–Reproductive Patterns

Knows if she/he is a girl/boy (feelings of maleness, femaleness)	Testicles examination
Basic language for body parts and functions	Breast examination
Direct teaching regarding sexuality	Genitalia
Response to questions	
Best friend	
Menarche	

X. Coping–Stress Tolerance Patterns

Response to stress changes	Problem solving/coping
New environment/people	observed
Illness	
Hospitalization	

(continued)

DISPLAY 16.6

Guidelines for Recording the Pediatric Database
Using Functional Health Patterns (continued)

	Objective Data

Frequent illness(es)
Experience of separation from parents
Occurrence of dependent behavior
Method of discipline
    Reaction
Response to criticism, correction
Family stressors
Community resources used by the family
XI. Value–Belief Patterns
Goals for future
What qualities are important in life
    Parents/child
Is religious belief important/supportive to family?
    Religion   Sunday school
	Varied health practices

Other Diagnostic Screening Tests   *Other Laboratory Tests*

DDST2
Preschool Readiness: Experimental Screening Scale
Draw-a-Person
Neonatal Perception Inventory
Anticipatory Guidance Need
Others

Summary Statement: (Cluster cues—Nursing diagnosis)

(Developed by Marita Hoffart, Associate Professor of Nursing, Minot State University, Minot, North Dakota)

CHAPTER 16   S U M M A R Y

The health assessment of newborns, infants, children, and adolescents requires a different approach from that used for adults and may require a different interpretation of the findings. Developmental screening in these age-groups is important to determine whether physical growth as well as cognitive and social abilities are proceeding as expected. Developmental screening tests such as the DDST2 are routinely administered to children younger than 6 years old to detect developmental delays.

The nurse should consider the child's fears, ability to follow directions, and physical abilities when conducting the physical assessment. Flexibility is required to accommodate each child's special needs. An interview/examination data collection tool for pediatrics is illustrated in Display 16-6.

This chapter presents assessment information regarding newborns, infants, young children, older children, and adolescents. An overall knowledge base for the assessment of children is presented by functional patterns. Modifications to examination procedures and deviation from adult findings are presented for each age group.

The nursing diagnosis that applies only to children is Altered growth and development. Other nursing diagnoses that affect children are family diagnoses, such as the following:

• Altered parenting
• Alterations in family process
• Ineffective family coping

Most other nursing diagnoses can be used for children; however, some may not be appropriate because of the normal maturational status of young children (e.g., Incontinence and Self-care deficit).

Critical Thinking

Assessment of infants, children, and adolescents requires special attention to developmental stages and associated behaviors. The nurse is often required to create approaches to optimize the process of data collection.

Learning Exercises

1. Identify and discuss the primary similarities in assessing children and adults.

2. Explain how you would assess sexual and reproductive functions in a sexually active 13-year-old girl. Create a script of the first few sentences you might say in this situation.

3. How would your response differ if the girl in item 2 was 17 years old? How would your response differ if the individual was male and not female?

4. You are conducting a well-baby examination of a 16-month-old. He is crying and clings to his mother when you approach him. Describe how you would respond.

BIBLIOGRAPHY

Ashwill, J., & Droske, S. (1997). *Nursing care of children: Principles and practice.* Philadelphia: Saunders.

Ballard, J., et al. (1991). New Ballard score: Expanded to include extremely premature infants. *Journal Pediatrics, 119,* 417.

Bayley, N. (1993). *Bayley scales of infant development: Manual* (2nd ed.). San Antonio, TX: The Psychological Corporation.

Bishop, B. (1976). A guide to assessing parenting capabilities. *American Journal of Nursing, 76*(11), 1784–1787.

Brazelton, P. (1973). *The neonatal behavioral assessment scale.* Philadelphia: Lippincott.

Burns, C. (1996). *Pediatric primary care: A handbook for nurse practitioners.* Philadelphia: Saunders.

Carpenito, L. (1992). *Nursing diagnosis: Application to clinical practice* (4th ed.). Philadelphia: Lippincott.

Carpenito, L. (1997). *Handbook of nursing diagnosis* (7th ed.). Philadelphia: Lippincott.

Clark, A.C. (1976). Recognizing discord between mother and child and changing it to harmony. *American Journal of Maternal-Child Nursing, 1*(2), 94–99.

Edelman, C., & Mandle, C. (1997). *Health promotion throughout the lifespan* (4th ed.). St. Louis: Mosby.

Erikson, E. (1963). *Childhood and society* (2nd ed.). New York: W.W. Norton.

Fowler, J. (1974). Toward a developmental perspective on faith. *Religious Education, 69,* 207–219.

Frankenburg, W., Dodds, J., Archer, P., Bresnick, B., Maschka, P., Edelman, N., & Shapiro, H. (1990). *Denver II: Screening manual.* Denver, CO: Denver Developmental Materials.

Hay, W., Grothuis, J., Hayward, A., & Levin, M. (1997). *Current pediatric diagnosis & treatment* (13th ed.). Stamford, CT: Appleton & Lange.

Kohlberg, L. (1981). *The philosophy of moral development: Moral stages and the idea of justice.* New York: Harper & Row.

Murray, R. & Zentner, J. (1997). *Health assessment and promotion strategies through the life span* (6th ed.). Stamford, CT: Appleton & Lange.

Peter, G. (Ed.). *1997 red book: Report of the Committee on Infectious Diseases* (24th ed.). Elk Grove Village, IL: American Academy of Pediatrics.

Piaget, J. (1969). *The theory of stages in cognitive development.* New York: Basic Books.

US Preventive Services Task Force. (1996). *Guide to clinical preventive services* (2nd ed.). Baltimore: Williams & Wilkins.

Wong, D. (1995). *Whaley and Wong's nursing care of infants and children* (5th ed.). St. Louis: Mosby.

ASSESSMENT GUIDELINES

Elder Interview (Health History)

Physical Examination

CHAPTER ORGANIZATION

Introductory Overview
- Assessment Focus
- Nursing Diagnoses

Knowledge Base for Assessment
- Difference Between Normal Aging and Pathology

- Difference Between Normal Aging and a Medication Side Effect
- Variability of Physical Aging
- Illness in Elderly Persons

INTRODUCTORY OVERVIEW

In the United States, the fastest-growing age group consists of those individuals older than 85 years. Over 33% of all health care dollars goes to provide care to individuals older than 65 years. Most individuals older than 65 years are active and healthy. At any given time, only 5% of elders are in nursing homes. With the older person, it becomes important for the nurse to distinguish between normal aging changes and signs of threats to health and functional ability. Contrary to common beliefs, disease is not a normal part of the aging process. Health-promoting activities have relevance to the elderly population, and elders receive benefit from health activities as do younger individuals. Individuals are not too old to stop unhealthy habits and learn new ones (Kolcabar & Wykle, 1994). Common chronic health problems in elders include arthritis, hypertension, heart disease, diabetes, orthopedic impairments, sinusitis, and visual impairments (such as cataracts) (Edelman & Mandel, 1998). Many of these conditions and their complications are preventable with lifestyle changes.

In many respects, the approach to assessing older persons is similar to that for observing and interviewing younger adults. Information obtained from the health history and physical examination is analyzed to evaluate functional status and to identify and monitor physical problems regardless of the person's age. Some procedures and techniques may need to be modified when the client is older, especially if the person is less mobile or has some limited sensory or cognitive capacities. In addition, the assessment data should be interpreted in light of functional abilities and physical changes relative to the normal aging process.

ASSESSMENT FOCUS

Judgments about health status and the ability to perform activities of daily living are based on a comprehensive assessment of an elderly individual. The individual's perceptions and misconceptions about aging and health greatly influence the functional capability and seeking of health care when needed.

Evaluations regarding health status are based on interview data, observations, and physical examination of the individual. In the very old or in those elders with compromising health conditions such as obstructive lung disease, the emphasis on health assessment may turn toward the physical ability to perform activities of daily living (ADLs, such as dressing, bathing, feeding, and toileting) and instrumental activities of daily living (IADLs, such as shopping, house cleaning, yard maintenance, and meal preparation).

The goals for assessing elders include the following:

- Obtaining perception about health status
- Assessing health status
- Identifying normal changes of aging
- Distinguishing between normal aging and health problems
- Assessing ability to perform ADLs and IADLS
- Assessing medication-taking habits

Nursing Diagnoses

No specific nursing diagnoses relate only to elders. Some nursing diagnoses do not relate to elders because of the normal aging process; these include Altered growth and development and Effective and Ineffective breast-feeding. Although we often think of elders as not having parenting responsibilities, more elders are continuing to provide care to adult children, dependent adult children (such as those with developmental disabilities and post–brain-trauma victims), and grandchildren (as either secondary or primary caregivers). Elders who obtain guardianship of grandchildren may experience intergenerational altered family process.

Elders, especially the very old (85 years and older), are at high risk for nursing diagnoses that relate to physical mobility impairment, self-care deficits, altered home management, altered health maintenance, incontinence, social isolation, and grief. Elders are also at risk for poisoning related to side effects of the numerous drugs they ingest. Next to very young children, elders are the highest-risk group for fire trauma and death. An elder with an acute illness is at great risk for complications such as pneumonia, which can be life-threatening.

With the very old, it is not difficult to identify possible nursing diagnoses. The difficulty is in applying critical decision-making processes to select those nursing diagnoses that are primary and those that are secondary.

KNOWLEDGE BASE
FOR ASSESSMENT

Difference Between Normal Aging and Pathology

Although the rate of decline may vary, irreversible physical decline is an inevitable consequence of aging. Most gerontologists agree that humans begin to experience universal and progressive decline in physiologic capacities from the third decade until death. For example, longitudinal studies of aging populations provide evidence for the following age-related changes in the pulmonary system: increased residual lung volumes, decreased alveolar surface available for gas exchange, and decreased diffusion capacity across the alveolar capillary membrane. Although these physiologic changes are considered normal in the aging person, they also may be associated with disease states. For example, long-term exposure to environmental pollutants or tobacco smoke may cause similar lung changes, in which case the lung tissue should be considered diseased rather than aged.

Tissue injury or alteration may be caused by organisms or by immunologic, chemical, or physical factors. For example, lung tissue may be irreversibly altered by the chemical and physical effects of tobacco smoke. Conversely, tissue alteration may have a genetic basis in that a key substance has been affected or omitted, such as occurs in panlobular emphysema, in which a hereditary deficiency of the protein alpha-1-antitrypsin occurs. Finally, tissue alteration may be caused by intrinsic degenerative processes occurring as spontaneous biological and chemical reactions that are thermodynamically controlled. If a degenerative change occurs in all members of a population, despite diet, lifestyle, or genetic makeup, the change should be regarded as an aging process. Such distinctions provide the key for distinguishing pathology from normal aging.

Occasionally, an age-related physiologic change cannot be distinguished from pathologic or lifestyle factors because one process may be superimposed on another. For example, cardiovascular function declines with age, yet age-related changes may be difficult to distinguish from cardiovascular deconditioning associated with a sedentary lifestyle. Often the difficulty may be that some findings are associated with disease in younger age groups but attributed to normal aging in the elderly.

Although aging processes should not be confused with disease processes, some physiologic aging processes, although not in themselves significant, may increase the older person's vulnerability during illness. For example, age-related declines in the pulmonary system are not causative factors for pneumonia, but pneumonia can be a more threatening illness for an older person because of age-related alterations.

Difference Between Normal Aging and a Medication Side Effect

There are few elders (even those 90 and older) who take no medication of any type, prescription or over-the-counter. Health care providers prescribe drugs to elders more than to any other age-group. Drugs commonly used by elders tend to have a narrow therapeutic range, with more side effects than drugs used for other age groups. Additionally, normal changes of aging in the kidneys, liver, gastrointestinal tract, and body fluid composition can result in toxic drug effects even if the prescribed dose is in the correct dose range. The effect of each drug separately may have been studied and is known; however, many elders experience polypharmacy (taking numerous drugs). Many elders take four prescription drugs a day (sometimes several doses of the drug are taken per day). The greater the number of medications taken by an elderly person, the greater the risk for unintended drug interactions and the greater the possibility that not all will be taken as prescribed. Reasons for not taking medications as prescribed include cost, side effects, complicated regimen (taking more than once a day), difficulty opening containers, inability to read labels, and forgetfulness.

Occasionally, the nurse may overlook a medication effect when assessing an elderly person because adverse drug effects often mimic changes erroneously associated with aging, such as hearing loss, visual blurring, altered thought processes, muscle rigidity, and tremors. Whenever behavior or cognition changes, the health care provider should obtain a detailed drug history that includes prescribed, borrowed, and over-the-counter drugs; administration schedule; and reasons for altering recommended schedules. Furthermore, it is important to realize that some common drug side effects, such as altered thought processes, are not normal age-related changes and require further evaluation. Computer programs are available to assist in analyzing medications taken by elders to identify risks and undesired interactions.

Variability of Physical Aging

Even in the absence of pathologic conditions or medication effects, physical changes associated with aging may be difficult to describe. Generally, more physical variability occurs in older persons than among younger ones. The aging process occurs at different rates and, in some cases, is modified. For example, skin wrinkling, an inevitable consequence of aging, can be affected by genetic tendencies, sun exposure, or cosmetic surgery. Chronology alone cannot be used to predict all age-related changes.

Variability exists between different age groups as well as among the same age groups. For example, many growth and development theorists classify all persons older than age 65 years as elderly or older adults, yet a 65-year-old person may differ greatly in physical appearance and abilities from a 90-year-old. There also may be no differences in the health and functional status of a 65-year-old person and a 90-year-old person.

Illness in Elderly Persons

Altered Presentations

Physical signs and symptoms of illness may differ between younger and older age groups. Because the older

TABLE 17.1   Altered Presentations in the Elderly

Problem	Classic Presentation in Young Patient	Presentation in Elders
Urinary tract infection	Dysuria, frequency, urgency, nocturia	Dysuria often absent; frequency, urgency, nocturia sometimes present. Incontinence, confusion, anorexia are other signs
Myocardial infarction	Severe substernal chest pain, diaphoresis, nausea, shortness of breath	Sometimes no chest pain, or atypical pain location such as in jaw, neck, shoulder. Shortness of breath may be present. Other signs are tachypnea, arrhythmia, hypotension, restlessness, syncope
Pneumonia (bacterial)	Cough productive of purulent sputum, chills and fever, pleuritic chest pain, elevated white blood count	Cough may be productive, dry, or absent; chills and fever, and elevated white count also may be absent. Tachypnea, slight cyanosis, confusion, anorexia, nausea and vomiting, tachycardia may be present.
Congestive heart failure	Increased dyspnea (orthopnea, paroxysmal nocturnal dyspnea), fatigue, weight gain, pedal edema, night cough and nocturia, bibasilar rates	All of the manifestations of young adult or anorexia, restlessness, confusion, cyanosis, falls
Hyperthyroidism	Heat intolerance, fast pace, exophthalmos, increased pulse, hyperreflexia, tremor	Slowing down (apathetic hyperthyroidism), lethargy, weakness, depression, atrial fibrillation, and congestive heart failure
Depression	Sad mood and thoughts, withdrawal, crying, weight loss, constipation, insomnia	Any classic signs, plus memory and concentration problems, weight gain, increased sleep

(Henderson, M. L. [1985]. Assessing the elderly (part II): Altered presentations. *American Journal of Nursing, 85*[10], 1103–1106)

person's signs and symptoms tend to deviate from the usual, diagnosis of some conditions may be more difficult. For example, ischemic-quality chest pain is one of the hallmarks of myocardial infarction. Elderly persons do not always experience this type of chest pain during myocardial infarction, the location of the pain is atypical, and they may report pain as abdominal instead of precordial. For some elderly persons experiencing acute myocardial infarction, dyspnea or nausea may be the only symptom.

Conversely, the older person may have symptoms typically associated with a pathologic process yet without associated pathology. For example, the older person may experience voiding frequency, nocturia, and urgency, which are classic symptoms of urinary tract infection. The person may be free of infection, however, and such symptoms may represent structural alterations of the genitourinary system. Confusion and incontinence may be the only indications of urinary tract infection in elderly persons. Table 17-1 shows additional variations in pathologic presentations in older persons.

Elderly individuals usually have multiple health problems. Exploring symptoms of one health problem may lead to another. For example, an elderly woman is slightly confused and dehydrated. On hydration the confusion clears, and it is discovered that dehydration is intentional in her efforts to control incontinence. Additionally, one health problem may hide another. For example, a person aphasic after a stroke may not be able to tell anyone about intermittent chest pain.

Physical Examination   Elder Assessment

GENERAL PRINCIPLES

Always address the person as "Mr." or "Mrs." unless requested otherwise.

Keep the person warm. The older person may feel cold more readily.

Vary positions if mobility is impaired to reduce fatigue.

Guard against fatiguing the person. If performing a complete assessment, the nurse may wish to perform segments at different appointments or times. Allowing the individual to provide a health history over 1 to 2 days and completing the comprehensive physical examination at two or more different times reduces fatigue and allows the individual to remember past events.

Ask questions slowly and face the elder (this assists with lip reading). Try to eliminate extraneous noise.

(continued)

Physical Examination   Elder Assessment (continued)

Allow the person time to answer; questions may necessitate him or her to think back 40 to 60 years.

If the person responds to a question inappropriately, perhaps he or she did not hear or understand. Conversely, the person may not understand a question but answer anyway. Rephrase questions when in doubt.

Adjust the sequence of history and examination to focus on the most relevant problems first.

Do not rush the person because this may contribute to feelings of fatigue and frustration and could alter normal findings.

A spouse or other significant person accompanying the elder may indicate a hearing or cognitive impairment.

The elderly individual may need assistance with undressing and getting up and down from an examination table.

COMPREHENSIVE ELDER ASSESSMENT INCLUDES

Interview (health history)
Diagnostic tests
Functional assessment
Physical assessment

EQUIPMENT

The nurse uses the same equipment to assess elders as a younger adult.

ASSESSMENT AIDS

Interview guidelines for all functional patterns
Functional assessment tools
Age-specific height and weight charts
Computer software for medication analysis

▼ ▼ ▼

G U I D E L I N E S

Assessment Guidelines   Elder Interview (Health History)

Procedure

For interviewing elders, the following items should be added to the pattern interview guides presented in earlier chapters.

1. **Health perception and health management**
   a. Immunization status: pneumonia, influenza, and tetanus

   b. Perception of health

   c. Safety practices:
   Use of smoke and carbon monoxide detectors

   Medications: what are they, what are they for, how taken, and storage

   d. Screening activities: what self-screening activities are performed and frequency of professional screening.

Clinical Significance

These additional items will enhance the nurse's assessment of an elderly person.

- Pneumonia and complications of influenza are leading killers of elderly individuals. Many cases of tetanus occur among elders with decubitus ulcers.
- The elderly individual will often focus on functional abilities rather than health problems. The person may not perceive the seriousness of certain health problems as long as activities of daily living are not disrupted.

- After children, elders experience the most trauma and death from fires.
- Polypharmacy is a major concern with elders because of untoward interactions. Many elders do not know what medication they are taking and why it was prescribed. Some elders cannot open childproof containers. Waivers can be signed at pharmacy to get non-childproof caps. However, they need to be stored out of children's reach.
- Refer to Display 17–1 regarding recommended screenings for elders.

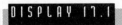

DISPLAY 17.1

Screening Recommendations for Elders

SCREENING

Blood pressure: every 1–2 years
Height and weight: annually
Fecal occult blood: annually or sigmoidoscopy: every
    3–5 years
Mammogram: every 1–2 years until age 70
Papanicolaou: if past negative until age 65
Vision screening: every 1–2 years
Hearing: every 1–2 years
Problem alcohol use: yearly
Skin cancer (those at risk): yearly

COUNSELING

Tobacco cessation
Alcohol use safety (avoiding while driving)
Fat and cholesterol intake
Balanced diet
Calcium intake (especially women)
Regular exercise

Fall prevention
Car restraint use
Smoke detectors
Hot water heater setting
CPR training for household members
Regular dental care
Avoidance of high-risk sexual behavior

IMMUNIZATIONS

Pneumococcal vaccine (booster possible every
    5 years, if at risk)
Influenza: yearly
Tetanus–diptheria booster: every 10 years
Hepatitis (only those at high risk)

CHEMOPROPHYLAXIS

Hormone replacement therapy (estrogen), post-
    menopausal women

Adapted from US Preventive Services Task Force. (1996). *Guide to clinical preventive services* (2nd ed.). Baltimore, MD: Williams & Wilkins.

▼ ▼ ▼

G U I D E L I N E S   *continued*   Elder Interview (Health History)

Procedure	Clinical Significance
2. Nutrition and metabolism	
a. Recent weight gain or loss	• Unintentional weight loss may indicate ill-fitting dentures, loss of appetite, inability to purchase or prepare meals, or health problems such as diabetes. Weight gain may be related to a reduced need for calories.
b. Complete Nutrition Screening of Elders form (see Chap. 6)	• This screening interview provides information regarding nutritional status and potential risk.
c. High- and moderate-risk diagnoses and medications (see Chap. 6)	• With advancing age, the individual is at greater risk for these health problems and medications to affect nutritional status.
3. Elimination	
a. Inquire into problems with incontinence.	• Due to weakness of pelvic floor and bladder muscles, stress and urge incontinence increase with age. Kegel's exercise remains useful, especially for stress incontinence.
b. Patterns of voiding	• Patterns may change related to reduced elasticity and size of bladder.
b. Inquire into problems with constipation.	• A frequent problem but usually related to reduced dietary fiber and fluid intake, increased inactivity, and use of constipating drugs.

▼ ▼ ▼

GUIDELINES *continued*   Elder Interview (Health History)

Procedure

4. Activity and exercise
   a. Inquire into functional ability to
   • Do household tasks
   • Prepare meals
   • Go shopping for food, etc.
   • Bathe
   • Get to toilet
   • Dress
   • Get in and out of chairs
   • Do yard work and house maintenance
   • Walk
   • Do desired activities
   • Drive a car
   See Display 17–2 for Functional Assessment Tool.
   b. Inquire into the frequency of falls.

Clinical Significance

• Activity and exercise is an important pattern for elders—functional abilities to manage ADLs and IADLs are dependent on mobility and cognition. Adaptive tools can assist elders in maintaining functional abilities (Fig. 17–1)
• Numerous health problems can interfere with an elderly individual's normal activities; these include arthritis, joint replacements, decreased lung capacity (COPD), cardiovascular problems, osteoporosis, and stroke. Inability to drive reduces independence, mobility, and ability to purchase needed items.

• Falls are the greatest cause of injury in those older than 70 years—fractures can result in immobility and even death.
• A more in-depth functional ability screening may be indicated if a problem is noted.

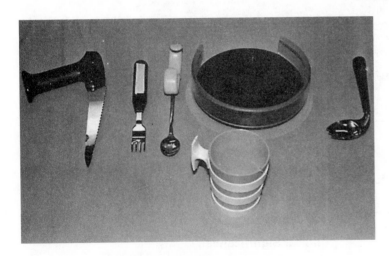

FIGURE 17.1 Adaptive eating utensils can help the older adult with a functional limitation to eat independently and maintain a healthy diet.

5. Cognition and perception
   a. Inquire into recent vision difficulty and last vision examination and use of corrective lenses.
   c. Inquire into hearing difficulty and whether hearing has been assessed and use of hearing aids.
   d. Inquire into recent sensory changes.

   e. Inquire into memory impairments.

   f. Inquire into ability to manage finances and pay bills.
   g. Inquire into ability to take medications correctly.

• At about age 40, near visual acuity is reduced related to decrease in accommodation (presbyopia).
• About age 40, hearing loss of high-frequency sounds begins (presbycusis); especially f/s/th/ch/sh sounds.
• With age, all senses decrease in sensitivity, including temperature, pain, smell, and taste.
• Many elders fear memory loss and Alzheimer's disease. This provides the opportunity to discuss fears and real concerns.
• The ability to manage finances and medications is a good indicator of cognitive abiiity and judgment and is important to functional ability.

DISPLAY 17.2

Functional Assessment: ADLs and IADLs

Use the following score for each activity:
1 = No help needed   3 = Some help needed
2 = Slight amount of help needed   4 = A lot of help needed
            5 = Completely dependent on others

ACTIVITIES OF DAILY LIVING

1. Able to dress (selecting, getting from closet/drawer, putting on clothes) _____
2. Able to go to toilet (getting to toilet, getting off and on, hygiene) _____
3. Able to control bladder and bowels_____
4. Able to bathe (getting into and out of shower/tub, washing) _____
5. Able to wash hair _____
6. Able to brush and comb hair _____
7. Able to do oral care (brush teeth, denture care) _____
8. Able to feed self _____
9. Able to transfer in and out of bed and in and out of chair by self_____
10. Able to walk by self or propel wheelchair 50 yards _____

INSTRUMENTAL ACTIVITIES OF DAILY LIVING

11. Able to use telephone _____
12. Able to shop for groceries_____
13. Able to prepare meals _____
14. Able to do own housework _____
15. Able to do minor home maintenance _____
16. Able to do own laundry_____
17. Able to manage finances, write checks _____
18. Able to handle personal business (will, taxes, etc.)__
    _____
19. Able to take own medications safely _____
20. Able to travel out of neighborhood _____
21. Able to make and keep appointments_____

Modified from Katz et al. (1963). Studies of illness in the aged: The Index of ADL: A standardized measure of biological and psychosocial function. *JAMA, 185,* 914–919; Lawton, M, & Brody, E. (1969). Assessment of older people: Self-maintaining and instrumental activities of daily living. *Gerontologist, 9*(3), 179–186; Mahoney, F., & Barthel, D. (1965). Functional evaluation: The Barthel index. *Maryland State Medical Journal, 14,* 62–68.

▼ ▼ ▼

 GUIDELINES   *continued*

Elder Interview (Health History)

Procedure

6. Sleep and rest
   a. Inquire into number of hours of sleep per night and number of awakenings per night.

   b. Number of naps per day

7. Self-concept
   Inquire into the individual's perception of self and potential threats.

8. Roles and relationships
   a. Inquire into adjustment to retirement.

Clinical Significance

• The amount of sleep needed per night might decrease (6–9 hours). Reduction in stage IV sleep declines with age, so elders may not feel rested. Nighttime awakening frequently occurs.
• Napping is frequent with elders and may interfere with night sleep if excessive (Floyd, 1996).

• Self-concept remains fairly stable throughout adulthood, although health problems such as a stroke or the loss of independence (can no longer drive a car) are threats to self-concept.

• Retirement is a big adjustment in the roles and relationships of an elderly person.

Procedure

b. Inquire into new roles or loss of roles and adjustment to these changes.

Clinical Significance

• The loss of roles through death or other situations can contribute to depression. New roles such as grandparenting can bring enjoyment (Fig. 17–2). However, a growing number of grandparents are primary care providers of grandchildren.

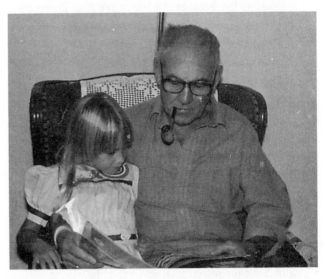

FIGURE 17.2 Grandparenting is a role nearly everyone enjoys.

c. Inquire into relationships with children and spouse.

• Elder abuse is a growing problem. Poor relationships with family members increase the risk of abuse/mistreatment.

9. Sexuality and reproductive function

a. Inquire into satisfaction with sexuality.

• Although reproductive ability decreases for both genders, sexuality and sexual satisfaction continue into old age. Each phase of the sexual response cycle may be prolonged.

b. Inquire into menopause and estrogen replacement therapy with women.

• Estrogen replacement therapy with or without progestin (should be used if uterus is present to reduce risk of uterine cancer) is beneficial in treating menopausal symptoms and may provide protection against cardiovascular disease, osteoporosis, and Alzheimer's disease.

▼ ▼ ▼

Procedure

10. Stress and stress responses
The interview guide in Chapter 14 is sufficient for interviewing elderly individuals.

11. Values and beliefs
Inquire into the presence of advance directives (living will) and desire for life support.

Diagnostic/Screening Studies

Procedure

No special diagnostic/screening tests are limited to elders. However, some diagnostic studies are more frequently used with elders.

See Display 17–2 for screening recommendations for people aged 65 years and older.

Functional Assessment Tools commonly used with elders include the following:

- Katz Index and Barthel Index

- Lawton Scale for instrumental activities of daily living
- Mini-Mental State Examination

- Geriatric Depression Scale

Clinical Significance

When using the Holmes and Rahe's Social adjustment scale, many elders have scores of 200 and above.

Values and beliefs evolve throughout life and are fairly stable in old age. Although many elders know what they want and what they don't want at the end of their life, these wishes frequently are not documented.

Clinical Significance

Laboratory values for some diagnostic test change with age (*i.e.,* erythrocyte sedimentation rate increases). However, most tests vary more because of gender than age when adulthood is achieved.

- Both of these measure activity of daily living independence. The Katz has 6 items and the Barthel 10 items.
- Nine-item instrument measuring IADLs
- Assesses cognitive status (orientation, attention, recall, and language); frequently used to screen for dementia
- A 15-item scale to identify risk for depression.

▼ ▼ ▼
GUIDELINES

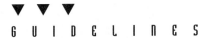

Assessment Guidelines   Physical Examination

Procedure

If an examination table is to be used, a step stool may be needed. Special geriatric examination tables are available that can be lowered closer to the floor and then raised as needed. When the person is on the examination table, ensure that he or she has adequate support. The elder may be more comfortable in a Fowler or semi-Fowler position.

1. Health perception and health management
   a. General appearance

   b. Observation of self-examination skills

2. Nutrition and metabolism
   a. Height and weight—Use weight chart for elders (see Displays 17-3 and 17-4)
   b. Midarm circumference, skinfold measurements

Clinical Significance

Many assessment findings for elders are the same as for younger adults presented in earlier chapters. Only those deviations from adult findings related to normal aging are presented here. Refer to previous chapters.

- Dress, grooming, hygiene, and lucidity of conversation can provide cues to the individual's ability to manage health care.
- Because of arthritis or other health problems, the individual may need assistance in modifying self-assessment skills.

- The individual may "shrink" 2–3 inches with age. Any weight change should be gradual.
- Adipose tissue decreases with age; therefore, these measurements decrease.

DISPLAY 17.3

Age- and Gender-Specific Values for Weight in Pounds (Kilograms)

AGE [YEARS]	PERCENTILE 5TH	50TH	95TH
Men			
65	138.0 (62.6)	175.0 (79.5)	224.9 (102.0)
70	131.6 (59.7)	168.7 (76.5)	218.5 (99.1)
75	125.2 (56.8)	162.3 (73.6)	212.3 (96.3)
80	118.8 (53.9)	155.9 (70.7)	205.9 (93.4)
85	112.4 (51.0)	149.5 (67.8)	199.5 (90.5)
90	106.0 (48.1)	143.1 (64.9)	193.1 (87.6)
Women			
65	112.9 (51.2)	147.3 (66.8)	192.0 (87.1)
70	108.0 (49.0)	142.4 (64.6)	187.2 (84.9)
75	103.2 (46.8)	137.6 (62.4)	182.5 (82.8)
80	98.5 (44.7)	132.7 (60.2)	177.7 (80.6)
85	93.7 (42.5)	127.9 (58.0)	172.8 (78.4)
90	88.8 (40.3)	123.2 (55.9)	168.0 (76.2)

From Chumlea, W., Roche, A., & Mukherjee, D. (1991). *Nutritional assessment of the elderly through anthropometry.* Columbus, OH: Ross Products Division, Abbott Laboratories.

DISPLAY 17.4

Average Weights for Height for Elderly Men and Women (estimated values)

HEIGHT [INCHES]	WEIGHT IN POUNDS					
	55—64 Y	65—74 Y	75—79 Y	80—84 Y	85—89 Y	90—94 Y
Men						
62	148	144	133	135	*	*
63	151	148	138	136	133	*
64	155	151	143	138	135	*
65	158	154	148	141	139	130
66	162	158	154	144	142	133
67	166	161	159	147	145	136
68	169	165	164	150	148	140
69	173	168	169	154	152	144
70	176	171	174	159	156	149
71	180	175	179	164	160	154
72	184	178	184	170	165	*
Women						
59	144	138	132	118	113	*
60	149	142	136	121	116	*
61	150	145	139	124	120	119
62	152	149	143	128	124	119
63	155	152	146	132	128	120
64	158	156	150	136	133	124
65	161	159	153	140	138	129
66	164	163	157	144	142	*
67	167	166	160	*	*	*
68	170	170	164	*	*	*

*Average weight not available.

Carnevali, D., & Patrick, M. (1979) *Nursing management for the elderly.* Philadelphia: Lippincott.

▼ ▼ ▼

 G U I D E L I N E S   *continued*   Physical Examination

Procedure

c. Skin: moisture
   Turgor
   Thickness
   Lesions

Clinical Significance

- Skin normally becomes drier (flaking may be common on limbs); turgor decreases as a result of reduced elasticity.
- Skin thins and may appear transparent—prone to skin tears.
- The following are common nonmalignant lesions of elders:
  Acrochordons (skin tags)—often appear on neck and chest.
  Sebaceous hyperplasia—yellowish papule with a central depression
  Sebaceous keratoses—raised, warty, pigmented (brown) lesions usually on trunk, face, and hands
  Senile lentigines (age spots)—brown macules found on areas with frequent sun exposure
  Cherry angiomas—small bright red lesion, may be raised, numbers increase after 40, usually on trunk

▼ ▼ ▼

G U I D E L I N E S *continued*   Physical Examination

Procedure

   d. Hair

   e. Nails

   f. Jaw and oral cavity

   g. Abdomen

   h. Thyroid and lymphatic system

3. Elimination
   a. Anus and rectum
      Sims' position may be the easiest position for this examination.

   b. Bowel sounds

   c. Urine

   d. Urinary bladder

Clinical Significance

- Hypopigmentation (gray) of hair, decrease in body and head hair; women may develop facial hair, men may develop coarse nasal, ear, and eyebrow hair.

- Increased brittleness, toenails may thicken, malformations increase, may turn yellowish.

- Temporomandibular joint may dislocate when mouth is open wide because of loss of ligament elasticity.

  Lips may wrinkle—elastin degeneration in the dermis and loss of the vermilion border may result in a pursed-lip appearance.

  Tongue—may become more fissured and dry, and papillae on lateral surface atrophy. Taste buds for salt and sweet decrease; those for bitter and sour remain constant. Ventral surface may have varicosities.

  Gums and teeth—Gums recede, and tooth roots are exposed; teeth may turn yellow. The newly exposed areas are at high risk for dental caries. Tooth loss is preventable although common due to gingivitis and bone reabsorption of jaw, making teeth loose.

  Oral mucosa may appear thin and paler than in younger adults. Dryness may be related to reduced salivation.

- All findings are similar to those for younger adults. Abdomen becomes rounder because of subcutaneous fat redistribution from extremities and face. Liver may extend below costal margin; this represents displacement secondary to increased lung distention and diaphragmatic flattening.

- Findings similar to those in younger adults

- Findings should be the same as with younger adults. The internal and external sphincter loses tone; rectal wall thins. Constipation and bowel incontinence are frequent problems but not normal.

- Peristalsis decreases with age; therefore, bowel sounds and quality also decrease.

- Specific gravity decreases related to reduced ability to concentrate urine.

- Difficult to palpate because of decreased size and reduced capacity. Incontinence common, especially in women, but not normal. Incontinence is a frequent cause of falls in the rush to get to the toilet. Urge incontinence (little warning before urge to void immediately) is more common than stress incontinence (associated with increased abdominal pressure) in elderly women.

▼ ▼ ▼

Procedure

4. Activity and exercise
   a. Heart—cardiovascular system

   b. Blood pressure—assess lying, sitting, and standing

   b. Respiratory system
      (1) Nose and sinuses

      (2) Lungs

   c. Bones, joints, and muscles

Clinical Significance

- Visible pulsation may be present above right clavicle, especially in women. The aorta elongates with age, and pulsation reflects blood movement in innominate artery, which moves up into the chest. Full jugular veins should disappear when supine. The heart sounds S1 and S2 may be less intense; S4 may be heard as ventricle becomes less compliant. Heart rate returns to resting state more slowly. Pulses may be more readily felt. Point of maximal impulse may be lateral to the midclavicular line; this is secondary to shoulder narrowing, kyphosis, and downward displacement of the heart. Amplitude may decrease as chest becomes more rigid. Systolic murmurs may be associated with calcification, fibrosis, and lipid accumulation on aortic or mitral valves, resulting in valve rigidity and incomplete closure. Diastolic murmurs are always abnormal in elders.
- Related to increased stiffness of aorta, blood pressure rises. Maximum 160/90 with no symptoms may be within normal limits. Orthostatic hypotension also increases with age and places elders at risk for falls; blood pressure should not drop more than 20 mm Hg with position change.
- Nose elongates due to cartilage formation. Membranes may appear dry. Greater difficulty distinguishing odors. Other findings are the same as in younger adults.
- Percussion of the lungs reveals more hyperresonance, which is secondary to increased residual lung volumes. Other findings should be similar to those in younger adults. Cough efficiency is reduced.
- Although the following are common, they may not be the result of normal aging. Anteroposterior chest diameter increases because of kyphosis, atrophy of respiratory muscles, and increased residual lung volumes. The transverse–thoracic diameter is decreased secondary to costal cartilage calcification. Chest expansion decreases with aging secondary to costal cartilage calcification, kyphosis, and atrophy of respiratory muscles. Breath sounds are diminished in intensity secondary to decreased ventilatory air flow.
- Muscle strength may decrease but should be bilaterally equal. Lumbar spine tends to flatten, causing the upper spine and head to tilt forward.

  Common but *not normal* findings include the following: Range of motion in some joints may be restricted owing to arthritis and similar disorders. Kyphosis occurs as a result of degenerative changes to disks. Gait may become smaller and speed slower. Elders are at risk for fractures (spine, wrist, and hip) related to bone reabsorption (osteoporosis).

▼ ▼ ▼

G U I D E L I N E S *continued*   Physical Examination

Procedure	Clinical Significance

Procedure

5. Cognition and perception

  a. Eyes and vision, ophthalmoscope—set diopter on 10–12

  b. Ears and Hearing
    Important to do Rinne and Weber tests to identify hearing loss and type

  c. Nervous system

  d. Cognitive function

6. Sleep and rest
  a. Sleep

7. Self-concept
  a. Self-concept

Clinical Significance

Assessment findings for cognition and perception are the same as for younger adults, except for:
- Loss of fat tissue causes eyes to appear sunken; lids may droop, resulting in inversion (entropion) or eversion (ectropion). Pupil diameter decreases and reaction slows. Increased sensitivity to glare. Owing to decreased tearing, eyes may be dry. There may be a lipid accumulation (*arcus senilis*) that causes a white–gray circle around cornea. Cornea may cloud with advanced age.

  Visual acuity: Visual acuity for far vision increases, and for near vision decreases. Ability to distinguish pastel colors, adapt to a dark or bright room, and accommodate to near objects (presbyopia) decreases, as does peripheral vision.

  Inner eye: Very little change is associated with normal aging; blood vessels may be minimally narrowed. The fundus may appear more yellow. Common but *not normal* changes: presence of cataracts, macular degeneration (lack of central vision), elevated eye pressure or cupping of optic disk (glaucoma), nicking of blood vessels.

- Outer ear elongates due to cartilage formation. Tympanic membrane may be whiter and thicker. Gradual and progressive hearing loss for 2–10 years. Difficulty is with understanding speech, not a reduction in hearing (presbycusis); caused by atrophy of organ of Corti. Cerumen is dryer.

- Except for the following, findings should be similar to those in younger adults.
  Muscle strength and agility may decrease. Deep tendon reflexes may be difficult to elicit, ankle jerks may be absent, vibratory sensation decreases.

- Findings should be similar to those in younger adults. Neurologic or systemic problems such as an infection or medication toxicity are the only reasons for abrupt loss of general intelligence (delirium). Short-term memory may decrease with age, but this is not associated with dementias. Depression is also a common but not a normal problem. Substantive memory loss and decline of cognitive function, as seen in Alzheimer's disease, are not a normal part of aging.

Findings should be similar to those in younger adults. Sleep may be more restless; there is less stage III and IV sleep and more night awakenings.

Findings should be similar to those in younger adults.

▼ ▼ ▼

GUIDELINES *continued*   Physical Examination

Procedure	Clinical Significance
8. Roles and relationships	Roles and relationships should be similar to those of younger adults.
a. Signs of abuse	• Elder abuse is an increasing problem. Signs of abuse include prolonged interval between trauma/illness and medical care; medication over or underuse, oversedation, poor nutritional status, dehydration, unexplained burns and abrasions, contusions and lacerations, bruises and hematomas, dislocation, fractures, decubiti, dehydration, and depression (Fulmer & O'Malley, 1987).
b. Signs of caregiver stress	• Many elders, especially women, suffer from caregiver stress. Signs of stress include fatigue, depression, decline in own health, insufficient time for IADLs and for self, anger, and social isolation.
9. Sexuality and reproductive function	
a. Female: the older woman may not be able to comfortably assume the lithotomy position and use the stirrups because of musculoskeletal changes. Modify the lithotomy position by allowing less knee flexion and foregoing the use of stirrups, or use a left lateral Sims' position. Vaginal size may decrease with advancing age, especially in nonparous women, so consider using a smaller vaginal speculum. Because of a decrease in size, the vagina may accommodate only one finger instead of two during bimanual palpation.	• Age-related changes in the external genitals occur secondary to estrogen depletion and include thinning and graying of the pubic hair, flattening and increased wrinkling of the labia majora, and decrease in size of the clitoris. The vagina becomes narrower because of fibrosis and reduced elasticity. The vaginal mucosa appears drier and paler, and rugae are less prominent. These changes are related to decreased secretory activity. The cervix decreases in size, and the os may appear smaller or stenotic. The uterus and ovaries decrease in size. A 50% decline in ovary size occurs by age 60 years, so the ovaries may not be palpable.
b. Male: If the man cannot tolerate the usual position (bending 90 degrees at the waist), examine from the left lateral Sims' position.	• Age-related changes in the appearance of the external genitals are related to depletion of sex hormones. The pubic hairs become thinner and grayer, the size of the penis and testes decreases, the consistency of the testes is less firm, and the scrotal sac becomes pendulous with fewer rugae. The prostate gland begins to enlarge at age 40 and places elderly men at risk for benign prostatic hypertrophy that can interfere with urine flow. The evaluation of hernias is similar in older and younger age groups.
c. Breasts	• In women, breasts become more elongated and flat with age. Granular tissue decreases. Any new lump is more likely to be due to cancer than any other etiology. Other deviations are the same as for younger woman. *Gynecomastia* may occur in men, related to hormone alterations or medication side-effect.
10. Stress and stress response	Stress response is the same in elders; however, elders often have fewer support systems—formal and informal—to assist with times of stress.
11. Values and beliefs	Values and beliefs usually remain stable in adulthood; religious/cultural rituals may become more or less important.

NDx

Documenting Elder Examination

90-Year-Old Woman Living Alone

S: No specific complaints, in excellent health, takes no medications, continues to mow lawn and plant vegetable garden. Friends provide transportation for shopping. Able to do own housework but not as well as a few years ago. Eats only two meals a day and coffee in the morning.

O: Only deviations from normal noted; see flow sheet for normals. Weight loss of 30 pounds in last year, 10 teeth upper and 10 lower, about half in poor repair. Oral mucosa dry. Hemoglobin 12.0 g.

A: Altered nutrition: less than body requirements as evidenced by weight loss. Possible cause: inadequate intake possibly complicated by tooth loss.

P: Return in 1 month to monitor weight. Refer to nutritionist and dentist. Make home visit in 2 weeks to evaluate environment and meal preparation in home.

Clinical Problems Related to Elder Examination

Elders experience numerous clinical problems and tend to have more health problems than any other age group. Few health problems escape elders. Elders can have developmental disabilities. There are numerous elderly individuals with mental retardation, Down syndrome, and cerebral palsy. Elders are susceptible to infectious diseases, including HIV/AIDS and other sexually transmitted diseases. Chronic disease tends to be prevalent in the elderly population. Some of the more life-threatening are cerebrovascular accidents, cancers, myocardial infarctions, and pneumonia and influenza. Neurologic problems that frequently occur in elders include Parkinson's disease, Alzheimer's disease, and cerebrovascular accidents.

The most common causes of death in older men are heart disease, cancers, accidents, cerebrovascular disease, and chronic obstructive pulmonary disease. The most common causes of death in older women are heart disease, cancers, cerebrovascular disease, diabetes, and accidents (USDHHS, 1992).

CHAPTER 17 SUMMARY

The comprehensive and focused assessment of older people is similar to assessments of younger people. Some modifications are required in collection and analysis of data due to physiologic changes related to the aging process. The aging process is highly variable, compounded by functional status and chronic illnesses. Polypharmacy also can contribute to health problems in elders.

A comprehensive assessment of elders includes the following:
- Obtaining information about perceptions of health status
- Assessing actual health status
- Identifying normal changes associated with the aging process
- Distinguishing between normal aging and health problems

- Assessing the ability to perform ADLs and IADLs (functional status)
- Assessing medication safety

Clinical problems suffered by elders are similar to those suffered by younger adults, but signs and symptoms may be altered. Except for three nursing diagnoses (Altered growth and development, Effective breast-feeding, and Ineffective breast-feeding), elders can have any of the human responses that nursing diagnoses are designed to address. All diagnostic test used in the assessment of adults can also be used with elders; however, tools have been developed to screen elders for functional ability, cognitive status, and depression. The challenge to nursing of elders is not to identify nursing diagnoses but to critically select those of primary importance to the well-being of elders.

Critical Thinking Exercise

1. An elderly woman with an elevated temperature and cough comes into the clinic for her first visit. You note that she is using a walker and appears to have arthritis. What would you assess during this visit? Why?

2. When assessing the health perception and health maintenance pattern, you discover that an 80-year-old male client has not had influenza, pneumonia, or tetanus-diphtheria immunizations. What would you tell him about the need for these immunizations and the special risks to elders of these diseases?

3. What would you say to a colleague regarding the need for assessment of the sexuality pattern in elders?

4. Discuss why functional assessment has importance in the comprehensive assessment of elders.

BIBLIOGRAPHY

Edelman, C., & Mandel, C. (1998). *Health promotion throughout the lifespan* (4th ed.). St. Louis: Mosby.

Eliopoulos, C. (1993). *Gerontological nursing* (3rd ed.). Philadelphia: Lippincott.

Floyd, J. (1995). Another look at napping in older adults. *Geriatric Nursing, 16* (3), 136–140.

Folstein, M., Folstein, S., & McHugh, P. (1975). Mini-mental state: A practical method for grading the cognitive state of patients for the clinician. *Journal of Psychiatric Research, 12,* 189–198.

Fulmer, T., & O'Malley, F. (1987). *Inadequate care of the elderly: A health care perspective on abuse and neglect.* New York: Springer.

Katz, S., et al. (1970). The index of independence in activities of daily living, progress in the development of the index of ADL. *Gerontologist, 10,* 23–28.

Kolcabar, K., & Wykle, M. (1994). Health promotion in long-term care facilities. *Geriatric Nursing, 15* (5), 266.

Lawton, M., & Brody, E. (1969). Assessment of older people: Self-maintaining and instrumental activities of daily living. *Gerontologist, 9* (3), 179–186.

Mahoney, F., & Barthel, D. (1965). Functional evaluation: The Barthel index. *Maryland State Medical Journal, 14,* 62–66.

Sheikh, J., & Yesavage, J. Geriatric depression scale (GDS): Recent evidence and development of a shorter version. *Clinical Gerontologist, 5* (1/2) 165–173.

US Department of Health and Human Services. (1992). *Health in the United States 1991 and prevention profile.* Washington, DC: US Government Printing Press.

US Preventive Services Task Force. (1996). *Guide to clinical preventive services* (2nd ed.). Baltimore: Williams & Wilkins.

Assessing in Special Situations

ASSESSMENT GUIDELINES

— Bedside Head-to-Toe Examination

— Chest Tubes

— Nasogastric Tubes

— Enteral Feeding Tubes

— Intravascular Pressure Monitoring

— Oxygen Therapy

— Urinary Catheters and Bladder Irrigation Systems

— Intravenous Therapy

— Cardiac Monitoring

— Pulse Oximetry

— Trauma

— Substance Abuse

— Bladder Retraining

CHAPTER ORGANIZATION

Introductory Overview

- Special Situations and Different Assessment Approaches

Different approaches to health assessment may be used depending on the setting, the condition of the patient, and the clinical situation in which the nurse practices. For example, approaches may differ with respect to the thoroughness of the physical examination. Previous chapters in this book have described detailed and comprehensive approaches to health assessment. Such approaches are important when establishing a broad clinical database. For example, the discussion of the eye examination in Chapter 9 addresses all aspects of the examination, including visual acuity testing, inspection and palpation, and the ophthalmoscopic examination. Similarly, the cardiovascular examination in Chapter 8 presents a detailed approach for evaluating heart sounds and pulses. In some situations, however, such comprehensive approaches are neither warranted nor practical, and a more focused database is sufficient for monitoring the person and for planning appropriate care. For example, a hospitalized patient who had an acute myocardial infarction will require ongoing, thorough evaluations of the cardiovascular and respiratory systems but may not have a need for a comprehensive eye examination. Data from the eye examination may contribute little or nothing to the plan of care for this patient. Furthermore, the nurse may not have sufficient time to conduct an all-inclusive, head-to-toe physical examination. Therefore, priorities need to be established to determine the most crucial components of history taking and examination, given the circumstances.

The purpose of this chapter is to present examination guidelines for special situations in which a comprehensive head-to-toe examination may not be practical or when specialized approaches may be indicated. The special situations discussed in this chapter include assessment of patients in acute care settings such as hospitals, assessment of victims of trauma, assessment of clients in chemical dependency care settings, and assessment of people in bladder-retraining programs. Obviously, there are many more situations in which the nurse would choose to modify or specialize the approach to health assessment. In these, as well as in the specific situations discussed in this chapter, the nurse should tailor history taking and examination to fit the individual and the situation. To plan an individualized approach to assessment in any special situation, the nurse should ask three questions:

What do I need to monitor most carefully for this person?
Why do I need to monitor these things?
How often should I evaluate this person?

SPECIAL SITUATIONS AND DIFFERENT ASSESSMENT APPROACHES

Four special situations and related assessment implications are presented in this chapter: acute care, trauma, chemical dependency, and bladder retraining. These situations were selected to illustrate important principles related to modifying the health assessment process. The acute care situation is a very common practice setting in which assessment must focus on detecting complications related to illness, treatment, or immobility in an efficient manner.

The discussion of trauma assessment illustrates a standardized approach that is used in a potentially life-threatening situation when minutes or even seconds really count. In a chemical dependency setting, special skills are required to assess a person who is typically denying their illness, may have altered cognitive functions, and may have multisystem physical disorders. Finally, the discussion of bladder retraining is included to illustrate the importance of assessment when planning a program of intervention for a specific health problem such as urinary incontinence.

Acute Care. The acute care setting usually refers to the hospital environment. Patients in acute care settings have health care needs because of acute illness, injury, surgical procedures, or special diagnostic procedures such as cardiac catheterization. Some outpatient settings, such as an outpatient surgical center or outpatient cardiac catheterization center, also may be considered acute care settings. Nonacute settings include places such as nursing homes, private homes, and clinics. However, specialized devices and equipment may be used in a nonacute setting. Assessment principles related to the use of devices in the acute care setting also can be applied to the use of such devices in nonacute settings.

In the acute care setting, as in other health care delivery settings, the nurse is required to balance quality care with efficiency. To do so, it is helpful to use systematic and consolidated approaches to assessment. One such approach is to modify the physical examination to focus on signs and symptoms indicating typical problems or complications associated with the person's acute illness, injury, or surgical or diagnostic procedure. Often in the acute care setting, the focus is on early detection of actual or potential problems so that any ill effects can be minimized. For example, after surgery, the nurse might examine the patient for signs and symptoms of shock, pain, and bleeding from the surgical site. Bedside assessment in the acute care setting requires a special approach (see Assessment Guidelines: Bedside Head-to-Toe Examination).

Another important consideration in the acute care setting is equipment that is part of the patient's treatment milieu. The nurse is responsible for assessing equipment or treatment devices for safe function as well as the patient's responses. Assessment of equipment requires special skill (see the Assessment Guidelines for selected types of equipment).

Trauma. Trauma consists of physical injuries or wounds caused by external force or violence. A person who experiences severe multisystem or major unisystem injury, the extent of which may result in death or major disability, is classified as having major trauma. The assessment of the victim of major trauma focuses on rapid detection and simultaneous treatment of life-threatening injuries. The approach to physical examination is therefore highly specialized, and the process is standardized to assure efficient attention to life-threatening problems (see Assessment Guidelines: Trauma).

Chemical Dependency. The chemical dependency setting refers to the clinical environment for the treatment of addiction to drugs or alcohol. Treatment may be provided on an inpatient or an outpatient basis. Special considerations are given to history taking in the chemical dependency setting. In addition to eliciting information pertaining to overall health status, special attention is given to the history and pattern of addiction. Considerable skill is required to elicit a history because the addicted person may typically deny his or her illness. However, special techniques may be helpful to penetrate the denial. The examination in this setting also requires special attention to cognitive function because the addicted person may have cognitive alterations as well as signs and symptoms of physical disorders associated with substance abuse (see Assessment Guidelines: Substance Abuse).

Bladder Retraining. Bladder retraining involves interventions to help a person regain control of urinary elimination. The success of any bladder-retraining program is directly related to the person's motivation and the nurse's ability to devise and implement an individualized retraining program. An individualized program begins with an accurate and thorough assessment of the person's urinary elimination patterns as well as any factors known to influence elimination patterns (see Assessment Guidelines: Bladder Retraining).

Nursing Observations Acute Care

GENERAL APPROACH

Patients in acute care settings are assessed, using physical examination techniques, on a regular basis; the frequency is determined by the patient's condition. Nurses usually conduct a focused or brief head-to-toe examination and inquire regarding any problems at the beginning of a shift. This enables the nurse to identify any immediate needs or problems and provides a baseline for making comparisons. A minimal bedside assessment includes consideration of general physical status, the safety and condition of the immediate environment, equipment being used for treatment, and psychosocial factors. Reassessment is conducted as needed based on the person's condition or policies of the hospital.

EVALUATING SUPPORTIVE EQUIPMENT AND PATIENT RESPONSES

Many patients in acute care settings require the use of supportive equipment during illness and recovery. Evaluation of equipment function and of the patient's response to equipment and associated treatments should be incorporated into the overall assessment process. Important assessment principles to keep in mind in relation to *any* type of equipment include the following:

- *Evaluate the person:* For example, if the patient has a chest tube, in addition to checking the equipment, auscultate breath sounds and palpate the chest for evidence of subcutaneous air.

(continued)

- *Be systematic:* Incorporate the assessment of equipment into the head-to-toe examination sequence. Observe the patient and move out along the connections of the device.
- *Reassess equipment function:* Evaluate equipment at least every 4 hours and as needed whenever a question occurs.
- *Evaluate safety:* Note where lines or tubes are in relation to side rails, whether connections are taped or otherwise secured appropriately, and whether intact grounds or third prongs are on electrical plugs. Some equipment is inspected routinely by biomedical departments for safety. This requirement may be indicated by attached stickers or tags.

Examination guidelines pertaining to equipment follow the bedside head-to-toe examination guidelines. The following types of equipment are discussed: chest tubes, nasogastric tubes, enteral feeding tubes, intravascular pressure monitoring systems, oxygen therapy systems, urinary catheters and bladder irrigation systems, intravenous therapy systems, cardiac monitoring systems, and pulse oximetry.

▼ ▼ ▼

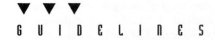

GUIDELINES

Assessment Guidelines Bedside Head-to-Toe Examination

Procedure	Clinical Significance
1. Inquire about general level of comfort and any immediate needs.	
a. Observe for pain, dyspnea, labored breathing, anxiety.	These symptoms usually require additional evaluation and intervention.
2. Perform a general survey.	
a. Note the following during the general survey: level of consciousness and mental status, the condition of the skin (color, edema, moisture), oral hygiene, and status of oral mucous membranes.	Any change in level of consciousness requires in-depth evaluation. Skin alterations may be noted secondary to immobility or changes in cardiovascular function.
b. Observe the safety of the immediate surroundings and environment.	Most safety risks can be eliminated by early detection.
c. Continue the general survey as you examine each body region. Survey each body region to detect obvious problems and threats to safety.	
3. Measure vital signs.	
a. Evaluate blood pressure (orthostatic if indicated), pulse, ventilatory (respiratory) rate, and body temperature.	Vital signs are general indicators of health status.
b. Compare the most current vital signs to baseline values.	Deviations from baseline values may indicate a change in health status. For example, as elevated temperature may be an indicator of infection.
4. Examine the anterior chest.	
a. Note the following: the ventilatory pattern, quality of the breath sounds, and quality of the heart sounds.	*Breath sounds:* The presence of crackles or wheezes may indicate underlying cardiac or pulmonary disease and deserves further investigation.
5. Examine the abdomen.	
a. Note the following: distention, tenderness, and quality of bowel sounds.	Hospitalized patients may have increased risk for ileus (indicated by absent bowel sounds) and constipation secondary to immobility.

▼ ▼ ▼

G U I D E L I N E S   *continued*   Bedside Head-to-Toe Examination

___

Procedure

6. **Survey the lower extremities.**

   a. Inquire about calf tenderness.
   b. Note any edema of the lower extremities and palpate to evaluate degree of pitting.
   c. Dorsiflex the foot to elicit Homans' sign.

7. **Palpate lower extremity pulses.**
   a. Palpate the posterior tibial pulse and the pedal pulse.

8. **Examine the back.**
   a. The person may be turned to the side or sit forward to expose the back. Note the skin condition, especially over bony prominences.
   b. Auscultate lung sounds over the posterior thorax. Note crackles or wheezes indicative of cardiovascular or respiratory problems.
   c. Percuss the lung fields, if indicated. For example, if the person has pneumonia, you may percuss for dullness caused by consolidation of mucus; if you suspect a pneumothorax, percuss for hyperresonance caused by air in the pleural space.

9. **Examine any other systems, symptoms, or functions as indicated by the person's condition.**
   a. For the person at risk for experiencing *shock,* evaluate the following:
      • Level of consciousness
      • Cardiovascular function—heart rate and rhythm, blood pressure, cardiac output
      • Pulmonary function—rate and quality of ventilations, arterial blood gases, breath sounds
      • Renal function—urine output, electrolytes, BUN, and creatinine
   b. For the person who is *immediately postoperative,* evaluate the following:
      • Vital signs—observe for rapid pulse, rapid respiratory rate, and lowered blood pressure
      • Level of consciousness
      • Pain
      • Pulmonary status—rate and quality of ventilations, ability to maintain airway
      • Wound/incision status—observe for bleeding, swelling

Clinical Significance

The lower extremities are monitored for indicators of adequate cardiovascular function and deep vein thrombosis.

Tenderness may indicate deep vein thrombosis.

Edema in lower extremities may indicate poor cardiovascular function.

If Homans' sign is present, the person will feel calf pain with dorsiflexion. Homans' sign is an indicator of deep vein thrombosis, but the reliability of this sign is questionable, because a positive Homans' sign is present in only 10% of all cases of deep vein thrombosis.

Diminished pulses are associated with impaired arterial perfusion.

Patients confined to bed have an increased risk for decubitus ulcers, which most frequently develop over bony prominences.

Level of consciousness, cardiovascular, pulmonary, and renal functions indicate the status of vital functions.

Frequency of assessment is based on stability of the patient.

These alterations may indicate shock secondary to bleeding, fluid loss, or other causes.

▼ ▼ ▼

Procedure

c. For the person reporting *distressing symptoms* (chest pain, dyspnea), conduct a complete analysis of the symptom.

   (1) Analyze *chest pain* as follows:
   - Have you experienced any chest pain (ache)?
   - *Description of the pain:* Burning, crushing, squeezing, heaviness, pressure, tightness, dull ache, heartburn, knife-like, stabbing, sharp, tearing, throbbing?
   - *Location (ask the person to point):* Substernal, abdomen, epigastric, shoulder(s), neck, jaw, arm(s), fingers, back?
   - *Onset of the pain:* When did you first notice the pain? Did it develop suddenly or gradually? How long does it last?
   - *Precipitating factors:* What were you doing when the pain occurred?
   - *Aggravating factors:* What made the pain worse? Deep breathing, coughing, moving, other factors?
   - *Intensity:* How would you rate the pain on a scale of 1 to 10, with 10 being the most severe pain?
   - *Relieving factors:* What helps alleviate the pain? Nitrates, rest, aspirin or acetaminophen, sitting upright, leaning forward, other?
   - *Other symptoms associated with chest pain:* Nausea, diaphoresis, palpitations, dizziness, dyspnea, other?

   (2) Analyze *dyspnea* as follows:
   - Have you experienced any difficulty breathing?
   - *Onset of dyspnea:* When did you first have difficulty?
   - *Aggravating factors:* What makes it worse? Activity (determine intensity of activity producing symptoms), lying flat, other?
   - *Relieving factors:* What helps alleviate the dyspnea? Sitting upright (specify how long it takes for relief), rest, oxygen, other?

valuate any wounds, intravenous lines, tubes, and any
her equipment in use (see Assessment Guidelines for
cific types of equipment).

Clinical Significance

Symptom analysis helps you identify the cause of the symptom and determine appropriate treatment.

Evaluation of these qualities of the pain is especially helpful when differentiating cardiac chest pain from pulmonary chest pain.

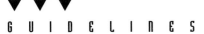

GUIDELINES

Assessment Guidelines   Chest Tubes

What to Consider Before You Begin

- Chest tubes may be inserted into the pleural space or mediastinal space to drain air, fluid, or blood, thus restoring normal lung function after surgery, trauma, or medical conditions.
- Chest tubes frequently are attached to a closed drainage system. The most popular systems operate on a water-seal principle. A water-seal system allows drainage *from* the chest but prevents air from moving back *toward* the chest.
- Either a bottle system or commercial disposable system (*e.g.,* Pleur-Evac) may be used to establish the closed drainage system and water seal.

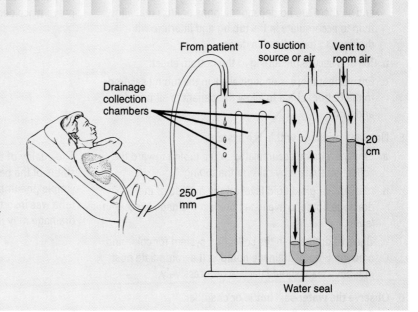

Procedure	Clinical Significance
1. Inspect, palpate, percuss, and auscultate the chest; note any respiratory distress.	
a. Observe for mediastinal shift, rapid shallow breathing, and cyanosis.	These signs and symptoms may indicate a tension pneumothorax that can result from chest tube obstruction.
b. Palpate around the chest tube insertion site.	The presence of subcutaneous air, indicated by palpation of a popping or crackling sensation, could indicate an air leak from the lung.
c. Auscultate breath sounds and percuss the chest.	Improvement in the quality of breath sounds indicates reexpansion of the lung. Loss of previously heard breath sounds may be a sign of tension pneumothorax.
2. Evaluate the dressing around the chest tube insertion site.	
a. Chest tubes usually are dressed with petrolatum gauze and sterile gauze covered by occlusive cloth tape.	The dressing provides extra protection against contamination, air leakage, and accidental dislodgement of the chest tube.
b. Note whether the dressing is clean, dry, and occlusive. Note any drainage or need for reinforcement.	
c. To prevent accidental dislodgement, tape the chest tube to the chest wall where it exits the occlusive dressing.	
3. Check the connection between the chest tube and the tubing to the drainage system.	The connection must be tight and taped securely to maintain a closed system and to prevent air leaks.

▼ ▼ ▼

G U I D E L I N E S   *continued*   Chest Tubes

Procedure	Clinical Significance

Procedure

4. **Note the placement of the drainage tubing.**
   a. Position the tubing so it will not be caught in side rails and so there are no dependent loops or links that allow fluid to accumulate in the tubing and interfere with drainage to the collection device.
   b. Coil and secure the tubing to the bottom sheet.
   c. Ensure that there is enough slack in the tubing secured to the bottom sheet to allow the patient to sit upright and turn.

5. **Note any drainage within the system.**
   a. Empty drainage accumulated in the tubing toward the collection system by milking the tubing.
   b. Mark the original fluid level on the outside of the drainage bottle to evaluate how fast drainage is accumulating.
   c. Observe drainage in the collection system for color and amount. Bloody drainage noted in the immediate postoperative state should decline progressively.

6. **Observe the water-seal bottle or chamber.**
   a. Ensure that the fluid level in the water-seal bottle or chamber is maintained at 2 cm.
   b. The fluid level in the water-seal bottle should fluctuate with respirations.

   c. Note any bubbling in the water-seal chamber. Determine the source of any leaks by clamping different points of the system. Start above the first connector and briefly clamp the chest tube; if bubbling stops, the source of the air leak is the lung. If the bubbling continues, the air leak is in the system. When the bubbling stops, the leak is proximal to the clamp.

7. **Observe the suction bottle (or chamber) and suction device.**
   a. If suction has been added to the system, determine whether the suction source is turned on and connections to suction are secure.
   b. Determine whether the correct amount of suction is being delivered to the system. If a bottle is used, the amount of suction is determined by the length of the pipet (in centimeters) beneath the water surface. If a disposable chest drainage unit is used, the amount of suction is determined by the height of the column of water (in centimeters) in the suction control chamber. If evaporation has occurred, additional water may need to be added to maintain the correct amount of suction.

Clinical Significance

Proper placement of tubing is essential to drain the system and prevent accidental dislodgment of the chest tube.

The quality of the drainage is evaluated relative to the clinical status of the patient. Little or no drainage is observed with a simple pneumothorax; bloody drainage is expected if the chest tube was inserted to drain a hemothorax. Sudden, bloody drainage may indicate active bleeding.

Evaporation may lower this level so that additional water may need to be added.

This fluctuation demonstrates patency between the pleural space and drainage system. Loss of fluctuation is associated with reexpansion of the lung, obstruction of the tubing, or malfunction of the suction.

Bubbling on expiration indicates that air is escaping from the pleural space. This is expected if the chest tube was inserted to treat a pneumothorax, but such bubbling should gradually diminish. *Note:* This type of bubbling will occur with inspiration if the patient is receiving positive-pressure ventilation. Continuous bubbling indicates a leak in the system.

Bubbling in the suction chamber indicates that the suction is on. The continuous suction mode is used rather than the intermittent mode. The bubbling should be gentle and continuous.

The typical range for water-seal suction is –20 to –30 cm of water.

▼ ▼ ▼

Assessment Guidelines   Nasogastric Tubes

What to Consider Before You Begin

- Nasogastric tubes are used to evacuate and decompress the stomach. They may also be used to assess gastric function, administer medication, and treat other problems.
- The two most common types of nasogastric tube are the single-lumen and the double-lumen sump tubes.
- The sump lumen of the double-lumen tube is a decompression vent to prevent blockage of the suction lumen.
- Tube sizes for adults range from 14 to 18 French.

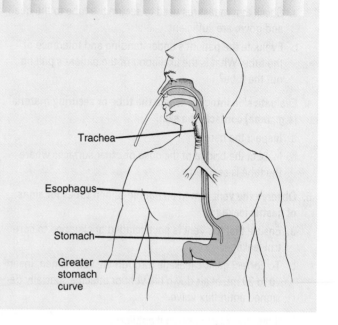

Trachea

Esophagus

Stomach

Greater stomach curve

Procedure

1. **Auscultate bowel sounds and note gastric distention and discomfort.**

   a. If the nasogastric tube is attached to suction, temporarily turn off the suction to avoid mistaking suction sounds for bowel sounds.

2. **Verify position of the tube in the gastrointestinal tract after insertion, as a routine assessment practice, and before instilling any solutions. Three methods are recommended for verifying the tube position:**

   a. Aspirate gastric contents by suction or syringe and check the pH of the aspirated fluid.

   b. Auscultate the gastric area while 30 mL of air is inserted into the tube. If the tube is in the stomach, a rush of air will be heard.

   c. Place the end of the tube under water to check for bubbling. Bubbling indicates that the tube is in the lung and should be removed immediately.

Clinical Significance

Nasogastric tubes may be inserted to drain gastric contents and may be removed when bowel sounds return.

Nasogastric tubes may be inserted to instill fluids and solutions. In this case, bowel sounds should be noted before using the tube. Gastric distension or discomfort may indicate blockage of the tube or dysfunction of the gastrointestinal tract.

A pH strip reading between 0 and 5 correlates with gastric placement. If the pH is greater than 6, the tube may have advanced into the small intestine.

The auscultatory method for checking placement is unreliable compared to the pH method.

▼ ▼ ▼

G U I D E L I N E S *continued*   Nasogastric Tubes

Procedure	Clinical Significance
3. **Determine whether methods to secure the tube are adequate.**	Secure the tube to help prevent accidental removal and unnecessary pressure on the nares.
a. Check that measures used to secure the tube to the head and gown are sufficient.	
b. Evaluate the patient's understanding and tolerance of the tube. What is the likelihood of the patient's pulling out the tube?	
4. **Evaluate skin integrity where the tube or securing material (*e.g.,* tape) contacts the skin.**	Tube contact with skin is a risk factor for pressure sore development.
a. Inspect the nares.	
b. Inspect the bridge of the nose or other surfaces where the tube is secured.	
5. **Observe the vent lumen on double-lumen tubes for signs of gastric leakage.**	
a. Ensure that the vent is not occluded or clamped to control leakage.	Clamping the vent lumen contributes to a buildup of negative pressure in the system.
b. To correct gastric leakage through the vent lumen, insert 20 to 30 mL of air down the vent or attach a specially designed antireflux valve.	
6. **Evaluate the suction setup if applicable.**	
a. Verify application of appropriate mode of suction— constant or intermittent.	
b. Verify application of the proper amount of suction—low, moderate.	
c. Note the quality of gastric secretions—color, amount.	
d. Determine whether the suction canister needs to be emptied or discarded.	

▼ ▼ ▼
GUIDELINES

Assessment Guidelines   Enteral Feeding Tubes

What to Consider Before You Begin

- Small-diameter silicone feeding tubes can be left in place comfortably and safely for several weeks to provide enteral nutrition for patients unable to eat.
- These tubes may be inserted blindly into the duodenum or introduced into the small intestine under fluoroscopy.
- Their small diameter and extreme flexibility require the use of a guide wire for placement.

Procedure

1. **Auscultate bowel sounds and note gastric distention and discomfort.**

2. **Aspirate stomach contents to determine amount of residual feeding solution.**
   a. Temporarily discontinue tube feedings if residual amounts are high.

3. **Determine whether methods to secure the tube and connections within the system are adequate.**

4. **Check pump function and the enteral feeding delivery system.**
   a. Verify prescribed delivery rate on the pump.
   b. Verify whether the prescribed solution is infusing.
   c. Note expiration date of the delivery system.

Clinical Significance

Active bowel sounds indicate intestinal activity that is necessary for digestion of tube feelings. Abdominal distention may indicate intolerance or inadequate digestion of tube feedings.

High amounts of residual feeding solution are associated with increased risk for aspiration. The method of aspirating from silicone tubes to determine residual feeding solution has been questioned. It is possible that the pliable silicone tube collapses when negative pressure is applied to aspirate. In this case, residual feeding solution could not be drawn back.

Secure the tube to prevent accidental removal and optimize patient comfort.

Continuous enteral feedings usually are delivered by volumetric pump to ensure delivery of a constant volume.

Delivery systems may be discarded and replaced every 1 or 2 days to prevent bacterial contamination, which contributes to diarrhea.

▼ ▼ ▼
GUIDELINES

Assessment Guidelines   Intravascular Pressure Monitoring

What to Consider Before You Begin

- Pressure monitoring systems are used to measure intravascular pressures continuously and to provide easy access for blood sampling.
- The system consists of an intravascular catheter, connecting tubing, one or two stopcocks, a continuous flush device, a transducer, and a monitor for reading pressures and waveforms.
- The most frequently monitored pressures are arterial blood pressure and pulmonary artery pressure.

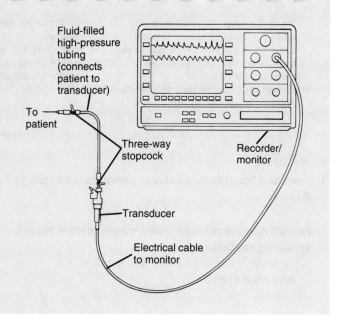

Fluid-filled high-pressure tubing (connects patient to transducer)

To patient

Three-way stopcock

Recorder/monitor

Transducer

Electrical cable to monitor

Procedure

1. **Evaluate neurovascular status distal to peripherally placed intravascular catheters. Common peripheral insertion sites include the radial, brachial, and femoral arteries.**
   a. Evaluate capillary refill time and quality of pulses distal to the catheter.
   b. Determine whether there is numbness, tingling, or loss of sensation distal to the catheter.
   c. If the pressure waveform is dampened, determine whether blood flow is obstructed by catheter malposition or a tight dressing.

2. **Evaluate the catheter insertion site and dressing.**
   a. Arterial puncture sites have the potential to bleed, so note any evidence of bleeding.
   b. Note whether the dressing is clean, dry, and occlusive. Note any drainage or need for reinforcement.

3. **Check the connecting tubing and stopcocks between the patient and the flush system.**
   a. Inspect junctions joining different pieces of tubing in the same system.
   b. Check that stopcocks are turned so the system is patent between the patient and transducer.

Clinical Significance

Neurovascular assessment is conducted to monitor the patient for thromboembolic complications.

Connections should be tight to maintain a closed system and prevent air leaks. Wet dressings may indicate leaks in the system.

An open system is necessary to prevent clotting and loss of pressure monitoring.

▼ ▼ ▼

G U I D E L I N E S   *continued*   Intravascular Pressure Monitoring

---

Procedure

   c. Inspect stopcocks and tubing for stasis of blood. If blood cannot be removed by flushing the system, consider replacing parts contaminated with blood.

   d. Examine the fluid in the pressure tubing for air bubbles.

4. **Note the saline flush solution bag.**

   a. Ensure that there is adequate volume in the bag. There is no alarm system associated with the system to note when the solution is low or gone.

5. **Balance and calibrate the system to atmospheric pressure if indicated.**

6. **Evaluate the pressure waveform on the monitor.**

   a. For intraarterial pressure monitoring, the arterial waveform is characterized by a rapid upstroke, a gradual downstroke, and a clear dicrotic notch (see Ch. 8, p. 315).

   b. For pulmonary artery monitoring, determine whether a pulmonary artery waveform is present.

   c. Determine whether the pulmonary artery waveform is dampened; if it is, determine possible causes (see *a*).

7. **Compare invasively obtained arterial blood pressure to auscultated cuff pressure.**

Clinical Significance

Blood provides a medium for bacterial growth.

Air bubbles should be removed because air will absorb some of the intravascular pressure before the pressure is sensed by the transducer. Air bubbles in the tubing result in underestimation of the systolic blood pressure and overestimation of the diastolic blood pressure.

Fluid is delivered under a pressure higher than the intravascular pressure to prevent backflow of blood. Patency of the system is maintained by the delivery of fluid under 300 mm Hg of pressure, which results in delivery of a small volume (usually 3 mL/hour) continuously through the catheter.

Balancing the system establishes a zero reference point that takes into account the effect of atmospheric (barometric) pressure.

If these components are not present or clear, the waveform is said to be absent or dampened. Possible causes include air in the system, obstruction of the catheter or tubing, and low blood pressure.

Other waveforms, such as a right ventricular waveform and a pulmonary artery wedge waveform, indicate malposition of the catheter. Corrective actions should be taken according to hospital protocols.

Direct invasive pressures are usually considered more accurate but comparable to blood pressures obtained by cuff.

The direct invasive pressure may be equal to or slightly higher than the cuff pressure.

If the cuff pressure is higher than the direct invasive pressure, there may be air in the system that is interfering with transmission of the blood pressure to the transducer.

▼ ▼ ▼
G U I D E L I N E S

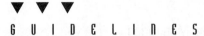

Assessment Guidelines   Oxygen Therapy

What to Consider Before You Begin

- Patients with acute or chronic cardiopulmonary dysfunction may require supplemental oxygen to increase oxygen loading in the lung and increase oxygen delivery to body tissues.
- The three most common oxygen delivery systems are the nasal cannula and simple face mask, which deliver oxygen at slow rates, and the heated nebulizer, which delivers oxygen at a higher flow rate. Heated nebulizer systems include a face mask, corrugated tubing, and a heated aerosol source.

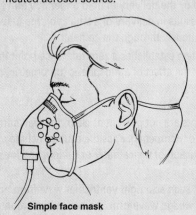

Simple face mask

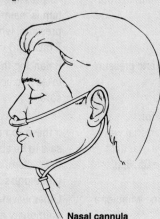

Nasal cannula

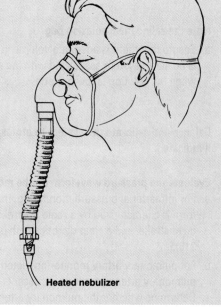

Heated nebulizer

Procedure

1. **Evaluate oxygenation status.**
   a. Observe the patient for restlessness, shortness of breath, and cyanosis.
   b. Evaluate results of arterial blood gases if available. Note whether blood gas values were measured on the current oxygen settings.

2. **Inspect skin surfaces contacting the oxygen delivery system.**
   a. *Nasal cannula:* Inspect the skin of the nares and ears for redness or impaired integrity. Examine the nasal mucosa for evidence of drying or bleeding.
   b. *Face mask:* Inspect the ears and the bridge of the nose for redness or breakdown.

Clinical Significance

These signs may indicate hypoxia. Indicators of oxygenation status on the arterial blood gases include Pao_2 and Sao_2.

Skin at tubing mask or cannula interface is at risk for pressure sore development.

▼ ▼ ▼

Procedure

3. **Verify proper placement of the nasal cannula or face mask.**

   a. Place a nasal cannula with the prongs in the nares. The prongs curve to fit along the floor of the nasal cavity.

   b. Ensure that the face mask fits snugly against the nose and chin with the head strap above the ears.

   c. Inspect the face mask of a heated nebulizer system during inspiration. If escaping mist disappears at the side vents of the mask, flow is inadequate. If the patient's inspiratory flow exceeds the nebulizer flow, the patient will entrain room air into the mask and decrease the oxygen percentage being inspired (Flo_2).

4. **Evaluate connecting tubing.**

   a. Ensure that all connections between tubing, flow meters, and oxygen delivery device are secure.

   b. Inspect the corrugated tubing of a heated nebulizer system from the mask to the reservoir bag. Drain any accumulated water to the reservoir bag. Empty the reservoir bag as needed.

5. **Evaluate the oxygen flow meter.**

   a. A nasal cannula usually delivers 6 L/min or less.

   b. A simple face mask usually is set at 5 L/min or higher to deliver the desired amount of oxygen.

   c. Turn the oxygen flow meter of a heated nebulizer system all the way up and turn the special dial to the ordered Flo_2 setting (0.40, 0.60, or 1.00). Liter flow must be maximal to ensure correct oxygen delivery and flow. An inline oxygen analyzer may be required for accurate measurement of the Flo_2.

6. **Evaluate the humidification system.**

   a. Check the fluid level in the humidifier or nebulizer bottle. Does sterile water need to be added?

   b. Humidifier bottles may be omitted from low-flow nasal cannula systems.

7. **Determine the temperature of the delivered gas (nebulizer system only).**

   a. Ensure that inspired gas is at body temperature.

   b. If inspired gas temperature is too high or too low, adjust the setting on the heating plate.

Clinical Significance

Proper placement assures optimal patient comfort and function of equipment.

System must be intact to assure delivery of prescribed amount of oxygen.

Water in nebulizer tubing can cause fluctuations in Flo_2 and can create an annoying gurgling sound.

The dial is set to deliver the prescribed amount of oxygen.

Lower flow rates are associated with carbon dioxide accumulation in the mask.

Water is added to some systems to humidify the patient's airway.

Proper temperature is maintained for patient comfort and to avoid tissue damage.

▼ ▼ ▼
GUIDELINES

Assessment Guidelines Urinary Catheters and Bladder Irrigation Systems

What to Consider Before You Begin

- Indwelling urinary catheters are inserted for a variety of reasons but generally have one purpose—to drain urine from the bladder.
- Indwelling urinary catheters are retained by virtue of a balloon that may contain 10 to 30 mL of water inserted to inflate the balloon inside the bladder after the catheter is in place.
- Irrigation is used to give medication or keep the bladder free from clots after surgery.
- Urine output may be monitored as frequently as every hour for evaluation of the patient's physiological status or to observe the patency of a continuous irrigation system.

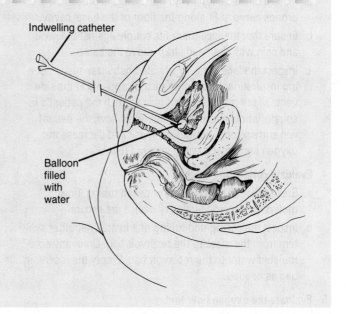

Indwelling catheter

Balloon filled with water

Procedure

1. **Note patency of the drainage system and placement of the drainage tubing and collection bag.**
   a. Inspect, palpate, and percuss the bladder to determine whether the bladder is distended.
   b. Observe for urine in the drainage tubing.
   c. Place the tubing so that it will not be caught in the side rails and so there are no dependent loops or kinks that allow urine to accumulate in it and interfere with drainage to the collection bag.
   d. Ensure that the catheter or tubing is taped in a manner to secure the catheter.
   e. Attach the collection bag to the bed frame (not the side rails), and ensure that it is off the floor.

2. **Evaluate skin surfaces near the catheter.**
   a. Inspect the urinary meatus for drainage or encrustations. Cleanse the meatal–catheter junction according to institution protocols.
   b. Inspect the meatal–catheter junction for urine leakage.

3. **Check the connections between the catheter and drainage/irrigation tubing. Check that all connections are tight.**

4. **Note the characteristics of urine flow from the bladder.**
   a. Observe the color, odor, presence of blood or sediment, and amount of urine.

Clinical Significance

If the bladder is distended, the drainage system may be obstructed.

Securing the catheter prevents unnecessary movement.

Bags attached to side rails can be inadvertently moved by repositioning side rails.

If urine leaks, a larger catheter may need to be inserted, the balloon may require more water, or the balloon may be ruptured.

Connections should be tight to ensure a closed system and to help prevent infection.

▼ ▼ ▼

Urinary Catheters and Bladder Irrigation Systems

Procedure

b. If continuous irrigation is being used after surgery, observe for active bleeding (dense, dark red drainage) and clots.

c. In continuous irrigation systems, determine the quantity of urine output. Measure the total output in the drainage system and subtract the amount of irrigation solution that was instilled.

5. **For continuous irrigation systems, evaluate the irrigation system.**

a. Check that the irrigating solution and flow rate correspond to physician's orders.

b. Irrigation flow rates are typically 40 to 60 mL/min to prevent postoperative clot development.

Clinical Significance

A patient with active bleeding requires additional evaluation.

▼ ▼ ▼

G U I D E L I N E S

Assessment Guidelines   Intravenous Therapy

What to Consider Before You Begin

- Intravenous (IV) therapy is initiated to provide hydration, medication, or nutrition.
- A needle or catheter is inserted either peripherally in the arms, legs, feet, or scalp, or centrally in a large vein such as the subclavian or jugular.

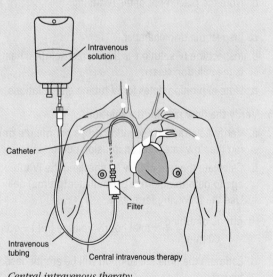

Central intravenous therapy

Procedure

1. **Evaluate the patient's fluid and electrolyte status.**

a. Examine the person for signs of overhydration or dehydration.

b. Review input and output data.

c. Review applicable laboratory data.

Clinical Significance

Evaluation is conducted to detect overall response to intravenous therapy, including adverse effects.

▼ ▼ ▼

GUIDELINES *continued*   Intravenous Therapy

Procedure	**Clinical Significance**

Procedure

2. **Evaluate the IV insertion site.**
   a. Inspect the site for signs of inflammation or infection—redness, warmth, swelling, tenderness, discharge. Note any redness or tenderness along the cannulated vein.
   b. Ensure that the dressing is clean, dry, and occlusive. Note the date of the last dressing change. Dressing policies vary among institutions.

3. **Check the connections and measures taken to secure the system.**
   a. Ensure that the connection between the IV needle or catheter and IV tubing is tight.
   b. Ensure that the IV needle or catheter and tubing is taped in a manner to prevent unnecessary movement or accidental removal.
   c. If an armboard is being used, ensure that it is stable and not compromising skin integrity or circulation.
   d. Check all other connecting sites in the system for tightness. Connecting sites may or may not be taped for additional security.

4. **Inspect the tubing and IV solution.**
   a. Check for air bubbles in the tubing.

   b. Note the placement of the IV tubing.

   c. Inspect the drip chamber.
   d. Inspect the IV solution. Is the correct solution hanging? Is the solution clear?
   c. Note expiration dates for IV tubing and solutions.

5. **Verify the flow rate for the solution.**
   a. Verify flow rates by counting drops per minute or reading the flow rate from an infusion pump.
   b. Calculate the rate of flow by checking the IV tubing package to determine drops per milliliter (gtt/mL) delivered. Use the following formula:

   $$\frac{\text{gtt/mL of tubing}}{60 \text{ min}} \times \text{total hourly volume (mL)} = \text{gtt/min}$$

   c. Estimate the time the solution will be empty based on flow rate.

6. **Evaluate infusion pump function if applicable.**
   a. Ensure that audible alarms are turned on. Most infusion pumps have an occlusion alarm to indicate when the maximum pressure that the pump will deliver has been violated.
   b. Inspect the electrical plug and ensure an intact ground wire.

Clinical Significance

Redness along the vein may indicate phlebitis.

A closed system is required to assure optimal function and minimize bacterial contamination.
Leakage of blood or fluid indicates a faulty connection.

Large air bubbles should be removed to minimize the risk of air embolism.
The tubing should be placed so it will not be caught in side rails, sheets, and so forth.
The drip chamber should be one-half to one-third full.

This calculation facilitates transition to the next solution.

Assessment Guidelines   Cardiac Monitoring

What to Consider Before You Begin

- Cardiac monitoring devices include telemetry or direct attachment to a cardiac monitor.
- Telemetry systems include chest electrodes and a radio transmitter. The transmitter is compact and usually secured to the patient's gown. The electrocardiographic (ECG) signal is transmitted to a central monitoring station via the transmitter. Patients with telemetry monitoring may be mobile.
- If the patient is attached directly to a cardiac monitor by wires and electrodes, the patient is confined to an area restricted by the length of the wires and cables.

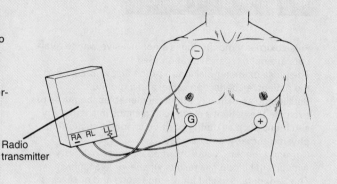

Radio transmitter

Procedure

1. **Verify the cardiac rhythm and the patient's response.**
   a. Identify the cardiac rhythm being recorded for the patient. Verify by telephone contact if remote telemetry monitoring is in effect.
   b. Note vital signs, level of consciousness, and quality of pulses.
   c. Auscultate the patient's apical pulse and compare that pulse rate with the pulse rate displayed by the cardiac monitor.
   d. Note the quality of the transmitted signal.

2. **Evaluate the areas of skin in contact with monitoring electrodes.**
   a. Inspect the skin around and under electrodes.

   b. Determine whether there is good contact between the electrode and skin.

3. **Evaluate wires and cables in the system.**
   a. Observe whether there is firm attachment of wires to the electrode snaps.
   b. Inspect the wires and cables for intact insulation (covering).
   c. Note whether wires are connected firmly to the telemetry transmitter or monitor cable block.
   d. Ensure that monitor cables are placed so the patient can move freely in bed.
   e. Ensure that the monitor cable is not draped over any piece of electrical equipment that may interfere with signal transmission.

Clinical Significance

These types of data indicate how the person is tolerating the displayed heart rhythm.

Indicates how well the actual heart rate correlates with the heart rate displayed by the monitor.

Excessive artifact may indicate patient movement or poor contact of the electrode with the skin. The QRS amplitude should be at least 5 mm to ensure accurate sensing of heart rate. A poor-quality signal in a telemetry system may indicate a low battery.

Conductive gel may irritate the skin and cause itching and redness after application.

Good contact is indicated if the electrode is secure, the gel beneath the electrode is moist, and the electrode is placed over fatty areas rather than bony or muscular areas. Electrodes may adhere poorly to moist or hairy skin surfaces.

This connection must be intact to transmit the ECG signal to the cardiac monitor.

Insulation prevents interference from other electrical equipment in the room.

▼ ▼ ▼
G U I D E L I N E S

Assessment Guidelines   Pulse Oximetry

What to Consider Before You Begin

- Pulse oximetry monitoring is a noninvasive way to evaluate arterial oxygen saturation (Sao_2).
- The pulse oximeter includes a probe that is attached to the patient, a connecting cable, and a monitor.
- Bedside pulse oximetry monitoring enables the nurse to evaluate the patient's oxygenation status in a variety of situations such as during position changes, suctioning, physical therapy, and exercise.
- Correlate the Sao_2 value obtained via pulse oximetry with arterial blood gas results whenever available.
- The Sao_2 data is useful for seeing trends and observing changes but therapeutic changes should be based on a complete clinical assessment not on a single number.
- Many types of pulse oximeters are available, but all have similar features for assessment purposes.

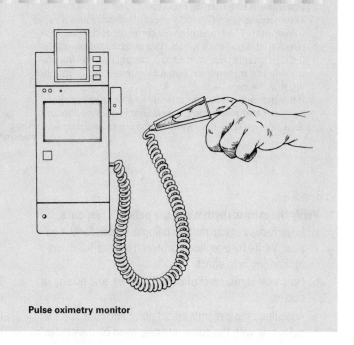

Pulse oximetry monitor

Procedure

1. **Evaluate the overall oxygenation status of the patient.**
   a. Note the Sao_2 value on the oximeter monitor.
   b. Note respiratory effort, skin color, and reports of dyspnea.

2. **Evaluate the skin surface in contact with the oximeter probe.**
   a. Assess the tissue perfusion under and around the probe.
   b. Evaluate the skin for irritation.

3. **Evaluate the quality of the waveform or readout on the monitor. If the quality is poor:**
   a. Determine whether the probe is secured adequately to the skin.
   b. Determine whether the probe needs to be cleaned. Cleanse the probe with isopropyl alcohol.
   c. Determine whether the area in contact with the probe is perfused adequately.

4. **Note the placement of the connecting cable.**

Clinical Significance

Increased respiratory effort, cyanosis, and dyspnea may indicate hypoxia.

The tissue must be perfused adequately for the oximeter to function.

Skin/equipment interface is at risk for impaired integrity.

Skin oils or other debris may interfere with light transmission.

Tubing should be placed so it is away from side rails and not interfering with patient movements.

Documenting the Bedside Physical Examination

It is important to maintain a record of the results of a bedside physical examination. Not only is the record a required legal document, it also serves as a means for comparing current findings with the patient's baseline or previous status. Because of the need for efficient documentation of frequent bedside assessments, as well as the status of equipment, many practitioners document in a manner that saves time. Flowsheets are widely used in clinical practice to document examination findings once an initial comprehensive admission database has been recorded. A typical practice is to develop flowsheets that allow a "charting by exception" method (see Chap. 2). Charting by exception consists of documenting only those findings defined as "abnormal." Because the definition of "normal" or "abnormal" may differ with different examiners, it is helpful to establish the criteria for "normal" findings in writing. Then when the nurse recognizes an exception to "normal," additional narrative charting is done to describe any significant findings.

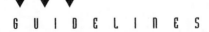

Nursing Observations   Trauma

GENERAL APPROACH   The initial assessment of the victim of major trauma is divided into the *primary survey* and the *secondary survey*. The primary survey focuses on the status of the person's airway, breathing, and circulation, and the secondary survey consists of a general head-to-toe evaluation to detect additional life-threatening injuries. The secondary survey is initiated only after completion of the primary survey. Based on the results of the primary and secondary survey, a trauma score can be calculated and recorded (see Assessment Guidelines: Trauma). The trauma score is used to make triage and transport decisions and to predict prognosis.

A trauma team is often used in emergency departments to evaluate and treat the victim of major trauma. The trauma team members usually have specific roles to perform in relation to assessment that have been predetermined by hospital protocols.

During the examination of a trauma victim, exposure of all body parts is essential. Clothing should be cut away rather than pulled over the head or over legs, which may aggravate musculoskeletal injuries such as C-spine fractures, pelvic fractures, or other bone fractures. Motorcycle helmets may be kept in place until x-rays have been evaluated for evidence of C-spine integrity. Once clothing is removed, care must be taken to keep the victim warm. Use of overhead warmers or light blankets may be helpful.

▼ ▼ ▼

GUIDELINES

Assessment Guidelines   Trauma

Procedure

Primary Survey:

1. **Perform the primary survey in 30 seconds (think "A-B-C's," or airway, breathing, circulation).**

2. **Determine airway status (obstructed or patent).**
   a. Ask the person his or her name.
   b. Move your head close to the victim's mouth. Listen for air movement and feel the person's breath against your cheek.

Clinical Significance

The primary survey must proceed rapidly to detect any life-threatening conditions and initiate simultaneous treatment.

A quick way to assess airway patency is to ask the person to speak. If person speaks, the airway is patent.

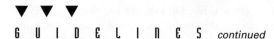

▼ ▼ ▼

G U I D E L I N E S *continued*   Trauma

Procedure	**Clinical Significance**

Procedure

c. If you do not detect air movement, try to establish a patent airway with mechanical maneuvers such as the jaw thrust or chin lift. *Do not* hyperextend the neck.

d. If necessary, clear debris from the airway manually or using suction.

3. **Evaluate breathing.**

a. Observe the rate, depth, rhythm, and symmetry of breathing. Expose the chest to optimize visualization.

b. Note the use of accessory muscles (trapezius muscles, scalenes, sternocleidomastoids).

4. **Evaluate circulation.**

a. Conduct a rapid survey, using the following techniques:

(1) Palpate the carotid pulse noting rate, quality, and rhythm.

(2) Measure capillary refill time. Squeeze nailbeds and count the number of seconds until blanching of the nailbed dissipates.

(3) Note the skin color.

(4) Survey for obvious bleeding.

Secondary Survey

1. **Perform the secondary survey in 5 to 10 minutes.**

2. **If the victim is conscious, ask about mechanism of injury, pain, numbness, tingling, and ability to move extremities.**

a. If the victim is unresponsive, obtain this information from others such as prehospital personnel or family members.

3. **Initiate a general survey and conduct a brief neurologic examination.**

a. Observe for guarding, stiffness, rigidity, or flaccidity. Note odors such as alcohol, gasoline, chemicals, urine, or feces.

Clinical Significance

Maintain neutral neck alignment until cervical spine injury has been definitively ruled out.

These actions may clear an obstructed airway.

Breathing may be significantly impaired after any of the following mechanisms of injury: striking a steering wheel, blunt or penetrating trauma to the thorax, falls or ejection from automobiles.

Use of accessory muscles indicates increased work of breathing. This is noted in life-threatening conditions such as pneumothorax, hemothorax, and thoracic musculoskeletal trauma.

Time does not permit blood pressure measurement during the primary survey.

If the carotid pulse is palpable, the systolic blood pressure is estimated to be at least 60 mm Hg (70 mm Hg for palpable femoral pulse; 80 mm Hg for palpable radial pulse).

Capillary refill time indicates the adequacy of tissue perfusion. Normal capillary refill times is less than 3 seconds.

Pallor is associated with shock.

The secondary survey is a brief head-to-toe examination to determine *all* injuries, not just the obvious ones.

These data provide additional information about more subtle and potentially life-threatening injuries.

Any of these positions may indicate injury. Odors may indicate need for special treatment or precaution. High alcohol levels could present neurologic concerns. Gasoline or chemical odors may signal need for decontamination. Urine or feces odor may indicate bladder or bowel incontinence and neurologic complications.

▼ ▼ ▼

G U I D E L I N E S   *continued*   Trauma

Procedure

b. Note the following neurologic indicators: eye opening; verbal response; motor response; pupil response to light, size and equality.

c. The Glasgow Coma Scale score may be calculated as follows:

Clinical Significance

Eye opening, verbal response, and motor response are assessed to determine the Glasgow Coma Scale score.

Glasgow Coma Scale scores can range from 3 to 15. A score of less than 8 indicates a poor prognosis. The Glasgow Coma Scale score is incorporated into calculation of the Trauma Score (see Table 18–1). The Trauma Score is used to estimate the severity of injury.

Glasgow Coma Scale

Finding	Score	Finding	Score
Eye Opening		**Best Motor Response**	
Spontaneous	4	Obeys commands	6
To voice	3	Purposeful movement (pain)	5
To pain	2	Withdraw (pain)	4
None	1	Flexion (pain)	3
Best Verbal Response		Extension (pain)	2
Oriented	5	None	1
Confused	4		
Inappropriate words	3		
Incomprehensible sounds	2		
None	1		

---

4. **Measure vital signs—pulse, respiratory rate, blood pressure, and body temperature.**

This set of vital signs serves as the baseline as you continue to evaluate and treat the victim.

5. **Inspect and palpate the head and the face.**

   a. Observe for lacerations and deformities.

   b. Examine the pupils for size, shape, equality, and reaction to light.

   Deviations from normal may indicate neurologic injury.

   c. Evaluate gross visual acuity by holding up fingers and asking victim to indicate how many fingers are being shown.

   d. Palpate the head and face for tenderness and crackling of subcutaneous emphysema.

   These are indicators of soft tissue injury.

   e. Check the mouth for drainage, foreign bodies, and broken teeth. Note alignment of jaw or bite.

   Any of these may compromise airway. Deformity may indicate jaw fracture.

   f. Note any drainage from nose or ears and test for glucose.

   Glucose-positive fluid represents cerebrospinal fluid.

6. **Inspect and palpate the neck.**

   a. Palpate the cervical spine and observe tenderness, spasm, or deformities.

   Suspect cervical spine injury in the presence of these findings or in any victim with a head injury.

   b. Observe for tracheal deviation.

   Associated with tension pneumothorax; requires immediate treatment.

▼ ▼ ▼

Procedure	Clinical Significance
c. Observe for penetrating injury, ecchymosis, and edema.	Internal bleeding may compromise airway.
d. Observe for pulsating or distended neck veins.	Distended neck veins indicate pump failure, which may be secondary to tension pneumothorax, myocardial contusion, air embolism, pericardial tamponade, or myocardial infarction.
7. Inspect and palpate the chest.	
a. Observe clavicular area for tenderness, hematoma, deformity, and subcutaneous emphysema.	These findings may indicate fractures or soft tissue injury.
b. Observe sternum and rib cage for tenderness, deformity, symmetry during breathing, and breathing effort.	Paradoxic movement with breathing indicates flail chest. Asymmetric movement is associated with pneumothorax or hemothorax.
c. Auscultate briefly for breath sounds and heart sounds. Observe for absent or reduced breath sounds and adventitious sounds.	
8. Inspect and palpate the abdomen.	
a. Observe for lacerations, ecchymosis, distension, guarding, and point tenderness.	
b. Measure abdominal girth if distention is observed.	Serial measurements will detect an increase in abdominal girth, which may indicate internal bleeding.
c. Ask the victim about any tender areas. Auscultate for bowel sounds and then lightly palpate, starting in nontender areas.	Avoid aggravating injury by identifying painful areas.
d. Do not palpate splenic area if pain is reported in that area.	An injured spleen is fragile and could rupture if palpated.
9. Inspect and palpate the pelvis.	
a. Gently palpate over the iliac crests and the symphysis pubis.	Pain or abnormal movement may indicate pelvic fracture.
b. Examine the urinary meatus for blood.	If blood is present, *do not* insert urinary catheter.
c. Examine the rectum, noting presence of blood and sphincter control.	Loss of sphincter tone indicates neurologic injury.
10. Inspect and palpate the extremities.	
a. Palpate peripheral pulses—radial, femoral, pedal.	Absent pulses indicate limb injury.
b. Observe for deformities, swelling, lacerations, sensory and motor function disturbances.	
11. Examine the back.	
a. Reach under and palpate the spinal processes.	The victim is usually not rolled over during the secondary survey to protect the integrity of the cervical spine.
b. Feel along the vertebral column for differences in spacing.	Separation or compression fractures of the spine may be felt as differences in spacing.
c. Observe for deformities and lacerations.	

NDx

Documenting the Trauma Survey

The primary and secondary trauma surveys are usually documented on flowsheets in the hospital's emergency department. An example of a trauma flowsheet is shown in Appendix G. Assessment data that do not fit into flowsheet categories may be documented elsewhere on the record in narrative form.

The person assigned to record events on the trauma flowsheet during a trauma resuscitation is usually a nurse with clinical background in trauma care. The recorder must have enough knowledge of trauma care to be able to integrate and summarize data in an accurate manner.

During a trauma resuscitation, it is critical that all details of the assessment be recorded concurrently with the collection of data. Documentation based on memory is usually not as reliable. If events are happening too rapidly for the recorder to adequately use the trauma flowsheet, a separate form may be used to record events as they happen. These data are then transcribed to the trauma flowsheet when time permits.

The Trauma Score

The Trauma Score is a numerical grading system for estimating the severity of injury. The score is composed of the Glasgow Coma Scale (reduced to about one-third total value) and measurements of cardiopulmonary function. The lowest score is 1, and the highest score is 16 (Table

18-1). Trauma victims with a trauma score of less than 10 have less than a 60% survival rate. The trauma score is usually incorporated into the trauma flowsheet as shown in Appendix G.

TABLE 18.1   The Trauma Score

Physical Sign	Value	Points
A. Respiratory rate	10–24	4
	25–35	3
	>35	2
	<10	1
	0	0
B. Respiratory effort	Normal	1
	Shallow or retractive	0
C. Systolic blood pressure	>90	4
	70–90	3
	50–69	2
	<50	1
	0	0
D. Capillary refill	Normal	2
	Delayed	1
	None	0
E. Glasgow Coma Scale	14–15	5
	11–13	4
	8–10	3
	5–7	2
	3–4	1

Trauma score = A + B + C + D + E

Nursing Observations   Chemical Dependency Settings

GENERAL APPROACH

The assessment of the addict seeking treatment will focus on the addiction history, family and social history, review and examination of major body systems that might be affected by substance abuse, and review of laboratory tests indicating the status of involved body systems. Because the addict may be at high risk for communicable diseases, additional diagnostic testing may be obtained as part of the admission laboratory profile. For example, the person may be tested for tuberculosis or for human immunodeficiency virus (HIV).

TYPICAL LABORATORY PROFILE

Liver enzymes
Complete blood count
Platelets
Urinalysis
Blood urea nitrogen
Blood alcohol levels
Toxicology screen

ASSESSING WITHDRAWAL FROM ALCOHOL

Patients who are initially admitted to a healthcare setting for detoxification from alcohol will be evaluated to determine the severity and optimal treatment of withdrawal symptoms. The Clinical Institute Withdrawal Assessment of Alcohol (CIWA-A) screening method can be used to determine the patient's status (see Displays 18-1 and 18-2).

(continued)

DISPLAY 18.1

Assessment Tool for Determining CIWA-A Score

Patient _____ Date_____

Time _____ Pulse or heart rate, taken for one minute _____

Blood pressure _____ / _____

NAUSEA AND VOMITING:

0   No nausea and no vomiting
1   Mild nausea with no vomiting
2
3
4   Intermittent nausea with dry heaves
5
6
7   Constant nausea, frequent dry heaves and vomiting

TREMOR—Arms extended and fingers spread apart, observation

0   No tremor
1   Not visible, but can be felt fingertip to fingertip
2
3
4   Moderate, with patient's arms extended
5
6
7   Severe, even with arms not extended

PAROXYSMAL SWEATS—Observation

0   No sweat visible
1   Barely perceptible sweating, palms moist
2
3
4   Beads of sweat obvious on forehead
5
6
7   Drenching sweats

ANXIETY—Ask, "Do you feel nervous?" Observation

1   No anxiety, at ease
2   Mildly anxious
3
4   Moderately anxious, or guarded, so anxiety is inferred
5
6
7   Equivalent to acute panic states, as seen in severe delirium or acute schizophrenic reactions

AGITATION—Observation

0   Normal activity
1   Somewhat more than normal activity
2
3
4   Moderately fidgety and restless

5
6
7   Paces back and forth during most of the interview, or constantly thrashes about

TACTILE DISTURBANCES—Ask, "Have you any itching, pins and needles sensations, any burning, any numbness, or do you feel bugs crawling on or under your skin?" Observation

0   None
1   Very mild itching, pins and needles, burning or numbness
2   Mild itching, pins and needles, burning or numbness
3   Moderate itching, pins and needles, burning or numbness
4   Moderately severe hallucinations
5   Severe hallucinations
6   Extremely severe hallucinations
7   Continuous hallucinations

AUDITORY DISTURBANCES—Ask, "Are you more aware of sounds around you? Are they harsh? Do they frighten you? Are you hearing anything that is disturbing to you? Are you hearing things you know are not there?" Observation

0   Not present
1   Very mild harshness or ability to frighten
2   Mild harshness or ability to frighten
3   Moderate harshness or ability to frighten
4   Moderately severe hallucinations
5   Severe hallucinations
6   Extremely severe hallucinations
7   Continuous hallucinations

VISUAL DISTURBANCES—Ask, "Does the light appear to be too bright? Is the color different? Does it hurt your eyes? Are you seeing anything that is disturbing to you? Are you seeing things you know are not there?" Observation

0   Not present
1   Very mild sensitivity
2   Mild sensitivity
3   Moderate sensitivity
4   Moderately severe hallucinations
5   Severe hallucinations
6   Extremely severe hallucinations
7   Continuous hallucinations

Assessment Tool for Determining CIWA-A Score (continued)

Patient _____ Date_____

Time _____ Pulse or heart rate, taken for one minute _____

Blood pressure _____ / _____

HEADACHE, FULLNESS IN HEAD—Ask, "Does your head feel different? Does it feel like there is a band around your head?" Do not rate dizziness or lightheadedness. Otherwise, rate severity.

0 Not present
1 Very mild
2 Mild
3 Moderate
4 Moderately severe
5 Severe
6 Very severe
7 Extremely severe

ORIENTATION AND CLOUDING OF SENSORIUM—Ask, "What day is this? Where are you? Whom am I?"

0 Oriented and can do serial additions
1 Cannot do serial additions or is uncertain about date
2 Disoriented for date by no more than 2 calendar days
3 Disoriented for date by more than 2 calendar days
4 Disoriented for place and/or person

Total CIWA Score _____
Rater's initials _____
Maximum possible score 67

Clinical Interpretation of CIWA-A Scores

CLINICAL INSTITUTE WITHDRAWAL ASSESSMENT OF ALCOHOL (CIWA-A)

Screen to be done every 2 hours with vital signs to assess patient's level of withdrawal from alcohol.

Score	Level of Withdrawal	Guidelines
0–19	Mild	Can manage without medication and utilize psychological support, oral rehydration, and symptomatic treatment with the 3Rs (reassurance of recovery, respect, and reality orientation)
20–25	Moderate	BP 150/100 mmHg Pulse 100–120 beats/min Temp. 100–101°F Administer sedation
26+	Severe	BP > 160/120 mmHg Pulse > 120 beats/min Temp > 101°F Increase sedation, potential for seizures

Discontinue CIWA-A after a score of 10 or less on three consecutive readings.

Nursing Observations   Chemical Dependency Settings (continued)

SPECIAL INTERVIEWING TECHNIQUES

Obtaining a history from the addicted person may be especially challenging because of the tendency of the addict to deny or attempt to hide his or her problems with substance abuse. One indication that the person may not be providing an accurate history is if the physical examination and laboratory profile indicate an advanced disease process but the person denies substance abuse. For example, if the liver is greatly enlarged and liver enzymes are elevated, the possibility of alcohol-induced cirrhosis of the liver should be considered.

It may be helpful to ask questions in a direct manner. For example, rather than asking, "Do you drink?", you may want to ask, "How many days out of seven do you drink?"

As you interview, focus on eliciting information pertaining to specific behaviors or symptoms rather than asking about general topics. For example, you might ask the person, "Do you ever wonder how you got home?" rather than asking, "Do you ever have blackouts?" Conversely, you may ask, "Do you ever notice your hands shaking in the morning?" rather than, "Do you have withdrawal symptoms?"

Know the Language

You will communicate better with the person abusing substances if you know any special jargon the person uses to refer to their habit. For example, common street terms for solvent inhalation include "huffing" or "sniffing." Jargon may vary, depending on terms used in the addict's peer group or social environment.

▼ ▼ ▼

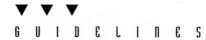

GUIDELINES

Assessment Guidelines   Substance Abuse

Procedure	Clinical Significance
1. Obtain a history pertaining to the pattern of abuse/addiction.	
a. Determine the following:	
• Substances being abused	Assume abuse of more than one substance until you have reason to believe otherwise.
• Last time the person used	
• Frequency of use	
• Age at first use	
• Quantity used	
• Blackouts	Blackouts are considered major indicators of alcohol dependence.
• Withdrawal symptoms	Withdrawal symptoms include tremors and seizures.
• Change in tolerance	Increased tolerance: More substance is required to produce desired effect.
	Decreased tolerance: May indicate a decline in the body's ability to metabolize the substance or decreased use of a substance.
• Legal problems	History of DUI (DWI): Consider that the person may have driven drunk many times before being cited.
2. Evaluate suicide risk. (See Chap. 14 for specific guidelines.)	Many abusive substances have depressive effects; the person also may experience despair/crisis because of related family, social, or job problems.

▼ ▼ ▼

Substance Abuse

Procedure

3. **Inquire about social and family history.**

   a. Determine the following:
      • Marital status
      • History of multiple marriages
      • Employment status
      • History of job loss
      • Educational background
      • Relationship with children

4. **Evaluate cognitive functions.** (See Chap. 9 for guidelines.)

5. **Review body systems most likely to be adversely affected by substance abuse.**

   a. Review the gastrointestinal system.

   b. Review the genitourinary system.

   c. Review the cardiovascular and respiratory systems.

   d. Review the nervous system.

6. **Conduct a complete physical examination.**

Clinical Significance

Family and social problems are common problems in this setting.

Cognitive functions may be altered in any person who abuses drugs or alcohol.

Problems associated with substance abuse: bleeding, ulcers, blood in stools, diarrhea, and loose stools.

Problems associated with substance abuse: venereal diseases, altered urinary patterns.

Problems associated with substance abuse: hypertension, chronic obstructive pulmonary disease, chest pain.

Problems associated with solvent inhalation: memory loss, loss of other cognitive functions.

Physical indicators associated with substance abuse: jaundice, ascites, pedal edema, dementia, nystagmus, gait alterations, neurologic alterations, bleeding tendencies.

Documenting the Assessment in the Chemical Dependency Setting

Most of the data obtained by applying the examination guidelines in this section will be recorded as part of the admission database for the person entering a treatment program for chemical dependency. Documentation of this information may be a one-time event rather than a series of sequential chart entries. Most facilities with chemical dependency services have standardized forms on which to record the admission database. An excerpt from one such form is shown in Figure 18-1. Physical examination findings should be recorded using guidelines presented elsewhere in this book.

Nursing Observations   Bladder Retraining

GENERAL APPROACH

Bladder retraining involves interventions to help a person regain control of urinary elimination. Restoring urinary continence not only helps to increase the person's self-esteem and independence, it also saves countless dollars. Urinary incontinence is a leading cause of admissions to long-term care facilities and may contribute to debilitating complications such as infection, loss of skin integrity, and calculi formation. Success rates of up to 75% have been reported for bladder retraining programs, but success depends on the person's motivation and on your ability to devise and implement an individual care plan. To develop an appropriate program, you must first accurately and thoroughly assess the urinary elimination pattern.

Date _____Time _____ Referred by _____ Informant: Patient

Name _____ DOB _____ Age_____

WHY ARE YOU HERE? _____

Aspects affecting impending withdrawal:

1. Drinking history: Date & time of last use _____ Amount _____

   What _____ Length of episode _____

   Pattern of drinking for last year _____

   _____

   _____

   _____

   _____

   In the past, what reactions have you experienced when you stopped drinking?

   _____Tremors _____ Blackouts _____ Pass outs _____ Other _____

   _____ DTs _____ Seizures _____ Hear or see things _____

2. Street drug history: for each drug, list age at first use, pattern over the last year; and date, time and amount of last use:

   _____

   _____

   _____

   _____

   Have you ever used needles?_____ Shared needles? _____

Psychosocial

1. What changes, if any, have you noticed as to the amount of alcohol/chemical it takes to bring about the effect you desire?

   _____More _____Less _____ Same

2. Have you ever been in legal difficulties because of drinking/using? ☐ Y   ☐ N When?_____

   What? _____

3. Have you been hospitalized for alcohol/drug abuse or received treatment? ☐ Y   ☐ N

   Date _____ Place _____

   Length of stay _____ Length of sobriety _____

4. Have you ever been under the care of someone for emotional, behavioral, or depression problems?

   Date _____ Place _____

   Diagnosis _____ Meds _____

5. Have you ever attempted suicide? ☐ Y   ☐ N   Can you tell me about it?_____

   _____

   Do you have a plan now?_____

   _____

   What do you expect to get out of treatment? (in patient's own words)

   _____

   _____

FIGURE 18.1   Chemical dependency data base. An excerpt from an admission data base in a chemical dependency setting illustrating the types of data obtained pertaining to drug/alcohol addiction (courtesy of UniMed Medical Center, Minot, ND.)

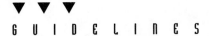

GUIDELINES

Assessment Guidelines   Bladder Retraining

Procedure

1. Identify any causes of incontinence that can be treated medically or surgically or by different nursing or self-care interventions.

2. Determine the person's response to loss of control of urinary elimination.
a. Determine whether the person feels helpless, frustrated, ashamed, or embarrassed.

3. Observe the voiding pattern in relation to fluid intake.
a. Maintain records for 3 days before implementing the bladder retraining program to obtain baseline data about the person's incontinence pattern. Check the person frequently for continence or incontinence, and record these data along with fluid intake data (see Display 18–3 for a tool for recording data).

4. Observe the person's response to trigger point stimulation.
a. Stimulate trigger points, by stroking the thigh, tapping the abdomen, or pulling on pubic hair.

5. Reassess the person's progress throughout the bladder retraining program.
a. If the person does not make progress during retraining, reassess for causes such as inadequate fluid intake or new stressors.

Clinical Significance

Conditions such as urinary tract infections must be resolved before initiating bladder retraining. Some anatomic abnormalities related to incontinence may respond to surgical treatment. For example, cystocele and urethrocele repair may eliminate stress incontinence. Stress and overflow incontinence (secondary to retention) may respond to interventions other than bladder retraining. For example, the person may benefit from exercises that strengthen the pelvic floor muscles or from intermittent self-catheterization.

The person may deny a bladder elimination problem. You must help the patient develop alternative coping strategies before implementing bladder retraining; otherwise, the person may refuse to participate. Cultivating self-esteem is essential for successful retraining. Encourage the person to participate in self-care activities, socialize, and wear his or her own clothes (rather than institution clothes), if appropriate.

Although time consuming, this particular assessment technique is a crucial component of successful bladder retraining for two reasons: First, you can ascertain bladder capacity. The time noted between incontinent episodes, especially during the night when the person is at rest emotionally and physically, indicates how often the person should be taken to toilet facilities during bladder retraining. Second, fluid intake data is important because fluid is needed to stimulate the micturition reflex. A daily fluid intake of 2500 mL is recommended for successful bladder retraining. A limited fluid intake is associated with urinary tract infections, constipation and impactions, and ineffective bladder contraction. However, in some people, such as those with congestive heart failure, fluid intake should be restricted.

Trigger point stimulation may stimulate the bladder to contract and empty, especially in reflex incontinence. Because different trigger points work differently among people, ascertaining methods that help is important for bladder retraining.

Because setbacks are common during bladder retraining, ongoing assessment is essential to identify situations requiring intervention.

DISPLAY 18.3

Bladder Retraining Assessment Tool

	TIME OF DAY	6 AM	8 AM	10 AM	12 AM	2 PM	4 PM	6 PM	8 PM	10 PM	12 PM	2 AM	4 AM
Day and Time	Wet												
	Dry												
Bedtime	Used urinal, commode, or bathroom												
	Amount												
Day and Time	Wet												
	Dry												
Bedtime	Used urinal, commode, or bathroom												
	Amount												
Day and Time	Wet												
	Dry												
Bedtime	Used urinal, commode, or bathroom												
	Amount												
Day and Time	Wet												
	Dry												
Bedtime	Used urinal, commode, or bathroom												
	Amount												

ND_x

Documenting the Bladder-Retraining Program

The documentation focus in a bladder-retraining program is to record data that best illustrate the person's urinary elimination pattern. Regular recording, such as every 2 hours, helps the nurse accurately identify the pattern (see Display 18-3). Once the pattern is well understood, interventions, such as planned toileting, are better planned and implemented.

CHAPTER 18 SUMMARY

Assessment of patients in the special situations addressed in this chapter requires specific selection and application of general assessment methods. This selection is influenced by the manner in which the following questions would be answered for a particular patient:
- What do I need to monitor most carefully for this person?
- Why do I need to monitor these things?

- How often should I evaluate this person?

Presented in this chapter are examination guidelines for the following types of special situations:
- The acute care setting
- Major trauma
- The chemical dependency setting
- Bladder retraining

Critical Thinking

Students are usually taught the particulars of health assessment in great detail, with emphasis on a comprehensive health history and complete physical examination. In practice, however, there may be times when a complete examination is neither indicated nor practical; also, the clinician may encounter situations requiring specialized assessment knowledge that may not have been acquired through a general discussion of assessment principles. Good judgment must be exercised to modify a lengthy and comprehensive assessment. Specialization is required for appropriate assessment in a number of clinical situations.

Learning Exercises

1. Describe an examination sequence and associated procedures you would select to evaluate a stable, postoperative patient on the morning of discharge from the hospital. Explain the essential components of this assessment.

2. Determine and discuss the primary differences between the secondary survey of a trauma victim and a complete head-to-toe physical examination.

3. You are caring for a patient who requires a type of equipment that you and other staff members are not familiar with. Explain how you would ensure that the equipment is functioning properly.

4. Identify and discuss the pros and cons of "charting by exception."

5. A patient admitted for treatment of alcoholism tells you that he does not drink and that his wife had him committed to win sympathy during divorce proceedings. Explain how you would respond.

6. Explain how you would use data about urinary elimination patterns in planning a bladder retraining program.

BIBLIOGRAPHY

Albrecht-Gallauresi, B. (1998). Device errors: Pulse oximeters. *Nursing, 28*(9), 31.

Burns, L., & Adams, M. (1997). Alcohol-history taking by nurses and doctors: How accurate are they really? *Journal of Advanced Nursing, 25*(3), 509–513.

Clarke, A. (1997). The nursing management of intravenous drug therapy. *British Journal of Nursing, 6*(4), 201–206.

Cobble, J.A. (1992). Trauma assessment. *Emergency, 24*(6), 24–28.

Colwell, C.B., & Smith, J. (1985). Determining the use of physical assessment skills in the clinical setting. *Journal of Nursing Education, 24*(8), 333–337.

Dougherty, L. (1997). Reducing the risks of complications in IV therapy. *Nursing Standards, 12*(5), 40–42.

Elder, A.N. (1991). Setting up and using a cardiac monitor. *Nursing, 21*(8), 4, 6.

Gallo, K. & Keane-Guercio, P. (1994). Emergency department assessment of the adult trauma patient. *STNS Journal of Trauma Nursing, 1*(1), 21–32.

Gallauresi, B.A. (1998). Pulse oximeters. *Nursing, 28*(9), 31.

Getliffe, K. (1996). Care of urinary catheters. *Nursing Standards, 11*(11), 47–50.

Hanna, D. (1995). Using pulse oximeters safely. *Nursing, 25*(7), 26.

Hokenson, P. (1994). Assessment of the patient at risk for acute alcohol withdrawal. *Med-Surg Nursing, 3*(3), 211–215, 217.

Keitz, J.E. (1989). Emergent assessment of the multiple trauma patient. *Orthopedic Nursing, 8*(6), 29–32.

Kiernan, M. (1997). Know how—IV insertion sites. *Nursing Times, 93*(37), 72–73.

Kosmos, C.A. (1989). Emergency nursing management of the multiple trauma patient. *Orthopedic Nursing, 8*(6), 33–36.

Lisant, P. (1991). *Substance abuse education in nursing curriculum modules. Module 1-3: Assessment of the adult client for drug and alcohol use.* Project SAEN, Volume 1, NLN Publication #15-2407, 151–247.

Martin, M.M. (1990). Assessing and planning care in substance abusing patients. *SCI Nurse, 7*(3), 76.

McConnell, E.A. (1997). Administering oxygen by mask. *Nursing, 27*(9), 26.

Metheny, N., Wehrle, M.A., Wiersema, L., & Clark, J. (1998). Testing feeding tube placement: Auscultation vs pH method. *American Journal of Nursing, 98*(5), 37–42.

Metheny, N., et al (1993). Effectiveness of pH measurements in predicting feeding tube placement: An update. *Nursing Research, 42*(6), 324–331.

Meusen, M. (1991). What do you think . . . bladder management. *Science of Nursing, 8*(2), 55.

Mergaert, S. (1994). S.T.O.P. and assess chest tubes the easy way. *Nursing, 24*(2), 52–53.

O'Hanlon-Nichols, T. (1996). Commonly asked questions about chest tubes. *American Journal of Nursing, 96*(5), 60–64.

Pettinicchi, T.A. (1998). Trouble shooting chest tubes. *Nursing, 28*(3), 58–59.

Sansivero, G.E. (1997). Taking care of PICCs. *Nursing, 27*(5), 28.

Stewart, E. (1998). Urinary catheters: Selection, maintenance, and nursing care. *British Journal of Nursing, 7*(19), 1152–1154, 1156, 1158–1161.

Sullivan, J.T., Sykora, K., Schneiderman, J., Naranjo, C.A., & Sellers, E.M. (1989). Assessment of alcohol withdrawal: The revised clinical institute withdrawal assessment for alcohol scale (CIWA-Ar). *British Journal of Addiction, 84*(11), 1353–1357.

Williamson, L. (1998). Postoperative care—1. *Nursing Times, 94*(11), 33A–33B.

Williamson, L. (1998). Postoperative care—2. *Nursing Times, 94*(12), suppl 1–2.

Winn, C. (1998). Complications with urinary catheters. *Professional Nurse, 13*(5), s7–s10.

Appendices

APPENDIX A

Recommended Daily Calorie Intake for Adults According to Body Weight and Activity Levels as Defined by the World Health Organization

Recommended Daily Calorie Intake for Adults According to Body Weight and Activity Levels as Defined by the World Health Organization

Body Weight (kg)	Lightly Active* (kcal)	Moderately Active[†] (kcal)	Very Active[‡] (kcal)	Exceptionally Active[§] (kcal)	Body Weight (kg)	Lightly Active* (kcal)	Moderately Active[†] (kcal)	Very Active[‡] (kcal)	Exceptionally Active[§] (kcal)
Men					**Women**				
50	2100	2300	2700	3100	40	1440	1600	1880	2200
55	2310	2530	2970	3410	45	1620	1800	2120	2480
60	2520	2760	3240	3720	50	1800	2000	2350	2750
65	2700	3000	3500	4000	55	2000	2200	2600	3000
70	2940	3220	3780	4340	60	2160	2400	2820	3300
75	3150	3450	4050	4650	65	2340	2600	3055	3575
80	3360	3680	4320	4960	70	2520	2800	3290	3850

*LIGHTLY ACTIVE

Men: Most professional men (lawyers, doctors, accountants, teachers, architects, etc.), office workers, shop workers, unemployed men.

Women: Homemakers in houses with mechanical household appliances, office workers, teachers, most professional women.

[†]MODERATELY ACTIVE

Men: Most men in light industry, students, building workers (excluding heavy laborers), many farmworkers, soldiers not in active service, fishermen.

Women: Most women in light industry, homemakers without mechanical household appliances, students, department store workers.

[‡]VERY ACTIVE

Men: Some agricultural workers, unskilled laborers, forestry workers, army recruits and soldiers in active service, mineworkers, steelworkers.

Women: Some farmworkers (especially in peasant agriculture), dancers, athletes.

[§]EXCEPTIONALLY ACTIVE

Men: Lumberjacks, blacksmiths, rickshaw pullers.

Women: Construction workers.

(After Whitney, E.N., & Cataldo, C.B. [1983]. *Understanding normal and clinical nutrition* (3rd ed.). St. Paul: West Publishing Co)

Recommended Daily Dietary Allowances (RDAs)

Food and Nutrition Board, National Academy of Sciences—National Research Council Recommended Dietary Allowances, Revised 1989*

Category	Age (yr) or Condition	Weight (kg)	Weight (lb)	Height† (cm)	Height† (in)	Protein (g)	Fat-Soluble Vitamins Vitamin A (mg RE)‡	Vitamin D (mg)§	Vitamin E (mg α-TE)‖	Vitamin K (mg)
Infants	0.0–0.5	6	13	60	24	13	375	7.5	3	5
	0.5–1.0	9	20	71	28	14	375	10	4	10
Children	1–3	13	29	90	35	16	400	10	6	15
	4–6	20	44	112	44	24	500	10	7	20
	7–10	28	62	132	52	28	700	10	7	30
Male	11–14	45	99	157	62	45	1000	10	10	45
	15–18	66	145	176	69	59	1000	10	10	65
	19–24	72	160	177	70	58	1000	10	10	70
	25–50	79	174	176	70	63	1000	5	10	80
	51+	77	170	173	68	63	1000	5	10	80
Females	11–14	46	101	157	62	46	800	10	8	45
	15–18	55	120	163	64	44	800	10	8	55
	19–24	58	128	164	65	46	800	10	8	60
	25–50	63	138	163	64	50	800	5	8	65
	51+	65	143	160	63	50	800	5	8	65
Pregnant						60	800	10	10	65
Lactating 1st 6 months						65	1300	10	12	65
Lactating 2nd 6 months						62	1200	10	11	65

*The allowances, expressed as average daily intakes over time, are intended to provide for individual variations among most normal persons as they live in the United States under usual environmental stresses. Diets should be based on a variety of common foods to provide other nutrients for which human requirements have been less well defined. See test for detailed discussion of allowances and of nutrients not tabulated.

†Weights and heights of Reference Adults are actual medians for the U.S. population of the designated age, as reported by NHANES II. The median weights and heights of those under 19 years of age were taken from Hamill et al. (1979) (see pages 16–17). The use of these figures does not imply that the height-to-weight ratios are ideal.

‡Retinol equivalents. 1 retinol equivalent = 1 μg retinol or 6 μg β-carotene. See text for calculation of vitamin A activity of diets as retinol equivalents.

§As cholecalciferol. 10 μg cholecalciferol = 400 IU of vitamin D.

‖α-Tocopherol equivalents. 1 mg d-α tocopherol = 1 α-TE. See text for variation in allowances and calculation of vitamin E activity of the diet as α-tocopherol equivalents.

¶1 NE (niacin equivalent) is equal to 1 mg of niacin or 60 mg of dietary tryptophan.

Reprinted with permission from Recommended Dietary Allowances, 10th edition, © 1989 by the National Academy of Sciences. Published by National Academy Press, Washington, DC.

RECOMMENDED DIETARY ALLOWANCES, USA

Summary Table: Estimated Safe and Adequate Daily Dietary Intakes of Selected Vitamins and Minerals*

Category	Age (yr)	Vitamins Biotin (μg)	Pantothenic Acid (mg)
Infants	0–0.5	10	2
	0.5–1	15	3
Children and adolescents	1–3	20	3
	4–6	25	3–4
	7–10	30	4–5
	11+	30–100	4–7
Adults		30–100	4–7

	Water-Soluble Vitamins						Minerals						
Vita-min C (mg)	Thia-min (mg)	Ribo-flavin (mg)	Niacin (mg NE)¶	Vita-min B₆ (mg)	Fo-late (μg)	Vita-min B₁₂ (μg)	Cal-cium (mg)	Phos-phorus (mg)	Mag-nesium (mg)	Iron (mg)	Zinc (mg)	Iodine (μg)	Sele-nium (μg)
30	0.3	0.4	5	0.3	25	0.3	400	300	40	6	5	40	10
35	0.4	0.5	6	0.6	35	0.5	600	500	60	10	5	50	15
40	0.7	0.8	9	1.0	50	0.7	800	800	80	10	10	70	20
45	0.9	1.1	12	1.1	75	1.0	800	800	120	10	10	90	20
45	1.0	1.2	13	1.4	100	1.4	800	800	170	10	10	120	30
50	1.3	1.5	17	1.7	150	2.0	1200	1200	270	12	15	150	40
60	1.5	1.8	20	2.0	200	2.0	1200	1200	400	12	15	150	50
60	1.5	1.7	19	2.0	200	2.0	1200	1200	350	10	15	150	70
60	1.5	1.7	19	2.0	200	2.0	800	800	350	10	15	150	70
60	1.2	1.4	15	2.0	200	2.0	800	800	350	10	15	150	70
50	1.1	1.3	15	1.4	150	2.0	1200	1200	280	15	12	150	45
60	1.1	1.3	15	1.5	180	2.0	1200	1200	300	15	12	150	50
60	1.1	1.3	15	1.6	180	2.0	1200	1200	280	15	12	150	55
60	1.1	1.3	15	1.6	180	2.0	800	800	280	15	12	150	55
60	1.0	1.2	13	1.6	180	2.0	800	800	280	10	12	150	55
70	1.5	1.6	17	2.2	400	2.2	1200	1200	300	30	15	175	65
95	1.6	1.8	20	2.1	280	2.6	1200	1200	355	15	19	200	75
90	1.6	1.7	20	2.1	260	2.6	1200	1200	340	15	16	200	75

		Trace Elements†				
Category	Age (yr)	Copper (mg)	Manganese (mg)	Fluoride (mg)	Chromium (μg)	Molybdenum (μg)
Infants	0–0.5	0.4–0.6	0.3–0.6	0.1–0.5	10–40	15–30
	0.5–1	0.6–0.7	0.6–1.0	0.2–1.0	20–60	20–40
Children and adolescents	1–3	0.7–1.0	1.0–1.5	0.5–1.5	20–80	25–50
	4–6	1.0–1.5	1.5–2.0	1.0–2.5	30–120	30–75
	7–10	1.0–2.0	2.0–3.0	1.5–2.5	50–200	50–150
	11+	1.5–2.5	2.0–5.0	1.5–2.5	50–200	75–250
Adults		1.5–3.0	2.0–5.0	1.5–4.0	50–200	75–250

*Because there is less information on which to base allowances, these figures are not given in the main table of RDA and are provided here in the form of ranges of recommended intakes.

†Since the toxic levels for many trace elements may be only several times usual intakes, the upper levels for the trace elements given in this table should not be habitually exceeded.

(Craven, R.F., & Hirnle, C.J. [1992]. Fundamentals of nursing. Philadelphia: J.B. Lippincott)

NUTRITION RECOMMENDATIONS FOR CANADIANS

Recommended Nutrient Intake Based on Age and Body Weight Expressed as Daily Rates

Age	Sex	Weight (kg)	Protein (g)	Vit. A (RE*)	Vit. D (μg)	Vit. E (mg)	Vit. C (mg)	Folate (μg)	Vit. B$_{12}$ (μg)	Cal-cium (mg)	Phos-phorus (mg)	Mag-nesium (mg)	Iron (mg)	Iodine (μg)	Zinc (mg)
Months															
0–4	Both	6.0	12†	400	10	3	20	25	0.3	250‡	150	20	0.3§	30	2§
5–12	Both	9.0	12	400	10	3	20	40	0.4	400	200	32	7	40	3
Years															
1	Both	11	13	400	10	3	20	40	0.5	500	300	40	6	55	4
2–3	Both	14	16	400	5	4	20	50	0.6	550	350	50	6	65	4
4–6	Both	18	19	500	5	5	25	70	0.8	600	400	65	8	85	5
7–9	M	25	26	700	2.5	7	25	90	1.0	700	500	100	8	110	7
	F	25	26	700	2.5	6	25	90	1.0	700	500	100	8	95	7
10–12	M	34	34	800	2.5	8	25	120	1.0	900	700	130	8	125	9
	F	36	36	800	2.5	7	25	130	1.0	1100	800	135	8	110	9
13–15	M	50	49	900	2.5	9	30$^{||}$	175	1.0	1100	900	185	10	160	12
	F	48	46	800	2.5	7	30$^{||}$	170	1.0	1000	850	180	13	160	9
16–18	M	62	58	1000	2.5	10	40$^{||}$	220	1.0	900	1000	230	10	160	12
	F	53	47	800	2.5	7	30$^{||}$	190	1.0	700	850	200	12	160	9
19–24	M	71	61	1000	2.5	10	40$^{||}$	220	1.0	800	1000	240	9	160	12
	F	58	50	800	2.5	7	30$^{||}$	180	1.0	700	850	200	13	160	9
25–49	M	74	64	1000	2.5	9	40$^{||}$	230	1.0	800	1000	250	9	160	12
	F	59	51	800	2.5	6	30$^{||}$	185	1.0	700	850	200	13	160	9
50–74	M	73	63	1000	5	7	40$^{||}$	230	1.0	800	1000	250	9	160	12
	F	63	54	800	5	6	30$^{||}$	195	1.0	800	850	210	8	160	9
75+	M	69	59	1000	5	6	40$^{||}$	215	1.0	800	1000	230	9	160	12
	F	64	55	800	5	5	30	200	1.0	800	850	210	8	160	9
Pregnancy (additional)															
1st Trimester		5	0	2.5	2	0	200	0.2	500	200	15	0	25	6	
2nd Trimester		15	0	2.5	2	10	200	0.2	500	200	45	5	25	6	
3rd Trimester		24	0	2.5	2	10	200	0.2	500	200	45	10	25	6	
Lactation (additional)		22	400	2.5	3	25	100	0.2	500	200	65	0	50	6	

*Retinol equivalents.

†Protein is assumed to be from breast milk and must be adjusted for infant formula.

‡Infant formula with high phosphorus should contain 375 mg calcium.

§Breast milk is assumed to be the source of the mineral.

$^{||}$Smokers should increase vitamin C by 50%.

Nutrition Recommendations: The Report of the Scientific Committee 1990, p. 204. Published by the authority of the Minister of National Health and Welfare.

Height and Weight Tables for Adults

Men						Women				
Height						**Height**				
Feet	Inches	Small Frame	Medium Frame	Large Frame		Feet	Inches	Small Frame	Medium Frame	Large Frame
5	2	128–134	131–141	138–150		4	10	102–111	109–121	118–131
5	3	130–136	133–143	140–153		4	11	103–113	111–123	120–134
5	4	132–138	135–145	142–156		5	0	104–115	113–126	122–137
5	5	134–140	137–148	144–180		5	1	106–118	115–129	125–140
5	6	136–142	139–151	146–164		5	2	108–121	118–132	128–143
5	7	138–145	142–154	149–168		5	3	111–124	121–135	131–147
5	8	140–148	145–157	152–172		5	4	114–127	124–138	134–151
5	9	142–151	148–160	155–176		5	5	117–130	127–141	137–155
5	10	144–154	151–163	158–180		5	6	120–133	130–144	140–159
5	11	146–157	154–166	161–184		5	7	123–136	133–147	143–163
6	0	149–160	157–170	164–186		5	8	126–139	136–150	146–167
6	1	152–164	160–174	168–192		5	9	129–142	139–153	149–170
6	2	155–168	164–178	172–197		5	10	132–145	142–156	152–173
6	3	158–172	167–182	176–202		5	11	135–148	145–159	155–176
6	4	162–176	171–187	181–207		6	0	138–151	148–162	158–179

(Source of basic data: 1979 Build Study, Society of Actuaries and Association of Life Insurance Medical Directors of America, 1980. Reprinted from Metropolitan Life Insurance Company, Medical Department, Health and Safety Education Division. Copyright 1900, 1900 Metropolitan Life Insurance Company)

TO APPROXIMATE YOUR FRAME SIZE

Bend arm upward at a 90-degree angle. Keep fingers straight and turn the inside of your wrist toward your body. Place thumb and index finger of your other hand on the two prominent bones on either side of the elbow. Measure space between your fingers on a ruler. (A physician would use a caliper.) Compare with tables below listing elbow measurements for medium-framed men and women. Measurements lower than those listed indicate small frame. Higher measurements indicate large frame.

ELBOW MEASUREMENTS FOR MEDIUM FRAME

Height in 1" Heels Men	Elbow Breadth	Height in 1" Heels Women	Elbow Breadth
5'2"–5'3"	2 1/2"–2 7/8"	4'10"–4'11"	2 1/4"–2 1/2"
5'4"–5'7"	2 5/8"–2 7/8"	5'0"–5'3"	2 1/4"–2 1/2"
5'8"–5'11"	2 3/4"–3"	5'4"–5'7"	2 3/8"–2 5/8"
6'0"–6'3"	2 3/4"–3 1/8"	5'8"–5'11"	2 3/8"–2 5/8"
6'4"	2 7/8"–3 1/4"	6'0"	2 1/2"–2 3/4"

Denver Developmental Screening Test II (DDST2) and Denver Articulation Screening Examination

GENERAL GUIDELINES FOR DDST2

1. Find the child's chronological age on the DDST2 form. Highlight the age line across the form (a ruler is helpful). For children who were born at least 2 weeks premature and are under age 2 years, chronologically subtract the number of weeks of prematurity from the chronological age to find the appropriate testing age.
2. Discuss the test with the parents. Explain that it is not an intelligence test but rather a means of evaluating the child's current level of development and that the child is *not* expected to pass every item.
3. Provide a quiet environment without distractions for testing. It is helpful to approach the screening test as a game. Introduce only one test at a time. Keep all equipment such as blocks and ball in the kit bag until needed because these often distract the child.
4. Test the child for each item intersected by the age line. Instructions for testing each item are provided with the test. Begin with "easy" items listed to the left of the age line to promote initial success and co-operation. The items that require a response from the parent may be asked first to allow both the parent and child to become more comfortable with the surroundings and the nurse.
5. Score items by writing on the form: "P" for *pass*, "F" for *failure*, "NO" for *no opportunity* to perform this skill (can only be used for report items), "R" for *refusal*, and "C" for *caution* (a "C" is always used in combination with an "R" or "F"). Be sure to refer to the back of the form any time a number appears by the skill.
6. Score the screening test by counting the number of delays and cautions identified.

Interpret the results as follows:

For Individual Items

Advanced: Passed an item completely to the right of the age line. The child has passed an item that most children do not pass until older.

Normal: Passed, failed, or refused an item intersected by the age line between the 25th and 75th percentile.

Caution: Failed or refused items intersected by the age line between the 75th and 90th percentile. This is used to note that the child is not performing a task that many younger children can perform.

Delay: Failed an item completely to the left of the age line; refusals to the left of the age line are delays since the refusal may be related to inability to perform the task.

For the Test with Recommendations for Follow-Up

Normal: No delays and no more than one caution for the entire test. Repeat routine screening at next well child assessment.

Abnormal: Two or more delays for the entire test. Refer for diagnostic evaluation.

Questionable: One delay and/or two or more cautions for the entire test. Rescreen in 3 months or at next well child assessment, whichever is first. Refer for diagnostic evaluation if rescreen is questionable or abnormal.

Untestable: This interpretation is based upon the number of refusals. If the number of refusals would equal an abnormal result, the child should be rescreened in 2 or 3 weeks before interpreting the results as abnormal. If the number of refusals equals questionable results, follow-up is the same as for questionable.

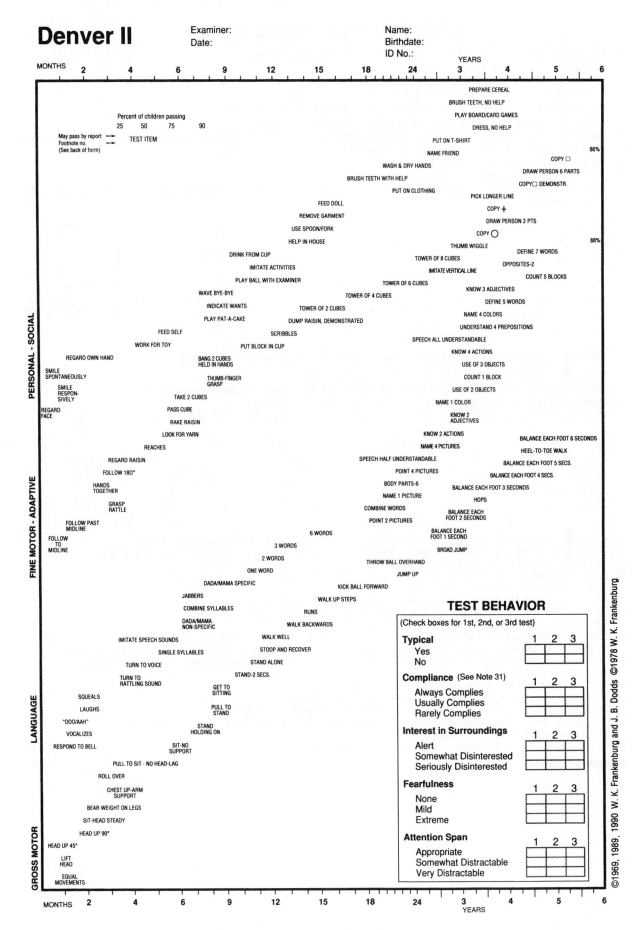

DIRECTIONS FOR ADMINISTRATION

1. Try to get child to smile by smiling, talking or waving. Do not touch him/her.
2. Child must stare at hand several seconds.
3. Parent may help guide toothbrush and put toothpaste on brush.
4. Child does not have to be able to tie shoes or button/zip in the back.
5. Move yarn slowly in an arc from one side to the other, about 8" above child's face.
6. Pass if child grasps rattle when it is touched to the backs or tips of fingers.
7. Pass if child tries to see where yarn went. Yarn should be dropped quickly from sight from tester's hand without arm movement.
8. Child must transfer cube from hand to hand without help of body, mouth, or table.
9. Pass if child picks up raisin with any part of thumb and finger.
10. Line can vary only 30 degrees or less from tester's line. $\diagup$
11. Make a fist with thumb pointing upward and wiggle only the thumb. Pass if child imitates and does not move any fingers other than the thumb.

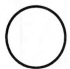

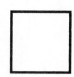

12. Pass any enclosed form. Fail continuous round motions.

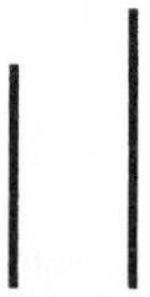

13. Which line is longer? (Not bigger.) Turn paper upside down and repeat. (pass 3 of 3 or 5 of 6)

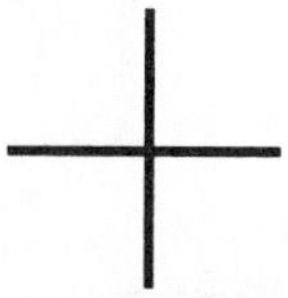

14. Pass any lines crossing near midpoint.

15. Have child copy first. If failed, demonstrate.

When giving items 12, 14, and 15, do not name the forms. Do not demonstrate 12 and 14.

16. When scoring, each pair (2 arms, 2 legs, etc.) counts as one part.
17. Place one cube in cup and shake gently near child's ear, but out of sight. Repeat for other ear.
18. Point to picture and have child name it. (No credit is given for sounds only.)
    If less than 4 pictures are named correctly, have child point to picture as each is named by tester.

 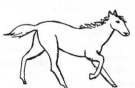 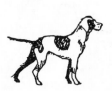 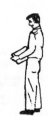

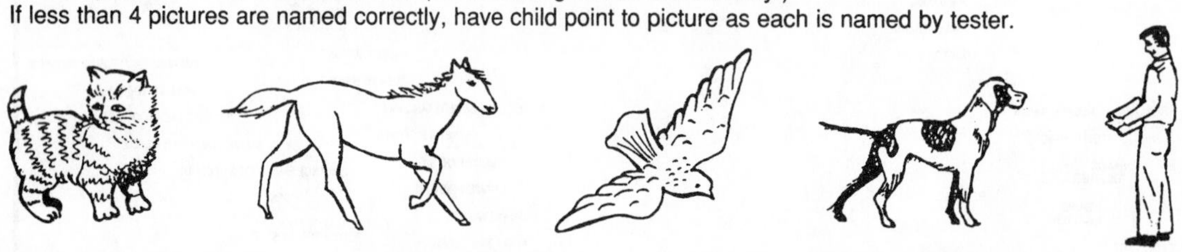

19. Using doll, tell child: Show me the nose, eyes, ears, mouth, hands, feet, tummy, hair. Pass 6 of 8.
20. Using pictures, ask child: Which one flies?... says meow?... talks?... barks?... gallops? Pass 2 of 5, 4 of 5.
21. Ask child: What do you do when you are cold?... tired?... hungry? Pass 2 of 3, 3 of 3.
22. Ask child: What do you do with a cup? What is a chair used for? What is a pencil used for?
    Action words must be included in answers.
23. Pass if child correctly places <u>and</u> says how many blocks are on paper. (1, 5).
24. Tell child: Put block **on** table; **under** table; **in front of** me, **behind** me. Pass 4 of 4.
    (Do not help child by pointing, moving head or eyes.)
25. Ask child: What is a ball?... lake?... desk?... house?... banana?... curtain?... fence?... ceiling? Pass if defined in terms of use, shape, what it is made of, or general category (such as banana is fruit, not just yellow). Pass 5 of 8, 7 of 8.
26. Ask child: If a horse is big, a mouse is __? If fire is hot, ice is __? If the sun shines during the day, the moon shines during the __? Pass 2 of 3.
27. Child may use wall or rail only, not person. May not crawl.
28. Child must throw ball overhand 3 feet to within arm's reach of tester.
29. Child must perform standing broad jump over width of test sheet (8 1/2 inches).
30. Tell child to walk forward, � heel-to-toe symbol⟩ heel within 1 inch of toe. Tester may demonstrate.
    Child must walk 4 consecutive steps.
31. In the second year, half of normal children are non-compliant.

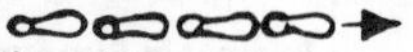

OBSERVATIONS:

Denver Articulation Screening Examination

(For children 2.5 to 6 years of age)

Instructions: Have child repeat each word after you. Circle the underlined sounds that he or she pronounces correctly. Total number of correct sounds is the raw score. Use charts on reverse side to score results.

NAME

HOSPITAL NO.

ADDRESS

Date: _____ Child's age: _____ Examiner: _____ Raw score: _____

Percentile: _____ Intelligibility: _____ Result: _____

1. table	6. zipper	11. sock	16. wagon	21. leaf
2. shirt	7. grapes	12. vacuum	17. gum	22. carrot
3. door	8. flag	13. yarn	18. house	
4. trunk	9. thumb	14. mother	19. pencil	
5. jumping	10. toothbrush	15. twinkle	20. fish	

Intelligibility (circle one): 1. Easy to understand   3. Not understandable
2. Understandable half of the time   4. Cannot evaluate

Comments:

Date: _____ Child's age: _____ Examiner: _____ Raw score: _____

Percentile: _____ Intelligibility: _____ Result: _____

1. table	6. zipper	11. sock	16. wagon	21. leaf
2. shirt	7. grapes	12. vacuum	17. gum	22. carrot
3. door	8. flag	13. yarn	18. house	
4. trunk	9. thumb	14. mother	19. pencil	
5. jumping	10. toothbrush	15. twinkle	20. fish	

Intelligibility (circle one): 1. Easy to understand   3. Not understandable
2. Understandable half of the time   4. Cannot evaluate

Comments:

Date: _____ Child's age: _____ Examiner: _____ Raw score: _____

Percentile: _____ Intelligibility: _____ Result: _____

1. table	6. zipper	11. sock	16. wagon	21. leaf
2. shirt	7. grapes	12. vacuum	17. gum	22. carrot
3. door	8. flag	13. yarn	18. house	
4. trunk	9. thumb	14. mother	19. pencil	
5. jumping	10. toothbrush	15. twinkle	20. fish	

Intelligibility (circle one): 1. Easy to understand   3. Not understandable
2. Understandable half of the time   4. Cannot evaluate

Comments:

(NK Frankenburg, University of Colorado Medical Center, Denver, 1971. Copyright © 1971. Amelia F. Drumwright)

To score DASE words: Note raw score for child's performance. Match raw score line (extreme left of chart) with column representing child's age (to the closest *previous* age group). Where raw score line and age column meet denotes percentile rank of child's performance when compared with other children that age. Percentiles above heavy line are *abnormal*, below heavy line are *normal*.

PERCENTILE RANK

Raw Score	2.5 yr	3.0 yr	3.5 yr	4.0 yr	4.5 yr	5.0 yr	5.5 yr	6 yr
2	1							
3	2							
4	5							
5	9							
6	16							
7	23							
8	31	2						
9	37	4	1					
10	42	6	2					
11	48	7	4					
12	54	9	6	1	1			
13	58	12	9	2	3	1	1	
14	62	17	11	5	4	2	2	
15	68	23	15	9	5	3	2	
16	75	31	19	12	5	4	3	
17	79	38	25	15	6	6	4	
18	83	46	31	19	8	7	4	
19	86	51	38	24	10	9	5	1
20	89	58	45	30	12	11	7	3
21	92	65	52	36	15	15	9	4
22	94	72	58	43	18	19	12	5
23	96	77	63	50	22	24	15	7
24	97	82	70	58	29	29	20	15
25	99	87	78	66	36	34	26	17
26	99	91	84	75	46	43	34	24
27		94	89	82	57	54	44	34
28		96	94	88	70	68	59	47
29		98	98	94	84	84	77	68
30		100	100	100	100	100	100	100

To score intelligibility:

	NORMAL	ABNORMAL
2.5 years	Understandable half of the time or easy to understand	Not understandable
3 years and older	Easy to understand	Understandable half of the time or not understandable

Test result: 1. Normal on DASE and intelligibility = *normal*
2. Abnormal on DASE or intelligibility = *abnormal**

If abnormal on initial screening, rescreen within 2 weeks. If abnormal again, child should be referred for complete speech evaluation.

Infant and Child Growth Charts

BOYS: BIRTH TO 36 MONTHS
PHYSICAL GROWTH
NCHS PERCENTILES*

NAME _____ RECORD # _____

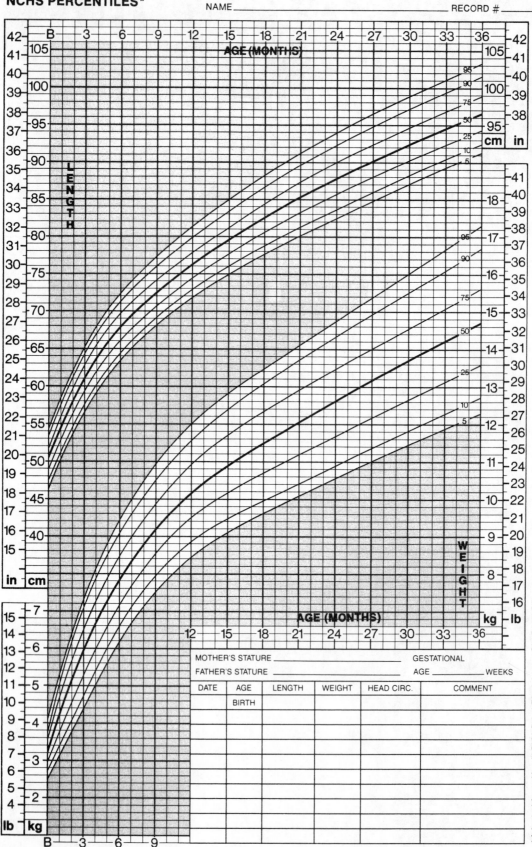

MOTHER'S STATURE _____ GESTATIONAL
FATHER'S STATURE _____ AGE _____ WEEKS

DATE	AGE	LENGTH	WEIGHT	HEAD CIRC.	COMMENT
	BIRTH				

*Adapted from: Hamill PVV, Drizd TA, Johnson CL, Reed RB, Roche AF, Moore WM: Physical growth: National Center for Health Statistics percentiles. AM J CLIN NUTR 32:607-629, 1979. Data from the Fels Longitudinal Study, Wright State University School of Medicine, Yellow Springs, Ohio.

© 1982 Ross Laboratories

BOYS: BIRTH TO 36 MONTHS
PHYSICAL GROWTH
NCHS PERCENTILES*

NAME _____

RECORD # _____

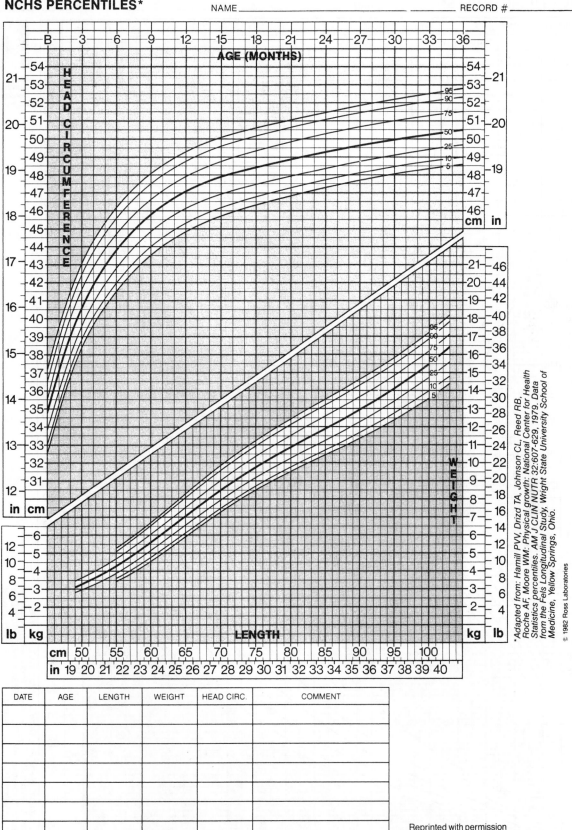

*Adapted from: Hamill PVV, Drizd TA, Johnson CL, Reed RB, Roche AF, Moore WM: Physical growth: National Center for Health Statistics percentiles. AM J CLIN NUTR 32:607-629, 1979. Data from the Fels Longitudinal Study, Wright State University School of Medicine, Yellow Springs, Ohio.

© 1982 Ross Laboratories

DATE	AGE	LENGTH	WEIGHT	HEAD CIRC.	COMMENT

Reprinted with permission
of Ross Laboratories

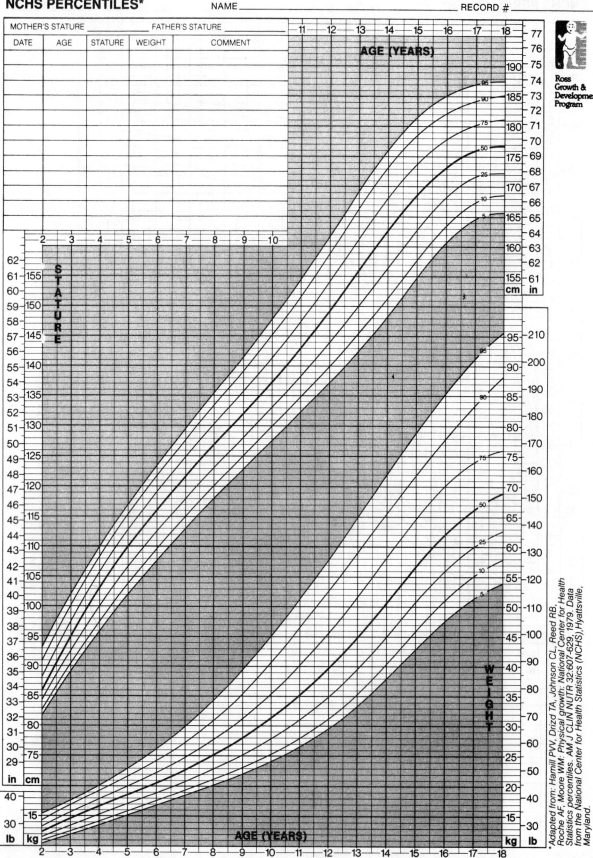

BOYS: 2 TO 18 YEARS
PHYSICAL GROWTH
NCHS PERCENTILES*

NAME _____   RECORD # _____

* Adapted from: Hamill PVV, Drizd TA, Johnson CL, Reed RB, Roche AF, Moore WM: Physical growth: National Center for Health Statistics percentiles. AM J CLIN NUTR 32:607-629, 1979. Data from the National Center for Health Statistics (NCHS), Hyattsville, Maryland.

© 1982 Ross Laboratories

Ross
Growth &
Development
Program

BOYS: PREPUBESCENT PHYSICAL GROWTH NCHS PERCENTILES*

NAME _____   RECORD # _____

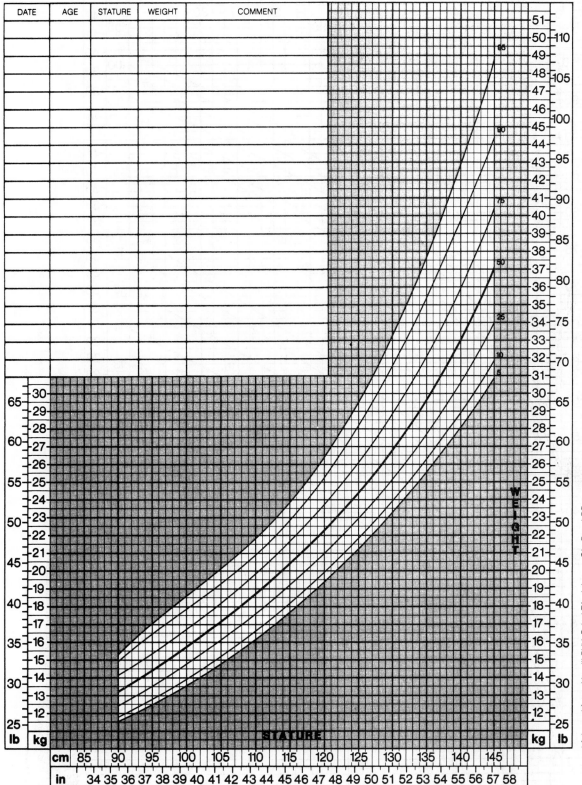

*Adapted from: Hamill PVV, Drizd TA, Johnson CL, Reed RB, Roche AF, Moore WM.: Physical growth: National Center for Health Statistics percentiles. AM J CLIN NUTR 32:607-629, 1979. Data from the National Center for Health Statistics (NCHS), Hyattsville, Maryland.

© 1982 Ross Laboratories

Reprinted with permission
of Ross Laboratories

GIRLS: BIRTH TO 36 MONTHS
PHYSICAL GROWTH
NCHS PERCENTILES*

NAME _____ RECORD # _____

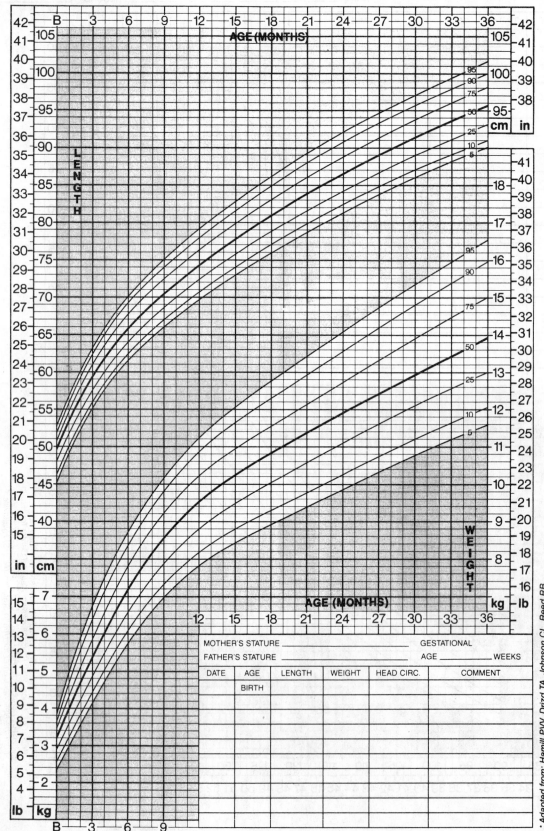

MOTHER'S STATURE _____ GESTATIONAL
FATHER'S STATURE _____ AGE _____ WEEKS

DATE	AGE	LENGTH	WEIGHT	HEAD CIRC.	COMMENT
	BIRTH				

* Adapted from: Hamill PVV, Drizd TA, Johnson CL, Reed RB, Roche AF, Moore WM: Physical growth: National Center for Health Statistics percentiles. AM J CLIN NUTR 32:607–629, 1979. Data from the Fels Longitudinal Study, Wright State University School of Medicine, Yellow Springs, Ohio.

© 1982 Ross Laboratories

GIRLS: BIRTH TO 36 MONTHS
PHYSICAL GROWTH
NCHS PERCENTILES*

NAME _____ RECORD # _____

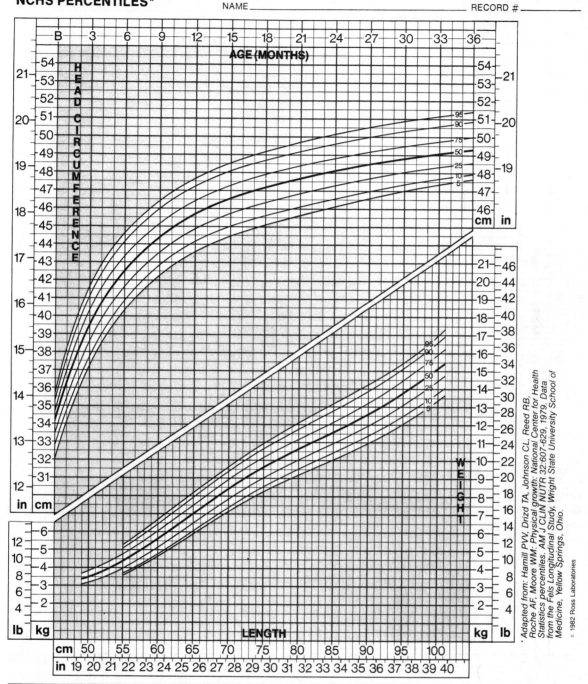

*Adapted from: Hamill PVV, Drizd TA, Johnson CL, Reed RB, Roche AF, Moore WM: Physical growth: National Center for Health Statistics percentiles. AM J CLIN NUTR 32:607-629, 1979. Data from the Fels Longitudinal Study, Wright State University School of Medicine, Yellow Springs, Ohio.

© 1982 Ross Laboratories

DATE	AGE	LENGTH	WEIGHT	HEAD CIRC.	COMMENT

Reprinted with permission of Ross Laboratories

GIRLS: 2 TO 18 YEARS
PHYSICAL GROWTH
NCHS PERCENTILES*

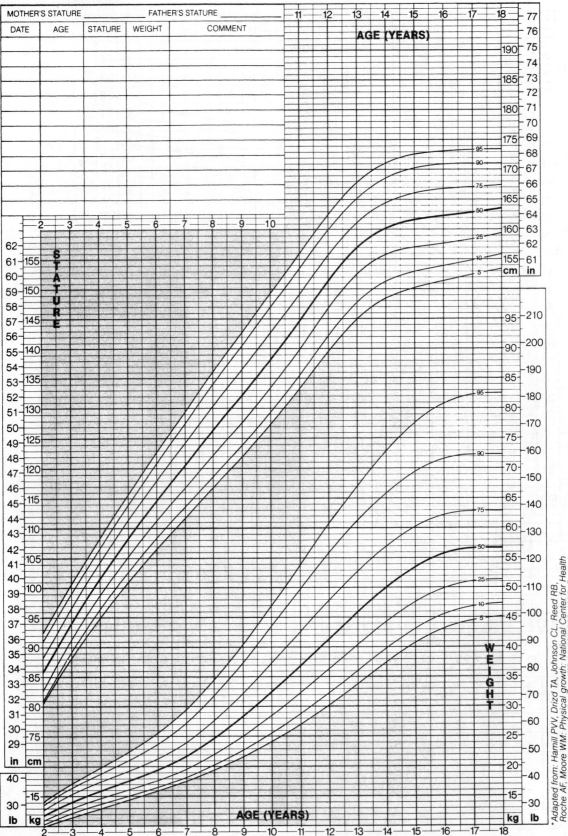

*Adapted from: Hamill PVV, Drizd TA, Johnson CL, Reed RB, Roche AF, Moore WM: Physical growth: National Center for Health Statistics percentiles. AM J CLIN NUTR 32:607-629, 1979. Data from the National Center for Health Statistics (NCHS), Hyattsville, Maryland.

© 1982 Ross Laboratories

**GIRLS: PREPUBESCENT
PHYSICAL GROWTH
NCHS PERCENTILES***

NAME _____ RECORD # _____

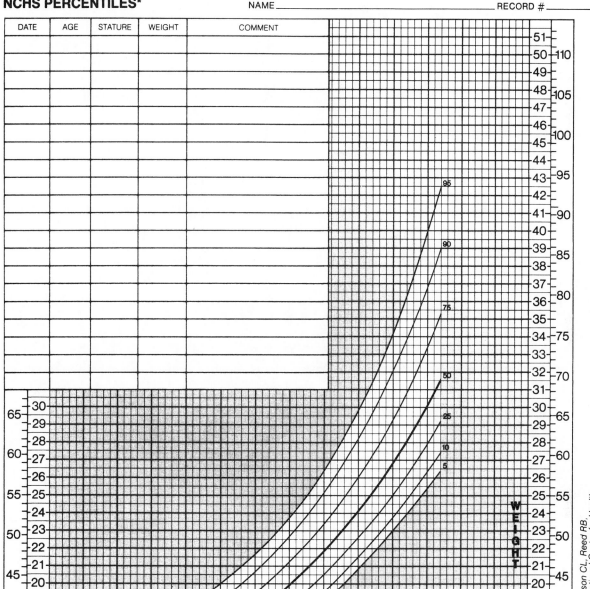

*Adapted from: Hamill PVV, Drizd TA, Johnson CL, Reed RB, Roche AF, Moore WM: Physical growth: National Center for Health Statistics percentiles. AM J CLIN NUTR 32:607-629, 1979. Data from the National Center for Health Statistics (NCHS) Hyattsville, Maryland.

© 1982 Ross Laboratories

Reprinted with permission of Ross Laboratories

Flowsheet for Documenting Assessment Findings in the Acute Care Setting

ASSESSMENT PARAMETERS: Circle appropriate word on assessment items. All abnormal findings must be elaborated on in additional charting.

DATE:	NIGHTS	DAYS	EVENINGS
NEUROLOGICAL: Alert and oriented x 3. Equal strength to extremities and coordinated movement. Speech clear. Swallowing intact.	WNL / Abnormal Unassesed _____	WNL / Abnormal Unassesed _____	WNL / Abnormal Unassesed _____
CARDIOVASCULAR: Regular apical pulse. Denies CP. Peripheral pulses palpable. No edema noted.	WNL Abnormal Telemetry Unassessed	WNL Abnormal Telemetry Unassessed	WNL Abnormal Telemetry Unassessed
RESPIRATORY: Resp. 10-24 per min. at rest. Resp. even and unlabored. Good air exchange. Lungs clear. Nail beds pink. Oxygen: Inspirometer/Tidal Volume:	WNL Abnormal Unassessed _____ _____	WNL Abnormal Unassessed _____ _____	WNL Abnormal Unassessed _____ _____
GASTROINTESTINAL: Abd. soft. Bowel sounds present x 4. No pain or tenderness with palpation. Diet tolerated without nausea or emesis. note NG, if applicable.	WNL / Abnormal / Unassessed _____ _____ _____	WNL / Abnormal / Unassessed _____ _____ _____	WNL / Abnormal / Unassessed _____ _____ _____
BOWEL ELIMINATION: Stool/Ostomy:	☐ Y ☐ N WNL Abnormal _____	☐ Y ☐ N WNL Abnormal _____	☐ Y ☐ N WNL Abnormal _____
GENITOURINARY: Able to empty bladder without dysuria. No bladder distension after voiding. Urine clear yellow to amber. No abnormal vaginal/penile drng. CBI's:	WNL / Abnormal Catheter Unassessed _____ _____	WNL / Abnormal Catheter Unassessed _____ _____	WNL / Abnormal Catheter Unassessed _____ _____
MUSCULOSKELETAL: Normal ROM to all joints. Absence of swelling or tenderness. No muscle weakness observed.	WNL Abnormal Unassessed	WNL Abnormal Unassessed	WNL Abnormal Unassessed
NEUROVASCULAR: Extremities pink, warm with normal mobility. No numbness or tingling reported. Peripheral pulses palpable. Neg. Homan's sign.	WNL _____ Abnormal_____ Unassessed _____ TEDS/Aces/SCD	WNL _____ Abnormal_____ Unassessed _____ TEDS/Aces/SCD	WNL _____ Abnormal_____ Unassessed _____ TEDS/Aces/SCD
INTEGUMENTARY: Skin W/D, pink. Note deviations from patients normal	WNL / Abnormal / Unassessed _____	WNL / Abnormal / Unassessed _____	WNL / Abnormal / Unassessed _____
WOUND: Dry/Intact: Changed: Wound Appearance:	_____ _____ _____	_____ _____ _____	_____ _____ _____
PHYSICAL COMFORT: Pain Medication: Time: Patient Response:	Severe/Moderate/Mild _____ _____ _____	Severe/Moderate/Mild _____ _____ _____	Severe/Moderate/Mild _____ _____ _____
Signature:			

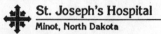 St. Joseph's Hospital
Minot, North Dakota

Medical/Surgical Flowsheet

881-2-560
1-92, 11-92

ASSESSMENT PARAMETERS: Circle appropriate word on assessment items. All abnormal findings must be elaborated on in additional charting.

DATE:	NIGHTS	DAYS	EVENINGS
NUTRITION: Placement Checked: Residual:	Tube Fdg? ☐ Y ☐ N N/A ☐ Y ☐ N Amt._____Time_____ Amt._____Time_____ Other_____	Tube Fdg? ☐ Y ☐ N N/A ☐ Y ☐ N Amt._____Time_____ Amt._____Time_____ Other_____	Tube Fdg? ☐ Y ☐ N N/A ☐ Y ☐ N Amt._____Time_____ Amt._____Time_____ Other_____
TUBES: Type: Location:	_____ _____	_____ _____	_____ _____
IV INFUSIONS: No reaction at site. No swelling or tenderness noted. Fluids infusing without difficulty Location:	WNL_____ Abnormal_____ IV/Lock/Dsg_____ _____	WNL_____ Abnormal_____ IV/Lock/Dsg_____ _____	WNL_____ Abnormal_____ IV/Lock/Dsg_____ _____
SLEEP/REST:	_____	_____	_____
ACTIVITY: Type: Assist of: Tolerance/gait:	_____ _____ _____ TCDB q2H ☐ Y ☐ N ☐ Self	_____ _____ _____ TCDB q2H ☐ Y ☐ N ☐ Self	_____ _____ _____ TCDB q2H ☐ Y ☐ N ☐ Self
SAFETY PRECAUTIONS: Side rails x2, bed low & locked, call light & table in reach, slippers & room in order	WNL	WNL	WNL
PATIENT EDUCATION/ DISCHARGE	re: _____ _____ Family present ☐ Y ☐ N	re: _____ _____ Family present ☐ Y ☐ N	re: _____ _____ Family present ☐ Y ☐ N
SPIRITUAL/ PSYCHOSOCIAL: Mood/Attitude:	_____ _____	_____ _____	_____ _____
SPECIAL EQUIPMENT:	K-pad CPM_____° Eggcrate Trapeze Other_____ _____	K-pad CPM_____° Eggcrate Trapeze Other_____ _____	K-pad CPM_____° Eggcrate Trapeze Other_____ _____
SIGNATURE:			

Nurses Notes: _____

_____

_____

_____

_____

_____

_____

_____

_____

_____

_____

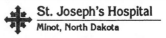

St. Joseph's Hospital
Minot, North Dakota

Medical/Surgical Flowsheet
881-2-560
1-92, 11-92

Trauma Flowsheet

T R A U M A	T E A M	MEMBERS	ETC PHYSICIAN	TRAUMA SURGEON	NEUROSURGEON	ANESTHESIA	CONSULT MD: TYPE:	CONSULT MD: TYPE:	ETC RN TRAUMA RN	MED RN / SURG RN	ICU RN	PASTORAL CARE
		Name										
		Time of arrival in ETC										

PRE-HOSPITAL DATA AND TREATMENT

DESCRIPTION OF INCIDENT

Time of Incident_____

Time of Arrival (ETA)_____

Trauma I activated ☐

FLUID RESUSCITATION PTA

TIME	FLUID TYPE	VOLUME	OUTPUT

MODE OF TRANSPORTATION
☐ Fire Rescue
☐ Police
☐ Ambulance
☐ Air Ambulance
☐ Self
☐ Other _____

TRANSPORT FROM
☐ Scene   ☐ Home
☐ Hospital _____
☐ Other _____

RESTRAINTS
☐ Seat Belt   ☐ NA
☐ Air Bags   ☐ Child Seat
☐ Air Bag & Belt   ☐ None
☐ Helmet   ☐ Unknown
☐ Padding/Protective Gear

MECHANISM OF INJURY
☐ Pedestrian
☐ Motor Vehicle Occupant
☐ Driver   ☐ Thrown from Vehicle
☐ Rollover
☐ Passenger - Front Seat
☐ Passenger - Back Seat
☐ Motorcycle
   ☐ Driver   ☐ Passenger
☐ Pickup Truck   ☐ Semi/Bus
☐ Gun Shotgun
   Calibre/Gauge_____
☐ Fall from Height_____feet
☐ Farming Accident
☐ Industrial Accident
☐ Burn
☐ Explosion
☐ Other_____
☐ Recreational Accident
   ☐ Bicycle
   ☐ All Terrain Vehicle (ATV)
   ☐ Horse
   ☐ Snow Ski
   ☐ Water Ski
   ☐ Tubing/Sledding
   ☐ Diving
   ☐ Other_____

VITAL SIGNS

TIME	BLOOD PRESSURE Manual Cuff	A/L or Autocuff	PULSE	RESP.	TEMP.	CARDIAC RHYTHM	OXIMETER	PUPILS R	L

TIME - Pre-Hospital/Medication-Dose-Route-Site By

PRE-HOSPITAL TREATMENT

1	Airway Inserted	13a	I.V._____gauge
2	Assisted Ventilation	14	Central Line
3	Bleeding Controlled	15	Intraosseous Access
4	Burn Care	16	P.A.S.G. Inflated
5	Cervical Immobilization	17	P.A.S.G. Not Inflated
6	CPR	18	N.G. Tube
7	Defib._____	19	O.B. Care
8	External Pacemaker	20	Oxygen - Mask
9	Cricothyroidotomy	21	Oxygen - Cannula
10	Endotracheal Intub.	23	Needle Thoracentisis
11	Esophageal Obturator	24	Spinal Immobilization
12	Turn on Side	25	Splinting
13	I.V._____gauge	26	Suctioning

REVISED TRAUMA SCORE

		GLASGOW		Pre-Hospital	Arrival in ETC	Discharge from ETC
C O M A S C A L E	A Eyes Open	Spontaneous	= 4			
		To Voice	= 3			
		To Pain	= 2			
		None	= 1			
	B Best Verbal Response	Oriented	= 5			
		Confused	= 4			
		Inapprop. Words	= 3			
		Incomprehen. Sounds	= 2			
		None	= 1			
	C Best Motor Response	Obeys Commands	= 6			
		Localizes to Pain	= 5			
		Withdraws to Pain	= 4			
		Abn. Flex.-decorticate	= 3			
		Abn. Ext.-decerebrate	= 2			
		Flaccid	= 1			

(A + B + C) = D GCS TOTAL_____

E Glasgow Conversion Score	13 - 15 = 4			
	9 - 12 = 3			
	6 - 8 = 2			
	4 - 5 = 1			
	> 4 = 0			

F Respiratory Rate	10 - 24/min 4			
	25 - 35/min 3			
	> 35/min 2			
	1 - 9/min 1			
	None 0			

G Systolic Blood Pressure No Pulse = no carotid pulse	90mmHG 4			
	70-89mmHg 3			
	50-88 mmHg 2			
	0 - 49 mmHg 1			
	No Pulse 0			

Trauma Score (E + F + G)			

_____
Recorder of Pre-Hospital Data

✠ **St. Joseph's Hospital**
Minot, North Dakota

Trauma Flow Sheet
Page One

678-1-018
2-93

PRIMARY ASSESSMENT

AIRWAY: ☐ Clear ☐ Obstructed ☐ Partially Obstructed
C-SPINE: ☐ Immobilized
BREATHING: ☐ Normal ☐ Labored ☐ Apneic
CIRCULATION: ☐ Pulse Present ☐ Cardiac Rate_____
                            Rhythm_____
HEMORRHAGE: ☐ None ☐ Location
NEURO: ☐ Alert ☐ Responds to Verbal stimuli
            ☐ Responds to Pain ☐ Unresponsive

LAB

		TIME DRAWN			TIME DRAWN
☐	CBC	_____	☐	BA	_____
☐	MD-20	_____	☐	T & S	_____
☐	UA	_____	☐	T & XM	_____
☐	PT/PTT	_____	☐	# OF UNITS	_____
☐	CPK	_____	☐	MISC	_____
☐	AMYLASE	_____	☐	MISC	_____
☐	BETA CG	_____	☐	ABG	_____
☐	TOX	_____	☐	EKG	_____

FLUID RESUSCITATION

TIME	NO.	IV FLUID-SITE-SIZE	BY	AMT. INF

Current Medications _____

_____

_____

Allergies _____

_____

PMHx _____

Menstrual Hx _____

Tetanus Status _____

Last Meal _____

Private MD _____

MEDICATION GIVEN

MEDICATION GIVEN	DOSE	ROUTE	TIME	TIME	GIVEN BY
Tetanus and Diphtheria Toxoids	0.5 CC	IM	N/A		

X-RAYS

STUDIES	PORTABLE	IN DEPT.	TIME IN	TIME OUT
☐ C-Spine	☐	☐	____	____
☐ Chest	☐	☐	____	____
☐ Pelvis	☐	☐	____	____
☐ Abdomen	☐	☐	____	____
Extremities - specify				
☐ #1_____	☐	☐	____	____
☐ #2_____	☐	☐	____	____
☐ IVP		☐	____	____
☐ CT HEAD		☐	____	____
☐ CT ABDOMEN		☐	____	____
Oral Contrast	☐ Yes	☐ No	_____cc	
Other - specify				
☐ #1_____	☐	☐	____	____
☐ #2_____	☐	☐	____	____

PROCEDURE

PROCEDURE	TIME	APPEARANCE/RESPONSE
O2		
Endotracheal intub.		
Cricothyroidotomy		
C-collar		
Backboard		
C-monitor		
I.V. access		
I.V. access		
Central I.V.		
Arterial line		
NG tube Size: ____		
Foley Size: ____		
Peritoneal lavage		
Chest tube size ____	Site:	
Chest tube size ____	Site:	

VITAL SIGNS

TIME	BLOOD PRESSURE Manual Cuff	A/L or Autocuff	PULSE	RESP.	TEMP.	CARDIAC RHYTHM	OXIMETER	PUPILS R	L	GCS E	V	M	Total

_____
M.D. Ordering Tests / Procedures

_____
Recorder of Page Two

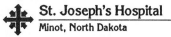

St. Joseph's Hospital
Minot, North Dakota

Trauma Flow Sheet
Page Two

678-1-018
2-93

SECONDARY ASSESSMENT

NEURO
- ☐ No Impairment
- Pupil Size in mm L _____ R _____

● ● ● ● ● · ·
7 6 5 4 3 2 1

(+) Reacts   (—) No Reaction   (c) Closed d/t edema

Evident Deficits _____
Evident Trauma _____

HEAD
- ☐ No Evident Trauma
- ☐ Check for Contacts Removed: ☐ Yes ☐ No ☐ N/A

Evident Trauma _____

NECK
- ☐ No Evident Trauma
- ☐ Spinal Immobilization

Evident Trauma _____

CHEST
- ☐ No Evident Trauma
- Breath Sounds _____
- Crepitus _____

Evident Trauma _____

ABDOMEN
- ☐ No Evident Trauma
- Bowel Sounds _____

Evident Trauma _____

PELVIS
- ☐ No Evident Trauma
- Blood at meatus: ☐ Yes ☐ No   Urine Color _____

Evident Trauma _____

EXTREMITIES
- ☐ No Evident Trauma
- Distal Pulses/Cap Refill _____

Evident Trauma _____

BACK
Evident Trauma _____

FRONT **BACK**

R   L   L   R

LEGEND

A	Abrasion	F	Fracture
Am	Amputation	Fb	Foreign Body
Av	Avulsion	GS	GSW/SGW
B	Burn	H	Hematoma
C	Ecchymosis	L	Laceration
E	Edema	S	Stab/Puncture

INTAKE AND OUTPUT

CRYSTALLOID	BLOOD	COLLOID	OTHER	OTHER	INTAKE
URINE	NG	CHEST	EBL	OTHER	OUTPUT

Total

DISPOSITION AND DISCHARGE PLAN

☐ DC ☐ TRANSFER ☐ ADMIT ☐ OR ☐ EXPIRED ☐ AMA
REPORT CALLED TO _____ RN ___ UNIT _____ TIME _____
TRANSPORT: ☐ SELF ☐ FAMILY/SO ☐ CAB ☐ WC ☐ GURNEY
OTHER ☐ _____
TRANSFER: ACCEPTING MD _____ TIME _____
ACCEPTING HOSPITAL _____
TIME OF DISCHARGE FROM ETC _____
CONDITION ON DC: ☐ SAME ☐ IMPROVED ☐ DETERIORATED ☐ EXPIRED

TIME	NURSING NARRATIVE

Nurse's Signature

✠ **St. Joseph's Hospital**
Minot, North Dakota

Trauma Flow Sheet
Page Three

678-1-018
2-93

INDEX

Note: Page numbers in *italics* indicate illustrations; those followed by *t* indicate tables; and those followed by *d* indicate display material.

A

ABCD formula, for skin cancer diagnosis, 199
Abdomen
  anatomy and physiology of, 211
  assessment of, 88–89, 211–224
    by auscultation, 212, 213, 216–217
    in bedside examination, 706
    clinical problems related to, 214–225
    documentation of, 214
    in elders, 697
    in elimination assessment, 263
    equipment for, 213
    in infant, 667
    by inspection, 215–216
    landmarks in, 211, *212*
    in newborn, 654–655
    nursing diagnoses for, 214
    in older child and adolescent, 676
    overview of, 213–214
    by palpation, 213, 220
    by percussion, 213, 217–220
    positioning for, 213
    preparation for, 213
    sequence in, 213
    in trauma survey, 726
    in young child, 672
  contours of, 215–216, *216*
  measurement of, 213
  peritoneum in, 212
  in pregnancy, 564d
  regions of, 211, *212*
  vasculature of, 212–213
Abdominal aorta, 212–213
Abdominal bruit, 217
Abdominal fluid, evaluation of, 223–224
Abdominal hernia, 215
Abdominal masses
  palpable, 221
  visible, 215–216, *216*
Abdominal muscles, 220
  spasm of, 224
Abdominal pain. *See also* Pain
  in appendicitis, 224
  in bowel obstruction, 224–225
  in diverticulitis, 224
  epigastric tenderness and, 214
  in gallbladder disease, 224
  in gastritis, 214
  on palpation, 221
  in paralytic ileus, 2257
  in peptic ulcer disease, 214–224
  in peritoneal injury, 212
  rebound tenderness and, 212, 221
Abdominal reflex, 411
Abducens nerve, 80, 402t, 403
Abduction, 340
Abscess, lung, 337
Absorption, of nutrients, 155
Abstract thinking, 386
Abuse, 509
  child, 506, 509
    assessment for, 506
    risk factors for, 130d
  elder, 509, 693, 700
  sexual, 526, 527d
  spousal, 509
    risk factors for, 130d
Accessory nerve, 402t, 406
Accident prevention, 128–131. *See also* Safety assessment
  for children, 631

Accommodation, pupillary, 423, 429
Acculturation, 611d
Achieved roles, 493
Achilles reflex, 410
Acne vulgaris, 190
Acoustic blinking reflex, 662t
Acoustic nerve, 402t, 405
Acquired immunodeficiency syndrome (AIDS), 550t. *See also* Human immunodeficiency virus (HIV) infection
Acrochordons, 696
Actinic keratosis, 199
Action inhibition, in coping, 591
Activities of daily living (ADLs), in elderly, 691, *691,* 692d
Activity and exercise
  aerobic capacity and, 284
  assessment of, 281–366
    in cardiac disease, 284–286
    cardiovascular assessment in, 291–292, 296–322, 365–366
    case study of, 365–366
    in children, 632
    clinical problems related to, 287–295
    data collection for, 282
    diagnostic studies in, 291–293
    focus for, 282
    guidelines for, 282
    interview and history taking in, 284–286, 288d, 289–290
    knowledge base for, 283–365
    metabolic equivalents in, 284–286, 285t
    musculoskeletal assessment in, 293, 338–366
    nursing diagnoses for, 287
    pattern assessment guidelines for, 284–285
    physical examination in, 284–286, 293–294
    physiologic basis for, 283–284
    respiratory assessment in, 325–338
    self-evaluation in, 286, 287d
  bladder elimination and, 249
  bowel elimination and, 245
  diet and, 157–158
  in elders, 691, 692d
  as functional health pattern, 9
  heart rate during, 283t, 283–284
  oxygen delivery during, 283
  physiologic response to, 283–284
  temperature variations and, 101
Activity and exercise assessment, in elderly, 691, 698
Activity intolerance, 287
Activity tolerance
  assessment of, 288d, 290
  classification of, 294
Acute care, assessment in, 704, 705–706
Acute gastroenteritis, 265
Acute pain, 397–398
Acute renal failure, 268
Adaptive aids, for elderly, 691, *691*
Adduction, 340
A-delta fibers, 393
Adherence, to prescribed health regimens, 127–128, 148–149
Adiadochokinesia, 421
Adnexa, 534
Adolescents. *See also* Children; Pediatric health assessment
  common health problems in, 678
  communication with, 32
  eating disorders in, 165, 180, 678
  as parents, 509

physical examination in, 675–678
  puberty in, 634, 634t, 635t
  relationships of, 636
  sexuality in, 634–635
  sleep patterns in, 633
  social development in, 636
Adult respiratory distress syndrome (ARDS), 337
Advanced practice nurse practitioner, 5
Adventitious breath sounds, 336d
Adynamic ileus, 225
Aerobic capacity, 284
Affect, flat, 389
African Americans. *See also under* Cultural; Culture
  health and illness concepts of, 612, 613
  health risks for, 614t
Age
  assessment of, 91
  body temperature and, 101
Age spots, 696
Aging. *See also* Elders
  normal
    vs. drug effects, 687
    vs. pathologic, 687
    variations in, 687
Agnosia, 416
Agoraphobia, 509
AIDS, 550t. *See also* Human immunodeficiency virus (HIV) infection
Airway clearance, ineffective, 337
Albumin, nutritional status and, 172
Alcohol use/abuse, *732*
  by adolescents, 674
  assessment in, 705, 727–731
  history in, 44–45, 730, *732*
  sexual function and, 525d
  skin changes in, 198
  sleep and, 464
Alert state, 382
Allen test, 317
Allergic contact dermatitis, 200
Allergies
  food, 165–166
  in infants, 661
Alpha-fetoprotein, prenatal test for, 530
Altered family processes, 506
Altered growth and development, 147
Altered health maintenance, 147
Altered nutrition:less than body requirements, 179–180
Altered nutrition:more than body requirements, 180
Altered parent-infant attachment, 507
Altered parenting, 506–507
Altered protection, 148
Altered sexuality pattern, 531–532
  in pregnancy, 569–570
Altered thought processes, 391
Altered tissue perfusion, 320–321
Alveolar-capillary membrane, 325, 330
Amblyopia, 670
Amnesia
  anterograde, 387
  retrograde, 387
Amniocentesis, 530
Amphiarthroses, 339
Amyl nitrate, sexual function and, 525d
Anabolism, 156
Anaerobic metabolism, 283
Anal canal, 268, *269*
  palpation of, 273

Anal examination, 264, 268–276, 273. *See also* Rectal examination
in elders, 697
in infant, 668
in newborn, 658
Analgesia, 422
Anal masses, 274
Anal sphincters, *239*, 240, 268, *269*
examination of, 273
Anal structure and function, 268, *269*
Anemia, 291
iron-deficiency, 172–173
Aneroid manometer, 116
Anesthesia, 417
Aneurysm, dissecting aortic, 294
Angel kisses, 659
Angina, 294
bedside assessment of, 708
Angiogram, 292
Angioma
cherry, 188, 696
spider, 188
Angry patients, interviewing of, 33–34
Ankle, examination of, 361–363
Anomic aphasia, 392t
Anorectal junction, 269, *269*
Anorexia nervosa, 165, 180, 674
Anterior chamber, 422, *423*
examination of, 430
Anterior spinocerebellar tract, 414
Anterior spinothalamic tract, 414–415
Anterograde amnesia, 387
Anthropometric assessment, 174–179
in children, 631–632
height measurement in, 174
in infant, 663
in older child and adolescent, 675
in young child, 670
length measurement in, in newborn, 647
weight assessment in, 165, 174–178. *See also* Weight
body mass index for, 175
in elders, 695, 695t, 696t
ideal body weight method for, 175
in infant, 663
life insurance tables for, 176
midarm muscle circumference in, 176–177, 178
in newborn, 647
in older child and adolescent, 675
triceps skinfold in, 177–178
weight range tables for, 158, 158d, 175
in young child, 670
Anticipatory grieving, 603
Antidepressants, sexual function and, 525d
Antihistamines, sexual function and, 525d
Antihypertensives, sexual function and, 525d
Antispasmodics, sexual function and, 525d
Anus. *See also under* Anal
examination of, 268–276
in elders, 697
in infant, 668
in newborn, 658
structure and function of, 268, *269*
Anxiety
acute, 92
vs. fear, 486–487
interviewing and, 34
Aorta, abdominal, 213
Aortic aneurysm, dissecting, 294
Aortic area, 302, *302, 303*
Aortic regurgitation, 310
Aortic stenosis, 310
Apgar score, 642, 642t, 644
Aphasia, 509
Broca's, 388, 392t, 509
differential diagnosis of, 392t
Wernicke's, 387, 392t
Aphthous stomatitis, 209
Apical area, 302, *302, 303*
Apical pulse, 110, *110,* 304
Apley's test, 361
Apnea, 114d
sleep, 459–460, 469
Apocrine sweat glands, 181, *181*
Appendicitis, 224
Apraxia, 388
Arcus senilis, 699
Areolae, 551
Arterial blood, pH of, 292
Arterial blood gas values, 292
Arterial insufficiency, 321
Arterial occlusion
acute, 322
skin changes in, 199
Arterial pulses. *See* Pulse(s)

Arteries, 297
Arteriogram, 292
Arthritis
degenerative, 364–365
rheumatoid, 365
Arthrography, 293
Ascites, 223–224
nutritional status and, 172, 178
Ascribed roles, 493
Asian Americans. *See also under* Cultural; Culture
health and illness concepts of, 612–613
health risks for, 614t
Aspiration
of foreign object, 338
high risk for, 146
Assessment. *See* Health assessment
Assimilation, 611d, 618
Asthenics, 93
Asthma, 337
Ataxia, 114d
Ataxic gait, 345d
Atherosclerosis
risk factors for, 130d
screening for, 138, 139
Athlete's foot, 200
Atonic bladder, 241
Atopic dermatitis, 668
Atopic eczema, 189
Atrial kick, 299
Atrial systole, 298–299
Atrioventricular node, 297, *298*
Atrioventricular valves, *299,* 299–300
Atrophy
muscle, 341
in malnutrition, 178
skin, 187, 336
Auditory meatus, 438, *439*
Aura, 381
Auricle, 438, *439*
Auscultation, 69. *See also specific structures auscultated*
of abdomen, 212, 213, 216–217
in blood pressure measurement, *113,* 113–115
of breath sounds, 334–335, 336d
of carotid artery, 315
of femoral artery, 315
of fetal heart sounds, 569
of heart, 298, 305–311. *See also* Heart, examination of; Heart sounds
of Korotkoff sounds, *113,* 113–115
over precordium, 305, 311
of pulse, 110. *See also* Pulse(s), assessment of
stethoscope for, 71, *71*
of voice transmission, 335
Auscultatory gap, 115
Awareness, 371, 385
Axilla, examination of, 86
Axillary nodes, 557
Axillary temperature, 103, 105. *See also* Body temperature

B

Babinski reflex, 412, 413, 662t
Baby. *See* Infant; Newborn
Back. *See also under* Spinal; Spine
assessment of, 86–87
in bedside examination, 706
in infant, 666
in newborn, 652
in trauma survey, 726
Bacterial infections, of skin, 199
Baekeland-Hoy Sleep Log, 459t
Balance, 379, 380
Ball and socket joints, 340
Ballottement
abdominal, 224
patellar, 360
Barbiturates, sexual function and, 525d
Barium enema, 251
Barlow's test, 655, 656
Barthel Index, 695
Bartholin's glands, 533
palpation of, 539–540
Basal cell carcinoma, 199
Basal metabolic rate (BMR), 155
Bayley Scales of Infant Development, 645
Beck Depression Inventory, 481
Bedside head-to-toe examination, 706–708
documentation of, 723
Bedtime habits, 463
Bedwetting, 247, 470
Behavior, assessment of, 92

Beliefs. *See* Values and beliefs
Bell's palsy, 405
Benign prostatic hypertrophy, 275, 700
Biceps reflex, 85, 409
Bilirubin, in newborns, 644
Bimanual palpation, 67, *67*
of bladder, for postvoid residual volume, 251, 263
of breast, 556
in pelvic examination, 544–546
in pregnancy, 563d
Binge eating disorder, 180
Biot's breathing, 114d
Birth control, 526
Birth defects, prenatal testing for, 530
Bitemporal hemianopsia, 438, *439*
Bladder
assessment of, in elderly, 697
atonic, 241
bimanual evaluation of, for postvoid residual volume, 251, 263
catheterization of, 718–719
distention of, 251, 263
hypotonic, 241, 276–277
lower motor neuron, 242, 276–277
reflex, 241, 276–277
structure and function of, 240, *240*
upper motor neuron, 241
Bladder elimination. *See* Urinary elimination
Bladder retraining, 705, 731–734
Bladder stones, 268
Bleeding
gastrointestinal, 266
nasal, 328
uterine, 528
Blepharitis, 432
Blindness. *See also* Vision impairment
night, 377
onset of, 377
unilateral, 438, *439*
Blind spot
pathologic, 377, 438
physiologic, 422
Blinking reflex, 662t
Blood, fecal occult, 253, 256, 266
test for, 257
Blood cells, in urine, 262
Blood pressure, 113–119
assessment of, 113–119
auscultatory gap in, 115
documentation of, 118
in elders, 698
flush method of, 666
guidelines for, *113,* 115–118
in infant, 666
Korotkoff sounds in, *113,* 113–115
in newborn, 653–654
in older child and adolescent, 676
in young child, 672
clinical problems related to, 119
diastolic, 113, 118
factors affecting, 115
high. *See* Hypertension
intravascular monitoring of, 714–715
low. *See* Hypotension
normal values for, 100t, 115
nursing diagnoses for, 118
in pregnancy, 564d
regulation of, 113
systolic, 113, 118
Blood pressure cuff, 115, 117
Body image, 478, 483
assessment of, 484
Body image disturbance, 486
Body language, 28–29, 30, 31
Body mass index (BMI), 175
Body righting reflex, 662t
Body structure, ethnic variations in, 612
Body systems approach, in physical examination, 6, 18, 61, 62t, 63t
Body temperature, 101–108
assessment of
documentation of, 107
equipment for, 103
guidelines for, 103–106
sites for, 103
axillary, 103, 105
clinical problems related to, 107
elevated, 101, 107–108
factors affecting, 101, *102*
low, 107
normal values for, 100t
normal variations in, 101, *102*
nursing diagnoses for, 107–108
oral, 103, 104–105

rectal, 103, 105
regulation of, 101
set point for, 101
tympanic membrane, 103, 105, 106
Body types, 93
Body weight. *See* Weight
Bohn nodules, 649
Boils, 199
Bonding, 636
Bone. *See also under* Musculoskeletal
formation of, 338–339, 339d
structure and function of, 338
types of, 338
Bone scintigraphy, 293
Bony labyrinth, 438
Boutonniere deformity, 355
Bowel elimination. *See also* Constipation; Diarrhea;
Stool
assessment of, 237–279
case study of, 276–277
clinical problems related to, 265–266
data collection for, 238
diagnostic studies in, 251
focus of, 237
interpretation of findings in, 263–264
interview and health history in, 242–247
knowledge base for, 238–239
nursing diagnoses for, 237–238, 264–265
in children, 632
diet and, 244–245
disorders affecting, 246
drugs and, 246–247
in elders, 690, 697
as functional health pattern, 9
functional status and, 245
painful, 264–265
pattern of, 243–244
physiology of, 239, 239–240
in pregnancy, 564d
self-care practices for, 244–245
Bowel incontinence, 265
case study of, 276–277
Bowel obstruction, 224–225
Bowel sounds, 212, 216–217
in elders, 697
in infant, 667
in newborn, 654
Brachial pulse, 85, 312
Brachioradialis reflex, 409
Bradycardia, 108
Bradypnea, 114d
Brain. *See also under* Cerebral
structure and function of, 371, *371*
Brain scan, 389
Breast
cancer of, 553, 554d
screening for, 137, 138, 141, 144d, 529
self-examination for, 137, 144d
cysts of, 554d
development of, 634, 634t
examination of, 86, 552–560
abnormal findings in, 554d-555d
clinical problems related to, 559–560
clock method for, 552, *552*
documentation of, 552–559
in elders, 700
focus for, 552
landmarks in, 552, *552*
in male, 559
in older child and adolescent, 676
procedures in, 553–559
quadrant method for, 552, *552*
fibroadenoma of, 554d
fibrocystic disease of, 554d
increased venous prominence in, 553, 554d
infection of, 555
Paget's disease of, 553, 555d
peau d'orange, 553, 554d
in pregnancy, 562d-563d
retraction signs in, 554d
structure and function of, 551–552, *551-553*
tumors of, 554d
Breast-feeding, 563d
effective, 532
ineffective, 532
Breast self-examination, 137, 144d
Breathing. *See also under* Respiration; Respiratory
anatomy and physiology of, 322–324, *322-324*
Biot's, 114d
Cheyne-Stokes, 114d
definition of, 111
Kussmaul's, 114d
mechanics of, 324–325
obstructive, 114d
Breathing pattern, ineffective, 337

Breath sounds, 334–335, 336d
adventitious, 336d
bronchial, 335
bronchovesicular, 335
vesicular, 335
Breech presentation, 570
Broca's aphasia, 388, 392t, 509
Broca's area, 371, *371, 372*
Brodman's areas, 415–416, *416*
Bronchial breath sounds, 335
Bronchial tumors, 338
Bronchitis
acute, 337
chronic, 337
Bronchophony, 335
Bronchovesicular breath sounds, 335
Bruits, 315, 321
abdominal, 217
in hyperthyroidism, 228
uterine, in pregnancy, 569
Bruxism, 470
Bulbocavernous reflex, assessment of, 253
Bulge sign, 360
Bulimia nervosa, 165, 180, 674
Bulla, 186
Bursae, 339
Bursitis, 365
elbow, 353
shoulder, 351

C

Cachexia, 91, 178
Café-au-lait spots, 659
Caffeine
sexual function and, 525d
sleep and, 463–464
Calculi, urinary, 268
Call-a Nurse programs, 131, 131d
Caloric needs, of children, 631
Caloric test, 405
Calorie count, 171
Cancer
breast, 553, 554d
screening for, 137–138, 139, 144d
self-examination for, 137, 144d, 526
bronchial, 338
cervical, 526
screening for, 139, 529
colorectal, 266
screening for, 138
gynecologic, 526
laryngeal, communication in, 509
oral cavity, 208, 211
oral lesions in, 210, 211
penile, 577
prostate, 266, 275
screening for, 139
sexuality and, 523
skin, 199
testicular, 575, 578
screening for, 137, 145d
self-examination for, 137, 145d
uterine, screening for, 529
Candidiasis, 199–200
oral, 210
vaginal, 549t, 551
Canker sore, 209
Cantharis, sexual function and, 525d
Capillary refill time, 197
Caput succedaneum, 647
Carbohydrates, 157d, 158, 160
Carbuncles, 199
Cardiac catheterization, 292
Cardiac chest pain, 294
Cardiac conduction system, 297, *298*
Cardiac cycle, 298–300, *299*
Cardiac enzymes, 291
Cardiac monitoring, 721
Cardiac output
decreased, 320
during exercise, 283t, 283–284
Cardiac valves, *299*, 299–300
Cardiovascular assessment, 296–322
arterial pulse assessment in, 300, 312–317
case study of, 365–366
clinical problems related to, 322
diagnostic studies in, 291–292
documentation of, 319–320
in elders, 698
equipment for, 301
general principles of, 300–301
heart and precordium examination in, 300–311.
See also Heart, examination of

neck vein assessment in, 300, 318–319
nursing diagnoses for, 320–322
physical examination in, 300–319
positioning for, 301
precordial landmarks in, 301–302, *302, 303*
preparation for, 301
pulse assessment in, 312–315, 316d
in trauma survey, 724
Cardiovascular disease
sexuality and, 523
skin changes in, 199
Cardiovascular system
anatomy and physiology of, *296-299*, 296–300
in stress response, 600
Caregiver role strain, 508, 594
Caregiver stress, 700
Carotid arteries, 84
auscultation of, 315
Carotid pulse, 312
Carpal tunnel syndrome, 356
Casts, urine, 262
Catabolism, 156
Cataplexy, in narcolepsy, 469
Cataracts, 430
Catecholamines, in stress response, 587–588,
590
Catheterization
cardiac, 292
in intravascular pressure monitoring, 714–715
in intravenous therapy, 719–720
for postvoid residual volume, 252
urinary, 718–719
Causalgia, 398
Cavernous hemangiomas, 659
Celiac artery, 212–213
Celiac disease, 266
Central neurogenic hyperventilation, 114d
Central venous pressure, 300
estimation of, 319
Cephalhematoma, 647
Cerebellar function, 416
assessment of. *See* Sensory and cerebellar assessment
Cerebral cortex
anatomy of, 371, *371*
areas of, 415–416, *416*
motor, 406, *407*
sensory, 415–416, *416*
Cerebral hemisphere dominance, 372
Cerebral tissue perfusion, chronic altered,
320–321
Cerumen, 438, 444
impaction of, 441, 442
removal of, 441
Cervical nodes, *229*, 231
examination of, 83
in young child, 672
Cervical spine. *See also* Neck
examination of, 349–350
Cervix, 533, *534*
cancer of, screening for, 138, 529
examination of, 90, 541–542
palpation of, 276, 544
in pregnancy, 563d
specimen collection from, 542–543
C fibers, 393
Chadwick's sign, 563d
Chalazion, 432
Charting. *See also* Documentation
problem-oriented, 15
Charting by exception, 94, 96d
Chart review, 11
Cheilitis, 208
Cheilosis, in malnutrition, 179, 203
Chemical dependency, *732*
in adolescents, 674
assessment in, 705, 727–731
history in, 44–45, 730, *732*
sexual function and, 525d
Chemotherapy, oral lesions in, 210, 211
Cherry angioma, 188, 696
Chest. *See also under* Thoracic
examination of, 86–88, 330–334
in bedside examination, 706
in elders, 698
in infant, 666
landmarks for, *323*, 323–324, *324*
in newborn, 652
in trauma survey, 726
in young child, 672
flail, 337–338
measurement of
in infant, 663
in newborn, 646
Chest expansion, 333

Chest pain
  anginal, 294
    bedside assessment of, 708
    cardiac, 294
    pulmonary, 294
Chest trauma, 337–338
Chest tubes, monitoring of, 709
Cheyne-Stokes respiration, 114d
Chicken pox, immunization schedule for, 630t, 638t, 639t
Child abuse, 506, 509, 668
  assessment for, 506
  risk factors for, 130d
  sexual, 526, 527d
Children
  activity and exercise in, 632
  age classifications for, 629
  cognitive development of, 632–633
  common health concerns and problems of, 629–631
  communication with, 32
  coping skills of, 635
  discipline of, 498, 502
  elimination in, 632
  growth and development of. See Anthropometric assessment; Development
  health assessment for. See Pediatric health assessment
  health promotion and health management for, 629–631
  immunizations for, 630, 630t, 638t, 639t
  interviewing of, 32, 36–37
  language development in, 633
  moral development in, 637
  nutrition in, 631–632
  physical examination of, 75, 76d
  preventive care for, 640d
  roles and relationships of, 635–636
  safety practices for, 143, 631
  screening for, 630–631
  self-concept of, 636–637
  sexual abuse of, 526, 527d
  sexual development in, 634t–635t, 634–635
  sleep patterns in, 457d, 458, 633
  socialization of, 498, 502
  spiritual development of, 637
  stress response in, 635
Chinese Americans. See also under Cultural; Culture
  health and illness concepts of, 612–613
  health risks for, 614t
Chin-lift maneuver, 203
Chlamydia
  in females, 549t
  in males, 577
Chloasma, 562d
Cholecystitis, 224
Cholesterol levels, assessment of, 173
Chordee, 573
Chorionic villus sampling, 530
Chronic arterial occlusion, skin changes in, 199
Chronic bronchitis, 337
Chronic obstructive pulmonary disease, 337
Chronic pain, 392, 400
Chronic venous insufficiency, skin changes in, 199
Chyme, 239
Cicatrix, 187
Cigarette smoking, sleep and, 463
Cimetidine, sexual function and, 525d
Circadian rhythms, temperature variations and, 101, 102
Circular communication, 495–496
Circulation. See also under Cardiovascular
  cardiac, 296–297, 297
Circumduction, 340
Classification, of health status, 19
Classification ability, 386
Claudication, 294–295
  intermittent, 321
Claw fingers, 355
Claw hammer toe, 363
Clinical database, 6
  components of, 12–13
  in diagnostic reasoning, 16–17
  health assessment interview in, 25–40
  health history in, 40–55
Clinical Institute Withdrawal Assessment of Alcohol (CIWA-A), 727, 728d-729d
Clinical problems, 10
Clinical record
  charting by exception in, 94, 96d
  problem-oriented, 15
  review of, 11
Clitoris, 533, 533
  in newborn, 657
  in older child and adolescent, 677

Closed-ended questions, 29
Clubbing, 196–197
Cochlea, 438, 440
Cognition
  assessment of, 386–388
  dimensions of, 371–372
Cognition and perception, as functional health pattern, 9
Cognition and perception assessment, 369–452
  aids for, 374
  case studies of, 450
  in children, 632–633
  cognitive function in, 386–388
  in cognitive impairment, 373
  comprehensive neurologic assessment in, 373
  cranial nerve assessment in, 401–406, 402t
  data collection for, 370–371
  diagnostic studies in, 389
  documentation of, 375–380
  ear examination in, 445–450
  in elders, 691, 699
  focus of, 370–371
  general approach in, 372–373
  hearing assessment in, 445–449
  interview and health history in, 376d, 377–381
  medication history in, 381
  mental status examination in, 373–374, 374d-375d, 382–390
  motor function assessment in, 406–413
  nursing diagnoses for, 371, 391, 412–413
  physical findings in, 389–391
  reflex assessment in, 408–413
    clinical problems related to, 412–413
    documentation of, 412, 412d
    nursing diagnoses for, 412–413
  screening, 373
  teaching and learning evaluation in, 380
  visual acuity testing in, 435–438
Cognitive appraisal of stressor, 588
Cognitive development, 632–633
Cognitive impairments, interviewing and, 33
Cold injury, 107
Colds, in infants, 661
Colic, 661
Colitis, ulcerative, 265
Collaborative problems, 10
Collateral relationships, 610
Colon
  cancer of, 266
    screening for, 138
  feces formation and evacuation in, 239, 239–240. See also Bowel elimination
  spastic, 266
Colonoscopy, 251
Color vision, assessment of, 436–437
Colostomy patients, sexual concerns of, 523
Comatose state, 383
Communication, 370, 495, 495–496. See also Language; Speech
  about sexuality, 518–519
  with angry patients, 33–34
  with anxious patients, 34
  aphasia and, 387–388, 392t, 509
  assessment of, 387–388, 502–503, 504
  body language in, 28–29, 30, 31
  with children, 32
  circular, 495–496
  with cognitively impaired patients, 33
  cultural factors in, 30, 31–32
  with depressed patients, 34
  with dying patients, 34–35
  with elders, 32–33
  emotional, 495–496
  eye contact in, 30, 31
  factors affecting, 496
  in family, 498, 501
  with hearing-impaired, 33
  impaired verbal, 391
  ineffective, 30–31, 496
  intercultural, 616d
  in interviewing, 28–31. See also Interview
    language barriers in, 31–32, 616
    listening in, 30
  with manipulative patients, 34
  with non-native speakers, 31–32
  nonverbal, 28–29, 30, 31, 388, 495
  open-ended questions in, 29
  patterns of, 495
  reflection in, 29
  with seductive patients, 34
  silence in, 30
  therapeutic, in interview, 28–31
  verbal, 495
    impaired, 508
  verbalization of implied ideas in, 29–30
Communication aids, 503

Communication processes, 371–372
Compliance, with prescribed health regimens, 127–128, 148–149
Comprehensive assessment, 12
  documentation of, 15
Computed tomography, in musculoskeletal assessment, 293
Computers, as health information source, 126, 128, 136
Conductive aphasia, 392t
Conductive hearing loss, 448d
Condyloid joints, 340
Condylomata acuminata
  in females, 547–551, 550t
  in males, 577
Cones, 422
Confabulation, 387
Confidentiality, in sexual assessment, 518–519
Congenital anomalies, prenatal testing for, 530
Congenital hypothyroidism, screening for, 644
Congestive heart failure
  case study of, 365–366
  in elders, 688t
Conjunctiva, 422, 423
  examination of, 427
Connective tissue, 183
Consciousness
  components of, 371
  level of, 371, 382–383
    Glasgow Coma Scale for, 373, 384, 725
Constipation, 214, 243, 244, 264–265. See also Bowel elimination
  causes of, 264, 265
  in elders, 690
  related to change in lifestyle, 264
  related to immobility, 264
  related to painful defecation, 264–265
  self-care practices for, 245
  signs of, 263
  stool in, 255, 264, 265
Contact dermatitis, 189, 200
Contraception, 526
Control, locus of, 135, 479, 590, 591d
  assessment of, 480, 485
  behavioral indicators of, 485t
Cooperative play, 636
Cooper's ligaments, 551
Coping, 584, 588–596
  definition of, 588–589
  effective, 592d
  emotion-focused, 584, 589–590
  ineffective individual, 601–603
  problem-focused, 584, 589
Coping and stress tolerance
  assessment of. See Stress and coping assessment
  in children and adolescents, 635
  as functional health pattern, 9
Coping Inventory for Stressful Situations, 596
Coping Scale, 596
Coping styles, 589–591, 595–596
Cornea, examination of, 427
Corneal light reflex, 404
  in newborn, 650
  in young child, 650
Coronal ridge, 570, 570
Coronary artery disease, screening for, 138, 139
Corpus cavernosum, 571, 571
Corpus spongiosum, 571, 571
Cortisol, in stress response, 587–588, 590
Costal angle, 323, 323
Costal margin, 323, 323
Cough, 295
Counseling, for health perception and health maintenance, 133d
Covert roles, 497
Cover/uncover test, 428, 670
Cowper's glands, 571, 571
Crackles, 336d
Cradle cap, 668
Cramps, muscle, 336
Cranial nerves
  anatomy and physiology of, 401, 402t
  assessment of, 79, 80, 83, 84, 401–406
    in newborn, 660–661
Cranium, examination of, 78–79
  in newborn, 647
Credé maneuver, 249
Cremasteric reflex, 411
Crepitus, 331
Crisis, 592
Critical indicators, for nursing diagnosis, 18
Crohn's disease, 265
Crust, 187
Cryptorchidism, 668, 673
Crystalline lens, 422, 423
  examination of, 430
  opacities of, 430

Cueing, in sensory assessment, 417
Cultural blindness, 611d
Cultural interview, 617d, 618–620
Cultural relativity, 611d
Cultural rituals, health-related, 613
Cultural sensitivity, 609–611
Cultural values, 608. *See also* Values and beliefs
Culture, 609
    biological variations and, 612
    characteristics of, 609
    communication and, 30, 31–32, 611, 616d
    definition of, 609
    definitions related to, 611d
    diet and, 612, 613
    dimensions of orientation in, 610–611
    environment and, 612
    health and, 611–614
    health and illness concepts and, 612–614
    personal space and, 611
    social organization and, 611–612
    stool, 254
    time sense and, 610, 611–612
Culture conflict, 611d
Culture imposition, 611d
Culture shock, 611d
Curandera/curandero, 613
Cushing's syndrome, 91
Cutis marmorata, 658
Cyanosis, 336
    nails in, 197
    in newborn, 658, 659
    oral mucosa in, 206
    skin in, 183, 336
        ethnic variations in, 612
Cyst, 186
    breast, 554d
    nabothian, 542
    pilonidal, 272
Cystocele, 540
Cystometrogram, 252

D

Dacryoadenitis, 426
Dacryocystitis, 426
Daily hassles, 595
Data
    definition of, 10
    objective, 11
    subjective, 11
Data analysis, 18–19
Database, clinical, 6
    components of, 12–13
    in diagnostic reasoning, 16–17
    health assessment interview in, 25–40
    health history in, 40–55
Data collection, 10–13
    comprehensive assessment in, 12, 13d
    coordination of, 35
    in diagnostic reasoning, 16–17
    documentation in, 13–15. *See also* Documentation
    focused assessment in, 12
    frequency of, 12
    functional health patterns in, 6–10, 38–40
    interview for, 11, 35. *See also* Interview
    methods of, 11
    physical examination in, 11. *See also* Physical examination
    prioritization in, 12
    review of records in, 11
    scope of, 11–12
    screening assessment in, 11–12. *See also* Screening
Deafness. *See* Hearing loss
Death and dying, discussion of, 34–35
Death practices, 619
Decerebrate posturing, 384
Decorticate posturing, 383
Decubitus ulcers
    assessment of, 191–194
    staging of, 191–193
    undermining (tunneling) in, 191
Deep palpation, 67, 67
Deep pelvic palpation, in pregnancy, 568
Deep tendon reflexes. *See* Reflex(es)
Deep vein thrombosis, Homan's sign in, 706
Defecation
    painful, 264–265
    physiology of, 240. *See also* Bowel elimination; Stool
Defecation reflex, 240, 243
Defense mechanisms, 599
Degenerative joint disease, 364–365

Dehydration, oral cavity in, 203–211
Dental hygiene, poor, 203
Denver Articulation Screening Examination (DASE), 633, 645
Depression
    assessment scales for, 481
    in elders, 688t, 695
    interviewing and, 34
Dermatitis, 199–200
    atopic, 668
    contact, 189, 200
    seborrheic, 189, 668
Dermatomes, 413, *414*
    assessment of. *See* Sensory and cerebellar assessment
    referred pain and, 413, *415*
Dermis, 181, *181*
Detrusor muscle, 240, 241
Development
    altered, 147
    assessment of
        in infants, 645
        in older children and adolescents, 645
        in young children, 645
    cognitive, 632–633
    language, 633
    motor, 632
    theories of
        Erikson's, 479, 636
        Fowler's, 615, 637
        Kohlberg's, 637
        Piaget's, 632–633
Developmental stages, of family, 497–498
Developmental tasks, 479
Diabetes mellitus
    oral changes in, 211
    sexuality and, 524
    skin changes in, 198
Diabetic retinopathy, 433
Diadochokinesia, 421
Diagnosis
    medical, 10, 19
    nursing, 6
Diagnostic reasoning, 15–19
    data collection in, 16–17
    data organization in, 17–18
    drawing conclusions in, 18–19
Diaper rash, 661, 668
Diaphragm, 325
Diarrhea, 214, 244, 265
    causes of, 265–266
    signs of, 265
    stool in, 255
    tube feeding and, 245
Diarthroses, 339
Diastole, 298, *299*
Diastolic blood pressure, 113, 118
Diet. *See also* Eating; Feeding; Food; Nutrition
    assessment of, 165–166, 169–173
    balanced, 156–160, 157d
        recommended dietary allowances and, 156
    bowel elimination and, 244–245
    cultural variations in, 612, 613
    guidelines for, 156d, 156–160
    religious beliefs and, 615
    therapeutic, 165
Diet history, 169
Digestion, 155
Digital rectal examination, 273–275
    in pelvic examination, 276
Diphtheria, immunization schedule for, 630t, 638t, 639t
Diplopia, 378
Dipstick tests, urine, 258
    for electrolytes, 262
    for pH, 261
Direct action, in coping, 590–591
Disc, herniated, 365
Discharge
    nipple, 558
    penile, 574
    vaginal, 539, 543
        in pregnancy, 563d
Discipline, of children, 498, 502
Disease(s). *See also* Illness
    classification and naming of, 19
    prevention of, 126–127
    risk factors for, 128d, 128–129, 130d
    susceptibility to, ethnic variations in, 612
Dissecting aortic aneurysm, 294
Distress, 584
Disturbances in role performance, 507
Diuretics, 250
    sexual function and, 525d
Diverticulitis, 224, 266
Divorce, single parent families and, 497

Dizziness, 379, 380
Documentation, 13–15
    charting by exception method of, 94, 96d
    guidelines for, 14–15
    of health history, 45–55
    narrative style for, 15, 16d, 46, 46d-48d, 94d-95d
    of physical examination, 74, 94, 94d-96d
    of pulse, 111
    purposes of, 13
    of respiratory rate and pattern, 113
    SOAP format in, 15
    standardized form for, 46, 48d-55d
Domestic violence, 509
    risk factors for, 130d
Doppler probe, 71, 71–72
    in blood pressure measurement, 115
Dorsalis pedal pulse, 314
Dorsal lithotomy position, 537, *538*
Dorsosacral position, 271, *271*
Double vision, 378
Drainage
    chest, monitoring of, 709–710
    wound, 191
Drawer sign, 361
Dress
    assessment of, 92–93
    cultural differences in, 621
Drug abuse, *732*
    by adolescents, 674
    assessment in, 705, 727–731
    history in, 44–45, 730, *732*
    sexual function and, 525d
Drug therapy
    adverse reactions to, history of, 45
    bladder elimination and, 250
    bowel elimination and, 246–247
    in elders, 687, 689
    history of, 44–45
    intravenous, 719–720
    mental status changes and, 381
    nutrition and, 168
    ototoxic, 379
    sexual function and, 525d
    sleep and, 464–465
Dry mouth, 207
Dullness on percussion, 68, 69t, 334
Duodenal ulcer, 214–224
Duration of sound
    in auscultation, 69
    in percussion, 69t
Dying patients, communication with, 34–35
Dysfunctional grieving, 603
Dysphagia, 210–211
Dyspnea, 295, 336
    bedside assessment of, 708
    nighttime, 463
Dyspnea index, for self-evaluation, 286
Dysuria, 248

E

Ear
    disorders of, 378–379, 445–449
    equilibrium and, 379
    examination of, 81–82, 378–379, 440–445
        documentation of, 441–442
        in infant, 664
        in newborn, 651
        in older child and adolescent, 675
        otoscopic, 72, 73
        procedures in, 443–445
        in young child, 671
    external
        examination of, 443
        structure of, 438, *439*
    inner, structure of, 438–439, *440*
    irrigation of, 441, *442*
    middle
        examination of, 443–444
        infection of, 442, 445–449
        structure of, 438, *440*
    structure and function of, 438–439
    swimmer's, 445
Ear canal, 438, *439*
Early Language Milestone Scale (ELM Scale), 633
Ear wax, 438
    impaction of, 441, 442
    removal of, 441
Eating, functional status and, 166
Eating behavior, in children, 631
Eating disorders, 165, 180, 674
Ecchymosis, 188
Eccrine sweat glands, 181, *181*
Echocardiography, 291
Eco-map, 494–495, *495*

Ectomorphs, 93
Ectopic area, 303, *303*
Ectropion, 432
Eczema, 189, 200, 668
Edema, 184–185
  breast, 554d
  grading of, 185d
  pulmonary, 338
  scrotal, 578
Effective breast-feeding, 532
Effective management of therapeutic regimen, 147–148
Egophony, 335
Ejaculation duct, 571, *571*
Ejection click, 308
Elbow, examination of, 353–354
Elderly families, 497
Elders. *See also* Aging
  abuse of, 509, 693, 700
    risk factors for, 130d
  activities of daily living in, 691, 692d
  assessment in, 686–701
    of activity and exercise, 691, 698
    clinical problems related to, 701
    of cognition and perception, 691, 699
    diagnostic and screening studies in, 694
    documentation of, 701
    of elimination, 690, 697–698
    focus for, 686
    general principles of, 688–689
    of health and health perception, 689, 695
    interview and health history in, 32–33, 36, 689–695
    knowledge base for, 687–688
    nursing diagnoses for, 686
    of nutrition and metabolism, 690, 695, 695t, 696t
    physical examination in, 695–700
    procedures in, 695
    of roles and relationships, 692, 700
    of self-concept, 692, 699
    of sexuality, 693, 700
    of sleep and rest, 692, 699
    of stress and coping, 694, 700
    of values and beliefs, 694, 700
  assessment of, interview and health history in, 32–33, 36
  body temperature in, 101
  bowel elimination in, 690
  causes of death in, 701
  cognitive function in, 691, 699
  communication with, 32–33
  degenerative joint disease in, 364–365
  depression in, 695
  drug therapy in, 687, 689
  health perception and management in, 689, 695
  hearing loss in, 378, 699
  illness in, 687–688, 688t
  in long-term care, stressors for, 589d
  medical history for, 41
  menopause in, 693
  normal vs. pathologic aging in, 687
  nutrition in, 690, 695
    screening for, 162d, 162–163
  physical examination of, 75
  roles and relationships of, 692–693
  safety assessment for, 143
  screening for, 690d
  self-concept of, 692
  sensory function in, 691
  sexuality of, 693
  skin in, 696
  sleep patterns in, 457d, 458, 692, 699
  social isolation of, 509
  urinary elimination in, 690
  vision impairment in, 438
Electrocardiography (ECG), 291
  in cardiac monitoring, 721
Electroencephalography (EEG), in sleep studies, 455, *455, 456*, 457, 465
Electromyography, 293
  in bladder elimination assessment, 253
  in sleep assessment, 455, *455*
Electronic thermometers, 103, 106
Electro-oculogram, 455, *455, 466*
Elimination. *See* Bowel elimination; Urinary elimination
Emboli, pulmonary, 338
Emotional communication, 495–496
Emotional expression, cultural factors in, 31–32
Emotion-focused coping, 584, 589–590
Emphysema, 337
Empyema, 337
Enacted roles, 492
Enculturation, 611d
Endocervical swab technique, 543
Endocrine system, in stress response, 587–588, *590*

Endomorphs, 93
Endophthalmos, 432
Enema, 245
  barium, 251
Engrossment, 636
Enteral feeding tubes, monitoring of, 713
Entropion, 432
Enuresis, 247
  nocturnal, 470
Environment, cultural variations in, 612
Environmental assessment, 129–131, 143
Environmental safety, 129–131, 143
Enzymes, cardiac, 291
Epicanthal folds, 432
Epidermis, 181, *181*
Epididymis, 571, *571*
  examination of, 575
Epididymitis, 578
Epigastric area, 303, *303*
Epigastric tenderness, 214
Epistaxis, 328
Epitrochlear nodes, 232
Epstein's pearls, 649
Equilibrium, 439
Equipment, for physical examination, 69–75, 70t, 70–73
Erb's point, 303, *303*
Erectile dysfunction, 577–578
Erikson's developmental theory, 479, 636
Erosion, 187
Erythema, 183
Erythema toxicum, 659
Erythrocytes, in urine, 262
Estrogen replacement therapy, 693
Ethmoid sinuses, 323, *323*
  examination of, 329–330
Ethnicity, 611d. *See also under* Cultural; Culture
  health and illness concepts and, 612–613
  health customs and rituals and, 613–614
  risk factors and, 613–614, 614t
Ethnocentrism, 611d
Eustachian tube, structure of, 438, *440*
Eustress, 584
Eversion, 340
Everyday Hassles Scale, 596, 598d
Excessive daytime sleepiness, 462
Excitement, in sexual response cycle, 517
Exercise. *See* Activity and exercise
Exercise tolerance
  self-assessment of, 286
  vital signs and, 287
Exercise tolerance test, 291
Exophthalmos, 432
Expiratory reserve volume, 325
Expressive aphasia, 388, 392t
Extension, 340
Extensor posturing, 384
External anal sphincter, *239,* 240, 268, *269*
  examination of, 273
External auditory meatus, 438, *439*
  examination of, 443
External hemorrhoidal plexus, 268, *269*
External inguinal ring, 571, *572*
External locus of control, 135, 480
External urinary sphincter, 240, *240,* 242
Exteroception, 408
Extraocular eye movements, 422
  assessment of, 427–428
  during sleep, 455–456, *456*
Extraocular muscles, examination of, 80
Extremities. *See* Lower extremity; Upper extremity
Eye
  age-related changes in, 438
  color of, in infant, 664
  disorders of, 377–378, 432–433
  examination of, 80, 377–378, 424–434
    abbreviations used in, 437d
    clinical problems related to, 438
    documentation of, 437d
    in elders, 699
    equipment for, 424
    focus of, 424
    general principles of, 424
    in infant, 663–664
    in newborn, 650
    nursing diagnoses for, 437–438
    in older child and adolescent, 675
    ophthalmoscopic, 72, *72,* 424, 429–434
    procedures in, 424–434
    pupil dilation for, 424
    in young child, 670
  muscles of, 422
  structure and function of, 422–423, *423*
  symmetry of, 425
Eyebrows, examination of, 425
Eye contact, cultural aspects of, 30, 31
Eyelashes, examination of, 425

Eyelids, examination of, 425
  in newborn, 650
Eye movements, 422
  assessment of, 427–428
  during sleep, 455–456, *456*

F

Face, examination of, 79, 91–92
  in newborn, 647
Face mask, oxygen, 716–717
Facial expression, cultural differences in, 621
Facial nerve, 79, 402t, 405
Faith development, 615, 615d
  in children, 637
Faith healers, 613
Fallopian tubes, 534, *534*
Family
  assessment of, 498, 501–502, 504–505. *See also* Roles and relationships assessment
  child-rearing and, 498, 502
  communication in, 498, 501
  concept of, 496
  decision-making in, 498
    cultural factors in, 32
  developmental stages of, 497–498
  elderly, 497
  functions of, 496
  merged, 497
  problems and concerns of, 498
  roles in, 497
  single parent, 497
  social relationships of, 502
  structure of, 496–497, *497*
    cultural variations in, 610
Family processes, 496–498, *497*
  altered, 506
Farsightedness, 423
  age-related, 691
  testing for, 435–438. *See also* Visual acuity, assessment of
Fasciculations, 336
Fasciculus cuneatus, 414
Fasciculus gracilis, 414
Fat
  dietary, 158d, 158–160
  fecal, 253, 255
Fatigue, 295
Fear, vs. anxiety, 486–487
Fecal fat, 253, 255
Fecal impaction, 265, 274
Fecal occult blood, 253, 256, 266
  test for, 257
Fecal urobilinogen, 254
Feces. *See* Stool
Feeding. *See also* Diet; Food; Nutrition
  enteral, monitoring in, 713
Feeding tubes, monitoring of, 713
Femoral artery, auscultation of, 315
Femoral hernia, 577
Femoral pulse, 313
Fencing response, *660*
Festinating gait, 345d
Fetal demise, 570
Fetal heart assessment, 569
Fetal position and lie, 567–568
  abnormal, 570
Fetal presentation, abnormal, 570
Fetal ultrasound, 530
α-Fetoprotein, prenatal test for, 530
Fever, 101, *107,* 107–108
Fiber, dietary, bowel elimination and, 244–245
Fibroadenoma, of breast, 554d
Fibrocystic disease, of breast, 554d
Filling cystometrogram, 252
Final common pathway, 406–408
Fingers
  deformities of, 355
  examination of, 355–356
    in newborn, 658
Finger-to-nose-to-finger test, 421
Fissure, 187
Fist percussion, 67, *68*
Flaccid response, 384
Flail chest, 337–338
Flaky paint dermatosis, 178, 198
Flat affect, 389
Flatness on percussion, 68, 69t
Fleabite rash, 659
Flexion, 340
Flexor posturing, 383
Floaters, 377, 438
Fluent aphasia, 392t
Fluid
  abdominal, 223–224
  in knee, 360

Fluid imbalance, oral cavity in, 203–211
Fluid intake
    bladder elimination and, 249
    bowel elimination and, 244
Fluid wave, abdominal, 223
Flush method, 666
Focused assessment, 12
Folk medicine, 136, 613, 618, 621
Folliculitis, 199
Fontanelles, examination of, 648, 663
Food. *See also* Diet; Feeding; Nutrition
Food allergies, 165–166
    in infants, 661
Food Diary, 171
Food Frequency Record, 171
Food intake history, 169
Food labels, 159d
    understanding of, 166
Food Pyramid, 156, *157*, 158
Foot. *See also* Lower extremity
    athlete's, 200
    examination of, 363
    in newborn, 655
Fordyce spots, 209
Foreign language speakers, interviewing of, 31, 616
Foreign object, aspiration of, 338
Foreskin, 570, *570*
Forms. *See also* Documentation
    for health history, 46, 48d-55d
Forward-sitting position, 301, *301*
Fovea centralis, 423
Fowler's stages of faith development, 615, 637
Fremitus, tactile, 332
Frenulum, penile, 570, *570*
Frontal lobe, 371, *371*
Frontal sinuses, 323, *323*
    examination of, 329–330
Frostbite, 107
Fully awake state, 382
Functional health patterns (FHPs), 6–10
    in diagnostic reasoning, 18
    in documentation, 38–40
    interview questions about, 38–40
    in physical examination, 62, 63t-65t
Functional incontinence, 267
Fundal height measurement, 561, 565–567
Fungal infections, of skin, 199–200
Furuncles, 199

G

Gag reflex, 206, 211, 405, 665
Gait
    abnormal, 93, 344, 345d-346d
    assessment of, 77, 93, 344
Gallbladder, inflammation of, 224
Gas exchange, 325
    impaired, 330–337
Gastric ulcer, 214–224
Gastritis, 214–225
Gastrocolic reflex, 240, 243
Gastroenteritis, acute, 265
Gastrointestinal hemorrhage, 266
Gastrointestinal motility, 212
Gastrointestinal system, in stress response, 600
Gastrostomy tubes, monitoring of, 713
Gate control theory, 393
Gender identification, 522
Gender identity, 516
Gender roles, 516–517, 522
General survey, 65, 706
    guidelines for, 77–93
Genital herpes
    in females, 547, 549t
    in males, 572
Genitals
    female
        examination of, 90, 534–551
            in bladder elimination assessment, 263–264
            clinical problems related to, 547–551, 548t-550t
            documentation of, 546–547
            in elders, 700
            equipment for, 535, *536*
            focus of, 534–535
            in infant, 667–668
            in newborn, 657–658
            in older child and adolescent, 676–677
            patient attitude toward, 536
            positioning for, 537–538, *538*
            preparation for, 536
            procedures in, 535–546
            in young child, 673
        in pregnancy, 563d
        structure and function of, 532–534, *533, 534*

    male
        development of, 634, 635t
        examination of, 90
            clinical problems related to, 572–578
            documentation of, 571–572
            in elders, 700
            in infant, 667–668
            in newborn, 657–658
            in older child and adolescent, 676–677
            procedures in, 573–576
            in young child, 673
        structure and function of, 570–571, *570–572*
Genital warts
    in females, 547–551, 550t
    in males, 577
Genitourinary tract, assessment of, in bladder elimination assessment, 263
Genogram
    in family assessment, 497, *497*, 501
    in risk assessment, 128, *129*
Genupectoral position, 270, *270*
Geriatric Depression Scale, 695
German measles, immunization schedule for, 630t, 638t, 639t
Gestational age assessment, 644
Gibbus, 347
Gingiva, 202
    disorders of, 203
    examination of, in newborn, 649
Glabellar reflex, 412, 413
Glans penis, 570, *570*
Glasgow Coma Scale, 373, 384, 725
Glaucoma, 378, 422, 431
    narrow angle, 433
    open angle, 433
Gliding joints, 340
Global aphasia, 392t
Glossitis, 203, 209
Glossopharyngeal nerve, 83, 402t, 405
Glucosuria, 262
Gluteal folds, examination of, 272
Gnosis, 416, 420
Goiter, 227
Goniometer, 342, *342*
Gonorrhea
    in females, 547, 548t
    in males, 572
Goodell's sign, 563d
Grandparenting, 693
Granulation tissue, 191
Graphognosia, 420
Grasp, 669
Grasp reflex, 412, 413
Gray matter. *See* Cerebral cortex
Great vessels, anatomy and physiology of, *296, 296–297, 297*
Grieving
    anticipatory, 603
    dysfunctional, 603
Groin, ringworm of, 200
Growth and development. *See also* Development
    altered, 147
Gums. *See* Gingiva
Gynecologic cancer, 526
Gynecologic examination, 534–551. *See also* Genitals, female, examination of
    digital rectal examination in, 276
    in elimination assessment, 264
    in pregnancy, 563d
Gynecologic surgery, 528
Gynecomastia, 700

H

Haemophilus influenzae pneumonia, immunization schedule for, 630t, 638t, 639t
Hair
    examination of, 182, 194–195
        in elders, 697
        in newborn, 647, 658
    lanugo, 647, 658
    in malnutrition, 178, 194, 197, 198
    in pregnancy, 564d
    pubic, 538, 573, 677
        development of, 634, 634t, 635t, 677
    structure and function of, 181
Hairy tongue, 209
Hall, Lydia, 5
Hallucinations, hypnagogic, in narcolepsy, 469
Hammer toe, 363
Hand. *See also* Upper extremity
    examination of, 355–356
        in infant, 669
        in newborn, 658
        in young child, 673

Hard palate
    examination of, 205
        in newborn, 648–649
    structure and function of, 202
Head, examination of, 78–79
    in infant, 663–665
    in newborn, 647–652
    in older child and adolescent, 675
    in trauma survey, 725
Headaches, 380
    in glaucoma, 378
Head circumference
    in infant, 663
    in newborn, 646
Head injuries, 381, 725
Head-to-toe approach
    in bedside examination, 706–708
    in physical examination, 61, 61d, 64d-65d, 77–91
Health
    cultural concepts of, 612–614
    definitions of, 124
Health assessment
    body systems format for, 6, 18
    comprehensive initial, 12
        documentation of, 15
    data collection in, 10–13. *See also* Data collection
    definition of, 4
    diagnostic reasoning in, 15–19
    documentation in, 13–15. *See also* Documentation
    expanded nursing roles and, 4–5
    focused, 12
    functional health patterns in, 6–10, 38–40
    health history in, 40–56. *See also* Health history
        history of, 4–5
    interview in, 25–40. *See also* Interview
    medical model of, 5
    nursing model of, 5
    pediatric. *See* Pediatric health assessment
    physical examination in, 59–98. *See also* Physical examination
    purpose of, 10
    screening. *See* Screening
    symptom analysis in, 37
    telephone triage and, 131, 131d
Health assessment processes, 10–19
Health behaviors, 127–128
    adherence, 127–128
    self-directed, 127
Health beliefs and practices
    cultural variations in, 612–614, 618
    religion and spirituality and, 614t, 614–615
Health care facilities, safety assessment for, 131, 143
Health history, 40–55
    definition of, 24
    documentation of, 45–55
        narrative-style, 15, 16d, 46, 46d-48d
        standardized form for, 46, 48d-55d
    interview for, 24–40. *See also* Interview
    medical, guidelines for, 40–44
    medication and substance use
        in cognition and perception assessment, 381
        guidelines for, 44–45
    overview of, 24–25
    primary sources for, 24–25. *See also* Interview
    questionnaire for, 24–25
    reproductive, 526
    review of systems in, 40–44
    sample questions for, 42–44
    secondary sources for, 25
    sexual, 520d-521d, 520–528
Health Locus of Control Scale, 480
Health maintenance, 126
    altered, 147
    definition of, 124
Health patterns
    dysfunctional, 10
    functional, 6–10
    potentially dysfunctional, 10
Health perception and health management
    adherence behavior and, 127–128
    assessment of, 125–150
        case examples of, 146
        components of, 132
        data collection for, 125
        documentation of, 145–146
        in elders, 689, 695
        focus for, 125–126
        interview and health history in, 125, 132, 133d-134d, 135–139
        knowledge base for, 126–131
        laboratory/X-ray evaluation in, 125, 138–139
        objectives of, 125
        physical examination in, 125, 132, 139–143
        via telephone, 131, 131d
    case study of, 149–150

Health perception and health management (*continued*)
  clinical problems related to, 149–150
  environmental safety and, 129–131, 143
  as functional health pattern, 9
  guidelines for, 132–145
  health maintenance and, 126
  health promotion and, 126
  nursing diagnoses for, 125–126, 146–150
  potential for injury and, 128–129
  prevention and, 126–127
  risk factors and, 128d, 128–129, 136–137
  screening and, 11–12, 126–127, 132
  self-directed health behaviors and, 127, 137–138
Health promotion, 126
Health records. *See also* Documentation
  problem-oriented, 15
  review of, 11
Health risks, 128–131
  environmental safety and, 129–131, 143
  potential for injury and, 128–129
  risk factors and, 128, 128d, 130d
Health-seeking behaviors, 148
Health status, classification and naming of, 19
Healthy People 2000, 126
Healthy personality, 480
Hearing
  assessment of, 82, 377–378, 446–449, 448d
    in elders, 699
    in newborn, 644, 652
  mechanisms of, 438–439
Hearing loss, 377–379
  communication in, 33
  conductive, 448d
  in elders, 691
  mixed, 448d
  sensorineural, 448d
Heart. *See also under* Cardiac; Cardiovascular
  anatomy and physiology of, *296–298,* 296–300
  blood flow through, 296–297, *297*
  electrical activity in, 297, *298*
  examination of, 300–311
    auscultation in, 305–311
    documentation in, 319–320
    in elders, 698
    guidelines for, 304–305
    in infant, 666
    in newborn, 653
    in older child and adolescent, 676
    palpation in, 304
    precordial inspection in, 304–305
    precordial landmarks in, 301–302, *302,* 304–305
    in young child, 672
  referred pain from, 414, *415*
Heart attack. *See* Myocardial infarction
Heart disease
  activity and exercise assessment in, 284–286
  case study of, 365–366
  risk factors for, 130d
  screening for, 138, 139
  sexuality and, 523–524
  skin changes in, 199
  stressors in, 586, 587d
Heart failure
  case study of, 365–366
  in elderly, 688t
Heart murmurs, 297, *297,* 309–311
  causes of, 297, *297*
  description of, 309–310
  in elders, 698
  in infant, 666
  in newborn, 653
  in newborns, 639
  types of, 310
Heart rate
  assessment of, 305
  exercise-induced maximal, 283t, 283–284
  fetal, 569
  in infant, 666
  in newborn, 653
  in older child and adolescent, 676
  self-evaluation of, 286
  in young child, 672
Heart rhythm, assessment of, 305
Heart sounds, 298, 299, *299*
  abnormal, 306d–318d. *See also* Heart murmurs
  auscultation of, 305–311
  in elders, 698
  fetal, 569
  in infant, 666
  in newborn, 653
  precordial landmarks and, 301–302, *302, 303*
  in pregnancy, 564d
  splitting of, 306d
  in young child, 672
Heated nebulizer, in oxygen therapy, 716–717

Heberden's nodes, 355
Hegar's sign, 563d, *564*
Height, measurement of, 174
  in infant, 663
  in older child and adolescent, 675
  in young child, 670
Height-weight tables, 158, 158d
Hemangiomas
  cavernous, 659
  strawberry, 659
Hematocrit
  in infant, 645
  normal values for, 173
  nutritional status and, 172–173
Hematoma, subungual, 196
Hemianopsia
  bitemporal, 438, *439*
  homonymous, 438, *439*
Hemiplegic gait, 345d
Hemodialysis, stressors in, 586, 588d
Hemoglobin
  in infant, 645
  normal values for, 173
  nutritional status and, 172–173
Hemoglobinopathy screen, in newborns, 644
Hemorrhage. *See also* Bleeding
  gastrointestinal, 266
  splinter, 196
Hemorrhoids
  external, 268, 274
  internal, 269, 274
Hepatic disorders, skin changes in, 198
Hepatitis, sexually transmitted, 550t
Hepatitis B, immunization schedule for, 630t, 638t, 639t
Hepatojugular reflux, 319
Hepatomegaly, in newborn, 654
Heritage consistence, 611d
Hernia
  abdominal, 215
  femoral, 577
  incarcerated, 215
  incisional, 215
  inguinal, 571, 572, *572,* 576, 577d
  reducible, 215
  umbilical, 215, 654, 667, 672
Herniated disc syndrome, 365
Herpes genitalis
  in females, 547, 549t
  in males, 572
Herpes simplex virus infection, cutaneous, 199
Herpes zoster, 190
High-density lipoproteins, 173
Hinge joints, 340
Hip
  disorders of, 669
  examination of, 357
    in newborn, 655–656
    in young child, 674
Hispanic Americans. *See also under* Cultural; Culture
  health and illness concepts of, 612, 613
History. *See* Health history
HIV infection, 550t
  in newborns, 639
  testing for, in newborns, 644
Holter monitor, 291
Homans' sign, 706
Home Observation for Measurement of the Environment (HOME), 130–131
Home safety assessment, 129–131, 143
Homonymous hemianopsia, 438, *439*
Hooking technique, 222
Hopelessness, 487
Hormone replacement therapy, 693
Hormones, in stress response, 587–588, *590*
Hospitalized patients, bedside examination of, 706–708
Hospitals, safety assessment for, 131, 143
Hot and cold illnesses, 613
Human immunodeficiency virus (HIV) infection, 550t
  in newborns, 639
  testing for, 644
Human papillomavirus infection, 550t
Hydrocele, 578, 657
Hygiene, assessment of, 92–93
Hymen, 677
Hypalgesia, 422
Hypercholesterolemia, 173
Hyperextension, 340
Hyperkalemia, 173
Hyperlipidemia, 173
Hypermetropia, 423
  testing for, 435–438. *See also* Visual acuity, assessment of
Hyperpigmentation, 183

Hyperpyrexia, 101, 107–108
Hyperresonance on percussion, 68, 69t, 334
Hypersthenics, 93
Hypertension, 119
  portal vein, 213, 223
  pregnancy-induced, 570
  risk factors for, 130d
Hypertensive retinopathy, 434
Hyperthermia, 101, 107–108
  malignant, 108
Hyperthyroidism, 226
  in elders, 688t
Hyperventilation, 114d
Hypesthesia, 417–418
Hyphemia, 430
Hypnagogic hallucinations, in narcolepsy, 469
Hypoalbuminemia, 172
Hypoesthesia, 417–418
Hypoglossal nerve, 83, 402t, 406
Hypokalemia, 173
Hypopyon, 430
Hypotension, orthostatic, 119, 320, 321
  in elders, 698
Hypothalamus, in temperature regulation, 101, 108
Hypothermia, 107, 108
Hypothyroidism, 226
  congenital, screening for, 644
Hypotonic bladder, 241, 276–277
Hypoxia, 336
Hysterosalpingography, 530

I

Ideal body weight (IBW), 175
Identification, 635
Ileus, paralytic, 225
Illness. *See also* Disease
  cultural concepts of, 612–614, 618
  in elders, 687–688, 688t
  prevention of, 126–127
  sick role in, 494
Imaging studies, in musculoskeletal assessment, 293
Immediate auscultation, 69
Immediate percussion, 67, *68*
Immunization schedule, 630, 630t, 638t, 639t
  for elderly, 690
Impaired gas exchange, 330–337
Impaired oral mucous membrane, 203–211
Impaired physical mobility, 364
Impaired social interaction, 508
Impaired verbal communication, 391, 508
Impetigo, 199
Impotence, 577–578
Incarcerated hernia, 215
Incisional hernia, 215
Incontinence
  bowel, 265
    case study of, 276–277
  urinary. *See* Urinary incontinence
Incus, 438, *439*
Indicators, for nursing diagnosis, 18
Indigenous healers, 613
Indirect percussion, 67, *68*
Individualistic relationships, 610
Indwelling urinary catheter, 718–719
Ineffective airway clearance, 337
Ineffective breast-feeding, 532
Ineffective breathing pattern, 337
Ineffective individual coping, 601–603
Ineffective management of therapeutic regimen, 147
Infant. *See also* Children; Pediatric health assessment
  common problems of, 661–663
  physical examination of, 75, 76d, 663–669
  sleep patterns in, 457d, 458, 633
  temperature regulation in, 101
Infant bonding, 636
Infections. *See also specific infections*
  ear, 442, 445–449
    in infants, 661
  high risk for, 146–147
  parasitic, stool examination in, 253, 256
  prevention of, 74–75
  respiratory
    in elders, 688t
    in infants, 661
  risk factors for, 130d
  sexually transmitted
    in females, 526, 547–551, 548t–550t
      laboratory diagnosis of, 529
    in males, 572–577
    in newborns, 639
    screening for, 142–143

skin, 199–200
urinary tract, 249, 267–268
in elderly, 688t
Infertility tests, 530
Information seeking, in coping, 591
Ingestion, 155
Inguinal area, examination of, 571, 575–576
Inguinal canal, 571, *572*, 576
Inguinal hernia, 571, 572, *572*, 576, 577d
Inguinal ligament, 571, *572*
Inguinal nodes, 232
Inhalation injury, 338
Initial insomnia, 462
Injury
high risk for, 147
prevention of. *See under* Safety
Inner self, 477–478
Insomnia, 461
initial, 462
persistent, 461
terminal, 462
transient, 461–462
Inspection, 62–66. *See also specific structures inspected*
Inspiratory reserve volume, 325
Instrumental activities of daily living (ADLs), in elders, 691, *691*, 692d
Instruments, for physical examination, 69–72, 70t, *70–73*
Integumentary system. *See also* Hair; Nails; Skin
anatomy and physiology of, 181, *181*
assessment of, 181–198
clinical problems related to, 198–200
documentation of, 182–198
nursing diagnoses for, 198
in malnutrition, 178
in pregnancy, 562d, 564d
in stress response, 600
Intensity, of sound
in auscultation, 69
in percussion, 69t
Intercostal spaces, 323, *323*
Intermittent claudication, 294–295, 321
Internal anal sphincter, *239*, 240, 268, *269*
Internal hemorrhoidal plexus, 268, *269*
Internal jugular vein pulsations, 300–301
Internal locus of control, 135, 479, 590, 591d
assessment of, 485
behavioral indicators of, 485t
cultural variations in, 612
International Classification of Diseases (ICD-10), 19
International Classification of Nursing Practice (ICPN), 19
Internet, health information on, 126, 128, 136
Interpersonal relationships. *See* Relationships
Interphalangeal joints, 355
Intervertebral disc, herniated, 365
Intervertebral joints, 340
Interview, 25–40
with angry patients, 33–34
case example of, 23d
with children, 32, 36–37
with cognitively impaired patients, 33
communication techniques in, 28–31. *See also* Communication
content of, 37–40
coordination of data collection for, 35
cultural considerations in, 31–32
with elders, 32–33, 36, 689–695
ensuring comfort in, 27
environment for, 35–36
establishing rapport in, 27
follow-up techniques in, 28
guidelines for, 35–40
in health perception and health maintenance assessment, 132, 133d–134d, 135–138
introductory phase of, 25, 26d, 27
language barriers in, 31–32, 616
medical model for, 27
nonverbal behavior in, 28–29, 30
nursing model for, 27
personalizing of, 28–29
presummary techniques in, 28
problem situations in, 33–35
process of, 25–28
purpose of, 25
statement of, 27, 36
questions in
closed-ended, 29
open-ended, 29
sample, 37–40
scope of, 35
structured, 25, 27–28
summary techniques in, 28
symptom analysis in, 37
termination phase of, 25, 26d, 28

working phase of, 25, 26d, 27–28
Intestinal obstruction, 224–225
Intestinal parasites, stool examination for, 253
Intraocular pressure, 422
Intrapsychic mode, in coping, 591
Intravascular pressure monitoring, 714–715
Intravenous pyelogram (IVP), 251
Intravenous therapy, 719–720
Intrinsic eye muscles, 422
Intubation
chest, monitoring in, 709
nasogastric, monitoring in, 711–712
Inversion, 340
Inverted nipples, 553, 554d
Iris, 422, *423*
examination of, 427
Iritis, 430
Iron-deficiency anemia, 172–173
Irrigation, of ear, 441, *442*
Irritable bowel syndrome, 266
Irritant contact dermatitis, 200
Ishihara plates, 436–437
Isolation aphasia, 392t

J

Jaeger chart, 435
Jaundice, 199
physiologic, 658
skin color in, 183
Jaw, examination of, 203, 204
Jaw opening techniques, 203
Jock itch, 200
Joint(s), 339–340. *See also under* Movement; Musculoskeletal
intervertebral, 340
movements of, 340
range of motion of, assessment of, 342, *342*, 343
synovial, *339*, 339–340
Joint capsule, 339
Joint position sense, 420
Judgment, 387
Jugular veins, assessment of, 87, 318–319
documentation of, 320
Jugular venous pulsations, 300–301, 318

K

Katz Index, 695
Keith-Wagner (KW) classification, 434
Keloid, 187
Keratosis, actinic, 199
Ketonuria, 262
Kidney
palpation of, 222
percussion of, 87
Kidney disease
oral changes in, 211
skin changes in, 198
Kidney failure, 268
Kidney stones, 268
Kleine-Levin syndrome, 470
Knee
examination of, 358–361
fluid in, 360
stability of, 361
Knee-chest position, 270, *270*
Kohlberg's moral development theory, 637
Korotkoff sounds, *113*, 113–115
KUB film, in bowel elimination assessment, 251
Kussmaul's breathing, 114d
Kwashiorkor, 172, 178
Kyphosis, 93, 347

L

Labia majora/minora, 533, *533*
examination of, 538
in infant, 657, 667–668
in newborn, 657
in older child and adolescent, 677
Lacrimal apparatus, 422, *423*
examination of, 425–426
in infant, 664
in newborn, 650
Landau reflex, 662t
Language. *See also* Communication; Speech
assessment of, 387–388
body, 28–29, 30
cortical control of, *371*, 371–372
development of, 633
Language barriers, in interviewing, 31, 616
Lanugo hair, 647, 658
Laryngeal cancer, communication in, 509
Lasegue's sign, 350
Lateral spinothalamic tract, 414–415

Lawton Scale, 695
Laxatives, 245, 247
Lazarus' Everyday Hassles Scale, 596, 598d
Learning, 371
Left lateral decubitus position, 301, *301*
Left lateral position, 270, *270*
Length, measurement of, in newborn, 647
Lens, crystalline, 422, *423*
examination of, 430
opacities of, 430
Leopold's maneuvers, 567–568
Letdown reflex, 532
Lethargic state, 382
Leukocytes, in urine, 262
Leukoplakia, 209
Levator ani muscles, 268, *269*, 534, *535*
palpation of, 273–274
Level of consciousness, 371, 382–383
Glasgow Coma Scale for, 373, 384, 725
Lice, 200
Lichenification, 187
Lichen planus, 190
Life insurance weight tables, 176
Life philosophy, 619
Light palpation, *66*, 66–67
Light reflex
corneal, 404
in newborn, 650
in young child, 650
pupillary, 81, 422, 429
in newborn, 650
Light touch sensation, 418
Limbs, measurement of, 342
Linea nigra, 562d
Linear relationships, 610
Lip
examination of, 206
ulcers of, 208
vesicles of, 208
Lipid profiles, 291
Lipids, serum, assessment of, 173
Listening, 30
Lithium carbonate, sexual function and, 525d
Lithotomy position, 271, *271*
Liver
enlarged, 219
in infant, 667
in newborn, 654
in older child and adolescent, 676
palpation of, 221–222
percussion of, 218–219
in young child, 654
Liver disease, skin changes in, 198
Liver span, measurement of, 218
Locus of control, 135, 479, 590, 591d
assessment of, 485
behavioral indicators of, 485t
Locus-of-control scales, 480
Loneliness, risk for, 507
Long-term care, stressors in, 589d
Looking glass self, 479
Lordosis, 93, 347
Lower abdominal reflex, 411
Lower extremity
examination of, 89
in bedside examination, 706
in newborn, 655
in trauma survey, 726
in young child, 674
measurement of, 342
Lower motor neuron, 406–408, *407*
Lower motor neuron bladder, 242, 276–277
Lower motor neuron disorders, 413, 413d
Lumbar puncture, 389
Lung
abscess of, 337
auscultation of, 334–335, 336d
borders of, 324, *324*
cancer of, 338
examination of
in elders, 698
in infant, 666
in newborn, 652–653
in older child and adolescent, 676
in young child, 672
structure and function of, 324, *324*
Lymphadenitis, 229, 230
Lymphadenopathy
generalized, 230
localized, 230
Lymphangitis, 229
Lymphatic system, 226–232
anatomy and physiology of, 226–229, *229*
assessment of, 229–232
Lymphedema, 229
Lymph nodes
axillary, 557

Lymph nodes (*continued*)
cervical, 83
in young child, 672
distribution of, 229, *229*
epitrochlear, 232
examination of, 83, 227–232
in young child, 672
of head and neck, *229*, 231
inguinal, 232
palpable, 230
popliteal, 232
shotty, 230
Lymphocyte count, nutritional status and, 172

M

Macula, examination of, 434
Macule, 186
Magnetic resonance imaging, in musculoskeletal assessment, 293
Malabsorption syndromes, 266
Malignant hyperthermia, 108
Malignant melanoma, 199
Malignant tumors. *See* Cancer
Malleus, 438, *439*
Malnutrition
in anorexia nervosa, 180
clinical findings in, 172, 178–179, 194, 197, 198
laboratory findings in, 172–173
oral cavity in, 203
risk factors for, 167
skin changes in, 178, 194, 197, 198
Malocclusion, 204
Mammogram, 138, 139, 141, 529
Mandibular division, of trigeminal nerve, 404
Manipulative patients, 34
Manometer, pressure, 116
Masseter muscle, 403
Mastitis, 555d
Mastoid air cells, 438
Maternal alpha-fetoprotein, 530
Maxillary division, of trigeminal nerve, 404
Maxillary sinuses, 323, *323*
examination of, 329–330
McDonald's sign, 563d
McGill Pain Questionnaire, 396
McMurray's test, 360
Measles, immunization schedule for, 630t, 638t, 639t
Measures of Perceived Exertion Scale, 286, 287d
Meconium stool, 658
Mediate auscultation, 69
Mediate percussion, 67–70, *68*
Medical diagnosis, 10, 19
Medical records. *See also* Documentation
problem-oriented, 15
review of, 11
Medication and substance use history, 44–45. *See also* Drug; Health history
in cognition and perception assessment, 381
Melanin, 183
Melanoma, malignant, 199
Membranous labyrinth, 438
Memory, 386–387
Menarche, 528, 634, 634t
Menisci, 339
Menopause, 528, 693
Menstrual cycle
temperature variations during, 101, *102*
vaginal discharge in, 539
Menstrual history, 528
Menstrual problems, 528
Menstruation, onset of, 528, 634, 634t
Mental status examination, 373–374, 374d-375d, 375d-376d, 382–390
awareness assessment in, 385
diagnostic studies for, 389
Glasgow Coma Scale in, 384
level of consciousness in, 382–383
memory assessment in, 386–387
motor responses in, 383–384
orientation assessment in, 385
physical findings in, 389–391
thought processes assessment in, 386
Mercury manometer, 116
Merged families, 497
Mesomorphs, 93
Metabolic equivalents (METs), 284–286, 285t
Metabolism, 155–156
anabolic, 155–156
anaerobic, 283
assessment of. *See* Nutrition and metabolism assessment
basal, 155

catabolic, 155–156
definition of, 155
Metacarpophalangeal joints, 355
Micturition. *See* Urinary elimination
Midarm circumference (MAC) measurement, 176–177, 178
Midsystolic click, 299–300, 308
Milia, 659
Mini-Mental Status Examination, 373, 374d-375d, 695
Mitral area, 302, *302, 303*
Mitral regurgitation, 310
Mobility. *See also* Movement
assessment of, 77, 93
Mongolian spots, 658
Moniliasis, vaginal, 549t, 551
Montgomery-Asberg Depression Rating Scale, 481
Moral development, in children, 637
Moro reflex, 662t
Mother-infant bonding, 636
Motor area, 371, *371*
Motor cortex, 406, *407*
Motor development, 632
in infant, 669
Motor function. *See also* Reflex(es)
anatomy and physiology of, 406–408, *407*
assessment of, 344–347
interview and health history for, 372–391
Mouth. *See* Oral cavity
Movement. *See also under* Motor
assessment of, 344–347
extraocular eye, 422
assessment of, 427–428
during sleep, 455–456, *456*
joint, 340
during sleep, 468
voluntary, 406
Mucocele, 208
Multiple sclerosis, sexuality and, 523–524
Mumps, immunization schedule for, 630t, 638t, 639t
Munchausen syndrome by proxy, 509
Murmurs, 297, *297*, 309–311
causes of, 297, *297*
description of, 309–310
in elders, 698
in infant, 666
in newborn, 639, 653
types of, 310
Murphy's sign, 224
Muscle
action of, 340
dysfunction of, 340–341
oxygen delivery to, 283
structure and function of, 340
Muscle atrophy, 341
in malnutrition, 178
Muscle cramps, 341
Muscle strains, 341
Muscle strength, assessment of, 343
in newborn, 660
Muscle tone, assessment of, 343
Musculoskeletal assessment, 338–366
clinical problems related to, 364–365
diagnostic studies of, 293–294
documentation of, 364
in elders, 698
focus for, 343
guidelines for, 341–344
in infant, 669
landmarks for, 342
measures and comparisons in, 342
in newborn, 660
nursing diagnoses for, 364
in older child and adolescent, 678
thorough vs. screening, 341–342
in young child, 673–674
Musculoskeletal pain, 295, 342–343
Musculoskeletal system
anatomy and physiology of, 338–341
in stress response, 600
Mydriatics, 424
Myelography, 293
Myocardial infarction
in elders, 688t
sexuality and, 523–524
stressors in, 586, 587d
Myoclonus, nocturnal, 470
Myopia, 423
testing for, 435–438. *See also* Visual acuity, assessment of

N

Nabothian cyst, 542

Nails
abnormalities of, 195–196
examination of, 182, 195–196
documentation of, 197
in elders, 697
in newborn, 658
in malnutrition, 178
structure and function of, 181
Naming systems, for health status, 19
NANDA (North American Nursing Diagnosis Association), 6, 19
NANDA Taxonomy I, Revised, 19
Narcolepsy, 469
Narcotics
abuse of. *See* Substance abuse
sexual function and, 525d
Narrative-style documentation, 15, 16d, 46, 46d-48d, 94d-95d
Nasal bleeding, 328
Nasal cannula, in oxygen therapy, 716–717
Nasal examination, 79, 327–328
in newborn, 650
Nasal polyps, 328
Nasal turbinates, 322, *322*
examination of, 328
Nasogastric tubes, monitoring of, 711–712
Natal tooth, 649, 665
Native Americans. *See also under* Cultural; Culture
health and illness concepts of, 612, 613
health risks of, 614t
Nature, relationship to, cultural variations in, 610
Nearsightedness, 423
testing for, 435–438. *See also* Visual acuity, assessment of
Nebulizer, in oxygen therapy, 716–717
Neck. *See also under* Cervical
examination of, 83–84, 349–350
in older child and adolescent, 675
in trauma survey, 725–726
in young child, 672
Neck righting reflex, 662t
Neck veins, assessment of, 87, 318–319
documentation of, 320
Needs, patient, classification system for, 19
Neglect, one-sided, 93, 290, 385, 391
Neonate. *See* Newborn
Nerves
cranial
anatomy and physiology of, 401, 402t
assessment of, 79, 80, 83, 84, 401–406
in newborn, 660–661
peripheral, 413, *414, 415*
abnormalities of, 379
Neuralgia, 398
trigeminal, 380
Neurologic assessment, 390. *See also* Cognition and perception assessment
comprehensive, 373
cranial nerve assessment in, 79, 80, 83, 84, 401–406
in elimination assessment, 264
Glasgow Coma Scale in, 725
motor function assessment in, 408–413
in newborn, 660
in trauma survey, 724–725
in young child, 674
Neurologic disorders, 380–381
in vitamin deficiencies, 179
Nevi, telangiectatic, 659
Newborn. *See also* Children; Pediatric health assessment
Apgar score for, 642, 642t
physical examination of, 646–661
sleep patterns in, 457d, 458, 633
Nicotine, sleep and, 463
Night blindness, 377
Nightingale, Florence, 4, 124
Nightmares, 469
Night terrors, 470
Nipple, 551
discharge from, 558
examination of, 553, 558
inverted, 553, 554d
Paget's disease of, 553, 555d
retraction of, 554d
supernumerary, 553
Nitrogen balance, nutritional status and, 172
Nociceptors, 392–393
Nocturia, 247, 463
Nocturnal enuresis, 470
Nocturnal myoclonus, 470
Nocturnal pain, 463
Nodule, 186
Nomenclature, for health status, 19
Noncompliance, 127–128, 148–149

Nonfluent aphasia, 388, 392t
Nongonococcal urethritis, 549t
Non-native speakers, interviewing of, 31, 616d
Nonspecific urethritis, 577
Nontraditional healers, 136, 613
Nontropical sprue, 266
Nonverbal communication, 28–29, 30, 31
  assessment of, 388
North American Nursing Diagnosis Association
  (NANDA), 6, 19
Nose. *See also under* Nasal
  examination of, 79, 327–328
    in newborn, 650
  structure and function of, *322,* 322–323
Numbness, 380
Numerical Rating Scales, for pain, 396, *396*
Nurse practitioner, 5
Nursing: A Social Policy Statement (ANA), 6
Nursing, transcultural, 611d. *See also under* Cultural; Culture
  communication in, 616d
Nursing assessment. *See* Health assessment
Nursing clinical database, 6
Nursing diagnoses, 6, 10
  for abdominal assessment, 214
  for activity and exercise, 282–283, 287
  for body temperature, 107–108
  for bowel elimination, 237–238, 264–265
  for cardiovascular assessment, 320–322
  classification of, 7d-8d
  clinical database for, 6
  for cognition and perception assessment, 371,
    391, 412–413
  for cranial nerve assessment, 401
  critical indicators for, 18
  defining characteristics for, 6
  definition of, 19
  development of, 6
  for elders, 686
  formulation of
    data collection in, 16–17
    data organization in, 17–18
    drawing conclusions in, 18–19
    steps in, 18–19
  for health perception and health management,
    125–126, 146–150
  indicators for, 18
  for integumentary assessment, 198
  for jaw and oral cavity assessment, 203–210
  for musculoskeletal assessment, 364
  for nutrition and metabolism, 155, 179–180
  for pain, 397–400
  for pediatric health assessment, 629
  for pregnancy assessment, 569–570
  for reflex assessment, 412–413
  for respiratory assessment, 330–337
  for roles and relationships assessment, 493,
    506–508
  for self-concept assessment, 486–487
  for sensory and cerebellar assessment, 412–413,
    422
  for sexuality and reproductive pattern assess-
    ment, 515–516
  for sleep and rest assessment, 455, 468–469
  for stress and coping assessment, 585, 601–603
  taxonomy of, 6, 19
  for urinary elimination, 266–267
  validation of, 19
  for values and beliefs assessment, 609, 620
  wellness, 125–126
Nursing process, 5, *9*
Nursing roles, expanded, 4–5
Nursing theory, 6
Nutrition. *See also* Diet; Eating; Feeding; Food
  altered
    less than body requirements, 179–180
    more than body requirements, 180
  in children, 631–632
  enteral, monitoring in, 713
  ethnic variations in, 612, 613
  functional status and, 166
  medical conditions and, 167
  medications and, 168
  socioeconomic factors in, 167
Nutritional deficiencies
  in anorexia nervosa, 180
  clinical findings in, 172, 178–179, 194, 197, 198
  laboratory findings in, 172–173
  oral cavity in, 203
  risk factors for, 167
  skin changes in, 178, 194, 197, 198
Nutritional guidelines, 156d, 156–160
Nutritional processes, 155–156
Nutritional requirements, 156
Nutrition and metabolism, as functional health pattern, 9
Nutrition and metabolism assessment, 154–235

anthropometric assessment in, 174–179. *See also*
  Anthropometric assessment
  in children, 631–632
  case study of, 233–234
  data collection for, 154–155
  definition of, 154
  diet assessment in, 165–166, 169–173
  documentation of, 161d-162d, 164
  in elders, 162, 163d
  focus for, 154–155, 233
  guidelines for, 160–179
  interview and health history in, 165–168
  knowledge base for, 155–160
  laboratory studies in, 172–173
  nursing diagnoses for, 155, 179–180, 233–234
  objectives of, 154
  overview of, 154
  pediatric, 631–632
  physical examination in, 160–163
    of integumentary system, 181–191
    of jaw and oral cavity, 200–211
  screening in. *See* Nutrition screening
Nutrition knowledge, assessment of, 166
Nutrition screening, 160, 161d–162d
  in elders, 162d, 162–163
Nystagmus, 427

O

Obesity
  binge eating disorder and, 180
  Pickwickian syndrome and, 179
Objective data, 11
Obstructive breathing, 114d
Obtunded state, 383
Obturator sign, 224
Occipital lobe, 371, *371*
Occult blood, fecal, 253, 256, 266
  test for, 257
Oculomotor muscles, 422
Oculomotor nerve, 80, 402t, 403
Odor, wound, 191
Olfaction, assessment of, 379
Olfactory nerve, 402t, 403
Oliguria, 260
One-sided neglect, 93, 290, 385, 391
Onychauxis, 196
Onychorrhexis, 196
Opening snap, 298, 307
Ophthalmoscope, 72, *72*
Ophthalmoscopic examination, 72, *72,* 424,
    429–434. *See also* Eye, examination of
  in infant, 663
  in older child and adolescent, 675
  in young child, 670
Opportunistic infections, risk factors for, 130d
Opthalmic division, of trigeminal nerve, 404
Optic disk, 422, *423*
  cupping of, 431
  examination of, 431
  swelling of, 422, 431
Optic nerve, 402t, 403, 422, *423*
Oral cavity
  anatomy and physiology of, 200–202
  in cancer, 210, 211
  cancer of, 208, 211
  in diabetes, 211
  disorders of, 208–210
  drug effects on, 210
  examination of, 82–83, 202–210
    documentation of, 203
    in elders, 697
    in infant, 665
    in newborn, 648–649
    in older child and adolescent, 675
    in young child, 671
    in malnutrition, 179
  mechanical trauma to, 210
  nursing diagnoses for, 203–210
  procedures in, 204–207
  in renal disease, 211
  in semiconscious/unconscious patient, 202–203
Oral hygiene, poor, 203
Oral mucous membrane
  dehydration of, 203–211
  examination of, 206–207
  impaired, 203–211
  structure and function of, 200, *200*
Oral temperature, 103, 104–105. *See also* Body temperature
Organ of Corti, 439
Orgasm, in sexual response cycle, 517–518
Orientation, 385
Oropharynx
  examination of, 205–206
  structure and function of, 202

Orthopnea, 295
Orthostatic hypotension, 119, 320, 321
  in elders, 698
Ortolani's test, 655, 656
Ossicles, 438, *440*
Osteoarthritis, 364–365
Ostomy patients, sexual concerns of, 523
Otitis externa, 445
Otitis media, 442, 445–449
  in infants, 661
Otorrhea, 379
Otoscope, 72, *73*
Otoscopic examination, 440–445. *See also* Ear, ex-
  amination of
  in infant, 652
  in newborn, 652
  in older child and adolescent, 675
  in young child, 652
Ototoxic drugs, 379
Ova and parasites, examination for, 253, 256
Oval window, 438, 439
Ovary
  palpation of, 545
  structure and function of, 534, *534*
Overt roles, 497
Oximetry, 292, *292*
Oxygen consumption, metabolic equivalents for,
    284–286, 285t
Oxygen delivery, to muscle, 283
Oxygen saturation (SO_2), 292
Oxygen therapy, 716–717

P

Paget's disease of breast, 553, 555d
Pain, 391–400
  abdominal
    in appendicitis, 224
    in bowel obstruction, 224–225
    in diverticulitis, 224
    epigastric tenderness and, 214
    in gallbladder disease, 224
    in gastritis, 214
    on palpation, 221
    in paralytic ileus, 2257
    in peptic ulcer disease, 214–224
    in peritoneal injury, 212
    rebound tenderness and, 212, 221
  acute, 92, 391–392, 397–398
  aggravating factors in, 400
  anatomy and physiology of, 392–393
  assessment of, 394–400, 418–419
    documentation of, 397
    nursing diagnoses for, 397–400
    nursing role in, 394–400
    perioperative, 394–396
    rating scales for, 395–396, *396*
  chest
    anginal, 294
    bedside assessment of, 708
    cardiac, 294
    pulmonary, 294
  chronic, 92, 392, 400
  claudication, 294–295
  communication of, 398–400
  deep, 419
  definitions of, 391–392
  dimensions of, 394, 395d
  in dissecting aortic aneurysm, 294
  dull, 418
  ear, 379
  effects of, 400
  expression of, cultural factors in, 31–32
  facial, 380
  intensity of, 398–399
  location of, 398
  musculoskeletal, 295, 342–343
  nocturnal, 463
  ocular, 378
  onset and chronology of, 399
  perception of, 418–419
  perceptual component of, 393
  in pericarditis, 294
  phantom, 398
  physiologic response to, 393
  postoperative, 394–396
  quality of, 399
  rectal, 244
  referred, 413, *415*
  relieving factors in, 399
  sensory component of, 392–393, *393*
  sharp, 418
  somatic, 398
  superficial, 418
  thalamic, 415
  theories of, 393

Pain (*continued*)
  types of, 398
  undertreatment of, 394
  on urination, 248
  visceral, 398
Painful stimuli, in level of consciousness evaluation, 382, 383
Pain-rating scales, 396, *396*, 399
Palate
  examination of, 205
  in newborn, 648–649
  structure and function of, 202
Pallor
  of oral mucosa, 206
  of skin, 183
Palmar grasping reflex, 662t
Palpation, *66, 66–67, 67. See also specific structures palpated*
  bimanual, 67, *67*
    of breast, 556
    in pelvic examination, 544–546
    in pregnancy, 563d
  light, *66, 66–67*
  Pawlik, 567
Papilledema, 422, 431
Pap smear, 138, 139, 521t, 529, 542
Papule, 186
Parachuting reflex, 662t
Paradoxical sleep, 458
Parallel play, 632
Paralysis
  sexuality and, 523–524
  sleep, 469
  unilateral, 380
Paralytic ileus, 225
Paranasal sinuses
  examination of, 329–330
  structure and function of, 323, *323*
Paraphasia errors, 388
Parasitic infestations, stool examination in, 253, 256
Parasomnias, 470
Parental role conflict, 507
Parent-infant attachment, altered, 507
Parenting, 498
  adolescent, 509
  altered, 506–507
  assessment of, 505
  discipline and, 498, 502
Paresthesias, 379, 380, 417
Parietal lobe, 371, *371*
Parkinsonian gait, 345d
Parotid glands, 200, *201, 204*
Partial pressure of carbon dioxide (pCO₂), 292
Partial pressure of oxygen (pO₂), 292
Parvor nocturnus, 470
Patch, 186
Patellar ballottement, 360
Patellar reflex, 85, 409–410
Patient and family education, 370
Patient needs, classification system for, 19
Patrick's sign, 351
Pattern(s)
  definition of, 9
  functional health, 6–10
    interview questions about, 38–40
Pattern theory, of pain, 393
Pawlik palpation, 567
pCO₂ (partial pressure of carbon dioxide), 292
Peau d'orange breast, 553, 554d
Pedal pulse, 89
Pediatric health assessment, 628–683. *See also* Children
  for activity and exercise, 632
  age classification for, 629
  clinical problems related to
    in infants, 661
    in newborns, 639
    in older children and adolescents, 674–678
    in young children, 674
  for cognition and perception, 632–633
  for coping and stress tolerance, 635
  data collection in, 628–629, 679d-682d
  diagnostic tests for, 644–645
  documentation of
    for infants, 641–661
    for newborns, 638–639
    for older children and adolescents, 674–678
    for young children, 674
  for elimination, 632
  focus for, 628
  for health perception and management, 629–631
  interview and health history in, 637–638, 642–644
  knowledge base for, 629–637
  nursing diagnoses for, 629
  for nutrition and metabolism, 631–632

overview of, 628–629
physical examination in
  of infants, 663–669
  of newborns, 646–661
  of older children and adolescents, 675–678
  of young children, 670–674
  recommendations for, 638d-640d
  for roles and relationships, 635–636
  screening in, 638d-640d, 644–645
  for sexuality and reproduction, 634–635
  for sleep and rest, 633
  standards for, 641d
Pediculosis, 200
Pelvic examination, 534–551. *See also* Genitals, female, examination of
  digital rectal examination in, 276
  in elimination assessment, 264
  in older child and adolescent, 676–677
  in pregnancy, 563d
Pelvic muscles, 534, *535*
  assessment of, 540
Pelvic ultrasound, 530
Pelvis, assessment of, in trauma survey, 726
Penis
  abnormalities of, 577
  anatomy of, *570*, 570–571
  cancer of, 577
  development of, 635t
  discharge from, 574
  examination of, 90, 573–574
    in infant, 667
    in newborn, 657
    in older child and adolescent, 677
    in young child, 673
Peptic ulcer, 214–224
Perceived roles, 492
Perception
  assessment of. *See* Cognition and perception assessment
  definition of, 370
  dimensions of, 372
Percussion, 67–69, *68,* 69t
  of abdomen, 213, 217–220
  of chest, 333–334
  dullness on, 68, 69t, 334
  hyperresonance on, 68, 69t, 334
  of kidney, 87
  of liver, 218–219
    in newborn, 654
  resonance on, 68, 69t
  of spleen, 220
    in newborn, 654
  of stomach, 220
  tympany on, 68, 69t
Pericardial friction rub, 308
Pericarditis pain, 294
Perineum, 533, *533*
  examination of, 272
Periodontal disease, 203
Peripheral nerves, 413, *414, 415*
Peripheral neuropathies, 379
Peripheral vascular disease, skin changes in, 199
Peripheral vision, assessment of, 436
Peristalsis, 212, 240
Peritoneum, 212
Perseveration, 388
Personal identity, 478, 482
Personal identity disturbance, 486
Personality, healthy, 480
Pertussis, immunization schedule for, 630t, 638t, 639t
Petechiae, 188
pH
  arterial blood, 292
  urine, 261
Phalen's sign, 356
Phantom pain, 398
Pharyngitis
  streptococcal, 210, 674
  viral, 210
Phenomenal self, 479
Phenylketonuria, screening for, 644
Philosophy of life, 619
Phimosis, 577
Physical abuse. *See* Abuse
Physical examination, 59–98
  abnormal findings in, 91–93
  annual, 126–127
  auscultation in, 69
  bedside, 706–708
  body systems approach in, 6, 18, 61, 62t, 63t
  definition of, 60
  documentation of, 74, 94, 94d-96d
  of elders, 75
  equipment and instruments for, 69–72, 69–75, 70t, *70–73*
  general approach in, 73–75

general survey in, 65, 77
guidelines for, 73–93
head-to-toe approach in, 61, 61d, 64d-65d, 77–91
  of infants and children, 75, 76d
inspection in, 62–66
interpretation of findings in, 61–62, 63t-65t
overview of, 60
palpation in, *66, 66–67, 67*
percussion in, 67–69, *68,* 69t
positioning for, 75
preliminary aspects of, 75
preparation for, 73–75
purpose of, 61
setting for, 73–74
Standard Precautions in, 74–75
techniques of, 62–69
in trauma, 705, 723–727
Physiologic jaundice, 658
Piaget's theory of cognitive development, 632–633
Pickwickian syndrome, 179
Piers-Harris Self-Concept Scale, 480
Pigmentation
  of hair, 194
  of oral mucosa, 206
  in renal disease, 199
  of skin, 181, 183
    assessment of, 183
    ethnic variations in, 612
Pilonidal cyst, 272
Piskacek's sign, 563d
Pitch
  in auscultation, 69
  in percussion, 69t
Pitting edema, 185d
Pityriasis rosea, 190
Pivot joints, 340
PKU (phenylketonuria), screening for, 644
Placing reflex, 662t
Plantar grasping reflex, 662t
Plantar reflex, 89, 411–412
Plaque, 186
Plateau, in sexual response cycle, 517
Play, 632, 636
Plethysmography, 291
Pleural friction rub, 336d
PLISSIT model, 514, 515t
Pneumatic otoscope, 440
Pneumonia, 337
  in elders, 688t, 689
  H. influenzae, immunization schedule for, 630t, 638t, 639t
Pneumothorax, 337
  tension, 337
pO₂ (partial pressure of oxygen), 292
Point of maximal impulse, 304
Poisoning, 674
Polio, immunization schedule for, 630t, 638t, 639t
Polypharmacy, 45
Polyps
  nasal, 328
  rectal, 274
Polysomnography, 455, *455,* 465
Polyuria, 250, 260
Popliteal nodes, 232
Popliteal pulse, 89, 313
Portal vein hypertension, 223
Portal veins, 213
Port wine stains, 659
Position
  dorsal lithotomy, 537, *538*
  knee-chest (genupectoral), 270, *270*
  left lateral, 270, *270*
  left lateral decubitus, 301, *301*
  lithotomy (dorsosacral), 271, *271*
  semi-Fowler's, 325
  Sims', 270, *270*
  squatting, 270, *271*
  standing, 270, *270*
  supine, 301, *301*
  tailor, 673
Positioning
  for blood pressure measurement, 116
  forward-sitting, 301, *301*
  for genital examination
    in older children and adolescents, 676
    in young children, 673
  for pelvic examination, 537–538, *538*
  for physical examination, 75
  for precordial examination, 301, *301*
  for rectal examination, *270,* 270–271, *271*
  for respiratory assessment, 325–326
Positron emission tomography (PET), 291
Posterior columns, 414
Posterior spinocerebellar tract, 414
Posterior tibial pulse, 89, 314
Postoperative pain, 394–396. *See also* Pain
Post-trauma response, 603

interview and health history for, 372–391,
408–413. *See also* Cognition and perception assessment; Musculoskeletal assessment; Reflex(es)
in mental status examination, 383–384
nursing diagnoses for, 412–413, 422
procedures in, 418–422
scope of, 416–417
Sensory aphasia, 387
Sensory association, 420–421
Sensory deprivation, 389
Sensory function
anatomy and physiology of, 413–416
cortical control of, 415–416
thalamus and, 415
Sensory overload, 389
Sensory-perceptual alteration, 391, 401
Sensory-perceptual alteration:hearing, 442
Sensory-perceptual alteration:visual,
437–438
Serous otitis media, 449
Sex education, 635
Sex roles, 516–517, 522
Sexual abuse, interview in, 526, 527d
Sexual assault victims, interview of, 526, 527d
Sexual assessment, terminology for, 519
Sexual development, 634, 634t
Sexual dysfunction
in females, 532
in pregnancy, 569–570
in males, 577–578
Sexual health, 516
Sexual history, 520d–521d, 520–528
Sexuality
adolescent, 634–635
definition of, 516
discussion of, 34, 518–519
drug effects on, 525d
emotional factors in, 518
health status and, 518, 522–524
in ostomy patients, 523
in pregnancy, 569–570
study of, 514
Sexuality and reproduction, as functional health
pattern, 9
Sexuality and reproductive pattern assessment,
513–581
case studies of, 578–580
data collection in, 515
in elders, 693, 700
equipment for, 520
focus for, 514–515
general principles of, 519–520
interview and history in, 520d–521d, 520–528
knowledge base for, 516–519
laboratory/X-ray studies in, 529–531
in males, 570–578
nursing diagnoses for, 515–516, 531–532
pediatric, 634–635
physical examination in, 532–546. *See also* Genitals
PLISSIT model and, 514, 515t
privacy and confidentiality concerns in, 518–519
procedures in, 529–531
terminology for, 519
Sexually transmitted diseases (STDs)
in females, 526, 547–551, 548t–550t
laboratory diagnosis of, 529
in males, 572–577
in newborns, 639
screening for, 142–143
Sexual response cycle, 517–518
Sexual response patterns, 517–518
Shortness of breath. *See* Dyspnea
Shotty node, 230
Shoulder, examination of, 351–353
Shoulder presentation, 570
Sickle cell test, in newborns, 644
Sick role, 494
Sims' position, 270, *270*
Single parent families, 497
Sinoatrial node, 297, *298*
Sinuses, paranasal
examination of, 329–330
structure and function of, 322–323, *323*
Skene's glands, 533
palpation of, 539
Skin
anatomy and physiology of, 181, *181*
appendages of, 181, *181*
assessment of, 182–190
clinical problems related to, 198–200
documentation of, 182–198
in elders, 696
in infant, 668
in newborn, 658–659
nursing diagnoses for, 198

in older child and adolescent, 676
atrophy of, 187, 336
cancer of, 199
color of, 181
assessment of, 183
ethnic variations in, 612
edema of, 184–185
flaky, 178, 198
hydration of, 183, 184
hygiene of, 184
infections and infestations of, 199–200
lesions of, 185–190
ABCD formula for, 199
distribution of, 189–190
malignant, 199
premalignant, 199
primary, 186
secondary, 187
types of, 186–188
vascular, 188
in malnutrition, 178, 194, 197, 198
pigmentation of, 181, 183
assessment of, 183
in pregnancy, 562d
in systemic disease, 198–199
temperature of, 184
texture and thickness of, 184
Skin tags, 696
anorectal, 272
Skin turgor, 184
Skull, examination of, 78–79
in newborn, 647
Sleep
alcohol and, 464
body movements during, 468
caffeine and, 463–464
definition of, 454, 455
disruptions of, 454
behavioral indicators of, 466
physical indicators of, 466–467
inhibitors of, 467
latency period in, 462
medications and, 464–465
non-REM, 455, *456, 457*
paradoxical, 458
patterns of, 456–458, *457*
promotors of, 467
REM, 455–456, *456, 457,* 458
REM rebound, 464
requirements for, 457d, 458
stages of, 455–456, 455–457, *456, 457*
teeth grinding in, 470
Sleep aids, 464
Sleep and bedtime habits, 463
Sleep and rest, as functional health pattern, 9
Sleep and rest assessment, 453–473
case study of, 470–472
clinical problems related to, 469–470
data collection for, 454–455
documentation of, 459–460
in elders, 692, 699
focus of, 454
general approach in, 458
interview and history in, 461–465
knowledge base for, 455–458
laboratory studies in, 455, *455,* 459, 465–466
measurement instruments for, 459, 459t
nursing diagnoses for, 455, 468–469
pediatric, 633
sleep log in, 458
Sleep apnea, 459–460, 469
Sleep attacks, 469
Sleep behaviors, observation of, 468
Sleep continuity, impaired, 462
Sleep deprivation, 469
cognitive signs of, 467
Sleep environment, 467
Sleepiness, excessive daytime, 462
Sleep log, 458, 459, 459t
Sleep measurement instruments, 459, 459t
Sleep paralysis, 469
Sleep pattern disturbance, 460–468, 468–469
Sleep patterns, 461
in elders, 457d, 458, 692, 699
in infants, 457d, 458, 633
in newborns, 457d, 458, 633
in older children and adolescents, 457d, 458, 633
in preschoolers, 633
Sleep rituals, 463
Sleep scales, 459, 459t
Sleep studies, 455, *455,* 459, 465–466
Sleepwalking, 470
Smell
assessment of, 379, 403
loss of, 403
Smoking, sleep and, 463
Snellen chart, 435, 437d

Snout reflex, 412, 413
SO_2 (oxygen saturation), 292
SOAP progress notes, 15
Social identity, 478, 482
Social interaction, 494–495. *See also* Relationships
impaired, 508
Social isolation, of elderly, 509
Social isolation/risk for loneliness, 507
Socialization, of children, 498, 502
Social Readjustment Rating Scale, 593–596, 596d
Social support, assessment of, 502
Socioeconomic status
access to care and, 614
health risks and, 614t
nutrition and, 167
Sodium
dietary intake of, 160
normal values for, 173
Soft palate
examination of, 205
in newborn, 648–649
structure and function of, 202
Somatic pain, 398
Somnambulism, 470
Spanish fly, sexual function and, 525d
Spastic colon, 266
Specimen
cervical, collection of, 542–543
stool, collection and handling of, 254
urine, 258
Speculum, vaginal, 535, *536,* 541
Speech. *See also* Communication; Language
assessment of, 92, 388
cortical control of, *371,* 371–372
cultural differences in, 621
development of, 633
hearing impairment and, 378
telegraphic, 388
Sperm antibody agglutination, 530
Spermatic cord, torsion of, 578
Sperm penetration assay, 530
Sphenoid sinuses, 323, *323*
examination of, 329–330
Sphygmomanometer, 115–116, *116*
Spider angioma, 188
Spinal accessory nerve, 84
Spinal cord injury, sexuality and, 523–524
Spinal cord sensory pathways, 413–415
Spinal nerve, 406
Spinal tap, 389
Spine
curvature of, 347–348
in newborn, 652
in young child, 673
examination of, 347–351
in bedside examination, 706
in infant, 666
in newborn, 652
in trauma survey, 726
Spinocerebellar tracts, 414
in pain transmission, 393, *393*
Spinothalamic tracts, 414–415
Spiritual development, in children, 637
Spiritual distress, 620
Spirituality. *See also* Religion; Values and beliefs
assessment of, 619–620, 621
definition of, 608
health beliefs and practices and, 614–615
Spiritual support, 620
Spiritual well-being, potential for enhanced, 620
Spirometry, 292
Spleen
palpation of, 222
percussion of, 220
in newborn, 654
Splinter hemorrhages, 196
Spooning, 195
Spousal abuse, 509
risk factors for, 130d
Sprue, nontropical, 266
Squamous cell carcinoma
of oral cavity, 208
of skin, 199
Squatting position, 270, *271*
Staging, wound, 191–193
Standard Precautions, in physical examination,
74–75
Standing position, 270, *270*
Stapes, 438, *439*
Startle reflex, 652, 662t
Stasis ulcers, 199, 321–322
Status, 493
Stensen's duct, 200, *201*
Stepping gait, 346d
Stepping reflex, 662t
Stereognosis, 420
Stereotype, 611d

Sternal angle, 323, *323*
Sternoclavicular area, 302, *302, 303*
Stethoscope, 69, 71, *71*
  in blood pressure measurement, 115
Sthenics, 93
Stomach, percussion of, 220
Stomatitis, 210, 211
  aphthous, 209
Stomatitis erythema, 206
Stones, urinary, 268
Stool. *See also under* Bowel; Fecal
  blood in, 253, 256, 266
  in bowel incontinence, 255, 265
  collection and handling of, 254
  color of, 254–255
  composition of, 256
  consistency and shape of, 255
  in constipation, 255, 264, 265
  in diarrhea, 255, 265
  examination of, 253–258
    documentation of, 258
    specimen collection and handling for, 254
  fat in, 253, 2554
  foreign objects in, 256
  formation and evacuation of, *239,* 239–240. *See also* Bowel elimination
  meconium, 658
  mucus in, 255
  in newborn, 658
  odor of, 256
  ova and parasites in, 253, 256
  urobilinogen in, 254
  volume of, 255
Stool culture, 254
Stool guaiac test, 257
Stork bites, 659
Strabismus, 428, 663, 670
Strains, muscle, 336
Strawberry hemangioma, 659
Strength, assessment of, 343
  in newborn, 660
Strep throat, 210, 674
Stress
  acute, 585
  caregiver, 508, 594, 700
  chronic, 585–586
  crisis and, 592
  definition of, 584
  indicators of, 599–600
  negative, 584
  overview of, 584
  perception of, 595
  positive, 584
  relocation, 507–508
  resolution of, 596
  role, 494
Stress and coping assessment, 583–605
  case studies of, 603–604
  clinical problems related to, 603
  documentation of, 601
  in elders, 694, 700
  focus for, 585
  general approach in, 592–593
  interview and history in, 593, 593d
  knowledge base for, 585–592
  measurement instruments in, 593–596
  nursing diagnoses for, 585, 601–603
  suicide potential and, 597–598, 601, 602
Stress Audit, 596
Stress incontinence, 266
  provocation testing for, 252
Stressors, 585–587
  appraisal of, 595
  classification of, 585–586, 586d
  cognitive appraisal of, 588
  environmental, 586d, 595
  in heart disease, 586, 587d
  in hemodialysis, 586, 588d
  identification of, 586–587, 587d–589d, 594–595
  physiologic, 586d
  psychological, 586d
  sociocultural, 586d
Stress response, 584, 587–588, *590*
  assessment of, 599–600
  in children and adolescents, 635
  documentation of, 601
Stress test
  exercise, 291
  for postvoid residual volume, 252
Stress ulcer, 588
Stretch marks, 562d
Striae, 215
Striae gravidarum, 562d
Stuporous state, 383
Stye, 432
Subclavian steal syndrome, 321

Subculture, 611d
Subcutaneous tissue, 181, *181*
Subjective data, 11
Sublingual glands, 200, *201,* 204
Submandibular glands, 200, *201,* 204
Substance abuse, *732*
  by adolescents, 674
  assessment in, 705, 727–731
  history in, 44–45, 730, *732*
  sexual function and, 525d
Substance use history, 44–45, 730. *See also* Health history
Subungual hematoma, 196
Sucking reflex, 662t
Sugar intake, 156d, 160
Suicide potential, assessment of, 597–598, 601, 602
Summation gallop, 307
Superficial reflexes. *See* Reflex(es)
Superior mesenteric artery, 213
Supernumerary nipples, 553
Supination, 340
Supine position, 301, *301*
Suppositories, rectal, 245
Suprapatellar pouch, 359
Suprasternal notch, 323, *323*
Surgery, gynecologic, 528
Swallowing
  impaired, 210–211
  phases of, 210–211
Swan neck deformity, 355
Sweat glands, 181, *181*
Swimmer's ear, 445
Symbolic interactionism, 479
Symptom analysis, 37
Synarthroses, 339
Syncope, 380
Synovial joints, *339,* 339–340
Syphilis
  in females, 547, 548t
  in males, 572
Systole, 298, *299*
Systolic blood pressure, 113, 118

T

Tachycardia, 108
Tachypnea, 114d
Tactile fremitus, 332
Tactile sensation
  assessment of, 379–380
  cortical control of, 415–416
Tail of Spence, 551, *552*
Tailor position, 673
Taste, assessment of, 379
Taste buds, 201
Taxonomy
  definition of, 6
  for nursing diagnoses, 6, 19
Teeth, 202, *202*
  care of, 203
  disorders of, 203
  eruption of, 665
  in infant, 665
  in newborn, 649, 665
Teeth grinding, nocturnal, 470
Telangiectasis, 188
Telangiectatic nevi, 659
Telegraphic speech, 388
Telemetry, 721
Telephone assessment, 131, 131d
Temperature, body. *See* Body temperature
Temperature sensation, 419
Temporal arteries, examination of, 78–79
Temporal lobe, 371, *371*
Temporal muscle, 403
Temporomandibular joint, examination of, 203, 204
Tenesmus, 244
Tension pneumothorax, 337
Tension reduction, 589–590
Terminal illness, discussion of, 34–35
Terminal insomnia, 462
Tertiary prevention, 127
Testicular self-examination, 137, 145d, 526
Testis, 571, *571*
  cancer of, 575, 578
    screening for, 137, 145d
    self-examination for, 137, 145d, 526
  examination of, 574–575
    in newborn, 657
    in older child and adolescent, 677
    in young child, 673
  undescended, 668, 673
Tetanus, immunization schedule for, 630t, 638t, 639t
Tetany, 336

Thalamic pain, 415
Thalamus, 415
Thallium scanning, 291
Therapeutic communication. *See also* Communication
  in interview, 28–31
Therapeutic diet, 165
Therapeutic regimen, management of
  effective, 147–148
  ineffective, 147
Therapeutic relationships, 495, 502
Thermometers, 103
  electronic, 103, 106
  glass, 103, 104–105
  tympanic, 103, 106
Thinking ability, 386–388
Thomas test, 358
Thoracic compliance, 325
Thoracic landmarks, *323,* 323–324, *324*
Thorax. *See* Chest
Thought processes, 371, 386–388. *See also* Cognition
  altered, 391
Thrombosis, deep vein, Homan's sign in, 706
Thyroid
  anatomy and physiology of, 225, *225*
  assessment of, 225–228
  examination of, 84
Thyroid disease, 226
  in elders, 688t
Thyroid hormones, 225
  screening for, in newborns, 644
Thyroid nodules, 228
Thyroxine (T_4), 225
  screening for, in newborns, 644
Tidal volume, 325
Time orientation, cultural variations in, 610, 612, 619
Tinea, 200
Tinel's sign, 356
Tine test, 139
  in children, 645
Tingling, 380
Tinnitus, 379
Tissue, oxygen delivery to, 283
Tissue perfusion, altered, 320–321
Toddler. *See also* Children; Pediatric health assessment
  common health problems in, 674
  physical examination of, 670–674
  sleep patterns in, 633
Toes, examination of, 363
Toilet training, 632
Tongue
  examination of, 204–205, 207
    in newborn, 649
  hairy, 209
  inflammation of, 209
  structure and function of, 201
Tonic neck reflex, *660,* 662t
Tonsils, examination of, 672
Tooth. *See* Teeth
Topognosia, 420
Torus palatinus, 208
Total incontinence, 267
Total lung capacity, 325
Total lymphocyte count, nutritional status and, 172
Touch
  assessment of, 379–380
  cortical control of, 379–380
  cultural variations in, 621
Toxemia of pregnancy, 570
Trachea, examination of, 331
Tracheostomy, communication with, 509
Tranquilizers, sexual function and, 525d
Transcortical aphasia, 392t
Transcultural nursing, 611d. *See also under* Cultural; Culture
  communication in, 616d
Transferrin, nutritional status and, 172–173
Transillumination
  of sinuses, 329–330
  of skull, in newborn, 647
  of testis, 574
Translators, 31
Transport, of nutrients, 155
Transverse lie, 570
Trauma, assessment in. *See also* Trauma survey
  assessment in, 705
  chest, 337–338
  head, 381
  risk factors for, 130d
Trauma score, 727t
Trauma survey, 723–727
  documentation of, 727
  primary, 12, 723–724